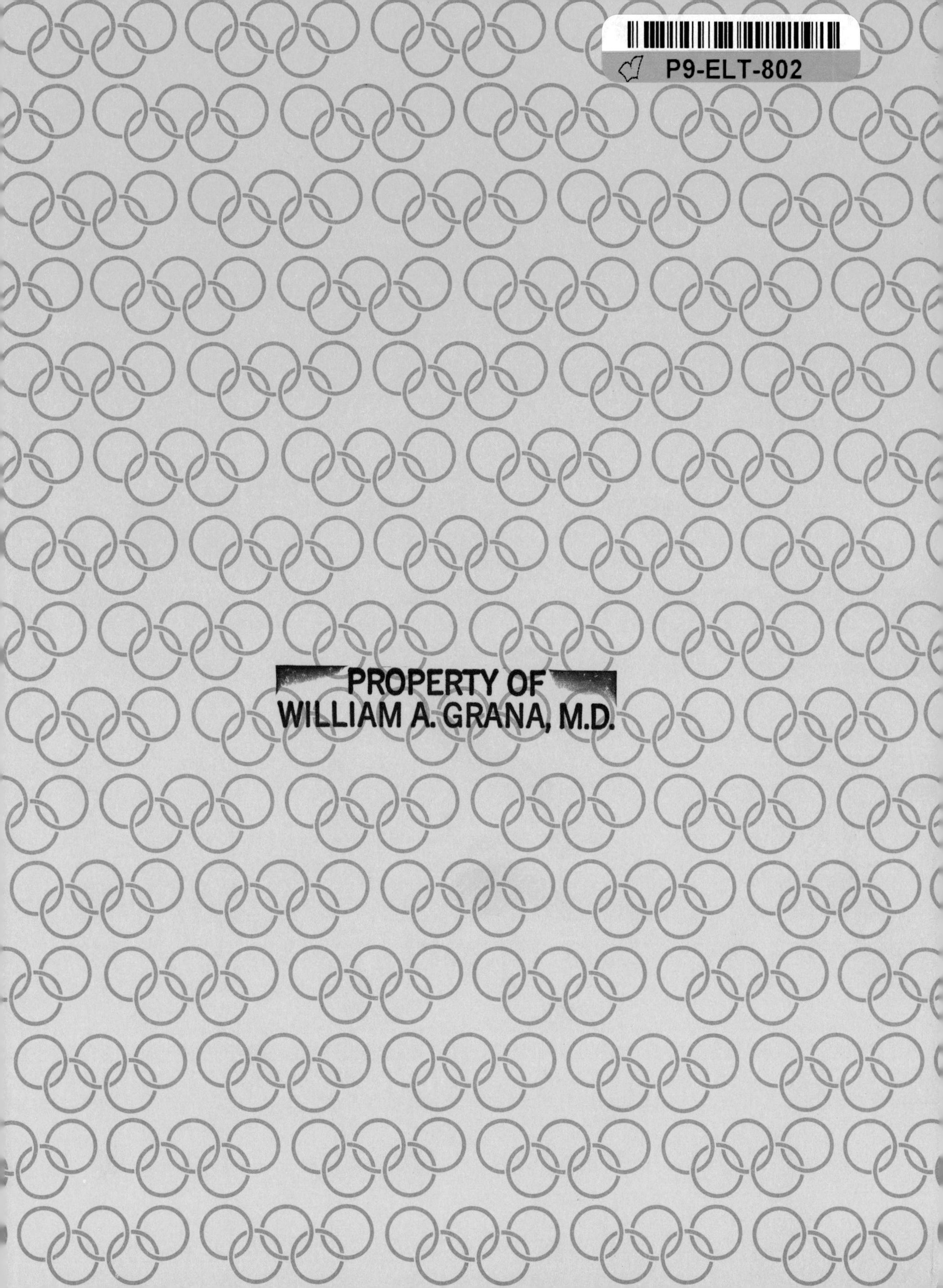

CLINICAL PRACTICE OF
SPORTS INJURY PREVENTION AND CARE

IOC MEDICAL COMMISSION

PUBLICATIONS ADVISORY SUB-COMMITTEE

Clinical Practice of Sports Injury Prevention and Care

VOLUME V OF THE ENCYCLOPAEDIA OF SPORTS MEDICINE

AN IOC MEDICAL COMMISSION PUBLICATION

IN COLLABORATION WITH THE

INTERNATIONAL FEDERATION OF SPORTS MEDICINE

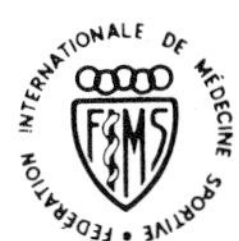

EDITED BY

P.A.F.H. RENSTRÖM

OXFORD

BLACKWELL SCIENTIFIC PUBLICATIONS

LONDON EDINBURGH BOSTON

MELBOURNE PARIS BERLIN VIENNA

Published by
Blackwell Scientific Publications
Editorial Offices:
Osney Mead, Oxford OX2 0EL
25 John Street, London WC1N 2BL
23 Ainslie Place, Edinburgh EH3 6AJ
238 Main Street, Cambridge
Massachusetts 02142, USA
54 University Street, Carlton
Victoria 3053, Australia

Other Editorial Offices:
Librairie Arnette SA
1, rue de Lille
75007 Paris
France

Blackwell Wissenschafts-Verlag GmbH
Düsseldorfer Str. 38
D-10707 Berlin
Germany

Blackwell MZV
Feldgasse 13
A-1238 Wien
Austria

First published 1994

Set by Setrite Typesetters, Hong Kong
Printed and bound in Great Britain
at the University Press, Cambridge

Part title illustrations by Grahame Baker

A catalogue record for this title
is available from the British Library

ISBN 0–632–03785–7

DISTRIBUTORS

Marston Book Services Ltd
PO Box 87, Oxford OX2 0DT
(*Orders*: Tel: 0865 791155
Fax: 0865 791927
Telex: 837515)

USA
Blackwell Scientific Publications, Inc.
238 Main Street, Cambridge, MA 02142
(*Orders*: Tel: 800 759–6102
617 876–7000)

Canada
Times Mirror Professional Publishing Ltd
130 Flaska Drive, Markham, Ontario L6G 1B8
(*Orders*: Tel: 800 268–4178
416 470–6739)

Australia
Blackwell Scientific Publications Pty Ltd
54 University Street, Carlton, Victoria 3053
(*Orders*: Tel: 03 347–5552)

Library of Congress
Cataloging-in-Publication Data

Clinical practice of sports injury prevention and care /
edited by P.A.F.H. Renström.
p. cm.
(The Encyclopaedia of sports medicine; v. 5)
'An IOC Medical Commission publication
in collaboration with the
International Federation of Sports Medicine'.
Includes bibliographical references and index.
ISBN 0–632–03785–7
1. Sports injuries. I. Renström, Per A.F.H.
II. IOC Medical Commission.
III. International Federation of Sports Medicine.
IV. Series.
(DNLM: 1. Athletic Injuries — prevention and control.
2. Athletic Injuries — therapy. 3. Sports Medicine.
QT13 E527 1988 v. 5)
RD97.C594 1994
617.1'027—dc20
DNLM/DLC for Library of Congress

Contents

Part 2: Sport-Specific Injuries: Prevention and Care

Part 2a: Team Sports

Part 2b: Individual Sports

List of Contributors

B.D. ADAMS MD, *Department of Orthopaedics, University of Iowa Hospitals and Clinics, Iowa City, IA 522 42–1088, USA*

P. AGLIETTI MD, *Department of Orthopaedics, University of Florence, 50139 Florence, Italy*

Å. ANDRÉN-SANDBERG MD PhD, *Department of Surgery, Lund University, S-221 85 Lund, Sweden*

J.R. ANDREWS MD, *American Sports Medicine Institute, 1313 Thirteenth Street South, Birmingham, AL 35205, USA*

F.J.G. BACKX MD PhD, *Janus Jongbloed Research Centre on Sports and Health, University of Utrecht, 3521 GG Utrecht, The Netherlands*

D. BARRAULT PhD, *National Institute of Sports, Rue de L'Epee, 89100 SENS, France*

W.F. BERGFELD MD, *Department of Dermatology, The Cleveland Clinic Foundation, Cleveland, OH 44195–5032, USA*

B. BERGLUND MD PhD, *Department of Medicine, Karolinska Hospital, S-104 01 Stockholm, Sweden*

P. DE BIASE MD, *Department of Orthopaedics, University of Florence, 50139 Florence, Italy*

A.L. BOLAND MD, *Department of Orthopaedic Surgery and Sports Medicine, Massachusetts General Hospital, Boston, MA 02114, USA*

J.P. BRAMHALL MD, *Team Physician, Texas A&M University, College Station, TX 77843, USA*

G. CAVALIERE MD, *Department of Sports Medicine, New York University Medical Center, New York, NY 10016, USA*

G. CERULLO MD, *Clinica Valle Giulia, Via G. de Notans, 00197 Rome, Italy*

K.-M. CHAN MD, *Department of Orthopaedics and Traumatology, Chinese University of Hong Kong, Prince of Wales Hospital, Shatin, NT, Hong Kong*

F.A. COMMANDRE MD, *Department of Sports Medicine, University of Aix-Marseille II, 13385 Marseille, Cedex 5, France*

M.R.J. COOLICAN MD, *Department of Orthopaedic and Traumatic Surgery, Royal North Shore Hospital of Sydney, St Leonards, Sydney, NSW 2065, Australia*

P. DALY MD, *Sports Medicine Unit, Massachusetts General Hospital, Boston, MA 02114, USA*

K.A. DECKER BS, *Mid-America Center for Sports Medicine, Wichita, KS 67214–4906, USA*

C.N. VAN DIJK MD, *Academic Medical Centre, Meibergdreef 9, 1105 AZ Amsterdam, The Netherlands*

J. EKSTRAND MD PhD, *Department of Orthopaedic Surgery, Linköping Medical Center, University of Linköping, 68 Klostergatan, S-582 23 Linköping, Sweden*

D.M. ELSTON MD, *Dermatology Service of Brooke Army Medical Center, Ft Sam Huston, San Antonio, TX 78234, USA*

E. FAXÉN RPT, *Department of Orthopaedics, East Hospital, Gothenburg University, S-416 85 Gothenburg, Sweden*

T. FOSTER MD, *Sports Medicine Unit, Massachusetts General Hospital, Boston, MA 02114, USA*

P.J. FOWLER MD, *Department of Orthopaedic Surgery, University of Western Ontario, London, Ontario N6J 5A5, Canada*

V. FRANCO MD, *Clinica Valle Giulia, Via G. de Notans, 00197 Rome, Italy*

C.B. FRANK MD, *Department of Surgery, University of Calgary, Calgary, Alberta T2N 4N1, Canada*

M. GOERTZEN MD PhD, *Dusseldorf Sports Rehabilitation Center, University of Dusseldorf, 4000 Dusseldorf, Germany*

W.A. GRANA MD, *Department of Orthopaedic Surgery and Rehabilitation, University of Oklahoma Health Sciences Center, Oklahoma City, OK 73104, USA*

N.D. GRIFFIS BS, *TOSA Medical, 1407 North Main, Rose Hill, KS 67133, USA*

J. HARVEY MD, *Orthopaedic Center of the Rockies, 2500 East Prospect Road, Fort Collins, CO 80525, USA*

R.J. HAWKINS MD, *The Steadman Hawkins Clinic, Vail Valley Medical Center, Vail, CO 81657, USA*

C.E. HENNING MD, *Mid-America Center for Sports Medicine, Wichita, KS 67214–4906, USA*

P. HØLMICH MD, *Department of Orthopedic Surgery, Gentofte Hospital, University of Copenhagen, 2900 Hellerup, Denmark*

T.M. HOSEA MD, *Robert Wood Johnson Medical School, New Brunswick, NJ 089021, USA*

S.Y.C. HSU MBBS, *Department of Orthopaedics and Traumatology, Princess Margaret Hospital, Shatin, NT, Hong Kong*

M. JÄRVINEN MD PhD, *Division of Orthopaedics and Traumatology, University Hospital, University of Tampere, 33520 Tampere, Finland*

D.H. JANDA MD, *Institute for Preventative Sports Medicine, Ann Arbor, MI 48107, USA*

R.J. JOHNSON MD, *McClure Musculoskeletal Research Center, Department of Orthopaedics and Rehabilitation, University of Vermont, Burlington, VT 05405, USA*

U. JØRGENSEN MD PhD, *Department of Orthopedic Surgery, Gentofte Hospital, University of Copenhagen, 2900 Hellerup, Denmark*

P. KANNUS MD PhD, *Tampere Research Station for Sports Medicine, The Urho Kaleva Kekkonen Institute for Health Promotion Research, SF-33500 Tampere, Finland*

J. KARLSSON MD PhD, *Department of Orthopaedics, East Hospital, Gothenburg University, S-416 85 Gothenburg, Sweden*

H. LAMENDIN SFOSS, *Laboratory of Cellular and Animal Biology, University of Orleans, BP 6759, 45067 Orleans, Cedex 2, France*

F. LATELLA MD, *Fiorentina Soccer Club, Piazza Fra G. Savonarola 6, 50132 Florence, Italy*

J. LLOYD PARRY MB BChir, *The Medical Equestrian Association, The Royal College of Surgeons, 35–45 Lincoln's Inn Fields, London WC2A 3PN, UK*

M. LYNCH MD, *Department of Orthopaedics, Norwalk Hospital, Norwalk, CT 06851, USA*

D. MCKENZIE MD PhD, *Division of Sports Medicine, The University of British Columbia, Vancouver V6T 1Z3, Canada*

G.R. MCLATCHIE MB, *Department of Surgery, General Hospital, Hartlepool, Cleveland TS24 9AH, UK*

W.J. MALLON MD, *Division of Orthopaedic Surgery, Duke University Medical Center, Durham, NC 27710, USA*

D.L. MANN MD, *6857 Gerrard Street, Powell River, British Columbia V8A 1S4, Canada*

D.F. MARTIN MD, *Department of Orthopaedic Surgery, Bowman Gray School of Medicine, Wake Forest University, Winston-Salem, NC 27157–1070, USA*

J.M. MARZO MD, *Sports Medicine Service, The Hospital for Special Surgery, 535 East 70th Street, New York, NY 10021, USA*

W. VAN MECHELEN MD PhD, *Department of Health Science, Vrije University and University of Amsterdam, 1105 AZ Amsterdam, The Netherlands*

L.J. MICHELI MD, *Department of Orthopaedics, Children's Hospital Medical Center, 319 Longwood Avenue, Boston, MA 02115, USA*

O. MICHELINI MD, *Radiology Department, Ospedale 'S Maria di Collemagio', 67100 L'Aquila, Italy*

J. MINKOFF MD, *Minkoff Orthopaedic Associates, 333 East 56th Street, New York, NY 10022, USA*

J.A. MITCHELL BS, *Hand Rehabilitation Center, University Orthopaedics, Burlington, VT 05401, USA*

K.W. MOORE MSc, *Department of Surgery, University of Calgary, Calgary, Alberta T2N 4N1, Canada*

D.L. MULLER MD, *McClure Musculoskeletal Research Center, Department of Orthopaedics and Rehabilitation, University of Vermont, Burlington, VT 05405, USA*

C.E. NICHOLS MD, *McClure Musculoskeletal Research Center, Department of Orthopaedics and Rehabilitation, University of Vermont, Burlington, VT 05405, USA*

R.P. NIRSCHL MD, *Virginia Sports Medicine Institute, 1715 N. George Mason Drive, Arlington, VA 22205, USA*

S. ORAVA MD PhD, *Hospital Meditori and Sports Medical Research Unit, Paavo Nurmi Centre, University of Turku, 20100 Turku, Finland*

F. DE PAULIS MD, *Radiology Department, Ospedale 'S Maria di Collemagio', 67100 L'Aquila, Italy*

G. PUDDU MD PhD, *Clinica Valle Giulia, Via G. de Notans, 00197 Rome, Italy*

J.I.B. PYNE MD, *McClure Musculoskeletal Research Center, Department of Orthopaedics and Rehabilitation, University of Vermont, Burlington, VT 05405, USA*

P. QUANG CHAU DIUFAMS, *Department of Sports Medicine, University of Aix-Marseille II, 13385 Marseille, Cedex 5, France*

P.A.F.H. RENSTRÖM MD PhD, *McClure Musculoskeletal Research Center, Department of Orthopaedics and Rehabilitation, University of Vermont, Burlington, VT 05405, USA*

A. SCALA MD, *Orthopaedic Department, Ospedale 'C. Forlanini', 00152 Rome, Italy*

D.F. SCARPINATO MD, *Suburban Orthopaedic Associates, 1974 Sproul Road, Broomhall, PA 19008, USA*

G. SERNI MD, *Fiorentina Soccer Club, Piazza Fra G. Savonarola 6, 50132 Florence, Italy*

R.J. SHEPHARD MD PhD, *School of Physical and Health Education, University of Toronto, Ontario M5S 1A1, Canada*

O.H. SHERMAN MD, *Minkoff Orthopaedic Associates, 333 East 56th Street, New York, NY 10022, USA*

B.G. SIMONSON MD, *Department of Sports Medicine, New York University Medical Center, NY 10016, USA*

J. SOBEL BS, *Virginia Sports Medicine Institute, 1715 N. George Mason Drive, Arlington, VA 22205, USA*

T.K.F. TAYLOR DPhil, *Department of Orthopaedic and Traumatic Surgery, Royal North Shore Hospital of Sydney, St Leonards, Sydney, NSW 2065, Australia*

J.S. TORG MD, *Sports Medicine Center, University of Pennsylvania, Philadelphia, PA 19104, USA*

P. VANUXEM DIUFAMS, *Department of Sports Medicine, University of Aix-Marseille II, 13385 Marseille, Cedex 5, France*

S.W. VEQUIST BS, *Mid-America Center for Sports Medicine, Wichita, KS 67214–4906, USA*

J. WATKINS PhD, *Faculty of Education, University of Strathclyde, Glasgow G13 1PP, UK*

G.G. WEIKER MD, *Department of Orthopaedic Surgery, The Cleveland Clinic Foundation, Cleveland, OH 44106, USA*

T.L. WICKIEWICZ MD, *The Hospital for Special Surgery, 535 East 70th Street, New York, NY 10021, USA*

S. WOTOWEY BS, *Orthopaedic Center of the Rockies, 2500 East Prospect Road, Fort Collins, CO 80525, USA*

R.R. WROBLE MD, *Sports Medicine Grant, 323 East Town Street, Columbus, OH 43215, USA*

K.M. YEAROUT BS, *Mid-America Center for Sports Medicine, Wichita, KS 67214–4906, USA*

G. ZACCHEROTTI MD, *Department of Orthopaedics, University of Florence, 50139 Florence, Italy*

H. ZAKARIAN, DIUFAMS, *Department of Sports Medicine, University of Aix-Marseille II, 13385 Marseille, Cedex 5, France*

B. ZARINS MD, *Sports Medicine Unit, Massachusetts General Hospital, Boston, MA 02114, USA*

Forewords

On behalf of the International Olympic Committee, I should like to welcome Volume V of the Encyclopaedia of Sports Medicine series. This new volume, which addresses the problem of injuries in sport, represents a continuation of the previous work in the series.

The Olympic Movement naturally has a duty to protect its athletes and uphold the true values of sport. Thanks to the continuous scientific research of our Medical Commission and its specially selected members, we are now able to provide athletes, trainers and team physicians with scientific means of injury prevention which we trust they will find useful in their daily sporting activities.

Juan Antonio Samaranch
Marqués de Samaranch

It is well known that athletes have to endure social, economic and national pressure to win, sometimes at all costs, which results in ethical and health problems for them.

The IOC Medical Code includes provisions relating to the medical care of athletes, and the IOC Medical Commission keeps a very close watch on the problem of injuries in élite sport.

This volume of the Encyclopaedia series includes a long chapter devoted to sport-specific injuries, prevention and care. To cite one example, in recent years the sport of boxing has repeatedly been at the centre of heated controversy. World opinion has been influenced by the seriousness of certain accidents which have been the focus of much attention. According to some studies, this sport is seemingly so dangerous that it should be banned, while others claim that it presents no greater risks than football.

Concerned about the ambiguities of this situation, the IOC is making every effort to study the dangers of boxing very carefully. In 1984, the IOC Medical Commission established a Special Commission on Boxing incorporating members of the International Amateur Boxing Federation's medical commission. Subsequently, this federation made important changes to its rules.

In 1980 we invited highly qualified representatives from a dozen medical academies worldwide to join the work of our special commission. The discussions have been lengthy, and the results of the scientific projects undertaken will provide valuable information and advice for preventing injuries, not just in boxing, but for élite sport in general.

Prince Alexandre de Merode
Chairman, IOC Medical Commission

Preface

Injury prevention must be given careful consideration by health professionals in the future. Today, there is a clear focus in sports medicine on the treatment and rehabilitation of the injured individual, but neither the prevention of injuries nor the recurrence of injuries is given high priority.

In spite of the great possibilities and importance of injury prevention, very little has been carried out during the years, both in research, education and practical sports activities. The first major step in prevention was taken by President Theodore Roosevelt as long ago as 1905. He told the American colleges 'to adjust the rules in American football to eliminate risks'. This had a great impact, although it took a long time before anything of significance happened. There are a few other landmark preventive activities that should be mentioned. One was Peterson's (1970) analysis of the injury rate in American football, which led to the elimination of cross-body blocking and, thereby, a substantial reduction in injuries. Another was the report of Pashby, Bishop and Easterbrook (1982) concerning protective eye wear during racquet sports, which led to a significant decrease in eye injuries and associated health care costs. Rule changes such as the introduction of helmets and face masks in non-professional ice hockey and head guards in non-professional boxing, have also reduced the incidence of injury dramatically. These changes are just a few positive landmarks, but there is much more that should be considered.

Most injuries can be prevented. Dramatic acute injuries are, of course, often difficult to prevent, but much can be done to improve the situation. Players and athletes should, in some sports, be required to use protective equipment to minimize the risk of injury. The rules in many sports could be changed so that they give maximum protection to the athletes. Most overuse injuries can also be prevented. The athlete can avoid training errors, eliminate unsafe practices, use proper equipment and correct malalignments and asymmetry of the kinetic chain.

The risk of injury varys from sport to sport and some injuries are sports-specific. Terms such as tennis elbow, jumper's knee, runner's knee or rider's strain, indicate this. Most of these injuries are preventable with the application of training modifications, improved equipment and rule changes. Every sport needs to be analysed for injury mechanisms and risks, but very little has been done so far. Ekstrand's (1983) work in football (soccer) is a good example of how injury mechanisms can be analysed; following which, intervention measures can be made to prevent injuries. It is, in other words, very important to understand the specific risks of a sport and thereby the injury mechanisms. Most of the Olympic sports have, in this volume, been analysed from the aspect of prevention as well as that of clinical care by authors who are involved in the different sports. Their work and analysis can hopefully be a stepping stone to further and deeper analyses of injury risks in different sports, making preventive intervention possible.

Injuries are often specific to anatomical location and tissues. These factors also determine the type of clinical care and rehabilitation. The ankle is, for example, subjected to ligament sprains, which usually heal with conservative treatment, while ligament injuries to the knee need surgery in 20% of cases. The rehabilitation after knee ligament injuries involves a comprehensive rehabilitation programme, which is concentrated on thigh muscle-strengthening exercises. The rehabilitation after ankle ligament injuries is focused on both strength training and proprioceptive exercises. As clinical practice varys with the anatomical location and the tissues involved, specific injuries at different locations on the body have also been analysed regarding prevention and care.

Prevention of injuries in sport has been difficult to carry out, mainly because there has been very little research on the efficacy of preventive measures. Even if there are well-substantiated studies, the athletic community has not enforced protective rules and the utilization of protective equipment. Tradition, inefficiency and cost seem to be common obstacles for the implementation of preventive measures. Improving and implementing rules in, for example, international football (soccer), may take years. Peak performance has highest priority for the individual athlete. Athletes do not, in general, want to implement equipment changes if this affects their performance in any way, Making new protective equipment compulsory may also be expensive. Sports clubs, schools and other organizations may not be able to absorb the additional costs.

The number of people participating in sports is ever increasing. The physical demands of different sports is also increasing and, thereby, the risk for injury. It will be necessary for the sports world to focus more on prevention and correct clinical care. By understanding the injury mechanisms and the risk for injury, prevention can be made effective. This requires, however, much more support from scientific studies, and for more education in injury prevention and clinical care in sports.

The 47 chapters in this book have been written by professionals who have expertise in the different sports and specific anatomical locations. It has been considered important that the authors have both a scientific background and extensive experience in order to analyse the means of injury prevention. Because of their varying backgrounds and experience, the authors have used different approaches; each chapter is characterized by the author's own experience and available research. We still lack scientific background to prevention of injuries in most sports, but this book includes what is known today.

I would like to thank the authors for their great contributions, Jane Andrew for her editorial skills and Carrie Beauchemin, my secretary, for her enormous energy in endless and time-consuming communications with the authors. I would also like to thank the IOC Medical Commission's Publications Advisory Sub-Committee for its support during this difficult task and Prince Alexandre de Merode for his encouragement.

Per A.F.H. Renström, *Burlington*
1993

Units of Measurement and Terminology*

Units for quantifying human exercise

Mass	kilogram (kg)
Distance	metre (m)
Time	second (s)
Force	newton (N)
Work	joule (J)
Power	watt (W)
Velocity	metres per second ($m \cdot s^{-1}$)
Torque	newton-metre (N·m)
Acceleration	metres per second^2 ($m \cdot s^{-2}$)
Angle	radian (rad)
Angular velocity	radians per second ($rad \cdot s^{-1}$)
Amount of substance	mole (mol)
Volume	litre (l)

Terminology

Muscle action: The state of activity of muscle.

Concentric action: One in which the ends of the muscle are drawn closer together.

Isometric action: One in which the ends of the muscle are prevented from drawing closer together, with no change in length.

Eccentric action: One in which a force external to the muscle overcomes the muscle force and the ends of the muscle are drawn further apart.

* Compiled by the Publications Advisory Sub-Committee, IOC Medical Commission.

Force: That which changes or tends to change the state of rest or motion in matter. A muscle generates force in a muscle action. (SI unit: newton.)

Work: Force expressed through a displacement but with no limitation on time. (SI unit: joule; note: 1 newton × 1 metre = 1 joule.)

Power: The rate of performing work; the product of force and velocity. The rate of transformation of metabolic potential energy to work or heat. (SI unit: watt.)

Energy: The capability of producing force, performing work, or generating heat. (SI unit: joule.)

Exercise: Any and all activity involving generation of force by the activated muscle(s). Exercise can be quantified mechanically as force, torque, work, power, or velocity of progression.

Exercise intensity: A specific level of muscular activity that can be quantified in terms of power (energy expenditure or work performed per unit of time), the opposing force (e.g. by free weight or weight stack) isometric force sustained, or velocity of progression.

Endurance: The time limit of a person's ability to maintain either an isometric force or a power level involving combinations of concentric and/or eccentric muscle actions. (SI unit: second.)

Mass: The quantity of matter of an object which is reflected in its inertia. (SI unit: kilogram.)

Weight: The force exerted by gravity on an object. (SI unit: newton; traditional unit:

kilogram of weight.) (Note: mass = weight/acceleration due to gravity.)

Free weight: An object of known mass, not attached to a supporting or guiding structure, which is used for physical conditioning and competitive lifting.

Torque: The effectiveness of a force to overcome the rotational inertia of an object. The product of force and the perpendicular distance from the line of action of the force to the axis of rotation. (SI unit: newton-metre.)

Strength: The maximal force or torque a muscle or muscle group can generate at a specified or determined velocity.

PART 1

TRAUMATIC AND OVERUSE INJURIES: PREVENTION AND CARE

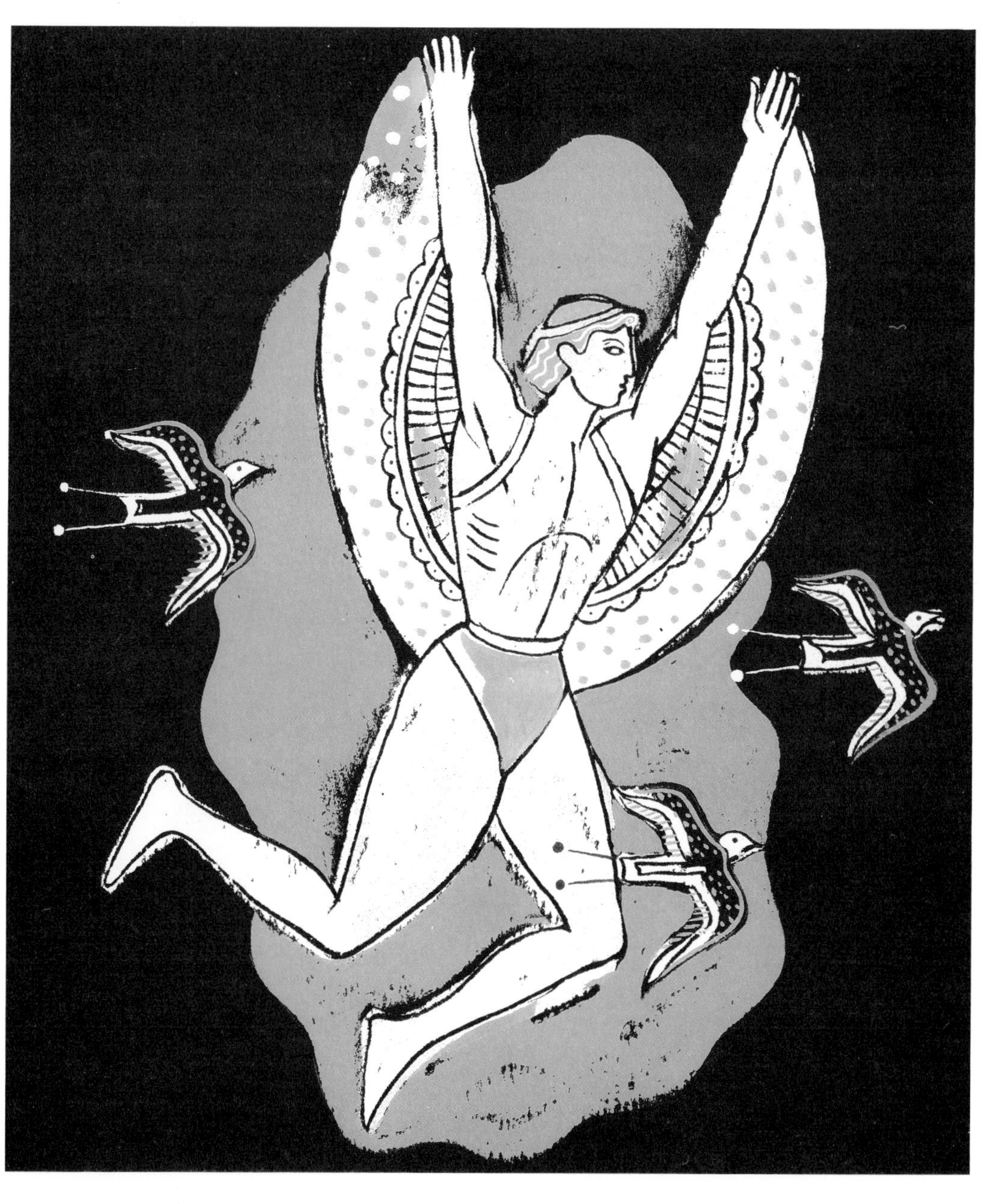

Chapter 1

Head Injuries

WILLEM VAN MECHELEN

'Wear a helmet. It's inconvenient, but so is not being able to think or talk because your head has been pounded into jelly.'
(Ballantyne, in Thompson *et al.*, 1989)

In order to rule out interpretation problems it is first necessary to define what is generally understood by head injuries.

In accordance with Thompson *et al.* (1989, 1990) a head injury can be defined as any injury to the forehead, scalp, ears, skull, brain and brain stem. Brain injuries are defined as being present in case of a concussion or more serious brain dysfunction, whereas facial injuries are defined as injuries to the area of the face beginning with the eyebrows and extending to the chin, mouth and teeth.

A distinction should be made between acute and chronic head injuries. Acute head injuries, with or without linear skull fracture, include 'a spectrum of disorders with concussions at its most benign end death caused by expanding intracranial mass lesions at its other end' (Lehman & Ravich, 1990). Chronic head injury, known as the punch-drunk syndrome (dementia pugulistica), is the result of the cumulative effects of repetitive episodes of 'minor' closed head injuries resulting in neuropathological, pathophysiological and abnormal neuropsychological findings (Lehman & Ravich, 1990; Tysvaer & Løchen, 1991).

This chapter will only deal with some aspects of head and brain injuries and their prevention by the use of helmets.

Acute head injuries

Incidence and severity

In the absence of information on the population at risk, it is not possible to produce incidence figures on acute head injuries. However, some authors do give clues about the extent of the problem.

Mueller and Blyth (1987) mention over a 40-year period (1945–1984) 433 direct fatalities as a result of head injuries in American football. Lehman and Ravich (1990) mention, without further information on their source, that in relation to sports in the USA acute closed head injuries account for some 6000 potentially preventable deaths and millions of episodes of less severe head injuries each year. They also note that, with regard to the risk on acute closed head injury, there are marked differences between various types of sport. It was noted by Wasserman and Buccini (1990) that head injuries account for approximately two-thirds of the hospital admissions and 85% of the deaths attributable to bicycle trauma. Thompson *et al.* (1989) state that in the USA, bicycling is enjoyed by more than 85 million people and that the most common cause of death (70–80% of all cases) and serious disability in bicycle accidents is head injury. In a case-control study they classified about 50% of registered bicycle-related head injuries as serious injuries at least resulting in unconsciousness of any duration, skull fracture or lethargy.

With regard to boxing, Blonstein and Clarke (1957) estimated that serious concussions occurred at one in every 100 contests. Over 60% of the boxing injuries received by 11 820 RAF amateur boxers during the 1960–1966 period were located at the head (Brennan, 1968, in Unterharnscheidt, 1985). In horse-riding about 25% of all injuries are located in the head/neck region many of them being serious (fracture and concussion) (Van Mechelen *et al.*, 1987). Sennerich (1988) registered 11.3% head injuries on a total of 1403 clinically treated sports injuries over a period of 7 years. In The Netherlands in 1985, 11% of head and face injuries were registered on a total of 21 614 emergency ward treated sports injuries (Stichting Consument en Veiligheid, 1986).

Injury mechanism

According to Bishop (1976) head and/or brain injuries are caused in a direct way by either a fall or by a collision between two players or a player and a wall, a goalpost, etc. Also a collision with a hockey puck, a baseball, etc. should be taken into account. The first category of impact is qualified as a low-velocity, blunt impact and the second as a high-velocity, penetrating impact (Bishop & Wells, 1990).

Also an indirect injury mechanism should be recognized in which a sudden acceleration of the head as a result of a sudden change of motion of the torso ('whiplash trauma') is the prime cause of head injury (Norman, 1983). A direct impact to the head may result in local skull deformation (possibly skull fracture) and subsequent intracranial pressure changes at the site of the impact as well at the opposite site ('contracoup lesion') and/or in rotatory or linear head movement, also leading to changes in intracranial pressure and to shear stress of the brain stem predominantly at the site of the foramen magnum, in this way leading to local, more generalized intracranial injury (Ommaya & Hirsch, 1971; Bishop, 1976; Mills & Whitlock, 1989). In the case of whiplash trauma, pressure changes in the brain and shear stresses will indirectly lead to more generalized diffuse brain damage (concussion, contusion and worse).

Whether or not direct or indirect impact will lead to head or brain injury depends largely on the magnitude of the impact, the site of the impact, the magnitude of acceleration and the impact time. In a literature review, Norman (1983) summarized various reported tolerances of the skull and brain:

1 Angular accelerations somewhere between 1800 and 3500 $rad \cdot s^{-2}$ are likely to produce cerebral concussion.

2 Average linear acceleration of the head up to at least 42 *g* and perhaps as high as 80 *g* for impacts against a yielding surface, are probably tolerable regardless of duration of the pulse; in addition to this it was noted that telemetered head accelerations from 40 to 230 *g* during American football did not produce any damage.

3 Skull fractures in human cadavers where produced by (i) an average acceleration of 112 *g*; (ii) a peak acceleration of 200 *g*; and (iii) an increased intracranial pressure of 207 kPa lasting 4 ms.

4 Linear or commuted skull fractures in cadavers were produced at kinetic energy levels ranging from 363 to 788 J.

5 The tolerance of the frontal bone of the human cadaver was found to be about 5782 N against a flat rigid surface and 3736 N against a rigid hemisphere with a 7.6 cm radius, whereas the back of the skull fractured under similar conditions at about 13 344 and 4181 N respectively.

6 The tolerance to the rate of change of acceleration (jerk) is dependent on the rise time of the pulse: for very short rise times (1 ms) and short total pulse duration the non-injurious jerk is very high ($10^5\ g \cdot s^{-1}$), as the rise time increases (e.g. to 100 ms) the non-injurious jerk level decreases to $10^2–10^3\ g \cdot s^{-1}$.

Head injury criteria

In the literature, various head injury criteria are described. The Wayne State Tolerance Curve (WSTC), the Gadd Severity Index (GSI) and the Head Injury Criterion (HIC) will be discussed briefly.

WSTC

The WSTC uses linear skull fracture combined with severe concussion as injury criterion (Gurdjian *et al.*, 1966). The curve represents a linear 'effective' acceleration–time relation based on the outcome of experiments with human cadavers and anaesthetized dogs. As effective acceleration originally an acceleration value of slightly greater then half the peak acceleration was taken, which was later interpreted as the average acceleration over the entire pulse (Bishop & Briard, 1984).

The WSTC (Fig. 1.1) is considered as a boundary curve by which impacts of a certain magnitude and duration can be classified as either safe or unsafe (Norman, 1983). However, there are some problems with the application of the WSTC as outlined by Gurdjian *et al.*, (1964), Goldsmith (1981), Norman (1983) and Bishop and Briard (1984).

1 The curve is based on a limited set of data involving frontal impact and linear accelerations ranging from 3 to 5 ms, therefore the criterion seems more valid for impacts of relatively short duration rather than long duration, whereas the criterion may be different for impacts at other sites of the head (temporal, occipital) due to local differences in energy-absorbing qualities.

2 There is a problem in assessing the average acceleration which makes the application of the criterion difficult.

3 The criterion does not address the occurrence of skull fracture due to contact processes that generate stresses in excess of the fracture limit.

4 The criterion does not apply for the consequences of rotational acceleration.

5 The criterion is a single boundary measure which recognizes only pass or fail in which failing represents skull fracture, but brain damage can occur with and without skull fracture and vice versa.

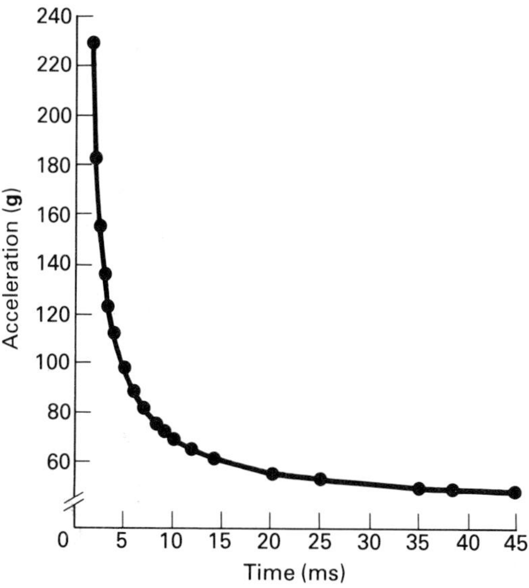

Fig. 1.1 The Wayne State Tolerance Curve.

GSI

In order to solve the problem of assessing the effective or average acceleration in the WSTC, Gadd developed the GSI as a generalization of the WSTC (McElhaney *et al.*, 1973). GSI is the integration of an acceleration–time ($a-t$) pulse experienced by simulated human heads due to impact (Hodgson, 1975) such that:

$$\text{GSI} = \int_{t_0}^{t_1} a^{2.5}\, \mathrm{d}t.$$

GSI is used in the automobile industry (Johnson *et al.*, 1975) and for the evaluation of American football helmets using a norm set by the National Operating Committee on Standards for Athletic Equipment (NOCSAE) (Hodgson, 1975; Reid & Reid, 1981). It is also used for the evaluation of various other sports helmets, such as bicycle helmets (Bishop & Briard, 1984), baseball helmets (Goldsmith & Kabo, 1982) and ice-hockey helmets (Bishop, 1977).

The criterion value for GSI was calculated from the WSTC and initially set at 1000 for concentrated frontal impacts and later modified to 1500 for non-concentrated, distributed impacts in which the hazard of skull fracture is removed (McElhaney *et al*., 1973; Hodgson, 1975; Bishop & Briard, 1984). According to Bishop and Briard (1984) the use of the NOCSAE football helmet standard has led a more effective football helmet. In research on the effectiveness of American football helmets Bishop *et al*. (1984), however, set the index at a more conservative value of 1200 for the evaluation of used football helmets under impact conditions using two arguments:

1 The GSI concussive threshold of 1500 was developed for frontal impacts, while other regions of the head may have lower tolerance.

2 Lowering the GSI index lowers the risk of a false-positive qualification of tested helmets.

A point of critique on the GSI derives from Reid *et al*. (1974) who state that the GSI is based on the assumption that the force required to produce a linear skull fracture in a cadaver head is equivalent to the force that will produce a concussion in a football player. This assumption is not valid according to Reid *et al*. In their opinion, skull fracture is rare in football, even in fatal head injuries and furthermore, concussion in football occurs in players wearing GSI passed helmets before and after impact. Bishop and Briard (1984) criticize the fact that the GSI does not give insight into the shape of the acceleration–pulse time curve.

HIC

HIC is also based on the WSTC and can be considered as an interpretation of the GSI that tries to overcome the problem of applying GSI in the case of long pulse head acceleration.

$$\mathrm{HIC} = \left[(t_2 - t_1)^{-1} \int_{t_1}^{t_2} a\,dt \right]^{2.5} (t_2 - t_1)$$

in which t_1 = an arbitrary time in the pulse, t_2 = for a given t_1 a time in the pulse that maximizes HIC, and a = resultant acceleration. The tolerable value for HIC is set at 1000 in part on the basis of volunteer response to long-duration pulses (McElhaney *et al*., 1973; Goldsmith, 1981). HIC was criticized by Goldsmith (1981) because (i) the criterion value of 1000 is questioned as being too low; (ii) HIC only addresses unidirectional acceleration excursions and cannot accommodate negative or oscillory acceleration values; and (iii) there is no correlation between the measures provided by HIC and a quantified injury scale.

Head protection

In various sports the head and brain are protected against impact by a helmet. A helmet is supposed to protect the brain and the skull from high-velocity, penetrating impacts and from lower velocity, blunt impacts. The effectiveness of helmets is evaluated in two ways:

1 By evaluating the biomechanical properties of a helmet upon impact.

2 By assessing the effectiveness of helmet use in epidemiological studies (e.g. the effect of wearing helmets on head injury incidence).

BIOMECHANICAL EVALUATION

Biomechanical evaluation of helmets is usually done by application of a drop test. A drop test can be described as a guided free fall under gravity of a helmet fitted on a standardized headform to strike a rigid anvil. Mostly, the headform is instrumented with an accelerometer. Upon impact acceleration–time curves can be produced. Depending on the testing protocol *g* peak or GSI are applied as evaluating criteria. In the previous paragraph, the NOCSAE standard is mentioned. The NOCSAE protocol involves drop test evaluation of helmets. It includes drop tests from three different drop heights, at six impact locations, under four different environmental conditions. As performance criterion GSI less than 1500 on a second drop at all locations under all conditions is used (Hodgson, 1975; Reid & Reid, 1981). Other standards applied for biomechanical evaluation of helmets are the 'standard hockey helmets' of the Canadian Standards Association (CSA) (Bishop, 1977; Norman, 1983), the bicycle helmet standard of the American National

Standards Institute (ANSI) (Wasserman & Buccini, 1990) and the British Standard BS 6473 for a horse and pony riders hat (Mills & Whitlock, 1989). Basically, these standards involve a drop test more or less similar to the NOCSAE test.

It should be recognized that the outcome of drop tests is influenced by the mechanical properties of the headform; there are, for instance, differences in impact response between a metal headform and a so-called 'humanoid' headform (Berger & Calvano, 1979).

It should also be recognized that with regard to approved helmets the response of helmets on a drop, regardless of drop height, is not uniform within helmets at different impact locations and between helmets at identical impact locations (Bishop, 1977, 1978; Bishop & Briard, 1984; Bishop *et al.*, 1984).

With respect to attenuating qualities of helmets, one should be aware of the fact that once the bottoming limit of a helmet liner is exceeded a rapid rise in acceleration will follow. Liners usually bottom when they are compressed to about 70% of their thickness (Norman, 1983). The drop height at which bottoming is reached is not identical for all helmets. It is therefore important to test helmets at a level severe enough to reveal differences between helmets if they exist (Bishop *et al.*, 1984). One should also be aware of the fact that in some drop tests the impact speed resulting from the applied drop height does not necessarily reflect player speed in specific sports situations. For instance, in the CSA protocol for ice-hockey helmets, impact speed is 3.4 $m{\cdot}s^{-1}$, while skating speed can run up to 11 $m{\cdot}s^{-1}$ (Norman, 1983). In the NOCSAE protocol, impact speed is 5.4 $m{\cdot}s^{-1}$ with 36.5 m (40 yd) running speed in American football varying from 7.3 to 8.2 $m{\cdot}s^{-1}$ (Hodgson, 1975).

The shock-absorbing quality of a helmet upon impact is largely dependent on the liner. From experiments by Bishop and Briard (1984) it seems clear that with respect to padded helmets, a polystyrene liner is superior to a polyfoam liner, though one should bear in mind that polystyrene does not rebound after impact thereby loosing its shock-absorbing effectiveness at second impact. This damage may not always be visible because of its location at the shell–liner interface. Next to padded helmets, suspension helmets are also used. In a study by Bishop *et al.* (1984), used padded helmets were found to be superior to used suspension helmets. The shock-absorbing qualities of the suspension helmets had diminished over time as a result of stretching of the suspension web.

With regard to helmet use it should be noted that neck injuries cannot be predicted from results of helmet drop tests due to the fact that the neck and head are not rigid and that they are as stiff or less stiff than a helmet. As a result of this, the shock-absorbing effect of a helmet is minimized, so the forces experienced by the neck are largely dictated by its own properties. Consequently, differences between helmets in drop tests do not indicate differences between helmets regarding cervical spine loading during head-first collision (Bishop & Wells, 1990).

EPIDEMIOLOGICAL EVALUATION

> 'Whether laboratory testing standards for helmets are appropriate or applicable to performance in the field is unknown'
>
> (Thompson *et al.*, 1989)

Only a few epidemiological studies on the effectiveness of sports helmets are known from the literature.

D'Abreu (1978) reports that in 1968 the Jockey Club and Betting Levy Board announced a number of preventive measures for jockeys taking part in horse-racing:

1 Hard hats were to be worn to prevent head and brain injuries.

2 Plastic supports were to be worn to prevent spinal injuries.

3 Plastic materials were to be used in the construction of fencing, etc. and projecting parts to be eliminated.

An analysis of the number of accidents during

races in 1967–1968 and 1973–1974 showed a reduction of 42% in the absolute number of head injuries and 70% in the absolute number of spinal injuries. The number of injuries for which no preventive measures were recommended, i.e. fractures of the extremities, remained virtually constant during this period.

Torg *et al.* (1979) noted a shift in head and neck injury pattern in American football between 1959 and 1977. In their opinion the number of serious head injuries had decreased due to enhanced protective capabilities of the helmet–face–mask unit, while the number of serious spinal injuries had increased due to increased use of the head as the primary point of contact in blocking, tackling and head butting. Mueller and Blyth (1987) describe the number of fatalities in American football due to head and neck injury from 1945 to 1984. They noted a major decrease in both numbers and percentages of head and cervical spine fatalities from 1975 to 1984. This decrease was attributed to changes of the football rules in 1976 that made it illegal to butt block, face tackle and spear. Also the introduction of the mandatory use of NOCSAE safety standard approved American football helmets in 1978 for colleges and in 1980 for high schools, was held responsible by Mueller and Blyth.

Although the effectiveness of helmets can, with some precaution, be judged from changes in injury pattern, one should keep in mind that it is hard to establish the 'true' effect of helmet use on injury statistics because of the complexity of interacting factors in the playing environment (Norman, 1983). A better way of studying the effectiveness of preventive measures is by a case-control study, although differences between 'cases' and 'controls' cannot be ruled out due to the retrospective nature of this kind of research (Walter *et al.*, 1985).

Wasserman and Buccini (1990) performed a retrospective study on the effect of ANSI-approved bicycle helmets amongst 191 recreational cyclists (57% were wearing such a helmet) who had reported a fall or who had struck their head in a cycling mishap. They found that helmet wearers in comparison to non-wearers suffered significantly fewer ($P < 0.01$) skull fractures (1% versus 11%) and facial soft tissue injuries (5% versus 18%). This difference was not explained by differences in age, gender or cause of mishap. There was no significant difference between the two groups in the proportion of concussion, facial fracture, neck injuries and injuries below the neck. However, it should be noted that the effect of helmet use may have been underestimated as a result of cyclists killed in accidents. Wasserman and Buccini state that their findings suggest that helmets afford protection from skull fractures and facial soft tissue injury when cyclists strike their head in cycling mishaps.

Thompson *et al.* (1989) performed a case-control study on the effectiveness of bicycle safety helmets. 235 case patients (those with head injuries from cycling seen in an emergency room) were compared with 433 emergency room controls (those with other cycling injuries seen in an emergency room) and with 558 population-based controls (those who had had an accident regardless of injury and medical care). When case patients were compared to emergency room controls, the calculated odds ratio (multiple logistic regression) for head injury was 0.26; 95% confidence limits (CL) 0.14–0.49. This ratio was adjusted for age, gender, household income, education level and amount of cycling per week. In comparison to the population controls, applying the same above mentioned adjustments, the odds ratio was 0.19 (95% CL 0.06–0.57). Similar calculations were made for brain injuries (concussions) giving comparable results. Thompson *et al.* (1989) concluded that their study provided convincing evidence of the effectiveness of bicycle helmets in preventing injury: riders who did not wear helmets had a significant 6.6-fold greater risk of head injury and a 8.3-fold greater risk of brain injury than riders who did. From the results of a similar case-control study, Thompson *et al.* (1990) concluded that bicycle helmets did not have an effect on the risk of serious facial injury. However, in this study helmets did appear to have a significant protective effect on injuries to the upper face (age, gender, cycling experience, injury severity, education, income and hospital adjusted odds ratio was 0.29; 95% CL 0.1–0.8).

Chronic head injury

Unterharnscheidt *et al.* (1985) noted from their tests on animals that a single blow, which in itself could cause concussion, produced no histological changes in the brain tissue. The situation was the opposite with light blows dealt in quick succession: in the long run the repeated blows caused degeneration of the brain tissue, without concussion.

The neuropathological findings in cases of repetitive chronic head injuries may include premature atrophic changes, hydrocephalus, cavum septum pellucidum, microscopic changes to the substantia nigra and other areas rich in neurotransmitters, and cortical scarring (Lehman & Ravich, 1990).

The delayed effects of repeated brain injuries are described in the literature as dementia pugilistica or 'punch-drunk syndrome'. This disorder is characterized by loss of psycho-intellectual and motor performance (Council Report, 1983). The syndrome occurs in between 17 and 55% of professional boxers; it is less common in amateurs (Ross *et al.*, 1983). Ross *et al.* (1983) demonstrated a positive correlation between the number of disorders found in ex-boxers in computerized tomographic (CT) scans and electroencephalogram (EEG) tests and the number of bouts fought. For other sports, no incidence figures of chronic brain damage are known.

With respect to boxing, Kaste *et al.* (1982) discovered the first symptoms of chronic brain damage (CT scan and EEG disorders, as well as impaired results on psychological tests) in 14 young (average age of 31 years) Finnish ex-champions. This means that damage probably starts in young boxers. Kaste stressed that these were champions, who took far fewer knocks than their less skillful fellow boxers. It is likely, then, that brain disorders would be more common among average boxers.

Schneider (1984) reports on the risk of brain injury from heading the ball in soccer. Biomechanical tests were carried out to ascertain the accelerations to which the head is subjected in heading a ball. From the experiments it was concluded that an acceleration limit of 55–65 *g* taken from the WSTC was not exceeded in the laboratory situation. After extrapolating the laboratory data to the field situation, it was concluded that here too the limit would not be exceeded, although it would be approached with ball velocities of about 22 $m \cdot s^{-1}$. With an increase in ball weight to 700 g, which can occur in wet weather, body weight under 50 kg and ball velocity higher than 22 $m \cdot s^{-1}$, the limit would be exceeded, yielding a risk of acute brain damage (which could be irreversible). The aim of the experiment by Schneider was to assess the danger of a single 'header'; the figures did not take the risk of repeated heading into account. Despite this fact, Schneider explicitly warned for possible negative long-term effects of heading a soccer ball with forces not exceeding the WSTC.

Schneider's fear seems confirmed by the outcome of a case-control study by Tysvaer and Storli (1989). In this study, an increased incidence of EEG disturbances amongst 69 first league soccer players (age 15–34 years) compared to matched controls was found. The disturbances were most pronounced in the youngest players. It was concluded that the higher incidence of EEG disturbances found in football players was most likely due to neural damage caused by repeated minor head trauma. In a second study on the same subject, Tysvaer and Løchen (1991) found a higher degree of neuropsychological impairment, as measured by various verbal and performance tests, in 37 former players of the Norwegian national soccer team in comparison to matched controls. According to the authors, the applied neuropsychological tests are highly efficient in differentiating persons with and without brain damage. They concluded that 'blows to the head by heading show convincing evidence of brain damage similar to that found in patients who sustained minor head injuries'.

Prevention of head injury

The most effective preventive measure with respect to acute and chronic brain injury in sports is probably to avoid any minor blow to the head. Since this measure does not seem realistic under all sporting conditions, other measures should be introduced. Lehman and Ravich (1990) suggested that all athletes should be warned about 'particularly dangerous maneuvers' that may involve blows to the head within each dangerous sport. Sportspersons should be taught to avoid such manoeuvres and be made aware of the fact that wearing approved helmets is a necessity in many of these sports. But they should also be made aware that wearing a helmet does not rule out all chances of acute or chronic brain damage and that wearing a helmet is not an excuse to seek dangerous situations. Nevertheless, the use of approved helmets should be encouraged in all sports sustaining the danger of head or brain injury (Fig. 1.2; see Fig. 24.1).

From the three studies on brain injury in soccer, although not explicitly mentioned, one may suggest the following preventive measures:

1 Ball weight should be constant and related to body weight.

2 Soccer players should perhaps be advised not to head the ball if it is travelling at a 'high' velocity.

3 Balls that are too hard or have become heavy with rain-water should be banned.

With regard to secondary and tertiary prevention, on-field evaluation of head injury is important. Guidelines are given by Lehman and Ravich (1990). Also some criteria for returning to competition after head injury are given. These criteria include:

1 Athletes who have sustained a severe head injury necessitating neurosurgical intervention should be restricted from participating in contact sports.

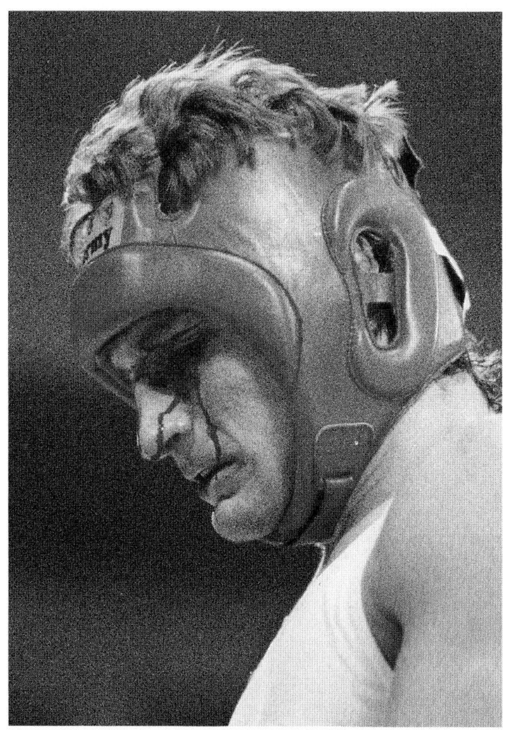

(a)

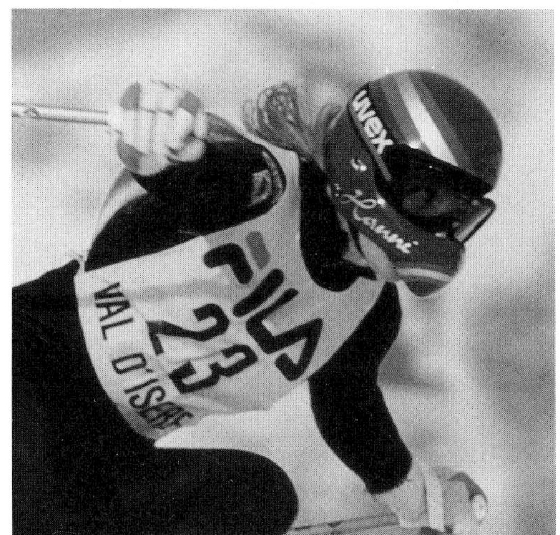

(b)

Fig. 1.2 Approved headgear helps to prevent serious head injuries, for instance in (a) boxing, and (b) skiing. (a) © IOPP/R. Kuntz, (b) © Allsport/R. Martin.

2 Athletes who have sustained a mild closed head injury usually may return to competition after a period of observation of 1 week and a normal neurological examination.

3 Athletes who have sustained a very mild closed head injury (no loss of consciousness) usually may return to competition after a brief period of sideline observation if completely asymptomatic.

References

Berger, R.E. & Calvano, N.J. (1979) Evaluation of product safety test methods: Protective headgear. *J. Safety Res.* **11**, 14–19.

Bishop, P.J. (1976) Head protection in sport with particular application to ice-hockey. *Ergonomics* **19**, 451–64.

Bishop, P.J. (1977) Comparative impact performance capabilities of ice hockey helmets. *J. Safety Res.* **9**(4), 159–67.

Bishop, P.J. (1978) Impact performance of ice hockey helmets. *J. Safety Res.* **10**(3), 13–129.

Bishop, P.J. & Briard, B.D. (1984) Impact performance of bicycle helmets. *Can. J. Appl. Sport Sci.* **9**, 94–101.

Bishop, P.J., Norman, R.W. & Kozey, J.W. (1984) An evaluation of football helmets under impact conditions. *Am. J. Sports Med.* **12**(3), 233–7.

Bishop, P.J. & Wells, R.P. (1990) The inappropriateness of helmet drop tests in assessing neck protection in head-first impacts. *Am. J. Sports Med.* **18**(2), 201–5.

Blonstein, J.L. & Clarke, E. (1967) Further observations on the medical aspects of amateur boxing. *Br. Med. J.* **16**, 362–4.

Council Report (1983) Brain injury in boxing (Council on Scientific Affairs). *JAMA* **249**(2), 254–7.

D'Abreu, F. (1978) The role of the specialized sports doctor in the prevention of injuries in sports. *Roy. Soc. Health J.* **98**(1), 27–9.

Goldsmith, W. (1981) Current controversies in the stipulation of head injury criteria. *J. Biomech.* **14**, 883–4.

Goldsmith, W. & Kabo, J.M. (1982) Performance of baseball headgear. *Am. J. Sports Med.* **10**(1), 31–7.

Gurdjian, E.S., Hodgson, V.R., Hardy, W.G. & Patrick, L.M. (1964) Evaluation of the protective characteristics of helmets in sports. *J. Trauma* **4**, 309–24.

Gurdjian, E.S., Roberts, V.L. & Thomas, L.M. (1966) Tolerance curves of acceleration and intracranial pressure and protective index in experimental head injuries *J. Trauma* **6**, 600–4.

Hodgson, V.R. (1975) National operating committee on standards for athletic equipment football helmet certification program. *Med. Sci. Sports* **7**, 225–32.

Johnson, J., Skorecki, J. & Wells, R.P. (1975) Peak acceleration experienced in boxing. *Med. Biol. Eng.* **13**, 396–404.

Kaste, M., Wilki, J., Saino, K., Kuurne, T., Katevuo, K. & Meurala, H. (1982) Is chronic brain damage in boxing a hazard of the past? *Lancet* **ii**, 1186–8.

Lehman, L.B. & Ravich, S.J. (1990) Closed head injuries in athletes. *Clin. Sports Med.* **9**(2), 247–61.

McElhaney, J.H., Stalnaker, R.L. & Roberts, V.L. (1973) Biomechanical aspects of head injury. In King & Mertz (eds) *Human Impact Response*, pp. 85–112. Plenum Press, New York.

Mills, N.J. & Whitlock, M.D. (1989) Performance of horse-riding helmets in frontal and side impacts. *Injury* **20**, 189–92.

Mueller, F.O. & Blyth, C.S. (1987) Fatalities from head and cervical spine injuries occurring in tackle football: 40 years' experience. *Clin. Sports Med.* **6**(1), 185–96.

Norman, R.W. (1983) Biomechanical evaluation of sports protective equipment. *Sport Sci. Rev.* **11**, 232–74.

Ommaya, A.K. & Hirsch, A.E. (1971) Tolerance for cerebral concussion from head impact and whiplash in primates. *J. Biomech.* **4**, 13–21.

Reid, S.E., Epstein, H.M., O'Dea, T.J., Louis, M.W. & Reid Jr, S.E. (1974) Head protection in football. *Sports Med.* **2**(2), 86–91.

Reid, S.E. & Reid Jr, S.E. (1981) Advances in sports medicine — Prevention of head and neck injuries in football. *Surg. Ann.* **13**, 251–70.

Ross, R.J., Cole, M., Thompson, J.S. & Kim, K.H. (1983) Boxers — Computed tomography, EEG, and neurological evaluation. *JAMA* **249**, 211–13.

Schneider, K. (1984) Das Risiko einer Hirnverletzung beim Fuβball-Kopfstoβ (Risk of brain injuries from kicking in football). *Unfallheilkunde* **87**, 40–2.

Sennerich, K.W.Th. (1988) Beitrag zur Epidemiologie der Sportverletzungen (The epidemiology of sports injuries). *Zeitschr. Sportmed.* **39**(4), 136–42.

Stichting Consument en Veiligheid (SCV) (1986) *PORS-sport 85, Jaaroverzicht 1985*. Uitgave van St. Consument en Veiligheid, Amsterdam.

Thompson, D.C., Thompson, R.S., Rivara, F.P. & Wolf, M.E. (1990) A case-control study of the effectiveness of bicycle safety helmets in preventing facial injury. *Am. J. Pub. Health* **80**(12), 1471–4.

Thompson, R.S., Rivara, F.P. & Thompson, D.C. (1989) A case-control study of the effectiveness of bicycle safety helmets. *New Engl. J. Med.* **320**(21), 1361–7.

Torg, J.S., Truex, R., Quedenfeld, Th.C. & Burstein, A. (1979) The National Football Head and Neck

Injury Registry. *JAMA* **241**, 1477–9.

Tysvaer, A.T. & Løchen, E.A. (1991) Soccer injuries to the brain, a neuropsychologic study of former soccer players. *Am J. Sports Med.* **19**(1), 56–69.

Tysvaer, A.T. & Storli, O.-V. (1989) Soccer injuries to the brain, a neurologic and electroencephalographic study of active football players. *Am. J. Sports Med.* **17**(4), 573–8.

Unterharnscheidt, F. (1985) Boxing injuries. In: R.C. Schneider, J.C. Kennedy, & M.L. Plant (eds) *Sports Injuries*, pp. 462–95. Williams & Wilkins, Baltimore.

Van Mechelen, W., Hlobil, H. & Kemper, H.C.G. (1987) *How can sports injuries be prevented?* NISGZ Publication No. 25E, The Netherlands.

Walter, S.D., Sutton, J.R., McIntosh, J.M. & Connolly, C. (1985) The aetiology of sports injuries. A review of methodologies. *Sports Med.* **2**, 47–58.

Wasserman, R.C. & Buccini, R.V. (1990) Helmet protection from head injuries among recreational bicyclists. *Am J. Sports Med.* **18**(1), 96–7.

Chapter 2

Cervical Spine Injuries in American Football

JOSEPH S. TORG

Epidemiological, pathological, biomechanical and cinematographic data on head and neck injuries occurring in American tackle football (called football from now on) have been compiled since 1971 by the National Football Head and Neck Injury Registry. Preliminary analysis performed in 1975 indicated that the majority of serious football cervical spine injuries were due to axial loading. Based on this observation, the National Collegiate Athletic Association (NCAA) and the National Federation of High School Athletic Associations (NFHSAA) implemented rule changes banning 'spearing' and the use of the top of the helmet as the initial point of contact in striking an opponent during a tackle or block. Between 1976 and 1987, as a result of these rule changes, the Registry has documented a dramatic decrease in both the total number of cervical spine injuries and those resulting in quadriplegia at both the high-school and college level. It is suggested that development and implementation of similar preventative measures based on clearly defined injury mechanisms would decrease injury rates in diving, Rugby, ice hockey, wrestling and other high-risk sports as well.

Cervical spine injuries

Athletic injuries to the cervical spine resulting in damage to the spinal cord are infrequent but catastrophic events. Accurate descriptions of the mechanism or mechanisms responsible for a particular injury transcend simple academic interest. Before preventative measures can be developed and implemented, identification of the mechanisms involved in the production of the particular injury is necessary. Due to the inability of the nervous system to recover significant function following severe trauma, prevention assumes a most important role when considering these injuries.

Injuries resulting in spinal cord damage have been associated with football (Schneider, 1966; King, 1967; Leidholt & John, 1973; Schneider & Richard, 1973; Dolan *et al.*, 1975; Funk *et al.*, 1975; Maroon *et al.*, 1979), water sports (Richman & Friedman, 1954; Schneider, 1955; Schneider *et al.*, 1956; Rogers, 1957; Whitley & Forsyth, 1960; Petrie, 1964; King, 1967; Garger *et al.*, 1969; Dall, 1972; Albrand & Walter, 1975; Kewalramani & Taylor, 1975; Stauffer & Kaufer, 1975; Albrand & Corkhill, 1976; Coin *et al.*, 1979; Gehweiler *et al.*, 1979; Mennen, 1981; Scher, 1981a, 1982b,c; Tator *et al.*, 1981; Allen *et al.*, 1982; Adelstein & Watson, 1983; Mawk, 1983; Dorwart & LeMasters, 1985; Haines, 1986), gymnastics (Schneider, 1955; Schneider & Kahn, 1956), wrestling (Cloward, 1980; Wu & Lewis, 1985), Rugby (Scher, 1978, 1981b; Carvell *et al.*, 1983; Silver, 1984), trampolining (Frykman & Hilding, 1970; Steinbruck & Paeslack, 1978; Hammer *et al.*, 1981; Torg & Das, 1984), and ice hockey (Tator & Edmonds, 1984; Tator *et al.*, 1984).

This study, through the use of epidemiological data, biomechanical evidence and cinematographic analysis, will:

1 Define and support the involvement of axial load forces in cervical spine injuries occurring in football.
2 Demonstrate the success of appropriate rule changes in the prevention of these injuries.
3 Emphasize the need for employment of epidemiological methods to prevent cervical spine and similar severe injuries in other high-risk athletic activities.

Comparison of head injury data from the period 1959–1963 to that obtained by the Registry for the years 1971–1975 demonstrated that both intracranial haemorrhages and intracranial deaths had decreased (Table 2.1). Schneider (1966) found 139 lesions (3.39 per 100 000) in which intracranial haemorrhages were a component, and 65 deaths (1.58 per 100 000) from craniocerebral injuries. The Registry documented 72 intracranial lesions (1.15 per 100 000), and 58 craniocerebral deaths (0.92 per 100 000) occurring between 1971 and 1975. These rates represent a 66% decrease for haemorrhages and a 42% decrease in craniocerebral deaths.

With regard to cervical spine injuries, Schneider (1966) reported 56 injuries (1.36 per 100 000) that involved a fracture and/or dislocation, and 30 with associated permanent cervical quadriplegia (0.73 per 100 000). The Registry documented 259 injuries (4.14 per 100 000) involving a fracture and/or dislocation of the cervical spine, and 99 cases (1.58 per 100 000) of cervical quadriplegia. These rates represented a 204% increase for cervical spine fractures–subluxations–dislocations, and a 116% increase for cases of cervical quadriplegia. While the rates of head injuries had decreased, the rates of cervical spine injuries with or without quadriplegia had increased dramatically from the data reported by Schneider (Table 2.1).

Three conclusions were made based on these findings:
1 The improved protective capabilities of modern helmets accounted for the decrease in head injuries between the two studies.
2 The improved protection of the head led to the development of playing techniques that used the top or crown of the helmet as the initial point of contact.
3 These head-first techniques placed the cervical spine at risk for serious injury. It was postulated that execution of head-first techniques increased the risk of neck injury by exposing the athlete's cervical spine to excessive axial loads, a force to which the cervical spine appears to be particularly susceptible.

These preliminary observations were reported at the annual meeting of the NCAA Football Rules Committee in February 1976. As a result, the following rules were instituted beginning with the 1976 season:
1 No player shall intentionally strike a runner with the crown or top of the helmet.
2 Spearing is the deliberate use of the helmet in an attempt to punish an opponent.

Table 2.1 In comparing the occurrence and rate of head and neck injuries in American football during two 5-year periods, 1959–1963 (Schneider, 1966) and 1971–1975 (National Football Head and Neck Injury Registry), a 66% decrease in the rate of intracranial haemorrhages and a 42% decrease in the rate of craniocerebral deaths between the two periods is noted. More significantly, the rate of cervical spine fractures, subluxations and dislocations increased 204% and the rate of cervical spine injuries associated with permanent quadriplegia increased 116%.

Year	Intracranial haemorrhages	Craniocerebral deaths	Cervical spine fractures–subluxations–dislocations	Permanent cervical quadriplegia
1959–1963	139 (3.39)	65 (1.58)	56 (1.36)	30 (0.73)
1971–1975	72 (1.15)	58 (0.92)	259 (4.14)	99 (1.58)

3 No player shall deliberately use helmets to butt or ram an opponent.
(*NCAA Football Rule Changes and/or Modifications*, 23 January 1976, rule 2, section 1, article 2-L, 2-N.) Similar rules were also adopted by the NFHSAA during the same year. The goal of these rule changes was to bring about changes in coaching and playing techniques in order to eliminate the use of the head as the initial point of contact in blocking and tackling.

Axial loading has been implicated as the primary mechanism producing severe cervical spine injuries in tackle football through review of epidemiological, biomechanical and cinematographic data compiled by the National Football Head and Neck Injury Registry. In the course of a contact activity, such as tackle football, the cervical spine is repeatedly exposed to potentially injurious energy inputs. Fortunately, however, most forces are effectively dissipated by the energy-absorbing capabilities of the cervical paravertebral musculature and the intervertebral discs through controlled spinal motion. However, the vertebra, intervertebral discs and supporting ligamentous structures can be injured when contact occurs on the top or crown of the helmet with the head, neck and trunk positioned in such a way that forces are transmitted along the vertical axis of the cervical spine. In this situation in which the cervical spine assumes the physical characteristics of a segmented column, motion is precluded in response to axial directed impacts, and the forces are directly transmitted to the spinal structures.

When viewed from the lateral perspective, with the neck in the neutral position, the normal alignment of the spine is one of extension because of the normal lordotic curve (Fig. 2.1). It is with 30° of neck flexion that the cervical spine is straightened (Fig. 2.2). With impact exerted along the longitudinal axis of a straight spine, loading of a segmented column occurs (Fig. 2.3a,b). At first, energy inputs are absorbed by the intervertebral discs and compressive deformation occurs. When maximum deformation is reached, continued energy input

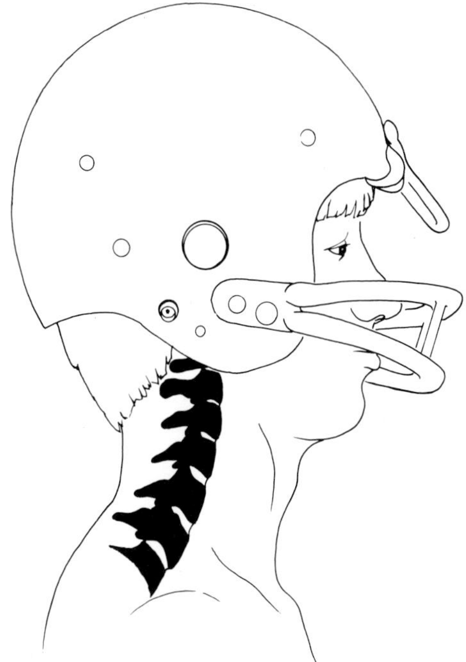

Fig. 2.1 When the neck is in a normal, upright, anatomical position, the cervical spine is slightly extended due to natural cervical lordosis. With permission from Torg *et al*. (1990).

results in angular deformation and buckling with failure of the intervertebral discs and/or bony elements. This results in subluxation, facet dislocation, or fracture–dislocation at one spinal level (Frankel & Burstein, 1970) (Fig. 2.3c,d,e).

Axial loading of the cervical spine occurs when the neck is slightly flexed, normal cervical lordosis is straightened, and the spine is converted into a segmented column. Assuming the head, neck and trunk components of a composite injury model to be in motion, rapid deceleration of the head occurs when it strikes another object, such as an opposing player, and results in the fragile cervical spine being compressed by the force of the oncoming trunk. Essentially, the head is stopped, the trunk is still moving, and the spine is crushed between the two. As mentioned, if the compression force is not dissipated by controlled

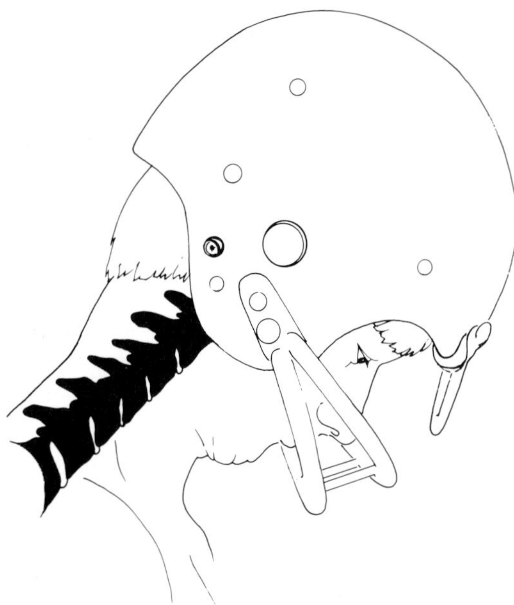

Fig. 2.2 When the neck is slightly flexed to approximately 30°, the cervical spine is straightened and converted into a segmented column. With permission from Torg *et al.* (1990).

motion in the spinal segments, fracture and/or dislocations results.

National Football Head and Neck Injury Registry

In order to obtain data on football-related injuries with associated neurological sequelae, the National Football Head and Neck Injury Registry was established. Initiated in 1975 as an ongoing registry, information was first collected retrospectively to 1971. Criteria for inclusion in the Registry were those head or cervical spine injuries that:

1 Required hospitalization for more than 72 h.

2 Required surgical intervention.

3 Involved a fracture, subluxation or dislocation.

4 Resulted in permanent paralysis or death.

Information was obtained by several methods. Project descriptions and injury report forms were mailed at the conclusion of each football season to the 40 000 members of

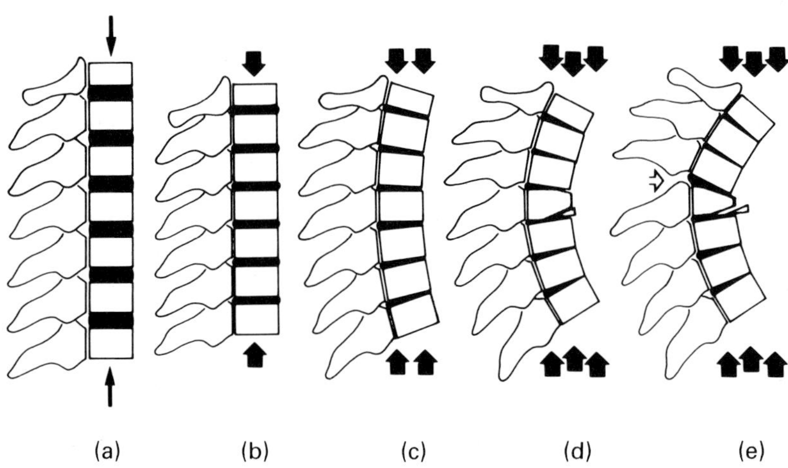

Fig. 2.3 Biomechanically, a straight cervical spine responds to an axial load force like a segmented column. Axial loading of the cervical spine first results in compressive deformation of the intervertebral discs. (a & b) As the energy input continues and maximum compressive deformation is reached, angular deformation and buckling occur. The spine fails in a flexion mode (c) with resulting fracture, subluxation or dislocation. (d & e) Compressive deformation to failure with a resultant fracture, dislocation or subluxation occurs in as little as 8.4 ms (Frankel & Burstein, 1970). With permission from Torg *et al.* (1990).

the National Association of Secondary School Principals and the 5000 members of the National Athletic Trainers Association. In addition, a newspaper/media-clipping service was contracted each year to identify those head and neck injuries reported in the press, radio or television. When an injury was reported, more detailed information was obtained from the athlete, parent and school officials. Pertinent medical and radiographic data from the physicians and hospitals responsible for the care of the athlete was also acquired. All the information collected on each athlete was reviewed for:

1 The mechanism of injury.
2 The pathological state of spinal and neural elements.
3 The type of treatment received.
4 The extent and duration of neurological deficit resulting from the injury.

Injury rates for intracranial haemorrhages, intracranial deaths, cervical spine fractures/dislocations/subluxations, and permanent quadriplegia were calculated for both high school and collegiate participants each year of the study.

When available, game films or videotapes of the injury were studied in order to determine the mechanism of injury and to calculate the force of impact. Cinematographic records were reviewed for 60 athletes with injuries resulting in neurological deficits. Stop-frame kinetic analysis, a method which allows estimation of the magnitude of injury-producing forces, was performed on 11 films of athletes sustaining injuries which resulted in quadriplegia. The force acting on the athletes head, cervical spine and trunk segment was calculated using the law of conservation of linear momentum. The orientation of the head, cervical spine and trunk segment of each athlete was analysed to determine the mechanism of injury.

A review of the biomechanical literature was undertaken to correlate the clinical observations documented from the Registry data with the experimental information on cervical spine injury mechanisms.

Results of Registry data

Analysis of the Registry data revealed definite trends in the incidence of head and cervical spine injuries occurring in both high-school and collegiate football. Intracranial haemorrhages demonstrated an apparent increase between the years 1976 and 1982 and then maintained a fairly constant rate for the duration of the study. The brief increasing trend was due to the improved diagnostic capabilities in identifying these lesions provided by the advent of computerized axial tomography. Intracranial haemorrhages resulting in death remained relatively constant throughout the study.

Fractures, subluxations and dislocations of the cervical spine demonstrated a progressive decrease between the years 1976 and 1987 (Fig. 2.4). The 1976 injury rates of 7.72 per 100 000 and 30.66 per 100 000 for high-school and college athletes, respectively, decreased to 2.31 per 100 000 and 10.66 per 100 000 during the subsequent 12 years (Table 2.2). These rates represented a 70% reduction in high-school injuries and a 65% reduction in college injuries. The largest single year drop occurred between 1977 and 1978, 2 years following the 1976 rule changes. During this year, high-school injury rates fell from 7.06 per 100 000 to 3.72 per 100 000, a 47% decrease, and college injury rates declined from 20.00 per 100 000 to 10.66 per 100 000, also a 47% decrease.

Cervical spine injuries resulting in quadriplegia consistently declined from a total of 34 cases in 1976 to five cases in 1984 (Fig. 2.5). In 1976, the injury rate was 2.24 per 100 000 at the high-school level and 10.66 per 100 000 at the college level (Table 2.1). In 1977, just 1 year following the rule changes, the rates dropped to 1.30 per 100 000, a 42% decrease, and 2.66 per 100 000, a 75% decrease, for high-school and college athletes respectively. The rates continued to decline at both the high-school and college level until 1984. In 1984, the injury rates had fallen to 0.40 per 100 000 for high schools, an 82% decrease, and to 0 per 100 000 for col-

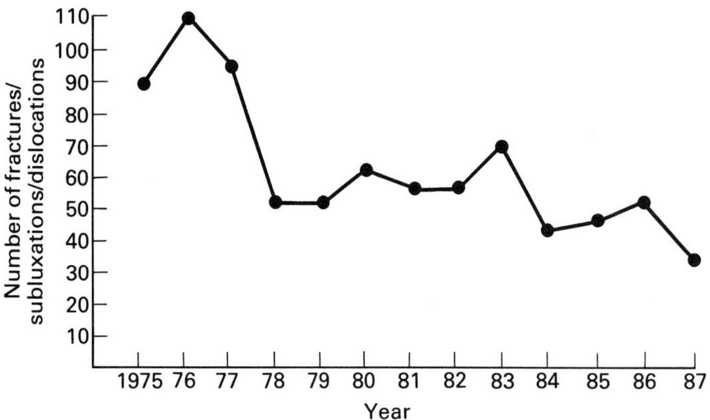

Fig. 2.4 The yearly incidence of cervical spine fractures–dislocations–subluxations for all levels of participation (1975–1987) decreased markedly in 1978 and continued to decline during the remaining 9 years as a direct result of the rule changes instituted in 1976 banning head-first blocking, tackling and spearing. With permission from Torg *et al.* (1990).

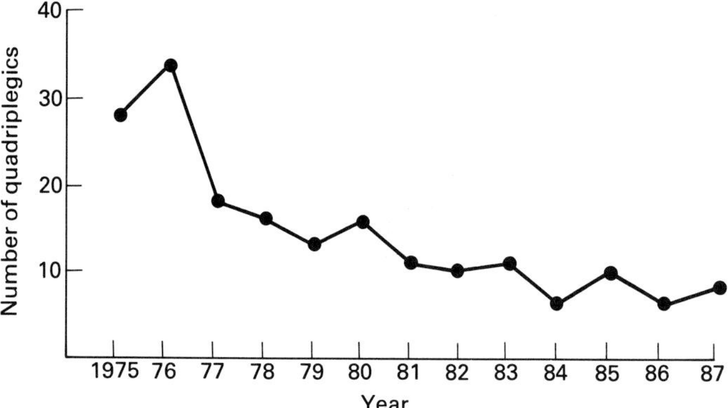

Fig. 2.5 The yearly incidence of permanent cervical quadriplegia for all levels of participation (1975–1987) decreased dramatically in 1977 following the initiation of the rule changes prohibiting the use of head-first tackling and blocking techniques. The number of injuries continued to decline until 1984, and were maintained for the remainder of the study. With permission from Torg *et al.* (1990).

leges, a 100% decrease. In 1985, the injury rates at both the high-school and college levels increased slightly from the low noted in 1984 and remained constant from 1985 to 1987 (Table 2.2).

Axial compression was identified as the mechanism causing the highest percentage of football cervical fractures–dislocations–subluxations with and without quadriplegia (Fig. 2.6). From 1971 to 1975, 39% of non-quadriplegia cervical spine injuries and 52% of the quadriplegia were attributed to this mechanism. During the years between 1976 and 1987, 52.5% of the quadriplegia and 49% of the non-quadriplegic cervical spine injuries were caused by the same mechanism.

Documentation of axial loading as the responsible mechanism of injury in the production of catastrophic football cervical spine injuries was obtained from the review of game films of actual injuries. Sixty films of injuries resulting in neurological deficits were available for study. Analysis of these films allowed determination of the mechanism of injury in 85% of the cases. In the 52 films in which it was possible to observe the mechanism of injury, it was determined to be axial loading in every instance. Stop frame analysis performed on 11 of these films determined that three distinct types of collisions existed. The first type was a direct collision in which two bodies travelled along the same straight line and in opposite directions prior to impact. The second type of collision was also direct but one in which a moving body hit another which was stationary. The third type was an oblique collision in which two moving bodies met at an angle. All eleven of the injuries were determined to be the result of head-first contact and all resulted

Table 2.2 12-year data for severe and catastrophic head and neck injuries occurring in American football at the high-school, college and professional/recreational levels. Rates in parentheses are per 100 000 participants based on participation numbers from the National Collegiate Athletic Association and the National Federation of State High School Athletic Associations for 11-man football.

Injury		1976	1977	1978	1979	1980	1981	1982	1983	1984	1985	1986	1987
Intracranial haemorrhage	High school	10	6	10	8	8	11	17	12	16	9	15	17
		(0.89)	(0.55)	(0.93)	(0.85)	(0.85)	(1.15)	(1.88)	(1.30)	(1.62)	(0.96)	(1.57)	(1.78)
	College	1	1	1	1	0	3	1	1	4	2	1	0
		(1.33)	(1.33)	(1.33)	(1.33)	4	(4.00)	(1.33)	(1.33)	(5.33)	(2.66)	(1.33)	
	Other	1	0	0	2		3	1	0	1	0	1	0
	Total	12	7	11	11	12	17	19	13	21	11	17	17
Craniocerebral deaths	High school	11	5	5	1	7	6	8	6	6	3	5	1
		(0.98)	(0.46)	(0.46)	(0.10)	(0.74)	(0.63)	(0.88)	(0.65)	(0.60)	(0.32)	(0.52)	(0.10)
	College	0	0		1	1	2	1	1	1	1	1	0
				0	(1.33)	(1.33)	(2.66)	(1.33)	(1.33)	(1.33)	(1.33)	(1.33)	
	Other	1	0	0	2	3	1	1	0	2	2	1	0
	Total	12	5	5	4	11	9	10	7	9	6	7	1
Cervical spine FX/DISL/SUBL	High school	86	76	40	42	52	49	46	60	36	32	36	22
		(7.72)	(7.06)	(3.72)	(4.47)	(5.54)	(5.16)	(5.10)	(6.50)	(3.65)	(3.43)	(3.78)	(2.31)
	College	23	15	8	7	9	8	6	7	5	6	11	8
		(30.66)	(20.00)	(10.66)	(9.33)	(12.00)	(10.66)	(8.00)	(9.33)	(6.66)	(8.00)	(14.66)	(10.66)
	Other	1	5	3	2	1	0	5	2	1	5	3	2
	Total	110	96	51	51	62	57	57	69	42	43	50	32
Permanent quadriplegia	High school	25	14	14	8	13	7	7	9	4	7	6	7
		(2.24)	(1.30)	(1.30)	(0.95)	(1.38)	(0.73)	(0.77)	(0.97)	(0.40)	(0.75)	(0.63)	(0.73)
	College	8	2	0	4	2	2	1	1	0	2	0	0
		(10.66)	(2.66)		(5.33)	(2.66)	(2.66)	(1.33)	(1.33)		(2.66)		
	Other	1	2	2	1	1	2	2	1	1	1	0	1
	Total	34	18	16	13	16	11	10	11	5	10	6	8

DISL, dislocation; FX, fracture; SUBL, subluxation.

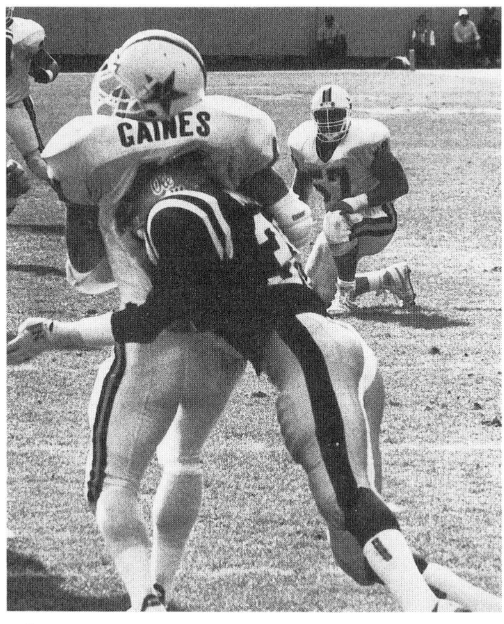

(a)

Fig. 2.6 Axial load mechanism. (a) With the advent of the polycarbonate helmet–face mask protective device, use of the top or crown of the helmet as the initial point of contact in blocking and tackling became prevalent. Contact is made, the head abruptly stops, the momentum of the body continues, and the cervical spine is literally crushed between the two. In this instance the fracture–dislocation transected the spinal cord.

in permanent cervical quadriplegia. Four of the injuries were type 1 collisions, three were type 2, and four were type 3. All 11 athletes were injured while tackling an opposing player.

The forces involved with the production of the 11 injuries was calculated based on the law of conservation of linear momentum. By determining the rate of change of the momentum of a body upon collision, the force of that collision can be determined. The impulse of a force ($F \times \Delta t$) is equal to the change of momentum that it produces ($mv_f - mv_i$) (where m = body mass, v = player velocity, f = final and i = initial). In a collision, the respective changes in momentum of the two bodies must be equal and opposite such that the total momentum of the system is unaltered by the impact. A sample calculation (Fig. 2.7) and the results for the 11 cases (Table 2.3) are presented. According to the data, the range of axial force which acted on the cervical spine during a direct collision resulting in cervical quadriplegia was approximately 400–800 kg F, and the oblique resultant force range was approximately 400–800 kg F, and the oblique resultant force range was approximately 400–700 kg F. This estimated force was similar to the forces calculated by Hodgson and Thomas (1980). They calculated

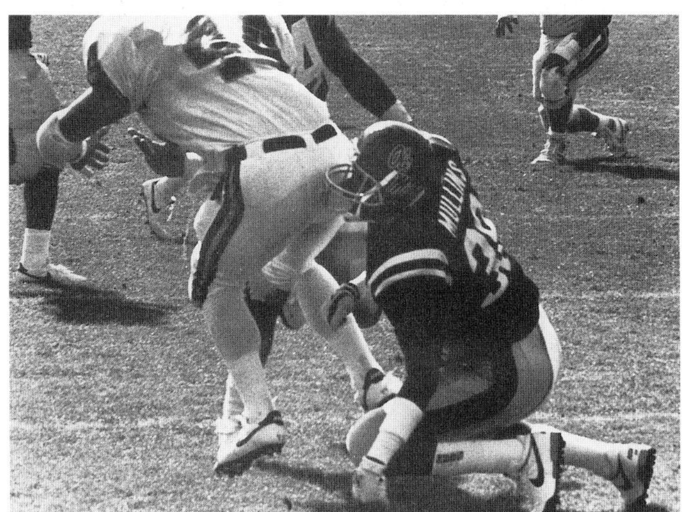

(b)

Fig. 2.6 (b) The injured player collapses, having been rendered quadriplegic.

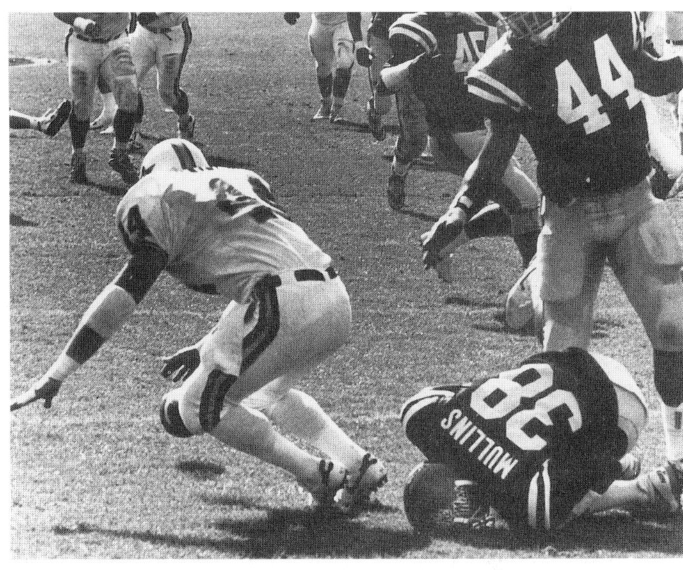

(c)

Fig. 2.6 (c) Further collapse is noted.

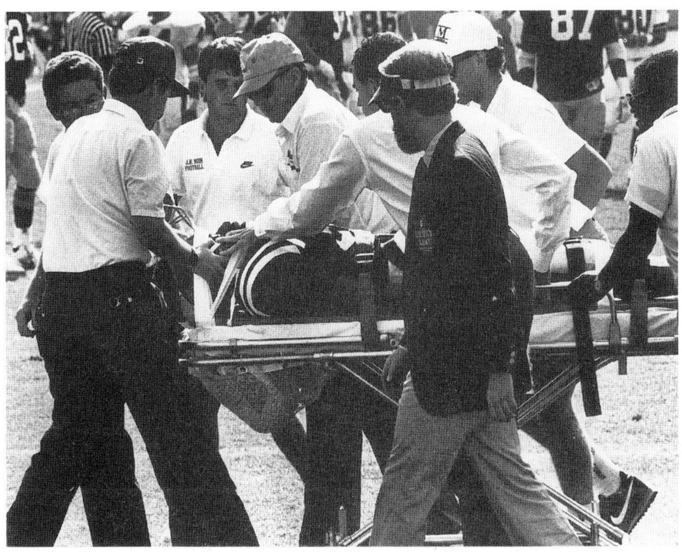

(d)

Fig. 2.6 (d) The player is evacuated on a spine board and stretcher. With permission from Torg (1982).

the estimated force of impact in axial loading cervical spine injuries from the work–kinetic energy point of view. The average force involved in each collision they studied was determined from the following formula:

$$\text{work} = F \times \Delta X = \tfrac{1}{2}\, mv^2$$

where X = stopping distance, m = body mass, and v = player velocity. Hodgson and Thomas concluded the average force acting on the neck was between 318 and 727 kg (700 and 1600 lb) F, a range nearly identical to that derived from stop frame analysis (Table 2.3).

wt = 84 kg
$V_i = 4.9\ \text{m·s}^{-1}$
$V_f = 0\ \text{m·s}^{-1}$
$t = 0.06$ s

According to Newton's second law and the concept of conservation of momentum,

$$F_1 = m_1a_1 = F_2 = m_2a_2$$
$$= \frac{(m_1v_{i1}) - (m_1v_{f1})}{t} = \frac{(m_2v_{i2}) - (m_2v_{f2})}{t}$$

$$\because v_{f1} = 0 = v_{f2}$$

$$\therefore F_1 = m_1\frac{v_{i1}}{t} = F_2 = m_2\frac{v_{i2}}{t}$$

Therefore,

$$F = \frac{(84\ \text{kg})\ (4.9\ \text{m·s}^{-1})}{0.06\ \text{s}}$$
$$= 6860\ \text{kg·m}^{-1}\text{·s}^{-2}$$
$$= 6860\ \text{N}$$

Since 1 kg force = 9.8 N,

$$F = \frac{6860\ \text{N}}{9.8\ \text{N·kg force}^{-1}} = 700.00\ \text{kg force}$$

700.00 kg force is the estimated axial force acting upon the victim's cervical spine during the injury producing impact. The same type of calculation is used to estimate the force of impact in type two collisions. In type three collisions, however the additional variable 0_i (angle of incidence) must be added into the calculation of momentum.

Fig. 2.7 Sample calculation using the law of conservation of momentum in order to estimate the force of impact values by stop frame analysis. With permission from Torg *et al.* (1990).

Discussion

Refutation of the 'freak accident' concept with the more logical principle of cause and effect has been most rewarding in dealing with the problem of football-induced cervical spine trauma and quadriplegia. Definition of the axial loading mechanism in which football players, usually defensive backs, make a tackle by striking their opponent with the top of their helmets has been key in this process. Implementation of rule changes and coaching techniques eliminating the use of the head as a battering ram have resulted in a dramatic reduction in the incidence of cervical spine injuries with or without quadriplegia between 1976 and 1987.

Although this data leads to the conclusion that axial loading is the predominant force involved in the production of athletic cervical spine injuries, classically, these injuries have been attributed to either hyperflexion or hyperextension mechanisms. Schneider (1966, 1973), the first researcher to catalogue head and neck injuries occurring in athletic competition, supported this traditional view. In his series of cervical spine injuries occurring in tackle football, he concluded that the most severe injuries to the cervical spine occur as a result of hyperflexion.

Table 2.3 Presentation of the estimated force of impact values for 11 axial loading injuries resulting in quadriplegia calculated in stop frame analysis. See Fig. 2.7 for a sample calculation of the estimated force of impact values.

	Case	Age	m (kg)	v_i ($m \cdot s^{-1}$)	v_f ($m \cdot s^{-1}$)	O_i (deg)	Est. force (kg F)
Type 1 collisions	1	19	84	4.90	0	—	700.00
	2	19	77	6.63	0	—	368.21
	3	17	75	5.08	0	—	667.96
	4	15	68	5.83	0	—	674.22
Type 2 collisions	5	17	80	6.10	0	—	829.89
	6	17	75	3.59	0	—	457.91
	7	16	75	3.39	0	—	432.40
Type 3 collisions	8	15	75	4.70	0	10	550.03
	9	15	64	3.81	0	90	439.85
	10	17	73	6.10	0	30	751.11
	11	17	73	5.08	0	90	501.71

m, Injured player's mass in kg; v_i, injured player's velocity in $m \cdot s^{-1}$ prior to impact; v_f, injured player's velocity in $m \cdot s^{-1}$ after collision; O_i, the incident angle for those collisions which were oblique; Est. force, estimated force calculated in stop frame analysis.

Schneider also mentioned that hyperextension may cause cervical lesions resulting in neurological damage. He did not list axial loading or vertex impact among the forces associated with football cervical spine neurotrauma.

Other authors have also used these mechanisms to account for a variety of catastrophic athletic cervical spine injuries. Carvell *et al.* (1983) (Rugby), Gehweiler *et al.* (1979) (diving), Leidhold (1973) (football), McNab (1964) (diving), McCoy *et al.* (1984) (Rugby), O'Carroll *et al.* (1981) (Rugby), Paley and Gillespie (1986) (general sports), Piggot and Gordon (1979) (Rugby), Scher (1982a) (Rugby), Williams and McKibbin (1978) (Rugby), and Wu and Lewis (1985) (wrestling). All proposed hyperflexion as the most frequent cause of serious cervical injuries in the activities they reviewed.

Others who, like Schneider, have emphasized both hyperextension and hyperflexion as the two dominant forces producing most types of cervical spine lesions with cord damage include Dolan *et al.* (1975) (football), Funk and Wells (1975) (football), and Silver (1984) (Rugby). Although some authors, such as Kazarian (1981) (general sports), Kewalramani and Taylor (1975) (diving), recognized that axial loading is associated with severe cervical spine injuries, they continued to emphasize the dominant role of hyperflexion and/or hyperextension forces in the production of these lesions.

Traditionally, axial loads have not been mentioned among the major forces contributing to cervical spine fractures, dislocations or fracture–dislocations occurring in athletes. Allen *et al.* (1982) (diving), Jackson and Lohr (1986) (general sports), King (1967) (football and diving), and Stauffer and Kaufer (1975) (diving) mentioned axial loading as a common mechanism but they stated that hyperextension and/or hyperflexion still accounted for a significant number of the lesions. As a direct result of the National Football Head and Neck Injury Registry data, the axial loading mechanism has been identified as the predominant mechanism of injury for athletic cervical spine injuries. In addition to the studies of Torg (1982), Torg and Das (1984), Torg *et al.* (1977, 1979a,b, 1984, 1985), Scher in diving (1981a) and Rugby (1981b), Tator and Edmonds (1984), Tator *et al.* in diving (1981) and ice hockey (1984), and Watkins (1986) in football demonstrated vertical impact and axial loading to be the major forces to consider when analysing cervical spine injuries in athletes.

A review of the literature pertaining to the biomechanics of cervical spine injuries yielded experimental support for the axial loading theory. Mertz *et al.* (1978), Hodgson and Thomas (1980), and Sances *et al.* (1984) measured stresses and strains within the cervical spine when axial impulses were applied to helmeted cadaver head–spine–trunk specimens. They were able to produce fractures of the lower cervical spine when the impulse was applied to the crown of the helmet. Hodgson and Thomas determined that direct vertex impact imparted a larger force to the cervical vertebra than forces applied further forward on the skull. Gosch *et al.* (1972) investigated three different injury modes, hyperflexion, hyperextension, and axial compression in their experiment involving anaesthetized monkeys and concluded that axial compression produced cervical spine fractures and dislocations. Maiman *et al.* (1983), Roaf (1960), and White and Punjabi (1978) demonstrated vertebral body fractures in the lower cervical spine due to the axial loading of isolated spinal units. Roaf (1960) subjected spinal units to forces differing in direction and magnitude, i.e. compression, flexion, extension, lateral flexion, rotation and horizontal shear. He stated unequivocally that he had never succeeded in producing pure hyperflexion injuries in a normal intact spinal unit, and concluded that hyperflexion of the cervical spine was an anatomical impossibility. Roaf was able to produce almost every variety of spinal injury with a combination of compression and rotation.

Bauze and Ardran (1978) postulated that axial loads were responsible for cervical spine dislocations as well as fractures. They demonstrated that failure of the facet joints and posterior ligaments occurred when axial loads were applied to cadaveric spines. When the lower portion of the spine was flexed and fixed, and the upper part extended and free to move forward, vertical compression produced bilateral dislocation of the facet joints without fracture. If lateral tilt or axial rotation occurred as well, a unilateral dislocation was produced. The forces observed were all less than those required for bony failure and allowed facet dislocation without associated bony pathology.

Conclusion

This study has delineated the important role that axial loading plays in the production of football cervical spine injuries. The author believes this mechanism is also responsible for similar injuries occurring in other collision sports. Whether it be a football player striking an opponent with the top or crown of the helmet, a poorly executed dive into a shallow body of water where the subject strikes his or her head on the bottom, or a hockey player checked into the boards head first, injury occurs as the fragile cervical spine is compressed between the rapidly decelerated head and the continued momentum of the body. Appropriate rule changes recognizing this mechanism have resulted in a marked reduction of football cervical injuries with and without quadriplegia. The success of the preventative measures advocated by the National Football Head and Neck Injury Registry leads to the suggestion that similar studies, directed towards the prevention of injuries rather than their treatment would almost likely decrease rates for many types of injuries in a wide variety of athletic activities. Continued research; development of clear and concise definitions of the responsible injury mechanisms based on sound biomechanical, epidemiological, and clinical evidence; education of coaches and players; and enforcement of rules is essential in order that the preventative measures may succeed.

References

Adelstein, W. & Watson, P. (1983) Cervical spine injuries. *J. Neurosurg. Nursing* **15**, 65–71.

Albrand, O.W. & Corkill, G. (1976) Broken necks from diving accidents: A summer epidemic in young men. *Am. J. Sports Med.* **4**, 107–10.

Albrand, O.W. & Walter, J. (1975) Underwater deceleration curves in relation to injuries from diving. *Surg. Neurol.* **4**, 461–5.

Allen, Jr, B.L., Ferguson, R.L., Lehman, R.T. & O'Brien, R.P. (1982) A mechanistic classification of closed, indirect fractures and dislocations of the lower cervical spine. *Spine* **7**, 1–27.

Bauze, R.J. & Ardran, G.M. (1978) Experimental production of forward dislocation in the human cervical spine. *J. Bone Joint Surg.* **60B**, 239–45.

Carvell, J.E., Fuller, D.J., Duthrie, R.B. & Cockin, J. (1983) Rugby football injuries to the cervical spine. *Br. Med. J.* **286**, 49–50.

Cloward, R.B. (1980) Acute cervical spine injuries. *Clin. Symp.* **32**, 2–32.

Coin, C.G., Pennink, M., Ahmad, D.W. & Keranen, V.J. (1979) Diving-type injury of the cervical spine: Contribution of computed tomography to management. *J. Computer Ass. Tomogr.* **3**, 362–72.

Dall, D.M. (1972) Injuries of the cervical spine. *S. Afr. Med. J.* **46**, 1048–56.

Dolan, K.D., Feldick, H.G., Albright, J.P. & Moses, J.M. (1975) Neck injuries in football players. *Am. Fam. Phys.* **12**, 86–91.

Dorwart, R. & LeMasters, D.L. (1985) Application of computed tomographic scanning of the cervical spine. *Orthop. Clin. N. Am.* **16**, 381–93.

Frankel, V.H. & Burstein, A. (1970) *Orthopaedic Biomechanics*. Lea & Febiger, Philadelphia.

Frykman, G. & Hilding, S. (1970) Hop pa studsmatta kan orska allvarliga skador (Trampoline jumping can cause serious injury). *Läkartidningen* **67**, 5862–4.

Funk, Jr, F.J. & Wells, R.E. (1975) Injuries of the cervical spine in football. *Clin. Orthop. Rel. Res.* **109**, 50–8.

Garger, W.N., Fisher, R. & Halfmann, H.W. (1969) Vertebrectomy and fusion for 'tear drop fracture' of the cervical spine: case report. *J. Trauma* **9**, 887–93.

Gehweiler, J.H., Clark, W.M., Schaaf, R., Powers, B. & Miller, M. (1979) Cervical spine trauma: The common combined conditions. *Radiology* **130**, 77–86.

Gosch, H.H., Gooding, E. & Schneider, R.C. (1972) An experimental study of cervical spine and cord injuries. *J. Trauma* **12**, 570–5.

Haines, J.D. (1986) Occult cervical spine fractures. *Postgrad. Med.* **80**, 73–7.

Hammer, A., Schwartzbach, A.L., Darre, E. & Osgaard, O. (1981) Svaere neurologiske skader some folge af trampolinspring (severe neurologic damage resulting from trampolining). *Ugeskrift Laeger* **143**, 2970–4.

Hodgson, V.R. & Thomas, L.M. (1980) *Mechanisms of cervical spine injury during impact to the protected head*, pp. 15–42. 24th Stapp Car Crash Conference.

Jackson, D.W. & Lohr, T. (1986) Cervical spine injuries. *Clin. Sports Med.* **5**, 373–86.

Kazarian, L. (1981) Injuries to the human spinal column: Biomechanics and injury classification. *Exerc. Sport Sci. Rev.* **9**, 297–352.

Kewalramani, L.S. & Taylor, R.G. (1975) Injuries to the cervical spine from diving accidents. *J. Trauma* **15**, 130–42.

King, D.M. (1969) Fractures and dislocations of the cervical spine. *Australia N. Zeal. J. Surg.* **37**, 57–64.

Leidholt, J.D. (1973) Spinal injuries in athletes: Be prepared. *Orthop. Clin. N. Am.* **4**, 691–707.

McCoy, G.F., Piggot, J., Macafee, A.L. & Adair, I. (1984) Injuries of the cervical spine in schoolboy rugby football. *J. Bone Joint Surg.* **66B**, 500–3.

MacNab, I. (1964) Acceleration injuries of the cervical spine. *J. Bone Joint Surg.* **46A**, 1797–9.

Maiman, D.J., Sances, A., Myklebust, J.B., Larson, J.L., Houterman, C., Chilbert, M. & El-Gatit, A.Z. (1983) Compression injuries of the cervical spine: A biomechanical analysis. *Neurosurgery* **13**, 254–60.

Maroon, J.C., Steele, P.B. & Berlin, R. (1979) Football head and neck injuries — An update. *Clin. Neurosurg.* **27**, 414–29.

Mawk, J.R. (1983) C7 burst fracture with initial 'complete' tetraplegia. *Minn. Med.* **66**, 135–8.

Mennen, U. (1981) Survey of spinal injuries from diving: A study of patients in Pretoria and Cape Town. *S. Afr. Med. J.* **59**, 788–790.

Mertz, H.J., Hodgson, V.R., Murray, T.L. & Nyquist, G.W. (1978) An assessment of compressive neck loads under injury-producing conditions. *Phys. Sportsmed.* **6**(11), 95–106.

O'Carroll, F., Sheenan, M. & Gregg, T.M. (1981) Cervical spine injuries in rugby football. *Irish Med. J.* **74**, 377–9.

Paley, D. & Gillespie, R. (1986) Chronic repetitive unrecognized injury of the cervical spine (high jumper's neck). *Am. J. Sports Med.* **14**, 92–5.

Petrie, J.G. (1964) Flexion injuries of the cervical spine. *J. Bone Joint Surg.* **46A**, 1800–6.

Piggot, J. & Gordon, D.S. (1979) Rugby injuries to the cervical cord. *Br. Med. J.* **i**, 192–3.

Richman, S. & Friedman, R. (1954) Vertical fracture of cervical vertebral bodies. *Radiology* **62**, 536–42.

Roaf, R. (1960) A study of the mechanics of spinal injuries. *J. Bone Joint Surg.* **42E**, 810–23.

Rogers, W.A. (1957) Fractures and dislocations of the cervical spine: An end-result study. *J. Bone Joint Surg.* **39a**, 341–76.

Sances, A.J., Myklebust, J.B., Maiman, D.J., Larson, S.J. & Cusick, J.F. (1984) Biomechanics of spinal injuries. *Crit. Rev. Biomed. Eng.* **11**, 1–76.

Scher, A.T. (1978) The high rugby tackle — An avoidable cause of cervical spinal injury? *S. Afr. Med. J.*

53, 1015–18.

Scher, A.T. (1981a) Diving injuries to the cervical spinal cord. *S. Afr. Med. J.* **59**, 603–5.

Scher, A.T. (1981b) Vertex impact and cervical dislocation in rugby players. *S. Afr. Med. J.* **59**, 227–8.

Scher, A.T. (1982a) 'Crashing' the rugby scrum — An avoidable cause of cervical spinal injury. *S. Afr. Med. J.* **61**, 919–20.

Scher, A.T. (1982b) Radiographic indicators of traumatic cervical spine instability. *S. Afr. Med. J.* **62**, 562–5.

Scher, A.T. (1982c) 'Tear-drop' fractures of the cervical spine — Radiologic features. *S. Afr. Med. J.* **61**, 355–9.

Schneider, R.C. (1955) The syndrome of acute anterior spinal cord injury. *J. Neurosurg.* **12**, 95–123.

Schneider, R.C. (1966) Serious and fatal neurosurgical football injuries. *Clin. Neurosurg.* **12**, 226–36.

Schneider, R.C. (1973) *Head and Neck Injuries in Football*. Williams & Wilkins, Baltimore.

Schneider, R.C. & Kahn, E.A. (1956) Chronic neurologic sequelae of acute trauma to the spine and spinal cord. Part I. The significance of the acute-flexion or 'tear-drop' fracture dislocation of the cervical spine. *J. Bone Joint Surg.* **38A**, 985–97.

Silver, J.R. (1984) Injuries of the spine sustained in rugby. *Br. Med. J.* **288**, 37–43.

Stauffer, E.S. & Kaufer, H. (1975) Fractures and dislocations of the spine. In C.A. Rockwood Jr & D.P. Green (eds) *Fractures*, Vol. 2. Lippincott, Philadelphia.

Steinbruck, J. & Paeslack, V. (1978) Trampolinspringen — Ein gefahrlicher Sport? (Is trampolining a dangerous sport?) *Munch. Med. Wochenschr.* **120**, 985–8.

Tator, C.H. & Edmonds, V.E. (1984) National survey of spinal injuries to hockey players. *Can. Med. Assoc. J.* **130**, 875–80.

Tator, D.H., Ekong, C.E.U., Rowed, D.A., Schwartz, M.L., Edmonds, V.E. & Cooper, P.W. (1984) Spinal injuries due to hockey. *Can. J. Neurol. Sci.* **11**, 34–41.

Tator, C.H., Edmonds, V.E. & New, M.L. (1981) Diving: frequent and potentially preventable cause of spinal cord injury. *Can. Med. Assoc. J.* **124**, 1323–4.

Torg, J.S., Otin, J.C. & Burstein, A.H. (1982) Mechanisms and pathomechanics of athletic injuries to the cervical spine. In J.S. Torg (ed) *Athletic Injuries to the Head, Neck and Face*, 2nd edn, pp. 139–54. Lea & Febiger, Philadelphia.

Torg, J.S. & Das, M. (1984) Trampoline-related quadriplegia: review of the literature and reflections on the American Academy of Pediatrics' position statement. *Pediatrics* **74**, 804–12.

Torg, J.S., Quedenfeld, T.C., Burstein, A., Spealman, A. & Nichols III, C. (1979a) National Football Head and Neck Injury Registry: Report on cervical quadriplegia 1971 to 1975. *Am. J. Sports Med.* **7**, 127–32.

Torg, J.S., Quedenfeld, T.C., Moyer, R.A., Truex, R., Spealman, A.D. & Nichols III, C.E. (1977) Severe and catastrophic neck injuries resulting from tackle football. *J. Am. Coll. Heath Assoc.* **25**, 224–66.

Torg, J.S., Truex, R., Quedenfeld, T.C., Burstein, A., Spealman, A. & Nichols, C. (1979b) The National Football Head and Neck Injury Registry report and conclusions. *JAMA* **241**, 1477–9.

Torg, J.S., Vegso, J., O'Neill, M.J. *et al.* (1990) The epidemiologic, pathologic, biomechanical and cinematographic analysis of football-induced cervical spine trauma. *Am. J. Sports Med.* **18**(1), 50–7.

Torg, J.S., Vegso, J.J., Sennett, B. & Das, M. (1985) The National Football Head and Neck Injury Registry. 14-year report on cervical quadriplegia, 1971 through 1984. *JAMA* **254**, 3439–43.

Torg, J.S., Vegso, J.S., Yu, A. & Gurtler, R. (1984) Cervical quadriplegia resulting from axial loading injuries: Cinematographic, radiographic, kinetic, and pathologic analysis. *Proceedings, Interim Meeting, American Orthopaedic Society for Sports Medicine*, 9 February 1984, Atlanta, Georgia.

Watkins, R.G. (1986) Neck injuries in football players. *Clin. Sports Med.* **5**, 215–46.

White III, A.A. & Punjabi, M.M. (1978) *Clinical Bio-Mechanics of the Spine*. Lippincott, Philadelphia.

Whitley, J.E. & Forsyth, H.F. (1960) The classification of cervical spine injuries. *Am. J. Roentgenol.* **83**, 633–44.

Williams, J.P.R. & McKibbin, B. (1978) Cervical spine injuries in rugby union football. *Br. Med. J.* **ii**, 1747.

Wu, W.Q. & Lewis, R.C. (1985) Injuries of the cervical spine in high school wrestling. *Surg. Neurol.* **23**, 143–7.

Chapter 3

Shoulder Injuries

WILLIAM J. MALLON AND RICHARD J. HAWKINS

Prevention of injuries to the shoulder requires warm-up before sports activities, flexibility and strength training in the preseason and maintained during the competitive season, proper techniques and equipment for the sports involved, and a knowledge of the injuries specific to each sport. A background on anatomy and biomechanics of the shoulder girdle will provide a better understanding of warm-up, strength training and flexibility training. Finally, the biomechanics and injuries specific to each sport and the techniques and training recommended to prevent them will be discussed.

Anatomy and biomechanics

To understand injuries to the shoulder joint complex, it is important to have an understanding of its normal anatomy and biomechanics. The shoulder joint consists of three joints and two articulations:

1 The glenohumeral joint.

2 The acromioclavicular joint.

3 The sternoclavicular joint.

4 The acromiohumeral articulation.

5 The scapulothoracic articulation.

In general, with movement of the shoulder, some motion will occur in all of the joints and articulations, although most often, discussion of motion at the shoulder is centred on motion at the glenohumeral and scapulothoracic joints.

The shoulder has the largest range of motion of any 'joint' in the body, and all of the above joints and articulations contribute to this motion. When performing sports, the joints are typically moved through extreme ranges of motion at very high angular velocities, thus predisposing to injuries (Sobel, 1986b) (Fig. 3.1). In addition, many overhead sports require multiple repetitions at this high velocity, which, with this wide range of motion, can lead to chronic injuries (Hawkins & Hobeika, 1983).

The shoulder during athletic use is not subject to the same loads as is the lower extremity during weight-bearing. In the hip and knee, joint reaction force is three to four times body weight during the single leg stance of gait and much higher during sprinting or jumping. Although the shoulder does not support the body weight while performing its activities, it is nevertheless under considerable stress. It has been shown that joint reaction force at the glenohumeral joint can approach 90% of body weight at 60–90° of abduction (Inman *et al.*, 1944; Freedman & Munroe, 1966). When combined with high angular velocities, extreme ranges of motion, and multiple repetitions of these motions, it is obvious that the shoulder is under great stress during certain athletic activities.

The acromiohumeral articulation is important in understanding the pathophysiology of certain athletic injuries to the shoulder. The articulation is often termed the supraspinatus outlet. It is unique in that it is the only place in

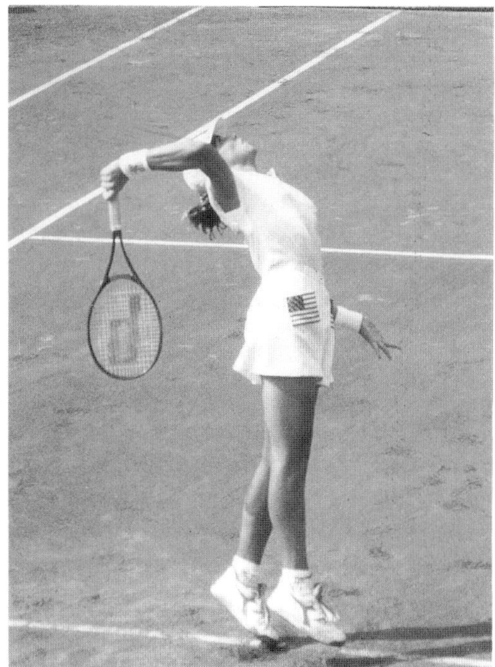

Fig. 3.1 During the tennis serve the shoulder is subjected to great stress. Courtesy of Dr P.A.F.H. Renström.

the body in which a muscle or tendon courses between two bones. In this case, the rotator cuff covers the top of the humeral head and, in turn, is covered by the undersurface of the acromion. In most activities, it is the supraspinatus tendon and muscle which is entrapped between acromion and humeral head, although in certain extreme positions, the subscapularis and infraspinatus (both rotator cuff muscles) may be entrapped within the supraspinatus outlet.

In addition to the tendons of the rotator cuff, the supraspinatus outlet includes the subacromial bursa and is bordered superiorly and medially by the coracoacromial ligament. When inflammation and oedema occurs within these structures, an impingement syndrome may develop in this space-limited area. As swelling and inflammation occurs, the outlet is filled to its limit and bony impingement on the structures within the outlet ensues (Hawkins & Kennedy, 1980; Hawkins & Hobeika, 1983). This can create a vicious cycle by causing further inflammation and oedema.

When swelling or muscle hypertrophy occurs in the supraspinatus outlet in an athlete, further repetition of overhead activity may increase the swelling or inflammation. This can lead to bony impingement and continued repetition may cause a tear of the rotator cuff (Hawkins & Hobeika, 1983).

In addition to injuries at the acromiohumeral articulation, athletes are also subject to instability of the glenohumeral joint. This is partly due to the unique anatomy of the glenohumeral joint which allows an almost global range of motion.

The head of the humerus articulates with the glenoid fossa to form the glenohumeral joint. The periphery of the glenoid fossa is bordered by the glenoid labrum, which is a fibrous thickening of the glenohumeral capsule. Compared to the hip joint, bony stability of the glenohumeral joint is almost nil. The femoral head is almost fully covered by the acetabulum, providing excellent architectural stability. In contrast, less than 30% of the surface of the humeral head is covered by the glenoid fossa, providing little intrinsic bony stability at this joint. With the addition of the glenoid labrum (which provides a modicum of additional support), the diameters of the glenoid surface are increased to 75% of the humeral head vertically and 67% in the transverse direction (Saha, 1973). However, this is often not enough to prevent instability from occurring in the glenohumeral joint.

The glenohumeral joint may thus dislocate and this can occur in any direction. Over 95% of dislocations occur anteriorly, with approximately 3% occurring posteriorly. Dislocations may recur and can become a recurrent problem for the athlete. The greatest prognostic factor in determining whether an anterior shoulder dislocation will become a recurrent problem is the age of the person who sustains the first-time dislocation; this probably relates to activity level. Recurrence rates of 90%+ are common when the first dislocation occurs in a person 20 years old or less. This is an age at which many adolescents are participating in sports and recurrent instability among athletes is common (Garth *et al.*, 1987).

In addition to frank dislocations, the shoulder may undergo subluxations or more subtle forms of anterior instability and these may also become troublesome (Garth *et al.*, 1987), often more disabling than dislocations. Because frank dislocation does not occur, the main symptom may be pain and the athlete may be unaware of the instability. This may delude the examining physician into failing to consider instability as a source of the pain (Garth *et al.*, 1987).

Finally, although recurrent anterior instability is the most common direction, some loose-jointed athletes develop a syndrome in which the glenohumeral articulation will be unstable in more than one direction. This is known as multidirectional instability (MDI) and is an especially invidious problem with which to deal.

Because of the lack of inherent bony stability in the glenohumeral joint, the joint relies on the soft tissues — joint capsule, ligaments and muscles — to provide stability. As athletes perform overhead activities through the extremes of motion, these soft tissues are often overworked and overstretched. In addition, repetitive motion in one direction affects structures on the opposite side of the joint and these soft tissues may then become contracted. It is felt that this combination of lax tissues on one side of the joint, and contracted tissues on the opposite side, may contribute to instability in the athlete by 'pushing' the humeral head asymetrically in the glenoid fossa. In addition to overwork and overstretch, the muscles of the shoulder joint are subjected to excessive loads and it is thought that this eccentric overload may cause tendinitis and degeneration.

Besides injuries to the acromiohumeral articulation and the glenohumeral joint, athletes may develop injuries to the acromioclavicular joint. In contrast to problems at the other joints, these tend to be acute, traumatic injuries, rather than overuse injuries (Norfray *et al.*, 1977; Kulund *et al.*, 1979; Pritchett, 1980; Canale *et al.*, 1981). An acromioclavicular dislocation (colloquially known as a 'shoulder separation') usually occurs from a direct blow to the top of the shoulder, while the arm is held at the side of the body. This is commonplace for contact sports such as American football, ice hockey, rugby football and lacrosse.

Chronic arthritic problems of the shoulder are rare among athletes. When they do occur it is almost exclusively in the acromioclavicular joint. This is usually secondary to an acromioclavicular dislocation in a contact sport. However, chronic degenerative changes in this joint can occur among weightlifters and ice-hockey players who have never sustained an acute, traumatic episode (Norfray *et al.*, 1977; Cahill, 1982; Silloway *et al.*, 1985).

Arthritic problems of the glenohumeral joint rarely occur in a young athletic population since these take several years to develop. When they do occur, they are likely to be secondary to a fracture of the humeral head, with secondary development of avascular necrosis of the humeral head or iatrogenically produced from surgical misadventure. This would likely preclude further participation in sports. Minor arthritic problems of this joint have been documented in pitchers (Bennett, 1959).

Athletic injuries to the sternoclavicular joint and scapulothoracic articulation can occur but are quite rare. It is important to remember, however, that contact trauma, either directly to the sternoclavicular joint or indirectly to the lateral aspect of the shoulder, can cause a dislocation of that joint, or a fracture of the inner clavicular physis. In fact, sports is the second most common cause of these injuries (after motor vehicle accidents) (Nettles & Linscheid, 1968). A posterior sternoclavicular dislocation can impinge upon the great vessels and trachea and can be a life-threatening situation. It is important to identify this situation accurately because treatment is prompt reduction of the joint (Nettles & Linscheid, 1968).

Warm-up

Warming up before playing any sports activity is felt to be critical to prevention of injury (Hawkins & Kennedy, 1980). However, there is little scientific evidence to support this traditional dogma which has been espoused for many years. Recently, the physiological benefits of warm-up have been studied for certain sports and in animal models.

Among runners, Ingjer and Strømme (1979) compared an active warm-up, passive warm-up (using hot showers) and no warm-up. They concluded that the active warm-up could substantially benefit athletic performance. In a review article, Bennett (1984) concluded that high body temperatures permitted rapid rates of muscle contraction. However, this may also only affect performance and not necessarily prevent injury.

Safran *et al.* (1988) used a rabbit model to study the effects of isometric preconditioning on muscular injury. They concluded that physiological warming by isometric preconditioning was of benefit in preventing muscular injury by increasing the elasticity and the length to failure of the muscle–tendon unit.

Strickler *et al.* (1990) also studied the effects of passive warming on muscle injury in a rabbit model. They concluded that passive warming increases the extensibility of the muscle–tendon unit and may thereby reduce its susceptibility to strain injury.

These results cannot be extrapolated directly to human performance and injury rates. It is difficult to study the effects of warm-up on athletes to determine its influence on injury prevention. Thus most of the studies have evaluated the effects of warm-up on performance. These two factors may be related, since improved performance may permit the athlete to put less stress on his or her body, thereby decreasing injury rates.

Using human runners, Ingjer and Strømme (1979) compared active warm-up, passive warm-up and no warm-up on oxygen uptake. They felt that the physiological effects of an active warm-up could be beneficial to athletic performance.

However, other studies have not supported these findings. Karpovich and Hale (1956) studied athletes performing a 402-m (440-yard) run and compared performance after deep muscle massage, superficial massage, and preliminary exercise. Though the variables are less controllable in this study than that by Strickler *et al.*, Karpovich and Hale concluded that neither deep nor superficial massage nor preliminary exercise improved performance.

Despite the lack of hard scientific evidence, most clinicians who treat significant numbers of athletes believe a thorough warm-up is very beneficial to both performance and injury prevention. Jobe and Moynes (1986) have stated that an effective warm-up is one in which the body temperature has been elevated sufficiently to make the athlete break into a sweat. Even before exercising the upper body, they advocate warming up by running, jogging or riding a stationary bicycle.

Typical warm-up regimens begin with some exercise which raises overall body core temperature. It would then be appropriate to stretch the body parts which will be used in the sport activity; in this case, the shoulders. Warm-up then finishes by actually performing the sport, first at a low intensity and then increasing to full speed or power shortly prior to starting the activity.

Conditioning to avoid injury

Conditioning must include flexibility and strength training of the shoulders as well as overall body conditioning (Jobe, 1979; Sobel, 1986a,b). Overall body conditioning is important because the kinetic chain typically begins with the legs and hips and transmits forces to the upper body, arms and shoulders. By strengthening the lower body and trunk, the overall kinetic chain is strengthened and stress can be lessened on the shoulder. This chapter will not discuss specific techniques of conditioning for body parts other than the shoulder, since other chapters deal with those areas.

Flexibility training

As with warm-up, precise scientific confirmation that proper flexibility training decreases injury rates and improves performance is lacking. Nevertheless, most clinicians present strong acecdotal evidence that a good stretching programme for the correct musculotendinous units will definitely lower injury rates.

It is important to appreciate that too much flexibility can become a liability. In someone who already possesses a lax glenohumeral joint capsule, further stretching may predispose to increased laxity and even joint instability (Sobel, 1986b). Thus a stretching programme must be individually designed for each athlete, stressing development of flexibility where it is lacking. Without specific goals, stretching can go on endlessly and harmfully or, on the other hand, can be undervalued and neglected because it becomes vague and seemingly purposeless (Sobel, 1986b).

In general, stretching for athletes with impingement problems may differ from those with instability problems. Also, different sports may preferentially develop or fail to develop certain muscles about the shoulder. Often flexibility training in these cases requires restoring balance to the shoulder by stretching the opposite muscle groups.

Matsen and Arntz (1990) have made the point that impingement may be exacerbated by a tight posterior glenohumeral joint capsule. Hawkins and Angelo (1990) have recently published a paper showing that a tight anterior repair can push the shoulder posteriorly. It is also becoming better understood that anterior sub-luxation may produce secondary impingement. In many athletes, there is a limitation of internal rotation manifested by a diminution of where the hitch-hiking thumb can reach in reference to the posterior anatomy compared to the normal side as well as limitation of crossed-arm abduction.

Exercises should be designed to stretch the posterior capsule and rotator cuff and these are depicted in Figs 3.2–3.4. These consist of crossed-arm adduction, elbow below the chin for posterior capsule, behind the head stretching for postero-inferior capsule and internal rotation stretching with the arm pulled behind the back. These are probably the most important stretches in shoulder rehabilitation. Other stretches such as external rotation–abduction are appropriate in certain situations, but should be used with caution since anterior subluxation can be worsened with this stretch. Similarly, in any patient who has impingement syndrome, stretching in forced elevation may aggravate this impingement (Fig. 3.4). Therefore, patients must be asymptomatic relating to instability and impingement before stretching in external

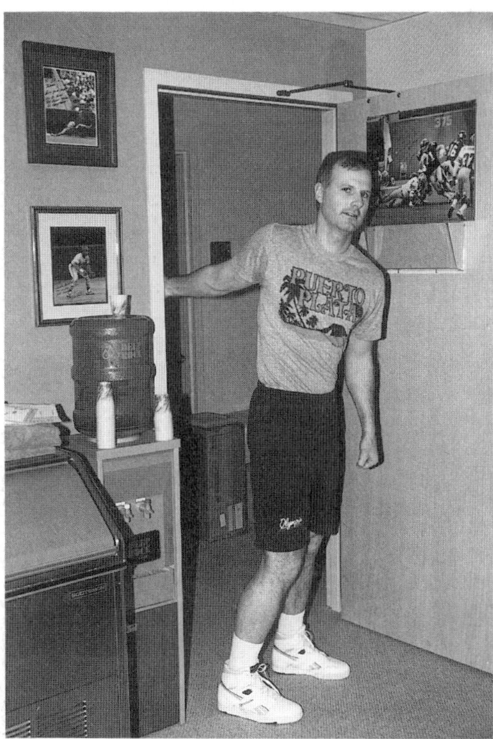

Fig. 3.2 Anterior rotator cuff stretching. Using a doorframe for resistance, the patient walks forward and turns the body slowly away from the shoulder being stretched.

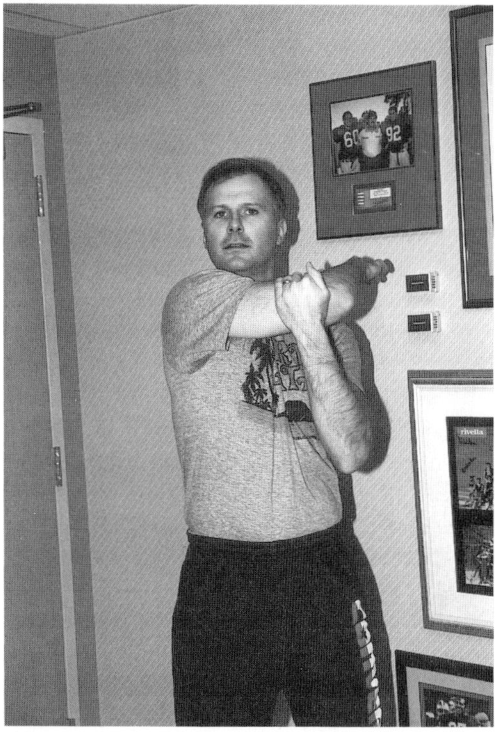

Fig. 3.3 Posterior rotator cuff stretching. The posterior cuff is stretched by gentle pressure from the opposite arm, as shown.

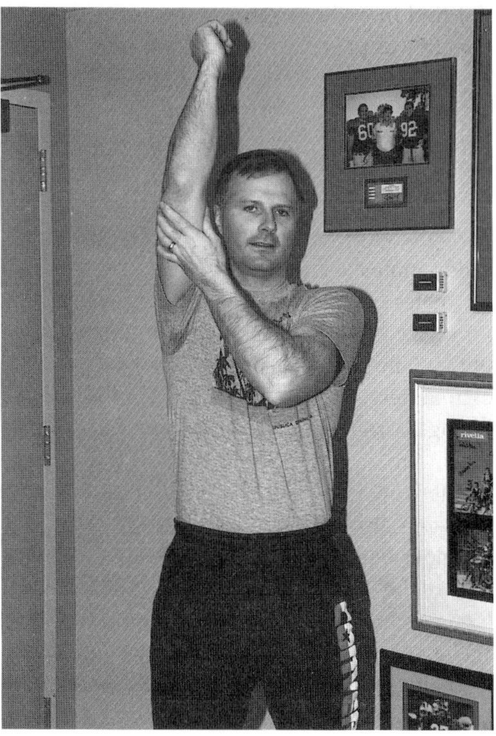

Fig. 3.4 Inferior rotator cuff stretching. The opposite arm applies gentle pressure to provide a stretch to the inferior cuff.

rotation–abduction, i.e. the anterior shoulder structures and in stretching in forward elevation, the supraspinatus under the acromion. An example of an exercise which will help develop flexibility in the external rotators of the shoulder is shown in Fig. 3.3 (Einhorn & Jackson, 1985). In throwing athletes, one must not overstretch the anterior capsule because of concern about contributing to anterior subluxation. External rotation can be stretched safely with the arm at the side.

The most common type of recurrent instability occurs in an anterior direction and the position which predisposes to instability is one of abduction and external rotation. Most flexibility programmes for anterior instability stress stretching the posterior capsule (Fig. 3.3).

There is a debate as to how stretching is best performed (Sady *et al.*, 1982). Types of stretches include static, ballistic and proprioceptive neuromuscular facilitation. Proprioceptive neuromuscular facilitation is a technique of therapeutic exercise which works muscles in diagonal patterns to take them from their fully lengthened state to their most shortened state (Sobel, 1986b). In general, no advantage has been proven for one method over the other in relation to developing shoulder flexibility. We recommend a slow, sustained stretch holding the position for several seconds at the point of slight discomfort.

In animal models, Taylor *et al.* (1990) have found that flexibility training by either static or cyclic (ballistic or repetitive static) methods can produce musculotendinous elongation. They did find in cyclic stretching that the maximum benefit was produced by the fourth stretch, and suggested limiting the amount of repetition as a consequence.

Strength training

Participation in various strength-training programmes has increased throwing velocity in males (Rowlands, 1963; Sullivan, 1970; Popescue, 1974; Thompson & Martin, 1978) but not in females (Deatrick, 1978). In lower extremities, preseason conditioning and strength training has produced lower injury rates, although this has not been well studied in the upper extremities. It is, however, emphasized by many authors writing about shoulder injuries (Kennedy *et al.*, 1978; Fowler, 1979; Jobe, 1979; Hawkins & Kennedy, 1980; Richardson *et al.*, 1980; Hawkins & Hobeika, 1983).

Cahill and Griffith (1978) reported lower knee injury rates among football players who underwent an extensive preseason conditioning programme consisting of cardiovascular, flexibility and strength training. Kraus (1976) has suggested that physical conditioning (including strength training) is an important factor in both the prevention of primary injury and in preventing reinjury (Maksud, 1989).

The normally weak external rotators are stressed in most programmes. Low-weight, high-repetition strengthening exercises can be conducted in the side-lying position to strengthen the external rotators (Fig. 3.5) or they may be strengthened in the upright position by using surgical tubing (Fig. 3.6) (Jobe & Moynes, 1986). The internal rotators can be developed by the exercises shown in Figs 3.7 & 3.8. Finally, the shoulder elevators are developed by variants of the lateral raise exercise. Jobe and Moynes (1986) have emphasized performing the lateral raise exercise as shown in Fig. 3.9 to isolate the supraspinatus and preferentially strengthen the rotator cuff. Emphasis is placed on eccentric contractions in these exercises. Eccentric overload seems to be aetiological in the cause of tendinitis and degenerative rotator cuff problems. It therefore makes sense to focus on eccentric strengthening about the shoulder which can be done with a rubber-band exercise as demonstrated in the illustrations or can be done as described in the next paragraph with isokinetic training. Recently Belle and Hawkins (1991) have demonstrated the role of eccentric strengthening and rehabilitation exercises and their importance.

Isokinetic training is felt to be ideal for developing strength and endurance because it allows specificity of muscle fibre recruitment and eccentric strengthening is more effectively employed with such equipment (Hawkins &

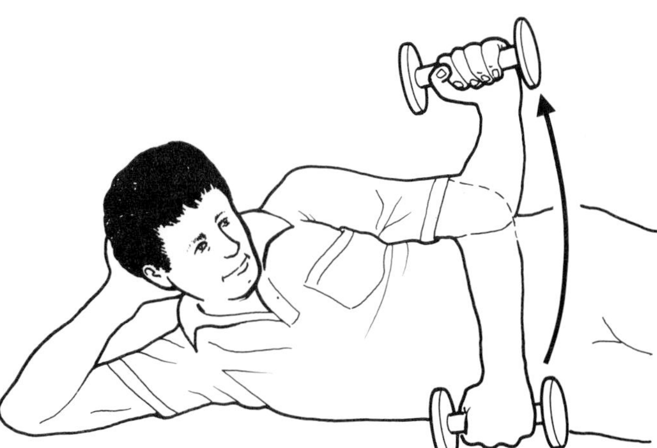

Fig. 3.5 Strengthening the external rotators. While lying on the side, the weight is elevated with the elbow maintained against the side. From Jobe & Moynes (1986).

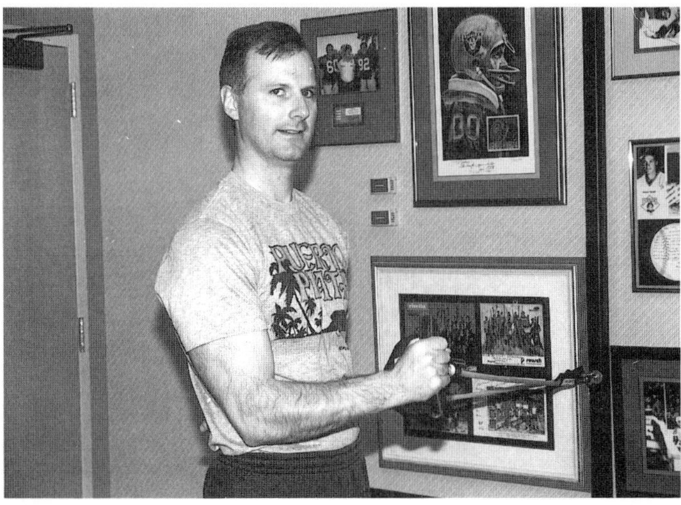

(a)

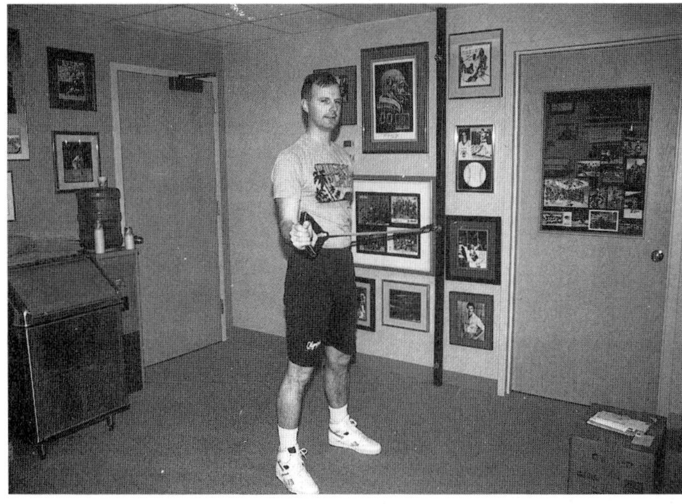

(b)

Fig. 3.6 Strengthening the external rotators, upright position. Surgical tubing is used and anchored on a fixed object for resistance. (a) Start; (b) finish.

Kennedy, 1980). Unfortunately, it requires the most expensive equipment. An alternative would be isotonic exercises or weight-training, with or without machines, with emphasis on the eccentric phase of motion (Einhorn & Jackson, 1985).

Because of the extreme range of motion required of the shoulder in most sports, careful strengthening at these extremes of motion is probably important for injury prevention (Sobel, 1986b).

The scapula has frequently been neglected in our rehabilitation strengthening programmes in the past. It is not uncommon in throwing athletes for subtle amounts of scapular winging to be present, particularly if there is any element of instability or impingement. It is therefore necessary in rehabilitation to focus on strengthening the scapular musculature such as the serratus, rhomboids and trapezius. In all shoulder rehabilitation programmes we employ push-ups with the arms adducted, upright (Fig.

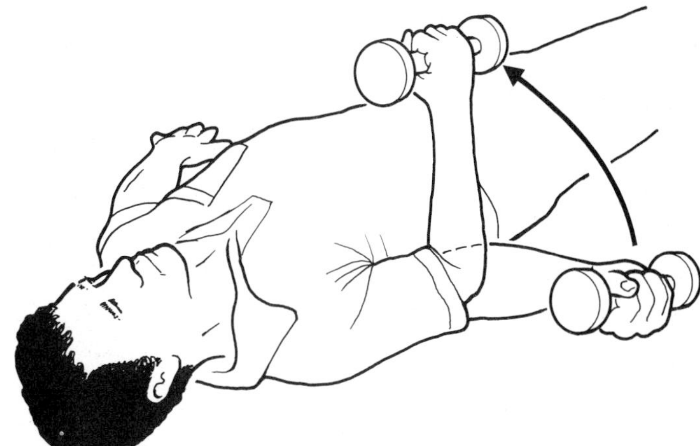

Fig. 3.7 Strengthening the internal rotators. While lying supine, the elbow is held against the side, and the arm is externally rotated. It is then brought to the midline of the body while the elbow remains against the side. From Jobe & Moynes (1986).

3.10) and bent over (Fig. 3.11), rowing exercises using tubing as resistance and shrugging exercises (Fig. 3.12). The push-ups are for serratus, rowing is for serratus and rhomboids, and the shrugging exercise is to strengthen the trapezius. All of these allow a stronger and more efficient functioning scapula to provide more normal shoulder rhythm.

Acute injuries

Acute injuries virtually always occur during contact sports such as American or Rugby football, ice hockey or lacrosse (Norfray *et al.*, 1977; Kulund *et al.*, 1979; Pritchett, 1980; Canale *et al.*, 1981; Silloway *et al.*, 1985). The most common injuries are usually acromioclavicular dislocations, glenohumeral dislocations, clavicular fractures and rotator cuff contusions.

Acromioclavicular dislocations usually occur from direct trauma to the tip of the shoulder in any of the above contact sports. Rarely, they occur from falling on an outstretched arm with a direct axial load to the arm and shoulder. They are prevented to some degree by proper shoulder pads. Lacrosse and hockey pads are less adequate in this regard than American football shoulder pads (Norfray *et al.*, 1977; Kulund *et al.*, 1979; Silloway *et al.*, 1985). However, because of the high rate of trauma to the shoulder in tackling and blocking, acromioclavicular dislocation remains one of the most common injuries to the shoulder in football (Pritchett, 1980; Canale *et al.*, 1981). Prevention of this injury is very difficult in football. Proper preseason conditioning to strengthen the shoulder girdle and adequate padding may lessen its occurrence.

Glenohumeral dislocations are most common in American football. They are the second most common shoulder injury in that sport (Pritchett, 1980; Canale *et al.*, 1981). They occur from one of three mechanisms.

1 The athlete lands on an outstretched arm which is abducted and externally rotated. The force of landing accentuates this position and contributes to the dislocation.

2 Football linemen or linebackers attempt to tackle or block a player with their arm well out to their side in a position of abduction and external rotation. When the opposing player strikes the arm in this position, it forces it farther, levering the humeral head out of the joint.

3 Dislocation may also occur from a direct blow with the force directed anteriorly.

Prevention of this injury requires the teaching of proper techniques. When landing from a fall, the player should attempt not to land on an outstretched arm, but to land on the shoulder,

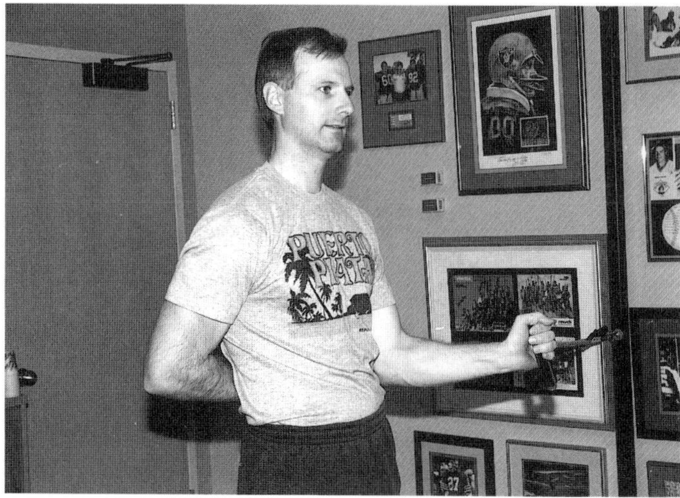

(a)

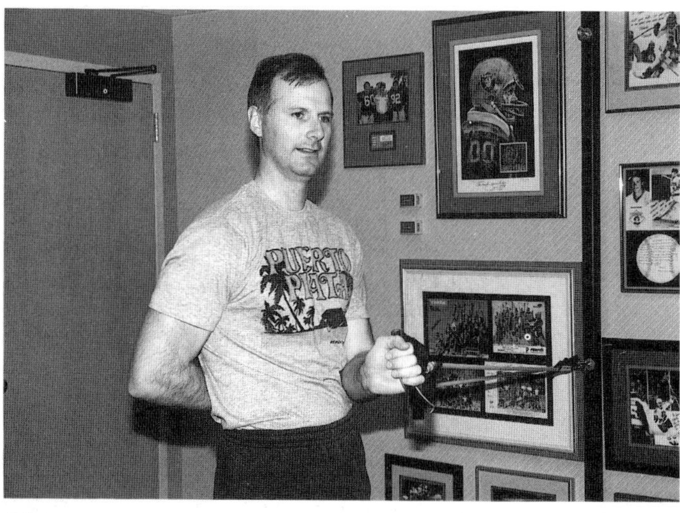

(b)

Fig. 3.8 Strengthening the internal rotators, upright position. Surgical tubing is used and anchored on a fixed object for resistance. (a) Start; (b) finish.

which is protected by pads, and roll whilst landing. When blocking or tackling, players must learn not to attempt this with their arms (which is actually illegal in certain cases), but to move their body quickly enough so they are in position to block or tackle with their body. Clavicle fractures may occur in any of the above-mentioned contact sports. Most direct stresses to the shoulder more commonly produce acromioclavicular dislocations in mature athletes. However, in lacrosse clavicle fractures do occur with some frequency (Kulund *et al.*, 1979; Silloway *et al.*, 1985). This occurs because lacrosse players frequently swing their stick across the top of a player's shoulder in an attempt to strip them of the ball. Although striking the player intentionally with the stick in such a manner is illegal, it occurs to some degree in all games. If the blow to the top of the shoulder is forceful enough, the direct trauma

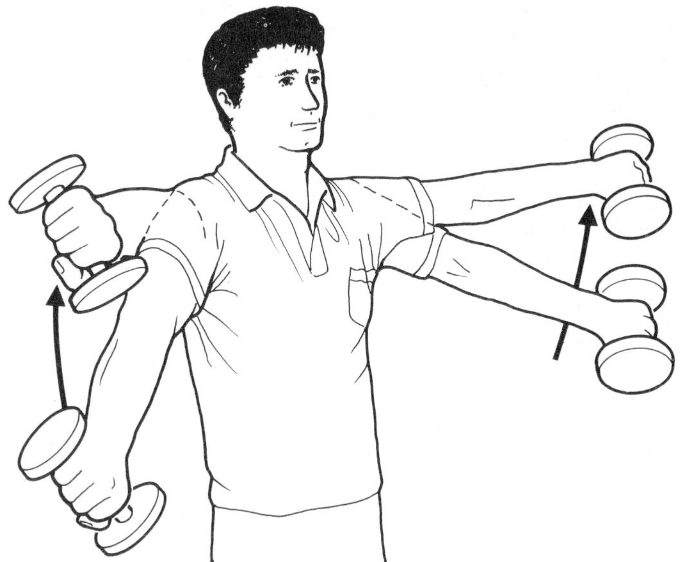

Fig. 3.9 Strengthening the supraspinatus (rotator cuff). This is a lateral raise exercise with the arms horizontally adducted about 30° when they are elevated to shoulder height. To fully isolate the supraspinatus, the arms should be rotated such that the thumbs point to the floor. This position can be achieved by imagining attempting to empty a can. From Jobe & Moynes (1986).

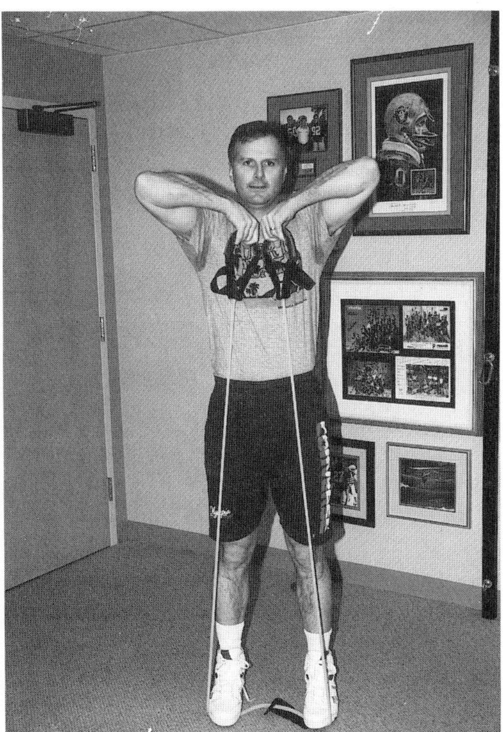

Fig. 3.10 Upright rowing exercise, finish position. The athlete begins this exercise with the hands at waist height and pulls straight upward to strengthen the trapezius and scapular stabilizers.

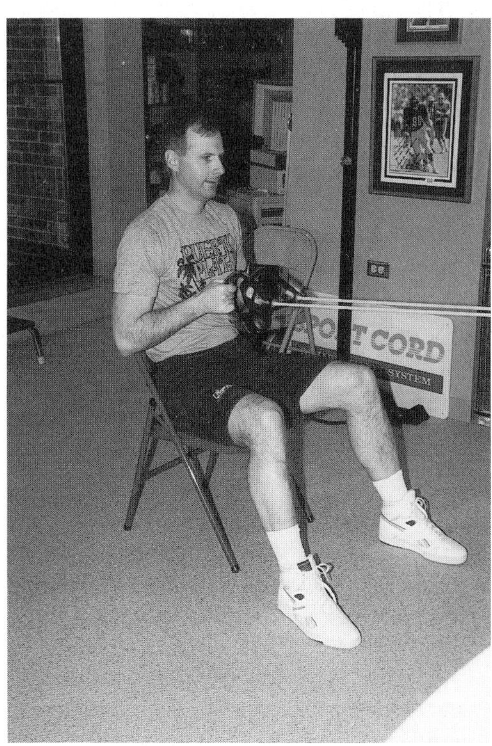

Fig. 3.11 Bent over rowing exercise. Also a scapular stabilizer (especially of the serratus and rhomboids), this exercise may be performed seated as shown or standing in a bent over position.

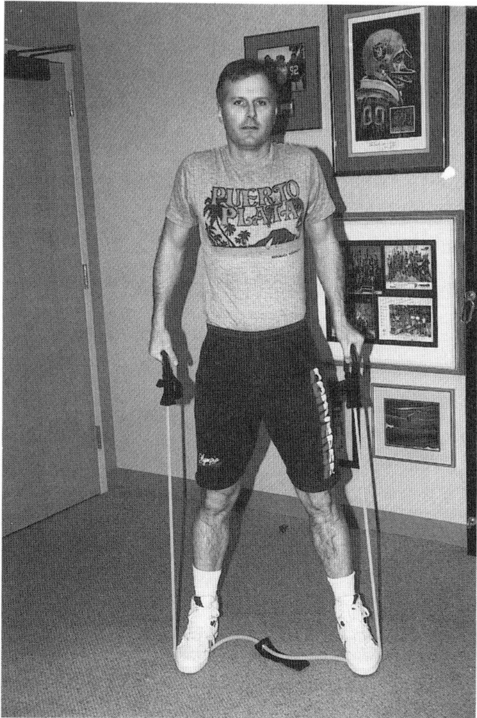

Fig. 3.12 Shoulder shrugs. In this exercise the athlete exercises primarily the trapezius by shrugging upward with the shoulders against the resistance of the tubing.

may fracture the clavicle (Kulund *et al.*, 1979; Silloway *et al.*, 1985).

Until recently, shoulder pads in lacrosse were not required by the National Collegiate Athletic Association (NCAA) and clavicular fractures were much more common. They are now required, but the pads are still much less bulky than football pads and provide little protection from a direct blow to the clavicle (Silloway *et al.*, 1985).

Prevention of this injury in lacrosse requires enforcement of the rules to stop players from striking opposing player's shoulders with their sticks. Well-padded shoulder pads with extra padding over the top of the clavicle would be helpful in preventing this injury (Kulund *et al.*, 1979). Norfray (1977) suggested that the design of shoulder pads for hockey could be improved and might help prevent injuries to the clavicle and acromioclavicular joint in that sport.

Chronic injuries — throwing sports

Biomechanics

Nicholas *et al.* (1977) analysed 63 sports and found that the throwing motion was by far the most common movement. The biomechanics of the throw have been studied extensively (Tullos & King, 1973; Atwater, 1979; Gainor *et al.*, 1980; Jobe *et al.*, 1983, 1984; Perry, 1983; Gowan *et al.*, 1987). The mechanism is usually separated into three segments: (i) wind-up (cocking); (ii) acceleration; and (iii) follow-through.

Cocking the arm results in positioning the humerus in 90° of abduction, and maximal horizontal extension and external rotation. This occurs in about 0.14 s. A torque of 17 000 kg·cm^{-1} across the anterior joint capsule has been calculated from motion analysis (Freedman & Munro, 1966). Cocking is perfomed primarily by the deltoid muscle with minimal participation by the rotator cuff, and it is terminated by the pectoralis major and latissimus dorsi (Jobe *et al.*, 1984).

Acceleration is initiated by the internal rotation force of the latissimus dorsi, and pectoralis major (sternal portion) (Perry, 1983; Jobe *et al.*, 1984). The biceps is noticeably quiet during acceleration (Jobe *et al.*, 1984). There is an almost instantaneous force reversal to reach a peak internal rotation torque of 17 000 kg·cm^{-1} within 0.01 s (Freedman & Munro, 1966; Gainor *et al.*, 1980). It was noted that acceleration had a relative lack of muscular activity on electromyelogram (EMG), despite the high torques generated (Jobe *et al.*, 1983).

Follow-through is a continuation of the arm's forward travel into internal rotation with the humerus horizontally flexed across the body. The posterior musculature of the rotator cuff provides an eccentric decelerating torque which equals the peak values for the other forces generated (Perry, 1983). This is the phase of most intense muscle activity on EMG (Jobe *et al.*, 1983, 1984; Pettrone, 1986).

This study of the biomechanics of the throw demonstrates the extreme velocities and torques developed. With the high demand of training and competition, any muscle or joint imbalance, along with poor techniques can result in injury.

Javelin throwing involves a motion which is similar to that of an overarm baseball pitcher (Bunn, 1972; Wickstrom, 1977). Atwater (1979) states that although release directly over the javelin thrower's head is stressed by coaches, this position is determined more by the lateral flexion of the trunk away from the throwing arm. Miller (1960) suggests that the proper javelin throw is more of a pulling motion over the shoulder with elbow extension providing the acceleration, accompanied by less external rotation (cocking) and internal rotation (acceleration) at the shoulder than a baseball throw. He found that the baseball motion among javelin throwers was associated with increased frequency of elbow injuries.

The volleyball spike involves a cocking, acceleration, follow-through motion which is similar to the baseball or javelin throw (Oka *et al.*, 1976). Oka noted that there are two types of cocking motion. In one, the humerus is elevated first in a forward flexion motion, while in the second, the humerus is kept below the acromion and swung back in horizontal extension before elevation (Oka *et al.*, 1976). Since the first style more closely mimics an impingement sign, it may be more advantageous to use the second technique to prevent impingement-related shoulder problems among volleyball spikers. The impact of the ball on the hand during the spike probably contributes to sudden eccentric overload of the cuff musculature.

Chronic injuries

Bennett (1959) was the first to study shoulder problems in baseball pitchers. Although the term did not exist at the time, he discussed an impingement-type problem in which the supraspinatus was frayed. He stated that tearing of the supraspinatus was rare among baseball pitchers. His main finding was of an osteoarthritic condition in which spurring developed on the postero-inferior segments of the glenoid. Barnes and Tullos (1978) noted this lesion in one-third of the 100 symptomatic baseball players they examined.

In general, throwers develop a change in their shoulder range of motion, with an increased external rotation and decreased internal rotation (at 90° abduction) (King *et al.*, 1969; Tullos & King, 1973). Garth *et al.* (1987) feel that this alteration in range of motion is indirect evidence of anterior capsular laxity and, along with muscle imbalance, may lead to instability.

Tullos and King (1973) felt that the cocking phase was associated mostly with tendon problems, such as biceps and triceps tendinitis. They felt that the acceleration phase was associated with stress fractures to the proximal humeral epiphysis among adolescents — the so-called 'Little Leaguer's shoulder'.

It is now believed that eccentric overload and fibre failure in the supraspinatus tendon frequently causes shoulder problems in the throwing athlete, and may result in secondary impingement. Anterior subluxation may present with impingement signs and cuff failure.

Prevention of injuries

The prevention of injury among athletes who use their shoulders extensively begins with conditioning in the preseason and continuing throughout the season (Jobe, 1979). This should include both flexibility and strength conditioning as discussed above. It is important to emphasize overall conditioning in addition to specific shoulder exercises (Jobe, 1979). This better conditions the legs and allows them to take stress off the shoulder during overhead movements.

Warming up prior to overhead use of the shoulder is critical to injury prevention (Jobe, 1979). Warm-up might begin with 10–15 min of some aerobic activity such as jogging to warm the entire body musculature. This should be followed by stretching the shoulder girdle as well as the back and legs. Only after this is done should the overhead activity begin. It should be initiated with short, low-intensity motion and only build up gradually to full-distance, high-speed motion.

The technique of pitching is a learned skill and may be related to the incidence of injuries. The degree to which a pitcher throws overhead or sidearm is often felt to be of critical importance in shoulder pathology. Atwater (1979) has performed extensive studies of the biomechanics of throwing. She has emphasized that the position of the arm overhead or sidearm is related more to the degree of trunk lean during the throwing motion than it is to the relative abduction of the glenohumeral joint. Atwater (1979), Gowan *et al.* (1987) and Jobe *et al.* (1983, 1984) compared EMG analysis of professional and amateur pitchers and found that the professionals use all their muscles in a more efficient manner during throwing.

No study has documented a higher rate of shoulder injuries among overhead athletes using one technique over another. However, it seems reasonable that any such athlete developing a shoulder problem should consider discussion of his or her mechanics with an experienced coach. It may be possible to design a technique which reduces stress on the shoulder, either by strengthening and using the legs more, or increasing the lateral/backward lean of the trunk.

Chronic injuries — swimming

Biomechanics

Competitive swimmers typically train between 10 000 and 25 000 $m \cdot day^{-1}$ for 6 or 7 days a week. It has been estimated that the typical competitive swimmer today puts each shoulder through 16 000 or more revolutions of motion each week (Richardson *et al.*, 1980; Johnson, 1986).

The basic action of swimming is to use the hand as a paddle pushing against the water to pull the body forward (Perry, 1983). The shoulder is subject to strain by three mechanisms: (i) high repetition rates; (ii) extremes of range used; and (iii) force requirement of a sustained propulsive effort (Perry, 1983).

Four major strokes are used in competition: (i) freestyle (crawl); (ii) butterfly; (iii) breaststroke; and (iv) backstroke. Freestyle, butterfly and backstroke all involve internal rotation and adduction during the pull-through and external rotation and abduction during recovery.

Chronic injuries

It has been estimated that 50–67% of national or world-class swimmers have had significant shoulder problems. They appear most frequently among sprinters, rather than distance swimmers (Richardson *et al.*, 1980; Johnson, 1986). There was also a high association of shoulder injuries and the use of hand paddles for added resistance while training (Kennedy *et al.*, 1978; Richardson *et al.*, 1980; Johnson, 1986). Richardson *et al.* (1980) noted a high incidence of impingement problems among freestylers, butterflyers and backstroke swimmers, and termed this 'swimmer's shoulder'.

Freestyle and butterfly are associated with high rates of impingement-like symptoms (Fowler, 1979). Backstroke may also cause impingement problems (Richardson *et al.*, 1980; Johnson, 1986) but often backstrokers will have symptoms of instability (Fowler, 1979; Johnson, 1986). Fowler feels that backstrokers rarely develop impingement syndromes (1979). The breaststroke provides relative immunity from shoulder problems.

Prevention of injuries

In present-day competitive swimming, there is a great deal of emphasis on weight-training (Richardson *et al.*, 1980). Richardson *et al.* state that in their experience, most swimmers feel this decreases their shoulder pain and has been associated with a decreased rate of shoulder injuries. Because of the tendency to emphasize internal rotation during the swim strokes, weight-training should aim to develop the external rotators as well in order to avoid unbalanced shoulder musculature (Fowler, 1979).

Avoidance of injury in swimming should begin with an adequate warm-up prior to swimming, followed by thorough stretching of the shoulder girdle. This should be followed by 20–30 min of easy swimming prior to any high-intensity work. Kennedy *et al.* (1978) have emphasized the need to change strokes frequently during work-outs to avoid overstressing one particular muscle group or area of the shoulder.

Richardson *et al.* (1980), Hawkins and Kennedy (1980), Johnson (1986) and Kennedy *et al.* (1978) have noted improvement in symptoms of shoulder pain by using strengthening and stretching exercises. Fowler has emphasized that a preseason conditioning programme consisting of flexibility and strengthening will prevent many shoulder problems (1979). He also felt that ballistic stretching was better than static stretching and recommended the swinging of Indian clubs as a method of ballistic stretching.

To decrease stress on the painful structures, swimmers may be able to obtain active rest by changing strokes frequently (Kennedy *et al.*, 1978). Hawkins and Kennedy (1980) have stated that a swimmer with shoulder problems may benefit by conversion to a sprinter, but this does not correlate with the findings of Richardson *et al.* (1980) that impingement syndrome was more common among sprinters.

Techniques which are emphasized by coaches are not to 'drop the elbows' during either pull-through or recovery. Dropping the elbows is the first sign of fatigue among swimmers and places the shoulders at risk for injury by requiring more shoulder external rotation, and placing the muscles of propulsion at a mechanical disadvantage (Richardson *et al.*, 1980).

Kennedy *et al.* (1978) have emphasized that a swimmer's shoulder range of motion may often be restricted in an insidious manner. They feel this predisposes to injury when the swimmer compensates by dipping the opposite shoulder, thereby placing his or her muscles at a mechanical disadvantage, forcing them to work harder. They did not feel that a higher arm entry (i.e. not dropping the elbows) would always alleviate this problem.

Many swimmers will breathe only to one side while swimming, often the dominant arm side. Shoulder pain frequently develops unilaterally among swimmers, and Richardson *et al.* (1980) found this to be common among swimmers who breathed only to one side. They felt that it was important for the swimmer to learn to breath on alternate sides.

The use of hand paddles as a training technique is common among national or world-class swimmers. Its use should be limited as it increases the stress on the shoulder during pull-through and is associated with a high rate of shoulder problems (Richardson *et al.*, 1980). In addition, it should never be used by any swimmer who has had or is recovering from shoulder injuries.

Chronic injuries — tennis

Biomechanics

Although the overhead strokes in tennis constitute a small portion of the total strokes used while playing tennis, they are felt to be responsible for most shoulder problems. Serves and overhead smashes are performed with an overhead throwing type motion which puts the shoulder at risk for both instability and impingement.

The tennis serve uses a motion that is very similar to that of an overhead throw (Perry, 1983). It is compared to the motion of a pitcher, but Dulany (1986) makes the point that the serve is an attempt to throw the arm up, more like the throw of an outfielder than a pitcher (Perry, 1983; Dulany, 1986). As with the throwing motion, posterior deltoid activity can be reduced by a prominent backward lean of the trunk, which leads to a correspondingly greater use of the anterior deltoid during the abduction phase of cocking (Atwater, 1979). Similar to the throwing motion, Van Gheluwe and Hebbelinck (1985) emphasize the high rates of angular velocities and rotatory torques developed during the tennis serve.

The added lever of the racquet and the impact of the ball may change the biomechanics of tennis compared to throwing. The backhand and forehand strokes can put excessive demand on the subscapularis and infraspinatus and result in tendinitis.

Injuries and prevention

Priest and Nagel (1976) have identified a deformity of the shoulder, termed 'tennis shoulder', which consists of a depression of the shoulder with concomitant hypertrophy of the muscles in the region. They felt that the depression produced a relative abduction of the arm, which predisposed to impingement among tennis players. They also felt that the shoulder depression may produce thoracic outlet syndrome and simulate scoliosis among tennis players.

As with throwers, injury prevention in tennis players begins with conditioning in the preseason and continuing throughout the season. This should include both flexibility and strength conditioning as discussed above.

Warming up prior to playing is critical to injury prevention (Jobe, 1979). This should begin with 10–15 min jogging or some other aerobic motion to increase core muscle temperature. This should be followed by stretching the shoulder girdle as well as the back and legs. Actual playing should be initiated with short, low-intensity strokes and only build up gradually to high-intensity stroking. This especially applies to overhead strokes.

Technique changes may avoid or decrease injury problems. The tennis player who has had a shoulder injury or is developing one may have less problems by more lateral and backward trunk lean to decrease the amount of active abduction and forward flexion required at the shoulder. In addition, softening and spinning the serve more may take stress off the shoulder joint (Dulany, 1986; Groppel, 1986).

During the groundstrokes (forehand, backhand), emphasis on proper positioning and footwork is important. This puts the player in position to make an efficient stroke without overstressing the upper extremity with an awkward stroke. This is in keeping with Groppel's statement (1986) that the goal of any racquet sport athlete is to be as efficient and effective as possible yet always minimize the potential for injury.

Chronic injuries — other sports

Cahill (1982) has described a chronic problem which is most prevalent among weightlifters. In this syndrome, the distal clavicle undergoes osteolysis. Though his population consisted entirely of males, this may be because at the time of his study, weightlifting among females was not a common athletic activity.

Cahill emphasized that the syndrome was most painful during overhead or forward pressing activities, such as the bench press or parallel bar dips. In addition, the syndrome developed most frequently among athletes who performed these types of movements excessively. We would recommend that athletes who develop pain near the acromioclavicular joint while weightlifting, which may indicate incipient distal clavicular osteolysis, abstain from pressing movements and substitute other motions in which the elbows remain below the shoulders and preferably that the elbows remain lateral to the shoulder. A substitute exercise for the pectoralis which satisfies this requirement would be cross-over pulley flies. It should be cautioned, however, that when performing this exercise with shoulder pain, the hands should not be brought to the midline at the bottom of the movement.

Acromioclavicular arthritis as a chronic injury is most often secondary to an old acromioclavicular dislocation. This arthritic type of problem with the acromioclavicular joint occurs frequently among ice-hockey players (Norfray *et al.*, 1977). They found that 45% of the hockey players they studied had roentgenographical abnormalities of the end of the clavicle. This is probably due to the high incidence of trauma to the lateral acromion during hockey games, and may be caused by recognized and unrecognized dislocations or subluxations of the acromioclavicular joint. Unfortunately, Norfray *et al.* (1977) felt that improved shoulder pads, which may help with the acute injury, would not help the chronic problem.

In gymnastics, the rings provide the greatest stress to the shoulders as extreme strength moves are often required with the arms held away from the body in a position of mechanical disadvantage. A syndrome termed ringman's shoulder has been described which appears to be a combination of eccentric muscular overload and impingement (Einhorn & Jackson, 1985).

When dealing with ringman's shoulder, rest is necessary but it is important to emphasize that rest does not mean total abstention from gymnastics. (This applies to all sports as well.) The rings can be excluded temporarily and the gymnast may work on floor routines, forearm strengthening and leg power exercises (Einhorn & Jackson, 1985). In addition, proper warm-up and conditioning, as for other sports, should be emphasized.

The shoulder is fourth in the incidence rates of injuries among professional golfers, after the back, elbow and wrist (McCarroll & Gioe, 1982). Most of the problems in golfer's shoulder relate to impingement syndromes. In addition to proper warm-up and conditioning, several technique changes may be beneficial. To decrease impingement it may be helpful to play with a slightly flatter swing. Overemphasis on this, however, may exacerbate the problem as a very flat swing requires increased internal rotation of the humerus. Standing a bit further from the ball and leaning over from the waist at address will give a slightly steeper shoulder turn which will allow an upright swing with decreased shoulder elevation.

Conclusion

The shoulder is commonly injured during athletics. This is related to the high stress placed upon it by extremes of range of motion, high angular velocities and torques during upper extremity motions, the mechanical disadvantage the shoulder muscles are placed at when the arm is held at the side, and the high rate of repetition of most overhead activities during training and competition.

Prevention of shoulder injuries requires strengthening and stretching the shoulder girdle during preseason and in-season conditioning programmes. All training sessions and competitive sports should be preceded by a thorough warm-up which includes aerobic warming, stretching the shoulder muscles, and low-intensity build up to the sport activity. Finally, prevention of injury to the shoulder requires knowledge of the biomechanics of each sport. Attention should be paid by the athlete and his or her coach to developing techniques for that sport which decrease stress on the shoulder.

References

Atwater, A.E. (1979) Biomechanics of overarm throwing movements and of throwing injuries. *Exerc. Sports Sci. Rev.* **7**, 43–85.

Barnes, D.A. & Tullos, H.S. (1978) An analysis of 100 symptomatic baseball players. *Am. J. Sports Med.* **6**(2), 62–7.

Belle, R.M. & Hawkins, R.J. (1991) Dynamic electromyographic analysis of the shoulder muscles during rotational and scapular strengthening exercises. In M. Post, B.F. Morrey & R.J. Hawkins, (eds) *Surgery of the Shoulder*, pp. 32–5. CV Mosby, St Louis.

Bennett, A.F. (1984) Thermal dependence of muscle function. *Am. J. Physiol.* **247**, 217–29.

Bennett, G.E. (1959) Elbow and shoulder lesions of baseball players. *Am. J. Surg.* **98**, 484–92.

Bunn, J.W. (1972) *Scientific Principles of Coaching*, 2nd edn. Prentice Hall, Englewood Cliffs, New Jersey.

Cahill, B.R. (1982) Osteolysis of the distal part of the

clavicle in male athletes. *J. Bone Joint Surg.* **64A**(7), 1053–8.

Cahill, B.R. & Griffith, E.H. (1978) Effect of preseason conditioning on the incidence and severity of high school football knee injuries. *Am. J. Sports Med.* **6**, 180–4.

Canale, S.T., Cantler, E.D., Sisk, T.D. & Freeman, B.L. (1981) A chronicle of injuries of an American intercollegiate football team. *Am. J. Sports Med.* **9**(6), 384–9.

Deatrick, D.J. (1978) The use of the Apollo exercise in improving softball throwing ability in 7th-grade girls. *Completed Research in HPER*, **20**, 102.

Dulany, R. (1986) Tennis strokes. In F.A. Pettrone (ed) *Symposium on Upper Extremity Injuries in Athletes*, pp. 47–58. CV Mosby, St Louis.

Einhorn, A.R. & Jackson, D.R. (1985) Rehabilitation of the shoulder. In D.R. Jackson (ed) *Techniques in Orthopaedics*, Vol. 4, *Shoulder Surgery in the Athlete*. Aspen, Rockville, Maryland.

Fowler, P. (1979) Symposium: shoulder problems in overhead-overuse sports — swimmer problems. *Am. J. Sports Med.* **7**(2), 141–2.

Freedman, L. & Munro, R.R. (1966) Abduction of the arm in the scapular plane. *J. Bone Joint Surg.* **48A**, 1503–10.

Gainor, B.J., Piotrowski, G., Puhl, J., Allen, W.C. & Hagen, R. (1980) The throw: biomechanics and acute injury. *Am. J. Sports Med.* **8**(2), 114–18.

Garth, W.P., Allman, F.L. & Armstrong, W.S. (1987) Occult anterior subluxations of the shoulder in noncontact sports. *Am. J. Sports Med.* **15**(6), 579–85.

Gowan, I.D., Jobe, F.W., Tibone, J.E., Perry, J. & Moynes, D.R. (1987) A comparative electromyographic analysis of the shoulder during pitching. *Am. J. Sports Med.* **15**(6), 586–90.

Groppel, J.L. (1986) The utilization of proper racket sport mechanics to avoid upper extremity injury. In F.A. Pettrone (ed) *Symposium on Upper Extremity Injuries in Athletes*, pp. 30–5. CV Mosby, St Louis.

Hawkins, R.J. & Angelo, R.L. (1990) Glenohumeral osteoarthosis: A late complication of the Putti–Platt repair. *J. Bone Joint Surg.* **72A**, 1193–7.

Hawkins, R.J. & Hobeika, P.E. (1983) Impingement syndrome in the athletic shoulder. *Orthop. Clin. N. Am.* **2**(2), 391–405.

Hawkins, R.J. & Kennedy, J.C. (1980) Impingement syndrome in athletes. *Am. J. Sports Med.* **8**(3), 151–8.

Ingjer, F. & Strømme, S.B. (1979) Effects of active, passive or no warm-up on the physiological response to heavy exercise. *Eur. J. Appl. Physiol.* **40**, 273–82.

Inman, V.T., Saunders, J.B. & Abbot, L.C. (1944) Observations on the function of the shoulder joint. *J. Bone Joint Surg.* **26**, 1–30.

Jobe, F.W. (1979) Symposium: Shoulder problems in overhead-overuse sports — thrower problems. *Am. J. Sports Med.* **7**(2), 139–40.

Jobe, F.W. & Moynes, D.R. (1986) *Thirty Exercises for Better Golf*. Champion, Inglewood, California.

Jobe, F.W., Tibone, J.E., Perry, J. & Moynes, D.R. (1983) An EMG analysis of the shoulder in throwing and pitching: A preliminary report. *Am. J. Sports Med.* **11**(1), 3–5.

Jobe, F.W., Tibone, J.E., Perry, J. & Moynes, D.R. (1984) An EMG analysis of the shoulder in throwing and pitching: A second report. *Am. J. Sports Med.* **12**(3), 218–20.

Johnson, D.C. (1986) The upper extremity in swimming. In F.A. Pettrone (ed) *Symposium on Upper Extremity Injuries in Athletes*, pp. 36–46. CV Mosby, St Louis.

Karpovich, P.V. & Hale, C.J. (1956) Effect of warming-up upon physical performance. *JAMA* **162**, 1117–19.

Kennedy, J.C., Hawkins, R.J. & Krissoff, W.B. (1978) Orthopaedic manifestations of swimming. *Am. J. Sports Med.* **6**(6), 309–22.

King, J.W., Brelsford, H.J. & Tullos, H.S. (1969) Analysis of the pitching arm of the professional baseball pitcher. *Clin. Orthop.* **67**, 116–23.

Kraus, H. (1976) *Proceedings of the American Medical Association's National Conference in the Medical Aspects of Sports*. 7th Congress, Chicago, pp. 98–103.

Kulund, D.N., Schildwachter, T.L., McCue, F.C. & Gieck, J.H. (1979) Lacrosse injuries. *Phys. Sportsmed.* **7**(5), 83–90.

McCarroll, J.R. & Gioe, T.J. (1982) Professional golfers and the price they pay. *Phys. Sports Med.* **10**, 54–70.

Maksud, M.G. (1989) Conditioning for sports. In A.J. Ryan & F.L. Allman (eds) *Sports Medicine*. Academic Press, San Diego, California.

Matsen, F.A. & Arntz, C.T. (1990) Subacromial impingement. In C.A. Rockwood & F.A. Matsen (eds) *The Shoulder*, pp. 623–46. WB Saunders, Philadelphia.

Miller, J. (1960) Javelin thrower's elbow. *J. Bone Joint Surg.* **42B**(4), 788–92.

Nettles, J.L. & Linscheid, R. (1968) Sternoclavicular dislocations. *J. Trauma* **8**(2), 158–64.

Nicholas, J.A., Grossman, R.B. & Hershman, E.B. (1977) The importance of a simplified classification of motion in sports in relation to performance. *Orthop. Clin. N. Am.* **8**, 499–532.

Norfray, J.R., Tremaine, M.J., Groves, H.C. & Bachman, D.C. (1977) The clavicle in hockey. *Am. J. Sports Med.* **5**(6), 275–80.

Oka, H., Okamoto, T. & Kumamoto, M. (1976) Electromyographic and cinematographic study of the volleyball spike. In P.V. Komi (ed) *International Series on Biomechanics: Biomechanics*, Vol. 5B, *Proceedings of the 5th International Congress*. University Park Press, Baltimore.

Perry, J. (1983) Anatomy and biomechanics of the shoulder in throwing, swimming, gymnastics and tennis. *Clin. Sports Med.* **2**, 247–70.

Pettrone, F.A. (1986) The pitching motion. In F.A. Pettrone (ed) *Symposium on Upper Extremity Injuries in Athletes*, pp. 59–63. CV Mosby, St Louis.

Popescue, M.G. (1974) Weight training and the velocity of a baseball. *Athletic J.* **55**, 105–6.

Priest, J.D. & Nagel, D.A. (1976) Tennis shoulder. *Am. J. Sports Med.* **4**, 29–42.

Pritchett, J.W. (1980) High cost of high school football injuries. *Am. J. Sports Med.* **8**(3), 197–9.

Richardson, A.B., Jobe, F.W. & Collins, H.R. (1980) The shoulder in competitive swimming. *Am. J. Sports Med.* **8**(3), 159–63.

Rowlands, D.J. (1963) The effect of weight-training exercises upon the throwing power and strength of college baseball players. *Completed Research in HPER*, **5**, 96.

Sady, S.P., Wortmann, M. & Blanke, D. (1982) Flexibility training: Ballistic, static or proprioceptive neuromuscular facilitation. *Arch. Phys. Med. Rehabil.* **63**, 261–3.

Safran, M.R., Garrett, W.E., Seaber, A.V., Glisson, R.R. & Ribbeck, B.M. (1988) The role of warm-up in muscular injury prevention. *Am. J. Sports Med.* **16**(2), 123–9.

Saha, A.K. (1973) Mechanics of elevation of the glenohumeral joint. Its application in rehabilitation of flail shoulder on upper brachial plexus injuries and poliomyelitis and in replacement of the upper humerus by prosthesis. *Acta Orthop. Scand.* **44**, 668–78.

Silloway, K.A., McLaughlin, R.E., Edlich, R.C. & Edlich, R.F. (1985) Clavicular fractures and acromioclavicular joint dislocations in lacrosse: Preventable injuries. *J. Emerg. Med.* **3**, 117–21.

Sobel, J. (1986a) Shoulder rehabilitation: rotator cuff tendinitis, strength training, and return to play. In F.A. Pettrone (ed) *Symposium on Upper Extremity Injuries in Athletes*, pp. 338–47. CV Mosby, St Louis.

Sobel, J. (1986b) Supplemental exercise program for throwing, swimming, and gymnastics. In F.A. Pettrone (ed) *Symposium on Upper Extremity Injuries in Athletes*, pp. 348–56. CV Mosby, St Louis.

Strickler, T., Malone, T. & Garrett, W.E. (1990) The effects of passive warming on muscle injury. *Am. J. Sports Med.* **18**(2), 141–5.

Sullivan, W.J. (1970) The effects of three experimental training factors upon baseball throwing velocity and selected strength measures. *Diss. Abst. Intl.* **31**, 2162A.

Taylor, D.C., Dalton, J.D., Seaber, A.V. & Garrett, W.E. (1990) Viscoelastic properties of muscle–tendon units: The biomechanical effects of stretching. *Am. J. Sports Med.* **18**(3), 300–9.

Thompson, C.W. & Martin, E.T. (1978) Weight training and baseball throwing speed. *J. Assoc. Phys. Ment. Rehab.* **78**(1), 29–31.

Tullos, H.S. & King, J.W. (1973) Throwing mechanism in sports. *Orthop. Clin. N. Am.* **4**(3), 709–20.

Van Gheluwe, A.T. & Hebbelinck, M. (1985) The kinematics of the service movement in tennis: a three-dimensional cinematographical approach. In D.A. Winter *et al.* (eds) *International Series on Biomechanics: Biomechanics*, Vol. 9B, *Proceedings of the 9th International Congress*. Human Kinetics, Champaign, Illinois.

Wickstrom, R.L. (1977) *Fundamental Motor Patterns*, 2nd edn. Lea & Febiger, Philadelphia.

Chapter 4

Elbow Injuries

KAI-MING CHAN AND STEPHEN Y.C. HSU

A great deal of elbow injuries in sports are related to the fundamental throwing act. The sports that are commonly associated with elbow injuries are baseball, Rugby, American football, tennis, badminton, squash, volleyball, basketball, handball, swimming and discus throwing. It is therefore of paramount importance to understand the actual throwing mechanism and its related stress on the elbow in order to understand the exact anatomical and pathological entities of the various elbow injuries (Atwater, 1977, 1979; Gainor *et al.*, 1980).

The throwing mechanism can be divided into three stages:

1 The wind up or the cocking stage.

2 The acceleration or forward motion stage.

3 The forward follow-through stage.

Wind-up and cocking stage

During the wind-up stage, the shoulder has to be hyperextended and externally rotated in an abducted position with the elbow flexed at an angle of 45°. At this point, the musculature in the flexor and extensor compartment around the elbow are tightly contracted and they are particularly prone to overuse injuries in repeated motion.

Acceleration or forward motion stage

From the end of the wind-up stage to the moment of ball release, this stage can be divided into two distinct phases. In the first phase, the shoulder and elbow are brought forward leaving the forearm and the hand behind in the situation that will create tremendous valgus stress upon the elbow causing distraction of the medial aspect of the elbow and compression of the lateral aspect (Fig. 4.1). In the second phase, the shoulder is internally rotated rapidly with a 'whip-like' action as the forearm and the hand are snapped forward. The injury may occur around the shoulder and upper part of the humerus.

Follow-through stage

This third stage starts with ball release and is characterized by the forearm rotated into pronation. The associated rotational and shearing force stresses the lateral side of the elbow and compresses on the posterior aspect.

In order to achieve maximum velocity on the throwing act, there is usually a great transference of the forward momentum of the whole body or torque to the throwing object using the arm as the lever arm. A greater force can also be achieved with the arm in this maximally extended position by unwinding the shoulder backward, by throwing sidearm and by maximum pronation in the follow-through. All these throwing techniques put tremendous stress on the elbow. Therefore, with the exception of the knee, the elbow is the most commonly encountered site for overuse injuries.

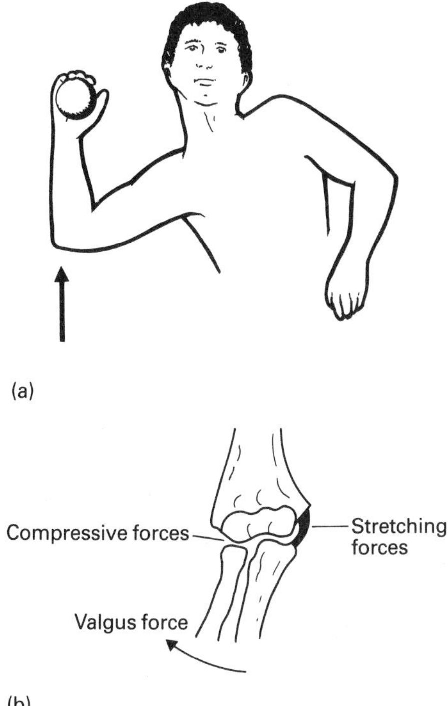

Fig. 4.1 Biomechanics of the throwing act. The elbow is in extreme valgus stress at the moment of cocking and acceleration stage leading to stretching of the medial structure and compression of the lateral structure.

Throwing injuries of the elbow in children and adolescents

This is an important category of throwing injuries to be considered in growing individuals because of the popularity of various competitive sports such as baseball amongst this age group. Much has been described throughout the literature on this condition of 'Little League elbow' (Bennett, 1959; Adams, 1965; Tullos & King, 1972; Kennedy & Willis, 1976). This is also applicable to other strenuous sports which demand intensive training at an early age such as gymnastics, tennis and other racquet sports.

The developmental stage of the elbow can be identified in three stages:

1 Before the appearance of all the secondary centres of ossification.

2 Before the fusion of the ossification centres in adolescents.

3 Before the completion of bone growth in young adults.

Types of throwing injuries

Schneider *et al.* (1985) have divided throwing injuries into three categories: medial, lateral and posterior injuries.

Medial injuries. The medial side of the elbow is often subjected to great distraction forces which cause injuries to the soft tissue and the bony structure. In children, before the completion of the appearance of the ossification centre, there may be disturbance with enlargement of the medial epicondyle and osteochondritic changes. In adolescents, before the fusion of the ossification centre, there may be avulsion fracture of the medial epicondyle with mechanical derangement of the joint due to displacement (Fig. 4.2). In young adults, after fusion of the medial epicondyle, there may be avulsion of the muscle and capsular structure with the associated formation of osteophytes.

Lateral injuries. Due to repetitive compression and shearing forces on the lateral side of the

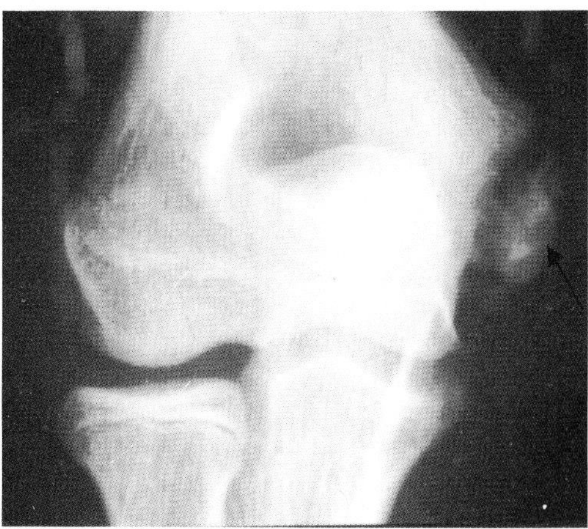

Fig. 4.2 Avulsion of the medial epicondyle (arrow) in an adolescent volleyball player.

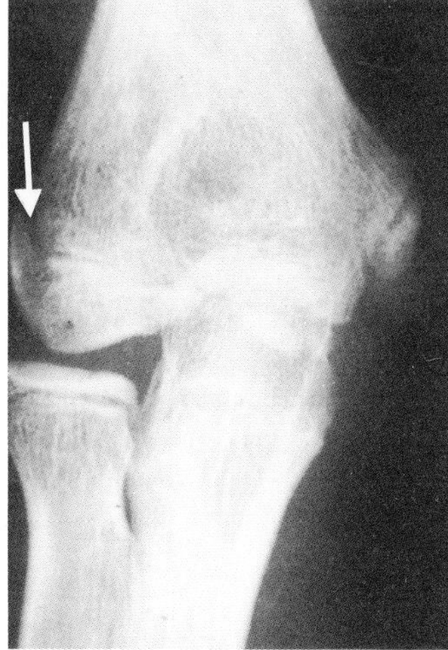

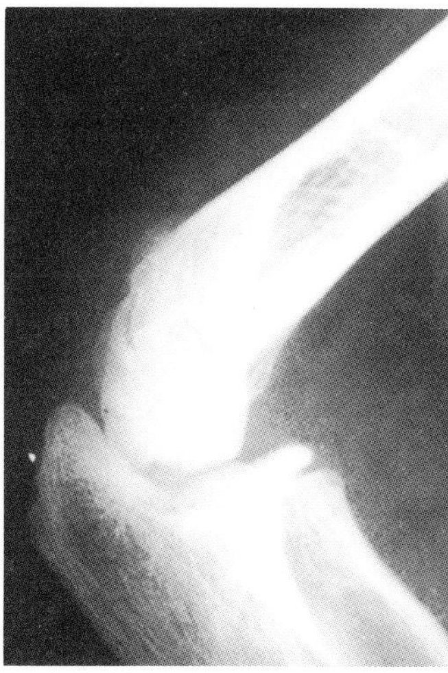

Fig. 4.3 Osteochondritis of the capitellum in a young pitcher with loose bodies formation.

elbow during childhood, there will be disturbance of growth of the head of the radius and the capitellum leading to enlargement and fragmentation (Fig. 4.3). During the adolescent period, the periphery of the ossification centre may be affected with subchondral necrosis and avulsion fracture with concomitant injury to articular cartilage and formation of loose bodies.

Posterior injuries. In children, there may be stress fractures and non-union of the olecranon epiphysis with ectopic bone formation around the olecranon tip and loose bodies formation.

Clinical features

Pain is usually the chief complaint from young patients and it occurs particularly during the act of throwing with concomitant swelling and stiffness after training and competition. Sometimes, a sensation of locking may be experienced during the act of throwing if there is mechanical derangement within the joint. In addition to the overuse symptoms, sometimes there may be presentation of acute pain right after a traumatic episode and this may indicate the possibility of an epiphyseal fracture.

Physical examination usually demonstrates specific local tenderness directly over the medial or the lateral epicondyle with demonstration of restriction of the range of motion.

At this point, it must be emphasized that a proper X-ray of the elbow should be taken to delineate the extent of the various injuries. Plain radiography is usually the first line of investigation which may show up the changes in the medial epicondylar epiphysis and the radial head or the distal capitellar epiphysis. More recently, the use of computerized tomographic (CT) scanning and magnetic resonance imaging (MRI) may enhance the diagnostic horizon at a much earlier stage.

Treatment and prevention

Treatment for these conditions is usually conservative, there are four important parameters in the whole management strategy:

Early recognition and adequate diagnosis. If the coach can bring the attention of the sports medicine physicians early, the condition is usually recognized at an early stage such that a full planning scheme of treatment can be instituted with modification of the training programme. This is an important message to be relayed to parents and the coaches in order to minimize progression of the overuse injury which may lead to permanent disability and

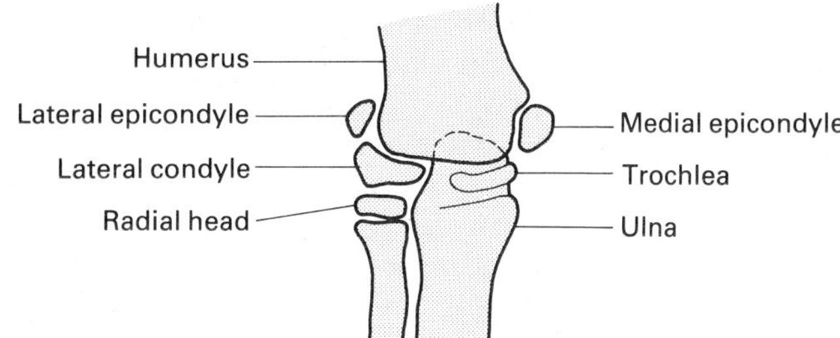

Fig. 4.4 Epiphyses of the elbow in a growing child.

perhaps jeopardize the athletic career of the child. A proper X-ray of the elbow should be taken to assess the possible bony lesion and special attention should be taken to identify all the epiphyses (Fig. 4.4).

Symptomatic relief may be achieved with adequate rest and temporary cessation of the throwing movement completely (usually for about 6–8 weeks). The use of various physiotherapy modalities such as ice, ultrasound, interferential therapy, magnetic therapy or laser therapy will help contain the associated inflammatory changes. For severe pain and possible fracture in the growing child, it may be sometimes necessary to immobilize the elbow in a brace or a cast.

It must be emphasized that the use of medication such as non-steroidal anti-inflammatory medication, or steroid injection should be avoided as far as possible in the growing athlete. During this period of treatment, the physiotherapist should institute a programme of muscle strengthening and stretching exercises to maintain the flexibility of the elbow and the overall tuning of the musculature. It is also customary to maintain an appropriate level of cardiorespiratory training with other kinds of exercise that do not demand heavy use of the elbow. Running treadmill or exercise bikes are appropriate alternatives in the management of upper limb overuse injuries.

Prevention — adjustment of training technique and progression of intensity. In pitching injuries, an experienced coach can usually alter the pitching style to take emphasis away from the sidearm throw or away from 'opening up too fast' thus relieving the symptoms of excessive stress. Recently, there has been much progress made in restricting the number of innings that may be pitched by Little League participants and also restricting the practising session. The parents and the coach should encourage proper counselling of the young athlete, otherwise some may continue to practise outside the confine of the League or may even join a second one. It should also be properly explained that the misconception of 'throwing through to discomfort' will only cause further, and maybe irrevocable, damage to the elbow.

Surgical treatment. If loose bodies are found in the elbow, they should be removed in order to avoid further mechanical derangement of the joint. It is now possible to utilize advances in arthroscopic surgery to remove loose bodies without a more traumatic open procedure. For loose fragments, it is sometimes necessary to excise the fragment and curette the base. The use of bone grafting for avascular changes in the capitellum has not been giving consistently good results. The replacement of loose fragments likewise yields unsatisfactory outcomes. It should be realized that any surgical intervention to an overused elbow in the adolescent may relieve the symptoms but at the very high price of the child not being able to return to his or her top throwing performance.

Fracture and dislocation in children and adolescents

As more and more children are involved in high-energy sports, it is not surprising to find that paediatric fracture is on the rise. The intuition of straightening the elbow when a child falls explains the high incidence of forearm and elbow fractures in this age group. Since the elbow is comprised of several important growth centres, it is small wonder that injuries around the elbow carry important implications in the subsequent growth of the upper limb.

Supracondylar fracture of the humerus

This constitutes the commonest fracture around the elbow in the paediatric age group (Fowles & Kessab, 1974). The child usually falls on an outstretched hand when the olecranon process is tightly locked into the olecranon fossa. Further extension would allow the elbow joint to lever backwards and break the supracondylar area just like the action of a bottle-opener. The result is an extension type of supracondylar fracture (Fig. 4.5) which is far more common than the flexion counterpart. This type of fracture is notoriously associated with brachial artery and peripheral nerve injuries. Failing to detect the former will lead to the much dreaded complication of Volkmann's ischaemic contracture in which the patient will have problems with opening the palm fully. The way to avoid this is to be vigilant at the acute phase and palpate the radial pulse before and after reduction of the fracture. The median, ulnar and radial nerves course through the elbow region and various combinations of nerve injuries have been reported.

Any attempt at anatomical reduction should consider the exact direction of displacement of the distal fragment. It is often displaced backwards, shifted medially, rotated into varus and even turned around the long axis of the humerus. Good remodelling can be expected if the reduction is less than perfect in the first two types of displacement but the persistence of the last two types of displacement tend to leave a permanent deformity. Most of these fractures can be treated successfully with close manipulation under general anaesthesia and fluoroscopic control. Subsequent stabilization usually relies on percutaneous K-wires (Fig. 4.6) or plaster of Paris. Open reduction is infrequently required and is only reserved for the irreducible fracture or presence of neurovascular compromise.

Fracture of the medial epicondyle of the humerus

A fracture of the medial epicondyle of the humerus (Fig. 4.7) is a fairly common fracture in the early teens. The exact mechanism is not

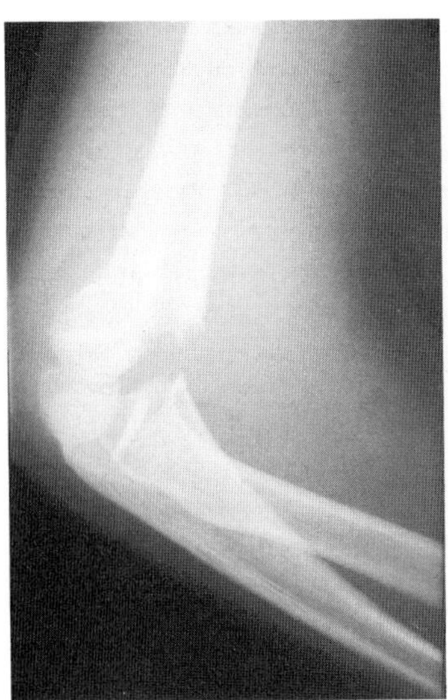

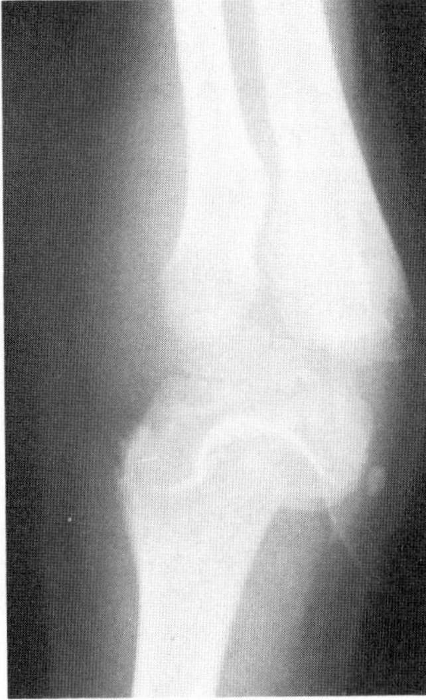

Fig. 4.5 Supracondylar fracture of the humerus.

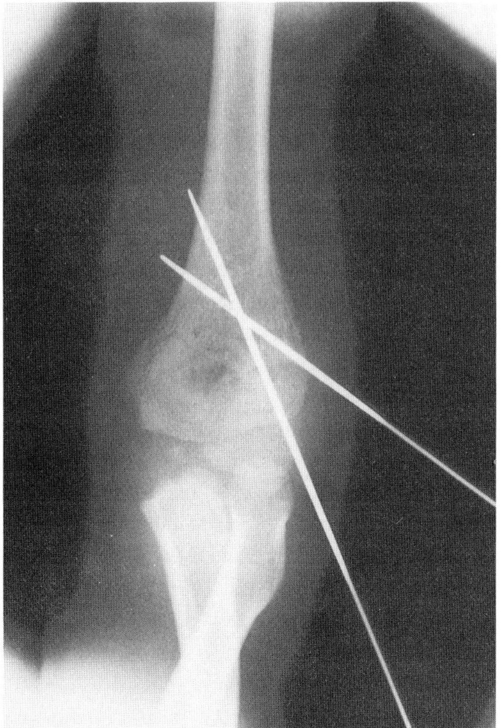

Fig. 4.6 Supracondylar fracture of the humerus treated with percutaneous K-wires.

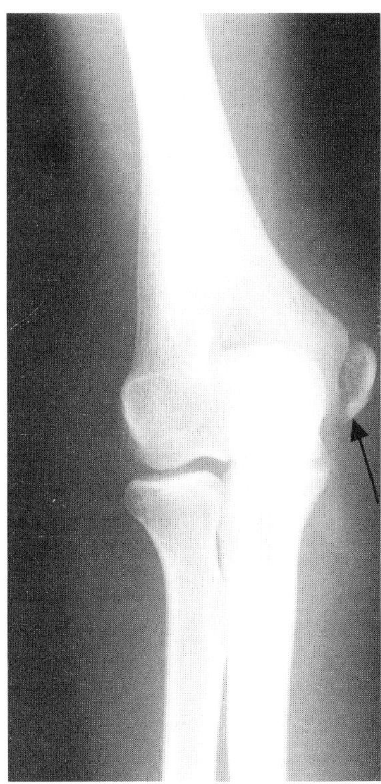

Fig. 4.7 Fracture of the medial epicondyle of the humerus.

entirely clear but is thought to be either due to an avulsion from forceful contraction of the common flexors or an avulsion by the ulnar collateral ligament during a dislocation of the elbow joint. Although it has been postulated to be the result of a direct posterior blow to the medial epicondyle, this is thought to be rare.

There is little argument about the treatment if the fracture is minimally or non-displaced. On the other hand, most authors would advise operative treatment if there is a concommitant ulnar nerve palsy or when there is entrapment of the fragment into the joint which is irretrievable by non-operative means. However, contention exists for the frankly displaced type. Some authors have suggested open reduction and internal fixation if the displacement is significant fearing that non-union (Ogden, 1982) may weaken the flexor muscles and attrition ulnar nerve injury may occur. These, however, have not been substantiated by clinical study. Hence, rest and early mobilization is the mainstay of treatment. The only exception to the rule may be an athletically active child with a clearly demonstrable valgus instability in whom operative fixation may be considered.

Dislocation of the elbow

Elbow dislocation is much less common in children than in adults (Henrikson, 1966). When it does occur, it is usually due to a fall that results in a hyperextension and valgus force that pushes the elbow into a posterolateral dislocation. The clinical presentation is obvious and the child usually comes in tears with a deformed elbow who refuses to move the joint at all. The diagnosis is easily confirmed by radiography.

Before a close reduction of an elbow dislocation is attempted, a careful neurovascular examination should be performed. Under heavy sedation or general anaesthesia, gentle close reduction will usually relocate the joint. There are various ways to reduce an elbow dislocation. One can apply a longitudinal force along the direction of the arm to disengage the dislocated articular surfaces followed by another longitudinal force along the direction of the forearm to relocate the joint into its original position. Others have used different thumbing techniques to push the joint into place. Whichever method one is adopting, it is mandatory for the surgeon to test the range of movement after reduction. Any crepitus or mechanical block is taken to mean an avulsion fracture of the medial epicondyle which has been entrapped into the joint until proven otherwise. A postreduction examination of the major nerves is essential to detect any traction or impingement injuries.

Fracture of the neck of the radius

Similar to dislocation of the elbow, the mechanism of injury is thought to be a fall on the outstretched hand forcing the elbow into extension and valgus. However, why it sometimes results in dislocation while at other times resulting in a fracture of the radial neck is not entirely clear. The radial head and neck is commonly found to tilt laterally. This tilting, if left uncorrected, may bring about limitation in rotation of the forearm. The correction may be achieved by either manipulation or the patient's own remodelling power, or both. Since the elbow habours several growth centres, it has great remodelling potential when the patient is young, Thus, one can accept a larger degree of tilt in younger patients. Conversely, the closer the patient is to skeletal maturity, the better the reduction should be before it is accepted.

Fracture of the olecranon

Fracture of the olecranon is uncommon in children. When it occurs, it is usually associated with other injuries around the elbow (Fahey, 1960). This fracture may result from an avulsion by the resisted and forceful contraction of the triceps or a fall that leads to a lateral or medial bending of the forearm when the elbow is being held in extension. Some of these fractures are minimally displaced or green-stick in type which can be adequately treated by conservative means. However, there are cases where the extensor mechanism of the elbow is lost which demand open reduction and internal fixation in order to avoid weakness of elbow extension in the future.

Throwing injuries of the elbow in adults

Throwing injuries in skeletally mature persons present a picture different from that of children and adolescents. It is customary to divide the sites of injuries into three categories: (i) medial; (ii) lateral; and (iii) posterior regions (Slocum, 1968). A fourth category, anterior elbow injuries, is also included here.

Types of throwing injuries

Medial injuries. The soft-tissue injuries include: (i) acute rupture of the common flexor origin; (ii) a chronic elongation of the medial collateral ligament with or without osteophytic formation due to prolonged traction; and (iii) ulnar nerve neuropathy.

Lateral injuries. In this area, the major trauma is due to compression. Therefore soft tissue injuries are less common than the medial side. However, there may be significant compression on the lateral condyle leading to post-traumatic type of hypertropic osteoarthritis with loose bodies formation. When there is excessive pronation in a repeated act, the overuse stretching may lead to lateral epicondylitis.

Anterior injuries. Anterior injuries include elbow contracture, pronator teres syndrome and entrapment of the median nerve.

Posterior injuries. Traction injuries may arise from overpull of the triceps on the tip of the olecranon leading to degenerative changes. An avulsion injury of the olecranon may lead to impingement on the olecranon giving rise to flexion deformity that limits full extension.

Clinical features

The athlete usually complains of pain and occasionally swelling in the elbow with limitation of motion particularly in full extension and pronation. Physical examination usually reveals local tenderness depending on the site of the overuse injury. Sometimes a small joint effusion and synovial hypertrophy can be felt along the joint line. In cases of medial collateral ligament laxity, there may be demonstrable instability on stress testing. Radiological examination is important to reveal the extent and the stage of the lesion. For example, an ossification of the medial collateral ligament can be identified. A gravity X-ray may reveal opening of the joint line on the medial site in the case of chronic ligamental instability. In acute rupture of the medial collateral ligament, medial instability can be demonstrated on valgus stress as well.

Treatment

In the early stage, conservative treatment usually suffices which includes rest, ice application and non-steroidal anti-inflammatory agent. The use of corticosteroid injection should be cautioned. If judiciously selected in acute cases, it may have an anti-inflammatory efficacy. However, repeated use of corticosteroids will only lead to further weakening of the ligamentous structures which may predispose to rupture.

Sometimes, traction spurs may fracture and demand surgical removal if they are painful. Loose bodies can now be removed successfully with arthroscopic techniques without major open surgery (Fig. 4.8). Chronic ligamental instability as revealed clinically and via stress radiography may demand elaborate reconstructive procedure.

Prevention

For competitive athletes such as a pitcher who demands high-intensity training, particularly in the throwing act, a well-structured programme of preventive measures must be instituted.

In the off-season period, the athlete should go through a conditioning programme with progressive resistance exercise of the entire body, and understand the proper utilization of body mechanics in order to exert a maximal biomechanical advantage of the throwing action. During pitching routine, there must be a careful planning of progression of intensity such as starting with 10 min of light throwing and progressing steadily to 15 min with increasing speed and distance. Passive stretching by the trainer and 'ice-down' treatment in between sessions are important.

There must be adequate provision of proper equipment such as protective cup, sufficiently warm clothing in cool weather and properly sized gloves.

Finally, a seasoned competitive athlete should be able to pick up an early 'body signal' of fatigue or overuse such that the training programme can be adjusted in consultation with the team physician, trainer and coach.

Medial elbow injuries

MEDIAL EPICONDYLITIS

The pathological entity is chronic irritation of the medial epicondyle with inflammation of the flexor muscle insertion. Usually an excessive valgus stress is the leading cause. There are a number of sports associated with medial epicondylitis:

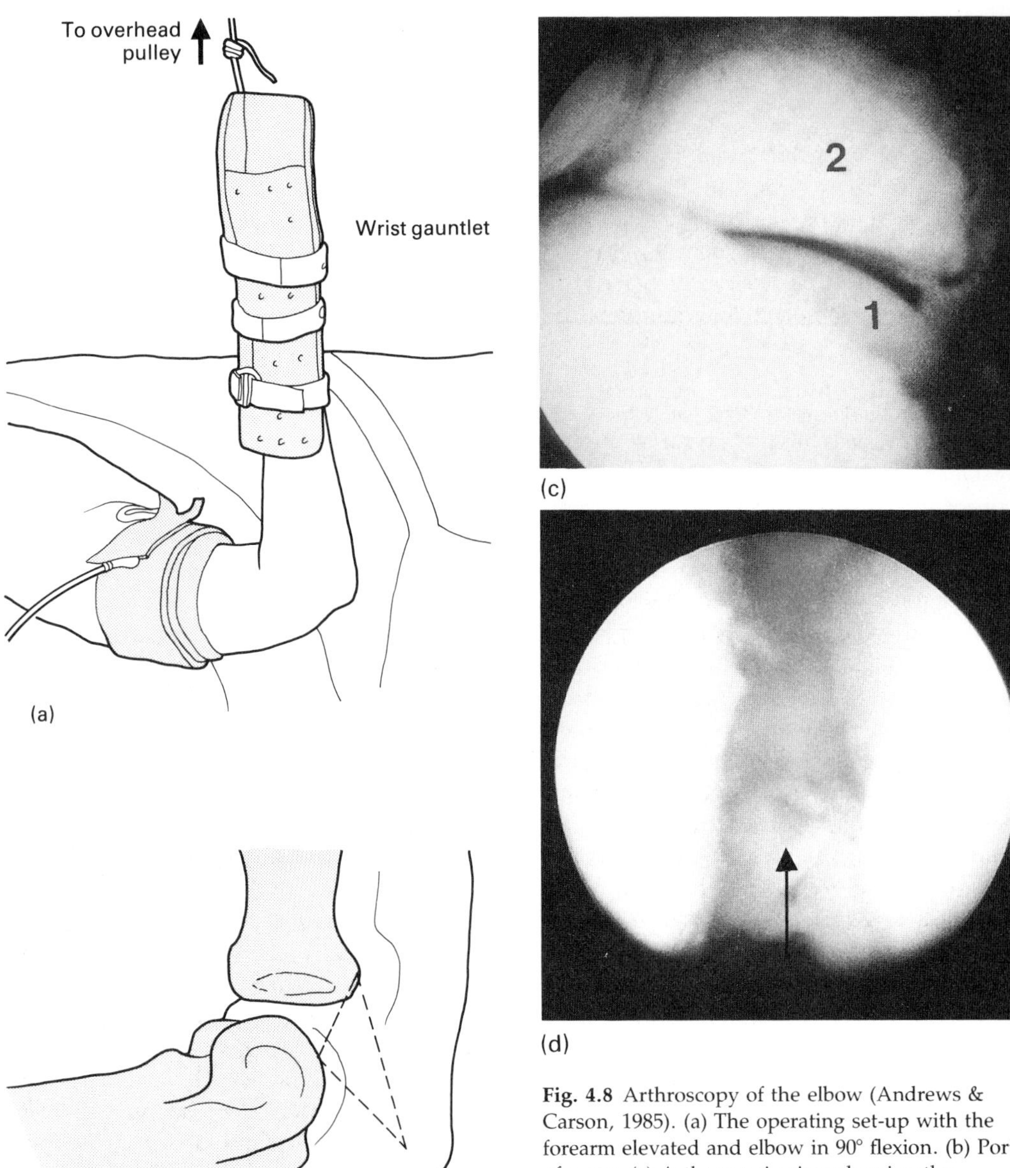

Fig. 4.8 Arthroscopy of the elbow (Andrews & Carson, 1985). (a) The operating set-up with the forearm elevated and elbow in 90° flexion. (b) Portal of entry. (c) Arthroscopic view showing the radiohumeral joint: (1) capitellum; (2) radial head. (d) Loose bodies in the elbow joint.

1 Golf. This is perhaps the commonest occurrence, hence the name 'golfer's elbow'. Usually this is related to using the golf club to hit the ground rather than the golf ball.

2 Baseball. Pitchers who use a great deal of forceful flexion while releasing the pitch may also have overstress of the medial epicondyle.

3 Tennis. Players who forcibly flex the wrist with service motion or hitting the forehand ground stroke may result in overuse of the forearm muscle group.

4 Other sports that put excessive stress on the

forearm flexor such as table tennis, squash and gymnastics may also present with medial epicondylitis.

Clinical features

The symptoms are similar to that of the commonly encountered tennis elbow or 'lateral epicondylitis' but the location is mainly at the inner aspect of the elbow with exquisite tenderness over the medial epicondyle when it is subjected to pressure or flexing the hand downward at the wrist against resistance.

Treatment and prevention

The time-honoured method of rest, ice, anti-inflammatory agents and various forms of physiotherapy can usually contain the problem. Forearm muscle stretching and strengthening exercises are advised once the acute symptoms are under control. The use of a forearm elbow belt may be helpful at times. Likewise, attention should be directed towards the specific technique of the sports or the use of various equipment in order to minimize the stress. Surgical intervention is not usually indicated unless there is uncontrolled persistent symptoms with radiological evidence of bony changes at the medial epicondyle. At surgery, it is often necessary to excise the granulation tissue and the scar due to the repeated overuse injury and to release the origin of the flexor muscle with a sliding procedure. Rehabilitation after this kind of surgery for medial epicondylitis may take a long time and the prognosis of returning to a top level of sports participation should be guarded.

ENTRAPMENT OF THE ULNAR NERVE

The ulnar nerve runs along the medial edge of the olecra just behind the medial epicondyle to the flexor muscles. In some racquet or throwing sports, the nerve may be unduly stretched or slip in and out of its normal groove with subsequent mechanical irritation (Fig. 4.9).

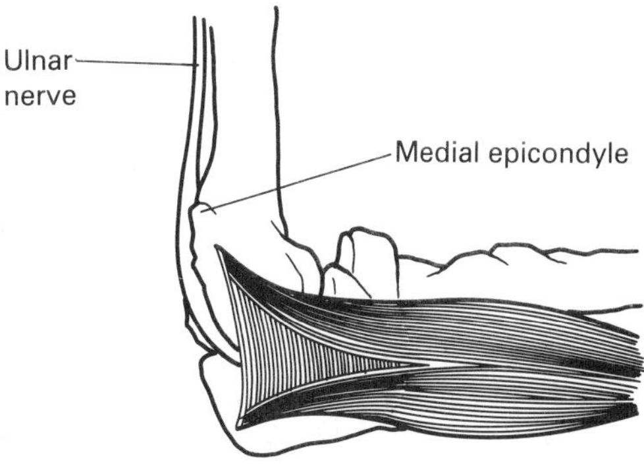

Fig. 4.9 Ulnar nerve entrapment. Neuropathy around the medial epicondyle.

Clinical features

Usually the athlete will experience pain and paraesthesia along the 4th and 5th finger and pain on the medial aspect of the elbow. There will be tenderness along the nerve on the medial and dorsal side of the elbow with a positive Tinel's sign.

Treatment and prevention

Early recognition of the condition is important as symptoms usually subside with adequate rest. Sometimes anti-inflammatory medication will be required together with a course of physiotherapy utilizing the various anti-inflammatory modalities.

If the symptoms tend to recur repeatedly or the extent of neurological impairment is significant, surgical intervention should be considered. At the operation, the nerve is frequently found to be embedded in chronically inflamed tissue or scar tissue. The ulnar nerve should be transposed anteriorly with excision of a segment of the intermuscular septum and freeing the nerve all the way up to Struthers' ligament. At the same time, careful inspection of the medial collateral ligament should be made. If there is chronic stretching and attenuation of the medial collateral ligament with demonstrable instability, it should be reconstructed and reinforced. Postoperatively, the patient is usually immobilized for about 3 weeks to allow tissue healing followed by early activity to encourage recovery of range of motion. Usually, after another 3 weeks, strengthening exercises can be instituted.

Lateral elbow injuries

LATERAL EPICONDYLITIS (TENNIS ELBOW)

Tennis elbow is perhaps the most commonly known condition in overuse injury of the elbow. Obviously, the sports involved are not confined to tennis alone as the name may imply. Other types of sports that may predispose to the occurrence of tennis elbow include table tennis, badminton, squash, golf and other non-sporting activities which require repetitive one-sided movement.

The main pathological entity is the repetitive trauma of the extensor muscle origin primarily the extensor carpi radialis brevis leading to fibrosis as a response to the chronic irritation. The other muscle group may also be involved such as the extensor digitorum communis, extensor radialis longus and the extensor carpi ulnaris. Due to the small area of the extensor origin, the force which develops in the muscles creates a high load per unit area thereby focusing the irritative trauma on a single spot. It has been estimated that about 45% of the athletes who play tennis daily or 20% of those who play twice a week may at certain stages suffer from lateral epicondylitis. Individuals over 40 are said to be more commonly involved.

Clinical features

There is usually pain over the lateral aspect of the elbow radiating upwards along the upper arm or downward along the outside of the forearm. Gradually, the athletes may feel weakness in the wrist and may have progressive difficulty in other activities of daily living such as lifting a cup, opening a door knob, wringing a wet towel or even shaking hands. There is usually a distinct tender spot of pressure over the lateral epicondylar area and the outer aspect of the elbow by extending the flexed middle finger against resistance. A further provocation test can be done with the hand dorsiflexed at the wrist against resistance and pain elicited over the lateral epicondyle. This sign is usually sufficient to justify a proper diagnosis of 'tennis elbow'. X-ray of the elbow usually shows no significant features but may be carried out to rule out other pathology such as loose bodies, fracture or rheumatic disorders.

Treatment

Conservative treatment is usually indicated in the early stage, including rest, ice, use of various physical modalities such as ultrasound, laser and interferential therapy to decrease the inflammation. The use of anti-inflammatory drugs should be guided by the physician. The traditional use of one to two corticosteroid injections is acceptable if the exercise regime is unsuccessful. However, it should be emphasized again that injudicious use of steroids may add further damage to the ligamental structure (Kennedy & Willis, 1976). Adequate rest should be instituted in the acute stage but exercises should start as early as possible. The use of an elbow brace around the elbow or a forearm brace to decrease the excursion of the muscle sometimes gives further relief from pain. Return to vigorous use of the forearm in sports should be gradually instituted.

Surgical intervention is only indicated when an active physiotherapy programme and various conservative regimes have failed to contain the symptoms. Release of the extensor muscle origin particularly the extensor carpi radialis brevis may be indicated together with excision of the scar tissue. Rehabilitation after surgery usually takes 2–3 months with gradual institution of a stretching programme and strengthening exercises to restore power. Competitive sports is usually allowed after 3–4 months.

Prevention

Prevention is the key to containing this problem and it can be broadly divided into intrinsic and extrinsic measures (Nirschl, 1973; Berg, 1977; Peterson & Renström, 1986).

Intrinsic measures:

1 The athletes should maintain a reasonable level of flexibility around the elbow and adequate muscle strength of both the extensor and the flexor groups.

2 Technical skill acquired by the athletes plays an important part in the preventive measures such as:

(a) good foot work so that the player can approach the ball correctly;

(b) the shoulder and the whole body should participate in the stroke such that breaking does not occur when the ball is hit; the stroke should be followed through and the wrist should be held firm;

(c) the use of a two-handed backhand taking stress off the extensor of the elbow particularly in female players may be a rewarding preventive measure.

Extrinsic measures:

1 Slow court surface helps decrease the velocity of the ball. Care must be taken particularly on fast court surfaces such as concrete as it may result in increasing load in the player's arm. The ball should be hit correctly with the racquet at the right spot and it should be light. Dead and wet balls are usually heavy.

2 The selection of the racquet string tension is important in that a tightly strung racquet tends to transmit excessive force across to the elbow. Gut strings give more resistance and less vibration than most nylon ones.

3 Correct sporting equipment should be selected for a casual player. The racquet should be light as a heavy racquet may cause increased load. The racquet should be well-balanced in manoeuvre and the recent introduction of graphite racquets with a large head and a larger sweet spot help reduce the stress transmitted to the elbow.

4 The size of the racquet grip should be carefully selected. A rough estimation is to measure the distance from the midpalm crease to the tip of the middle finger which give a fairly adequate estimation of the size of the grip suitable for the particular athlete.

ENTRAPMENT OF THE RADIAL NERVE

The deep-seated branch of the radial nerve which arises just below the elbow in the outer part of the medial compartment of the forearm may sometimes be trapped as it passes through a narrow channel in the supinator muscle. This may give a clinical picture quite similar to that of tennis elbow but the tenderness is located below and in front of the lateral epicondyle and the athletes will feel pain at the point where the forearm is supinated and the wrist is extended. The treatment is in accordance with the general principle of nerve entrapment with rest and anti-inflammatory medication. Only very rarely will symptoms be severe enough to indicate operative intervention to release the entrapped radial nerve (Fig. 4.10).

Anterior elbow injuries

ELBOW CONTRACTURE

In throwing sports, repeated microtrauma may produce stretching and minor tear of the capsular structure in front of the elbow joint. Prolonged overuse may lead to progressive contracture of the elbow. Athletes initially may experience pain in front of the elbow followed by inability to extend fully. Usually it takes 2–3 days of rest before he or she can return to full extension. But as the contracture sets in, there may be permanent loss of full extension. It is therefore important to recognize this problem at an early stage so that the pathology is reversible. An established elbow contracture at later stages responds very poorly to surgical intervention.

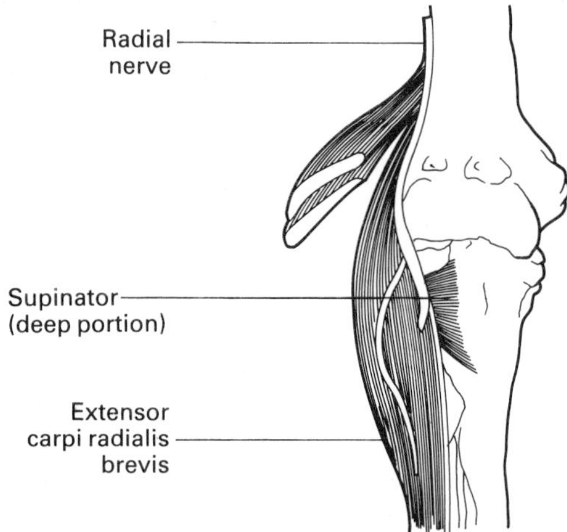

Fig. 4.10 Radial nerve entrapment. Neuropathy around the supinator.

PRONATOR TERES SYNDROME

This is a condition in which a hypertrophied pronator teres is compressed by the lacertus fibrosis. The athlete will feel heavy and fatigue in the forearm after excessive use and progressive pain may set in. Conservative treatment will usually suffice; but if the symptom is recurrent, release of the lacertus fibrosis is quite rewarding.

ENTRAPMENT OF THE MEDIAN NERVE

The median nerve as it passes through the front of the elbow joint through the pronator teres, may be trapped in overuse. The athlete may feel pain in the middle of the anterior aspect of the elbow with numbness in thumb as well as the second, third and the radial half of the 4th finger. Pain may be elicited by pronation of the lower arm against resistance and weakness demonstrated in palmar flexion of the hand. The treatment for this kind of nerve entrapment is on similar lines as the other entrapment neuropathies.

Posterior elbow injuries

OLECRANON IMPINGEMENT SYNDROME

In the repeated throwing act, the impingement of the medial aspect of the olecranon process against the wall of the olecranon fossa may produce degenerative changes and loose bodies in the posterior aspect of the elbow joint. Clinically, the athlete will experience pain in the elbow and symptoms of catching and locking. The X-ray will reveal the presence of the degenerative changes at the tip of the olecranon with osteophyte formation and loose bodies in the olecranon fossa. This is a condition that clearly demands surgical removal of the loose bodies together with excision of a portion of the tip of olecranon to allow better fitting into the olecranon fossa.

TRICEPS TENDINITIS

Chronic irritation of the insertion of the triceps into the olecranon is a common feature in athletes who lift excessive weights or participate in explosive events such as shotput. The pathological entity is similar to that of patella tendinitis and lateral epicondylitis.

The athlete will experience exquisite pain at the back of the elbow and tenderness at the insertion of the tricep. Conservative treatment usually consists of rest, ice and non-steroidal anti-inflammatory agents in the acute phase. When the symptoms have become incapacitating, surgical intervention may be advisable. The triceps tendon can be explored with a view to excising the area of chronic irritation with granulation together with readjustment of the insertion of the triceps into the olecranon and reattachment. The postoperative management is similar to other surgical procedures with gradual restoration of the range of motion and progressive resistive exercises to improve muscle strength and functional return to athletic activities.

OLECRANON BURSITIS

Certain sports that are associated with repeated abrasion of the elbow such as wrestling, judo, basketball, rugby, volleyball and team handball, ice hockey and orienteering, may lead to persistent irritation of the olecranon bursa sometimes with acute bleeding leading to swelling and inflammation. The athletes usually feel pain and have swelling over the tip of the elbow if there is an acute episode of bleeding. For inflammatory bursitis, the pain and swelling is usually gradual and insidious.

There is a clear need for protection of the elbow in certain contact sports to avoid repeated abrasion (Fig. 4.11). The acute bleeding usually subsides with pressure bandage, ice and sometimes aspiration. Bursitis may be controlled with anti-inflammatory medication and physiotherapy.

If the bursa has become a nuisance at the peak of the athletic career, it may be advisable to have the olecranon bursa excised together with trimming of the tip of the degenerative part of the olecranon process. The result is usually very gratifying and the athlete can return to the previous level of athletic activity.

Fracture and dislocation in adults

Although fractures and dislocations around the the elbow are less common than overuse injuries in sports, they certainly carry a far more significant consequence and sequel in the long run. Such injuries usually result from high traumatic energy and are seldomly missed in the acute phase. Most of the contact sports and sports that involve high kinetic energy are responsible for most of the fracture–dislocations. Because of the muscle attachments and the anatomical configuration of the elbow, most of these injuries are inherently unstable and would warrant early surgical intervention and stabilization. This is more so when the fracture involves the articular surface of the joint. Perfect anatomical reduction and stabilization will minimize the complications of stiffness.

Intra-articular fracture of the lower humerus

An intra-articular fracture of the lower humerus (Fig. 4.12) usually involves a high-energy trauma. Rarely, it is due to a direct force from below the olecranon process but more often, it is due to an indirect force from falling on an outstretched hand forcing the olecranon upwards and thus splitting the lower humeral articular surfaces into pieces. Because of the different muscle attachment to these shattered pieces, they are bound to be widely separated resulting in severe deformity of the elbow (Wickstrom & Meyer, 1967).

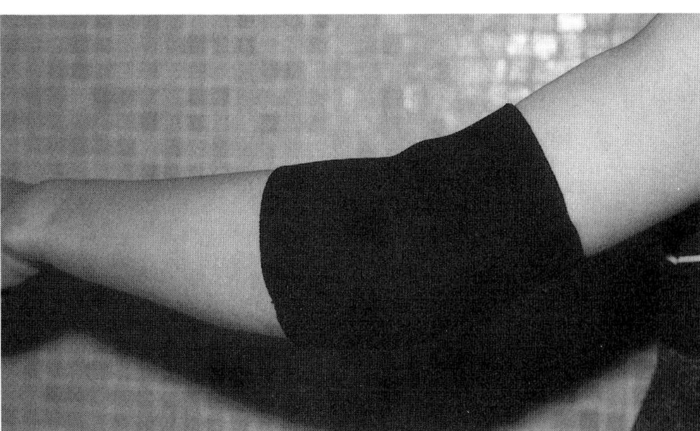

Fig. 4.11 A protective brace around the elbow to avoid contusion and friction injury.

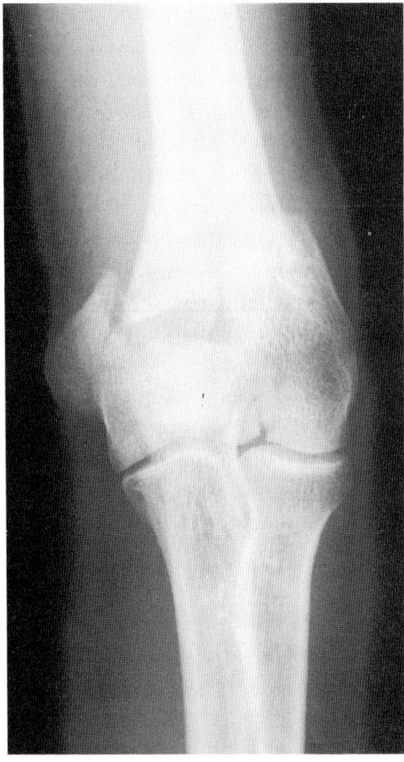

Fig. 4.12 Intra-articular fracture of the lower humerus in an adult.

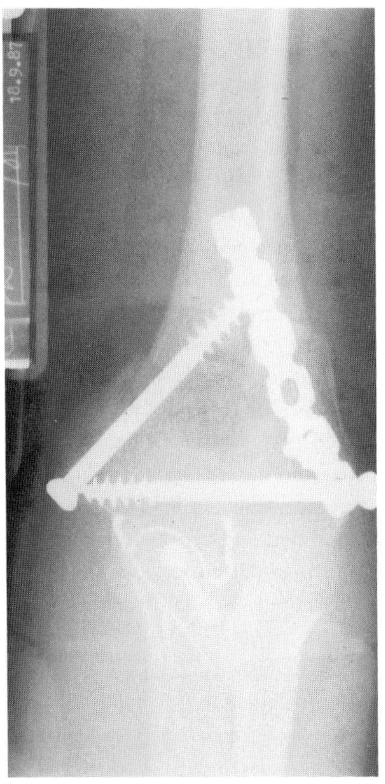

Fig. 4.13 Radiographic appearance after open reduction and internal fixation of the fracture in Fig. 4.12.

No matter what type of treatment is offered, the key to a successful outcome after such a severe injury is to move the elbow joint as early as possible. Unless the displacement of the fracture fragments is minimal, most surgeons would not hesitate to perform an open anatomical reduction and internal fixation in order to allow early mobilization (Fig. 4.13). Nevertheless, the fracture is at times so comminuted as to be not reconstructable, in which cases the surgeon may opt to offer a skeletal traction while still allowing the elbow to move early (Brown & Morgan, 1971).

Dislocation of the elbow

Dislocation of the elbow is fairly common in sports ranking the second commonest after shoulder dislocation. The commonest mode of injury is falling on an outstretched hand with the elbow in extension and abduction (DeLee *et al.*, 1984). Because of the long lever arm of the forearm, the semilunar notch is levered backwards and laterally. Although it is the joint which falls out of place, the blunt of the trauma falls on the collateral ligaments, the capsule as well the brachialis and the triceps muscles. Elbow dislocation may appear trivial and it is not uncommon for some non-clinicians with some sports injury experience to reduce one in the field. However, it is of the utmost importance to bring the injured athlete to an experienced orthopaedic surgeon who should be able to detect any associated complications. These complications include vascular compression, neurological deficit and the presence of any associated fractures. Missing any of these complications may have a dire consequence on the eventual outcome.

Most elbow dislocations can be closely reduced under general anaesthesia or deep sedation. However, it is mandatory for the surgeon to test the range of movement after a close reduction. Any locking or crepitus may denote the presence of occult fractures or soft tissue impingement that would warrant a closer scrutiny of the radiographs or even a surgical exploration. After a successful close reduction, the elbow is protected for about 3 weeks during which time active graduated exercises may be started under supervision. At no time should the elbow be passively stretched or else the daunting complication of myositis ossificans may set in.

Fracture of the olecranon

Although the olecranon may be fractured by a direct fall onto the olecranon process, most of the time it is an avulsion fracture from forceful contraction of the triceps muscle (Waxman & Geshelin, 1947). The direct consequence of which is the creation of an intra-articular fracture and the loss of the extensor mechanism of the elbow. Both of these demand an operative reduction and rigid internal fixation, thus allowing early mobilization and faster rehabilitation. Various types of fixative devices have been recommended which include rods, plates, screws and wires but the best is probably tension bend wiring. This device allows compression at the fracture site whenever the elbow goes into flexion.

Fractures of the radial head and neck

Most of these fractures result from a fall on the outstretched hand when the elbow is in an abducted position. The severe compression at the lateral compartment of the elbow joint forces the convex capitellum into the concave radial head thereby either shattering it or forcing it into valgus. Fractures with marked displacement are easily detected by conventional radiographs. Nevertheless, those with little displacement are often missed and passed off as 'contusion of elbow'. Associated injuries are not uncommon and should be carefully looked for. These include tearing of the medial collateral ligament, avulsion fracture of the medial humeral epicondyle, ulnar nerve palsy, dislocation of the elbow and fracture of the olecranon.

Controversy exists as to the best mode of treatment for this seemingly straightforward fracture. Most surgeons would choose the conservative treatment if there is little or no displacement. Prosthetic replacement of the radial head is reserved for comminuted and non-reconstructable fractures. However, for the intermediate ones, there is a variety of options that include leaving it alone, throwing the fragment away or fixing it at all costs. No matter which form of treatment is adopted, early mobilization is advised because stiffness of the elbow is almost unavoidable.

Fracture of the medial epicondyle of the humerus

This type of fracture is much less common in adults than in children or adolescents. When it does occur, it is often associated with dislocation of the elbow. Therefore when an elbow dislocation is reduced, it is mandatory to rule out an intra-articular entrapment of the fractured medial epicondyle (Sisk, 1980). When this is found to be the case, it becomes an absolute indication for retrieval from the joint which often requires surgery. For simple fracture of the medial epicondyle, most would advocate a conservative approach unless there is definite evidence of ulnar nerve entrapment.

References

Adams, J.E. (1965) Injury to the throwing arm. *Calif. Med.* **102**, 127.

Andrews, J.R. & Carson, W.G. (1985) Arthroscopy of the elbow. *Arthroscopy* **1**, 97–107.

Atwater, A.E. (1977) Biomechanical analysis of different pitches delivered from the windup and stretch positions. *Med. Sci. Sports* **9**, 49.

Atwater, A.E. (1979) Biomechanics of overarm throwing movements and of throwing injuries. *Exerc. Sports Sci. Rev.* **7**, 43.

Bennett, G. (1959) Elbows and shoulder lesions of baseball players. *Am. J. Surg.* **98**, 484.

Berg, K. (1977) Prevention of tennis elbow through conditioning. *Phys. Sportsmed.* **5**, 110.

Brown, R.F. & Morgan, R.G. (1971) Intercondylar T-shaped fractures of the humerus. *J. Bone Joint Surg.* **5313**, 425–9.

DeLee, J.C., Green, D.P. & Wilkins, K.E. (1984) Fracture in adults. In C.A. Rockwood & D.P. Green (eds) *Fractures and Dislocations of the Elbow*, 2nd edn, Vol. 1, pp. 601–18. Lippincott, Philadelphia.

Fahey, J.J. (1960) Fractures of the elbow in children. *American Academy of Orthopaedic Surgeons Instructional Course Lectures*, Vol. 17, pp. 13–46. CV Mosby, St Louis.

Fowles, J.V. & Kassab, M.T. (1974) Displaced supracondylar fractures of the elbow in children. *J. Bone Joint Surg.* **56B**, 490–500.

Gainor, B.J., Piotrowski, G., Puhl, J., Allen, W.C. & Hagen, R.(1980) The throw: biomechanics and acute injury. *Am. J. Sports Med.* **8**, 114–18.

Henrikson, B. (1966) Supracondylar fracture of the humerus in children. *Acta Chir. Scand.* 369.

Kennedy, J.C. & Willis, R.B. (1976) The effects of local steroid injections on tendons: a biomechanical and microscopic correlative study. *Am. J. Sports Med.* **4**, 11–21.

Nirschl, R.P. (1973) Tennis elbow. *Orthop. Clin. N. Am.* **4**, 787.

Ogden, J.A. (1982) *Skeletal Injury in the Child*. Lea & Febiger, Philadelphia.

Peterson, L. & Renström, P. (1986) *Sports Injuries — Their Prevention and Treatment*, pp. 207–20. Martin Dunitz, New York.

Schneider, R., Kennedy, J. & Plant, M. (1985) *Sports Injuries — Mechanisms, Prevention and Treatment*, pp. 715–22. Williams & Wilkins, Baltimore.

Sisk, T.D. (1980) Fractures. In A.S. Elmonson & A.M. Grenshaw (eds) *Campell's Operative Orthopaedics*, 6th edn. CV Mosby, St Louis.

Slocum, D.B. (1968) Classification of elbow injuries from baseball pitching. *Texas Med.* **64**, 48.

Tullos, H.S. & King, J.W. (1972) Lesions of the pitching arm in adolescents. *JAMA* **220**, 264.

Waxman, A. & Geshelin, H. (1947) Fractures of the olecranon process due to muscle pull with the forearm in hyperextension. *Calif. Med.* **66**, 358–9.

Wickstrom, J. & Meyer, P.R. (1967) Fractures of the distal humerus in adults. *Clin. Orthop. Rel. Res.* **50**, 43.

Further reading

Adams, J.E. (1965) Injury to the throwing arm (a study of traumatic changes in the elbow joints of boy baseball players). *Calif. Med.* **102**, 127.

Attenborough, C.G. (1956) Remodelling of the humerus after supracondylar fractures in childhood. *J. Bone Joint Surg.* **35B**, 386–95.

Bennett, G.E. (1941) Shoulder and elbow lesions of the professional baseball pitcher. *JAMA* **117**, 510–14.

DeHaven, K.E. & Evarts, C.M. (1973) Throwing injuries of the elbow in athletes. *Orthop. Clin. N. Am.* **4**, 801–8.

Evans, E.M. (1953) Supracondylar-Y fractures of the humerus. *J. Bone Joint Surg.* **35B**, 381–5.

Jobe, F.W., Stark, H. & Lombardo, S.J. (1986) Reconstruction of the ulnar collateral ligament in athletes. *J. Bone Joint Surg.* **68A**, 1158–63.

Kilfoyle, R.M. (1965) Fractures of the medial condyle and epicondyle of the elbow in children. *Clin. Orthop. Rel. Res.* **41**, 43.

Larson, R.L. & McMahan, R.O. (1966) The epiphyses and the childhood athlete. *JAMA* **196**, 607–12.

Lavine, L.S. (1953) A simple method of reducing dislocations of the elbow joint. *J. Bone Joint Surg.* **35A**, 785–6.

Liang, L.K. (1970) A review of recent supracondylar fractures of the humerus in children. *Singapore Med. J.* **11**, 264.

Norwood, L.A., Shook, J.A. & Andrews, J.R. (1981) Acute medial elbow ruptures. *Am. J. Sports Med.* **9**, 16–19.

Purser, D.W. (1954) Dislocation of the elbow and inclusion of the medial epicondyle in the adult. *J. Bone Joint Surg.* **36B**, 247–9.

Salter, R.B. & Harris, W.R. (1963) Injuries involving the epiphyseal plate. *J. Bone Joint Surg.* **45A**, 587–622.

Tivnon, M.C., Anzel, S.H. & Waugh, T.R. (1976) Surgical management of osteochondritis dissecans of the capitellum. *Am. J. Sports Med.* **4**, 121–8.

Unverferth, L.J. & Olix, M.L. (1973) The effect of local steroid injections on tendon. *Am. J. Sports Med.* **1**, 31.

Wadsworth, T.G. (1976) Screw fixation of the olecranon. *Lancet* **ii**, 1118–20.

Wilson, F.D., Andrews, J.R., Blackburn, T.A. *et al.* (1983) Valgus extension overload in the pitching elbow. *Am. J. Sports Med.* **11**, 83–8.

Woods, G.W. & Tullos, H.S. (1977) Elbow instability and medial epicondyle fractures. *Am. J. Sports Med.* **5**, 23–30.

Chapter 5

Hand and Wrist Injuries

JOYCE A. MITCHELL AND BRIAN D. ADAMS

Injuries to the hand and wrist may account for as much as 20% of all injuries sustained during sports activities (Allieu, 1988). The percentages of injuries vary from one sport to another, with those such as handball reported to be as high as 30%, and football as low as 10% (Thiebault, 1980). Accurate statistics are difficult to collect because initial treatment of injuries is often provided on site and many athletes do not seek medical care by a specialist. Epidemiological studies which are available may not necessarily give a true overall picture of hand and wrist injuries in sport. Some surveys only include traumatic or acute injuries, excluding overuse or chronic problems. Others include injuries only in amateur sports. Surveys may also reflect a higher proportion of injuries for sports that are popular within that survey's geographical area. This could provide inaccurate representation of other sports that otherwise make up a considerable portion of the general sports population. There are some less common sports that are never represented in the overall percentage producing an underestimated figure for athletic hand and wrist injuries.

The frequency of sport-related trauma to the hand and wrist depends on the extent of involvement of the upper extremities within a specific sport and the amount of exposure or contact to which they are subjected during participation. Vulnerability to injuries is increased when the hand is used to divert or absorb the initial impact of balls or opponents (i.e. handball, football). Higher incidences of injury also occur in sports in which falling onto the ground with outstretched hands is common (i.e. rugby, skiing). In some sports, the hand may be used as a weapon (i.e. karate, boxing), while in others it is used for protection (i.e. boxing). Repetitive motion, sustained grasp, extreme positions, and overloading or weight-bearing on the hands and wrists are particular activity patterns which increase the risk of injury (i.e. tennis, windsurfing, gymnastics, weightlifting). In sports which specifically require greater dexterity, precise movements, or sensory feedback, use of protective gear is impossible (i.e. rockclimbing). The use of certain equipment may impose additional risks (i.e. skiing). Even sports which require little or no use of the hands may still inflict injury (i.e. soccer, skating). In most cases, however, the hand is required in some way and loss of function would be detrimental to the athlete's performance.

Many sports are associated with specific hand or wrist injuries due to particular patterns of use. Although some injuries are unavoidable, in many cases preventive measures may be employed. It would be difficult to generalize prevention for all sports. Providing such general guidelines would be like giving a protocol for the management of all hand injuries. Therefore, this chapter will address preventive measures within specific sports. The problems most common to each sport will be outlined. However, it should be noted that some types of injuries described may also occur in other sports. The objective is to provide a review of commonly exhibited hand and wrist injuries within selected athletic activities, identify the mechanisms of injury, highlight the evaluation and treatment, and discuss ways to minimize the risk of these injuries.

Ulnar neuropathy in cyclists

Ulnar nerve compression at the wrist or hand level is a frequently cited problem for both racing and touring cyclists (Eckman *et al.*, 1975; Hoyt, 1976; Weiss, 1985; Jackson, 1989). 'Handlebar palsy' was described by Smail in 1975 following a personal experience on a long-distance bicycle journey in 1896 when bicycles were still fairly new (Destot, 1896). Recently, the incidence of this problem has been estimated to be around 5–20% in amateur cyclists (Weiss, 1985; Jackson, 1989); specific statistics for ulnar nerve compression in competitive cyclists were not available in these studies.

The ulnar nerve is vulnerable to pressure at the palm due to its anatomical exposure to external mechanical forces. The ulnar nerve descends to the hand after the dorsal cutaneous branch divides proximal to the wrist. This branch provides sensation to the dorsal ulnar aspect of the hand. The main branch of the ulnar nerve enters the hand along with the ulnar artery through the canal of Guyon. This tunnel is formed by a thin ligament which connects the pisiform and the hook of the hamate. It lies superficially and is covered only by the hypothenar aponeurosis. The nerve bifurcates within this canal into the superficial branch, which is primarily sensory, and the deep branch, which innervates intrinsic muscles of the hand. The superficial branch exits the canal and then travels deep to the palmaris brevis muscle, which is the nerve's only protective cover distal to the canal. It then continues subcutaneously to provide sensation to the volar ulnar aspect of the palm and to the ulnar ring and the small fingers. The deep branch of the ulnar nerve winds around the hook of the hamate and courses between the abductor digiti minimi (ADM) and the flexor digiti minimi (FDM) muscles, which it supplies. It then penetrates and innervates the opponens digiti minimi (ODM) and proceeds along the deep palmar arterial arch to innervate other intrinsic muscles within the hand.

Since the ulnar nerve is situated superficially and ulnarly in the hand, it becomes susceptible to pressure where much of the cyclist's body weight is transmitted into the hands against the handlebars (Fig. 5.1). Smail stated that the most advantageous riding position which permits the strongest pedalling and transfers the weight from the cyclist's ischia, requires about one-third of the body weight to be supported by the palms of the hands (Smail, 1975). Prolonged hyperextension of the wrists which places the ulnar nerve and artery on stretch may also be a contributing factor. Vascular compromise or trauma within Guyon's canal may also produce compression symptoms. Ulnar neuritis may be further aggravated by vibration due to the road surface.

'Handlebar palsy' has been used throughout literature but is an unfortunate term since it implies muscle weakness. In actuality, ulnar nerve compression may present itself with sensory disturbances alone. Shea and McClain have classified ulnar neuropathy in the hand into three specific syndromes according to the location of the lesion and the resulting clinical symptoms (Shea & McClain, 1969). Type 1 syndrome involves motor weakness of the ulnar innervated muscles in the hand in combination with a sensory deficit to the volar ulnar side of the palm and the ulnar ring and the small fingers. Sensation on the dorsal ulnar aspect of the hand remains intact. This distinguishes it from compression more proximal to the dorsal cutaneous branch. Type 1 syndrome is caused by compression of the nerve just proximal to the canal or within the canal before the nerve divides. Type 2 involves weakness of the hand muscles innervated by the deep branch of the ulnar nerve. Sensation supplied by the superficial branch is spared. Compression of this type occurs at the motor branch where it exits

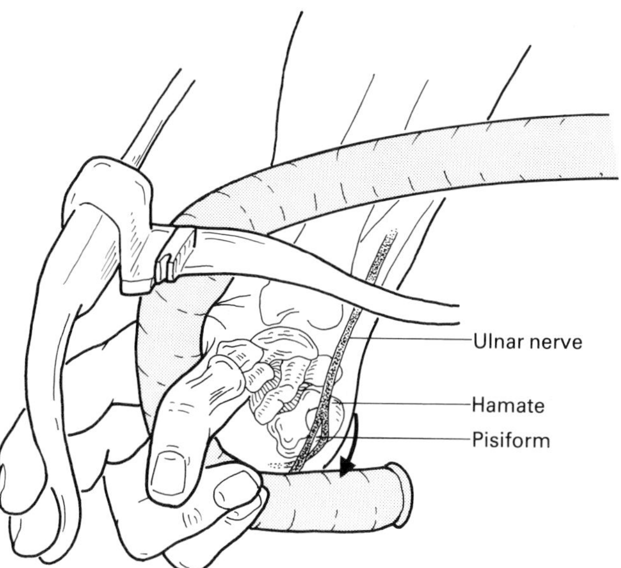

Fig. 5.1 Compression of the ulnar nerve against the handlebar.

the canal in the area of the hook of the hamate between the ADM and FDM muscle origins or as it courses through the ODM. Pressure may also occur further as the nerve crosses the palm under the flexor tendons and over the metacarpals. Type 3 syndrome involves sensory deficit only. Again, this is isolated to the volar ulnar aspect of the palm and the ulnar one and a half fingers. There is no motor deficit. Compression of the superficial branch occurs within the canal or distal to the canal along the superficial path on the ulnar side of the palm.

Ulnar nerve compression may present itself in any of the above forms in the cyclist. Complaints include paraesthesias, numbness, hypothenar pain and tenderness, diminished grip strength or decreased dexterity. The symptoms may be intermittent or persistent. Evaluation should include history of the sport or recreational activities and vocation (as one's occupation may also contribute to the condition). General medical history should be assessed to rule out other problems, such as diabetes or arthritis, that may involve peripheral nerve disturbances. A sensory examination will assist in determining the level of compression. Manual muscle test will also indicate the level and severity of the lesion. Atrophy of the intrinsic muscles, especially the hypothenar eminence and the first dorsal interosseous, may be evident if the problem is long standing. A positive Tinel's sign over Guyon's canal may be present. A definitive diagnosis should be made through electromyography and nerve conduction studies, including measurements of both sensory and motor amplitude and latencies distal to the wrist. These will rule out proximal lesions, localize the site of compression within the hand, and determine the degree of injury. Roentgenograms, including the carpal tunnel view, may also be necessary to identify any fractures or bone displacements which may impinge on the nerve. Various other hand conditions may predispose one or contribute to ulnar nerve injury or compression (Shea & McClain, 1969) but may not be detectable without invasive means.

Once ulnar nerve compression has been diagnosed, conservative treatment may produce reversible results. This includes immobilization of the wrist in neutral to 30° extension, anti-inflammatory medication and rest from cycling and any other contributing activities until full recovery is noted.

If the problem is severe or persistent and does not respond to the above, then surgical decompression may be necessary. Full exploration of the nerve at its lesion site should be undertaken following incision of the ligament.

Preventive measures may be taken by cyclists who are aware of the problem as well as by those who must prevent recurrence after developing the problem. This primarily entails modification and use of special equipment. Many authors have reported good results when cyclists followed certain recommendations (Hoyt, 1976; Burke, 1981; Jackson, 1989). Padded gloves should be worn to give added protection to the palms of the hands. The gel type (Spenco*) is designed to absorb shock, vibration and friction. Worn-out gloves should be replaced. Handlebars padded with foam or gel are also available in bike shops. Larger sized handlebars or padded tape applied around the bars may help to decrease the pressure exerted onto the palms. The angle of the handlebars, especially with straight handlebars, should be checked for comfort. Handlebar extensions and various handlebar configurations may be attached to or replace the dropped handlebars of road bikes or the straight bars of mountain bikes. These allow one to vary the hand positions providing intermittent relief to different points on the hand. Certain handlebars (i.e. Aero Handlebars†) are made with padded armrests and extensions for the clasped-hand position. Although these were designed for their aerodynamic advantage during time trials and triathlons, they also relieve the hands of prolonged pressure. However, these are illegal in racing for their obvious 'bull horn' configuration rendering them dangerous in accidents (United States Cycling Federation, 1991). These should not be used by amateurs who are uncomfortable with positioning the hands away from the brake levers. Whether the regular straight or dropped handlebars are used or any of the other alternatives are chosen, hand positions should be changed frequently. Proper placement of the brake levers also deserves attention so that friction is minimized over the ulnar side of the palm during use.

Proper bicycle fit is probably the most significant aspect in preventive measures (Gardiner, 1975; Hoyt, 1976; Burke, 1981). Each person should be measured for custom fit of the bicycle. Although this is never a problem for the competitive or avid cyclist, the recreational cyclist may not be aware of its importance. Purchasing a bicycle from a department store where one might be steered by poor advice should be avoided as should acquiring a second-hand bicycle. Proper fit is crucial in distributing body weight evenly, especially in bicycles with dropped handlebars which require a hunched-over riding position. Less than one-third of the body weight should be supported by the hands on the handlebars. This is achieved by considering several factors. The frame size should barely allow one to straddle the top horizontal bar with the feet flat on the ground in road bikes. Approximate 5 cm (2 in) from the bar to the crotch is allowable for mountain bikes. This initial step will allow for proper setting of the saddle and handlebars. The saddle should be horizontal. Too much forward tilt of the saddle may cause anterior slippage of the body off the seat, putting excessive weight onto the hands and causing the cyclist to continuously push the body back with the hands. The saddle should be adjusted to a height which allows full knee extension during the downstroke of the pedal. The handlebars should then be level with the saddle. The distance from the nose of the saddle to where the handlebar attaches to the stem should equal the distance from the elbow to the fingertips. Adjustments may be made by sliding the seat forward or backward (as long as full knee extension is still attainable) or by choosing the appropriate stem length. While in the riding position, one should be able to visually make a line through the handle-

* Spenco Biosoft Cycling Gloves from Spenco Medical Corp., Waco, Texas, USA.

† Aero Handlebars from Profile for Speed Inc., Chicago Illinois, USA.

bar stem and the front hub. If the stem falls behind the hub, there is probably too much forward pressure. Bike shop employees should be able to properly fit a bicycle to an individual. One system often used is the Fit Kit (New England Cycling Academy) in which torso, arm and leg measurements are incorporated.

Even with stringent compliance with these guidelines, it is not known whether total prevention is possible in all individuals. Further studies are needed to determine what length of time a position may be maintained before symptoms arise or how often hand positions must be changed. Other questions that need to be addressed include the thickness and material of glove or handlebar padding that is required to avert problems effectively. Despite the lack of conclusive evidence, the above recommendations may help to diminish the risk of developing ulnar nerve compression or at least delay it.

Finger injuries in rock climbers

Rock climbing has become an increasingly popular sport. National and world competitions engage extreme climbers who undertake climbs that were considered highly difficult, if not impossible, just over a decade ago. With the development of safer equipment and the advancement of techniques, the risk of injury due to falls has decreased. However, as the standards of technical difficulty have increased, acute and chronic soft tissue injuries of the hand have subsequently multiplied. Only recently have hand injuries in rock climbers been studied. The hand has been identified as the most frequently injured region in competition rock climbers (Bollen, 1988). The ring and long fingers are the most commonly involved digits as they bear the most weight during power moves on small holds.

A2 pulley injuries

Injury to the A2 pulley of the flexor tendon sheath of the ring finger has been cited as the most common hand injury, constituting 26% of competitive climbers (Bollen & Gunson, 1990). This injury may occur when the climber falls or slips while hanging onto a small hold or when pulling the body up on a small hold. The configuration of the fingers most often used during these manoeuvres, known as 'crimping', is with the proximal interphalangeal (PIP) joints flexed and the distal interphalangeal (DIP) joints extended (Fig. 5.2). The fingerholds may only be about 0.5 cm wide. This places immense strain on the A2 pulley, leading to a partial or complete tear. Gradual stretching of the pulley may also occur with the prolonged or repetitive stress of climbing.

Injury to the A2 pulley usually generates pain and swelling over the volar aspect of the proximal phalanx. The pain may persist for several months. On examination, 'bowstringing' of the flexor tendons with resisted flexion may be elicited.

The A2 pulley is one of the most important pulleys within the finger flexor mechanism. The transverse fibres of this pulley form a thickening over the fibro-osseous tunnel through which the flexor tendons glide. These fibres insert directly along both sides of the lateral shaft of the proximal phalanx. The A2 pulley, along with the A4, provides the

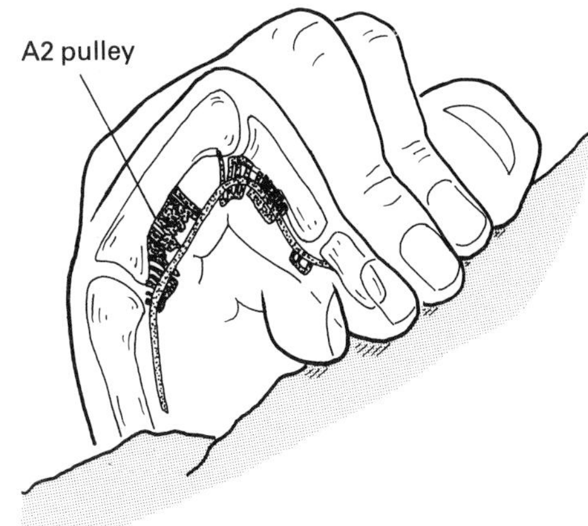

Fig. 5.2 Position of fingers on a small hold which produces strain on the A2 pulley.

strongest resistance of all the pulleys against the pulling force of the flexor tendons and hence are the most efficient in directing the flexor tendons in the axis of the phalangeal row. Loss of the A2 pulley will cause bowstringing and subsequently reduce grip strength.

Primary repair of the A2 pulley in a rock climber has been reported, but follow-up information on long-term results with resumption of the sport was not addressed (Tropet *et al.*, 1990). Surgical reconstruction of the A2 pulley is possible but may not withstand the amount of exertion required by further rock climbing (Lin *et al.*, 1989). Surgery may not necessarily be required in minor tears. Support of the A2 pulley using firm taping may be all that is needed during healing. It is therefore imperative that early detection of this injury be followed by adequate rest from all resistive activities.

Taping around the proximal phalanges, especially the third and fourth, is recommended during climbing or training on finger boards and climbing walls. This helps to provide external support to the flexor tendons. Rings are contraindicated and should be removed as they may directly cause other traumatic injuries if they catch on holds in the rock when falling or slipping. Although studies have not been conducted to determine the number of injuries sustained by those who utilize taping, one would expect that this would at least reduce the degree of injury. Bollen and Gunson (1990) are currently performing a study to determine the theoretical protection that taping can provide. The long-term effects in regards to functional limitations of those who have already acquired serious injury to the A2 pulley and continue to climb fanatically are yet to be studied.

Maximal upper extremity strength and endurance is needed for a rock climber who must hold and help pull his or her body weight up nearly vertical rock walls, and sometimes even past overhangs. A routine exercise programme should include resistive exercises for the forearm flexor muscles. This may include hand grippers and special devices (Digiflex*) which develop isolated finger flexion strength. Wrist flexion and extension strength is also important. This type of conditioning programme will reduce fatigue and help avoid slipping or falling. Training on finger boards and climbing walls will help improve one's climbing technique.

Proximal interphalangeal joint contractures

It has also been reported that 24% of climbers develop PIP joint flexion contractures of approximately 15°, again most commonly in the ring finger followed by the long finger (Bollen & Gunson, 1990). It is postulated that joint inflammation caused by abnormally high loading of those fingers give way to contractures as the fingers are allowed to rest in the normally flexed position. Dynamic splinting (i.e. LMB Spring Finger Extension Assist Splint†) may correct these deformities if recognized and treated early enough. However, this problem is best avoided by stretching the fingers into extension after a hard climb. Awareness of this problem is therefore of utmost importance in preventing permanent deformities of the PIP joints.

Ulnar collateral ligament (UCL) injury in skier's thumb

Acute rupture of the UCL of the metacarpophalangeal (MP) joint of the thumb is a common injury in skiing (Carr *et al.*, 1981). It is also prevalent in contact sports and in sports in which falling onto the hands is likely (McCue, 1982; McCue & Garroway, 1985). This injury in skiing was first noted by Petitpierre in 1939 (Petitpierre, 1939). Skier's thumb has also been referred to as 'gamekeeper's thumb' throughout

* Digiflex from I.M.C. Products Corp., Westbury, New York, USA.

† LMB Spring Finger Extension Assist Splint from Rehabilitation Technologies Inc., Luis Obispo, California, USA.

the literature. However, the original description of this problem involved chronic stretching of the UCL leading to ulnar MP joint laxity in the thumbs of gamekeepers (Campbell, 1955). This was due to the repetitive method they used for killing hares. The majority of those patients complained of pinch weakness and achiness, while others were without complaints. This chronic condition is actually a different scenario from that of the acute injury. Therefore it is preferrable to use the term 'skier's thumb' when describing an acute injury of the UCL of the thumb MP joint.

Traumatic injury to the UCL complex is the second most frequently occuring injury overall (9.5%) and the most frequently reported upper extremity injury (37.1%) in downhill skiing (Carr *et al.*, 1981). Investigations of current trends in ski injuries have shown that the relative frequency of cases of skier's thumb within all ski injuries is increasing. This is due to the decline of lower extremity injuries, not to an increase in the absolute number of skier's thumb incidents. However, the studies also revealed that out of 405 skiers interviewed, 25% had sustained thumb injuries while skiing in the past, but only a quarter of these sought medical attention. This could indicate that UCL injury may actually have the highest incidence of all skiing injuries.

The mechanism of UCL injury in skiing is a fall onto the snow with the thumb forced into abduction and hyperextension (Fig. 5.3). As the skier instinctively tries to break the fall with an outstretched hand, retention of the pole within the first web space traps the thumb into this vulnerable position, creating the fulcrum for injury.

Conventional use of the ski pole is with the hand passed through the strap and locked down on the grip. This allows the skier to plant the pole harder by pulling down on the strap with the hand without sustaining a tight grip. Such a technique makes discarding of the pole difficult during a fall. Avoiding the use of ski poles with straps was recommended so that the pole can disengage from the hand during a fall

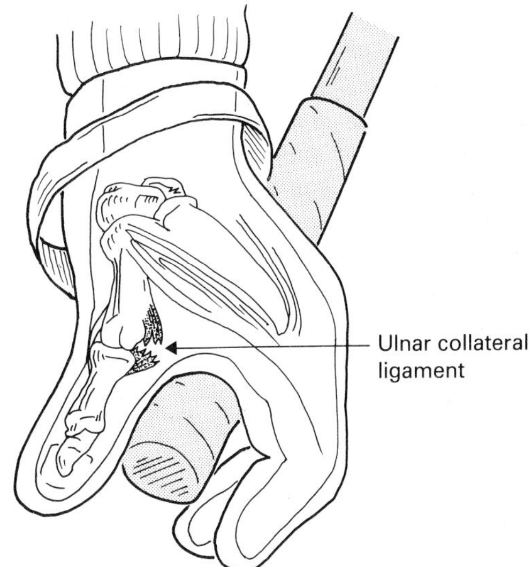

Fig. 5.3 Rupture of the ulnar collateral ligament caused by a fall onto the hand with retention of the ski pole.

(Browne *et al.*, 1976). Ski pole manufacturers, who attributed the blame to the strap itself as the cause of pole retention, introduced the 'new grip' ski poles. These were made with molded hand grips on platforms or with a break-away 'saber' handle. However, these did not solve the problem as the pole still maintained its position in the hand during a fall. A variety of thumb injuries were reported with use of these poles (Primiano, 1985). In fact, it was found that these poles were associated with a higher incidence of UCL injury (Carr *et al.*, 1981; Van Dommelen & Zvirbulis, 1989). An investigation on ski pole grip revealed that 81% of skiers used poles with straps (Carr *et al.*, 1981). 52% went through the strap and locked down on their grip, 24% went straight through the strap, and 5% kept their hands outside of the straps. Skiers receiving thumb injuries using each grip technique were 25, 21 and 5% respectively. The 19% of skiers who used the 'new grip' poles made up 27% of the thumb injuries.

The MP joint is unique in its anatomy and functional biomechanics. Stability of this joint is required for both power grip and pinch. The proper collateral ligaments and accessory collateral ligaments, joint capsule, volar plate and the encompassing intrinsic musculature and aponeurosis all contribute to this indispensable stability. Normal mobility of the thumb MP joint varies greatly in individuals (Palmer & Louis 1978). Some may hyperextend the joint while others lack full extension. Flexion may range from 5 to 115°. Lateral motion is less than that of the fingers since greater stability is an essential function of this joint in the thumb. Radial deviation may range from 0 to 30° in the extended position and 0 to 15° in full flexion. The radial deviation that is available enables the thumb to grasp around large objects further than what the carpometacarpal (CMC) joint would allow alone in the abducted position. It is the stability here that provides the counterforce to radial stress during strong grip and pinch.

The superficial layer of the thumb MP joint consists of the dorsal aponeurosis, whose transverse fibres expand to connect to the medial and lateral sesamoid bones, and the volar plate, which connects the sesamoid bones volarly. The adductor aponeurosis is the thick fibrous portion of the dorsal aponeurosis that extends from the volar plate and medial sesamoid bone to the extensor pollicus longus (EPL) tendon as it passes through the thumb to the dorsal hood. The adductor pollicus muscle contributes fibres to this portion of the aponeurosis and continues on into the triangular expansion which then inserts into the EPL tendon distal to the MP joint. Deep to the dorsal aponeurosis is the joint capsule which is reinforced by the collateral ligaments. The oblique fibres of the UCL proper originate from the MP head tubercle and insert into the volar ulnar aspect of the proximal phalanx base near the insertions of a portion of the adductor pollicus fibres and the volar plate. The transverse fibres of the ulnar accessory collateral ligament (ACL) arise from the MP head and insert into the medial border of the volar plate and medial sesamoid bone.

The adductor aponeurosis, via the adductor pollicus muscle, provides active stabilization of the joint but is not resistant to abduction by passive forces. Stener (1962) demonstrated in fresh cadaver studies that incision of the adductor aponeurosis produced no change in lateral stability. On the other hand, severance of the UCL with an intact adductor aponeurosis gave way to ulnar instability. When the UCL proper was incised and the ACL was preserved, the stability of the joint was maintained in the extended position but then greater than normal abduction was possible in the flexed position. Severance of the ACL produced even greater instability. Furthermore, incision of the volar plate created total instability. Palmer and Louis (1978). Supported this in another cadaver study which confirmed that the position of greatest stability is full flexion (Table 5.1). When the MP joint is flexed, the UCL proper becomes taut and the ACL, volar plate and adductor aponeurosis loose. In extension, the reverse is true.

Of the UCL injuries reported in skiing accidents, 34.8% were reported to be grade 1, representing microscopic tear of the UCL fibres without loss of integrity (Carr *et al.*, 1981).

Table 5.1 Average radial deviation (cadaver study). From Palmer & Louis (1978).

Position of MP joint	Structures intact (°)	AA cut (°)	DC cut (°)	UCL proper cut (°)	ACL and VP cut (°)
Full extension	4	7	12	28	>90
Flexed 15°	9	10	14	32	>90
Full flexion	0	0	2	42	>90

AA, adductor aponeurosis; ACL, accessory collateral ligament; DC, dorsal capsule; MP, metacarpophalangeal; UCL, ulnar collateral ligament; VP, volar plate.

Grade 2, which is partial tear of the fibres without compromise of integrity but with elongation of the fibres, made up 47%. Grade 3 is a complete rupture, usually at its distal end near its insertion onto the proximal phalanx. These injuries made up 18.2%. It was also revealed that 23.3% involved a fracture. The most common of these injuries in the younger athlete who has not reached skeletal maturity is the Salter–Harris 3 fracture in which the ulnar corner of the proximal phalanx epiphysis is avulsed with the UCL (Rosenberg *et al.*, 1991).

Displacement of the torn proximal flap of the UCL may occur after a rupture. Initially the adductor aponeurosis covers the UCL. Once the ligament ruptures with forced abduction of the thumb, the torn proximal end passes the proximal edge of the adductor aponeurosis as this migrates distally. The ligament then becomes trapped superficially when the proximal phalanx returns to its original position. This was described by Stener (1962) and is now known as the Stener lesion. He found this to be true in 64% of cases. This type of lesion will not heal without surgical intervention to reapproximate the two ends.

Thorough examination of the athlete with potential joint injury is critical in order to make an accurate diagnosis and establish early and appropriate treatment. Neglect in seeking medical treatment or failure to provide precise evaluation may lead to serious consequences in which severe and permanent functional impairment may occur, primarily pinch weakness and ulnar instability when the thumb is stressed in abduction.

Following UCL injury, the patient may complain of localized tenderness or pain over the ulnar aspect of the MP joint with associated swelling. One may also have volar or dorsal pain. Palpating the joint to localize the area of pain will assist in determining the direct area of trauma. Injured structures on the ulnar aspect of the joint may involve the UCL proper, adductor aponeurosis, ACL, dorsal capsule or the volar plate.

Much controversy exists regarding what the diagnostic assessment should comprise. It is agreed upon in the literature that once a UCL injury is suspected according to the patient's complaints and history of injury mechanism, roentgenograms (postero-anterior, lateral and oblique) should be taken to determine whether an avulsion fracture is present. Physical examination should not take place before this is performed as iatrogenic displacement of an aligned proximal phalanx fracture may change a non-operative case into one requiring surgery. If a non-displaced avulsion fracture is detected, cast immobilization is appropriate. If it is a displaced fracture, surgery may be required.

If the X-ray excludes bony involvement, some advocate follow-up with clinical examination by assessment of joint stability. Radial stress testing of the joint is performed in extension and flexion. It is compared with the contralateral joint to determine the normal amount of laxity and thus to avoid misinterpretation. Digital anaesthesia may be used if necessary. To assess ulnar MP joint stability, the thumb is placed into opposition to lock the CMC joint in a position which will reduce rotation of the first metacarpal. The metacarpal is secured with one hand taking care to prevent rotation of the bone while the proximal phalanx is radially deviated with the other hand. Lateral stress is applied in full extension and varying degrees of flexion depending on the author (Palmer & Louis, 1978; Rettig & Wright, 1989). Instability at 0° extension indicates loss of integrity of the ACL and volar plate. Instability in flexion indicates discontinuity of the UCL proper. Some even advocate stress radiographs as an adjunct to clinical stability assessment to confirm the degree of joint angulation. However, the criteria for resolving complete soft-tissue rupture is also controversial. Depending on the author, absence of an end-point, 10–35° difference in angulation in various degrees of flexion compared to the normal side, more than 30–45° angulation with the MP joint in full flexion, more than 30% subluxation of the proximal phalanx, may constitute a grade 3 injury.

Some authors advocate the utilization of an arthrogram as the diagnostic tool for UCL tear once avulsion fracture has been ruled out (Bowers & Hurst, 1977). This not only determines complete rupture of the UCL, but also differentiates a rupture with ligament ends in apposition from a Stener lesion. Lack of this definitive diagnosis may be why some patients in the literature yielded good results with casting (those without a Stener lesion) while others did so poorly (those with displaced ligament with interposition of adductor aponeurosis). Vigorous stress testing for joint stability is disputed as one may create a Stener lesion out of a previously non-displaced UCL, thereby requiring surgical repair in a patient who could have been treated conservatively. Only gentle radial stress is applied to verify pain with stress.

Grade 1 or 2 sprain of the UCL is probable if there is no leakage of radiographic dye from the joint capsule. Escape of the contrast medium through a small rent in the ligament into the surrounding tissue represents a complete rupture with non-displaced ends. Leakage through a larger tear may denote a Stener lesion. If the arthrogram is inconclusive, then other methods of evaluation may be used. However, with experience, utilization of the arthrogram can often provide the correct diagnosis.

Grade 1 may only require a forearm or hand-based splint until pain and tenderness subside, or taping (thumb spica or check-rein) to prevent further injury during healing. Grade 2 may require cast immobilization for 3–4 weeks. If the injury is grade 3 with ligament ends in apposition, then cast immobilization is appropriate for approximately 4–6 weeks. When surgical repair is indicated, it should be performed within the first few weeks following acute injury. It is not absolutely necessary to undergo this immediately, therefore the skier who is on vacation may choose to have his or her surgical care delayed until the return home provided the athlete is given adequate cast protection for the remainder of the vacation. However, surgery should not be delayed too long due to possible ligament contracture that would make secondary reconstruction necessary.

Following injury, the athlete may resume skiing and most sports activities during the course of healing with cast or splint protection. The thumb spica cast or splint should be applied without producing radially deviating forces onto the proximal phalanx and without allowing ulnar deviation of the first metacarpal by the first dorsal interosseous muscle which may achieve indirect abduction of the MP joint. This is achieved by incorporating the thumb web space sufficiently. Opposition of the thumb should be avoided as this will cause abduction at the MP joint. The MP joint should be flexed approximately 30° and the interphalangeal (IP) joint approximately 20°. The IP joint should be included for return to skiing or else the cast becomes a fulcrum for injury. The cast or splint that is forearm-based provides proximal stabilization for increased protection. Some have treated patients with a modified thumb spica cast allowing for wrist mobility following UCL injury or repair (Primiano, 1986). However, this type of cast has not been subjected to sports activities.

A fibreglass cast is sufficiently rigid to allow return to skiing with minimal risk of reinjury. A splint is not adequate immobilization and protection because it does not conform uniformly to the hand. Splints may be indicated for further protection during physical activities once a cast has been removed or when less protection is needed, such as with a grade 1 injury. A thermoplastic material with high rigidity and good draping characteristics is important in achieving a conforming fit while ensuring the greatest safety. The material can be remolded or adjusted as swelling changes. While perforated material may provide ventilation to the skin, it also weakens the structure at points of high stress. The splint may be secured with elastic wrap or Velcro straps. When more reliable security is needed during competition, cloth adhesive tape should be used.

If the patient wishes to participate in other sports as well, regulations should be checked as some competition or team sports rules do not allow hard surface protective devices because of the danger to others. Rules may also vary within the different levels of a particular sport. A soft playing cast made of silicone may be fabricated for certain sports when approved by the physician and allowed by the local official and governing regulations (Bassett *et al.*, 1979). Participation without protective devices is usually allowed approximately 8–12 weeks following treatment of a grade 2 or 3 injury.

Bilateral hand-based thumb spica splints may be fabricated for wear under ski gloves for those who wish to take extra precautions during downhill skiing. These should be custom made. Again, the IP joint should be included for skiing and the thumb web space and ulnar border of the palm incorporated to provide stability against rotational forces. The splints should be held in place with elastic wrap or tape. One should be wary of factory prefabricated splints as these are usually made of less rigid material, are difficult to fit adequately, and may expose the IP joint to potential trauma.

The ski pole itself has been implicated as the mechanism of injury (Carr *et al.*, 1981). This was deduced from subjective information and observation that many other sports activities result in falls onto the outstretched hands but result in fewer UCL injuries. That only 5% of skiers who gripped poles outside of the straps acquired injury is a strong argument for use of this technique. It is therefore recommended that the 'new grip' ski poles not be used. Straps on the poles should either be removed or held around the outside of the pole. This will allow the pole to separate from the hand prior to striking the snow. Skiers should be advised to discard the pole deliberately during a fall. The inconvenience of climbing up the slope to retrieve the discarded pole should outweigh the risk of injury. This has been taught to ski racers by some instructors for many years. Ski instructors at resorts should incorporate this as a safety factor when teaching novice skiers.

Eisenberg *et al.* (1990) are currently researching a sports thumb protection system which is already being marketed by a ski glove manufacturer*. It was designed to protect the thumb MP joint from collateral ligament injury. The protective device is incorporated into the ski glove. It allows all normal motions of the thumb but prevents abnormal ulnar stress. The eccentric hinge design allows comfortable flexion of the thumb. In their preliminary studies, they documented 170 000 man days skiing (MDS) with no reported thumb injuries compared to one thumb injury per 8000 MDS. This could be very promising if further research also produces good results. This type of protection would be more likely used by skiers of all levels of expertise since it is incorporated into a commonly used piece of equipment. The glove does not affect the skier's technique and is always prepared in case of an accidental fall.

Perineural fibrosis in bowler's thumb

The ulnar digital sensory nerve of the thumb is commonly traumatized in bowlers due to direct mechanical compression. This leads to a painful neuroma which can become incapacitating. This is an otherwise rare entity. Siegel noted this problem in bowlers in 1965 and others have subsequently reported it (Marmor, 1966; Howell & Leach, 1970; Dobyns *et al.*, 1972; Dunham *et al.*, 1972; Minkow & Bassett, 1972).

The problem evolves when the hard edge of the thumb hole in the bowling ball causes friction over the ulnar digital nerve at the base of the thumb during delivery (Fig. 5.4). This subcutaneous nerve lies superficial to the ulnar sesamoid bone at the MP joint, making it susceptible to injury with direct repetitive pressure. Subsequent scarring entraps the normally mobile nerve causing it to be tethered by its cutaneous branches. The nerve then becomes unable to escape from irritating pressures. Normally, callus formation allows mobility

* Thumbsaver Ski Glove from Kombi Ltd, Naugatuck, Connecticut, USA.

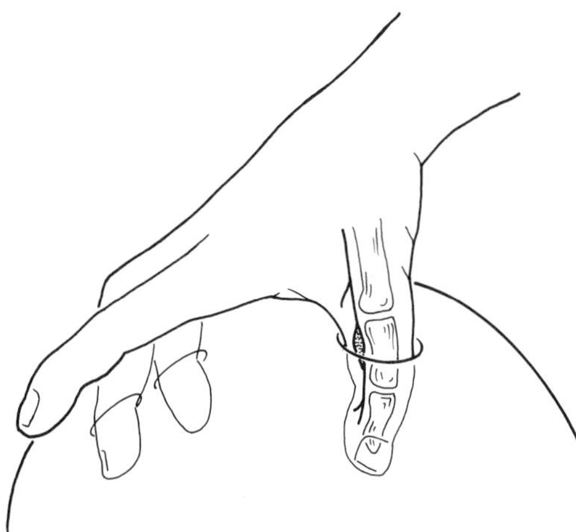

Fig. 5.4 Neuroma of the ulnar digital nerve caused by friction against the rim of the thumb hole.

of the underlying nerve and protects it from injury.

The bowler will usually complain of localized tenderness and pain at the site of compression. A fusiform mass can usually be palpated. Percussion over the volar ulnar aspect of the MP crease may produce distal paraesthesias. The bowler may also exhibit hypaesthesias or a sensory deficit.

Best results are achieved with early recognition and treatment. Initial care of the painful neuroma should always be conservative. This includes a desensitization programme and temporary cessation of bowling. Splinting is not recommended as this could possibly contribute further to compression of the nerve due to slippage of the splint during functional activities (Rayan & O'Donoghue, 1983). When bowling is continued, technique or equipment modifications must be made. Most bowlers spontaneously make changes in their technique when discomfort or pain is noticed. If the problem progresses despite alterations or if the bowler persists without modifications, recovery becomes more difficult and prolonged. If the severe or chronic condition is unresponsive to conservative attempts, surgery may be indicated. Neurolysis of the ulnar digital nerve with excision of the thickened epineurium should be performed. Transposition of the nerve to a more dorsal ulnar protected position may also be necessary. Even following operative treatment, modifications must be made upon resumption of the sport.

Contributing factors leading to bowler's thumb include the use of a heavy or oversized ball, a wide or improper bore spread and poor delivery technique. Preventive measures include changing the position of the thumb hole into more abduction and extension, which decreases the pressure on the ulnar base of the thumb. A three-quarter grip technique, in which the thumb is not fully inserted into the hole, may also help. Other suggestions include contouring the hole edge, redrilling larger holes and applying padding.

Acute and chronic injuries in golfing

Despite popular belief, golf is a physically demanding sport. Both the repetitive nature of the required motions and the level of exertion contribute to wrist and hand injuries in this sport. The left wrist is the most frequently injured body part in professional golfers, making up 23.9% of all injuries (McCarroll, 1985, 1990). It is the second most frequent upper extremity injury in recreational golfers, accounting for 8.7% of all injuries. The left hand (in right-handed golfers) is the second most frequent upper extremity injury in professionals (7.1% of overall injuries) and the fourth in non-professionals (5.4% of overall injuries).

The biomechanics of the golf swing are broken into three parts (McCarroll, 1985, 1990). During take-away, the golfer takes the grip position on the club. In the right-handed golfer, this means that the left hand is on the upper end of the club, with the end of the handle resting against the proximal ulnar aspect of the palm. Both wrists are ulnarly deviated. As the body rotates with the back swing, the left wrist deviates radially and the right wrist extends dorsally. At the impact phase, the accelerating force of the down swing causes the left wrist and hand to be thrust into the ball. The right wrist maintains its position in maximal extension. During follow-through, the wrists, especially the left, are forced into ulnar deviation while the thumbs maintain their grasp around the handle.

Although injury may occur in any of the above phases, the wrist is most commonly affected during the take-away and impact phases (McCarroll, 1990). The hand is usually afflicted in the impact phase. The mechanics of golfing injuries are usually related to the swing. Upper extremity injuries in professional golfers are most commonly caused by the repeated stress of practice (21.4% of cases) but can also result from poor swing mechanics (14.4% of cases). The latter is usually the most frequent cause is recreational golfers. Other mechanisms of injury include hitting tree roots or taking a large divot.

There are various wrist and hand problems derived from golfing. However, this section will address only two that are unique to this sport.

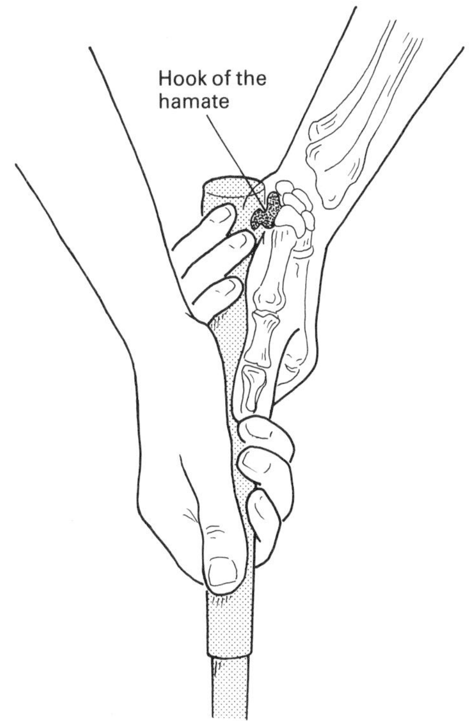

Fig. 5.5 The hook of the hamate protrudes toward the end of the golf club.

Hook of the hamate fracture

The hook of the hamate is subject to injury in golfers. A case of such an injury sustained by a golfer was reported in 1972 (Torisu, 1972) and many other reports have followed (Stark *et al.*, 1977; Watson & Rogers, 1989; McCarroll, 1990). Incidences of this injury in other sports which involve swinging a racquet or striking a ball (i.e. tennis, baseball) have also been reported (Stark *et al.*, 1977; Parker *et al.*, 1986). Fractures of the hamate hook are rare outside of sports. The percentage of this injury within golfers is unknown.

The hook of the hamate is a long, thin bone which protrudes volarly from the body of the hamate into the hypothenar eminence. When the golfer grips the club, the end of the handle rests against the proximal ulnar aspect of the non-dominant hand, coming into contact with the hook of the hamate (Fig. 5.5). Fracture of the hook, usually at its base, occurs when the end of the club strikes the hook at the end of a swing or at the time of impact with the ball. It can also occur when the golfer accidently strikes the ground or a tree root causing forces to be transmitted directly to the hook through the club. A contributing mechanism may involve violent contraction of the flexor carpi ulnaris (FCU) muscle which inserts onto the hook through the pisohamate ligament. However, since an avulsion fracture at the base of the 5th metacarpal, onto which the FCU tendon also inserts, does not occur simultaneously, this is not considered to be the primary cause.

Following a hook of the hamate fracture, the golfer will complain of wrist pain or ache and a weak grip, which is usually caused by pain inhibition. Diffuse swelling may be noted in the hypothenar area. Severe tenderness to firm pressure over the hook, which is situated approximately 2–3 cm along a line from the pisiform prominence to the base of the index finger, is a strong indicator of fracture. Active wrist and finger motion is usually non-painful, even when making a full fist. However, gripping around an object elicits pain. The golfer can usually recall the onset of symptoms. When hook of the hamate fracture is suspected, roentgenograms should be obtained, including antero-posterior, lateral, oblique and carpal tunnel views of the wrist. If these are negative, then a bone scan or computerized tomography may be pursued if this fracture is still strongly suspected.

This injury is frequently misdiagnosed as wrist sprain or tendinitis. It is important to identify this fracture through precise evaluation as complications may evolve from such an injury. The ulnar nerve which passes ulnarly to the hook of the hamate through Guyon's canal may become irritated or compressed, resulting in sensory or motor impairment (Howard, 1961; Baird & Friedenberg, 1968; Shea & McClain, 1969). The flexor digitorum profundus (FDP) tendons to the ring and small fingers traverse radially to the hook of the hamate. A fractured hook may cause these tendons to rupture (Crosby & Linscheid 1974; Stark *et al.*, 1977).

If the acute fracture is non-displaced, a short arm cast including the ring and small fingers should be applied for 4–6 weeks. There is a high incidence of non-union with this type of fracture, however, because of the contraction of the muscular attachments onto the loose fragment (FDM and ODM via the transverse carpal ligament and the FCU via the pisohamate ligament). There is also decreased blood supply to the hook. If the fracture is displaced or non-union occurs, excision of the hook may be indicated. Return to golfing may then be resumed once scar tenderness diminishes. Bone grafting and internal fixation may be performed for treatment of non-union hook fractures to reduce sensitivity in the hypothenar area and to preserve the pulley effect of the hook on the FDP tendons of the ring and small fingers allowing for maximum power grip in the ulnarly deviated position (Watson & Rogers, 1989). It is 3 months before the athlete can return to golfing following this procedure, but the long-term benefits may outweigh the decrease in strength or increase in recovery time.

De Quervain's tenosynovitis

An overuse syndrome that is associated with golfing (McCarroll, 1990) as well as racquet sports and bowling (Easterbrook & Cameron, 1985; Hunter & Poole, 1987) is de Quervain's tenosynovitis. This problem is common in sports which involve repetitive wrist motion. De Quervain's tenosynovitis is inflammation of the abductor pollicus longus (APL) and extensor pollicus longus (EPL) tendons at the level of the wrist where they pass through the first dorsal compartment *en route* to the thumb. The first dorsal compartment is the most radial of the six extensor compartments of the wrist. The APL and EPL tendons each pass through a synovial sheath, which helps to reduce friction between the tendons, compartment and radius. Both tendons share the same fibro-osseous tunnel. The compartment is formed by the osseous groove in the radial styloid at its floor and the extensor retinaculum forming the cover. The extensor retinaculum serves as a pulley to the tendons to direct their line of pull. It is unyielding to stretch in extreme positions, particularly ulnar deviation. Repetitive motion, especially ulnar deviation with a thumb grasp, can cause inflammation of the tendons within this restricted space. As the inflammatory cycle persists, the enlarged, swollen tendons must pass through the swollen, constricted tunnel. This causes extreme pain upon wrist motion or with use of the thumb. In severe cases, this can produce 'triggering' of the tendons.

Tenderness and swelling should be noted over the radial styloid. The golfer may complain of pain radiating into the thumb or travelling proximally into the forearm along the course of the tendon. The pain may be inhibitory, causing decreased pinch strength. Pain may be elicited with resisted thumb extension. A posi-

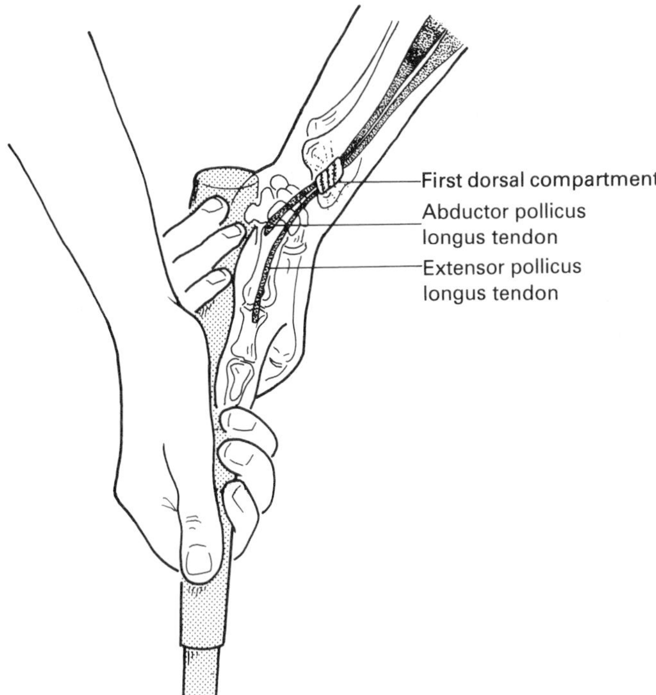

Fig. 5.6 De Quervain's tenosynovitis caused by repetitive ulnar deviation of the wrist during the golf swing.

tive Finkelstein's test is the diagnostic indicator. This manoeuvre is performed by tucking the thumb into the fisted fingers and forcibly deviating the wrist into ulnar deviation. A positive sign is marked by exquisite pain over the radial styloid. This manoeuvre is similar to the mechanics of swinging a golf club (Fig. 5.6).

This condition must be identified and treated early in order to reduce the chances of chronic symptoms which are difficult to treat. Initial signs of an acute onset of de Quervain's tenosynovitis should be addressed conservatively. This includes ice, medication and a removable thermoplastic splint. The splint should position the wrist in the neutral to extended position, avoiding ulnar deviation. The thumb IP joint should be left free to move as the EPL tendon which serves this joint passes through a separate compartment (the third dorsal compartment) and thus does not contribute to this problem during its function. The purpose of the splint is to rest the hand from irritating activities so that inflammation of the synovium may be reduced. Once symptoms have resolved, a gradual return to activities is emphasized. Careful monitoring for recurrence is important. In resistant cases, steroid injections along with rest may be necessary. If conservative treatment is unsuccessful, surgical decompression may be indicated. When releasing the compartment, septa between the APL and EPL tendons, and multiple APL slips should be recognized in order to ensure adequate decompression. The hand is then splinted for up to 3 weeks with gradual progression of the range of movement and strengthening. Golfing may be resumed in 6–8 weeks.

Prevention of wrist injuries in golfing

The Nirschl R-U Wrist Brace* may be used to prevent de Quervain's tenosynovitis or hinder exacerbations of this overuse syndrome

* Nirschl R-U Wrist Brace from Medical Sports Inc., Arlington, Virginia, USA.

(Wright, 1991). This brace was designed to support the wrist and prevent extreme motions, especially into ulnar deviation. This, or other similar splints, can serve as a good training device for modification of swing technique.

Professional golf instructors can teach proper mechanics of the golf swing to avoid undue stress on the wrists and hands. Also, use of proper equipment is important. The club professional can assist in selecting the appropriate size and shape of grip handle to facilitate proper swing mechanics and alleviate tortional stress during impact.

The Bio-Curve Grip* was designed with a 19° bend in the handle, placing the apex at the base of the non-dominant long finger (McCarroll, 1990; Cahalan *et al.*, 1991). This ergonomic handle was intended to decrease the torsional stress to the arm and hand. A study has indicated that this type of handle provides greater resistance to torque allowing the wrist to attenuate the force of impact during a swing, which is especially important when taking a divot or striking a tree root (Cahalan *et al.*, 1991). The ulnar bend of the club and conforming grip of the handle provides improved positioning, requiring less ulnar deviation of the wrist. Both normal and symptomatic golfers have reported improved grip and decreased shock transmitted from the club to the hands. While use of this club may potentially prevent wrist and hand problems in golfers, including de Quervain's tenosynovitis and fracture of the hook of the hamate, it does not affect club head speed, impact force by the golfer or accuracy of the point of impact, and therefore does not have a greater mechanical advantage over the straight club. However, the Bio-Curve Club has not been approved for use by the United States Golf Association (1990). Further studies should be conducted to assess any wrist or hand problems among those who use the Bio-Curve Club over a long period of time to clinically confirm this injury prevention hypothesis.

* Bio-Curve Golf Club from Chicago Golf and Sport, Clearwater, Florida, USA.

The importance of conditioning should not go unmentioned. This involves both stretching and strengthening exercises. Stretching helps to maximize flexibility and range of motion of the joint and to increase the resting length of the musculotendinous unit. Strengthening will facilitate more powerful strikes and enable better control of the swing. The upper extremity that undergoes a routine conditioning programme which improves flexibility and strength will better withstand the stress of repetitive swinging of the club and the forceful striking of the ball, thus reducing the risk of injury.

Wrist pain in gymnasts

Gymnastics is a popular sport world-wide, with an increasing number of participants noted in the last two decades. A variety of wrist injuries, both acute and chronic, osseous and soft tissue, have evolved from participation in this sport. In a recent study, 87.5% of male and 55% of female collegiate gymnasts were reported to have experienced wrist pain during practice or competition, the majority of those having pain for longer than 4 months (Mandelbaum *et al.*, 1989). Wrist injuries in gymnasts are attributed to the types of stresses endured, including repetitive motion, high impact loading, axial compression, torsional force and distraction. This is combined with positions which almost always involve forced hyperextension of the wrist, but also include loading in positions of radial and ulnar deviation. The mechanisms of loading the wrist in end-point positions transforms the wrist into a weight-bearing joint in which the hand may be used as a fulcrum around which the body rotates (Fig. 5.7). Since this is the inherent nature of the sport, wrist pain is often regarded as a consequence of the sport. It is not uncommon for gymnasts to neglect their pain for fear of losing time from the sport. Some only seek medical attention when they become unable to participate in the

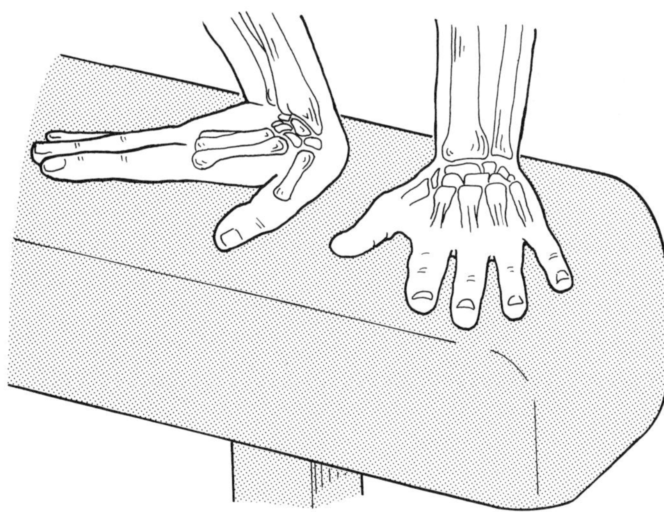

Fig. 5.7 Weight-bearing of the upper extremities during gymnastics may cause a variety of wrist problems.

activities. Peter Kormann, an Olympic medallist in gymnastics, stated that 'All gymnasts work out and compete with ongoing problems in their upper extremities. These problems are only considered serious injuries when the gymnast can no longer compete' (Aronen, 1985).

Gymnastics demands a high level of participation at an early age. Entry into gymnastics for the élite male is about 9 years of age, with peak level of competition at 22, and retirement at 24. The female initiates the sport at about 6 years of age, with peak involvement at 16, and retirement from active participation at 18. This involves the most important years of skeletal growth and development. Training time is approximately 1–3 $h \cdot week^{-1}$ in the United States Gymnastics Federation (USGF) class 4, or preparatory level, and graduating to 15–30 $h \cdot week^{-1}$ in class 1, or élite level. The percentage of injuries is proportionate to the amount of time spent training and the class level of performance. This is due to increased exposure time to risk of injury, higher skill levels required and greater degree of difficulty of routines with the changes in performance standards. The intensity of competition may also create immense psychological pressure on the gymnast.

Men's events include floor exercise, vault, rings, high bar, parallel bars and the pommel horse; the latter is associated with the greatest incidence of wrist injuries in men. These events all involve compressive loading of the wrist with the addition of rotational force in the pommel horse and vault events, and traction in the rings and high bar events. Women's events include balance beam, uneven parallel bars, vault and the floor exercise, which contributes to the greatest number of wrist injuries in women. These also involve compression as well as rotation during the vault and traction with the uneven parallel bars. With the difference in peak participation and performance demands, different injury patterns are noted in male and female gymnasts.

Injuries to the wrists are numerous (Linscheid & Dobyns, 1985; Dobyns & Gabel, 1990; Weiker, 1990) and, therefore, will be mentioned only briefly. Since knowledge of wrist anatomy and biomechanics has increased during the last two decades, injuries now have more accurate diagnoses, instead of such terms as 'wrist sprain'. Injuries may be acute, but more often there is an insidious onset of symptoms. With continued stress on the wrist, these become more severe and chronic in nature.

Evaluation should include an accurate history and thorough physical examination. Information such as total number of hours per week of gymnastic participation, progression of pain, points of maximal tenderness and areas of pain associated with motion and loading should be assessed. Routine roentgenograms (anteroposterior and lateral) should be taken and inspected for ulna variance, changes in the distal radius and ulna physes, articular surface irregularities, sclerosis and fractures. Conservative treatment consisting of rest, medication, activity modification and immobilization as necessary should be attempted first. If pain persists after 6 weeks, then an arthrogram or magnetic resonance imaging (MRI) should be obtained to rule out a triangular fibrocartilage complex (TFCC) tear, loose bodies and ligament instabilities. Some possible wrist injuries in gymnasts are listed below.

Distal radius physeal stress reaction

A widened and irregular distal radius physis, cystic changes, irregularity of the metaphyseal margin of the growth plate, and haziness of the physis may be seen radiographically. This stress reaction is due to poorly mineralized cartilage at the metaphyseal side of the growth plate. It is caused by repetitive microtrauma which disrupts the metaphyseal vascular network producing ischaemia. This can possibly result in permanent deformities. Axial compression and torsional loading may be responsible for this. Symptoms include dorsal wrist pain, swelling and tenderness on the dorsal aspect of the distal radius intensified by hyperextension of the wrist. Treatment involves cessation of gymnastics until symptoms resolve and splint immobilization in severe cases.

Distal radius and ulna physeal stress reaction

This stress reaction is similar to the one above, but is instead caused by distraction of the wrist with contribution by the use of dowel grips, which allows more complex manoeuvres on the bars. Normally when hanging or swinging on the bars, the wrist and finger flexor and extensor muscles carry most of the load in tension while at the same time applying a compressive force to the distal radius physis. Use of the dowel grips requires less muscle contraction by passively applying force to the wrist and thereby allowing increased distraction forces to be applied to the distal radius physis. Pain can be reproduced with axial traction.

Distal radius physeal arrest

Premature closure of the growth plate of the distal radius due to repetitive loading of the wrist with subsequent relative overgrowth of the ulna may be a permanent result of stress reaction. The ulna growth plate normally closes before the radius. Symptoms include chronic dorsal wrist pain. Radiographs may reveal growth plate closure of the distal radius, increased volar angulation of the distal radius articular surface and ulna positive variance. Ulna shortening may be performed surgically if necessary.

TFCC tears

Tear of the TFCC, usually at the point of insertion at the sigmoid notch of the distal radius, is common in older gymnasts due to the high frequency of ulna-positive variance and increased ulnar-sided transmission of force from repetitive weight-bearing. Arthrography or MRI will confirm the diagnosis. Arthroscopic debridement often renders good results. Repair is possible in some peripheral tears. Simultaneous ulna shortening may prevent further injury to the TFCC as well as restore the normal load transmission across the wrist.

Scaphoid stress fracture

Stress fracture of the scaphoid is a rare entity. It is caused by repetitive compressive loading of the wrist in extension, such as with handstands. Forearm muscle fatigue may also contribute because decreased support is provided causing greater stress concentration on the scaphoid. This leads to a stress reaction across the waist of the scaphoid. Symptoms include chronic wrist pain without an acute injury, tenderness directly over the scaphoid exacerbated with hyperextension and radial deviation. Radiographs may reveal sclerosis at the waist early on and later a fracture. Treatment involves short arm cast immobilization until significant radiographic healing is noted.

Scaphoid impaction syndrome

Impaction of the dorsal rim of the scaphoid against the dorsal lip of the radius is caused by forced hyperextension of the wrist. Tenderness over the dorsal scaphoid is noted. Pain is reproduced with hyperextension. Radiographs may reveal a small ossicle or hypertrophic ridge at the dorsal scaphoid rim. Rest and avoidance of hyperextension may relieve symptoms. Otherwise, surgical removal of the opposing surfaces may be necessary.

Ulnar impaction syndrome

Ulnotriquetral abutment is common especially with use of the pommel horse. When the wrist is subjected to repetitive radial and ulnar deviation forces while the wrist is hyperextended and the forearm is pronated, there is an increased load transmission through the ulnar aspect of the wrist. Biomechanical studies have shown that in the neutral forearm position, the ulna bears 15% of applied loads (Af Ekenstam *et al.*, 1984). There is little change of this in extension or flexion, but at 25° of ulnar deviation, this increases to 24%. Additional load transmission to the ulna is seen at 75° of forearm pronation with an increase to 37%. Ulnar loading is also greater in wrists with ulna-positive variance. Such ulnar load stresses may result in TFCC tears, ulnotriquetral ligament attrition, chondromalacia, subchondral sclerosis, and subchondral cyst formation of the opposing articular surfaces of the lunate, triquetrum or ulna.

Symptoms include tenderness over the proximal lunate and triquetral area intensified by forced ulnar deviation and anteroposterior translation of the ulnar head with the wrist in ulnar deviation. Radiographs may reveal an ulna-positive variance. Conservative treatment is attempted first with rest, medication and modification of training. If this is unsuccessful, 4–6 weeks of immobilization and cessation of gymnastics should be prescribed. If the pain still does not resolve, then an arthrogram or MRI should be obtained to determine the integrity of the TFCC and intercarpal ligaments. Arthroscopy and distal ulna shortening may be indicated.

Lunotriquetral impingement

Impingement of the dorsal lunate and triquetral rims may be caused by repetitive hyperextension and ulnar deviation of the wrist. Associated problems may include radiolunate impingement, triquetrohamate impingement, and lunotriquetral ligament tears and dissociations. Symptoms include tenderness over the involved joint exacerbated by extension and ulnar deviation. Rest should be tried before surgical intervention.

Chondromalacia

Chondromalacia of the radioscaphoid, lunotriquetral, ulnolunate, triquetrohamate and capitolunate joints are usually seen in association with other wrist injuries.

Capsulitis

Synovitis of the dorsal wrist capsule is marked by chronic, diffuse dorsal wrist tenderness, mild swelling and warmth. This is probably the result of dorsal impaction with hyperextension of the wrist. Radiographs are normal. Rest, ice, and anti-inflammatory medication may be sufficient.

Ganglia

Ganglion cysts originating from the scapholunate interval are not uncommon in the gymnast. Occult dorsal ganglia may easily be overlooked since there is a diversity of problems which produce dorsal wrist pain. Cysts of more than 2 mm may be detected by ultrasonography. Percutaneous punctures and splint immobilization may help, but the recurrence rate is high in the gymnast. Surgical excision may be performed along with treatment of other associated problems.

Carpal instability

A variety of carpal instabilities may occur in gymnasts, including both dissociative and non-dissociative types. In the gymnast, these are usually associated with abnormalities within the involved region. Carpal instability has a poor prognosis for continuation of gymnastics whether treated or not.

Prevention of wrist injuries in gymnastics

Several measures which may help to prevent overuse injuries to the distal radius physis and problems associated with ulna-positive variance have been outlined (Mandelbaum, 1991). The gymnast should have biannual X-rays of the wrist to detect widening of the physis and ulna-positive variance. Overloading of the wrists should be avoided during the younger years with a gradual increase through the years. Wrist stretching exercises to increase flexibility and strengthening exercises, especially of the forearm flexors, to improve control of the wrist's tendency to hyperextend should be performed before and after each workout at all ages. The amount of wrist loading during workouts should be cyclically progressive so that periodic healing can occur. Support and swinging activities should be alternated during practice. The wrists should be positioned in neutral during a round-off. Foam beam covers and padded vaults should be used to absorb the shock of impact. An ulnar variance wrist brace, which is undergoing experiment, may help to distribute and transfer loads while limiting the amount of wrist extension (Mandelbaum, 1991). Splints, such as the Lion's Paw Splint*, may be used to prevent hyperextension of the wrists (Wright, 1991).

Conclusion

The hands and wrists of athletes are subjected to a multitude of stresses and mechanical forces which lead to injury. The literature is limited in regards to the prevention of these injuries. General guidelines include avoidance of hazardous movements or positions, use of protective devices or taping, proper use of the equipment and conditioning. Most important is the early recognition of injuries, especially those due to overuse, and of certain detrimental patterns of use within each sport so that modification can avert or reverse problems.

Prevention should be an integral component of training and education in all sports. Taking extra precautions or using prevention techniques during sports is not always considered by the athlete until an injury is sustained. Many athletic group members are aware of common injuries but lack proper medical and professional advice in the prevention of these injuries.

Research in the area of hand injury prevention should be encouraged in order to reduce the number of injuries within specific sports. It would also contribute to the development of proper athletic techniques, safer equipment and protective devices. Specialized knowledge of sports, biomechanics and mechanisms of injury are required in the development of prevention, including equipment and modifications to technique. Although certain risks will always remain in sports, appropriate research can minimize their impact.

* Lion's Paw Splint from RBJ Athletic Specialists, Spanish Fork, Utah, USA.

References

Af Ekenstam, F.W., Palmer, A.K. & Glisson, R.R. (1984) The load on the radius and ulna in different positions of the wrist and forearm. *Acta. Orthop. Scand.* **55**, 363–5.

Allieu, Y. (1988) The sportsman's hand. In R. Tubiana (ed) *The Hand*, pp. 925–39. WB Saunders, Philadelphia.

Aronen, J.G. (1985) Problems of the upper extremity in gymnasts. *Clin. Sports Med.* **4**, 61–71.

Baird, D.B. & Friedenberg, Z.B. (1968) Delayed ulnar–nerve palsy following a fracture of the hamate. *J. Bone Joint Surg.* **50A**, 570–2.

Bassett, F.H., Malone, T. & Gilchrist, R.A. (1979) A protective splint of silicone rubber. *Am. J. Sports Med.* **7**, 358–60.

Bollen, S.R. (1988) Soft tissue injuries in extreme rock climbers. *Br. J. Sports Med.* **22**, 145–8.

Bollen, S.R. & Gunson, C.K. (1990) Hand injuries in competition climbers. *Br. J. Sports Med.* **24**, 16–18.

Bowers, W.H. & Hurst, L.C. (1977) Gamekeeper's thumb: Evaluation by arthrography and stress roentgenography. *J. Bone Joint Surg.* **59A**, 519–24.

Browne, E.Z., Dunn, H.K. & Snyder, C.C. (1976) Ski pole thumb injury. *Plast. Reconstr. Surg.* **58**, 19–23.

Buck, P.G., Sophocles, A.M. & Beckenbaugh, R.D. (1982) Unique aspects of downhill ski injuries. Part 2: diagnosis and acute management of specific injuries. *Orthopaedics* **5**, 444–55.

Burke, E.R. (1981) Ulnar neuropathy in bicyclists. *Phys. Sportsmed.* **9**, 53–6.

Cabrera, J.M. & McCue, F.C. (1986) Nonosseous athletic injuries of the elbow, forearm and hand. *Clin. Sports Med.* **5**, 681–700.

Cahalan, T.D., Cooney, W.P., Tamai, K. & Chao, E.Y.S. (1991) Biomechanics of the golf swing in players with pathologic conditions of the forearm, wrist and hand. *Am. J. Sports Med.* **19**, 288–93.

Campbell, C.S. (1955) Gamekeeper's thumb. *J. Bone Joint Surg.* **37B**, 148–9.

Carr, D., Johnson, R.J. & Pope, M.H. (1981) Upper extremity injuries in skiing. *Am. J. Sports Med.* **9**, 378–83.

Crosby, E.B. & Linscheid, R.L. (1974) Rupture of the flexor profundus tendon of the ring finger secondary to ancient fracture of the hook of the hamate. *J. Bone Joint Surg.* **56A**, 1076–8.

Destot, M. (1896) Paralysie cubitale par l'usage de la bicyclette. *Gaz. Hôp.* **69**, 1176–7.

Dobyns, J.H. & Gabel, G.T. (1990) Gymnast's wrist. *Hand Clin.* **6**, 493–505.

Dobyns, J.H., O'Brien, E.T., Linscheid, R.L. & Farrow, G.M. (1972) Bowler's thumb: Diagnosis and treatment. *J. Bone Joint Surg.* **54A**, 751–5.

Dunham, W., Haines, G. & Spring, J.M. (1972) Bowler's thumb (ulnovolar neuroma of the thumb). *Clin. Orthop.* **83**, 99–101.

Easterbrook, W.M. & Cameron, J. (1985) Injuries in racquet sports. In R.C. Scneider, J.C. Kennedy, & M.L. Plant (eds) *Sports Injuries: Mechanisms, Prevention and Treatment*, pp. 553–71. Williams & Wilkins, Baltimore.

Eckman, P.B., Perlstein, G. & Altrocchi, P.H. (1975) Ulnar neuropathy in bicycle riders. *Arch. Neurol.* **32**, 130–1.

Eisenberg, J.H., Redler, M.R. & McCarthy, J.C. (1990) *Sports thumb protection system.* Presented at the 45th Annual Meeting, American Society for Surgery of the Hand, Toronto, Canada.

Gardiner, K.M. (1975) More on bicycle neuropathies (letter). *N. Engl. J. Med.* **292**, 1245.

Howard, F.M. (1961) Ulnar nerve palsy in wrist fractures. *J. Bone Joint Surg.* **43A**, 1197–201.

Howell, A.E. & Leach, R.E. (1970) Bowler's thumb. *J. Bone Joint Surg.* **52A**, 379–81.

Hoyt, C.S. (1976) Ulnar neuropathy in bicyle riders (letter). *Arch. Neurol.* **33**, 372.

Hunter, S.C. & Poole, R.M. (1987) The chronically inflamed tendon. *Clin. Sports Med.* **6**, 371–88.

Jackson, D.L. (1989) Electrodiagnostic studies of median and ulnar nerves in cyclists. *Phys. Sportsmed.* **17**, 137–48.

Lin, G.T., Amadio, P.C., An, K.N., Cooney, W.P. & Chao, E.Y.S. (1989) Biomechanical analysis of finger flexor pulley reconstruction. *J. Hand Surg.* **14B**, 278–82.

Linscheid, R.L. & Dobyns, J.H. (1985) Athletic injuries of the wrist. *Clin. Orthop.* **198**, 141–51.

McAuley, E., Hudash, G., Shields, K. *et al.* (1987) Injuries in women's gymnastics: The state of the art. *Am. J. Sports Med.* **15**, 124–31.

McCarroll, J.R. (1985) Golf. In R.C. Scneider, J.C. Kennedy & M.L. Plant (eds) *Sports Injuries: Mechanisms, Prevention and Treatment*, pp. 290–4. Williams & Wilkins, Baltimore.

McCarroll, J.R. (1990) Evaluation, treatment and prevention of upper extremity injuries in golfers. In J.A. Nicholas & E.B. Hershman (eds) *The Upper Extremity in Sports Medicine*, pp. 883–90. CV Mosby, St Louis.

McCue, F.C. (1982) The elbow, wrist and hand. In D.N. Kulund (ed) *The Injured Athlete*, pp. 295–329. Lippincott, Philadelphia.

McCue, F.C. & Garroway, R.Y. (1985) Sports injuries to the hand and wrist. In R.C. Scneider, J.C. Kennedy & M.L. Plant (eds) *Sports Injuries: Mechanisms, Prevention and Treatment*, pp. 743–63. Williams & Wilkins, Baltimore.

Mandelbaum, B.R. (1991) Gymnastics. In B. Reider (ed) *Sports Medicine: The School-age Athlete*, pp. 415–28. WB Saunders, Philadelphia.

Mandelbaum, B.R., Bartolozzi, A.R., Davis, C.A., Teurlings, L. & Bragonier, B. (1989) Wrist pain syndrome in the gymnast: Pathogenic, diagnostic and therapeutic considerations. *Am. J. Sports Med.* **17**, 305–17.

Marmor, L. (1966) Bowler's thumb. *J. Trauma* **6**, 282–4.

Melone, C.P. (1990) Fractures of the wrist. In J.A. Nicholas & E.B. Hershman (eds) *The Upper Extremity in Sports Medicine*, pp. 419–56. CV Mosby, St Louis.

Minkow, F.V. & Bassett, F.H. (1972) Bowler's thumb. *Clin. Orthop.* **83**, 115–17.

Mogan, J.V. & Davis, P.H. (1982) Upper extremity injuries in skiing. *Clin. Sports Med.* **1**, 295–308.

Mogan, J.V. & Lavalette, R. (1986) Arthrography for MCP joint injuries of the thumb. *Tech. Orthop.* **1**, 27–30.

Netter, F.H. (1987) *The CIBA Collection of Medical Illustrations*, Vol. 8, Part 1. CIBA-Geigy, New Jersey.

Palmer, A.K. & Louis, D.S. (1978) Assessing ulnar instability of the metacarpophalangeal joint of the thumb. *J. Hand Surg.* **3A**, 542–6.

Parker, R.D., Berkowitz, M.S., Brahms, M.A. & Bohl, W.R. (1986) Hook of the hamate fractures in athletes. *Am. J. Sports Med.* **14**, 517–73.

Petitpierre, M. (1939) *Die Wintersportsverletzungen* (Winter Sports Injuries). Enke-Verlag, Stuttgart.

Pianka, G. & Hershman, E.B. (1990) Neurovascular injuries. In J.A. Nicholas & E.B. Hershman (eds) *The Upper Extremity in Sports Medicine*, pp. 691–722. CV Mosby, St Louis.

Pitner, M.A. (1990) Pathophysiology of overuse injuries in the hand and wrist. *Hand Clin.* **6**, 355–64.

Posner, M.A. (1990) Hand injuries. In J.A. Nicholas & E.B. Hershman (eds) *The Upper Extremity in Sports Medicine*, pp. 495–594. CV Mosby, St Louis.

Press, J.M. & Wiesner, S.L. (1990) Prevention: conditioning and orthotics. *Hand Clin.* **6**, 383–92.

Primiano, G.A. (1985) Skier's thumb injuries associated with flared ski pole handles. *Am. J. Sports Med.* **13**, 425–7.

Primiano, G.A. (1986) Functional cast immobilization of thumb metacarpophalangeal joint injuries. *Am. J. Sports Med.* **14**, 335–9.

Rayan, G.M. & O'Donoghue, D.H. (1983) Ulnar digital compression neuropathy of the thumb caused by splinting. *Clin. Orthop.* **175**, 170–2.

Rettig, A.C. & Wright, H.H. (1989) Skier's thumb. *Phys. Sportsmed.* **17**, 65–75.

Rosenberg, T.D., Franklin, J.L. & Paulos, L.E. (1991) Skiing. In B. Reider (ed) *Sports Medicine: The School-Age Athlete*, pp. 673–88. WB Saunders, Philadelphia.

Shea, J.D. & McClain, E.J. (1969) Ulnar nerve compression syndromes at and below the wrist. *J. Bone Joint Surg.* **51A**, 1095–103.

Siegel, I.M. (1965) Bowling-thumb neuroma (letter). *JAMA* **192**, 263.

Smail, D.F. (1975) Handlebar palsy (letter). *N. Engl. J. Med.* **292**, 322.

Stark, H.H., Jobe, F.W., Boyes, J.H. & Ashworth, C.R. (1977) Fracture of the hook of the hamate in athletes. *J. Bone Joint Surg.* **59A**, 575–82.

Stener, B. (1962) Displacement of the ruptured ulnar collateral ligament of the metacarpo-phalangeal joint of the thumb. *J. Bone Joint Surg.* **44B**, 869–79.

Thiebault, J. (1980) Le risque sportif: Etude de 43093 dossiers concernant 57 disciplines (sport amateur). *Rev. Franc. Dom. Corp.* **6**, 319–52.

Torisu, T. (1972) Fracture of the hook of the hamate by a golfswing. *Clin. Orthop.* **83**, 91–4.

Tropet, Y., Menez, D., Balmat, P., Pem, R. & Vichard, P. (1990) Closed traumatic rupture of the ring finger flexor tendon pulley. *J. Hand Surg.* **15A**, 745–7.

United States Cycling Federation (1991) *Rulebook*. USCF, 1750 E. Boulder St, Colorado.

United States Golf Association (1991) *Rules of Golf*. USGA, Liberty Corner Road, New Jersey.

Van Dommelen, B.A. & Zvirbulis, R.A. (1989) Upper extremity injuries in snow skiers. *Am. J. Sports Med.* **17**, 751–3.

Watson, H.K. & Rogers, W.D. (1989) Nonunion of the hook of the hamate: An argument for bone grafting the nonunion. *J. Hand Surg.* **14A**, 486–90.

Weiker, G.G. (1990) Upper extremity gymnastic injuries. In J.A. Nicholas, & E.B. Hershman (eds) *The Upper Extremity in Sports Medicine*, pp. 861–82. CV Mosby, St Louis.

Weiss, B.D. (1985) Nontraumatic injuries in amateur long distance bicyclists. *Am. J. Sports Med.* **13**, 187–92.

Wright, H.H. (1991) Hand therapists set the pace in sports medicine. *J. Hand Ther.* **4**, 37–41.

Further reading

Amadio, P.C. (1990) Epidemiology of hand and wrist injuries in sports. *Hand Clin.* **6**, 379–81.

Aulicino, P.L. (1990) Neuromuscular injuries in the hands of athletes. *Hand Clin.* **6**, 455–66.

Bogumill, G. (1990) Anatomy of the forearm, wrist and hand. In J.A. Nicholas & E.B. Hershman (eds) *The Upper Extremity in Sports Medicine*, pp. 373–98. CV Mosby, St Louis.

Gieck, J.H. & Mayer, V. (1986) Protective splinting for the hand and wrist. *Clin. Sports Med.* **5**, 795–807.

Hankin, F.M. & Peel, S.M. (1990) Sport-related fractures and dislocations in the hand. *Hand Clin.* **6**, 429–53.

Hilfrank, B.C. (1991) Protecting the injured hand for

sports. *J. Hand Ther.* **4**, 51–6.

Isani, A. & Melone, C.P. (1986) Ligamentous injuries of the hand in athletes. *Clin. Sports Med.* **5**, 757–71.

Jennings, J.F. & Peimer, C.A. (1990) Ligamentous injuries of the wrist in athletes. In J.A. Nicholas & E.B. Hershman (eds) *The Upper Extremity in Sports Medicine*, pp. 457–82. CV Mosby, St Louis.

Koman, L.A., Mooney, J.F. & Poehling, G.G. (1990) Fractures and ligamentous injuries of the wrist. *Hand Clin.* **6**, 477–91.

Mayer, V.A. & McCue, F.C. (1990) Rehabilitation and protection of the hand and wrist. In J.A. Nicholas & E.B. Hershman (eds) *The Upper Extremity in Sports Medicine*, pp. 619–58. CV Mosby, St Louis.

Stener, B. (1981) Acute injuries to the metacarpophalangeal joint of the thumb. In R. Tubiana (ed) *The Hand*, pp. 895–903. WB Saunders, Philadelphia.

Wilgis, E.F.S. & Yates, A.Y. (1990) Wrist pain. In J.A. Nicholas & E.B. Hershman (eds) *The Upper Extremity in Sports Medicine*, pp. 483–94. CV Mosby, St Louis.

Chapter 6

Spinal Injuries

LYLE J. MICHELI AND MICHAEL LYNCH

There is good evidence that participation in sports and organized exercise is increasing throughout the world. Active sports participation in the USA alone in the mid-1970s was estimated at 150 million people (Nicholas, 1978; Torg, 1991). As the number of participants increases, sports-related injuries will almost certainly increase. The proportion of these athletic injuries to the spine, as opposed to the remainder of the musculoskeletal system, is relatively low.

Most sports-specific reviews show that less than 10% of all injuries include the spine (Spencer & Jackson, 1983). The impact of these injuries can vary from the nagging back strain of the football lineman, to the potential career-ending development of spondylolisthesis in the élite gymnast, to the potentially life-ending cervical spine dislocation in the rugby forward. While the neck strains and the backaches of athletes differ from their workplace and traffic accident counterparts with regard to motivational factors, their diagnoses and therapies can remain just as obscure and frustrating for athlete and physician alike.

As in any area of sports medicine or medicine in general, efforts aimed at prevention of injury remain the most effective and economically sound means of intervention when they are successful. Unfortunately, for a variety of reasons, the spine is a difficult area in which to implement preventive measures. Much research has gone into the prevention of low back pain in the workplace. Efforts addressing physical fitness of the worker, design of the workplace, and studies of lifting have had some success in reducing the incidence of back injury, but the results are by no means overwhelming (Bishop & Wells, 1990; Hall *et al.*, 1990; Walsh & Schwartz, 1990). The axial nature of the spine itself makes it difficult to implement protective measures, bracing or padding. In addition, its axial site and function often places it at risk for secondary injury in activities involving the limbs in athletics.

A review of the present literature on prevention of spinal injuries in sports shows predictable patterns. Just as in the non-athletic population, the thoracic region is rarely involved in spinal injury. The lumbar and cervical regions are the primary sites of athletic spinal trauma, owing to their increased mobility and accessibility. Because injuries to the cervical and lumbar region are quite different with respect to types of injury, degree of spinal cord involvement, and sport-specific incidence of injury, they will be discussed separately. There are five major types of preventive intervention:

1 Rules or policy changes.
2 Equipment.
3 Education.
4 Exercise.
5 Preparticipation evaluation.

These preventive medicine interventions will be discussed with reference to specific areas of the spine and as they have been implemented in specific sports.

Injury surveillance

There is an additional element which must be present if any intervention is to prevent injury effectively or decrease its severity in sports: an injury surveillance system. While endorsed by a great variety of sports organizations, the systematic monitoring and categorizing of sports injuries by injury site, severity and factors related to injury, such as player position, stage in the game or practice, etc., is difficult to implement. The reasons for this include the fact that properly designed and monitored systems are time-consuming and expensive. Additionally, there is often little appreciation of the importance of surveillance systems to coaching staff and team personnel. They are, therefore, often of low priority.

Determination of the efficacy of any preventive medicine intervention is totally dependent on having an accurate injury surveillance system in place before, during and after any of the above interventions have occurred.

Needless to say, injury surveillance systems are particularly important in sports where there is risk of death or catastrophic injury to the head or spine. This includes most body contact sports. A number of sports governing organizations, including the National Collegiate Athletic Association (NCAA) (1992), now recommend injury surveillance by their members. The quality of this monitoring, however, is not known.

Cervical spine injury

Rules/policy changes

Determination of the mechanics of injury which result in cervical spine injuries in sport is essential before protective rule changes are instituted. Aside from the unique occurrence of severe hyperflexion leading to bilateral facet dislocation, encountered in a rugby forward when a scrum collapses, most cervical spine injuries in sports are now believed to be the result of axial loading applied to the vertex of the head. As Scher (1981) reports, when the neck is slightly flexed, the spine is straight, and axial forces that exceed the energy-absorbing capability of the structures involved will lead to cervical spine flexion and dislocation. This theory is further supported by Bauze and Arden (1978), who experimentally reproduced this mechanism with cadaver models. These studies have also been supported by retrospective reviews of specific injuries that confirm that the primary mechanism of injury is a blow to the vertex of the head. Logically, rules and policy changes which prevent these types of dangerous contacts should result in further prevention of injury.

This hypothesis is supported by changes observed in American grid iron football. In 1976, rules specifically prohibiting intentionally striking an opponent with the crown of the helmet were instituted. Following the institution of these 'spearing' rules, significant decrease in the incidence of surgical spine injury and quadriplegia was observed. Data from 1975, the season prior to the initiation of the rule changes, showed an incidence of 16.8 catastrophic spinal injuries per 100 000 participants at the college level. Despite a slight increase in 1976, the levels continued to decrease, reaching a low by 1984 of $3.9 \cdot 100\,000^{-1}$ at the high-school level and $6.6 \cdot 100\,000^{-1}$ at the college level. Fortunately, the incidence of permanent quadriplegia as a result of these spine injuries showed a similar decline (Torg *et al.*, 1987). While this decline is encouraging, much more can and should be done to prevent injury in this sport. Coaching education to eliminate dangerous tactics during practice and training and strict enforcement of existing game rules by referees and officials could further reduce these injuries.

In Rugby football, a number of independent studies have noted an apparent increase in the incidence of cervical spine injuries in the game. Scher (1987), in his extensive review of the subject, defined several mechanisms of injury, all of which are amenable to rule and policy changes. These injuries were categorized into scrum injuries, injuries sustained while making a tackle, injuries sustained while being tackled, and injuries sustained in rucks and mauls.

Deliberate crashing of the scrum or a 'hard set-in' certainly can lead to axial loading injuries. A second mechanism of injury may be that of hyperflexion. The collapsing scrum is unique for the unprotected position of the hooker, who, with both arms locked to the props, is unable to control the position of his or her head and, should the scrum collapse and continue to move forward behind the hooker, a severe hyperflexion injury can ensue. Injuries sustained while tackling an opponent probably closely mirror the American football counterpart in that avoidance of the slightly flexed position while performing a tackle should prevent this.

Scher's recommendations include (i) staggering the scrum set-in so that there is no posterior driving force to the initial front row at the time of set-in; (ii) strict adherence to the avoidance of intentional collapsing of the scrum and severe penalty thereof; (iii) outlawing the high tackle; (iv) emphasis on teaching safe methods of tackling; and (v) closer adherence to limiting loose ruck play, during which time varied forces can be applied to the ball handler, tacklers and those setting in late. As recently recommended by the International Rugby Board, rugby is a game which must be played while 'on your feet'. In a ruck or maul where one or more players have left their feet and are sprauled around the ball, play must be stopped by the referee. One can only hope that the implications of these regulations will have the success encountered in American football.

It must be noted that rule changes which are instituted to decrease the incidence of cervical spine injury may result in increased risk of injury at other sites. For example, the progressive modifications and design changes of American football helmets from 1920 through 1960 did decrease the incidence of intracranial injury in this sport, particularly with the introduction of the hardshell plastic helmet. These changes in helmet design may have unintentionally resulted in the subsequent higher incidence of cervical spine injury, as the well-protected head was brought into dangerous play more frequently (Reid & Reid, 1981; Torg, 1991).

A more recent and quite similar phenomenon has occurred in ice hockey. Tator (1987), in his retrospective review of 55 sport-related and recreation-related spinal cord injuries between 1948 and 1973 in Canada, found none that were related to hockey. However, a review conducted in 1982, subsequently identified 42 cases of major spinal injury due to hockey (Tator, 1987). This apparent dramatic rise in incidence correlated with the increased use of rigid helmets and face masks while playing hockey. Factors such as diminished vision from the face mask, increased use of the head in play, and alteration of the centre of gravity of the head from the position of the helmet were all implicated in contributing to this increase. Following documentation of this increased incidence, stricter enforcement of rules against boarding and cross-checking was called for. In the 42 cases researched by Tator, 17 were the result of a push or a check, 13 of these coming from behind. In 25 of the 42, the head struck the board with an axial loading mechanism (Tator, 1987).

Another sport in which implementation of a specific rule has served to bring about reduction in the incidence of cervical spine injury and quadriplegia is that of gymnastics, and specifically trampoline-induced injuries in gymnastics training. Torg's review (1987) of the literature presented convincing evidence that the majority of catastrophic spine injuries were associated with the use of the trampoline and the mini-trampoline. Of the 114 injuries reviewed, many were sustained by experienced, expert and élite trampolinists. The American Academy of Pediatrics initially called for banning the use of trampolines at grammar school, high-school and college levels. This stand was subsequently modified to a position recommending a highly supervised and limited use.

This intervention is believed to bear prime responsibility for the dramatic decline in catastrophic gymnastic injuries noted in recent years. It is difficult to assess presently whether these stern recommendations will keep the incidence of catastrophic injury low, but certainly it must be recognized that the trampoline and the mini-trampoline, often used to assist training for vaulting events in gymnastics and in diving, may be dangerous, and their use should be limited to training with experienced coaches using approved safety devices and spotting techniques.

Another area in which a high incidence of cervical spine injury occurs is that of the water sports, especially diving. Torg (1991) points out that most sport-related injuries associated with diving are preventable by enforcement of regulations against diving in specific areas and posting of warnings. Indeed, a review by Shields *et al.* (1978) of spinal cord injuries admitted to Ranch el Los Amigos Hospital in 1974 revealed that the vast majority were related to recreational water-related activities. Continuing attention to regulations avoiding this can aid further in reducing incidence.

Equipment

As indicated in the introduction, the axial spine is a difficult area to brace and/or protect. The cervical spine is not amenable to any form of rigid immobilization, as this would render participation in almost all athletic events impossible. Some efforts have been made in American football to modify shoulder pads with neck rolls in an effort to limit the range of motion of the neck. These are probably more effective against the brachial plexus stretch injury or 'burner' than they are against severe cervical spine injury. But, certainly, attention to well-fitting helmets that do not go too low in the posterior aspect of the neck and well-fitting shoulder pads that will block the extremes of range of motion of the neck may help to decrease cervical spine injury (Schneider *et al.*, 1985; Watkins *et al.*, 1990).

The introduction of new types of protective equipment must be carefully monitored. As noted above, the introduction of helmets and face masks in hockey may have resulted inadvertently in an increased incidence of cervical spine injury. Similarly, the addition of the face mask to the football helmet provides a very effective handle for a would-be tackler or a lever arm for neck flexion for a player striking the ground face first. Strict enforcement of face mask rules in grid iron football has partially obviated this risk (Reid & Reid, 1981; Torg, 1991).

Much of the research in football helmet design had been directed to protecting the cranium and brain from injury. It has been recently noted that these testing mechanisms, while setting minimum standards for intercranial injury, do not provide information on the helmet's ability to protect the cervical spine (Bishop & Wells, 1990). In the past, recommendations have been made to replace the rigid plastic football and ice-hockey helmets with foam or semirigid helmets in an effort to decrease the potential for injury to opponent or wearer from striking with the head as a battering ram. It is difficult to predict whether any such modifications might also decrease the incidence of cervical spine injury. Much more research is needed into the relationship between helmet composition and design as related to the potential for cervical spine injury.

Education

The role of preparation and education of coaches and athletes for athletic competition cannot be overemphasized. Certainly, all participants, parents and coaches should be aware of the potential catastrophic injuries associated with various sports.

The development of effective reporting mechanisms on the incidence of head and neck injuries in football resulted in successful implementation of the rule changes outlined in the previous section (Reid & Reid, 1981; Torg, 1991). Tator's efforts to implement a similar reporting system in Canada to monitor the incidence of cervical spine injuries has resulted in public awareness of the problem and has stimulated leagues, coaches and hockey organizations to develop educational programmes for players and coaches. His observations that it is actually more dangerous to play ice hockey in Canada than it is to play football in the USA mobilized the ice hockey medical community in Canada (Torg, 1987). Once again, the importance of injury monitoring systems to every phase of injury prevention, including education, is evident.

An example of this, which parallels the rule changes in football are Scher's recommendations (1987) for rules changes and altered playing techniques in the sport of Rugby. He points out that players should be made aware of the dangers of charging into rucks and that coaches should emphasize the correct position of the head when the player is making a tackle. High tackles and diving tackles are exceedingly hazardous and late tackles should be avoided at all costs. Similarly, all players must be educated about the tragic consequences of scrum collapse.

Educational intervention may be the only effective means of preventing cervical spine injury in water sports. Shields *et al.* (1978) reported in a retrospective review of 1600 patients that the majority of catastrophic injuries to the cervical spine occurred during water sports. Torg (1991) emphasizes that the majority of these sport-related injuries can be prevented, specifically those involving diving accidents, and presents a series of eight guidelines. The following guidelines can be observed for safe diving:

1 Do not dive into water which is shallower than twice your height.
2 Do not dive into unfamiliar water. Know the depth and be sure the water is free of submerged objects.
3 Do not assume water is deep enough. Familiar rivers, lakes, bays and swimming holes change levels. Remember at low tide there is 1.8–2.4 m (6–8 ft) less depth than at high tide.
4 Do not dive near dredging or construction work. Water levels may change; dangerous objects may lie beneath the surface.
5 Do not dive until the area is clear of other swimmers.
6 Do not drink and dive. Alcohol distorts judgement.
7 Do not permit or indulge in horseplay while swimming and diving.
8 Do not dive into the ocean surf of front beaches.

Exercise

Resistive exercises to strengthen the muscles of the neck and upper torso are frequently recommended to prevent cervical spine injury. There is, unfortunately, no epidemiological data which supports this recommendation. Certain biomechanical observations, however, at other sites indirectly support this recommendation. Studies of impact absorption about the knee and lower extremity suggest that the musculature and soft tissues absorb a high proportion of the force applied to the extremity (Lukoschek *et al.*, 1986). Works of Reid and Reid emphasize the need for continued training and learned habitual responses to loads. The athlete either performing a tackle or being tackled, can initiate what should be a programmed response in an effort to 'bull' the neck and thereby protect the cervical spine. They recommend that the continued training of athletes to perform perfectly skilled movements results in the successful repression of undesired contractions and delays in spinal readjustment and decrease motor recruitment that might place their neck in danger (Reid & Reid, 1981).

Preparticipation evaluation

Determination of host factors which could contribute to an increased risk of cervical spine injury in sports has received increased interest in recent years.

Albright *et al.* (1985) noted unexpectedly high

incidence of previous neck injury and radiographical changes in the cervical spine found in candidates for the grid iron football team at the University of Iowa. Torg (1991), in a recent review, summarized both congenital and acquired anatomical or structural abnormalities of the cervical spine which appear to increase the risk for cervical spine injury in sport. He particularly emphasized the history of previous neck injury in the preparticipation evaluation as well as careful attention to any limitations of range of motion on the physical examination (Torg & Glasgow, 1991).

Lower back injury

Rules

Unlike the cervical spine, specific rules changes to prevent injury to the lumbar spine are less obvious. While the vast majority of injuries to the cervical spine are acute and single event occurrences, injuries to the lumbar spine in athletes are far more commonly the result of repetitive microtrauma, resulting in stress or fatigue injuries.

Unlike the cervical spine, these occur in both contact and non-contact sports. Sports such as gymnastics, ballet, figure skating, hockey, football, weightlifting, wrestling and rowing are the events that primarily make up the occurrences of low back pain (Jackson *et al.*, 1976; Garrick & Requa, 1980; Goldberg, 1980; Semon & Spengler, 1981; Micheli, 1983; Cannon & James, 1984; Hall, 1986; McCarroll *et al.*, 1986; Ireland & Micheli, 1987; Hresko & Micheli, 1990). Sward *et al.* (1990) notes that of 142 top athletes in Sweden, the incidence of low back pain ranged from 5 to 85%, depending on the sport. Ferguson *et al.* (1974) reported an incidence of 48% of back pain in 25 football linemen. On assessing the aetiology of this pain, there is little to suggest rule changes that might decrease this incidence. There have been suggestions, based on clinical reviews of injury, to establish a minimum age at which heavy contact sports and hyperextensile sports such as gymnastics and weightlifting should be initiated, but no sports governing body has yet instituted such rules (Ciullo & Jackson, 1985).

Equipment

Thermoplastic lumbar corsets of polypropylene or polyethylene have been used successfully for the treatment of existing spondylolysis or spondylolisthesis and similar disorders of the lumbar spine and to serve as protective equipment to prevent further injury (Micheli *et al.*, 1980; Steiner & Micheli, 1985) (Fig. 6.1). Much more research is needed to study the design and composition of lumbar spinal braces and techniques for preventing deconditioning while bracing is used.

Education

Participants and coaches in sports which have increased risk of lumbar spine injury should be educated in preventive techniques. Repetitive hyperextension, flexion, and torsional forces from the thoracolumbar spine are associated with stress or fatigue injuries (Wiltse, 1962; Wiltse *et al.*, 1975; Hutton *et al.*, 1977; Cyron & Hutton, 1978; Jackson, 1979; O'Neil & Micheli, 1989). As outlined above, sports such as ballet (Micheli, 1983; Ciullo & Jackson, 1985; Ireland & Micheli, 1987), football (Ferguson *et al.*, 1974; McCarroll *et al.*, 1986; Hresko & Micheli, 1990), hockey (Hresko & Micheli, 1990), weightlifting (Granhed & Morelli, 1988; Sward *et al.*, 1990), and, of course, rowing (Howell, 1984; Hensinger, 1985), are all associated with overuse and stress-induced posterior element failure. The independent variables that contribute individually or in combination include poor technique, poor conditioning and abnormal anatomy. Poor technique is reflected in insufficient warm-up and inadequate technical supervision. For example, with dance and gymnastics, this would be the too rapid advancement to more difficult events and tasks without the necessary increases in strength

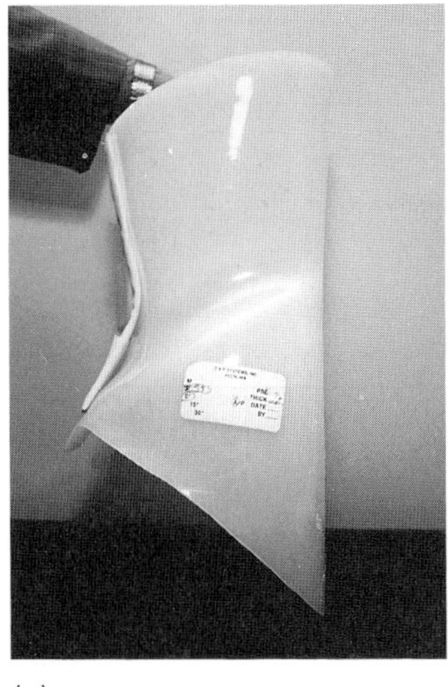

(a)

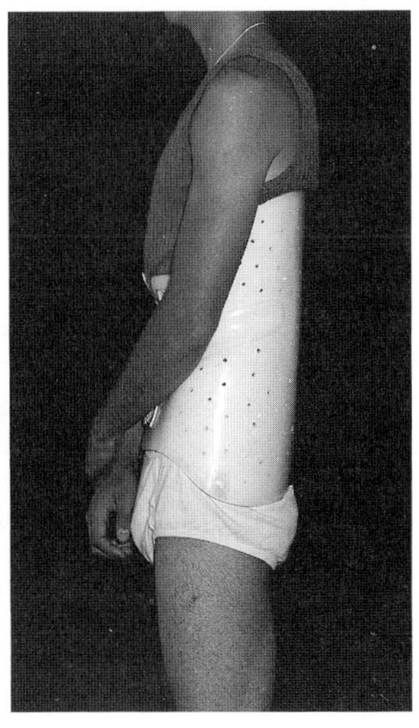

(b)

Fig. 6.1 A thermoplastic anti-lordotic lumbar brace (a) can be worn by the young athlete in competition to prevent further injury while treating the primary condition (b).

and flexibility (Micheli, 1983; Hresko & Micheli, 1990).

Goldberg (1980) reported low levels of abdominal strength in young gymnasts and recommended supplemental abdominal strengthening exercises. In addition, gymnasts should be educated in the dangers of hyperlordosis, such as the hyperlordotic posture effected at the end of a layout technique (Fig. 6.2).

The athlete engaged in sports with a high risk of back injury should be educated to seek qualified medical assessment early, in order to prevent progression to more severe tissue injury. A high proportion of back pain in young athletes engaged in sports with repetitive extension of the spine is due to overuse injury to the posterior elements of the spine, particularly the pars interarticularis. If detected early by newer imaging techniques such as computerized bone scan (SPECT), at the stage of early stress reaction, complete stress fracture of the bony elements can be avoided (Bellah *et al.*, 1991).

Further, relatively simple educational intervention measures to help avoid lumbar injury in athletes can vary from the proper placement of mats in gymnastics (Garrick & Requa, 1980; Goldberg, 1980), to reducing the exaggerated lordosis of a bicyclist who rides too upright by correctly positioning his or her seat (Sheets

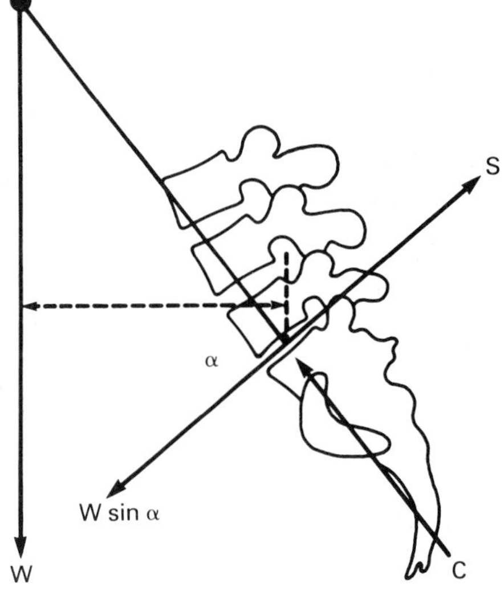

Fig. 6.2 Increased lordosis of the lumbar spine, with increased lumbosacral angle (α), increases the shear stress on the lumbar spine (W sin α) and increases the risk of back injury.

& Hochschuler, 1990), to strong emphasis on proper technique in weightlifters so that they can maximize the load-sharing capabilities of the spine which has been proven to undergo extremely high stresses during weightlifting activities (Greene *et al.*, 1985; Granhed *et al.*, 1987) (Fig. 6.3).

While these educational interventions may help prevent lumbar spine injuries in sports, a study of industrial injuries by Snook *et al.* (1978) suggested that education in proper lifting ergonomics was less important than simply avoiding excessive loads by workers.

Exercise

While little work has been done to evaluate the effectiveness of exercise in preventing cervical spine injuries, some work has been done in the role of exercise in preventing low back pain. Most of this work is not sports-related. Cady *et al.* (1985) studied 1652 firefighters and showed a clear correlation between the level of physical fitness and an exercise programme which prevented the incidence of low back injury. Jackson and Brown (1983) reviewed studies which proposed exercise as a treatment for low back pain and concluded that 'a paucity of information exists concerning these exercises and the management of patients with low back pain.'

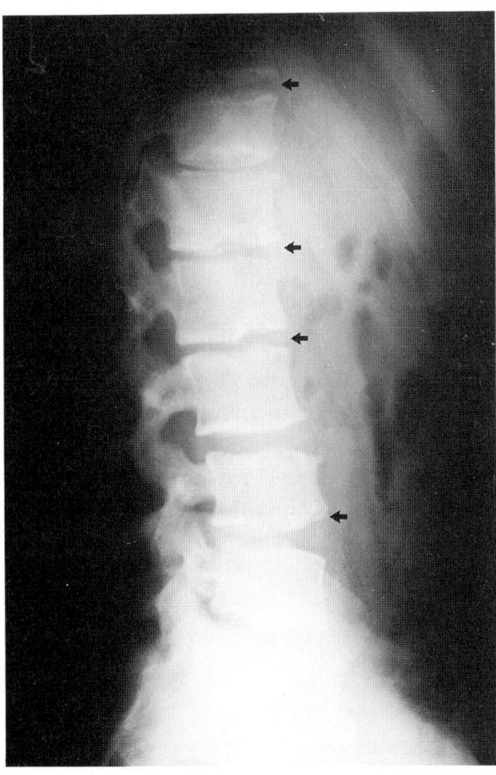

Fig. 6.3 Multiple sites of apophyseal wedging are seen in this lateral radiograph of the lumbar spine in a 22-year-old collegiate oarsman with low back pain.

Many exercise regimens utilized in clinical practice are unsubstantiated. Exercise to improve mobility has a sound scientific basis but lacks specific parameters when applied to the clinical setting. Nonetheless, there is a widely held belief that specific exercises in sports are important in preventing injury (Jackson *et al.*, 1976; Micheli, 1983).

Proper weightlifting technique and posturing in weightlifting and gymnastics can effectively reduce the forces across the lumbosacral spine (Gracovetsky, 1990). Lack of selective conditioning may contribute to abnormal compensatory lordotic posturing in these events (Granhed & Morelli, 1988; Arvidson & Micheli, 1990). Specific attention must be paid to strengthening the abdominal musculature with pelvic tilts and modified sit-ups, preinjury, rather than as rehabilitation efforts (Cannon & James, 1984; Hall *et al.*, 1990; Hresko & Micheli, 1990). It has been further stated that coaching techniques and the intensity of practice sessions with regards to gymnastics probably play a greater role in injury prevention than any other factor (Hresko & Micheli, 1990; R.A. Yancey & L.J. Micheli, unpublished data).

A general flexibility and strengthening programme can be hypothesized to 'probably' preclude many of the minor lumbar spine injuries from occurring. Adequate stretching prior to exercise will aid in increased flexibility in most athletes. Prone press-ups, hamstring stretching and lateral side-bending are all excellent warm-up exercises.

With the development of more effective ways

to strengthen the back, and in particular the extensors of the lumbar spine, studies to evaluate the role of this intervention in injury prevention as well as rehabilitation after injury must be done (Pollock *et al.*, 1989). A recent study comparing the effects of isometric and isokinetic exercises has confirmed a marked increase in lumbar spine strength in individuals previously felt to be adequately fit (Pollock *et al.* 1989). Perhaps with more focus on these events, we can more adequately assess the role of exercise.

Preparticipation evaluation

Rules requiring a complete preparticipation evaluation by a qualified, fully licensed physician should be enforced. The preparticipation should include screening for any pre-existing back disorders. Gait, leg length, symmetry, thoracic kyphosis, scoliosis and sacral lengthening should all be viewed. Attentiveness to hyperextension testing should be implicated to assess pre-existing spondylolysis or spondylolisthesis. The tightness of the lumbodorsal fascia and hamstrings are observed throughout range of motion by degree of mobility. Finally, the Fabere test is performed to assess sacroiliac function (Micheli, 1984; Rooks & Micheli, 1988; R.A. Yancey & L.J. Micheli, unpublished data).

Careful attention must also be given to the presence of either thoracolumbar kyphosis or scoliosis. With the diagnosis of scoliosis, the major definitive investigation should be to document the degree and to rule out any aetiological factor other than the idiopathic. One must establish whether or not there is a congenital component, and this is essential in a screening programme to determine whether or not an individual is capable of participating in contact sports. Congenital scoliosis which can be associated with diastematomyelia, spinal cord abnormalities and renal abnormalities is an important finding and needs to be worked up thoroughly prior to participation. Certainly, cervical abnormalities such as the Klippel–Feil syndrome, atlantoaxial instability and os odontoid are important findings that could preclude participation in contact sports (Torg & Glasgow, 1991; R.A. Yancey & L.J. Micheli, unpublished data).

It is of interest to question the incidence of thoracolumbar kyphosis in the trained athlete. It has been hypothesized that vigorous athletic training in the skeletally immature does not result in an increase in sagittal spine curvature, though others have argued this fact. Scheuermann noted in his initial description of Scheuermann's disease (in Wassman, 1951) that it occurred in a well-muscled teenage male who developed back pain after shoveling clay in the summer and demonstrated irregular vertebral endplates, narrowing of the intervertebral disc spaces, and wedging of the adjacent vertebrae. Wassman's survey of army recruits showed that dorsal lumbokyphosis was eight times more common than in 'lads from the country' (Wassman, 1951). The demonstration of the severe forces and activities such as weightlifting, which can reach 10 times the gravitational force due to body weight on the lumbar spine, may have an effect on the immature adolescent spine (Greene *et al.*, 1985; Granhed *et al.*, 1987).

Swimming sports with its spine compression caused by muscle force repetitive exercises may similarly predispose the back to abnormalities (Wilson & Lindseth, 1982). Studies are presently underway to evaluate the spines of active athletes in their adolescent days with the use of surface photography in an effort to determine whether these individuals are predisposed to spinal abnormalities (E.M. Wojtys, personal communication). These could serve as guidelines in the future for levels of training allowed at various ages with regards to weightlifting and, for example, gymnastics participation.

Conclusion

It is relatively clear that much work remains to be done in the area of prevention of spinal injury in regards to athletics. Although most major advances have been in the area of preventing cervical spine injury through the implementation of rule changes and equipment changes, much work needs to be done in evaluating the role of sport-specific exercise to eliminate the incidence of back pain in these high-risk activities. We should continue to encourage participation in spine injury reporting systems as these have served as excellent sources of information so that effective preventative measures can be undertaken. As the level of participation in all forms of athletics, specifically the recreational variety, continue to increase, injuries to the spine may also increase unless effective measures to decrease the risk of these injuries are implemented.

References

Albright, J.P., McAuley, E., Martin, R.K., Crowley, E.T. & Foster, D.T. (1985) Head and neck injuries in college football: an eight-year analysis. *Am. J. Sports. Med.* **3**(3), 147–52.

Arvidson, E.B. & Micheli, L.J. (1990) Spine and trunk problems in athletes. *Curr. Opinion Orthop.* **1**(3), 361–4.

Bauze, R.J. & Ardran, G.M. (1978) Experimental production of forward dislocation in the human cervical spine. *J. Bone Joint Surg.* **60B**(2), 239–45.

Bellah, R.D., Summerville, D.A., Treves, S.T. & Micheli, L.J. (1991) Low-back pain in adolescent athletes: detection of stress injury to the pars interarticularis with SPECT. *Radiology* **180**(2), 509–12.

Bishop, P.J. & Wells, R.P. (1990) The inappropriateness of helmet drop tests in assessing neck protection in head-first impacts. *Am. J. Sports. Med.* **18**(5), 201–5.

Cady, Jr, L.D., Thomas, P.C. & Karwasky, R.J. (1985) Program for increasing health and physical fitness of fire fighters. *J. Occup. Med.* **27**(2), 110–14.

Cannon, S.R. & James, S.E. (1984) Back pain in athletes. *Br. J. Sports Med.* **18**(3), 159–64.

Ciullo, J.V. & Jackson, D.W. (1985) Pars interarticularis stress reaction, spondylolysis, and spondylolisthesis in gymnasts. *Clin. Sports Med.* **4**(1), 95–110.

Cyron, B.M. & Hutton, W.C. (1978) The fatigue strength of the lumbar neural arch in spondylolysis. *J. Bone Joint Surg.* **60B**(2), 234–8.

Ferguson, R.J., McMaster, J.H. & Stanitski, C.L. (1984) Low back pain in college football linemen. *Am. J. Sports Med.* **2**(2), 63–9.

Garrick, J.G. & Requa, R.K. (1980) Epidemiology of women's gymnastics injuries. *Am. J. Sports Med.* **8**(4), 261–4.

Goldberg, M.J. (1980) Gymnastics injuries. *Orthop. Clin. N. Am.* **11**(4), 717–26.

Gracovetsky, S. (1990) The spine as a motor in sports: Application to running and lifting. In S. Hochschuler (ed) *The Spine in Sports*, pp. 11–30. Hanley & Belfus, Philadelphia.

Granhed, H., Jonson, R. & Hansson, T. (1987) The loads on the lumbar spine during extreme weight lifting. *Spine* **12**(2), 146–9.

Granhed, H. & Morelli, B. (1988) Low back pain among retired wrestlers and heavyweight lifters. *Am. J. Sports Med.* **16**(5), 530–3.

Greene, T.L., Hensinger, R.N. & Hunter, L.Y. (1985) Back pain and vertebral changes simulating Scheurmann's disease. *J. Pediatr. Orthop.* **5**(1), 1–7.

Hall, S.J. (1986) Mechanical contribution to lumbar stress injuries in female gymnasts. *Med. Sci. Sports Exerc.* **18**(6), 599–602.

Hall, S.J., Lee, J. & Wood, T.M. (1990) Evaluation of selected sit-up variations for the individual with low back pain. *J. Appl. Sports Sci. Res.* **4**(1), 42–6.

Hensinger, R.N. (1985) Back pain in children. In D.S. Bradford & R.N. Hensinger (eds) *The Pediatric Spine*, pp. 41–60. Thième, New York.

Howell, D.W. (1984) Musculoskeletal profile and incidence of musculoskeletal injuries in lightweight women rowers. *Am. J. Sports Med.* **12**(4), 278–82.

Hresko, M.T. & Micheli, L.J. (1990) Sports medicine and the lumbar spine. In Y. Floman (ed) *Disorders of the Lumbar Spine*, pp. 879–94. Aspen, Baltimore.

Hutton, W.C., Stott, J.R.R. & Cyron, B.M. (1977) Is spondylolysis a fatigue fracture? *Spine* **2**(3), 202–9.

Ireland, M.L. & Micheli, L.J. (1987) Bilateral stress fracture of the lumbar pedicles in a ballet dancer. *J Bone Joint Surg* **69A**(1), 140–2.

Jackson, D.W. (1979) Low back pain in young athletes: Evaluation of stress reaction and discogenic problems. *Am. J. Sports Med.* **7**(6), 364–6.

Jackson, C.P. & Brown, M.D. (1983) Is there a role or exercise in the treatment of patients with low back pain? *Clin. Orthop.* **179**, 39–45.

Jackson, D.W., Wiltse, L.L. & Cirincione, R.J. (1976) Spondylolysis in the female gymnast. *Clin. Orthop.* **117**, 68–73.

Lukoschek, M., Boyd, R.D., Schaffler, M.B., Bur, D.B. & Radin, E.L. (1986) Comparison of joint degeneration models. Surgical instability and repetitive impulse loading. *Acta Orthop Scand.* **57**(4), 349–53.

McCarroll, J.R., Miller, J.M. & Ritter, M.A. (1986) Lumbar spondylolysis and spondylolisthesis in college football players. A prospective study. *Am J. Sports Med.* **14**(5), 404–6.

Micheli, L.J. (1983) Back injuries in dancers. *Clin.*

Sports Med. **2**(3), 473–84.

Micheli, L.J. (1984) Preparticipation evaluation for sports competition: musculoskeletal assessment of the young athlete. In V.C. Kelley (ed) *Practice of Pediatrics*, Vol. 10, pp. 1–9. Harper & Row, Philadelphia.

Micheli, L.J., Hall, J.E. & Miller, M.E. (1980) Use of modified Boston brace for back injuries in athletes. *Am. J. Sports Med.* **8**(5), 351–6.

National Collegiate Athletic Association (1992) NCAA injury surveillance system summary. In *1992–93 NCAA Sports Medicine Handbook*. NCAA, Kansas.

Nicholas, J.A. (1978) What sports medicine is about. *Conn. Med.* **42(1)**, 4–8.

O'Neil, D.B. & Micheli, L.J. (1989) Postoperative radiographic evidence for fatigue fracture as the etiology of spondylolysis. *Spine* **14**, 1342–55.

Pollock, M.L., Leggett, S.H., Graves, J.E., Jones, A., Fulton, M. & Cirulli, J. (1989) Effect of resistance training on lumbar extension strength. *Am. J. Sports Med.* **17**, 624–9.

Reid, S.E. & Reid, Jr, S.E. (1981) Advances in sports medicine. Prevention of head and neck injuries in football. *Surg. Ann.* **13**, 251–70.

Rooks, D.S. & Micheli, L.J. (1988) Musculoskeletal assessment and training: the young athlete. *Clin. Sports Med.* **7**(3), 641–77.

Scher, A.T. (1987) Rugby injuries of the spine and spinal cord. *Clin. Sports Med.* **6**(1), 87–99.

Scher, A.T. (1981) Vertex impact and cervical dislocation in rugby players. *S. Afr. Med. J.* **59**(7), 227–8.

Schneider, R.C., Peterson, T.R. & Anderson, R.E. (1985) Football. In R.C. Schneider, J.C. Kennedy & M.C. Plant (eds) *Sports Injury Mechanics, Prevention, and Treatment*, pp. 1–61. Williams & Wilkins, Baltimore.

Semon, R.L. & Spengler, D. (1981) Significance of lumbar spondylolysis in college football players. *Spine* **6**(2), 172–4.

Sheets, C.G. & Hochschuler, S.H. (1990) Considerations of cycling for persons with low back pain. In S.H. Hochschuler (ed) *The Spine in Sports*, pp. 125–31. Hanley & Belfus, Philadelphia.

Shields, Jr, C.L., Fox, J.M. & Stauffer, E.S. (1978) Cervical cord injuries in sports. *Phys. Sportsmed.* **6**, 71.

Snook, S.H., Campanelli, R.A. & Hart, J.W. (1978) A study of three preventive approaches to low back injury. *J. Occup. Med.* **20**(7), 478–81.

Spencer, C.W. & Jackson, D.W. (1983) Back injuries in the athlete. *Clin. Sports Med.* **2**(1), 191–215.

Steiner, M.E. & Micheli, L.J. (1985) Treatment of symptomatic spondylolysis and spondylolisthesis with the modified Boston brace. *Spine* **10**(10), 937–43.

Sward, L., Hellstrom, M., Jacobsson, B. & Peterson, L. (1990) Back pain and radiologic changes in the thoraco-lumbar spine of athletes. *Spine* **15**(2), 124–9.

Tator, C.H. (1987) Neck injuries in ice hockey: A recent, unsolved problem with many contributing factors. *Clin. Sports Med.* **6**(1), 101–14.

Torg, J.S. (1987) Trampoline-induced quadriplegia. *Clin. Sports Med.* **6**(1), 73–85.

Torg, J.S. (1991) Injuries to the cervical spine and cord resulting from water sports. In J.S. Torg (ed) *Athletic Injuries to the Head, Neck and Face*, 2nd edn, pp. 157–73. Lea & Febiger, Philadelphia.

Torg, J.S. & Glasgow, S.G. (1991) Criteria for return to contact activities following cervical spine injury. *Clin. J. Sport Med.* **1**(1), 12–26.

Torg, J.S., Vegso, J.J. & Sennett, B. (1987) The National Football Head and Neck Injury Registry: 14-year report on cervical quadriplegia (1971–1984). *Clin. Sports Med.* **6**(1), 61–72.

Walsh, N.E. & Schwartz, R.K. (1990) The influence of prophylactic orthoses on abdominal strength and low back injury in the workplace. *Am. J. Phys. Med. Rehab.* **69**(5), 245–50.

Wassman, K. (1951) Kyphosis jeuvenalis Scheuermann — An occupational disorder. *Acta. Orthop. Scand.* **21**, 65–73.

Watkins, R.G., Dillin, W.H. & Maxwell, J. (1990) Cervical spine injuries in football players. In S.H. Hochschuler (ed) *The Spine in Sports*, pp. 157–74. Hanley & Belfus, Philadelphia.

Wilson, F.D. & Lindseth, R.E. (1982) The adolescent 'swimmer's back'. *Am. J. Sports Med.* **10**(4), 174–6.

Wiltse, L.L. (1962) The etiology of spondylolisthesis. *J. Bone Joint Surg.* **44A**(3), 539–60.

Wiltse, L.L., Widell, E.H. & Jackson, D.W. (1975) Fatigue fracture: The basic lesion in isthmic spondylolisthesis. *J. Bone Joint Surg.* **57A**(1), 17–22.

Chapter 7

Groin and Hip Injuries

PER A.F.H. RENSTRÖM

Groin injuries in athletes are being recognized as one of the most difficult problems in sport, and prevention is, therefore, of utmost importance. The symptoms associated with chronic groin injuries are often diffuse and uncharacteristic. These injuries usually constitute a major diagnostic and therapeutic challenge, the success of which depends on a correct diagnosis. It is necessary to establish a broad, differential background, and to have a good knowledge about the different risks for injuries in the groin area in order to work out an adequate preventive programme.

Groin injuries are not uncommon in sports such as fencing, ice hockey, skating, skiing, hurdles, high jump, horse-riding, team handball and soccer. A prospective study of soccer injuries in Göteborg, Sweden, revealed that 5% of all injuries were localized in the groin region (Renström & Peterson, 1980) (Fig. 7.1). A survey of 6347 karate participants reported a 2.5% incidence of groin strain in spite of the high risk of exposure to such injury in this sport. The participants were, however, young high-school students (Estwanik *et al.*, 1990).

The most common injuries in the groin area in sports are muscle–tendon problems involving adductor longus, rectus femoris, rectus abdominis and iliopsoas (Renström, 1992). Pain in the groin can also have many other causes which are discussed below. A correct diagnosis is the key to successful care if prevention fails.

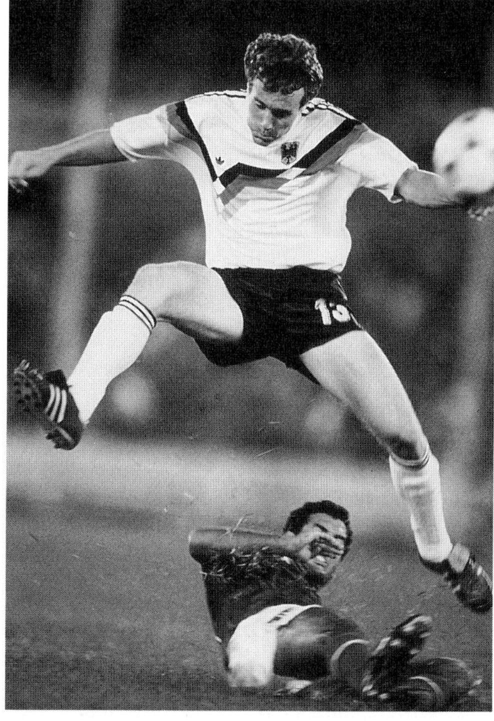

Fig. 7.1 The physical activities involved in playing soccer result in a high proportion of groin injuries. © Allsport/R. Cheyne.

Strain of the adductor longus

The adductors of the hip joint include adductor longus, adductor magnus, adductor brevis and pectineus muscles. The gracilis and the lower fibres of gluteus maximus can also act as adductors. It is, however, mainly the adductor longus, which is injured in connection with most sports (Fig. 7.2).

The mechanism behind injuries to the adductor longus can be traumatic such as a powerful abduction stress during simultaneous adduction of the leg when passing or shooting the ball in soccer, or overuse such as repetitive abduction of the free leg in skating or cross-country skiing. The injury mechanism should be carefully analysed as it is helpful in securing a correct diagnosis. Extrinsic factors such as training methods, training camp routines, running surfaces and shoes should be discussed. Awareness of injury mechanism and risk factors is important in the prevention and care of these injuries.

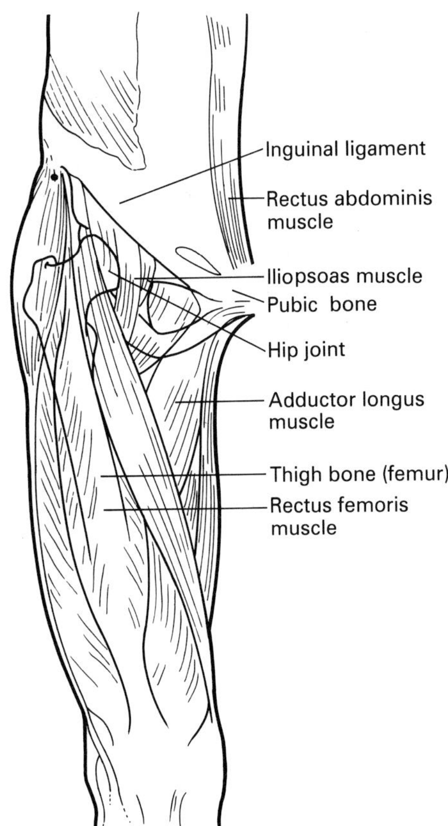

Fig. 7.2 Location of the muscles and tendons most often injured in the groin area. With permission from Peterson & Renström (1985).

The adductor longus injury is often a strain at the muscle–tendinous junction or at the origin of the tendon–muscle insertion on the pubic bone. Complete muscle tears or grade III strains are most commonly located in the distal muscle tendinous junction located towards the insertion on the femur (Peterson & Renström, 1985).

HISTORY AND SYMPTOMS

A grade I or II acute strain of the muscle will cause pain which feels like a sudden stab with a knife in the groin area. If the injured athlete tries to continue activity, this intense pain recurs. Locally, there is haemorrhage and swelling which may not be seen until a few days after the injury. The diagnosis can be made on the injury history, localized tenderness and the difficulties of contracting the muscle.

In chronic cases, the symptoms often begin insidiously. The pain can be more or less diffuse, or localized over the tendon area of the adductor longus. With time, as the injury gets more chronic, there is a tendency for the pain to radiate out distally along the medial aspect of the thigh and/or proximally towards the rectus abdominis. A history of a groin injury should include an analysis of the pain distribution into the groin, abdomen, scrotum, perineum, back and buttocks. There can be pain on coughing or sneezing. The tenderness will generally become more diffuse and uncharacteristic with time. Tenderness may also be present over the insertion of the rectus abdominis to the pubic bone. The distance between the origin of the adductor longus and the rectus abdominis, is very short and chronic inflammatory changes can sometimes involve both tendon insertion areas at the same time.

The radiating pain may be associated with stiffness which often decreases during and after some warming-up and will, after some time, disappear completely. The pain, however, usually reappears with greater intensity after continued activity. There is a risk that the athlete will be caught in a vicious so-called pain cycle. If the athlete does not break this pain cycle by rest, there is a great risk for chronic pain and a very difficult, clinical problem will arise.

In chronic or subchronic cases, the symptoms are often vague and diffusely located. The most common symptom is pain during exercise, but the symptoms can vary and be multiple. The symptoms and their frequency in a follow-up study of athletes with groin pain (Renström & Peterson, 1980) are seen in Table 7.1.

DIAGNOSIS

The diagnostic examination should be complete. The injured athlete should first be examined by inspection in a standing position to evaluate the alignment of the extremities. Palpation for hernias should also be carried out. The patient can, thereafter, be examined in the supine position when hip joint motion and flexibility tests of the groin and hip muscles can be carried out. Resistive contraction tests of the knee extensors, knee flexors, abdominal muscles, hip rotators, extensors and flexors should be carried out as well as of hip adductors and abductors. If there is an adductor longus injury, pain will be elicited at the area of the adductor longus tendon–muscle injured area by resisting leg adductors. There may be pain on passive stretching at full passive abduction of the hip. Tenderness on palpation is localized to the injury site at the origin of the adductor longus tendon or at the muscle–tendinous junction. The rest of the groin area should be routinely palpated including lymph nodes, inguinal canals, scrotum, etc. Neurological examination of the lower leg should be carried out. In the prone position, the back can be examined with palpation of the spinous processes and muscles, as well as sacroiliac joints. It is important to carry out a rectal examination in athletes with a long history of groin pain. In the side position it is possible to evaluate the trochanteric area.

Complementary investigations are often necessary. Routine X-rays of the pelvis and the hip joint should always be taken. Sometimes bone scan, magnetic resonance imaging (MRI) and computerized tomography (CT) scan are indicated. If there is a history of a hernia, herniography (Ekberg *et al.*, 1981) can be of value. Arthroscopy of the hip is technically difficult and is rarely indicated, but has been used in the diagnosis of disorders of the hip and in the treatment of loose bodies. Laboratory tests can be indicated especially if there is a suspicion of a tumour or an infection. Sometimes, diagnostic local injections are carried out on the suspicion of nerve entrapment or neuromas.

Table 7.1 Symptoms caused by groin muscle–tendon injuries in 53 athletes. With permission from Renström & Peterson (1980).

	Adductor longus injuries (n = 34)	Rectus abdominis injuries (n = 12)	Other groin tendon–muscle injuries (n = 7)
Pain at rest	21	4	3
Pain during exercise	30	9	8
Stiffness initially	19	5	3
Stiffness after exercise	23	3	5
Stiffness in the morning	21	5	5
Tenderness	21	4	6
Weakness in the extremities	4	0	3

CARE AND PREVENTION

Treatment can start once the diagnosis is established. The programme must be well planned. The treatment includes three phases (Grimby & Thomeé, 1988; Thomeé, 1994):

1 Acute treatment of pain and swelling to decrease muscle inhibition.

2 Exercise of strength, flexibility and endurance.

3 Return to sports.

The first phase

This includes immediate rest until a diagnosis is secured. Crutches are recommended in the initial phase. Ice can be applied to the injured area, and if possible compression. The injured part should not participate in activities which may cause pain.

Anti-inflammatory medication may be used for short periods. This treatment will relieve the symptoms especially pain and morning stiffness, but can also mask the seriousness of an injury.

The negative effects of inhibition should be minimized and, therefore, the pain must be controlled by medication together with careful and gradual mobilization. Muscle exercises should start as early as possible, but they must be well monitored. The training should start with careful, isometric contractions without resistance with a few seconds contraction time followed by isometric contractions against resistance (Fig. 7.3), the limit being pain. Range-of-motion exercises and gentle stretching can start gradually but carefully in acute and subacute cases. In chronic injuries without major strains or disruptions, early stretching is valuable (Fig. 7.4). Dynamic training initially without resistance and then with increasing resistance may be started when they can be carried out without pain. It is important not to overtrain.

The second phase

This starts when the athlete has regained full range of motion and can activate the muscle groups. The main goal is to regain full muscle volume. Different training equipment can now be used (Fig. 7.5).

Predisposing factors should be corrected (Zimmerman, 1988). Specific muscle weakness of the groin, especially of the adductor group, abdominal and low back muscles should be corrected, as well as poor flexibility of the groin and low back region.

After the initial phase, heat is usually valuable especially when the muscle training starts.

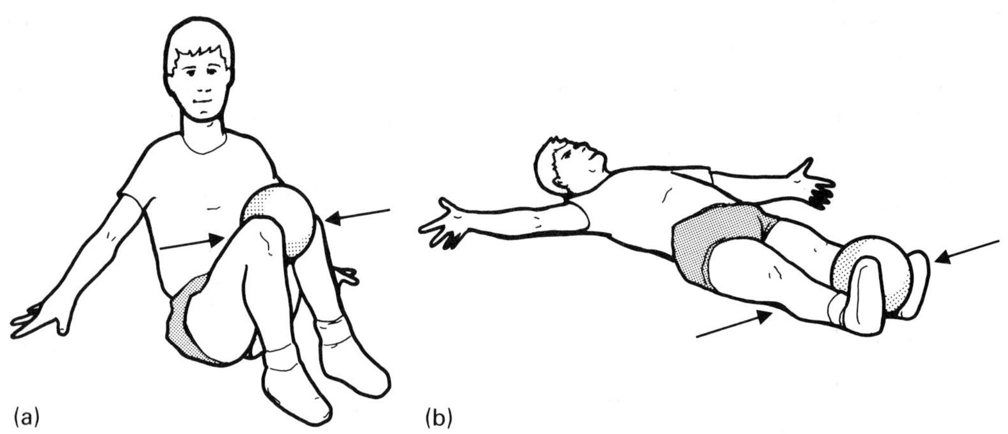

Fig. 7.3 Isometric exercises: (a) with knees bent; and (b) with knees straight.

Local heat can be given with hot packs, etc. Special heat retainers of neoprene can be used like trousers during the training programme (Fig. 7.6). Heat will increase the extensibility of the collagen in tendons and muscles and thereby be beneficial for continued rehabilitation.

If the aforementioned treatment has not been successful or prevented proper rehabilitation for 2–4 months, an injection of local anaesthetic with or without corticosteroids in the tendon periosteal area may be tried. This infiltration should be given into the most painful and tender areas of the origin of the tendon, but not into the tendon itself. This treatment should be combined with 1–2 weeks of active rest and may give lasting effects. Cortisone injection in this area should, however, only be given on strict indications by experienced personnel.

The third phase

This can start when normal concentric and slow eccentric strength have been achieved (Thomeé, 1994). Exercise for coordination, speed, etc., are now important as well as functional exercises (Fig. 7.7).

General conditioning can often be maintained with cycling and backstroke swimming depending on the injury. Running can be allowed if the athlete can do this without pain. Cutting in soccer training should not be started until dynamic training with maximal resistance and running can be carried out without pain. The return to sports should be gradual. The programme should be discussed with both coaches and athletes.

A variety of conservative treatment methods are often tried in chronic groin problems indicating the difficulty of the problem.

SURGERY

Surgical treatment of groin injuries is seldom indicated. When there is a complete tear of a muscle–tendon unit, which has a significant function or has no or few agonists of importance to compensate for the loss of function, surgery should be considered. It can also be indicated when there is a major strain or injuries with intramuscular haematomas affecting the function and interfering with the healing process. Surgical treatment of chronic groin problems has been increasingly common when conservative methods have been unsuccessful. The duration of the problems before surgery has often been more than 6–12 months.

During surgery of chronic adductor problems, the patient is in the supine position with the knees in 90° of flexion and the hip in 45° of hip flexion. The adductor longus tendon is then easily exposed to palpation and inspection. Sometimes there is a very short tendon, or no tendon at all, and the muscle inserts into the bone. The tendon may then be opened longitudinally, and in some patients pathological granulation tissue may be found. The pathological lesion should be excised in the fibre direction to healthy tissue until normal fibres appear in the area. When this is the case, careful side-to-side adaptations of the tendon should be carried out with resorbable sutures. In cases with no findings in the tendon, a tenotomy at the origin of the adductor longus can be carried out. Sometimes the adductor longus can insert into the pubic bone directly with the muscle which is then released. Good results have been reported with surgery (Hermans & Verwiel, 1983; Martens *et al.*, 1987).

Postoperatively, weight-bearing is allowed within the limitation of pain. Range of motion exercises and isometric muscle training starts early. After 3 or 4 weeks, bicycling with low resistance can be started. Running can be allowed after 8 weeks and athletes can often go back to full activity in 10–12 weeks. There may sometimes be some remaining tenderness over the operated area, which may require a long time to resolve. The success of the surgical treatment of muscle–tendon injuries in the groin depends on a correct diagnosis, an atraumatic surgical technique and an optimal postoperative rehabilitation.

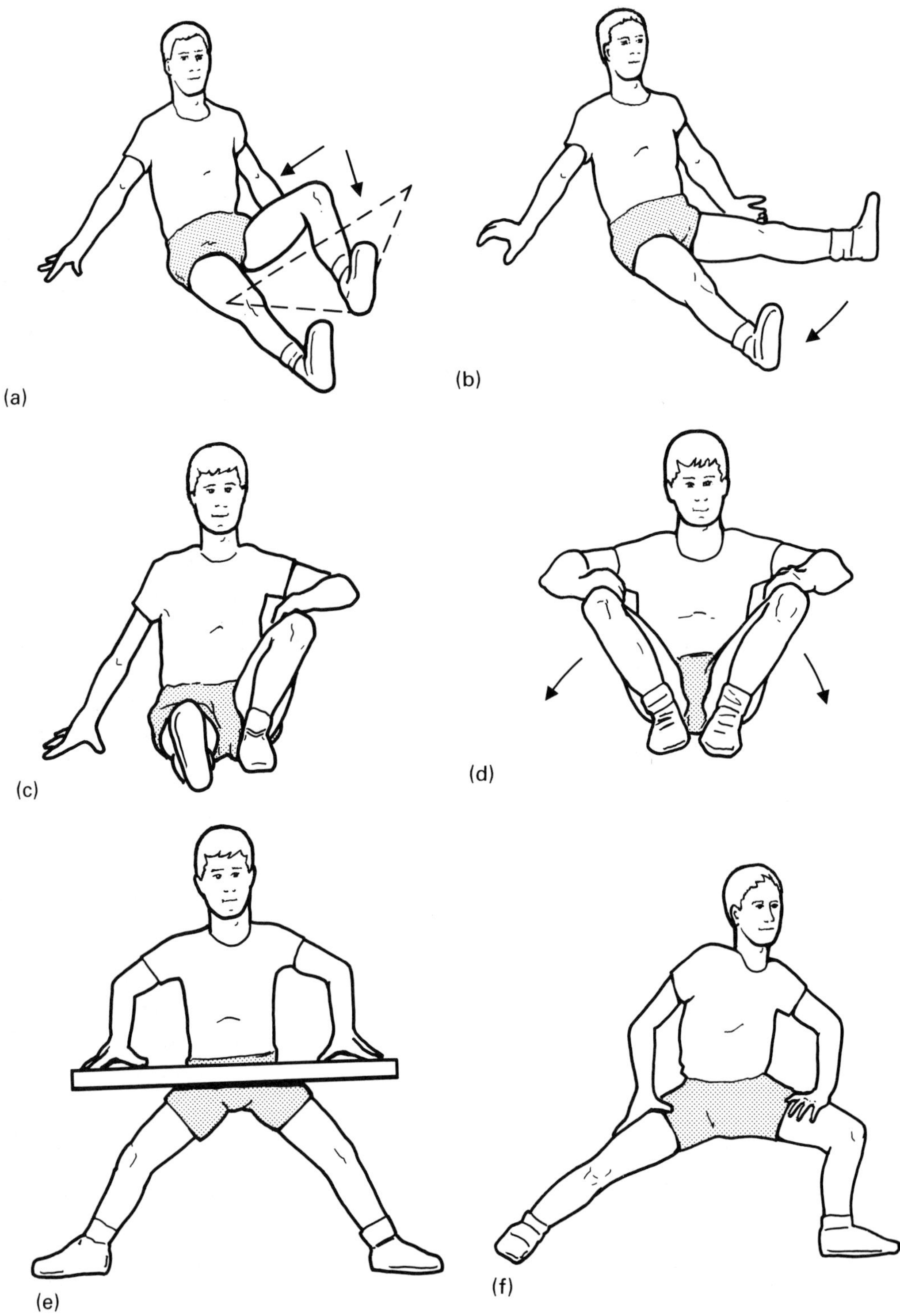
(a)
(b)
(c)
(d)
(e)
(f)

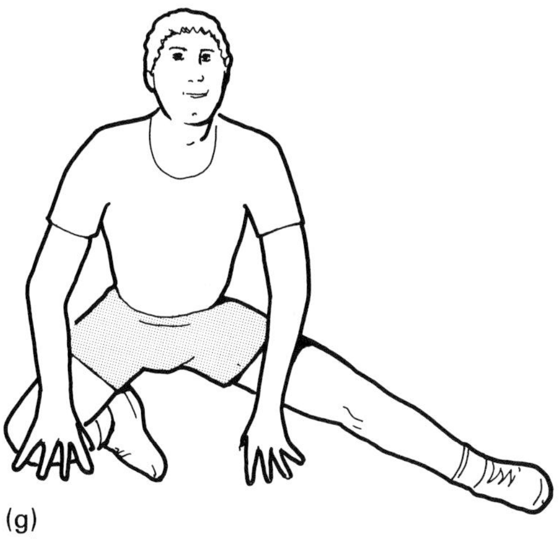

Fig. 7.4 (*Opposite and above*) Range-of-motion and stretching exercises: (a) with knees bent; (b) with knees straight; (c) with one leg; (d) with two legs; (e and f) standing; and (g) kneeling.

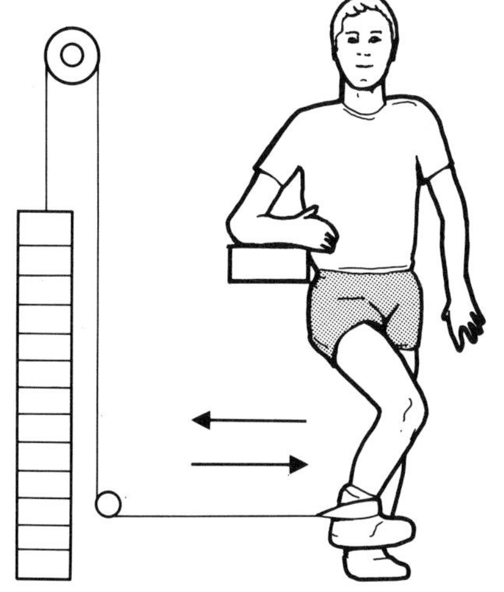

Fig. 7.5 Dynamic exercises, standing or seated doing straight leg pulls.

HEALING TIME

In a follow-up study, the time for return to sports was found to be very long for athletes with subchronic or chronic groin injuries (Renström & Peterson, 1980). 42% of the athletes with groin muscle–tendon injuries could not return to physical activity until more than 20 weeks after the time of injury (Table 7.2).

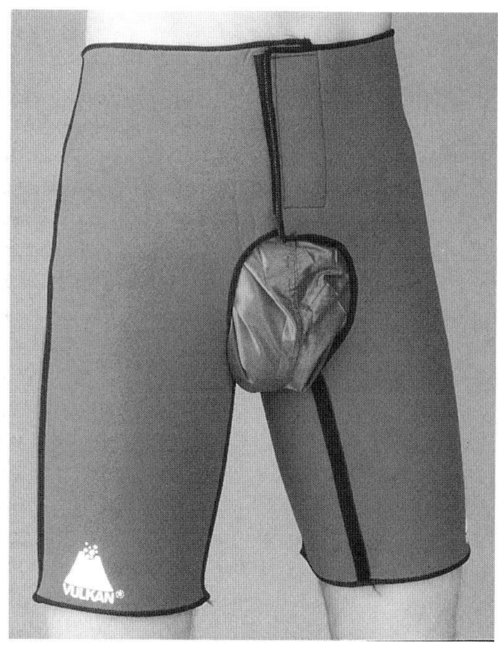

Fig. 7.6 Heat retainers keep the groin area warm, which is valuable as prevention.

CARE AND PREVENTION

Preventive training including strength training and stretching of the adductors, is essential and should be included in every training occasion and warming-up as an integrated part. The value of preventive training of the groin tendons and muscles is well documented in soccer (Ekstrand, 1982). Careful preventive training will decrease the number of injuries.

It is important to stress that these injuries should be treated with great respect. Groin tendon injuries, which are poorly treated, will become chronic. They are then extremely difficult to treat, and may result in the inability of the athlete to continue with his or her main sports.

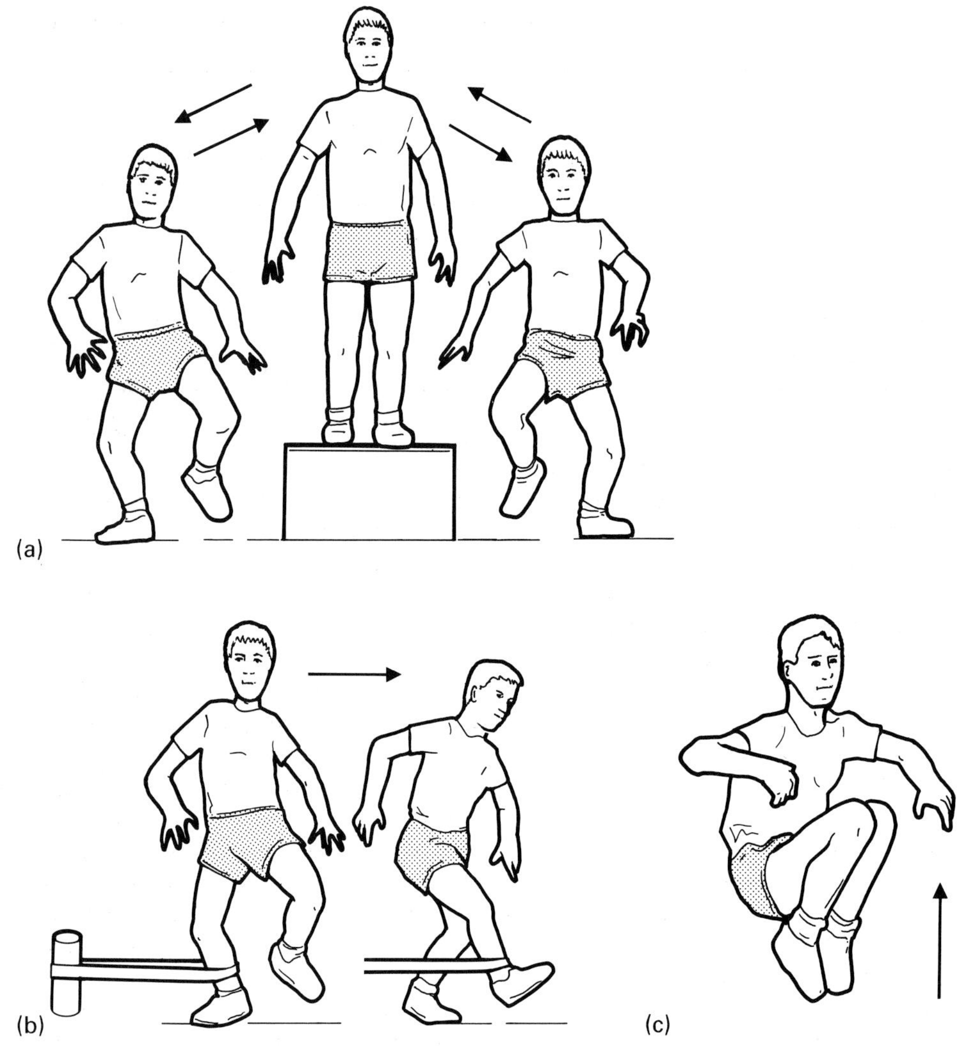

Fig. 7.7 Functional exercises: (a) side jumps; (b) side jumps with or without resistance; and (c) jumping exercises.

Complete rupture of the adductor longus

A grade III strain or complete rupture may be sustained by a powerful abduction trauma during simultaneous adduction of the leg, e.g. two players kicking the ball at the same time (Symeonides, 1972). An incomplete, partial rupture of the adductor longus is usually located in the muscle–tendinous junction, or at the pubic origin (Fig. 7.8). If the ability to contract the muscle is lost, a complete disruption of the fibres may be suspected. Complete disruption may occur without causing much discomfort or pain and occurs most commonly at the muscle–tendinous junction towards the insertion of the femur.

Peterson and Stener (1976) reported seven cases of old complete disruptions of the adductor longus at the insertion of the femur. They

Table 7.2 Return to physical activity for 53 athletes with groin muscle–tendon injuries. With permission from Renström & Peterson (1980).

	Adductor longus injuries (n = 34)	Rectus abdominis injuries (n = 12)	Other groin tendon–muscle injuries (n = 7)
Less than 1 week	0	0	0
1–4 weeks	8	3	1
5–8 weeks	6	3	1
9–12 weeks	4	1	1
13–20 weeks	2	0	0
More than 20 weeks	14	5	4

were referred on the suspicion of tumour. Five of these seven patients had noted a growing mass and this increase in size is probably due to a compensatory hypertrophy of the avulsed muscle–tendon as it has to work with the disadvantage of a shortened distance between its origin and new insertion created by scar tissue. Clinical examination must always include analysis of the trauma, inspection, palpation of function and testing, with and without resistance.

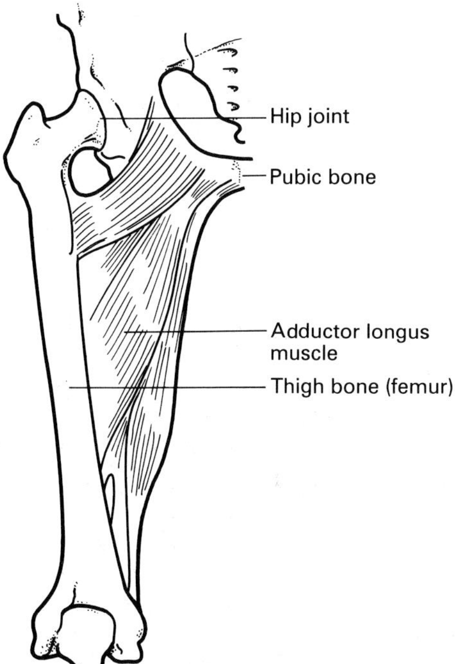

Fig. 7.8 Partial rupture of the adductor longus. With permission from Peterson & Renström (1985).

CARE

When acute, the athlete should treat the injury with rest, cold, compression and elevation. Thereafter, the treatment principles as discussed above concerning strain of the adductor longus should be used. The athlete should, however, be careful with stretching of the muscles and instead use isometric exercises to the level of pain. Surgical treatment should be considered in fresh complete disruptions. Old complete disruptions can usually be treated conservatively with muscle exercises and stretching after being differentiated from soft-tissue tumours.

Strain of the rectus femoris

Rectus femoris muscle and its tendon originates just above the acetabulum and inserts as the patella tendon at the tibial tuberosity. The rectus femoris muscle flexes the hip and is an extensor of the knee.

The rectus femoris is the muscle about the hip joint most commonly susceptible to disruptions (Lotke, 1973). These disruptions are usually located more distally on the thigh. Chronic strain injuries are often located at the

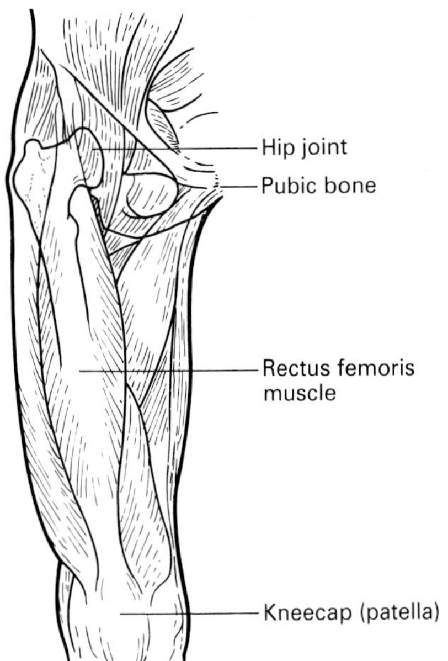

Fig. 7.9 Strain of the rectus femoris. With permission from Peterson & Renström (1985).

origin just above the hip joint (Fig. 7.9), and may occur during intensive training with shooting in soccer or repeated sprint training. During skating, the rectus femoris is heavily activated and may be overused.

Pain may be experienced from the area anterior of the acetabulum and may radiate to the anterior hip and groin area. The athlete may experience pain by resisted flexion of the hip joint or resisted extension of the knee joint. Tenderness on palpation may be experienced over the origin of the tendon approximately 8 cm distal of the anteriosuperior spine. Proximal rectus femoris injuries may cause haemorrhage, which later may result in calcification on X-ray examination.

CARE AND PREVENTION

When there is an acute or a chronic strain, conservative treatment as outlined for injuries of the adductor longus should be used. A careful stretching programme of the muscle should be included in every training session in the warm-up for competition in sports such as soccer, ice hockey, skating and fencing.

Strain of the rectus abdominis

Rectus abdominis muscle–tendon inserts on the pubic bone. The short distance to the origin of the adductor longus should be noticed. Weightlifters, pole vaulters and serving tennis players are subjected to these injuries which most commonly are located at the muscle–tendinous junction or in the tendon or at the insertion on the pubic bone where localized tenderness may be expected.

The strain in the muscle may be caused by overloading and a very sharp pain is located at the insertion or the junction at the moment the injury occurs. Recurrent pain at the insertion area or in the tendon when loading and contracting the abdominal muscles by elevating the legs and head from a supine position will indicate the diagnosis.

A strain in this muscle–tendinous unit can be difficult to differentiate from an intra-abdominal process, e.g. appendicitis. Typical for a strain is the localized tenderness and that the pain is more intensive as the injured athlete contracts the muscles compared to when the abdomen is relaxed. The localization of the pain is also different.

CARE AND PREVENTION

The treatment is usually conservative and is principally the same as for adductor longus strain. This injury may readily become chronic and has stopped top-level athletes from continued physical activity. In long-lasting therapy-resistant cases, surgery may, therefore, be necessary.

Athletes such as tennis players should include stretching and muscle exercises of the abdominal muscles in their training. If they have a tendency towards problems during the serve, perhaps the serving technique should be looked over, and the twisting motion should be decreased.

Strain of the iliopsoas

Iliopsoas muscle–tendon inserts at the lesser trochanter and is a strong flexor of the hip joint. Injuries to the iliopsoas muscle–tendon unit may be sustained by repeated flexing of the muscles of the hip or by forceful flexion of the hip joint against resistance. Strain in the iliopsoas tendon may occur after weightlifting, snow running, uphill running, intensive shooting training in soccer and after sit-ups, etc. The same pain cycle as experienced in adductor longus strain may also be present here.

Iliopsoas strain is usually located at the insertion of the lesser trochanter. There may be local tenderness in the anteriomedial thigh area overlying the attachment to the lesser trochanter. This area is difficult to palpate. It may be possible to locate it when palpating bimanually over the medial aspect of the femur. Pain is elicited by flexing the hip joint against resistance with the hip flexed at 90°, or on passive stretching with hyperextension of the hip, or internally rotating the femur.

CARE AND PREVENTION

The treatment is, in principle, the same as for adductor longus strain. These injuries often heal with conservative treatment. Runners who run very much uphill or on sand beaches, or rowers, need to include stretching of this muscle in their programme. Neoprene heat retainers can be used in cold weather as part of a prevention programme.

Injuries to other groin muscles and tendons

Other groin muscles like sartorius, gracilis, tensor fasciae latae and gluteus medius may also be injured. It is important to decide where the pain is located and together with a muscle function test this will give the diagnosis. In principle, the prevention and care is the same as in strain of the adductor longus.

Other causes for groin pain

It is the physician's responsibility to establish a specific diagnosis. The history and a thorough analysis of the type and quality of groin pain can be of great value. The patient can experience a sudden, severe pain, which can indicate an acute injury. The patient can have a continuous dull aching pain, or a chronic low-grade pain often worse at night indicating different types of chronic injuries. The patient can also have referred pain suggesting nerve involvement. The pain can be of throbbing character indicating intra-abdominal problems. Genitourinary, spasmodic pain can also be present. Vascular pain should direct the examination towards evaluation of the circulation.

Groin pain may have many causes such as different types of fractures including stress fractures, hip joint changes, bursitis, nerve entrapment, hernias, intra-abdominal processes, prostatitis, urinary infections, gynaecological disorders, inflammation of the pelvic joints, sciatic nerve pain, tumours, etc. (Renström, 1980).

Fractures

Fractures of the femoral neck and in the trochanteric region are common in elderly people, but may also be seen in younger athletes and adolescents. Acetabular or pelvic fractures are rare in athletes. They are usually caused by a direct contusion trauma in, for example, skating or skiing when falling on the ice or hard-packed snow. Femoral neck fractures usually require surgery, but the frequency of complications is high in the young person.

Fatigue or stress fractures may occur in the femoral neck and shaft, or on the inferior pubic bone. They may be seen after a sudden change in training routines, or a repetitive loading in long- and middle-distance runners and joggers and are now becoming an increasing problem. These injuries should be prevented. When pain is elicited by exercise or motion of the hip joint and if pain is experienced after exercise, the examiner should not be satisfied with a negative X-ray, but use other diagnostic procedures such as a bone scan. A bone scan may be positive after 2–8 days and will secure the diagnosis. An X-ray may be repeated after 3 weeks interval and callus formation may then be found. Stress fractures of the femoral neck sometimes require surgery. The treatment is otherwise conservative. Stress fractures can be prevented by using a well-monitored training programme, adequate equipment, turf and shoes.

Avulsion fractures may occur in adolescents from any of the muscular or tendon insertions in the groin area. The most common locations are the anterosuperior and inferior spines of the ilium, ischium, lesser trochanter and occasionally the greater trochanter. Clinical examination will reveal localized pain and tenderness and the history usually includes muscular trauma. The function of the involved muscle–tendon attachment will be painful and active motion against resistance will cause pain to the area involved in both types of injuries. An X-ray examination will establish the diagnosis. Depending on the age, the occupation and degree of dislocation of the fracture, the treatment will vary. If the distance between the avulsed fragment and its origin is large, surgery is recommended in order to restore normal anatomy. Young athletes should include stretching in their exercise programme when their muscles start to grow in volume. This will give a better balance, and may be preventive.

Hip joint changes

According to Cailliet (1978) there are four specific structures about the hip joint that may elicit pain: (i) the fibrous capsule and its ligaments; (ii) the surrounding muscles; (iii) the bony periosteum; and (iv) the synovial lining of the joint. Pain in the hip region must be differentiated as to which tissues are involved. The most painful condition of the hip joint is degenerative joint disease — osteoarthrosis. Degenerative joint disease is considered primary when it is the result of aging alone, but is secondary when trauma or disease are involved.

Pain in the hip joint may be an early symptom of localized changes in the joint such as arthrosis–arthritis, or osteochondritis dissecans or loose bodies. In rare cases, the outer rim of the joint–labrum or limbus can be avulsed and the torn end can rotate into the joint. These injuries may produce a sharp and catching pain during exercise and often persistent pain after exercise. Pain elicited by rotation in the hip joint indicates an intra-articular lesion and requires an X-ray. Sometimes CT scan or MRI is necessary to establish a diagnosis. Arthroscopy can be of value especially when loose bodies are present. Hip pain should lead to restrictions in athletic activity to prevent further deterioration.

The most common cause of painful hip in children is transient synovitis or capsulites. This is assumed to be a benign self-limiting condition seen in children less than 10 years of age. This condition should be differentiated from serious lesions such as congenital dislocation of the hip, Legg–Calvé–Perthes disease, osteomyelitis, bone disorders, osteoid osteoma, tuberculosis, pyogenic and rheumatoid arthritis, etc. Two important hip conditions in adolescents are slipped capital femoral epiphysis and osteochondritis dissecans coxae, which both will give pain to the groin area.

Inflammation in pelvic joints

Inflammatory conditions may be seen in the joints of the symphysis and sacroiliac joints. Sacroiliitis is not uncommon in outdoor winter sports. Sacroiliitis can also be a symptom in a generalized disease such as rheumatoid arthritis or Bechterew disease. Pain and/or discomfort may radiate out in the groin, to the hip joint or to the thigh. Changes in the sacroiliac joints may be present without the athlete feeling any pain. The symptoms may be vague and most pronounced in the morning. Long intervals without symptoms may be present. The diagnoses are made by clinical examination and with the aid of CT scan.

CARE AND PREVENTION

The treatment consists of anti-inflammatory medication and physical therapy. Athletes participating in winter sports should use warm clothes and sometimes heat retainers. They should dress properly immediately after their activities, as they are sweaty and will quickly become cold.

Osteitis pubis

Some athletes have pain localized to the pubic bone caused by inflammation due to mechanical strain from trauma, abnormal motion or shear stress resulting in osteitis pubis. This lesion can occur with or without pubic instability. The pain can be combined with tenderness over the symphysis area. On X-ray, there are sometimes bony changes occurring 2–3 weeks after onset of symptoms. If such changes are not present, investigation with bone scan can sometimes be positive. In some cases, changes in the pubic bone on X-ray can be found without the athlete having any problems, i.e. the X-ray changes can be secondary findings.

CARE

The treatment of osteitis pubis is rest from painful activities and a minimum of 6–8 weeks of rest is needed to be effective. Anti-inflammatory medication, local corticosteroid injections and range of motion exercises are often used. Surgery is rarely needed. Osteitis pubis is a self-limited condition that heals with rest. The main differential diagnosis is osteomyelitis. In contrast to osteomyelitis, osteitis pubis is usually bilateral, has no sequestrum and a negative culture.

Bursitis

There are at least 13 permanent bursae present in the hip region and they are often localized between tendons and muscles and over bony prominencies. It is possible to divide the pathological conditions of bursae into traumatic and inflammatory conditions (Renström & Peterson, 1980).

Traumatic bursitis

The traumatic bursitis can be called haemorrhagic bursitis, or haemobursa. The most common cause of haemorrhagic bursitis is either a direct trauma such as a fall against the bursa, e.g. during skating against the ice, or an indirect trauma through a strain in a passing tendon with haemorrhage. In a haemorrhagic bursa a haemorrhage is formed and this will initiate a chemical inflammation. If the haemorrhage is extensive and not treated adequately, the blood will coagulate and eventually fibrinous adhesive tissue and fibrin bodies will be formed in the bursa. These adhesions or free bodies will produce a chronic inflammatory bursitis with recurrent problems.

CARE AND PREVENTION

The treatment of the acute haemorrhagic bursitis should be evacuation of the haematoma in order to prevent chronic bursitis. The superficial trochanteric bursa is often subject to direct trauma with a haemorrhagic bursa and bursitis as a result. In this case, a fluctuation over the bursa may be palpated. With an injection needle, the haematoma may be aspirated in the acute case. If the condition becomes chronic, surgical excision of the bursa is often the treatment of choice. Traumatic bursitis can often be prevented by using padding such as knee padding, or padding in the pants such as that used by goal keepers in soccer and team handball.

Inflammatory bursitis

The inflammatory bursitis may be divided into friction bursitis, chemical bursitis and infection bursitis. Friction bursitis may be caused by repeated frequent movements of a muscle–tendon against a bursa, for example, iliopsoas against the iliopectineal bursa. The iliopectineal bursa is located anterior to the hip joint and dorsal to the iliopsoas tendon and is the largest synovial bursa in the whole body and it is communicating with the joint in about 15% in adults. This bursa may be the location for inflammation whether isolated or combined with iliopsoas pathology. Iliopectineal bursitis may give a feeling of tenderness and swelling in the middle of the groin which might spread across the inguinal ligament.

On the lateral proximal femur, inside of the iliotibial band, there is a superficial bursa. Between the tendons to the gluteus medius and tensor fascia latae and behind the greater trochanter there is a deeper located bursa. Both these bursae may be the location for an inflammation because of maltreated haemorrhage. Malalignment with increased pronation with compensatory internal leg rotation can cause overload in this region. Trochanteric bursitis will cause pain and tenderness just lateral to the greater trochanter or just posterior to the prominence. The pain can radiate down along the outside of the thigh and be diagnosed as referred pain from herniated disc lesions in the lumbar spine. Pain may be elicited by rotation of the hip joint. Careful palpation around the lateroposterior aspect of the trochanter region will show localized tenderness.

The chemical bursitis which is sustained after a chemical irritation of products and seen after inflammation or degeneration in tendon tissue is not common in the groin. The infection bursitis may be septic or caused by a bacterial immigration through lacerated skin and can occasionally be seen over the trochanteric region.

CARE AND PREVENTION

Local treatment consists initially of cold packs and rest. After the acute phase, cortisone infiltration might give relief. Orthotics is sometimes of value. This condition can be long-lasting and surgery is sometimes indicated.

Friction bursitis should be prevented. It is important to choose a suitable running surface and avoid running on the camber of the road. Cambered running will cause short/long-legged running with overuse of the leg closest to the ditch. This will cause functional leg length discrepancy and stretch the iliotibial band, and thereby increase the risk for trochanteric bursitis. Avoidance of training errors is a very important part of prevention of trochanteric bursitis, which is an injury that is difficult to treat and can generate frustration.

Snapping hip

Snapping hip usually occurs from snapping either a thickened posterior border of the iliotibial band, or the anterior border of the gluteus maximus over the greater trochanter, which produces a secondary trochanteric bursitis. It is treated as a trochanteric bursitis, but sometimes surgery is indicated in a patient with continuous symptoms.

An 'internal' deep snapping hip can result when the iliopsoas tendon snaps over the iliopectineal eminence (Nanziata & Blumenfeld, 1951). This deep snapping is more intensive than the superficial snapping. Iliopsoas bursography has been used by Jacobsen and Allen (1990) to demonstrate a sudden jerking movement of the iliopsoas tendon between the anteroinferior iliac spine and iliopectineal eminence usually combined with pain and an audible snap. Surgical treatment by lengthening of the tendon has relieved the symptoms.

Intra-articular causes of snapping hip symptoms include synovial chondromatosis, loose bodies, osteochondritis dissecans, osteocartilaginous exostosis, labral tear or inverted labrum (Grana & Kalenack, 1991). MRI, CT scan or hip arthroscopy will help to secure the diagnosis.

Nerve entrapment

Peripheral nerves may become entrapped after direct trauma or inflammatory conditions. Nerves most commonly affected are the ilio-inguinal, genitofemoral and lateral cutaneous femoral nerves. Anterofemoral, obturatorial and iliohypogastric nerves may also be involved. These conditions are not common.

The ilioinguinal nerve transmits sensations from a proximal part of the penis and the base of the scrotum respectively labium major and parts of the medial side of the thigh. These sensations may be elicited by intensive abdominal muscle training leading to entrapment of the nerve when it passes through the abdominal muscles through the different layers. Pain in these areas should lead to suspicion of engagement of the nerve. The intensity and character of the pain vary. It is usually possible to show hyperaesthesia which is demonstrated by drawing a needle across the skin from a non-painful area to a painful area. The diagnosis is confirmed by a blockade of the nerve with local anaesthetics. If the pain is severe, there is an indication for surgical treatment.

The genitofemoral nerve is divided into two parts (i) ramus genitalia, which transmits sensations from labium major/scrotum; and (ii) ramus femoralis which gives sensations from the skin of the thigh just distal to the ilio-inguinal ligament. The symptoms are the same as was mentioned for the ilio-inguinal nerve.

A sensory mononeuritis of the lateral cutaneous nerve of the thigh is called paraesthetic neuralgia. The posterior branch transmits cutaneous sensations from the superior lateral part of the buttock and the anterior branch, which is the most important clinically, pass through the fascia latae through a small canal and transmits sensations and occasionally there is a hyperaesthesia. Usually, there is no history of any trauma, but factors like tight belts or corsets, or long periods of acute hip flexion may engender this condition. Posture exercises which decrease lordosis are considered valuable. Anti-inflammatory medicine is often indicated. Surgical decompression may be necessary.

Referred groin pain

Pain from the spine may arise from facet joint changes, arachnoiditis, intervertebral disc prolapse or spinal stenosis, and radiate out to the groin and down the thigh. Sciatic pain, such as L4 syndrome can be present in addition to groin radiating pain. Spine referred pain can also be caused by Scheuermann's disease, or lumbosacral abnormalities such as spondylolysis or spondylolisthesis.

Hernias

Inguinal and femoral hernias are quite common and may produce pain, radiating diffusely around the groin. Examination for hernias should be included in all cases of groin pain. Hernias should be suspected in patients with persistent groin pain despite adequate treatment and physical therapy.

The patients should be examined with the patient standing. An indirect hernia appears at the external ring and may extend into the scrotum. A direct hernia appears as a diffused bulge in the medial part of the inguinal canal (McLatchie, 1994). An inguinal hernia is above and medial to the pubic tubercle. A femoral hernia is below and lateral to the pubic tubercle. Herniorrhaphy is carried out in adults with good results. The patient can begin walking immediately, but serious athletic training should not start until 5–6 weeks after surgery. The recurrence rate is less than 1% at 5 years (Develin, 1982).

There are athletes with incipient groin hernias which become worse after strenuous physical activity, but it is clinically difficult to secure a diagnosis. To visualize these, Gullmo (1980) and Ekberg *et al.* (1981) have described a method which they have called herniography.

They have given contrast intraperitoneally making it possible to visualize changes interpreted as hernias as the contrast was sinking down in a deep sac. This technique has made it possible to diagnose some incipient hernias. Smedberg *et al.* (1985) have reported on an investigation comprising of 101 painful groins in which 23 athletes had bilateral symptoms. Before herniography, a hernia was palpated in only 7.9% of the groins with pain. Hernias were found at herniography in 84.2% of the symptomatic groins and in 49.1% of the asymptomatic groins. 63 cases of hernia surgeries were performed and the herniographic and the operative diagnoses corresponded well. Altogether, 69.8% of the operated patients were cured by hernia repair and another 20.6% were improved. Strain of the adductor muscle–tendons was the most frequent diagnosis in those not cured by surgery and among the non-operated cases. The athlete can usually return to conditioning a few weeks after surgery, but should not return to strength training until at the earliest 8–10 weeks after surgery.

Of interest to sports medicine is a generalized weakness of the muscular fascial apparatus in the groin, which has been called groin insufficiency (Ekberg, 1994). This bulging occurs particularly in the medial inguinal fossa and is due to weakness of the transversalis and soleus fascia. There is no proper hernial sac, but merely a broadening of the fossa in medial directions. This phenomenon can be verified by herniography and has been described in soccer players, and may be due to chronic trauma.

Other hernia formations may cause groin pain such as hydrocoele and varicocoele. Torsion of the testes may also cause groin pain.

Regional inflammations and infections

The iliopsoas muscle–tendon may be affected in some cases of appendicitis. The muscle may contract and the reflex spasm will result in the hip being held in flexion and external rotation. The obturator internus muscle, which is covered by a relatively dense fascia may also be irritated by pelvic inflammation especially a pelvic abscess. This will lead to pain in internal rotation of the hip joint.

Prostatitis and urinary infections are not uncommon in young athletes participating in winter sports. There may be pain diffusely radiating around the groin. Prostatitis is diagnosed by definite evidence of inflammation in the expressed prostatic secretion, culture positive in segmented urine, and/or prostatic secretion (Abrahamson & Westlin, 1985), and an abnormal prostate revealed by rectal examination. Rectal palpation should be included in the examination of groin pain. Proper clothing is important as prevention.

Gynaecological disorders may cause pain radiating to the groin. Such changes may be inflammatory changes, sexual diseases and tumours.

Rheumatological diseases may include rheumatoid arthritis, ankylosis, spondylitis, zero negative arthropathy, Reiter's syndrome and gout.

Bone infections giving groin pain may include osteomyelitis and tuberculosis.

Tumours

Tumours are not uncommon in the groin area and we have seen several cases where the pain at first was experienced in the groin area in connection with a soccer game or similar event. The pain was often considered to be caused by strain in the groin muscles and tendons. After 1–3 months, the patients are referred to orthopaedic departments because of persistent pain or tumour-suspect findings on X-ray. Chondrosarcomas, malignant schwannomas, osteosarcomas, Ewing's sarcoma, etc., have been diagnosed often at a late stage. Persistent pain in the groin region should be carefully investigated in order to exclude a tumour and a radiology examination should always be included at an early stage in patients with diffuse groin pain. MRI or CT scan will secure the diagnosis and allow proper care.

Conclusion

Groin injuries often cause long-lasting problems. Prevention is, therefore, of utmost importance. Most soccer and ice-hockey teams, as well as skaters and fencers, have integrated groin muscle stretching and flexibility training into their training and warm-up programmes as prevention.

Groin injuries in athletes continues, however, to be a rather common problem and they give the athlete and his or her medical advisor great diagnostic and therapeutic problems (Hess, 1980; Renström & Peterson, 1980; Schneider, 1980; Smodlaka, 1980; Muckle, 1982; Zimmerman, 1988; Estwanik *et al.*, 1990). These injuries are difficult to diagnose and difficult to treat as the symptoms may be very diffuse and uncharacteristic. Successful treatment of groin injuries depends on the correct diagnosis, which is based on a thorough knowledge of the differential diagnostic possibilities in the groin area. A multidisciplinary approach is very valuable when using a physician team with experience of different aspects of groin pain (Ekberg *et al.*, 1988). Team work is often the best way to successful care and outcome.

Athletes participating in sports with a high incidence of groin problems, should focus on prevention as most of the muscle–tendon injuries in the groin can be prevented. These injuries are usually very difficult to treat. A successful outcome depends on an early correct diagnosis. Groin injuries constitute a real challenge to doctors active in sports medicine and orthopaedics. The focus should be on prevention, proper diagnosis and care.

References

Abrahamson, P.A. & Westlin, W. (1985) Symphysitis and prostatitis in athletes. *Scand. J. Urol. Nephrol.* **19**(Suppl. 93), 42.

Cailliet, R. (1978) *Soft Tissue Pain and Disability*. FA Davies, Philadelphia.

Develin, H.B. (1982) Hernia. In R.C.G. Russell (ed) *Recent Advances in Surgery*, Vol. 11, pp. 209–23. Churchill Livingstone, Edinburgh.

Ekberg, O. (1994) Herniography in athletes with groin pain. In P. Renström & S. Hermans (eds) *Groin Injuries in Sports*. Karger, Basel (in press).

Ekberg, O., Blomquist, P. & Olsson, S. (1981) Positive contrast herniography in adult patients with obscure groin pain. *Surgery* **89**(5), 532–5.

Ekberg, O., Persson, N.A., Abrahamson, P.A. *et al.* (1988) Longstanding groin pain in athletes — A multidisciplinary approach. *Sports Med.* **6**, 56–61.

Ekstrand, J. (1982) *Soccer injuries and their prevention*. Dissertation, University of Linköping, Sweden.

Estwanik, J.J., Sloane, B. & Rosenberg, M.A. (1990) Groin strain and other possible causes of groin pain. *Phys. Sportsmed.* **18**(2).

Grana, W. & Kalenack, A. (1991) *Clinical Sports Medicine*. WB Saunders, Philadelphia.

Grimby, G. & Thomeé, R. (1988) Principles of rehabilitation after injuries. In A. Dirix, H.G. Knuttgen & K. Tittel (eds) *The Olympic Book of Sports Medicine*, pp. 489–502. Blackwell Scientific Publications, Oxford.

Gullmo, A. (1980) Herniography. The diagnosis of hernia in the groin and incompetence of the pouch of Douglas and pelvic floor. *Acta Radiol.* **361**(Suppl.), 1–76.

Hermans, G.P.H. & Verwiel, L.A.M. (1983) Ergenbnisse einer neuen Operationstechnik zur Behandlung von Adduktor–Tendopathhien bei Sportlern (A new surgical technique in the treatment of adductor tendon injuries in atheletes). In *Sportverletzungen und Sportschaden*, pp. 65–6. George Thieme Verlag, Stuttgart.

Hess, H. (1980) Leistenschmerz — Etiologie, Differential diagnose und terapeutische Moglichkeiten (Overuse injuries — aetiology, differential diagnosis and treatment possibilities). *Orthopade* **9**, 186–9.

Jacobson, T. & Allen, W.T. (1990) Surgical correction of the snapping iliopsoas tendon. *Am. J. Sports Med.* **18**(5), 470–4.

Lotke, P.A. (1973) Soft tissue lesions affecting the hip joints. In R. Tronzo (ed) *Surgery of the Hip Joint*, pp. 368–77. Springer, New York.

McLatchie, G.R. (1994) The presentation and management of the symptoms relating to the groin. In P. Renström & S. Hermans (eds) *Groin Injuries in Sports*. Karger, Basel (in press).

Martens, M.A., Hansen, L. & Mulier, J.C. (1987) Adductor tendinitis and musculus rectus abdominous tendonopathy. *Am. J. Sports Med.* **15**(4), 353–6.

Muckle, D.S. (1982) Associated factors in recurrent groin and hamstring injuries. *Br. J. Sports Med.* **16**(1), 37–9.

Nanziata, A. & Blumenfeld, J. (1951) Cadeva a resorte. A proposite de una variedad (Hip elasticity with regard to variety). *Prensa Med. Argentina* **38**, 1997–2001.

Peterson, L. & Renström, P. (1985) *Injuries in Sports*. Martin Dunitz, London.

Peterson, L. & Stener, B. (1986) Old total rupture of the adductor longus muscle. *Acta Orthop. Scand.* **47**, 653–7.

Renström, P. (1992) Muscle tendon injuries in the groin. *Sports Med.* **11**(4), 815–33.

Renström, P. & Peterson, L. (1980) Groin injuries in athletes. *Br. J. Sports Med.* **14**, 30–6.

Schneider, P.G. (1980) Liestenschmerz: Operative therapiemoglichkeiten (Groin pain: surgical treatment possibilities). *Orthopade* **9**, 190–2.

Smedberg, S.G.G., Broome, A.E.A., Gullmo, A. *et al.* (1985) Herniography in athletes with groin pain. *Am. J. Surg.* **140**, 378–82.

Smodlaka, V.N. (1980) Groin pain in soccer players. *Phys. Sports Med.* **8**(8), 57–61.

Symeonides. P.P. (1972) Isolated traumatic rupture of the adductor longus muscle of the thigh. *Clin. Orthop. Rel. Res.* **88**, 64–5.

Thomeé, R. (1994) Conservative treatment of muscle tendon injuries around the groin. In P. Renström & S. Hermans (eds) *Groin Injuries in Sports*. Karger, Basel (in press).

Zimmerman, G. (1988) Groin pain in athletes. *Australian Fam. Phys.* **17**(12), 1046–52.

Chapter 8

Muscle Injuries

MARKKU JÄRVINEN

Muscle injuries, contusions and strains, are common traumas in sports medicine and their incidence varies from 10 to 55% of all injuries in different sport events (Franke, 1980; Zarins & Ciullo, 1983; Sandelin, 1988). Muscle injury can occur in different forms depending on the trauma mechanism: the lesions can be lacerations, contusions or strains (Ryan, 1969; Millar, 1979). Sharp injury leading to a major trauma of the muscle is very rare in sports. Very often muscle can be injured in sport activities by excessive compressive force, such as a direct blow; this is a contusion. If excessive tensile force is applied, the muscle is overstretched, causing a strain. Distraction strains often occur in a muscle which works across two joints, i.e. the quadriceps muscles, which extend the knee and flex in the hip joint. Because both of these functions cannot normally occur at the same time controlled by a sensitive neuromuscular system, momentary incoordination, especially on fatigue, can be followed by muscle strain (Ryan, 1969; Renström, 1985).

Muscle contusions are common in all contact sports events and strains usually occur in sprinting and jumping and they are often located in superficially lying muscles, i.e. rectus femoris, semitendinosus and gastrocnemius, etc. The most common muscle strains are not complete but partial ruptures of the muscular tissue and the pathological lesions are often located in the region near the myotendinous junction (Millar, 1979; Almekinders & Gilbert, 1986; Garrett *et al.*, 1987). The capacity of the muscle–tendon unit to resist stretching plays an important role when muscle strain occurs. When contracted muscle is stretched, the failure load is higher before rupture than in relaxed muscle and all factors decreasing the tensile properties of muscle increase the risk of strain under stretching (Garrett *et al.*, 1987).

The prevention of soft tissue injuries is based on the understanding of many issues, such as injury risks, injury mechanism, pathology in injured tissue, healing mechanisms, treatment and rehabilitation principles and their effects on injured tissue, all kinds of preventive training systems, warming up, correct use of adequate equipments and pads, correct and balanced training, etc. The successful prevention programme is based on the understanding the biology of the healing muscle injury.

Classification of muscle injuries

The symptoms of muscle injury, strain or contusion, depend on the quality, intramuscular or intermuscular, of the haematoma or on the severity of the strain, and therefore the muscle injuries are often graded into three degrees (O'Donoghue, 1970). In mild (first degree) strain, only minimal tear of muscle fibres exists with low level of inflammation, swelling and discomfort during movements and there is no or only minimal loss of strength and restriction of movements. However, mild strain may be very distressing to the athlete. In moderate (second degree) strain, there has been actual damage to the muscle, there is not a complete disruption of muscle, but there is definite loss of strength. In severe (third degree) strain, the tear usually includes a total tear of the muscle–tendon unit and complete tear often means the total lack of function of the muscle–tendon unit.

Ryan's (1969) classification of quadriceps strain applies to all muscles and can be utilized as a subclassification.

Grade I is a tear of few fibres with fascia remaining intact.

Grade II is a tear of moderate number of fibres with fascia remaining intact (localized haematoma).

Grade III is a tear of many fibres with partial tearing of the fascia (diffuse bleeding or ecchymosis).

Grade IV is a complete tearing of the muscle and fascia (Fig. 8.1).

Clinical examination is initially carried out with an analysis of the cause of the injury. Thereafter close inspection and careful palpation of the involved muscles is made. The most important test is often the functional test with or without resistence.

Two different types of haematomas can be identified because of the different principles of treatment and prognosis; (i) intramuscular; and (ii) intermuscular haematomas (Fig. 8.2). Intramuscular haematomas may be caused by a muscle strain or bruise. The haematoma is limited by the intact muscle fascia epimysium. If the epimysium is intact, the blood flow is retained within the muscle which leads to an increase in the intramuscular pressure which

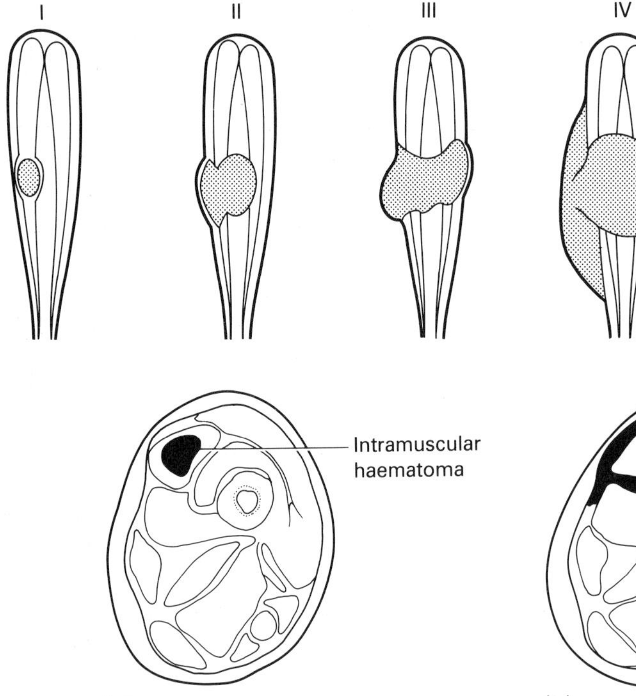

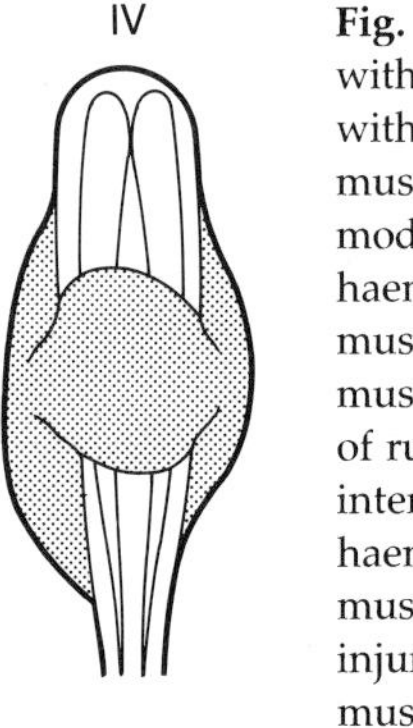

Fig. 8.1 A grade I muscle injury with a tear of some muscle fibres with an intact fascia. A grade II muscle injury with a tear of moderate muscle fibres and haematoma with an intramuscular spread. A grade III muscle injury with large amount of ruptured muscle fibres, large intermuscular spread of haematoma with ruptured muscle fascia. A grade IV muscle injury with a complete tearing of muscle and fascia.

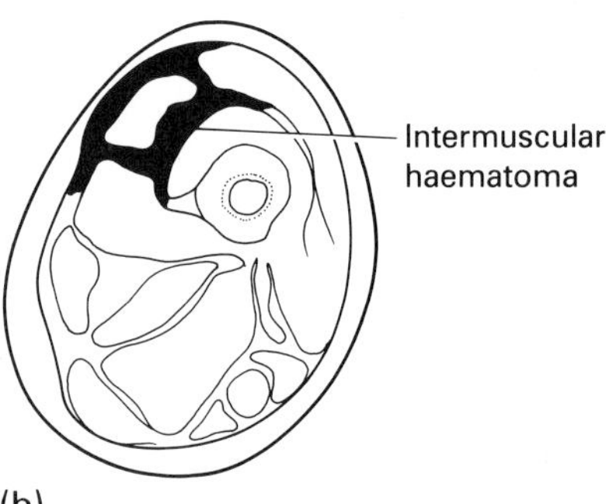

Fig. 8.2 Schematic presentation of (a) an intramuscular and (b) an intermuscular haematoma. The intramuscular haematoma remains inside the intact muscle fascia often combined with increased intramuscular pressure. Intermuscular haematoma is spread into intermuscular spaces without increasing the pressure inside the muscle.

compresses and limits the haematoma. There is pain and loss of function. Intermuscular haematomas may develop in the interfascial and interstitial spaces when the muscle fascia is also involved. The haematoma may spread into the intermuscular spaces without increase the pressure inside the muscle. A combination of intramuscular and intermuscular haematomas is not common. The symptoms are the same as described in muscle tears (Renström, 1985). Direct contusion is known to damage the deepest fibres adjacent to the bone, if the muscle is relaxed during contusion, because the pressure is transmitted from the superficial layer to the deeper muscle layers as though these were fluid compartments until the pressure wave is stopped at the bone level, so that the adjacent muscle layer is compressed against the bone and damaged (Benazzo *et al.*, 1989). Contusion to the contracted muscle is followed by a more superficial lesion than that of relaxed muscle.

Diagnosis of muscle injuries

Clinical diagnosis of strain and haematoma may be simple in cases where a history of contusion or muscle strain is accompanied by objective evidence of swelling and/or ecchymosis distal to the lesion. Small haematomas and those deep in the muscle mass are more difficult to diagnose clinically and their extend must be determined by instrumental investigation (Benazzo *et al.*, 1989). Ultrasonography, computerized tomography (CT) and magnetic resonance imaging (MRI) can be used for this purpose. Ultrasonography is currently the examination of choice for the anatomical definition of the muscle injury. It is both inexpensive and easy to perform and the instrumentation is available in most places (Laine & Peltokallio, 1991). The whole course of the repair of muscle injury can be followed very well by ultrasonography (Lehto & Alanen, 1987).

Biology of the repair of muscle injury

In the connection of mechanical muscle injury after retraction of disrupted muscle fibres followed by a gap filled with haematoma, the events of repair process can be classified into three phases:

1 Inflammation phase is characterized by haematoma formation, muscle tissue necrosis and degeneration as well as inflammatory cell reaction.

2 Repair phase consists of phagocytosis of damaged tissue, regeneration of striated muscle, production of connective tissue scar and capillary ingrowth.

3 Remodelling phase consists of maturation of regenerated muscle, contraction and reorganization of scar tissue and recovery of functional capacity of repaired muscle (Fig. 8.3) (Järvinen, 1976c; Allbrook, 1981; Carlson & Faulkner, 1983; Lehto, 1983; Hurme, 1991).

Within the first days, the macrophages phagocytose the necrotic muscle tissue in the injury gap and proximal and distal stumps of disrupted muscle fibres. Removal of necrotic debris is a start to regeneration activating the satellite cells into myoblasts along the periphery of preserved basal lamina cylinders (Carlson & Faulkner, 1983; Hurme *et al.*, 1991a). Simultaneously with regeneration of muscle tissue, the haematoma is gradually replaced by proliferating fibroblasts and extracellular matrix components to restore the integrity of the connective tissue (Järvinen, 1975; Lehto *et al.*, 1986). At the same time the regeneration of muscle fibres proceeds with an attempt to re-establish the contact between the ruptured ends of muscle fibres. These two reparative processes are supportive, but also competitive. The connective tissue transmits contraction force across the gap, which allows the use of injured limb before the repair is complete. In major muscle trauma proliferation of fibroblasts can rapidly lead to excessive formation of dense scar tissue, which is a mechanical barrier inhibiting complete regeneration of muscle fibres across the traumatic cap (Järvinen, 1975; Lehto *et al.*,

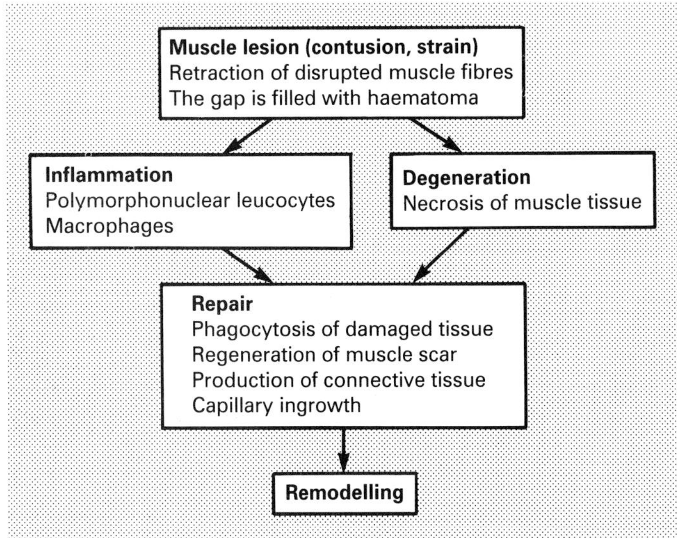

Fig. 8.3 Summary of events in healing muscle injury.

1985a). In the early phase of muscle injury it is important to limit the haematoma as small as possible to prohibit an excessive scar formation.

In the early phase of healing, the regeneration of muscle tissue is dependent on the ingrowth of capillaries to the injured area (Carlson, 1970; Järvinen, 1976a). Following injury, new capillaries sprout from the surviving trunks of blood vessels towards the centre of the injury (Järvinen, 1976a). The ingrowth of new capillaries to the injured area plays an important role in the oxygen supply necessary for an adequate energy metabolism in repairing tissue (Jozsa *et al.*, 1980). Histochemical studies (Snow, 1973) indicate that the fusion of myotubes requires aerobic metabolism. The young myotubes have a scarcity of mitochondria and a moderately increased activity of succinic acid dehydrogenase indicating aerobic metabolism via the citric acid cycle, but strongly increased activity of lactic acid dehydrogenase and glucose-6-phosphate dehydrogenase, which are indicators of anaerobic glycolysis and pentose phosphate shunt, respectively (Snow, 1973; Järvinen & Sorvari, 1978).

The adhesion of regenerating muscle fibre to the extracellular matrix is similar as the adhesion of myofibres to the myotendineal junction allowing both growth of the muscle cells across the scar and their use before regeneration is completed (Hurme & Kalimo, 1992). At the moment of the injury, the intramuscular nerve branches may also be damaged and since a muscle fibre receives its neural input at one location only, at the neuromuscular junction, the part of the fibre distal to the injury loses its neural input. Muscle fibre regeneration continues to the myotube phase without nerve supply, but atrophy is followed, if no reinnervation exists (Caplan *et al.*, 1988; Hurme *et al.*, 1991c).

The sequence of connective tissue proteins plays an important role and reflects the particular function that each carries out during muscle wound healing (e.g. fibronectin in fibroblast trapping, type III collagen in plasticity and flexibility and type I collagen in tensile strength) (Lehto, 1983; Hurme *et al.*, 1991b). In the early phase of healing (during the first 2 days) fibronectin, abundant in the trauma area, is derived mainly from plasma. The production of fibronectin by fibroblasts starts a little later and is closely followed by type III collagen. The early active synthesis of type III collagen and fibronectin is decreased after 1 week and the production of type I collagen by fibroblasts is activated somewhat later and remains elevated at least 3 weeks (Hurme *et al.*, 1991b).

The tensile strength of the scar after injury is based on the mechanical stability of the collagen fibres of which the scar is composed. The mechanical stability of the collagen fibre is largely based upon the formation of intermolecular cross-links between the constituent molecules. The presence of two major cross-links in muscle collagen has been demonstrated and during the development of the granulation tissue following muscle injury, considerable changes in the cross-linking were observed (Lehto, 1983; Lehto *et al.*, 1985b). The ratio of the two cross-links does not normalize before 6 weeks after injury and the normal cross-link pattern in intramuscular collagen 6 weeks after injury may indicate that a certain minimum of healing time is needed before the connective tissue possesses sufficient tensile strength.

The mechanical characteristics of healing muscle are closely related to the morphological changes described earlier. During the first week of healing, the injury site was the weakest point during passive stretching in experimental conditions (Järvinen, 1976b). After the first week, the rupture often occurred quite proximal to the injury. In the rat gastrocnemius muscle the rupture site in the intact muscle was most often in the muscle belly (Barfred, 1971; Järvinen, 1977). On the other hand, Nikolau *et al.* (1987) found the muscle–tendon junction to be the weakest point in the stretched muscle–tendon unit. They used tibialis anterior muscle, which apparently has a different structural organization and amount of connective tissue to gastrocnemius muscle, in which the proportion of muscle tissue is greatest and connective tissue is minimal in the muscle belly. In the contracted muscle, the muscle–tendon junction is in general the point of rupture when stretched and the force necessary to sustain a rupture is nearly twice as much as in muscles pulled to failure under passive tension (Garrett *et al.*, 1987).

Effect of mobilization and immobilization on the healing process

Early mobilization is regarded as the method of choice today in the treatment of muscle ruptures and contusions because of the smaller amount of complications and disabilities compared with treatment by immobilization (Knight, 1985; Renström, 1985; Benazzo *et al.*, 1989).

The superiority of early mobilization as a treatment regimen has first presented by Woodard (1954) in clinical practice, but today, experimental evidence on the superiority of mobilization exists (Järvinen, 1976a,b,c; Lehto, 1983). These experimental studies indicate that early mobilization is followed by a more rapidly and intensively occurring muscle regeneration, capillary ingrowth, vast production of granulation tissue and scar and parallel orientation but poor penetration of muscle fibres through the connective tissue scar (Järvinen, 1975, 1976a; Lehto *et al.*, 1985a, 1986) (Table 8.1).

Tensile properties of injured muscle returned in a relatively short time to the level of uninjured muscle under mobilization treatment, but immobilization has a tendency to decrease the tensile properties and strength throughout the immobilization period (Järvinen, 1976b, 1977).

However, a sufficient period of immobilization after the injury, about 5 days for a rat muscle, is needed to achieve a stage when the newly formed granulation tissue covers the injured area with a tensile strength high enough to resist the forces caused by mobilization treatment and to prevent reruptures in the early phase of healing (Lehto, 1983; Lehto *et al.*, 1985a).

Immobilization following injury limits the size of the connective tissue area formed within the site of injury; the penetration of muscle fibres through the connective tissue is not so much prohibited than in mobilized muscles, but their orientation is more complex and not parallel with the uninjured muscle fibres. When mobilization is started after a

Table 8.1 Effect of mobilization and immobilization on the healing of muscle injury (Lehto & Järvinen, 1991).

	Mobilization	Immobilization
Inflammatory cell reaction (day 1–2)	Intensive	Mild
Number of myotubes (day 3–5)	Numerous	Scanty
Capillary ingrowth (day 5–14)	Rapid and intensive	Delayed and moderate
Scar formation (day 5–14)	Starts slightly delayed but with high intensity	Starts undisturbed and progresses steadily but with moderate intensity
Gain of tensile strength (day 7–42)	Rapidly to normal or near to normal level	Slowly; normal level not achieved

short period of immobilization, a better penetration of muscle fibres through the connective tissue is found and the orientation of regenerated muscle fibres is aligned with the uninjured muscle fibres (Järvinen, 1975; Lehto *et al.*, 1985a).

The trends of these experimental studies are clear; short immobilization following injury is needed to accelerate formation of the granulation tissue matrix. The length of immobilization is, however, dependent on the grade of injury and should be optimized so that scar can bear the forces directed on it without rupture.

Mobilization, on the other hand, is followed by a rapid gain of original tensile strength of the muscle and good results in penetration and orientation of the regenerating muscle fibres, in resorption of connective tissue scar and recapillarization of the damaged area. Another important object of mobilization — in sport clinical practice especially — is to avoid muscle atrophy, which rapidly follows in prolonged immobilization.

Treatment of muscle injuries

Immediate treatment

Treatment of contusion and strain injuries with the formation of a haematoma must be immediate. It must be integrated with and promote the biological stages of muscle regeneration. Therapeutic managements should be focused to keep the circumstances in the injured tissue so that the quickest and most functionally effective regeneration is possible and to avoid and limit all irregularities in the healing process, which would impair the functional efficiency of the injured muscle (Benazzo *et al.*, 1989). The immediate treatment consists of rest, ice, compression and elevation. The aim is to reduce the formation of haematoma and interstitial oedema to shorten the tissue ischaemia and thus accelerate regeneration.

This treatment should be started as soon as possible by trainer or athlete. The idea is to control bleeding. The maximal compression bandage (cutaneous pressure about 85 mmHg) eliminates and reduces effectively the formation of an intramuscular haematoma (Thorsson *et al.*, 1987). Cold application on the injured area (ice packs) for 15–20 min should take place at intervals of 30–60 min. This kind of cooling is followed by a 3–7° decrease in the intramuscular temperature (Kellett, 1986). Massage should not be used until 1 week has passed (10–14 days in cases of serious muscle injury) (Benazzo *et al.*, 1989). Elevation decreases the inflow of blood to the injury site and increases the venous return to the heart. Rest of 1–3 days should be used and nonsteroidal anti-inflammatory medication should be started immediately after the injury. After 2–3 days, the contractile ability of the injured muscle should be controlled and, if it does not improve from the original postinjury level, a large intramuscular haematoma or total rupture of the muscle may be present and surgical intervention is necessary.

Ultrasound treatment is useful 2–3 days after the injury. It has a beneficial effect in the initial stage of regeneration, since the micromassage provided by its high-frequency sound waves serves to relieve pain. 10–15 sessions lasting 10–15 min are recommended.

Treatment after 3 days

After 3 days, the diagnosis is often clear. After the initial treatment, minor partial ruptures and minor intramuscular haematomas should be supported with elastic bandages and the conservative treatment consists of early mobilization with special muscle exercises for an injured muscle.

1 Isometric training without load and later with increased load within the limits of pain should be started initially.

2 Thereafter, isotonic training with and without load carefully and controlled should be performed.

3 Isokinetic, dynamic training with minimal load should be started also early, but this training requires special equipment.

4 Local heat or contrast treatment with cold and heat may be of value, accompanied with passive and active stretching of the affected muscle carefully in the limits of pain.

The purpose of stretching is to distend the scar tissue, while it is still plastic, but already strong to prevent functionally disabling retraction. The painless elongation must be reached gradually by stretching for periods of 10–15 s at first and then proceeding to 1 min (Renström, 1985; Benazzo *et al.*, 1989).

In the strength training after injury it should be remembered that warming up is important. The training should be all-round and the strength training should be combined with flexibility training.

In the final phase, sport-specific training under the supervision of a coach or trainer should be started. If the symptoms caused by the injured muscle fail to improve, it is necessary to reconsider the possibility of intramuscular haematoma and tissue damage, and a clinical re-examination should be carried out. Measurement of intramuscular pressure, puncture and aspiration of the injured area (if fluctuation is present), a soft-tissue X-ray or an ultrasonography examination, and sometimes surgical intervention may be necessary. Surgical treatment is often necessary in large intramuscular haematomas, in third-degree strain or tear in muscles which have few or no agonist muscles (muscles with the same function) and in second degree strains with more than half of the muscle belly torn (Renström, 1985).

Heterotopic bone formation, myositis ossificans, is the most serious complication after muscle injury. A single, severe or repeated injury may be the cause of myositis ossificans. Especially the muscle contusions with large haematoma close to the bone are suspicious. Also, too vigorous mobilization and rehabilitation is asserted as the cause of this complaint (Jackson & Feagin, 1973).

Preventive aspects of muscle injuries

The common opinion is that 'people are not interested to injury prevention. The possibilities to prevent sports injuries are limited'. These opinions cannot be accepted today in modern sports traumatology. Ekstrand (1982) could demonstrate in his thesis in Sweden that in soccer, the prophylactic programme including supervision by doctor and physiotherapist reduced the injuries by 75%; and in the hands of coaches the same programme reduced the injuries by 50%. As regards the prevention of sports injuries, health information and education should for the time being concern itself in particular with (Hlobil *et al.*, 1987):

1 The risks inherent in various sports.

2 The importance of 'disciplined' sports activities.

3 The use of protective equipment.
4 The importance of general preventive measures, e.g. stretching exercises, warming up, cooling down and taping.
5 Impressing an understanding of injury mechanism.

In muscle injury prevention, the use of protective equipment is of special importance to prevent bruising and contusions. In Ekstrand's study (1982), all traumatic lower leg injuries affected players using inadequate or no shinguards. Strain more commonly affected players with muscle tightness. Therefore active and passive stretching, warming up and cooling down as well as strengthening of muscles are of special importance in the prevention of muscle injuries.

Overall conditioning is very important. Conditioning is thought to result in muscle hypertrophy accompanied by increased vascularity with better circulation and supply of nutrients and thus less fatigue. Training is important to condition those muscles particularly involved in the activity and to gain proper technique, since limited technique can also lead to injury. Strengthening is important, because higher energy input and increased capacity to store so-called elastic energy under the lengthening phase of muscle prohibits the injury. Strength must also be balanced between antagonist muscle groups. If quadriceps muscles are over 10% stronger than the hamstrings, there exists an increased risk of hamstring strain under maximal work. These factors in muscle injury prevention must all be addressed far in advance of competition in order to be effective (Safran *et al.*, 1989). Warm-up reduces the muscle viscosity to promote smoother enzymatic enhancement of contraction, and relaxes muscles neurally. When warm-up is combined with stretching, the elasticity of muscle is temporarily increased requiring a greater force and degree of lengthening to tear muscle (Safran *et al.*, 1988). Stretching should always be performed after warm-up to reduce the possibility of injury from stretches and to increase extensibility and flexibility. The stretch should be slow, relaxed and graceful — both passive and active — and the stretch is performed slowly until muscle tightness, but no pain, is felt (Safran *et al.*, 1989).

Rehabilitation after injury should be a way of preventing an injured athlete recovering 'incompletely' and thus restarting his or her sporting activities at the preinjury level too soon. A rehabilitation programme cannot be regarded as having been completed until (i) the athlete is free from pain; and (ii) muscle strength and extensibility has returned to about preinjury level.

Conclusion

Muscle injury in its clinical manifestations — lacerations, contusions or strains — should be initially thoroughly examined to estimate the degree of damage. Ultrasonography may be very helpful in diagnosis. After first aid treatment with rest, compression, cold and elevation, the therapy can be tailored depending on the grade of injury, of which the complete ruptures should be operated on. The conservative treatment is based on the knowledge and understanding of the biological background of the healing processes in the muscle. The experimental studies have clearly shown that short immobilization following injury is needed to accelerate formation of the granulation tissue matrix. The length of immobilization is, however, dependent on the grade of injury and should be optimized so that the forming scar can bear the pulling forces directed on it without rupture. Mobilization, on the other hand, is required for the gain of original strength of the muscle and for good end results in penetration and orientation of the regenerating muscle fibres, and furthermore in resorption of the connective tissue scar and recapillarization of the damaged area. Another important aim of mobilization — in sport clinical practice especially — is to avoid atrophy, loss of strength and extensibility of the muscle, which is rapidly followed by prolonged immobilization (Lehto

& Järvinen, 1991). Careful active rehabilitation after muscle injury to prohibit reinjury and preventive management to avoid injuries are important in all sport activities.

References

Allbrook, D. (1981) Skeletal muscle regeneration. *Muscle Nerve* **4**, 234–45.

Almekinders, L.C. & Gilbert, J.A. (1986) Healing of experimental muscle strains and the effect of non-steroidal anti-inflammatory medication. *Am. J. Sports Med.* **14**, 303–8.

Barfred, T. (1971) Experimental rupture of Achilles tendon. *Acta Orthop. Scand.* **42**, 406–28.

Benazzo, F., Barnabei, G., Monti, G., Ferrario, A. & Jelmoni, G.P. (1989) Current thinking on the pathogenesis, progression and treatment of muscle haematomas in athletes. *Ital. J. Sports Traumatol.* **11**, 273–304.

Caplan, A., Carlson, B., Faulkner, J., Fischman, J. & Garrett Jr, W. (1988) Skeletal muscle. In S.L-Y. Woo & J.A. Buckwalter (eds) *Injury and Repair of the Musculoskeletal Soft Tissues*, pp. 213–91. American Academy of Orthopaedic Surgeons Symposium, Georgia.

Carlson, B.M. (1970) Histological observations on the regeneration of mammalian and amphibian muscle. In A. Mauro, S.A. Shafiq & A.T. Milhorat (eds) *Regeneration of Striated Muscle and Myogenesis*, pp. 38–72. Exerpta Medica, Amsterdam.

Carlson, B.M. & Faulkner, J.A. (1983) The regeneration of skeletal muscle fibers following injury: A review. *Med. Sci. Sports Exerc.* **15**, 187–96.

Ekstrand, J. (1982) *Soccer injuries and their prevention*. Medical dissertation No. 130, Linköping University.

Franke, K. (1980) Verletzungen und Fehlbelastungsfolgen im Bereich der Sehnenansätze, Sehnen und Muskeln (Injuries and failures of tendons and muscles). In K. Franke (ed) *Traumatologie des Sports*, pp. 46–70. VEB Verlag Volk und Gesundheit, Berlin.

Garrett Jr, W.E., Safran, M.R., Seaber, V., Glisson, R.R. & Ribbeck, B.M. (1987) Biomechanical comparison of stimulated and nonstimulated muscle pulled to failure. *Am. J. Sports Med.* **15**, 448–54.

Hlobil, H., Mechelen, W van. & Kemper, H.C.G. (1987) *How can Sports Injuries be Prevented?* National Institute for Sports Health Care, The Netherlands.

Hurme, T. (1991) *Regeneration of injured skeletal muscle. An experimental study in rats*. Thesis, University of Turku, Finland.

Hurme, T. & Kalimo, H. (1992) Adhesion in skeletal muscle during regeneration. *Muscle Nerve* **15**, 482–9.

Hurme, T., Kalimo, H., Lehto, M. & Järvinen, M. (1991a) Healing of a skeletal muscle injury. An ultrastructural and immunohistochemical study. *Med. Sci. Sports Exerc.* **23**, 801–10.

Hurme, T., Kalimo, H., Sandberg, M., Lehto, M. & Vuorio, E. (1991b) Localization of type I and III collagen and fibronectin production in injured gastrocnemius muscle. *Lab. Invest.* **64**, 76–84.

Hurme, T., Lehto, M., Falck, B., Tainio, H. & Kalimo, H. (1991c) Electromyography and morphology during regeneration of muscle injury in rat. *Acta Physiol. Scand.* **142**, 442–56.

Jackson, D.W. & Feagin, J.A. (1973) Quadriceps contusions in young athletes. *J. Bone Joint Surg.* **55A**, 95–105.

Järvinen, M. (1975) Healing of a crush injury in rat striated muscle. 2. A histological study of the effect of early mobilization and immobilization on the repair processes. *Acta Pathol. Microbiol. Scand. A* **83**, 269–82.

Järvinen, M. (1976a) Healing of a crush injury in rat striated muscle. 3. A microangiographical study of the effect of early mobilization and immobilization on capillary ingrowth. *Acta Pathol. Microbiol. Scand. A* **84**, 85–94.

Järvinen, M. (1976b) Healing of a crush injury in rat striated muscle. 4. Effect of early mobilization and immobilization on the tensile properties of gastrocnemius muscle. *Acta Chirurg. Scand.* **142**, 47–56.

Järvinen, M. (1976c) *Healing of a crush injury in rat striated muscle. With special reference to treatment by early mobilization and immobilization*. Thesis, University of Turku, Finland.

Järvinen, M. (1977) Immobilization effect on the tensile properties of striated muscle: An experimental study in the rat. *Arch. Phys. Med. Rehabil.* **58**, 123–7.

Järvinen, M. & Sorvari, T. (1978) A histochemical study of the effect of mobilization and immobilization on the metabolism of healing muscle injury. In F. Landry & W.A.R. Orban (eds) *Sports Medicine*, pp. 171–81. Symposia Specialists Inc., Florida.

Jozsa, L., Reffy, A., Demel, Z. & Szilagyi, I. (1980) Alterations of oxgyen and carbon dioxide tensions in crush-injured calf muscles of rat. *Zeitschr. Exper. Chirurgie Forsch.* **13**, 91–4.

Kellet, J. (1986) Acute soft tissue injuries — a review of the literature. *Med. Sci. Sports Exerc.* **18**, 489–500.

Knight, K.L. (1985) Guidelines for rehabilitation of sports injuries. *Clin. Sports Med.* **4**, 405–16.

Laine, H.R. & Peltokallio, P. (1991) Ultrasonographic possibilities and findings in most common sports injuries. *Ann. Chirurgiae Gynaecol.* **80**, 127–33.

Lehto, M. (1983) *Collagen and fibronectin in a healing skeletal muscle injury. An experimental study in rats under variable states of physical activity.* Thesis, University of Turku, Finland.

Lehto, M. & Alanen, A. (1987) Healing of a muscle trauma correlation of sonographical and histological findings. *J. Ultrasound Med.* **6**, 425–9.

Lehto, M., Duance, V.C. & Restall, D. (1985a) Collagen and fibronectin in a healing skeletal muscle injury. An immunohistochemical study of the effects of physical activity on the repair of injured gastrocnemius muscle in the rat. *J. Bone Joint Surg.* **67B**, 820–8.

Lehto, M. & Järvinen, M. (1991) Muscle injuries' healing and treatment. *Ann. Chirurgiae Gynaecol.* **80**, 102–9.

Lehto, M., Järvinen, M. & Nelimarkka, O. (1986) Scar formation in a healing skeletal muscle injury. A histological and autoradiographical study in rats. *Arch. Orthop. Traum. Surg.* **104**, 366–70.

Lehto, M., Sims, T.J. & Bailey, A.J. (1985b) Skeletal muscle injury — molecular changes in the collagen during healing. *Res. Exp. Med.* **185**, 95–106.

Millar, A.P. (1979) Strains of the posterior calf musculature ('tennis leg'). *Am. J. Sports Med.* **3**, 172–4.

Nikolaou, P.K., MacDonald, B.L., Glisson, R.R., Seaber, A.V. & Garrett Jr, W.E. (1987) Biomechanical and histological evaluation of muscle after controlled strain injury. *Am. J. Sports Med.* **15**, 9–14.

O'Donoghue, D.H. (1970) Principles in the management of specific injuries. In D.H. O'Donoghue (ed) *Treatment of Injuries to Athletes*, pp. 43–100. WB Saunders, Philadelphia.

Renström, P. (1985) Muscle injuries in sport. In *Sports Medicine in Track and Field Athletics*, pp. 17–28. Proceedings of the First IAAF Medical Congress, Espoo, Finland, 1983. Lehtikanta Oy, Kouvola.

Ryan, A.J. (1969) Quadriceps strain, rupture and charlie horse. *Med. Sci. Sports* **1**, 106–11.

Sandelin, J. (1988) *Acute sports injuries. A clinical and epidemiological study.* Thesis, University of Helsinki, Finland.

Safran, M.R., Garrett Jr, W.E., Seaber, A.V., Glisson, R.R. & Ribbeck, B.M. (1988) The role of warm-up in muscular injury prevention. *Am. J. Sports Med.* **16**, 123–9.

Safran, M.R., Seaber, A.V. & Garrett Jr, W.E. (1989) Warm-up and muscular injury prevention. An update. *Sports Med.* **8**, 239–49.

Snow, M.H. (1973) Metabolic activity during the degenerative and early regenerative stages on skeletal muscle. *Anat. Rec.* **176**, 185–204.

Thorsson, O., Hemdal, B., Lilja, B. & Westlin, N. (1987) The effect of external pressure on intramuscular blood flow at rest and after running. *Med. Sci. Sports Exerc.* **19**, 469–73.

Woodard, C. (1954) What is active treatment? In C. Woodard (ed) *Sports Injuries*, pp. 1–14. Max Parrish & Co, London.

Zarins, B. & Ciullo, J.V. (1983) Acute muscle and tendon injuries in athletes. *Clin. Sports Med.* **2**, 167–82.

Chapter 9

Traumatic Knee Injuries

KEN W. MOORE AND CYRIL B. FRANK

In a 1980 study, conducted in the USA, injuries to the knee and ankle accounted for 25% of all injuries and 35% of all health costs (Pritchett, 1980). Also in the USA, the annual number of knee injuries caused by skiing in 1982 was found to be 120 000 (Pope, 1982). The number caused by American football was estimated at between 100 000 and 130 000 (Torg & Quendenfeld, 1974). That year, knee injuries were declared a national health problem (Torg & Quedenfeld, 1974). These statistics, as well as knowledge that the incidence of knee injuries appears to be increasing, have spurred medical and sport officials to look for optimal preventive measures.

The incidence of traumatic knee injuries in certain sports is extremely high. Howe and Johnson (1982), for example, examined the incidence of ski injuries in Vermont from 1972 to 1981 and found 27.8% were to ligaments of the knee. Others have found that this incidence ranges from 20 to 24.7% (Moritz, 1959; Ellison *et al.*, 1962; Haddon *et al.*, 1962; Gutman *et al.*, 1974; Young *et al.*, 1976; Tapper, 1978; Edlund *et al.*, 1980; Johnson *et al.*, 1982). In American football, five high school studies found that the knee represented 12.7–36.5% of the injuries (Pritchett, 1980, 12.7%; Hale & Mitchell, 1981, 13%; Moretz *et al.*, 1978, 22%; Olson, 1979, 36.5%; Culpepper & Niemann, 1983, 22.2%). In racquet sports (squash and racquetball) knees can represent up to 55% of all injuries (Marans *et al.*, 1988). Eriksson (1976), reported that in Sweden the sports which had the greatest number of knee injuries were skiing and soccer. As a percentage of total injuries in four soccer studies, knee injuries ranged from 12 to 20% (Nilsson & Roaas, 1978, 14%; Sullivan *et al.*, 1980, 12%; Ekstrand, 1982, 20%; Albert, 1983, 18%). This rate is lower than American football but since soccer is the most popular sport in the world, with over 22 million participants annually (Keller *et al.*, 1987), the total number of knee injuries attributable to soccer worldwide are probably higher than any other sport. If only 1% of soccer players were injured, this would represent over 200 000 injuries per year.

These rather dramatic statistics clearly emphasize the need for a better understanding of exactly why and where knee injuries occur, and how they can be prevented. In this chapter we will endeavour to classify different types of injuries, identify a number of 'risk factors' which appear to contribute to their prevalence, and thereby propose a number of areas in which knee injury prevention can be focused.

Injury mechanisms

While any structure in or around the knee can be injured, ligament injuries appear to be particularly common and unusually debilitating for an athlete. We will therefore concentrate our review primarily on the causes, assessment and prevention of ligamentous knee injuries, keeping in mind that many of the principles which we discuss are also likely applicable to other injuries.

Biomechanical aspects

In order to assess possible preventative measures for knee ligament injuries, an awareness of the mechanisms by which they are caused is essential. The directions and magnitudes of the forces involved and their effect on the structures of the knee can lend some understanding to possible preventative measures. A knowledge of knee anatomy and biomechanics is also essential. It is beyond the scope of this chapter to review these matters in detail, as they are covered elsewhere in this book, but we will present at least an overview which provides some baseline information.

The knee consists of two distinct joints, (i) the patellofemoral; and (ii) the tibiofemoral joint. The former is the articulation between the patella and femur while the latter is the articulation between the tibia and the femur. While both can be injured, it is really the tibiofemoral joint which is damaged in most cases. The dual function of stability and mobility which is demanded of this joint are normally met by the complex interaction of the ligaments, capsule, cartilage and bones. It is this interaction which is destroyed by damage to any or all of the components, but particularly by damage to one of the four major ligaments: (i) the medial collateral ligament (MCL); (ii) the lateral collateral ligament (LCL); (iii) the posterior cruciate ligament (PCL); and (iv) the anterior cruciate ligament (ACL) (Fig. 9.1).

Any of these four ligaments can be damaged by a combination of extrinsic and intrinsic forces. These forces can be generated by either external agents (such as contact with another player, or a post, which we classify as 'contact injuries'), or purely by forces generated by the individual himself or herself (e.g. a sudden twist to avoid contact or simply a sudden violent muscle contraction itself). These we will classify as 'non-contact injuries'. The mechanisms of both contact and non-contact injuries will be reviewed separately.

Contact injuries

Contact injuries are the result of an external force directed at or near the knee. The position of the knee, the direction of the force, its magnitude and its point of application will determine which knee structures will be injured. These factors, plus the stiffnesses and strengths of the

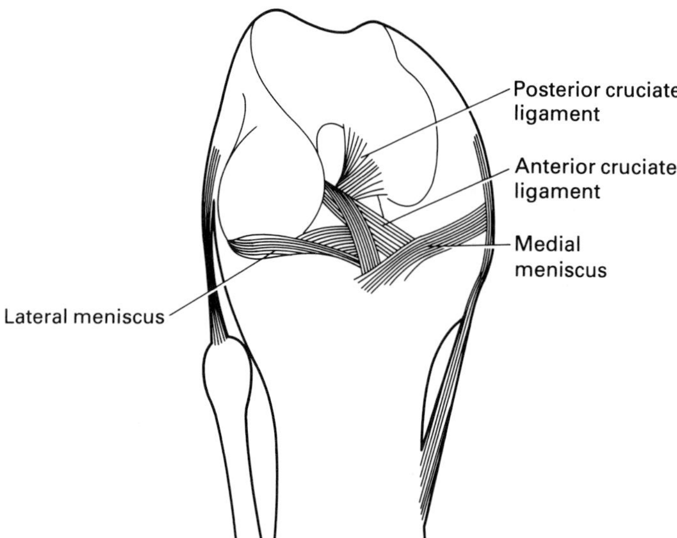

Fig. 9.1 Schematic representation of the four knee ligaments viewed from the front with the knee flexed and the patella removed.

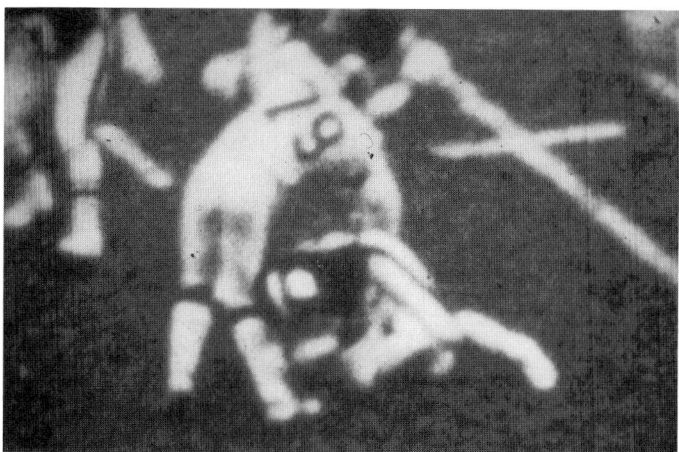

Fig. 9.2 Valgus injury to a football player. Courtesy of Dr R. Jackson.

tissues involved, will determine how much damage will occur to structures in and around the joint. Particular mechanisms, however, are associated with damage to particular structures.

One of the most common knee injuries is a tear of the MCL. This is typically caused by a valgus force (that is, a force applied to the lateral side of the leg) when an athlete has his or her foot fixed to the ground and the knee is at or near full extension (Fig. 9.2). This force causes tension in the MCL as the distance between the femur and the tibia on the medial side is forced to increase. With greater forces, other tissues begin to fail. The MCL and medial capsule are the first structures to tear, followed by the ACL, and possibly the medial meniscus. If the knee is almost fully extended, there is also a possibility of tearing the PCL instead of, or along with, the ACL.

A varus force (that is a force which is applied to the medial side of the knee) is far less common because the medial side of the knee is protected to some degree by the opposite leg. However, if a varus force does occur, the results can be similar, but opposite, to a valgus blow. The LCL and the lateral capsular restraints plus the cruciates may be damaged by this type of blow (Fig. 9.3).

The ACL can therefore be damaged in combination with other ligaments, but it can also be torn almost in complete isolation. This could happen theoretically when an anteriorly directed force contacts the tibia and causes it to move forward in relation to the femur, such as when an athlete is being tackled or hit from behind at the knees. The ACL can also be

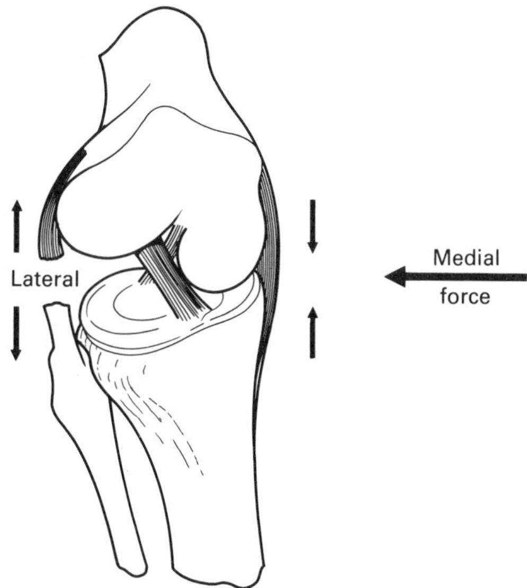

Fig. 9.3 Schematic representation of the relatively rare situation in which lateral structures (lateral cruciate ligament) will fail in tension from a so-called varus injury to the knee. The anterior cruciate ligament will be the next structure damaged if the lateral opening continues, particularly if there is any rotation superimposed.

damaged with forced hyperextension of a knee such as when a knee is bent backwards.

Injury to the PCL can occur with hyperextension or simply when a posteriorly directed force contacts the tibia, such as that which can occur when the knee is driven backwards or when it contacts the ground very hard while bent at 90°.

Non-contact injuries

Non-contact injuries to knee ligaments are also very common in sports. They occur when an athlete is changing directions such as in football, Rugby, soccer, basketball or skiing, when there is usually a combination of quadriceps deceleration, valgus and external rotation forces on a slightly flexed knee (Zarins & Nemeth, 1985). The athlete often hears a 'pop' and the knee feels as if it has momentarily 'gone out of place', due to failure of one or more ligaments. In fact, this is probably the most common mechanism of 'isolated' ACL disruption in sports. In skiing it can occur with either internal or external rotation (Feagin & Lambert, 1985). A second mechanism by which the ACL can be injured without any external contact occurs when a skier suffers a sudden internal rotation of the hyperflexed knee (Johnson, 1988). A third occurs when a skier with such a flexed knee begins to fall backwards and compensates with a large stabilizing quadriceps contraction (Hauser & Schaff, 1987). Secondary failure forces in the ACL apparently develop during such a quadriceps contraction since ski bindings do not typically release from this direction of force. Finally, the cruciates can be damaged by a non-contact hyperextension, such as that which can occur if an athlete steps into a hole, or lands under poor control from a jump.

Even this brief review suggests that there are numerous mechanisms which can cause injuries to knee ligaments and thus many mechanisms which would have to be prevented to stop them. Some would appear to be easier to prevent than others but, as will become apparent in subsequent sections, virtually none are totally preventable except perhaps by total avoidance of high-risk sports.

Risk factors

Intrinsic factors

Many intrinsic factors (factors which are inherent to the athlete) are key elements in the prevention of the mechanisms of knee injury noted above. While such factors are difficult to quantify, their importance should nonetheless be stressed since they clearly do influence both the incidence and likely the severity of many types of injuries.

PHYSICAL CONDITION

Conditioning of an athlete clearly plays a major role in the prevention of injuries. Feagin *et al.* (1987) noted a 'biphasic' pattern of injury risk after 2 or more hours of skiing. They found that injuries often happen just before lunch, or late in the day, often 'on the run which was going to be their last'. Young *et al.* (1976) similarly demonstrated that injury rates increase late in the ski day and also targeted fatigue as a major contributing factor. Karlsson *et al.* (1978) found a considerable loss of strength associated with fatigue and the glycolytic response to exercise. Eriksson (1976) performed muscle biopsies on skiers throughout the day and found up to 75% of the glycogen stores had been used by the end of it, indicating significant muscle fatigue. The inexperienced skier, when fatigued in this way, will usually be unable to use more thigh muscle force to maintain their balance so they attempt to relax their quadriceps by increased knee extension and increased hip flexion. Unfortunately, this position places the skier at higher risk due to decreasing the mechanical advantage of the quadriceps and preventing hip rotation. If the tibia is then forcibly rotated, injuries to the ligaments (e.g. ACL) can occur.

Skiers in particular should be aware that

endurance conditioning is a very important preventative measure. Endurance training by running, cycling or cross-country skiing, therefore, has been suggested by many authors to increase conditioning levels for that sport in particular.

While many other sports do not exhibit the clear relationship between injury potential and fatigue seen in skiing, some suggestions have been made that conditioning does decrease injury rates in other sports as well. For example, Cahill and Griffith, in a 1978 study, compared the effect of a preseason conditioning programme on the knee/ankle injury rates for American high-school football players and found that the incidence of injury declined from 6.8% (1969–1972) to 4.1% (1973–1976).

FLEXIBILITY, COORDINATION AND PROPRIOCEPTION

Other intrinsic qualities of an athlete which may decrease their chances of an injury are increased flexibility, coordination and proprioception. Just as greater muscle strength and endurance can help to counteract some potentially damaging forces, it seems likely that increased flexibility, body control, and position sense can also enable the knee to either avoid those forces or to absorb them. Any means of improving these qualities would therefore be a relatively simple means of prevention.

MUSCLE BALANCE

Muscle balance, or really correction of any 'imbalance' (i.e. abnormal ratios of flexors versus extensors) has been proposed as another factor in potentially limiting knee injuries. The balance between hamstring strength and quadriceps strength may affect joint positions or joint forces, and thus create situations in which certain structures are at risk. Feagin and Lambert (1985) for example, have speculated that there may be a predisposition to cruciate ligament injury in the athlete whose hamstrings are deficient. However, Grace *et al*. (1984) found no statistical difference between a group of uninjured athletes and a group of injured athletes for 10 different measures of muscle imbalance. They actually found a trend in nine of the measures for the non-injured athletes to have more imbalance. Ekstrand and Gillquist (1982) on the other hand found a significant effect of pre-existing quadriceps weakness in non-contact injuries. However, they also stated that a large number of the athletes who sustained these injuries also had ligamentous laxity caused by previous knee injuries. Knapik *et al*. (1991) also found an apparent relationship between muscle imbalance and increased lower extremity injuries. In that series, athletes experienced more injuries if they had knee flexor or hip extensor imbalances of 15% or more. While not exactly clear cut, there is at least some evidence to suggest that appropriate 'muscle balancing' may have at least some preventive value.

JOINT STABILITY

There is some data to suggest that unstable knee joints are more prone to injury than normal knees (Ekstrand & Gillquist, 1982). This is obviously true in post-traumatic unilateral instabilities where one knee has been rendered more unstable than the other by a previous injury. However, both knee joints may also be 'unstable' (as compared with so-called 'normals') due to congenital factors, and it is much less clear if such joints are actually predisposed to injuries or not. Nicholas (1970), for example, concluded that professional American football players with 'increased joint laxity' are more prone to suffer knee injuries. Glick (1971), however, found no difference in the frequency of knee injuries sustained by college football players with 'loose' or 'tight' joints. Johnson *et al*. (1979) on the other hand found that women usually have more laxity in their knee joints, and therefore are more prone to MCL sprains than men. They also found individuals with tighter ligaments sustained more grade III MCL sprains. Klein (1974) also associated a high incidence of knee injuries among high-school football players with increased ligament flexibility due to pubertal growth patterns.

Collectively, though, it can be said that studies which have addressed the relationship between joint laxity and the risk of injury have not been able to find a definitive relationship. They do suggest, that there may be some optimal range of laxity which provides the least risk of injury in certain ages or in a certain gender. At this point in time, though, this remains unknown.

OTHER FACTORS

In some sports, it appears that the potential for serious knee injury may increase with age. Keller *et al.* (1987) presented evidence showing that soccer injury rates increase with age. Senior and professional athletes were 15–30 times as likely to sustain injuries than youths. Goldberg *et al.* (1984) also found similar results in American football where the injury rate steadily increased in junior football from ages 13 to 17. Johnson *et al.* (1980) had somewhat contradictory results, concluding that younger skiers are prone to more injuries than the older skier. Similar to others, however, they found that older skiers had more severe injuries. While some of these effects may truly be due to aging of tissues, some could also be attributed to increases in the intensity of sports with maturation.

As with aging, some injury differences have also been shown between genders. In the study by Keller *et al.* (1987), female youths sustained twice as many injuries as their male counterparts. Johnson *et al.* (1980) similarly pointed out that female skiers seemed to have more injuries to the lower extremity than males and that they were predisposed to more grade I MCL injuries (Johnson *et al.*, 1979). As with aging, it is difficult to relate injuries to the gender of the athlete alone, but these trends are certainly suspicious.

SUMMARY AND RECOMMENDATIONS

While some factors which we have listed obviously cannot be controlled (e.g. aging, gender), some presumably can. In particular, training can improve the strength, power, muscle balance, endurance and flexibility of the athlete. Coordination and proprioception likely can be improved by the repetition of specific drills. We therefore suspect that implementation of appropriate training programmes can therefore be useful in preventing injuries.

Acquired factors

In addition to the eight so-called intrinsic factors noted above, there are a number of other risk factors which are 'acquired' throughout an athlete's career which may also affect their potential of suffering a knee injury.

EXPERIENCE, TECHNIQUE AND SKILL

There is very little technical or scientific information concerning how experience, technique and skill influence an athlete's risk of injury. In skiing, Johnson *et al.* (1980) found that experienced skiers are less prone to injuries than inexperienced skiers. In Canadian football, Jackson *et al.* (1991) found athletes in their first 2 years to have 5.8 times the number of injuries than players with more than 2 years of professional experience. Experienced athletes seem to be less prone to injury since their techniques are likely more advanced, giving them greater control of their body position and helping them avoid situations where injuries are more probable. While this logic is intuitively appealing, it of course remains speculative.

PLAYING POSITION

Some sports have playing positions which are more susceptible to injury than others. For example, in American football it has been shown that players who play along the offensive line, defensive line and linebackers are more prone to injuries than other positions (Stitler *et al.*, 1990; Jackson *et al.*, 1991). In soccer, two studies (McMaster & Walter, 1978; Ekstrand & Gillquist, 1983) found no difference between the injury rate for any positions except for the goaltender (who had a lower rate). However, in a different study of young soccer players (Sullivan *et al.*, 1980) the goaltenders had an increased rate of injury. Since positions cannot simply be avoided to prevent injuries, preventive measures should instead be focused at other risk areas.

COACHING

Coaching is a relatively abstract factor which likely influences many of the variables already addressed in this chapter, as well as a few more. There are very few people who have more influence over an athlete than the coach. An athlete's coaching will influence the athlete's physical condition and the development of his or her skill level. Unfortunately, a large variety of coaching methods are used for conditioning and skill development, making it difficult to assess their impact in any scientific way.

One of the few ways in which clear effects of coaching on injury rates have been documented are in varying amounts of contact which coaches plan in American football practices. Mueller and Blyth (1974) examined the difference in injury rates between regular football practices (48.8%) and practices which had limited contact (41.7%). They also found dramatic differences in the injury rate between different football drills. Practice games provided injury rates which were over twice as large as the worst drill. Cahill and Griffith (1979) found similar results. A number of studies have also, not surprisingly, found that there is a dramatic increase in the number of injuries in game situations compared to practice situations (Mueller & Blyth, 1974; Moretz *et al.*, 1978; Cahill & Griffith, 1979; Jackson *et al.*, 1991). Again, coaches can control intensity of practices, drills and games, thereby indirectly controlling relative injury exposure rates. A coach who insists on having continual full contact drills and scrimmaging will almost certainly be subjecting the players to an increased chance of injury.

Another preventative measure that coaches can control is the players regard for the rules. Many rules have been instituted to help protect a player's knees, however, coaches can certainly influence their priority and implementation.

SUMMARY AND RECOMMENDATIONS

In the area of acquired factors, prevention therefore involves both the athlete and the coach emphasizing practices which decrease the injury potential of the athlete. Coaches also need to assist the players in developing the proper techniques and observation of rules which will minimize the athlete's potential for injury.

Extrinsic factors

We define extrinsic factors as those which are completely external to the athlete. They are therefore factors over which both athletes and coaches actually have the least control. These relate to the surfaces, rules, equipment and loads which occur during their sport.

SHOE–SURFACE INTERFACE

One extrinsic factor which influences leg injuries in running sports is the shoe–surface interface. An important component of the mechanism of any knee injury is the relative fixation of the foot to the ground. The choice of footwear, the type of playing surface and the playing conditions may clearly affect the incidence or severity of the knee injuries via their effects on this fixation. While many athletes generally attempt to attain maximal foot grip, there is some evidence in American football that combinations of the shoe and surface creating the highest frictional properties seem to result in the greatest number of injuries (Nigg & Segesser, 1988). In 1971, Torg and Quedenfeld compared the frequency and severity of knee injuries for American high-school football players wearing conventional football shoes (with seven 19-mm cleats) and a soccer-type shoe (14 9.5-mm cleats). They found a greater frequency and severity of injuries in the group wearing the conventional shoe and postulated that the shoe which contains longer cleats causes the foot to become more fixed to the ground.

Optimizing frictional behaviour to allow reasonable performance without destructive forces being allowed to develop would thus be ideal in minimizing the number of injuries. This could be achieved by modifying either the shoes or the surfaces to allow 'just the right amount of slip'.

Mueller and Blyth (1974) compared injury rates on American football fields which had been completely resurfaced with those fields which were not resurfaced and found 30% lower rates on resurfaced fields. They therefore concluded that the condition and upkeep of fields is very important and can dramatically affect the injury potential on the field. Poor field conditions have also been assessed as contributing to injuries in two soccer studies (Sullivan *et al.*, 1980; Ekstrand & Gillquist, 1983) in which conditions were judged to contribute to 25% of all injuries.

There have been a number of studies which have compared the injury rates on artificial turf (Morehouse & Morrison, 1975) to the rate on natural grass. Nigg and Segesser (1988) compiled numerous studies from American football and found that for knee and ankle injuries, 41 seasons worth of data showed that artificial turf caused more injuries than grass, 45 seasons showed approximately the same number of injuries, and 14 seasons showed more injuries on grass. Skovron *et al.* (1990) also concluded from a major review that play on artificial turf presented a higher relative risk of injury to the knee and lower extremities in general. Jackson *et al.* (1991) on the other hand found 50% more injuries for a professional football team on natural grass compared to artificial turf over 12 years. Collectively, however, these studies generally appear to at least partially condemn artificial turf as having higher injury rates in football. This is not clear cut, though, and requires ongoing investigation.

RULES

Many sport governing bodies have tried to make revisions in their rules in an attempt to decrease the number of knee injuries to their participants. American football is probably the best example of a sport which has continually attempted to change its rules to limit injuries (e.g. elimination of blocking below the waist and clipping).

EQUIPMENT

Much of the sports equipment of the 1990s is devised to limit injuries. The knee, however, is difficult to protect. It has a great range of motion and with its 6° of freedom its movement during athletics is nearly unlimited. It can, however, be at least partly protected either indirectly by equipment modifications — such as through shoes, boots, bindings or skis — or directly, such as through attempted bracing or taping.

Ski bindings and boots

The development of modern equipment has had a large impact on the number of injuries which occur in skiing. Injuries to the foot and ankle have decreased significantly likely since the modern ski boot totally encapsulates the ankle and foot like a protective cast. However, knee injuries in skiing remain high and still represent around 20% of all injuries in that sport.

Mote (1987) examined the forces which are involved in skiing and found that even during normal skiing, forces which are transmitted through the knee are capable of injuring it. He also stated that even proper use of bindings permits forces of sufficient magnitude to cause injuries, since mechanical release bindings cannot be set below an injury force threshold which will still permit skiing. Bindings are, by definition, therefore, set at a point known to be above where the athlete can ski safely.

Bouter *et al.* (1989) supported these findings that bindings are often set too high by documenting that bindings often did not release when a knee injury occurred (males 38%, females 54%). A German study (Hauser, 1989), though, suggested that more than 50% of bindings were just badly adjusted and that the incidence of lower extremity equipment-related injuries was 3.5 times less for a group of skiers who had their bindings adjusted 'optimally'.

Further research is still needed to develop a binding system which is responsive to the actual forces and moments which will affect the knee (Maxwell & Hull, 1989). The optimal release forces should be evaluated to determine how the bindings should be adjusted and should account for variable muscular forces which are used to counteract the skiing forces. If such a system were available, at least some ski-induced knee injuries could be prevented.

Knee braces and taping

The use of adhesive strapping in sport has been used to attempt to prevent injuries, and to facilitate safe controlled use of a knee during rehabilitation. However, the only demonstrable effect of such taping has been to limit joint range (McLean, 1989). It is unknown whether such minimal restrictions actually decreases knee injuries or not.

A second common method of attempting to reduce knee injuries has been the use of knee braces. There are two types of braces which are currently used — the 'prophylactic brace' and the 'functional brace'. Each will be reviewed separately.

Prophylactic bracing. A prophylactic brace is worn on healthy knees in an attempt to prevent or reduce the severity of any injuries to them. This type of brace was first developed by Anderson (Anderson *et al.*, 1979) to reduce injuries to the MCL caused by valgus impact forces, so it typically consists of upright supports which connect the thigh and calf padded shells to a hinge in the centre (Fig. 9.4).

The arguments that such a brace should reduce the damaging strains on the medial side of the knee, plus some testimonials, social pressures and aggressive marketing by brace companies resulted in a dramatic increase in the use of these braces, including their mandatory use by some college and professional football teams in the 1980s. However, scientific evidence for their efficacy was lacking, prompting many recent longitudinal studies (Table 9.1). Of the 16 recent studies which we could find, 10 concluded that the braces were effective, five that the braces were either harmful or had no effect, and one concluded that more work had to be done to address the question.

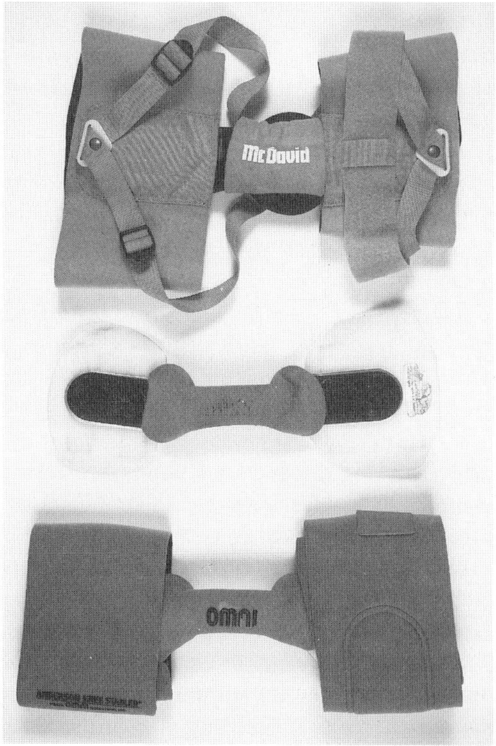

Fig. 9.4 Three examples of prophylactic knee braces which are available commercially.

Table 9.1 Summary of longitudinal clinical studies analysing prophylactic bracing.

Year	Authors	Time period	Subjects	Results	Conclusion
1979	Anderson *et al.*	1 year	9 pro FB players	WB no injuries	Effective
1984	Randall *et al.*	7 years	Iowa State FB	Fewer injuries, fewer surgeries	Effective
1985	Hansen *et al.*	4 years	USC FB	WB 5% injured, NB 11% injured	Effective
1985	McKelvie	2 years	10 NCAA FB teams	WB 50% decrease in injuries	Effective
1985	Moser	1 year	24 NCAA FB teams	—	Effective
1985	Schriner	1 year	25 HS FB	WB no injuries, NB 4.1% injuries	Effective
1985	Taft *et al.*	7 years	NC FB	Same no. of injuries, 70% less surgeries	Effective
1986	Curran *et al.*	1 year	78 NCAA FB teams	30 teams — fewer injuries, 2 teams — more injuries	Effective
1986	Hewson *et al.*	8 years	Arizona FB	No difference	No effect
1987	Garrick & Requa		[Analysis of six longitudinal studies]		Undeclared
1987	Rovere *et al.*	4 years	Wake Forrest FB	WB 7.5% injuries, NB 6.1% injuries	Increased injuries
1987	Teitz *et al.*	2 years	132 NCAA FB teams	—	No effect or harmful
1988	Grace *et al.*	1 year	Albuquerque HS FB	WB more injuries	Increased injuries
1990	Stitler *et al.*	2 years	West Point intramural FB	Fewer injuries	Effective
1990	Zemper	2 years	30 College FB teams	No change	No effect
1991	Jackson *et al.*	12 years	1 Pro FB team	WB 33% fewer injuries	Effective

FB, football; HS, high school; NB, no brace; NC, North Carolina; NCAA, National Collegiate Athletic Association; USC, University of Southern California; WB, wearing brace.

In analysing these studies, a number of uncontrolled variables were identified, including: (i) differences in playing surfaces; (ii) athletic shoes; (iii) knee injury history; (iv) application of braces; (v) brace assignment; (vi) athletic exposure; (vii) yearly injury fluctuations; (viii) changes in rules or coaches during the duration of the study; and (ix) changes in the assessment or management of injuries. The study which controlled at least five of these factors was performed by Stitler, at West Point (Stitler *et al.*, 1990), in which 1396 cadets were studied during the period 1986–1987 intramural football season. Results suggested that these braces significantly reduced the number of injuries, but not their severity; perhaps implying that braces worked better in some people than others, and that prophylactic braces likey do not have much of a mechanical effect, particularly at higher loads.

Interestingly, several recent biomechanical studies support the speculation that prophylactic braces provide little or no actual mechanical protection to the knee (Table 9.2). Baker *et al.*

Table 9.2 Results of biomechanical studies investigating prophylactic bracing.

Year	Authors	Methods	Results	Conclusion
1986	Paulos *et al.*	Valgus forces applied to braced cadaver knee and brace	Braces much less still than knee; no effect on joint force opening or ligament tension	Braces do not protect knee from valgus forces
1987	Baker *et al.*	Fixed foot, abduction, external rotation	Brace did not reduce stresses in knee	Braces not effective
1987	France *et al.*	Surrogate knee was used to evaluate six brace types	Brace was ineffective when knee was at more than 30° flexion or if unconstrained	Only one brace safe; brace best for high-mass, low-velocity forces
1987	Paulos *et al.*	Valgus forces applied to cadaver knee	Braces not effective in protecting MCL at low rate valgus forces	Braces ineffective
1989	Baker *et al.*	Valgus force supplied to cadaver knee	Some protection to the MCL at full extension but very little with added flexion or rotation	Braces provide limited protection
1989	Paulos *et al.*	Lateral impact forces applied to surrogate knee	Braces decreased the peak ACL force more than the peak MCL force	Braces that increase the time of impact protect ACL
1991	Daley *et al.*	Used surrogate knee to test different brace parameters	Best brace design had thickest and longest uprights and the longest hinges	—
1991	Erickson *et al.*	Measured the decrease in strain in the MCL with braces	Found impact forces to be 50% lower but strain to be only slightly lower	Braces act as shock absorbers
1988	France *et al.*	[Developed a surrogate model of the knee to test braces]		
1988	Van Hoeck *et al.*	[Developed a surrogate model of the knee to test braces]		

ACL, anterior collateral ligament; MCL, medial collateral ligament.

(1987, 1989) simulated injuries caused by two mechanisms: (i) a rotational force with the foot flexed; and (ii) a valgus load with the foot fixed, and found that braces were totally ineffective against the rotational forces, and were only somewhat successful in limiting valgus forces at full knee extension. France *et al.* (1987) used a surrogate knee also to determine that these braces were effective only at less than 30° of flexion. Paulos *et al.* (1987) likewise found that such braces afford some protection to valgus forces at those angles. Erickson *et al.* (1991), however, used a strain transducer to determine the MCL strain during valgus force and found only minimal decreases in strain in the ligaments of braced knees. On the other hand, using a surrogate knee, Paulos *et al.* (1989) found that peak ACL force decreased more than the peak MCL force when braces were applied, suggesting that perhaps braces are more effective for some ligaments than others.

Despite some optimistic signs, these mechanical studies collectively indicate that the current prophylactic brace designs are likely inadequate in protecting the knee. However, when combined with the longitudinal studies, which seem to indicate that they have some value, it is clear that some controversy about their use remains. More research is necessary to try to determine exactly what these braces do, and to develop braces which are able to provide more protection.

Functional braces. The second type of brace is the so-called functional knee brace, first designed by Castiglia in 1972 (Nicholas, 1983). These braces are designed to control ligament deficiencies in patients with unstable joints, thus preventing further injury. In particular, they attempt to limit extension, decrease anterior tibial translation and prevent excess anterolateral tibial rotation in the ACL-deficient patient or to prevent varus or valgus forces in collateral deficiencies. Such braces consist of a combination of rigid bar supports, soft tissue confinement shells, derotation straps and various hinge designs (Fig. 9.5).

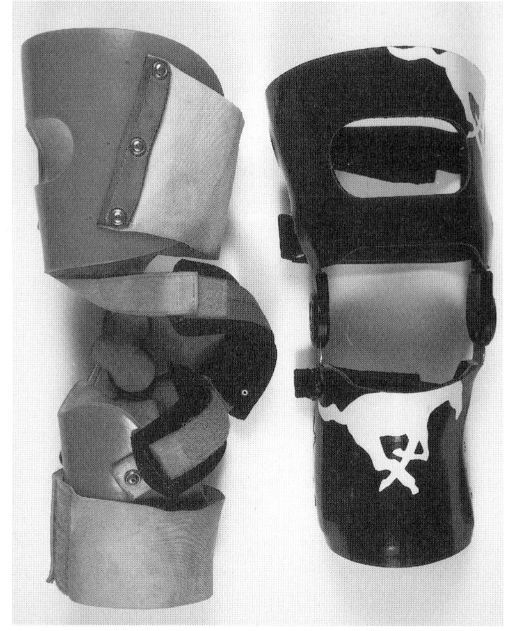

Fig. 9.5 Examples of two commercially available 'functional' or 'therapeutic' knee braces.

Biomechanical tests of functional braces suggest that they are effective in partially protecting knee ligaments but that the different brace designs exhibit a great variance in their effectiveness (Table 9.3). Baker *et al.* (1987), Carlson and French (1989) and Regalbuto *et al.* (1989) all indicate that the design (length of struts, soft tissue confinement, hinge type and hinge position) is very important in determining brace performance. Wojtys *et al.* (1990) found that braces reduce anteroposterior translation (20.5%) and rotation (12.5%) of the tibia. Other authors have similarly found that these braces limit these movements (Colville *et al.*, 1986; Baker *et al.*, 1987, 1989; Mishra *et al.*, 1988; Zogby *et al.*, 1989) but some indicate that as the load increases, the effectiveness of the brace diminishes (Beck *et al.*, 1986; Mortensen *et al.*,

Table 9.3 Biomechanical studies of functional knee braces.

Year	Authors	Methods	Results	Conclusion
1986	Beck *et al.*	Compared ability to control anterior tibial translation	Braces decreased translation but amount varied depending on brace design and force level	Greater forces decreased brace effectiveness, large variance between braces
1986	Colville *et al.*	Studied laxity in ACL-deficient subjects with and without a brace	Brace decreased rotary instability and resistance to displacement. No effect on maximal subluxation of tibia	91% of patients were pleased with the braces

Table 9.3 *Continued.*

Year	Authors	Methods	Results	Conclusion
1987	Arms *et al.*	Strain transducers were applied to AM band of ACL	Braces increased strain by 1–2% but did not reduce strain in ACL during an anterior tibial load	Preload not significant, not effective in reducing strain due to anterior loads
1987	Baker *et al.*	Evaluated braces to determine if they could provide medial stability	With fixed foot, abduction and external rotation the braces did protect the MCL	Best braces had a combo of double upright supports, crossed struts and rigid soft tissue confinement
1987	Coughlin *et al.*	Compared effect of braces on return to activity after ACL injury	Ability to return influenced most by injury severity	Knee brace use assisted in return to participation
1988	Mishra *et al.*	Compared brace effectiveness in ACL-deficient knees and normals	Reduced knee flexion ROM, pivot shift grade and mean laxity	Different brace types performed very differently
1988	Mortensen *et al.*	Movement in ACL-deficient cadaver knees was tested in knee braces	Reduction in AP laxity; depends on force and brace type. No effect or over constraint in rotations	Braces control AP translation of tibia, but effectiveness decreases at higher loads
1989	Baker *et al.*	Lateral impact force on knee of cadaver with fixed foot	Braces were able to limit abduction and rotation in MCL	Braces were effective in reducing stresses from these forces
1989	Carlson & French	Compared brace ability to protect knee from valgus force	8-fold difference in different braces ability to protect knee	Brace length and rigidity must both be proper for braces to be effective
1989	Lunsford *et al.*	Compared eight braces in response to valgus, varus and rotational forces	Braces varied in their ability to control these forces	Effectiveness of braces is extremely variable
1989	Regalbuto *et al.*	Compared hinge designs and forces which occur in brace	Forces depend on flexion angle, forces varied with hinge placement	Position of hinge is more important than hinge design
1989	Zogby *et al.*	Compared brace performance in ACL-deficient knees during tibial anterior displacement	Found significant differences in performance between different brace designs	Significant differences between braces
1990	Beynnon *et al.*	Measured strain in the ACL (i) at 30° with anterior shear; (ii) during flexion	Brace reduced strain during anterior shear, difference in strain during flexion ROM	Braces are somewhat effective
1990	Wojtys *et al.*	Compared brace types ability to control tibial rotation and translation	Braces decrease AP translation 20.5%, decrease rotation 12.5%, more effective at 30° than 60° of flexion	Functional braces are effective but very variable between designs

ACL, anterior cruciate ligament; AM, anteromedial; AP, anteroposterior; MCL, medial collateral ligament; ROM, range of motion.

1988). Arms *et al.* (1987), in an *in vitro* study, found functional bracing to have little ability to decrease strain during extrinsic anterior tibial loads. Beynnon *et al.* (1990), in an *in vivo* study, however, found some strain decrease during anterior shear tests. They also examined the bracing effect on ACL strain through normal knee extension–flexion and found that such strain was not altered.

Collectively these studies do show some effects of functional braces on at least partly limiting bony displacements and/or ligament strains at the knee. Their effectiveness, however, is probably limited at higher loads (at least, *in vitro*). Their true effectiveness in the clinical situation, of course, remains unknown.

SUMMARY AND RECOMMENDATIONS

The knee is a very difficult joint to protect. Prophylactic braces may have some benefits but, as most researchers conclude, 'they cannot be recommended at this time'. Future research into designs and materials may change this recommendation. Functional braces, on the other hand, have been shown to decrease bony displacements in unstable knees at low loads, and thus do appear to at least partly protect the knee from reinjury. Further improvements in functional knee bracing may also allow more athletes with ligament-deficient knees to participate more safely in all sports. Continued research in the design of knee braces and all sports equipment is essential in order to decrease the number of knee injuries which now occur.

Previous injuries

The final category of risk factors that we will discuss refers to people who, for a variety of reasons, have already sustained some injury. They are therefore, by definition, at risk to reinjure themselves. Certain measures can be taken to minimize the risk and these will be discussed briefly below.

APPROPRIATE DIAGNOSIS OF KNEE INJURIES

An important element in the prevention of traumatic knee injuries is their early and accurate diagnosis. While a large number of injuries are clearly 'primary' (i.e. no previous history of an injury), many are also 'secondary' (i.e. in people having had a previous injury which was either not assessed, assessed inadequately and/or not treated to prevent recurrence). While accurate diagnosis and thorough treatment does not guarantee that a new traumatic episode will not occur, common sense dictates that such intervention should have important preventive value. For that reason we will review briefly how ligamentous injuries of the knee are assessed.

Without question, the Lachman test for ACL injury (Torg *et al.*, 1976) is the single most important physical examination test in assessing a ligament-injured knee. Despite its broad use and obvious value, there are unfortunately still some physicians and/or therapists who do not appreciate its subtleties or its importance in determining if an athlete's knee is functionally stable or not. This creates situations in which athletes still return to competition prematurely — facing a strong likelihood of reinjury. This situation should be almost completely preventable if trainers, therapists and physicians make a point of erring on the side of conservatism if any doubt exists — asking for further examinations to determine whether or not some instability exists.

In order to perform an appropriate Lachman test, readers should review relevant articles on the subject (Torg *et al.*, 1976; Frank, 1986), and practice the test extensively. Subjective impressions of abnormal anterior tibial translation, either by a detection of 'a soft endpoint', or by more definite tibial displacement (as compared with a normal knee) should alert the medical team to a possible problem (Fig. 9.6). *Any* side-to-side difference in this test should be interpreted as positive until proven otherwise and patients appropriately coun-

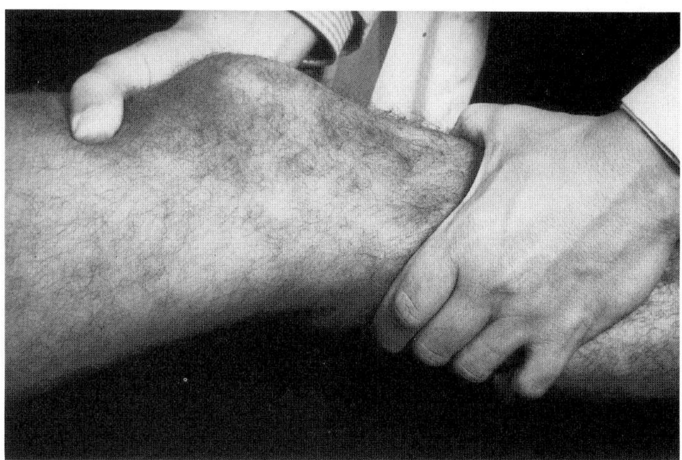

Fig. 9.6 A Lachman test of the left knee. Hand positions and force directions are critical in performing an appropriate test. Any side-to-side difference is interpreted as a positive test until proven otherwise.

selled and protected before returning to activity. Therapy and bracing may be able to prevent a recurrence in which irreparable damage may be done.

Other ligament tests are also obviously of benefit in diagnosing ligament injuries, and they *too* must be practised to be useful (Hughston *et al.*, 1976). The variety of tests for anterolateral rotatory instability (Losee *et al.*, 1978; Galway & MacIntosh, 1980; Larson, 1983) can also reveal an ACL injury if performed in an appropriate way on a compliant, relaxed patient. These tests, though, can be masked by muscle forces and are therefore subject to misinterpretation.

It should suffice to say that all tests for both collateral and cruciate ligaments are important in revealing all aspects of a potential knee instability. If physical examination tests are equivocal, then further investigations are warranted, including repeat examinations, examinations by radiological means (magnetic resonance imaging), examination under anaesthesia and arthroscopy. Prevention of injury recurrence demands a thorough investigation and optimal treatment of any instability prior to the athlete's safe return to sport.

KNEE REHABILITATION

As noted above, knee injuries can occur when attempting to return to sport with an ongoing injury (pain, weakness or instability), or after incomplete rehabilitation. Assuming that an accurate diagnosis can be made, it is mandatory that the athlete does not return to competition until he or she is as close to peak performance as possible. In most cases, this will involve what can be called 'aggressive conservative measures' (therapeutic modalities, physiotherapy and bracing or taping), but in some cases, surgery will be required. Following surgery, specific protocols must be followed in order to optimize healing (Arvidsson & Eriksson, 1988) and to minimize any iatrogenic disease (e.g. atrophy from immobilization, etc.).

Rehabilitation protocols are increasingly injury-specific and sport-specific and to attempt to list them, therefore, is impractical. It should suffice to say that textbooks have been and are being written on such rehabilitation protocols for a variety of common sports injuries. The fundamental aspects of each protocol generally involve: (i) early control of symptoms and inflammation; (ii) return of range of motion; (iii) strengthening (including power and endurance); (iv) proprioceptive training (including balance and coordination); and (v) sport-specific training (e.g. running, cutting, jumping, throwing, etc.). Attention to detail in making certain that the athlete can actually perform expected activities at a level close to that encountered in competition, but under controlled circumstances (i.e. in the therapy clinic), will minimize the risks of reinjury. Appropriate rehabilitation is therefore a cornerstone of knee injury prevention.

Overall recommendations

1 Increased emphasis by athletes, trainers, physicians and coaches on maximizing physical conditioning, strength, flexibility and muscle balance.

2 Increased emphasis by coaches on proper skill development and the use of drills and scrimmages which cause the fewest number of injuries.

3 Increased monitoring of the rules by the sport governing bodies to continue updating rules of their games which will limit injuries.

4 Continued research into the optimization of both knee braces and sports equipment (particularly ski equipment). Standards being set for all protective sports equipment.

5 Continued research towards identification of the ideal shoe–surface frictional parameters for different sports.

6 Early identification, aggressive treatment and total rehabilitation of knee injuries prior to the return to sport.

7 Injury-specific and sport-specific rehabilitation.

Acknowledgments

The authors gratefully acknowledge the financial support of the Alberta Heritage Foundation for Medical Research, the Canadian Arthritis and Rheumatism Society and the Medical Research Council of Canada.

References

Albert, M. (1983) Descriptive three year data study of outdoor and indoor professional soccer injuries. *Athletic Training* **18**, 218–20.

Anderson, G., Zeman, S.C. & Rosenfeld, R.T. (1979) The Anderson knee stabler. *Phys. Sportsmed.* **7**, 125–7.

Arms, S., Donnermeyer, D., Renström, P. *et al.* (1987) The effect of knee braces on anterior cruciate ligament strain. *Orthop. Trans.* **11**(2), 341–2.

Arvidsson, I. & Eriksson E. (1988) Counteracting muscle atrophy after ACL injury: scientific bases for a rehabilitation program. In J.A. Feagin, (ed) *The Crucial Ligaments*, pp. 451–64. Churchill Livingstone, New York.

Baker, B.E., VanHanswyk, E., Bogosian, S.P. *et al.* (1987) A biomechanical study of the static stabilizing effect of knee braces on medial stability. *Am. J. Sports Med.* **15**(6), 566–70.

Baker, B.E., VanHanswyk, E., Bogosian, S.P. *et al.* (1989) The effect of knee braces on lateral impact loading of the knee. *Am. J. Sports Med.* **17**(2), 182–6.

Beck, C., Drez, D., Young, J. *et al.* (1986) Instrumented testing of functional knee braces. *Am. J. Sports Med.* **14**(4), 253–6.

Beynnon, B., Wertheimer, C., Fleming, B. *et al.* (1990) An *in vivo* study of the anterior cruciate ligament strain biomechanics during functional knee bracing. *Transactions of the Orthopaedic Research Society 36th Annual Meeting,* **15**(1), 223.

Bouter, L.M., Knipschild, P.G. & Volovics, A. (1989) Binding function in relation to injury risk in downhill skiing. *Am. J. Sports Med.* **17**(2), 226–33.

Cahill, B.R. & Griffith, E.H. (1978) Effect of preseason conditioning on the incidence and severity of high school football knee injuries. *Am. J. Sports Med.* **6**, 180–4.

Cahill, B.R. & Griffith, E.H. (1979) Exposure to injury in major college football. A preliminary report of data collection to determine injury exposure rates and activity risk factors. *Am. J. Sports Med.* **7**, 183–5.

Carlson, J.M. & French, J. (1989) Knee orthoses for valgus protection. *Clin. Orthop. Rel. Res.* **247**, 175–92.

Colville, M.R., Lee, C.L. & Ciullo, J.V. (1986) The Lenox Hill brace. *Am. J. Sports Med.* **14**(4), 257–61.

Coughlin, L., Oliver, J. & Berretta, G. (1987) Knee bracing and anterolateral rotatory instability. *Am. J. Sports Med,* **15**(2), 161–3.

Culpepper, M.I. & Niemann, K.M.W. (1983) High school football injuries in Birmingham, Alabama. *Southern Med. J.* **76**, 873–8.

Curran, R.D. & Linquist, D.S. (1986) *Statistical analysis of the effectiveness of prophylactic knee braces.* Unpublished paper, Department of Mechanical Engineering, Duke University.

Daley, B.J., Ralston, J.A., Brown, T.D. *et al.* (1991) Prophylactic knee brace parametric design evaluation in a surrogate knee model. *Transactions of the Orthopaedic Research Society 37th Annual Meeting,* **16**(1), 185.

Davies, G.J., Wallace, L.A. & Malone, T. (1980) Mechanisms of selected knee injuries. *Phys. Ther.* **60**(12), 1590–5.

Edlund, G., Gedda, S. & Hemborg, A. (1980) Knee injuries in skiing: A prospective study from northern Sweden. *Am. J. Sports Med.* **8**, 411.

Ekstrand, J. (1982) *Soccer injuries and their prevention.* Medical Dissertation No. 130, Linkoping University, Sweden.

Ekstrand, J. & Gillquist, J. (1982) The frequency of muscle tightness and injuries in soccer players. *Am. J. Sports Med.* **10**, 75–78.

Ekstrand, J. & Gillquist, J. (1983) The avoidability of soccer injuries. *Int. J. Sports Med.* **4**, 124–8.

Ellison, A.E., Carroll, R.E. & Haddon, W. (1962) Skiing injuries. Clinical study. *Publ. Health Rep.* **77**, 985.

Eriksson, E. (1976) Sports injuries of the knee ligaments: their diagnosis, treatment, rehabilitation, and prevention. *Med. Sci. Sports* **8**(3), 133–44.

Erickson, A., Yasuda, K., Beynnon, B. *et al.* (1991) A dynamic evaluation of the effectiveness of prophylactic knee braces. *Transactions of the Orthopaedic Research Society 37th Annual Meeting*, **16**(1), 186.

Feagin, J.A. & Lambert, K.L. (1985) Mechanism of injury and pathology of anterior cruciate ligament injuries. *Orthop. Clin. N. Am.* **16**(1), 41–5.

Feagin, J.A., Lambert, K.L., Cunningham, R.R. *et al.* (1987) Consideration of the anterior cruciate ligament injury in skiing. *Clin. Orthop. Rel. Res.* **216**, 13–18.

France, E.P., Paulos, L.E., Cawley, P.W. *et al.* (1988) Development and validation of an instrumented surrogate limb for use in lateral impact testing. *Orthop. Trans.* **12**(2), 443.

France, E.P., Paulos, L.E., Jayaraman, G. *et al.* (1987) The biomechanics of lateral knee bracing. *Am. J. Sports Med.* **15**(5), 430–8.

Frank, C. (1986) Accurate interpretation of the Lachman test. *Clin. Orthop. Rel. Res.* **213**, 163–6.

Galway, H.R. & MacIntosh, D.L. (1980) The lateral pivot shift: A symptom and sign of anterior cruciate ligament insufficiency. *Clin. Orthop. Rel. Res.* **147**, 45–50.

Garrick, J.G. & Regua, R.K. (1987) Prophylactic knee bracing. *Am. J. Sports Med.* **15**(5), 471–6.

Glick, J.M. (1971) A study of ligamentous looseness in football players and its relation to injury. *Abbott Proc.* **1**, 34–9.

Goldberg, B., Rosenthal, P.P. & Nicholas, J.A. (1984) Injuries in youth football. *Phys. Sportsmed.* **12**(8), 122–30.

Grace, T.G., Skipper, B.J., Newberry, J.C. *et al.* (1988) Prophylactic knee braces and injury to the lower extremity. *J. Bone Joint Surg.* **70A**(3), 422–7.

Grace, T.G., Sweetser, E.R. & Nelson, M.A. (1984) Isokinetic muscle imbalance and knee joint injuries. *J. Bone Joint Surg.* **66A**, 734–40.

Gutman, J., Weisbuch, J. & Wolf, M. (1974) Ski injuries in 1972–1973: a repeat analysis of a major health problem. *JAMA* **230**, 423.

Haddon, W., Ellison, A.E. & Carroll, R.E. (1962) Skiing injuries: epidemiological study. *Publ. Health Rep.* **77**, 975.

Hale, R.W. & Mitchell, W. (1981) Football injuries in Hawaii 1979. *Hawaiian Med. J.* **40**, 180–3.

Hansen, B.L., Ward, J.C. & Diehl, R.C. (1985) The preventive use of the Anderson knee stabler in football. *Phys. Sportsmed.* **13**(9), 75–81.

Hauser, W. (1989) Experimental prospective skiing injury study. In R.J. Johnson (ed) *Skiing Trauma and Safety: Seventh International Symposium*. American Society for Testing and Materials, Philadelphia.

Hauser, W. & Schaff, P. (1987) Ski boots: biomechanical issues regarding skiing safety and performance. *Int. J. Sport Biomech.* **3**, 326–44.

Hewson, G.F., Mendini, R.A. & Wang, J.B. (1986) Prophylactic knee bracing in college football. *Am. J. Sports Med.* **14**(4), 262–6.

Hofmann, A.A., Wyatt, W.B., Bourne, M.H. *et al.* (1984) Knee stability in orthotic knee braces. *Am. J. Sports Med.* **12**(5), 371–4.

Howe, J. & Johnson, R.J. (1982) Knee injuries in skiing. *Clin. Sports Med.* **1**(2), 277–88.

Hughston, J.C., Andrews, J.R., Cross, M.J. *et al.* (1976) Classification of knee ligament instabilities. Part I. *J. Bone Joint Surg.* **58A**, 159–72.

Jackson, R.W., Reed, S.C. & Dunbar, F. (1991) An evaluation of knee injuries in a professional football team — risk factors, type of injuries, and the value of prophylactic bracing. *Clin. J. Sport Med.* **1**, 1–7.

Johnson, R.J. (1988) Prevention of cruciate ligament injuries. In J.A. Feagin (ed) *The Crucial Ligaments*, pp. 349–56. Churchill Livingstone, New York.

Johnson, R.J. & Ettlinger, C.F. (1982) Alpine ski injuries: changes through the years. *Clin. Sports Med.* **1**, 181–96.

Johnson, R.J., Ettlinger, C.F. & Campbell, R.J. (1980) Trends in skiing injuries. *Am. J. Sports Med.* **8**, 106–13.

Johnson, R.J., Pope, M.H., Weisman, G. *et al.* (1979) The knee injury in skiing. A multifaceted approach. *Am. J. Sports Med.* **7**, 321–7.

Karlsson, J., Eriksson, A. & Forsberg, A. (1978) *The Physiology of Alpine Skiing*. United States Ski Coaches Association, Stockholm, Sweden.

Keller, C.S., Noyes, F.R. & Buncher, C.R. (1987) The medical aspects of soccer injury epidemiology. *Am. J. Sports Med.* **15**(3), 230–7.

Klein, K.K. (1974) Muscular strength and the knee. *Phys. Sportsmed.* **2**, 29–31.

Knapik, J.J., Bauman, C.L., Jones, B.H. *et al.* (1991)

Preseason strength and flexibility imbalances associated with athletic injuries in female collegiate athletes. *Am. J. Sports Med.* **19**(1), 76–81.

Knutzen, K.M., Bates, B.T., Schot, P. *et al.* (1987) A biomechanical analysis of two functional knee braces. *Med. Sci. Sports Exerc.* **19**(3), 303–9.

Larson, R.L. (1983) Physical examination in the diagnosis of rotatory instability. *Clin. Orthop. Rel. Res.* **172**, 38–44.

Losee, R.E., Johnson, T.R. & Soutwick, W.O. (1978) Anterior subluxation of the lateral tibial plateau. A diagnostic test and operative repair. *J. Bone Joint Surg.* **60A**, 1015–30.

Lunsford, T.R., Lunsford, B.R., Greenfield, J. *et al.* (1989) Response of eight knee orthoses to valgus, varus and axial rotation loads. *J. Prosthet. Ortho.* **2**(4), 274–88.

McKelvie, R.W. (1985) *An investigation of the relative frequency and severity of knee injuries occurring to intercollegiate football players in the Mid-American conference wearing and not wearing an Anderson knee stabler.* Thesis, Bowling Green State University.

McLean, D.A. (1989) Use of adhesive strapping in sport. *Br. J. Sports Med.* **23**(3), 147–9.

McMaster, W.C. & Walter, M. (1978) Injuries in soccer. *Am. J. Sports Med.* **6**, 354–7.

Marans, H.J., Kennedy, D.K., Kavanagh, T.G. *et al.* (1988) A review of intra-articular knee injuries in racquet sports diagnosed by arthroscopy. *Can. J. Surg.* **31**, 199–201.

Maxwell, S.M. & Hull, M.L. (1989) Measurement of strength and loading variables on the knee during alpine skiing. *J. Biomech.* **22**(6), 609–24.

Mishra, D.K., Daniel, D.M. & Stone, M.L. (1988) The use of functional knee braces in the control of pathologic anterior knee laxity. *Transactions of the Orthopaedic Research Society 34th Annual Meeting,* **13**, 518.

Morehouse, C.A. & Morrison, W.E. (1975) *The artificial turf story: a research review.* Penn State University Health, Physical Education and Recreation Series No. 9.

Moretz, A., Rashkin, A. & Grana, W.A. (1978) Oklahoma high school football injury study: a preliminary report. *J Oklahoma Med. Assoc.* **71**, 85–8.

Moritz, J.R. (1959) Ski injuries. *Am. J. Surg.* **98**, 495.

Mortensen, W.W., Foreman, K., Focht, L. *et al.* (1988) An *in vitro* study of functional orthoses in the ACL disrupted knee. *Transactions of the Orthopaedic Research Society 34th Annual Meeting,* **13**, 520.

Moser, K.R. (1985) *Analysis of the use of valgus knee braces in selected intercollegiate football programs.* Unpublished paper, College of Education, Ohio University.

Mote, C.D. (1987) The forces of skiing and their implication to injury. *Int. J. Biomech.* **3**, 309–25.

Mueller, F.N. & Blyth, C.S. (1974) North Carolina high school football injury study: equipment and prevention. *J. Sports Med.* **2**, 1–10.

Nicholas, J.A. (1970) Injuries to knee ligaments: relationship to a looseness and tightness in football players. *JAMA* **212**, 2236–9.

Nicholas, J.A. (1983) Bracing the anterior cruciate ligament deficient knee using the Lenox Hill derotation brace. *Clin. Orthop. Rel. Res.* **172**, 137–42.

Nigg, B.M. & Segesser, B. (1988) The influence of playing surfaces on the load on the locomotor system and on football and tennis injuries. *Sports Med.* **5**, 375–85.

Nilsson, S. & Roaas, A. (1978) Soccer injuries in adolescents. *Am. J. Sports Med.* **6**, 358–61.

Olson, O.C. (1979) The Spokane study: high school football injuries. *Phys. Sportsmed.* **7**(12), 75–82.

Paulos, L.E., Drawbert, J.P., France, P. *et al.* (1986) Lateral knee braces in football: do they prevent injury? *Phys. Sportsmed.* **14**(6), 119–24.

Paulos, L.E., France, E.P. & Cawley, P.W. (1989) Impact biomechanics of lateral knee bracing: the anterior cruciate ligament. *Transactions of the Orthopaedic Research Society 35th Annual Meeting,* **14**, 220.

Paulos, L.E., France, E.P., Rosenberg, T.D. *et al.* (1987) The biomechanics of lateral knee bracing. *Am. J. Sports Med.* **15**(5), 419–29.

Pope, M.H. (1982) The biomechanics of tibial shaft and knee injuries. *Clin. Sports Med.* **1**(2), 229–39.

Pritchett, J.W. (1980) High cost of high school football injuries. *Am. J. Sports Med.* **8**, 197–9.

Randall, R., Miller, H. & Shurr, D. (1984) The use of prophylactic knee orthoses at Iowa State University. *Orthot. Prosthet.* **37**(4), 54–7.

Regalbuto, M.A., Rovick, J.S. & Walker, P.S. (1989) The forces in a knee brace as a function of hinge design and placement. *Am. J. Sports Med.* **17**(4), 535–43.

Renström, P. (1984) Swedish research in sports traumatology. *Clin. Orthop. Rel. Res.* **191**, 144–59.

Rovere, G.D., Haupt, H.A. & Yates, C.S. (1987) Prophylactic knee bracing in college football. *Am. J. Sports Med.* **15**(2), 111–16.

Schriner, J.L. (1985) The effectiveness of knee bracing in preventing knee injuries in high school athletes. *Med. Sci. Sports Exerc.* **17**(2), 254.

Skovron, M.L., Levy, I.M. & Agel, J. (1990) Living with artificial grass: A knowledge update. *Am. J. Sports Med.* **18**(5), 510–13.

Stitler, M., Ryan, J., Hopkinson, W. *et al.* (1990) The efficacy of a prophylactic knee brace to reduce injuries in football. *Am. J. Sports Med.* **18**(3), 310–15.

Sullivan, J.A., Gross, R.H. & Grana, W.A. (1980)

Evaluation of injuries in youth soccer. *Am. J. Sports Med.* **8**, 325–7.

Taft, T.N., Hunter, S.L. & Funderburk, C.H. (1985) Preventative lateral knee bracing in football. *Transactions of the American Orthopedic Society for Sports Medicine 11th Annual Meeting.*

Tapper, E.M. (1978) Ski injuries from 1939 to 1976: the Sun Valley experience. *Am. J. Sports Med.* **6**, 114.

Teitz, C.C., Hermanson, B.K., Kronmal, R.A. *et al.* (1987) Evaluation of the use of braces to prevent injury to the knee in collegiate football players. *J. Bone Joint Surg.* **69A**(1), 2–8.

Torg, J.S., Conrad, W. & Kalen, V. (1976) Clinical diagnosis of anterior cruciate ligament instability in the athlete. *Am. J. Sports Med.* **4**, 84–93.

Torg, J.S. & Quedenfeld, T. (1971) Effect of shoe type and cleat length on incidence and severity of knee injuries among high school football players. *Res. Q.* **42**, 203–11.

Torg, J.S. & Quedenfeld, T. (1974) The shoe–surface interface and its relationship to football knee injuries. *J. Sports Med,* **2**, 261–9.

Van Hoeck, J.E., Brown, T.D. & Brand, R.A. (1988) A surrogate model of prophylactic knee brace performance under dynamic valgus load. *Orthop. Trans.* **12**(2), 412.

Wojtys, E.M., Loubert, P.V., Samson, S.Y. *et al.* (1990) Use of a knee-brace for control of tibial translation and rotation. *J. Bone Joint Surg.* **72A**(9), 1323–9.

Young, L.R., Oman, C.M. & Crane, H. (1976) The etiology of ski injury: An eight-year study of the skier and his equipment. *Orthop. Clin. N. Am.* **7**, 13.

Zarins, B. & Nemeth, V.A. (1985) Acute knee injuries in athletes. *Orthop. Clin. N. Am.* **16**(2), 285–302.

Zemper, E.D. (1990) A two-year prospective study of prophylactic knee braces in a national sample of college football players. *Sports Training Med. Rehab.* **1**, 287–96.

Zogby, R.G., Baker, B.E., Seymour, R.J. *et al.* (1989) A biomechanical evaluation of the effect of functional braces on anterior cruciate ligament instability, using the Genucom knee analysis system. *Transactions of the Orthopaedic Research Society 35th Annual Meeting,* **14**, 212.

Chapter 10

Overuse Knee Injuries

JOHN M. MARZO AND THOMAS L. WICKIEWICZ

The proliferation of sports participation over the past decade has brought with it an increase in the number of overuse injuries of the knee. Many sports have running activities as their basis, from the repetitive rhythmical motion of the jogger to the sudden start and stop activities of the racquet sports player. With the knee as the pivotal joint between the upper body mass and the ground reaction, it is not unexpected that an increase in injuries in this particular joint has been seen.

Injuries may be defined as belonging to one of two broad categories, macrotrauma and microtrauma. Macrotrauma is defined as a specific event with force of a sufficient level to cause damage to an otherwise normal structure. Microtrauma are cumulative events, each individual event at a subthreshold level to cause injury. When applied over a sufficient duration or of sufficient intensity, then some form of injury will develop. With the repetitive stresses of running, impact loading from jumping or the torsional stresses from pivoting manoeuvres, it is not uncommon that overuse injuries will develop about the knee.

In a normal running motion, the biomechanics of the lower extremity play an important role in the development of some overuse syndromes about the knee. At heel strike, the supinated foot begins a rapid reversal to hindfoot and subtalar pronation. At this time, there is an obligatory internal rotation of the tibia which takes place. Concomitantly, activity can be seen in the quadriceps to allow for an eccentric contraction and thus slow knee flexion. This has the effect of both stabilizing the knee, as well as the dissipation of shock. If there is any biomechanical aberration there will be a greater likelihood of injury to the structures about the knee. An example would be hyperpronation of the foot causing excessive internal tibial rotation. In addition, abnormalities of the structures above the knee may have an ill effect. Tightness of biarthrodial structures such as the rectus femoris or hamstring muscles may result in an overload of forces at the level of the knee. Bony malalignments such as increased femoral anteversion, leg length discrepancies, abnormalities of the lumbar spine such as scoliosis, increased lumbar lordosis or abnormal pelvic obliquities may also predispose to biomechanical overload at the knee.

In the initial physical examination of an individual who presents with a painful knee as a result of sports participation, it is important to look for any of these abnormalities. Examination should begin with the patient sufficiently disrobed as to allow visualization of the entire lower extremity and lower back and pelvis. The examiner should make a visual inspection of overall alignment and note whether abnormal varus valgus or recurvatum attitude is present at the knee. The tibial torsion should be assessed, as well as checking for appropriate flexibility of the triceps surae and appropriate subtalar motion.

Careful attention should also be directed at an appropriate history. In many individuals, the biomechanical arrangement of the lower extremities and low back is normal and the cause for the overuse may be related to errors in training technique, improper foot wear, surface conditions or muscular fatigue. Appropriate treatment depends on identifying the cause of the injury and affecting appropriate change. In the case of biomechanical abnormalities, appropriate prosthetic or orthotic balancing may be required. Training regimens may need to be modified or even suspended temporarily.

Patellofemoral joint

Biomechanics

The patella aids extension by increasing the distance of the quadriceps mechanism from the axis of knee flexion and extension. By increasing the lever arm of the knee extensors, the patella increases the torque of extension by as much as 50%. By increasing the efficiency of the quadriceps, the same amount of work can be performed with lower energy demand. The patella is also important in transmitting the quadriceps force to the distal femur and proximal tibia. Articular cartilage has a very low coefficient of friction and a low compressive stiffness (Mow *et al.*, 1984). The articular cartilage of the patella is the thickest cartilage in the entire body and its form reflects the important role it plays in facilitating extensor function (Fig. 10.1). The compressive forces on the articular cartilage of the patella have been shown to be relatively constant throughout the range of motion. As the knee is flexed from full extension, the patellofemoral joint reaction force increases. At the same time, the contact area between the patella and the trochlea of the femur increases, so the force per unit area remains relatively constant. The patella also acts to centralize the input from the four components of the quadriceps mechanism. This aids in decreasing the possibility of subluxation or dislocation of the patella and helps control the retinacular tension around the knee. Finally, the patella acts as a bony shield to knee trauma

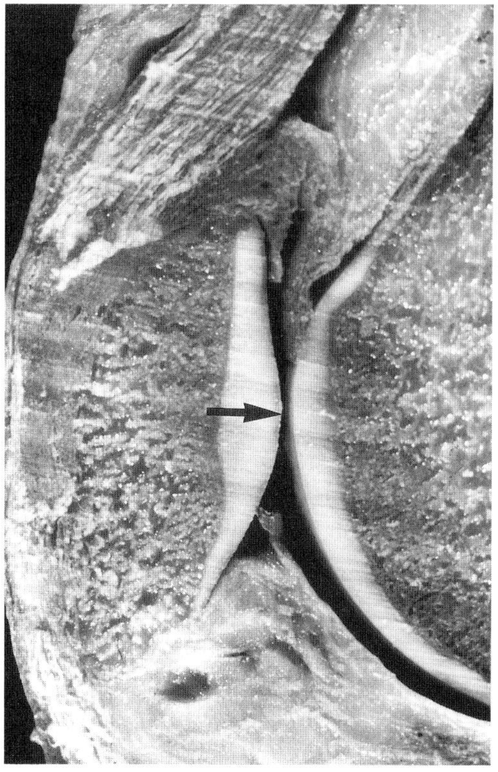

Fig. 10.1 The thickness of the articular cartilage reflects the high compressive forces experienced by the patellofemoral articulation. During level walking the resultant compressive force (arrow) reaches 0.5 times body weight. Forces while ascending and descending stairs reach 3.3 times body weight.

from an anterior direction and gives a cosmetic appearance to the anterior knee.

Normal knee valgus produces an angle between the line of pull of the quadriceps and the line of the patellar tendon, the Q angle (Fig. 10.2). The pull of the quadriceps produces a laterally pointing vector that increases as the Q angle increases. External rotation of the tibia near terminal extension, the 'screw home mechanism', causes lateralization of the tibial tubercle, increasing the lateral force on the patella. These laterally directed forces are resisted by the anterior projection of the lateral femoral condyle, the medial retinaculum and the vastus medialis obliquus muscle. Soft tissue structures

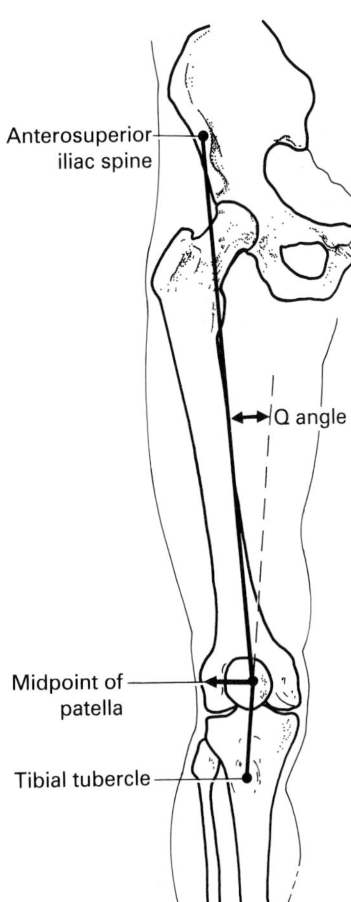

Fig. 10.2 The Q angle is measured between a line from the anteror superior iliac spine to the centre of the patellar, and another from the tibial tubercle to the centre of the patella. The Q angle produces a valgus vector during the terminal degrees of knee extension (arrow).

in the lateral side of the knee that resist medially directed forces are the lateral retinaculum, vastus lateralis and the iliotibial tract. These medial and lateral soft tissue restraints should be in balance to provide for normal patellar tracking (Fig. 10.3). The patella articulates with the supratrochlear fat pad in full extension. The patella is drawn into the femoral trochlea from a lateral direction and articular contact is made during the first 10° of flexion. From 20 to 30° of flexion, the patella becomes more prominent as it rides along the prominence of the trochlea. Beyond 30° the patella settles into the deepening of the groove and instability is relatively uncommon beyond this degree of flexion.

History and symptoms

A detailed history of the onset and progression of patellofemoral problems should be carefully obtained from each patient. Insidious onset of anterior knee pain, especially bilateral in location, suggests the patellofemoral mechanism as a cause. Traumatic events may cause acute onset of symptoms, as in patellar dislocations.

Patients with patellofemoral pain often describe a constant aching or throbbing sensation that is aggravated by prolonged sitting or bending. The pain may be sharp at times, provoked by activities such as ascending or descending stairs. Sports that involve activities that generate high patellofemoral joint reactive forces, like basketball and volleyball, may also aggravate symptoms. There may be reflex inhibition of the quadriceps musculature that produces a sense of giving way in the knee. While not true giving way from instability as in ligamentous injuries of the knee, this may occasionally lead to falls. Other patients may report locking of the knee, but upon closer questioning will usually describe a catching sensation during attempts at extending a loaded knee. These episodes of locking are usually transitory, and relatively easy to distinguish from true locking due to meniscal or other mechanical block. Some patients complain of pain associated with a grating sensation eminating from the anterior knee during flexion–extension. This crepitus is not, however, present in all patients with patellofemoral pain. When it is present, it does not necessarily cause pain. Swelling is not usually a major element of the clinical presentation, but may be present in some patients with patella chondromalacia or true patella instability.

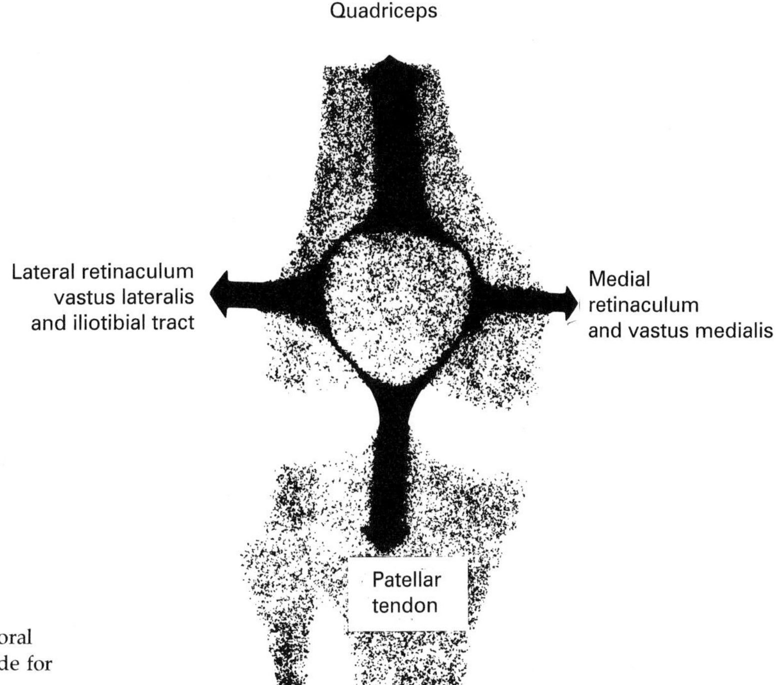

Fig. 10.3 The anatomical restraints of the patellofemoral joint must balance to provide for normal patella tracking.

Physical examination

The physical examination inspects the patient's overall extremity alignment in the anteroposterior (AP) and lateral planes. Visual assessment can be very helpful in the clinical evaluation of patellar alignment. The patient should walk several times to observe gait, with special attention to the presence of knee valgus or pes planus. Observe both legs for the presence of symmetry, atrophy, skin or other dystrophic changes. Elbow and knee recurvatum, and the thumb-to-forearm test can also be used as a measure of general ligamentous laxity.

With the patient supine and the knee in full extension with a relaxed quadriceps, the patellofemoral joint is palpated and the location of tenderness, e.g. medial retinaculum or inferior patella pole, is noted. Gentle medial displacement of the patella may aid in eliciting lateral retinacular tenderness by placing slight tension on the lateral retinaculum. It also helps to gauge the tension of the retinaculum itself, since excessive tightness may be associated with patellar tilt. Attempts to manually depress and elevate the patellar facets will give the examiner a clinical index of the tension of the medial and lateral retinaculae. The lateral restraints should normally allow the patella to be tilted so the medial facet is parallel to the horizontal plane in a supine patient. The patella can be grasped and moved mediolaterally to assess the resting tension of the retinacular tissues, and to distinguish which direction cause symptoms. The patella should be passively moved within the trochlea in an attempt to reproduce symptoms from an articular source of pain, but one should be careful not to pinch the suprapatellar synovial membrane since this is uniformly painful.

It is important to observe patellar tracking throughout the entire range of motion. Tightening of the quadriceps muscles with the knee extended normal produces a proximal and lateral movement of the patella in a 2 : 1 ratio. It should be apparent if lateral movement is excessive. With the patient in a sitting position, observe the patella as it tracks through a 0–90° arc of motion. Active flexion and extension of the knee may reveal noticeable lateral or medial movement of the patella. The patella should track smoothly throughout the range of motion with no sudden movement on exit from or entry to the femoral trochlea. The patella becomes engaged in the femoral trochlea at about 30° of knee flexion. A patella that shifts into the trochlea after 30° of flexion usually is entering from an excessively lateral position and does so with a distinctly brisk motion.

The Q angle with the patient supine helps gauge the alignment and the Q angle at 90° of flexion is helpful in detecting a tibial tubercle that lies in excessive external rotation. Dysplasias with subsequent patella instability tend to have low Q angles and patella pain syndromes with chondromalacia high Q angles. These, however, are trends, and the Q angle may not have a direct correlation with anterior knee pain.

The examination is completed by performing the routine manoeuvres for testing the ligaments and menisci to avoid missing a diagnosis of knee instability. It is absolutely essential that the correct diagnosis be made if one is to expect a treatment programme to be successful.

Radiography of the patellofemoral joint

A standard AP view is used to detect loss of cartilage joint space in the medial and lateral compartments, and should be taken during weight-bearing. The AP view may detect other problems that coexist with a patellofemoral disorder, or indicate a separate diagnosis such as a tumour or osteochondritis dissecans. Since the patella normally sits laterally with the knee in full extension, the standing AP radiograph is not particularly useful for assessing alignment of the patella with the femur.

The standard lateral view may be taken during standing or supine with the knee flexed 20–30° to place the patellar tendon under some tension. This allows assessment of the relationship of the patella to the femur. Blumensaat (1938) has described the normal relationship of the patella to a radiodense line which marks the ventral border of the intercondylar fossa (Fig. 10.4). Elevation of the patella above an extension of this line has generally been regarded as indicative of patella alta, which is felt to increase the likelihood of patellar instability. The method of Insall and Salvati (1971) does not rely on precise positioning of the knee. It consists of determining the ratio of patellar tendon length to the greatest diagonal length of the patella (Fig. 10.5). A value above the upper limit of 1.2 indicates patella alta. Standard lateral views may reveal patellar sclerosis or osteophyte formation, but provides little information regarding patellar alignment.

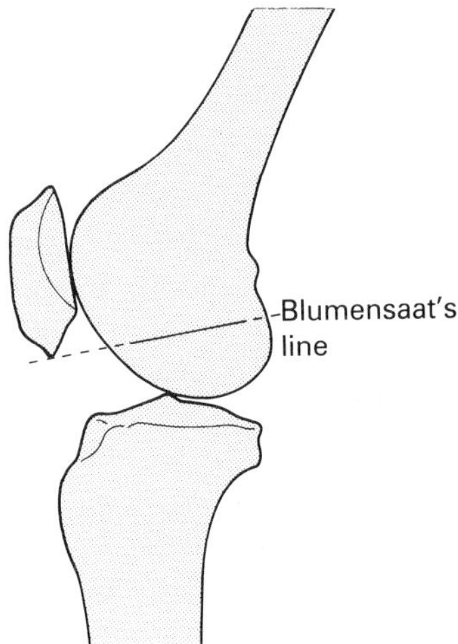

Fig. 10.4 Blumensaat's line is drawn along the dome of the intercondylar fossa of the femur. If the inferior pole of the patella lies above this line, patella alta is present.

Standard tangential axial views of the patellofemoral joint provide information regarding the condition of the articular cartilage surfaces. The tangential view described by Laurin *et al.* (1978) is useful in detecting subtle tracking abnormalities. On the 20° tangential view Laurin found that 97% of normal controls had a lateral patellofemoral angle that opened laterally, while those with subluxation showed

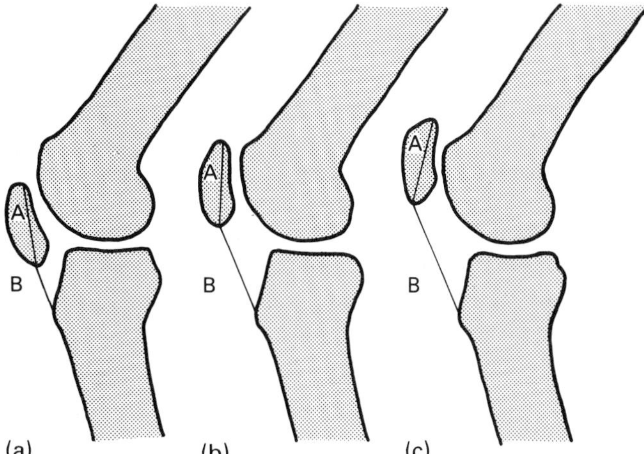

Fig. 10.5 The Insall–Salvati method for determining patellar height relates the greatest diagonal length of the patella to the length of the patellar tendon. A normal ratio (A : B) is 1.0. (a) Patella infera; (b) normal patella; and (c) patella alta.

parallel lines or an angle opening medially (Fig. 10.6) (Laurin *et al.*, 1979). This view is a good screening tool for detecting abnormal patellar tilt. The tangential view described by Merchant *et al.* (1974) is obtained by flexing the leg 45° over the end of the table and angling the tube 30° from the horizontal. Merchant reported measuring the patellofemoral congruence angle, and noticed that normal congruence at 45° is −6 +/− 11°. The angle must be less than 16° to be within the limits set by this method (Fig. 10.7). The congruence angle measured from this view is useful as an indicator of patellar centralization, and subluxation or dislocation, as opposed to patellar tilt. As long as radiographs allow one to differentiate tilt and subluxation from normal alignment, other imaging modalities are not needed.

To define more precisely patellar tracking and patellar tilt, computerized tomography (CT) scanning offers the advantage of sequential images at progressive degrees of flexion (Schutzer *et al.*, 1986; Fulkerson *et al.*, 1987). The posterior femoral condyles provide a much more consistent reference for measuring tilt. The patellar tilt angle is the relationship of the

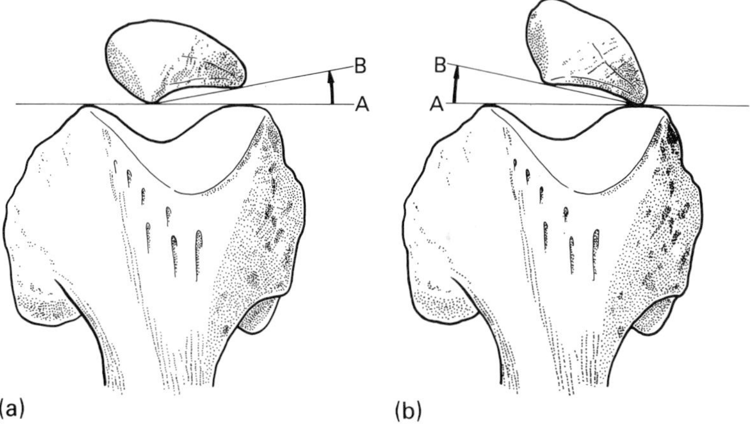

Fig. 10.6 The lateral patellofemoral angle is determined by drawing one line across the femoral condyles and a second line along the lateral facet of the patella. If the two lines diverge laterally, the patellar position is normal. If the two lines are parallel or converge laterally, a patella tilt is suspected. (a) Medial aspect; (b) lateral aspect.

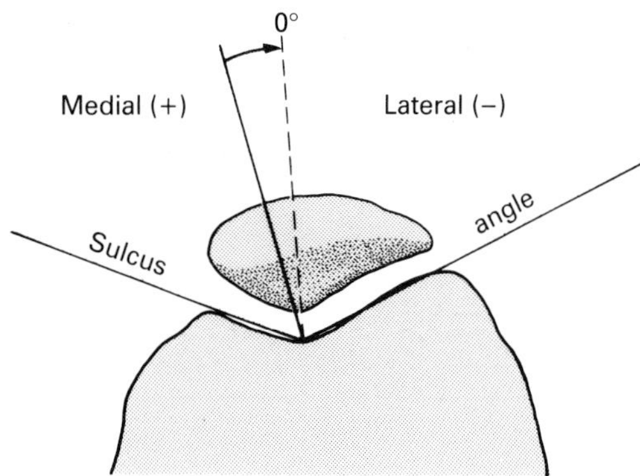

Fig. 10.7 The congruence angle is constructed by first bisecting the sulcus angle (the angle formed by two lines drawn from the deepest point of the femoral sulcus to each of the femoral condyles). The angle between this line and a second line from the sulcus to the lowest point on the articular ridge of the patella is the congruence angle (arrow). An angle greater than +16° indicates patellar subluxation.

posterior condyle reference line to that of the lateral patellar facet (Fig. 10.8). Using CT, one can note a variety of different tracking patterns which are not as well defined using standard radiographs (Schutzer *et al.*, 1986; Inoue *et al.*, 1988). With the use of contrast, CT is more able to evaluate the condition of the patellar and trochlear cartilage (Fig. 10.9) (Boven *et al.*, 1982). In this regard, CT scan with contrast is a much better imaging modality since the contour of the articular surface of the patella does not exactly coincide to the underlying osseous contour.

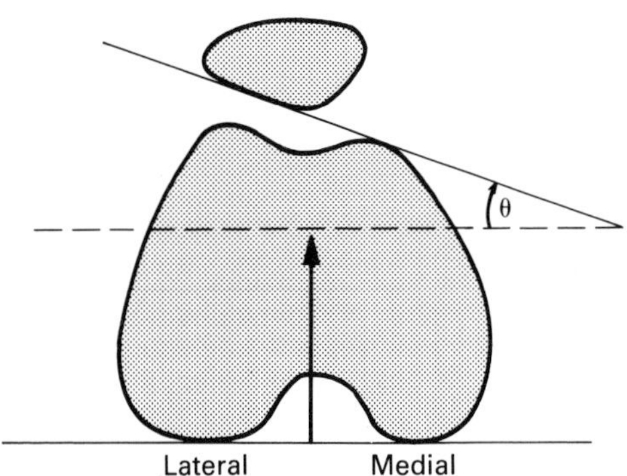

Fig. 10.8 The patellar tilt angle is that between lines drawn across the posterior femoral condyles and the lateral facet. This angle should always be 7° or greater in a normal patient.

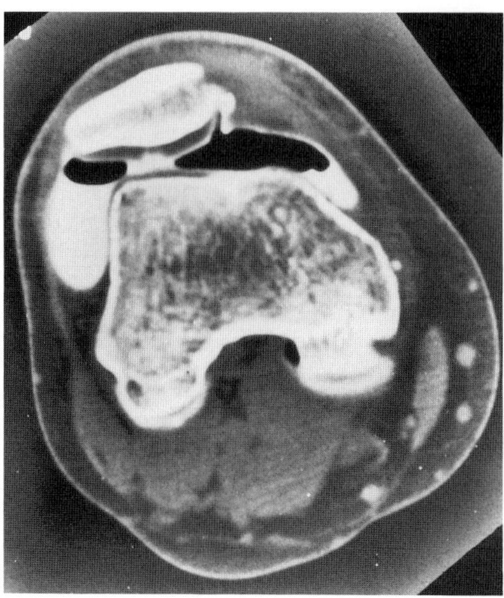

Fig. 10.9 Computed tomography with contrast is useful to evaluate the articular cartilage of the patellofemoral joint. This image shows dye within the cartilage of the patella, indicating articular wear.

Magnetic resonance imaging (MRI) offers advantages similar to CT scanning, with the additional benefit of better visualization of the cartilage surfaces of the patella and trochlea (Wojtys *et al.*, 1987; Yulish *et al.*, 1987). Contrast agents are not generally needed with this imaging modality.

In evaluating patients with resistant anterior knee pain, bone scan may be helpful to detect areas of osseous remodelling in response to excessive articular or subchondral loading. It will also indicate occult disease that has escaped conventional radiographic diagnosis.

Arthroscopy has proven to be a very valuable tool in assessing the appropriate operative treatment for a patient with patellar malalignment in whom conservative treatment has failed. Arthroscopy affords the best assessment of the articular surfaces and may allow decision-making with regard to which operation to select.

Excessive lateral pressure syndrome (ELPS)

CLINICAL FEATURES

This syndrome may proceed from soft tissue pain related to adaptive changes in the lateral retinaculum, to pain from patellar articular cartilage changes. It is important to emphasize examining the patella for the amount of 'play' or passive motion that is present. Patients with chronic lateral tilt develop adaptive shortening of the lateral retinacular tissues and concomitant relative lengthening of the medial retinacular tissues. In this group it is most common to find restricted passive movement to the medial side due to associated lateral patellar retinacular shortening. Tenderness along the tight lateral retinaculum is a fairly typical finding on physical examination of a patient with excessive lateral restraints (Fulkerson, 1982, 1989). With knee flexion the tension on the lateral structures increases, and can cause compression of small nerves, resulting in pain and tenderness (Fulkerson *et al.*, 1985). The lateral retinaculum may be thick, indurated and tight on palpation. Medial retinacular tenderness, however, may also be present due to either stretching of these tissues or medial patellar facet articular changes.

Chronic patellar tilting leads to lateral patellar facet degeneration from overloading, and medial facet degeneration due to the absence of contact pressures necessary for healthy articular cartilage. Isolated patellar tilt without subluxation may lead to early advancing patellofemoral arthrosis (Fulkerson & Shea, 1990). When articular cartilage changes have occurred, patients begin to experience crepitation with movement. Some patients respond to the release of products from cartilage wear by producing synovial fluid, and knee effusion is commonly seen as an element of this syndrome.

PREVENTION OF ELPS

In an individual in whom the anatomical risk factors for ELPS, as mentioned above are delineated, certain measures may be of help in the prevention of this syndrome. Careful attention should be placed on stretching exercise, especially of the quadriceps and lateral structures. Footwear which emphasizes shock absorption may help reduce some of the compressive load on the patellofemoral joint at heel strike in the individual who must run longer distances in their training regimen. Attention should be directed at carefully icing down the lateral structures following activity. Mobilization techniques of the patella may provide some protection against the development of this syndrome, but it must be cautioned that there is no clinical study, to date, to prove the efficacy of such techniques as preventive measures.

TREATMENT

The mainstay of treatment for ELPS is physical therapy (Grana & Kriegshauser, 1985; Fisher, 1986; Henry, 1989). Patients with ELPS may respond to non-operative treatment that focuses on mobilizing the lateral retinaculum and strengthening the vastus medialis. Special attention is directed to stretching of the lateral retinaculum and the iliotibial tract. Stretching of the hip adductors, hamstrings and heel cords are also part of the programme (Fig. 10.10). Strengthening exercises are designed to emphasize the vastus medialis obliquus muscle and are initiated using the weight of the limb. Weightlifting is progressed over a 2–3 month period. Quadriceps isometrics, straight leg raising, and hip adductor/abductor exercises are also emphasized (Fig. 10.11). Resistance exercises of the quadriceps through the 90° to full extension arc are avoided.

Patellar taping techniques have shown successful results when correctly performed (McConnell, 1986). The success of this technique relies on decreasing the amount of pain enough for a patient to enter a rehabilitation

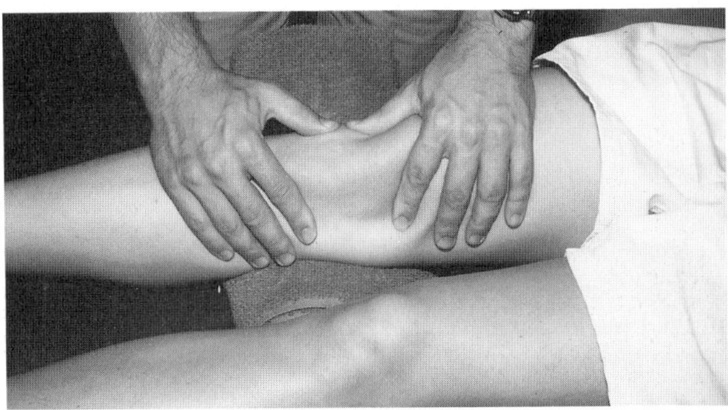

(a)

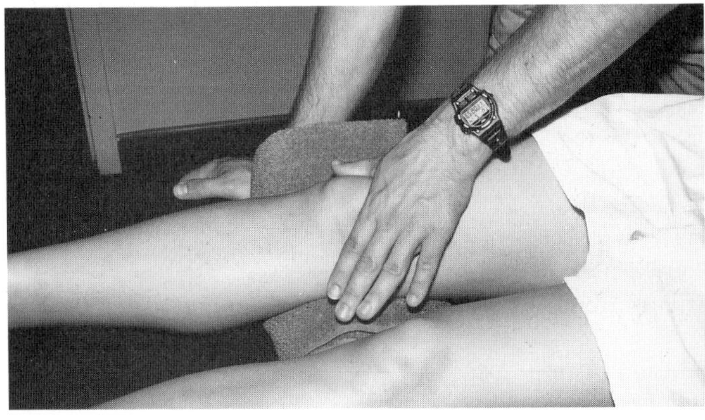

(b)

Fig. 10.10 Stretching of the lateral retinacular tissues (a) and the iliotibial tract (b), are integral to successful non-operative treatment of the excessive lateral pressure syndrome.

programme that will provide long-term benefit. Heat before each session of therapy and ice afterward will help relieve pain in the retinacular structures. We have not found other modalities like ultrasound, iontophoresis or laser to be of particular benefit in our patients. Anti-inflammatory medication may help in the acute phase. A local injection, directed at a specific source of pain may be useful as a diagnostic and therapeutic measure.

An integral, but often disregarded part of the rehabilitation of anterior knee pain is avoidance of activities that aggravate the condition. Cross-training may be an effective way to accomplish maintenance of general fitness, while resting the patellofemoral joint. The patient can gradually return to their desired activity after a 2–3-month asymptomatic interval. A practical maintenance programme must be initiated if long-term benefit is expected.

Patients that do not respond to 6–9 months of non-operative treatment should benefit from lateral retinacular release in most cases (Larson *et al.*, 1978; McGinty & McCarthy, 1981; Krompinger & Fulkerson, 1983; Schonholtz, 1987). The best results will be in the group that does not have evidence for lateral facet arthrosis as seen on preoperative studies, or during arthroscopy at the time of release. The release allows more appropriate tracking of the patella, reduces the abnormal tilt of the patella, and decreases the lateral patellar contact force.

Patellar subluxation

Patellar subluxation can occur in either direc-

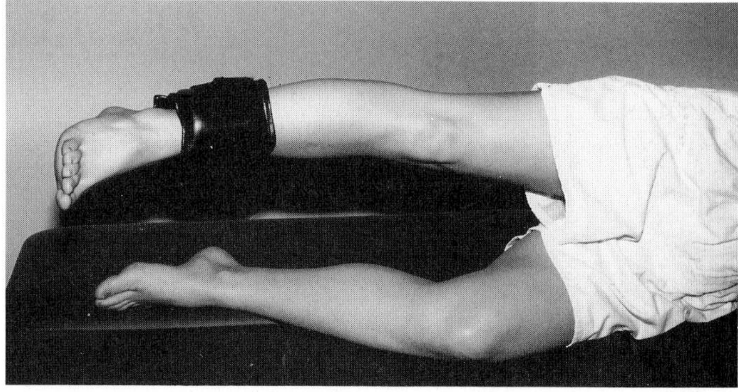

(a)

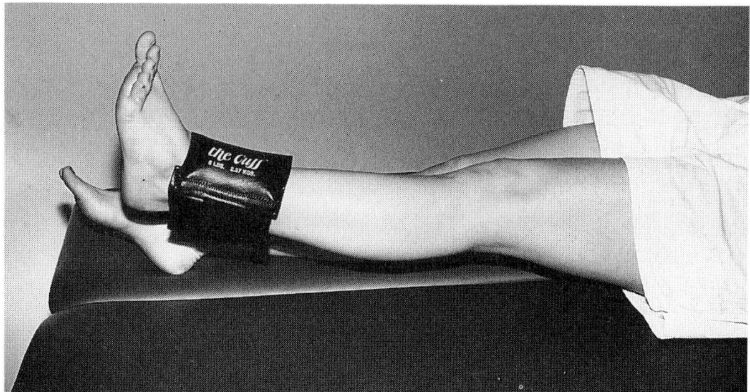

(b)

Fig. 10.11 Isometric exercises are added to the therapy, and weights are increased over a 2–3-month period.

tion as a result of patellar hypermobility. Medial subluxation is rare, but may occur in those patients with generalized ligamentous laxity, diseases of collagen like Marfan's syndrome or Down's syndrome, and in some neuromuscular diseases. Secondary medial subluxation may occur after overzealous surgical lateral retinacular release, or over medialization of the extensor mechanism proximally or distally (Radin, 1986b; Hughston & Deese, 1988). Recurrent subluxation is usually episodic with relatively asymptomatic intervals between events.

CLINICAL FEATURES

Patients with abnormal patellar tracking will experience a sense of instability, or 'giving way' of the knee during early knee flexion as a result of transient lateral movement of the patella. This is often associated with pain in the anterior knee. These episodes cause the patient to be apprehensive in performing activities. Episodes of giving way may be accompanied by subsequent effusions. While true locking of the knee is not usual, the momentary subluxation may clinically mimic a torn meniscus. Patients may complain of stiffness, especially after prolonged sitting with the knee flexed. This may limit a patient's ability to ride in a car or sit through a movie, and has been termed the 'movie theatre sign'. Usually, crepitus is not a dominant symptom early in the disease, but may become a problem as articular cartilage wear takes place. Patients with suspected patellar subluxation should be examined for generalized ligamentous laxity, alignment of the lower extremities and Q angle, proximal or distal resting position of the patella, and quadriceps bulk. Lower extremity geometry that contributes to abnormal patellar tracking includes increased Q angle, increased femoral anteversion, excessive external tibial torsion, and exaggerated heel pronation.

The anterior knee pain associated with this syndrome is typically poorly localized, and may be located at the medial or lateral retinaculum, the quadriceps tendon or the patellar ligament. The absence of joint line tenderness helps to distinguish patellar subluxation from a meniscal tear, since the history may be similar in these two conditions. The patella may illustrate excessive mobility on physical examination and the patient may have apprehension with lateral patellar displacement by the examiner. Muscle atrophy may be present as a relatively late physical finding. It is important to observe the tracking pattern of the patella throughout the entire range of motion, with special attention in the 10–20° range, as this is when the patella enters and exits the femoral trochlea.

TREATMENT

Initial management of patellar subluxation is with quadriceps rehabilitation and the use of a patellar support brace or patellar taping. Orthotics may be of use to improve lower extremity alignment in those patients in whom it is abnormal. Diligent and compliant patients who fail 6 months of conservative treatment, and continue to have symptoms and significant disability become surgical candidates.

Surgical management of patellar subluxation includes lateral retinacular release, more extensive proximal extensor mechanism realignment, or proximal and distal realignment. Lateral retinacular release is of particular value when preoperative studies have shown patellar tilt to be present. The procedure can be carried out by either arthroscopic or more traditional limited open methods. However, lateral release alone may not always correct subluxation. Proximal extensor mechanism realignment is of value when subluxation is present after lateral release. If patellar articular changes are present, operative treatment must aim to restore both alignment and to reduce pressure on the degenerated articular cartilage surface(s). Anterior or anteromedial transfer of the tibial tubercle relieves symptoms in many patients (Maquet, 1976; Fulkerson, 1983; Radin, 1986a,b).

Patellar dislocation

CLINICAL FEATURES

Complete dislocation of the patella represents one end of the spectrum of severity of patellofemoral instability. Lateral dislocation is far more common than medial dislocation, but the latter may occur in some neuromuscular disorders, or in general ligamentous laxity. The patient who experiences a complete dislocation of the patella is usually aware that such an event has occured. They will often describe the event as a 'knee dislocation', since they will have observed the obvious deformity of the patella lying outside the trochlear groove. The diagnosis is easily made if a closed reduction is required, but often reduction has been spontaneous, or has been done by the patient or other person at the scene. The dislocation may be the result of significant trauma, vigorous activity or a trivial movement. The patient may have pre-existing anterior knee pain as an element of the patellar malalignment syndrome, but this is not a consistent finding. In these patients, the severity of the event and subsequent symptoms are usually of greater magnitude than following an episode of subluxation.

In a patient who presents with the patella in a dislocated position, the diagnosis is obvious. If the patella is reduced, the knee will appear swollen and the patient will have considerable apprehension of the prospect of a knee examination. The knee should be examined in the position that is comfortable for the patient. The contralateral limb should be examined for overall alignment, patellar tracking, and patellar mobility. The patient should also be examined for generalized ligamentous laxity. Range of motion in the involved leg will be limited because of the swelling, pain and the possibility that an osteochondral fracture has resulted in a loose body within the joint. There may be some confusion as to whether other injury to the knee has occurred, such as anterior cruciate or meniscal tear. Gentle palpation should assess for tenderness at the retinacular structures and the joint lines. Tests for ligamentous instability are gently carried out. It will become apparent that the medial retinaculum is tender, and there is apprehension during any attempt at lateral displacement of the patella. The lateral retinaculum may or may not be tender.

RADIOGRAPHY

Radiographs are a mandatory component of the evaluation of a patient who has suffered a patellar dislocation. Anteroposterior, lateral, notch and tangential views are needed to rule out the presence of an associated osteochondral fracture of the patella or lateral trochlea, as well as evidence of other injury or coexistent disease. Other imaging modalities are usually not needed, and are of limited value unless one is looking for injury to other intra-articular structures like the menisci or cruciate ligament.

TREATMENT

Closed reduction of a dislocated patella is accomplished by manual reduction of the patella with the knee fully extended and the quadriceps relaxed. As mentioned, reduction may have occurred spontaneously with active or passive knee extension shortly after the event. A non-operative approach to the first time dislocator will result in successful outcome between 50 and 75% of the time (Cofield & Bryan, 1977; Larson & Lauridsen, 1982; Cash & Hughston, 1988). It has been our approach to immobilize the knee in a mildly compressive dressing to allow healing of the medial retinaculum in cases of traumatic dislocation. Straight leg raising and quadriceps isometric exercises are encouraged during this phase of treatment. Following this period, a standard programme of quadriceps rehabilitation is begun, and patients returned to regular activities with the aid of a patellar support brace when quadriceps control has been re-established.

If the radiographs indicate that an osteochondral fracture has occurred, we feel that arthroscopic examination should be carried out in the acute setting. If the fragment is of substantial size, a limited lateral arthrotomy is carried out to reduce anatomically and pin the fragment, and a lateral retinacular release is performed at the same time. If the fragment is small (less than 1 cm), arthroscopic removal is appropriate. If the patient has a history of anterior knee pain due to patellar malalignment, especially patellar tilt, arthroscopic lateral release may be beneficial.

In patients with recurrent patellar dislocations, the acute management is not significantly different. In general, the patient with recurrent dislocations will, however, have more severe malalignment, and subsequently, more damage to the lateral trochlear and patellar articular surfaces. More extensive surgery in the form of proximal and distal realignment may be necessary in this group. Success in preventing further episodes of dislocation is reported to be better than 80% in several series (Cerrullo *et al.*, 1988; Riegler, 1988; Turba, 1989). When patellar arthrosis is present, distal realignment alone may be performed using one of several reported techniques (Maquet, 1976; Cox, 1982; Fulkerson, 1983).

Medial plica syndrome

The medial patellar plica is a variably thick synovial fold that courses from the suprapatellar plica to the patellar fat pad. As it does so, it crosses the medial femoral condyle in the region of the anterior horn of the medial meniscus. Normally, this structure is small and inconsequential, but it may become thick and fibrotic if repeated impingement on the femoral condyle occurs. The symptoms are often difficult to distinguish from those of other anterior knee pain syndromes. The most helpful finding is tenderness with palpation along the medial femoral condyle in a fully flexed knee. Infrequently, the patient may experience snapping of the medial plica across the femoral condyle, and when present makes the diagnosis easy. Selective injection of local anaesthetic into the medial plica may help in localizing pain to this structure.

Non-operative treatment of a pathological medial plica includes local ice, rest, oral anti-inflammatory medication and a quadriceps rehabilitation programme. If symptoms persist, arthroscopic resection of the plica is a simple procedure, and when performed appropriately will be met with high success in relieving symptoms (Jackson *et al.*, 1982; Broom & Fulkerson, 1986).

Osgood–Schlatter disease

In 1903, Osgood and Schlatter independently described a disorder of the developing tibial tuberosity caused by recurrent trauma. Termed Osgood–Schlatter disease to recognize both men, this entity occurs most commonly in adolescents between 11 and 15 years of age. Boys are affected more often than girls, and onset often follows a period of rapid growth. A common history is activity involving kicking, jumping or squatting as a major component. Although usually unilateral, bilateral involvement has been reported in as much as 25% of cases.

The pathogenesis is traumatically induced disruption of the patellar ligament along its site of attachment to the tibial tubercle. This disruption can occur at either the cartilagenous or osseous stage of the developing tuberosity. Clinical signs are pain, tenderness and local soft-tissue swelling of various severity. Pain is usually temporally related to activity, and is relieved by rest.

Radiological abnormalities depend on the age of the patient and the stage of the disease. Since the tibial tuberosity lies slightly lateral to the midline of the tibia, a lateral projection should be taken with the lower extremity in slight internal rotation. In equivocal cases comparison views are important. Interpretation of the X-rays depends on an understanding of the normal pattern of ossification of the tibial tuberosity. In the acute phase, soft-tissue swelling in front of the tibial tuberosity may be significant, and low KV, and xeroradiography may be useful in this setting. If the tuberosity is entirely cartilagenous, no changes will be detected initially, but repeat X-rays several weeks later may show single or multiple ossific densities, and/or an avulsed fragment. In an older child, where the ossification centre has developed, radiodense foci can be seen, as well as surface irregularities where fragments of cartilage and bone have been avulsed. In the chronic phase, soft-tissue swelling has diminished, and displaced pieces of bone may increase in size due to either enchondral ossification or callus formation. The fragments can unite with one another or to the underlying tibial tuberosity. In fact, the radiographic appearance may return to normal, although usually some of the ossific fragments persist at the site of previous disease. A late finding may be the persistence of a large ossicle at the proximal aspect of the tibial tubercle, which may cause discomfort from a bursa that forms between the mobile ossicle and the tubercle (Fig. 10.12).

Treatment of Osgood–Schlatter disease ranges from none to complete immobilization. In the acute phase, rest, crutches, ice and anti-inflammatory medications are recommended. Upon resolution of symptoms, a complete quadriceps rehabilitation programme is initiated. Return to activity and sports is governed by the symptoms. Future episodes are similarly treated. The condition is usually self-limited, resolving completely with skeletal maturity. Occasionally, surgical exploration and excision of loose fragments, a bursa or an ossicle is necessary in a refractory case after skeletal maturity.

Complications and sequelae of this disease include non-union of the bone fragment, genu recurvatum, avulsion of the patellar ligament,

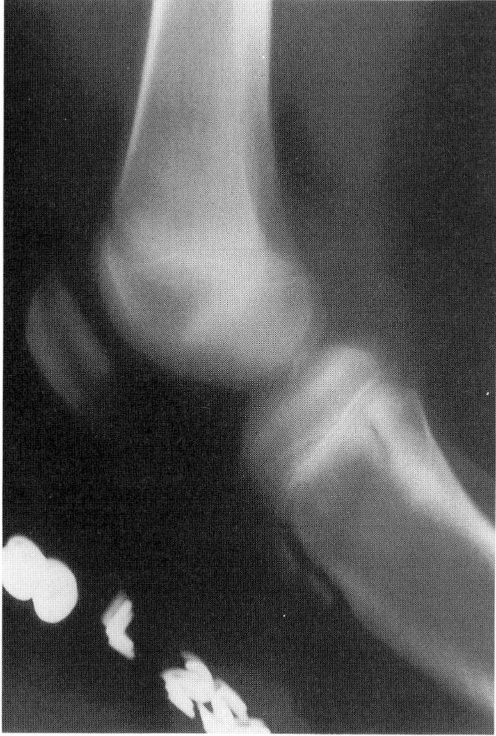

Fig. 10.12 A late radiographic finding of Osgood–Schlatter disease is the presence of an ossicle at the proximal aspect of the tibial tubercle.

patellar subluxation and chondromalacia. The normal tibial tuberosity growth plate does not seem to be affected by this disease, and premature closure with resultant genu recurvatum is a rare occurrence. Delayed distal displacement or excessive distal displacement of the tuberosity could cause patella alta or patella baja, respectively.

Sinding-Larson–Johansson disease

Sinding-Larson and Johansson independently described a disorder of the lower pole of the patella caused by recurrent trauma. The syndrome is most common in adolescent boys between the ages of 10 and 14 years. The clinical findings are pain, tenderness and swelling over the lower pole of the patella, accompanied by the typical radiographic appearance of osseous fragmentation in this area. Pain and tenderness are aggravated by activity involving running or jumping, and generally relieved by rest. Treatment of this condition is similar to that of Osgood–Schlatter disease. The natural history is resolution of symptoms in 3–12 months. The lesion is probably related to a traction of contusion injury followed by calcification and ossification, and in this respect is very similar to Osgood–Schlatter disease. The fragments may eventually coalesce into the inferior pole of the patella, so that late radiographs may show a normal appearing patella.

Bursitis

A bursa is a synovial lined cleft or sack lubricated by synovial fluid which functions to allow movement of one structure on another. Many bursa exist about the knee. The prepatellar bursa lies between the skin on the front of the knee and bony surface of the front of the patella. It functions to allow movement of the skin over the patella during flexion and extension movements of the knee. Other bursa exist between tendons and bone: the superficial infrapatellar bursa; between tendon and tendon: the bursa of the pes anserine; between tendon and ligament: the biceps femoris and the fibular collateral ligament; and between tendon and capsule: the semimembranosus and the medial and lateral heads of the gastrocnemius.

Bursitis is an inflammatory response in the synovial lined sack. It can have as its aetiology an inflammatory condition such as crystal disease or rheumatological manifestation, an infectious aetiology or a reaction process. In addition, the bursitis can be either acute or chronic in nature. Reactive bursitis may take place as a result of either macrotrauma or microtrauma. In cases of chronic bursitis, the synovial lining and wall of the bursal sack will become diseased causing thickening of these walls. At times, calcific precipitates may form within the walls of the bursa. In this disease state, the normal homeostatic mechanism which controls the amount of fluid production becomes adversely affected and may lead to a chronically swollen bursa.

Prepatellar bursitis

The prepatellar bursa, because of its location, is the one which is most likely to be injured due to macrotrauma. In any direct blow to the knee whether it be striking an opposing player, striking a hard object, such as a wall of a hockey rink or the ground may traumatize the bursa walls causing an acute haemorrhagic bursitis. Within moments, the bursal sack will fill with blood leading to a painful mass in the prepatellar region. In the examination of such an individual the differential diagnosis includes making sure that the response is not intra-articular. A haemarthrosis should be easily distinguished from a prepatellar collection. Prevention of prepatellar bursitis, which is traumatically induced, is directly dependent on appropriate padding of the region. In sports situations, where the participant is at risk for direct blow injury to the front of the knee, appropriate padding can play an integral role in the prevention of this phenomenon. Often the athlete will feel encumbered by any kind of padding or constrictive device and therefore have an aversion to using such devices. The athlete must be appropriately educated to the fact that protective equipment can play an integral role in the prevention of injury without affecting performance and should therefore be encouraged to use appropriate protection. The treatment of such a traumatic bursitis includes immediate ice application, compression and modification of activity so as to prevent immediate recurrent trauma.

In some situations, the individual may be allowed to continue to participate with appropriate padding in the prepatellar region. In situations in which the swelling is massive, pain relief may be obtained by aspiration of the bursa. Great care must be taken with special attention to strict aseptic technique as the blood-filled bursa is a perfect culture medium and an infectious prepatellar bursitis is a known complication of aspiration of a blood-filled bursa. Similarly, injections of steroids into the bursa causes an increased risk for subsequent infection.

With appropriate conservative care, haemorrhagic bursitis will mostly respond quickly, and the individual, when the knee range of motion is full, may return to participation with appropriate padding to protect the prepatellar region. Once the acute event resolves, there may be some residual thickening of the bursal walls that becomes palpable under the skin.

In situations where there is repeated trauma, the bursitis can become a chronic problem. In this setting, the fluid will have changed in character from blood to that of an exudate. Because of the thickening of the bursal wall and diseased lining, the bursa is unable to regulate the normal fluid production and resorption leading to a chronic bursitis. In this setting, one attempt may be made at aspiration and cortisone injection with appropriate care taken as mentioned above. If this is insufficient and if the bursa is large enough to warrant further treatment, surgical excision of the chronically inflamed tissues may be performed.

Although it is uncommon to see an acute bursitis unless there has been some element of a direct blow to the front of the knee, other conditions may be the cause. In a spontaneous bursitis without history of direct trauma, the differential diagnosis includes an infectious process or an inflammatory bursitis. If the clinical situation warrants it, (i.e. an acutely swollen, painful erythematous bursa) an aspiration for crystal analysis and appropriate cultures must be performed.

In chronic bursitis it is not uncommon that the constant grinding of the prepatellar skin against dirty objects such as the ground will drive bacteria through the dermis and then secondarily infect an otherwise sterile benign reactive bursitis. An infectious bursitis is a condition which requires immediate treatment with appropriate antibiotics and perhaps surgical decompression. A true inflammatory bursitis will respond well to treatment with non-steroidal medication.

Pes anserinus bursa

The tendons of the sartorius gracilis and semitendinosis wrap around the medial side of the knee just below the tibial metaphyseal flare and lie just below the tibial tubercle. These medial hamstring tendons have become collectively known as the pes anserinus. A bursal sack exists to lubricate the motion of the tendons one upon the other. At times, because of chronic overuse, a bursitis will develop in this region. Biomechanical abnormalities such as increased knee valgus, external rotation of the tibia or excessive tightness of the hamstring musculature have been implicated as being potential causes for this event. The differential diagnosis includes an intraosseous problem in the tibial metaphysis such as stress fracture, osteonecrosis of the medial tibial plateau or transient osteoporosis. At times, a benign tumour such as an osteochondroma will be present and by virtue of its presence cause a reactive bursitis. Evaluation includes a thorough diagnostic work-up including X-ray and at times, imaging studies such as a bone scan or MRI. Treatment includes standard modalities, such as rest, ice, non-steroidal medication when indicated, and gentle stretching and strengthening for the hamstring musculature. A biomechanical malalignment may need to be addressed by orthotic balancing of the foot.

Semimembranosus bursitis

The semimembranosus insertion is broad and spreads out on the medial side of the knee. A large tendon, it's direct head of insertion is on the posterior medial aspect of the tibia just below the joint line. A bursal separation between the tendon and surrounding medial head of the gastrocnemius and capsule exists and can at times become involved in a chronic bursitis. The diagnosis is made by localized pain on resisted flexion of the knee and direct tenderness over the insertion of the semimembranosus tendon into the posterior aspect of the tibia. The differential diagnosis is similar to that in pes anserinus bursitis and evaluation is similarly performed. Treatment is also very similar. When refractory, an injection of cortisone may be performed when other more conservative measures have failed.

Iliotibial band friction syndrome

Bursae also exist below subfascial planes. The most well known example is that which lies under the iliotibial tract and the prominence of the lateral femoral condyle. With activities such as running, there is constant movement of the iliotibial tract over this bony prominence which may lead to irritation in the bursa. Excessive foot pronation leading to excessive internal tibial rotation, as well as tightness of the tensor fascia lata muscle–tendon unit have been implicated as causing this problem.

The individual will present with pain quite specific to the lateral side of the knee in the region of the prominence of the lateral femoral condyle. When acute, subfascial crepitus may be felt. The differential diagnosis includes pathology of the lateral compartment of the knee, especially injury to the lateral meniscus. In the latter, the tenderness is often quite specific to the lateral joint line, whereas in the iliotibial band friction syndrome, the maximal point of tenderness is more proximal.

Prevention of this injury is dependent on appropriate education of the athlete. He or she must be encouraged to perform appropriate flexibility and stretching techniques both prior to and following sports participation. Care must be taken to equalize leg lengths, both true anatomical discrepancies as well as functional leg length differences, such as always running in the same direction on the side of the road, and thereby causing an inequality of leg length due to the underlying surface. Appropriate orthotic balancing of the hypermobile foot can also be preventive in the development of this syndrome.

Conservative treatment includes correction of the biomechanical abnormality, stretching of the tensor fascia lata and lateral knee structures, and subsequent strengthening. When refractory to conservative measures, a corticosteroid injection may be performed. If the condition becomes refractory, surgery may be performed. Surgical procedures are aimed at reducing the tautness of the iliotibial tract either by Z-band lengthening, simple sectionings of the anterior portion or an actual excision of a portion of the band to decompress the area.

Tendinitis

Tendinitis may exist as a component of several conditions. There is a true inflammatory tendinitis which may be present about tendons which are enclosed within synovial sheaths and pass around bony structures or under fibrous retinaculum. The synovial lining of the tendon sheath may manifest a true inflammatory response with an outpouring of either transudate or exudate containing inflammatory cells, and may be reactive due to overuse, direct trauma or inflammatory conditions. A second process may develop within the substance of the tendon itself which represents a degenerative process and not a true inflammatory response. Tendon response to chronic overload will initially be that of microscopic breakdown of the collagen with changes in the surrounding matrix. In more severe cases, a mucoid degeneration will take place with the central portion of the tendon being replaced by a jelly-like mucinous deposit. Most conditions of 'chronic tendinitis' present about the knee represent this latter phenomenon.

Patellar tendinitis

Chronic tendinitis of the infrapatellar ligament is better known as 'jumper's knee'. In the vast majority of movements in sports, the quadriceps functions in an eccentric manner. In the early phase of disease, the tendon will be painful and tender to the touch without any obvious deformity. With more severe trauma, a swelling in the substance of the tendon may develop. At times, the gross appearance of the tendon will still remain normal, or slightly enlarged. With more severe degeneration a mucinous replacement of the central portion of the tendon will take place. Once at this stage, surgical intervention is often required. At surgery, the degenerative portion of the tendon is excised with reconstruction of the remaining tendon. In the infrapatellar ligament, this degeneration has a propensity to occur either at the inferior pole of the patella or distally at the insertion onto the tibial tubercle.

Initially, the athlete will complain of pain after activities. With increasing severity, the pain will become present during the sport itself. With further progression, pain becomes present even during periods of inactivity. On examination, the pain can be elicited during active concentric extension and with direct pressure over the affected tendon. The examiner should feel for a fullness or swelling in the tendon itself. X-ray evaluation should be performed to rule out any intratendinous calcification. MRI examination may be helpful in the evaluation of this problem. The reaction in the tendon is due to excessive load and not biomechanical abnormality. Treatment must therefore address modifying the loads. This is most easily done by modifying the individual's activities. Adjunctive modalities such as ice, ultrasound and non-steroidal medications may be of some benefit. Stretching of the quadriceps mechanism is important, as well as re-education with eccentric strengthening exercises. Care should be taken to avoid concentric strengthening especially with isokinetic devices which may have a propensity to further irritate the tendon. Injections of corticosteroids are contraindicated in this condition, since direct steroid injection into the tendon will weaken the tendon and may result in patellar tendon rupture. When the disease process has progressed to the point of significant swelling in the tendon, surgical intervention is usually required.

There have been several reports in the literature of individuals, especially powerlifters, suffering ruptures of the infrapatellar ligament. Of note has been the high association of anabolic steroid use with this injury. Whether anabolic steroids truly have a detrimental effect on tendons or whether the steroids indirectly act by allowing more aggressive and stressful behaviour on the part of the individual as the cause for the tendon degeneration and rupture, is unclear.

Quadriceps tendinitis

In a similar fashion, degenerative changes may take place at the insertion of the quadriceps tendon into the superior pole of the patella. The pathogenesis of this is very similar to that which is seen in the infrapatellar tendinitis but the quadriceps tendon condition tends to be less common in a young athlete. In the older individual quadriceps tendon ruptures are common but this is often on the basis of degenerative disease with aging of the tendon. As in the above discussion, corticosteroidal injections into this region are contraindicated.

Stress fractures

Stress fractures can occur around the knee due to microtrauma of sports. They are not as common as stress fractures of the tibial shaft but should be included in the differential diagnosis of the painful knee in the endurance athlete. When present, they are most commonly located in the tibia at the flare of the metaphysis. Local tenderness on examination will be present and the differential diagnosis includes any soft-tissue overload such as the conditions discussed earlier in this chapter. The diagnosis is made on the basis of either X-ray findings or positive imaging studies, such as an MRI or bone scan.

Prevention, once again, primarily falls into the area of patient education. The athlete must be instructed on appropriate training techniques, which graduate the stress which the lower extremity sees during training and competitive events. In the female athlete it is especially important to be aware of the individual's menstrual status as amenorrhoea with it's attendant hormonal imbalance may lead to a relative osteopenia and make the individual more prone to the development of stress fracture syndrome. Careful histories must be obtained and appropriate records of dietary intake and, if necessary, appropriate gynaecological intervention performed so as to minimize the risk that the female athlete develops as a result of amenorrhoea. Treatment includes activity modification until the acute symptoms resolve and then adaptations in training techniques to allow for a graduated return to full activity.

Degenerative joint disease

Common concern among the lay public is whether the repeated microtrauma of sports will in any way predispose the individual to degenerative joint disease later in life. There has been no clinical study which has proven that repetitive stresses normally incurred in sports will in any way be the cause for osteoarthritis later in life. If there is pre-existing degenerative change in the joint then it is not uncommon for it to become irritated and symptomatic due to the repetitive microtrauma of sports. Individuals who have had macrotrauma to the knee such that they have lost part of the meniscal component of the knee may be more at risk if they lead a very vigorous sporting lifestyle than in someone who becomes more sedentary after such an injury. Such statements, however are speculative as there are no long-term studies which have proven that such an occurrence takes place.

The health-care practitioner must use his or her own judgement in counselling individuals who have undergone meniscectomy or who have existing degenerative disease with regard to their sports participation. Prevention of further degeneration in the knee becomes dependent on the practitioner educating the athlete of the potential worsening of this condition and carefully monitoring the response of the joint to training and competition. Appropriate padding in the shoe, surface selection for long training runs, appropriate muscle rehabilitation and flexibility training may all play a role in the ability of the lower extremity to absorb shock and thereby act as a protector of the joint. If the athlete develops progressive discomfort and pain, and especially if effusions develop, then modification in exercise intensity must be undertaken. In the otherwise normal knee, however, the routine trauma of sports seems to be well tolerated.

References

Blumensaat, C. (1938) Die Lageabweichungen and Veirunkengun der Kniescheibe. *Ergel. Chir. Orthop.* **31**, 149–223.

Boven, F., Bellemans, M.A., Gevits, J. & Potvliege, R.A. (1982) A comparative study of the patellofemoral joint in axial roentgenogram, axial arthrogram, and computed tomography following arthrography. *Skel. Radiol.* **8**, 179–81.

Broom, J.M. & Fulkerson, J.P. (1986) The plica syndrome. A new perspective. *Orthop. Clin. N. Am.* **17**, 279–81.

Cash, J. & Hughston, J. (1988) Treatment of acute patellar dislocation. *Am. J. Sports Med.* **16**, 244–50.

Cerullo, G., Puddu, G., Conteduca, F., Ferretti, A. & Mariani, P. (1988) Evaluation of the results of extensor mechanism reconstruction. *Am. J. Sports Med.* **16**, 93–6.

Cofield, R. & Bryan, R. (1977) Acute dislocation of the patella. Results of conservative treatment. *J. Trauma* **17**, 526–31.

Cox, J.S. (1982) Evaluation of the Roux–Elmslie–Trillat procedure for knee extensor realignment. *Am. J. Sports Med.* **10**, 303–10.

Fisher, R.L. (1986) Conservative treatment of patellofemoral pain. *Orthop. Clin. N. Am.* **17**, 269–2.

Fulkerson, J.P. (1982) Awareness of the retinaculum in evaluating patellofemoral pain. *Am. J. Sports Med.* **10**, 147.

Fulkerson, J.P. (1983) Anteromedialization of the tibial tuberosity for patellofemoral malalignment. *Clin. Orthop.* **177**, 129–33.

Fulkerson, J.P. (1989) Evaluation of peripatellar soft tissues and retinaculum in patients with patellofemoral pain. *Clin. Sports Med.* **8**, 197–202.

Fulkerson, J.P., Schutzer, S.F., Ramsby, G.R. & Bernstein, R.A. (1987) Computerized tomography of the patellofemoral joint before and after lateral release or realignment. *Arthroscopy* **3**, 19–24.

Fulkerson, J.P. & Shea, K.P. (1990) Current concepts review. Disorders of patellofemoral alignment. *J. Bone Joint Surg.* **72A**, 1424–9.

Fulkerson, J.P., Tennant, R., Jaivin, J. & Grunnet, M. (1985) Histological evidence of retinacular nerve injury associated with patellofemoral malalignment. *Clin. Orthop.* **197**, 196.

Grana, W.A. & Kriegshauser, S.F. (1985) Scientific basis of extensor mechanism disorders. *Clin. Sports Med.* **4**, 247–57.

Henry, J.H. (1989) Conservative treatment of patellofemoral subluxation. *Clin. Sports Med.* **8**, 261–78.

Hughston, J. & Deese, M. (1988) Medial subluxation of the patella as a complication of lateral retinacular release. *Am. J. Sports Med.* **16**, 383–8.

Inoue, M., Shino, K., Hirose, H., Horibe, S. & Ono, K. (1988) Subluxation of the patella: Computed tomography analysis of patellofemoral congruence. *J. Bone Joint Surg.* **70A**, 1331.

Insall, J. & Salvati, E. (1971) Patella position in the normal knee joint. *Radiology* **101**, 101–4.

Jackson, R., Marshall, D. & Fujisawa, Y. (1982) The pathological medial shelf. *Orthop. Clin. N. Am.* **13**, 307–12.

Krompinger, J. & Fulkerson, J. (1983) Retinacular release for intractable lateral retinacular pain. *Clin. Orthop.* **179**, 191–3.

Larson, E. & Lauridsen, F. (1982) Conservative treatment of patellar dislocations. *Clin. Orthop.* **171**, 131–6.

Larson, R.L., Cabaud, H.E., Slocum, D.B., Jones, S.L., Keenan, T. & Hutchinson, T. (1978) The patellar compression syndrome: Surgical treatment by lateral retinacular relase. *Clin. Orthop.* **134**, 158–67.

Laurin, C.A., Dusault, R. & Levesque, H.P. (1979) The tangential X-ray investigation of the patellofemoral joint. X-ray technique, diagnostic criteria and their interpretation. *Clin. Orthop.* **144**, 16.

Laurin, C.A., Levesque, H.P., Dusault, R., Labelle, M. & Peides, J.P. (1978) The abnormal lateral patellofemoral angle. *J. Bone Joint Surg.* **60A**, 55.

McConnell, J. (1986) The management of chrondromalacia patella: A long-term solution. *Austral. J. Physiother.* **32**, 215–33.

McGinty, J.B. & McCarthy, J.C. (1981) Endoscopic lateral retinacular release. A preliminary report. *Clin. Orthop.* **158**, 120–5.

Maquet, P. (1976) Advancement of the tibial tuberosity. *Clin. Orthop.* **115**, 225–30.

Merchant, A.C., Mercer, R.L., Jacobsen, R.H. & Coal, C.R. (1974) Roentgenographic analysis of patellofemoral congruence. *J. Bone Joint Surg.* **56A**, 1391.

Mow, V., Holmes, M. & Lai, W. (1984) Fluid transport and mechanical properties of articular cartilage. A review. *J. Biomech.* **17**, 372–4.

Radin, E.L. (1986a) Anterior tibial tubercle elevation in the young adult. *Orthop. Clin. N. Am.* **17**, 297–302.

Radin, E.L. (1986b) The Maquet procedure — anterior displacement of the tibial tubercle. Indication, contraindication, and precautions. *Clin. Orthop.* **213**, 241–8.

Riegler, H.F. (1988) Recurrent dislocations and subluxations of the patella. *Clin. Orthop.* **227**, 201–9.

Schonholtz, G. (1987) Lateral retinacular release of the patella. *Arthroscopy* **3**, 269–72.

Schutzer, S.F., Ramsby, E.R. & Fulkerson, J.P. (1986) Computed tomographic classification of patellofemoral pain patients. *Orthop. Clin. N. Am.* **17**, 235–48.

Turba, J. (1989) Formal extensor mechanism reconstruction. *Clin. Sports Med.* **8**, 297–317.

Wojtys, E., Wilson, M., Buchwalter, K., Braunstein, E. & Mantel, W. (1987) Magnetic resonance imaging of knee hyaline articular cartilage and intraarticular pathology. *Am. J. Sports Med.* **15**, 455–63.

Yulish, B.S., Montanez, J., Goodfellow, P.B., Bryan, P.J., Mulopulos, G.P. & Modic, M.T. (1987) Chondromalacia patellae: Assessment with MR imaging. *Radiology* **164**, 763–6.

Chapter 11

Sport-Specific Knee Injuries

CHARLES E. HENNING,* N. DEAN GRIFFIS, STEVEN W. VEQUIST, KIM M. YEAROUT AND KRISTA A. DECKER

One of the most devastating injuries to an athlete is a torn anterior cruciate ligament (ACL). The ACL is the primary restraint to anterior tibial displacement (Marshall & Baugher, 1980; Daniels *et al.*, 1981) by providing an average 86% of the total resisting force in the functional position of the knee during weight-bearing (Butler *et al.*, 1980). Without a functional ACL, athletes develop degenerative arthritis, are unable to participate in high-level lateral movement sports, and must maintain lifetime restrictions in order to extend the functional life of the knee (Johnson *et al.*, 1974; Feagin & Lambert, 1980; Lynch *et al.*, 1983; McDaniel & Dameron, 1983; O'Brien, 1989). When the ACL is surgically reconstructed, the athlete is restricted from most athletic participation for up to 1 full year.

While much work has been done on description of mechanism of injury and developing better techniques for treating a torn ACL, little work has been done on injury prevention of the 'not hit' ACL injuries (Abbott & Kress, 1969; Peterson, 1970, 1973; Eriksson, 1976; Feagin *et al.*, 1978; Feagin & Lambert, 1985). For the purpose of this study, a hit is defined as any contact the athlete encountered during the injury that made it impossible to utilize the injury prevention techniques that will be discussed later in this report. Feagin (1979) points out that non-contact ACL injuries are more frequent than contact injuries.

This study aimed to identify specific play situations and the associated technique involved in an ACL injury. Modified player techniques for these situations are recommended to decrease the incidence of not hit ACL injuries. The coaches and players can relate better to injury-producing play situations than to the techniques.

Previous studies have shown an interaction between the contraction of the quadriceps loading a posterior sloping patellar tendon and the loading of the ACL through the anterior shear force of the tibia (DeLorme, 1956; Lindahl & Movin, 1967; Johnson & Pope, 1978; Daniels *et al.*, 1981; Henning *et al.*, 1985; Paulos *et al.*, 1986; Renström *et al.*, 1986; Kain *et al.*, 1988; D.L. MacIntosh, personal communication). In 1956, DeLorme introduced the idea of a quadricep contraction being antagonistic to the ACL. Others have confirmed that the posterior slope of the patellar tendon results in an anterior tibial displacement force when the quadriceps contract. As the knee flexes, the posterior slope decreases and the anterior tibial displacement force decreases thus reducing the load through the ACL by the quadricep/cruciate interaction (Lindahl & Movin, 1967; Johnson & Pope, 1978; Daniels *et al.*, 1981; Henning *et al.*, 1985; Paulos *et al.*, 1986; Renström *et al.*, 1986).

Figure 11.1 illustrates the quadricep/cruciate interaction. Figure 11.1a shows 10° of flexion

* The authors of this chapter would like to dedicate it to Charles E. Henning, who unfortunately died during publication.

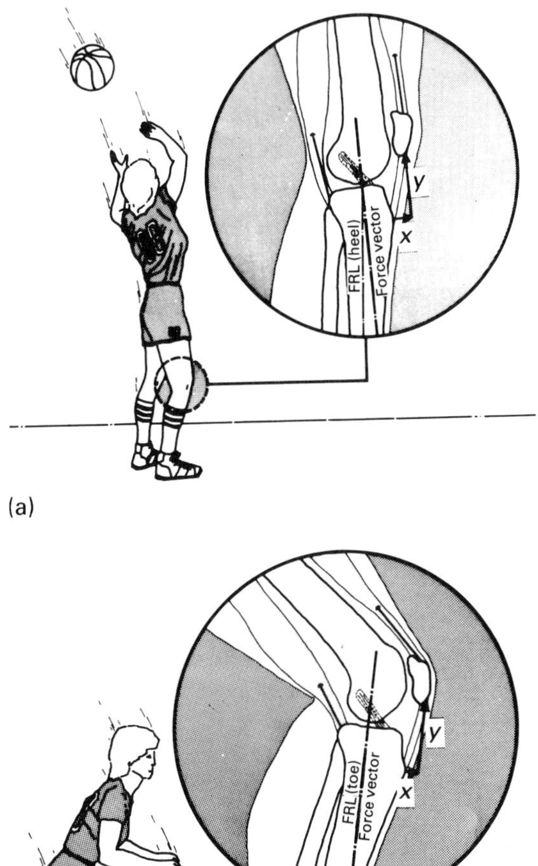

Fig. 11.1 (a) *Bad technique*. Knee is at 10° of flexion. The floor reactive line is the force from foot contact to axis of joint. The force vector line is a perpendicular force from the tangent of the femur and tibia. The two resulting forces of the patellar tendon during quad contraction are the vertical (y) which is parallel to the force vector that extends the knee, and the horizontal (x) which translates the tibia anteriorly. More anterior sheer force occurs with greater extension. (b) *Good technique*. Knee is at 60° of flexion. The floor reactive line and the force vector line are at the same force. The horizontal force vector is shorter thus less anterior sheer force of the tibia occurs.

and Fig. 11.1b 60° of flexion. A force vector line was drawn perpendicular to the tangent of the compression point between the femur and tibia to illustrate the joint compression force. A second line illustrates the floor reaction line between the point of foot contact and the compression point of the knee. In Fig. 11.1a, the total for these two forces are at different angles (adding to anterior tibial displacement load) and in Fig. 11.1b they are (not adding to anterior tibial displacement load) parallel.

The posterior slope of the patellar tendon from the patella to the tibial tuberosity has two resultant forces. The vertical force vector (force y) is parallel to the joint compression force, and extends the knee. The horizontal force (force x) is the perpendicular vector that causes the anterior shear force of the tibia on the femur. This force directly loads the ACL.

The anterior shear is much greater at 10° than at 60° flexion. Measurements of the vertical component to anterior shear ratio were obtained from X-rays at 10° of flexion, the vertical vector measured 65 mm and the horizontal measured 19 mm (a 1 : 0.29 ratio). At 60° of flexion, the vertical vector measured 65 mm and the horizontal measured only 12 mm (a 1 : 0.185 ratio). This study demonstrates that a 1.5 × greater anterior shear force of the tibia on the femur at 10° than at 60° flexion, which is consistent with the studies previously described (Lindahl & Movin, 1967; Daniels *et al.*, 1981; Henning *et al.*, 1985; Paulos *et al.*, 1986; Renström, 1986).

If the athlete is to reduce ACL loading via the quadricep–cruciate interaction during a specific play situation, it is necessary to prevent the knee from being in a straight or near straight position when a forceful concentric or eccentric quadricep contraction occurs. The most common sports involved in ACL injury as well as the associated injury techniques are listed in Table 11.1. Although some are not Olympic sports, they are listed so as to give the athletes a means of comparing injury risk.

Table 11.1 Injury-producing situations for the anterior cruciate ligament (n = 673). Hit versus not hit: 534 (79%) not hit; 133 (20%) hit; and 6 (1%) unknown.

					Injury technique						
Injury situation	Total		Not hit	Hit	PAC	SKL	OSS	TWS	HYP	BND	OTR
Basketball	180		152	28	44	52	31	9	6	0	10
Football (North American)	154	2*	77	75	50	7	6	5	2	0	9
Snow skiing	70		68	2	2	2	1	6	3	25	29
Baseball	64		57	7	20	6	14	2	4	0	11
Soccer	61		51	10	22	7	8	2	6	0	6
Volleyball	28		28	0	1	14	3	3	1	0	6
Track	13		13	0	1	7	0	0	2	0	3
Wrestling	12		7	5	2	0	0	2	0	0	3
Rugby	9		6	3	0	1	1	2	1	0	1
Racquetball	8		8	0	3	2	1	1	1	0	0
Cheerleading	6		6	0	0	4	0	2	0	0	0
Gymnastics	6		6	0	0	5	0	0	1	0	0
Bike riding	6		6	0	0	2	0	2	1	0	1
Other sports and accidents	56	4*	49	3	2	11	3	5	4	0	28
Total	673	6	534	133	147	120	68	41	32	25	107
%		1	79	20	22	18	10	6	5	4	16
All sports excluding North American football — Total	519	4*	457	58							
All sports excluding North American football — %		1	88	11							

* Not known if hit or not hit.

BND, bindings; HYP, hyperextended; OSS, one step stop; OTR, other; PAC, plant and cut; SKL, straight knee landing; TWS, twist.

Injury-producing techniques

From 1971 to 1987, research performed at the Mid-America Center for Sports Medicine in Wichita, Kansas shows that the majority of the ACL 'not hit' injuries involved three common injury-producing deceleration techniques (plant and cut, straight knee landing, and one step stop) (Table 11.1). The combination of the powerful quad contraction on the straight leg and the flexion force on the knee from the deceleration of forward momentum, producing ACL loading by the quadricep–cruciate interaction with the most common injury technique in all sports being the plant and cut.

Plant and cut

The plant and cut is a manoeuvre that involves sudden deceleration on a straight or near straight leg with intent to change direction in one step. It is often done in an attempt to elude a defender and make a quick change of direction. For example, an offensive player will attempt to make a turn to the right. As the player approaches the defensive opponent, the offensive player suddenly decelerates by planting the outside (left) foot with the left knee in a near straight position (less than 30°) and cuts or turns towards the inside (right) foot (Fig. 11.2a). As the player decelerates in one step for the turn with the knee in the near straight position, the quads are forcefully contracting eccentrically producing the quadricep–cruciate interaction.

Straight knee landing and vertical take-off

The straight knee landing technique is the result of a player landing from a jump with the legs too straight or failing to bend the knees throughout the landing as in the follow-through steps producing the quadricep–cruciate interaction (Fig. 11.3a).

ACL injury may also result from a take-off directly from a running stride (with no preparation step). The knee is straighter and all the conversion of horizontal momentum to vertical momentum is done by decelerating and taking off in a single step. An eccentric quadriceps contraction is followed immediately by a concentric contracture resulting in a greater force on the ACL through the quadricep–cruciate interaction.

One step stop

The third most common injury-producing technique is the one step stop. The one step stop is often combined with the player attempting to stop and reverse direction in one step. For example, a soccer player attempts to approach an offensive player at full speed. As the offensive player gets closer, the defender tries to stop in one step in order to play defence — producing a high-loading quadricep–cruciate interaction (Fig. 11.4a).

Improved player techniques

Due to the high association of ACL injury involving one or more of these three techniques, improved techniques were introduced to help reduce the chance of an ACL tear without compromising player performance.

Accelerated rounded turn

The plant and cut was modified into an accelerated rounded turn. The turn is actually begun on the inside foot (foot towards the direction of the turn), called the preparation step. The turn is continued on the outside foot with the player accelerating through the turn. As the player masters this drill, instruction is given to incorporate this into competitive situations. The offensive player approaches the defender at one-half to three-quarter speed (see Fig. 11.2b). When about 2 m from the defender and ready to make a move, the offensive player will accelerate past the defender. The offensive player makes a preparation step on the inside foot, while rounding the turn and accelerating past the defender (avoiding deceleration). Strong

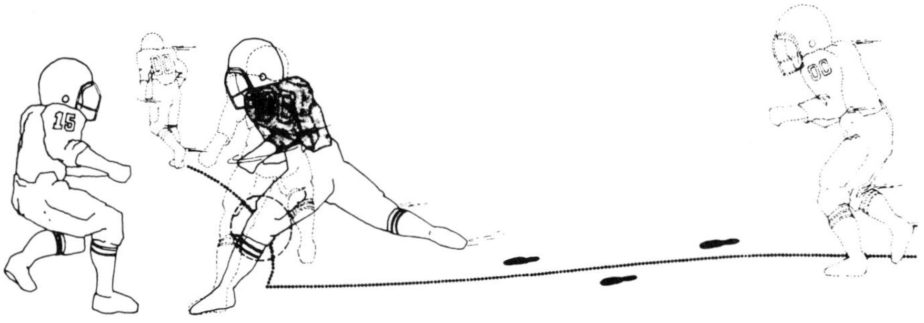

(a)

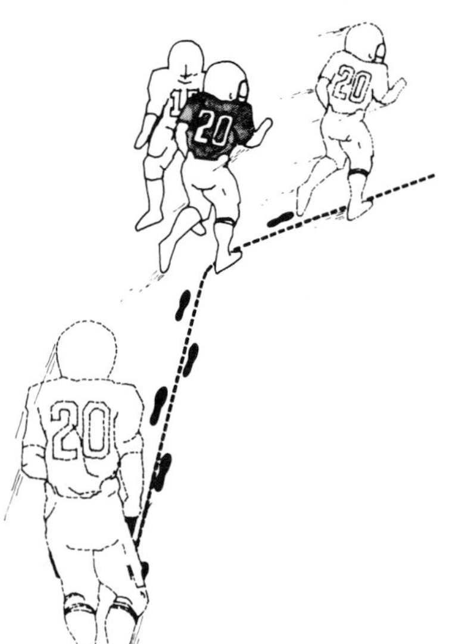

(b)

Fig. 11.2 (a) Bad technique: plant and cut. (b) Good technique: accelerated rounded turn.

arm motion and moderate stride lengths aid in the acceleration. The key to performing this safely and effectively is to initiate the turn off the inside foot and accelerate past the defender. When the athlete is accelerating through the turn, the magnitude of the quadricep–cruciate interaction force is reduced (see Fig. 11.1a).

Bent knee vertical landing and two step vertical take-off

The straight knee landing was modified to the bent knee landing (Fig. 11.3b). With landing from a running jump, common in sports such as basketball and volleyball, it is important each player be instructed to land from a jump shot, lay-up, block shot, spike, jump ball or rebound with the knees bent and continue to bend them as they land and take at least one more step in the same direction before stopping or turning.

The moving two step vertical take-off is the normal form that the athlete would use for shooting or defending a lay-up in basketball or spiking a volleyball. The right-handed player uses the right foot for the complete 'preparation step' to 'gather themselves' and the 'in control' vertical take-off is from the left foot.

The athlete decreases the quadriceps–cruciate interaction by continuing to bend the knees through the landing and by making the complete two step vertical take-off. It is important that the athlete, in this situation, be made aware of the 'intent' factor involved. In other words, when a player is attempting to make a sudden transition from horizontal or vertical deceleration to vertical acceleration in one step, they often do so without allowing the recovery from deceleration to occur. This 'intent' to make a sudden transition is considered an out of

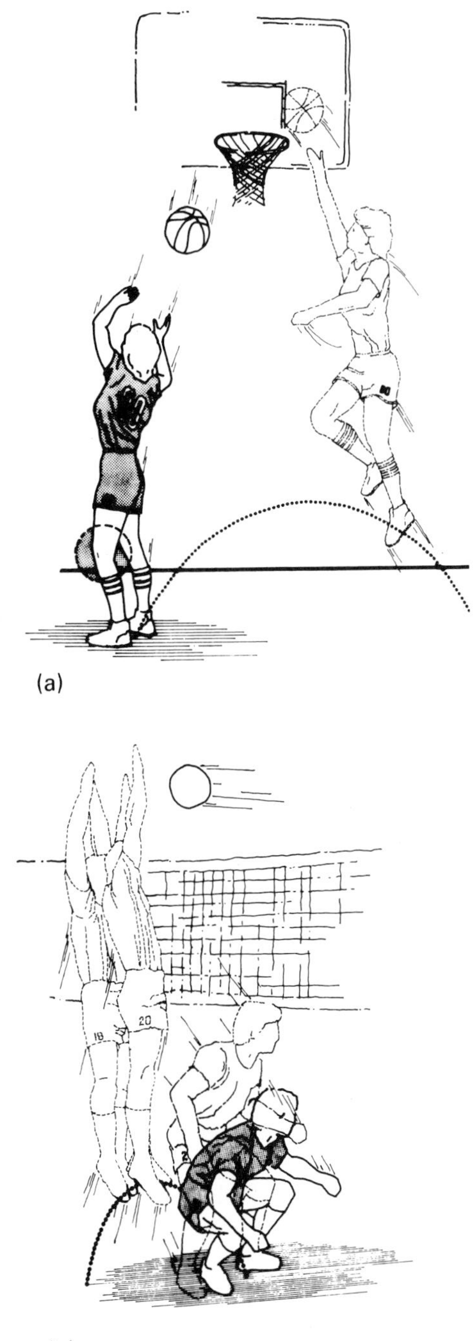

Fig. 11.3 (a) Bad technique: straight knee landing. (b) Good technique: bent knee landing.

control move and produces extreme, injury-producing quadricep–cruciate interaction loads.

Three step stop and block turn

The one step stop was modified to a three step stop that is used when a player needs to come to a stop or change direction (see Fig. 11.4b). For example, a soccer player is in a situation which requires sudden deceleration to defend an offensive player. The improved player technique allows the player to reduce the forward momentum by lowering the centre of gravity and bending the knees while decelerating in at least three steps. As the player lowers his or her centre of gravity by bending the knees, the quadricep–cruciate interaction produces lower ACL loads. The player is now in a position of good balance and prepared for any directional change. Gradual deceleration over three steps instead of sudden deceleration in one step also decreases the energy dissipated per step.

Another technique than can be used for reversing direction is the block turn. This is used when the athlete takes a preparation step, turning in by pivoting on the same foot, and landing on all fours to a sprint starting stance. The athlete then pushes off similar to a sprinter in track pushing out of the blocks. This is a safe means of changing direction 180° and much faster than the three step stop or even the injury-producing one step stop.

ACL injuries in specific sports

When attempting to develop an injury-prevention programme, it is important to emphasize those play situations responsible for most of the ACL injuries. To do this, the injury-producing play situation of that particular sport must be identified. This differs from the injury technique in that it is the actual event the athlete was conscious of doing at the moment of the injury. The injury technique is the bio-

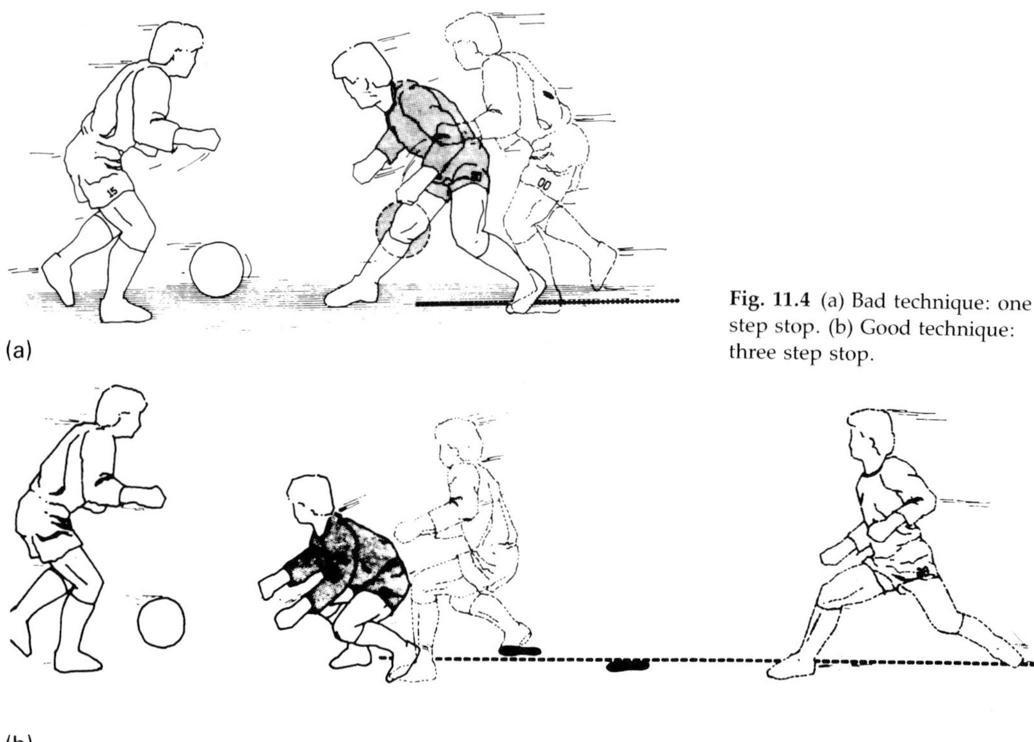

Fig. 11.4 (a) Bad technique: one step stop. (b) Good technique: three step stop.

mechanical result of the mechanism the athlete was using at the time of injury. It is important that the ACL injury-producing play situation is identified by the coach and athlete in order to modify the player technique effectively. Drills should emphasize the injury-prevention techniques.

Basketball is listed as the sport responsible for the most injuries to the ACL; a large portion of this chapter is therefore spent on this sport. Many of the injury situations in basketball are similar to those in other sports. Tables with injury situations and techniques that the athlete might have used to prevent an injury are listed for the Olympic sports most commonly responsible for ACL injuries. These tables and descriptions are designed to aid the athlete and coach with an easy 'at a glance' style for learning the injury situation and injury-prevention techniques.

Basketball

Basketball ranks as the highest ACL injury-producing sport with 27% of the total ACL tears in our clinic. This is perhaps due to the constant change of direction as well as the large amount of jumping and landing. The most common injury techniques are the straight knee landing (29%), plant and cut (24%), and the one step stop (17%). The lay-up, shifting on defence and the rebound attempt are the top three injury situations in basketball (Table 11.2).

Since the lay-up is the most common ACL-producing injury situation in basketball and the straight knee landing is the most comon injury technique, drills should overexaggerate the bent knee landing while doing the lay-up. It is also important that the athlete should not overextend the knee while looking back for the shot. This can cause the athlete to lose awareness in space and result in an overextended

Table 11.2 Injury-producing situations for the anterior cruciate ligament in basketball (men and women) (n = 180).

					Injury technique						
Injury situation	Total	(%)	Not hit	Hit	PAC	SKL	OSS	TWS	HYP	OTR	Improved player technique
Lay-up	22	(12)	20	2	4	8	4	0	1	3	BKL, TSS, BLT
Shifting on defence	22	(12)	20	2	10	1	5	1	1	2	ART, TSS, BLT
Rebound attempt	19	(11)	15	4	0	8	4	3	0	0	BKL, TSS
Dribbling	18	(10)	15	3	5	2	4	3	0	1	ART, TSS
Block shot attempt	15	(8)	15	0	3	10	2	0	0	0	BKL
Jump for a loose ball	15	(8)	14	1	0	10	2	0	1	1	BKL
Loose ball	12	(7)	9	3	1	5	2	0	1	0	BKL
Jump shot	10	(6)	9	1	3	3	3	0	0	0	BKL, TSS
Trying to stop	9	(5)	8	1	4	0	4	0	0	0	TSS, BLT
Other	9	(5)	9	0	2	0	1	2	1	3	
Plant and fake	7	(4)	7	0	7	0	0	0	0	0	ART, BLT
Landing from a jump	7	(4)	4	3	1	3	0	0	0	0	BKL
Hit	7	(4)	0	7	0	0	0	0	0	0	
Bad pass recovery	4	(2)	4	0	1	2	0	0	1	0	BKL, BLT
Posting up	2	(1)	2	0	2	0	0	0	0	0	ART, TSS
Setting a pick	2	(1)	1	1	1	0	0	0	0	0	ART
Total	180		152	28	44	52	31	9	6	10	
%			84	16	24	29	17	5	3	6	

ART, accelerated rounded turn; BKL, bent knee landing; BLT, block turn; HYP, hyperextended; OSS, one step stop; OTR, other; PAC, plant and cut; SKL, straight knee landing; TSS, three step stop; TWS, twist.

leg. Instead, the athlete should land with the legs bent and continue bending throughout the landing. For the situation which requires the player to get back to the ball quickly, the lay-up can be completed by turning in midair towards the basket and landing in a bent knee position, or in a position similar to a block turn. Both would enable the athlete to accelerate back to the ball safely.

SHIFTING ON DEFENCE

Defensive shifting is a very aggressive and unpredictable part of basketball competition. Since the defensive player does not know what to expect from the offensive player, the defender is often caught off guard and may overextend the leg in an attempt to get to the ball. It is important to drill the athletes to play defence in a bent knee position. That is, have the defenders lower their centre of gravity by bending their knees, and discourage any overstride when trying to play defence. This is considered a good defensive position but all too often as the players tire or get caught by surprise, they overextend the leg or play poor defence in an upright position. It is also important to instruct the athletes to push off from the inside foot (foot towards the direction of the turn).

Another injury-producing technique while shifting on defence is stopping in one step. It is often the case that a defender will attempt to change direction in one step. This injury-producing situation should be replaced with the three step stop. For example, in a situation where the defender is forced to run up on the offensive player, the defender should lower his or her centre of gravity and continue to lower it whilst reducing forward momentum in at least three steps. A good drill for this is the defensive triangle. The defender is placed in the centre and three offensive players form a triangle approximately 4.5 m (15 ft) apart. The idea of the drill is to pass the ball from player to player, trying to keep it from the defender. The defender must use the three step stop technique. The offensive player should hold the ball for a few seconds before passing it so as to give the defender time to run and perform the three step stop correctly.

DRIBBLING

While dribbling the ball, a player will often try to elude a defender by planting and cutting in the opposite direction, especially when they are out of control. When the dribble is practised, each player should concentrate on control and the use of good injury-prevention technique such as making the rounded turns off the inside foot and decelerating with the three step stop (Table 11.2).

North American football

Football is considered by many to be more of a collision sport than a contact sport. Each play results in multiple collisions with contact at various body parts. Athletes have to be able to react quickly (Fig. 11.5). Knees are perhaps most susceptible to injury since they are exposed without protection and are at a level where a lot of contact occurs. Even with this considered, approximately 50% of all ACL injuries in North American football occur without contact at the knee (Table 11.3). This might suggest that ACL injury prevention would have a place in a high-contact sport such as football. Although North American football is not an Olympic sport, it is addressed due to the high incidence of ACL injury (Table 11.3).

Baseball and softball

Baseball and softball are closely related. Due to the similarities of the two sports, they will both be classified as baseball for this project. Baseball is a sport that involves very little contact. Only 11% of the total ACL tears in baseball occurred as the result of a hit (Table 11.4).

BASE RUNNING

The leading injury situation for ACL tears in

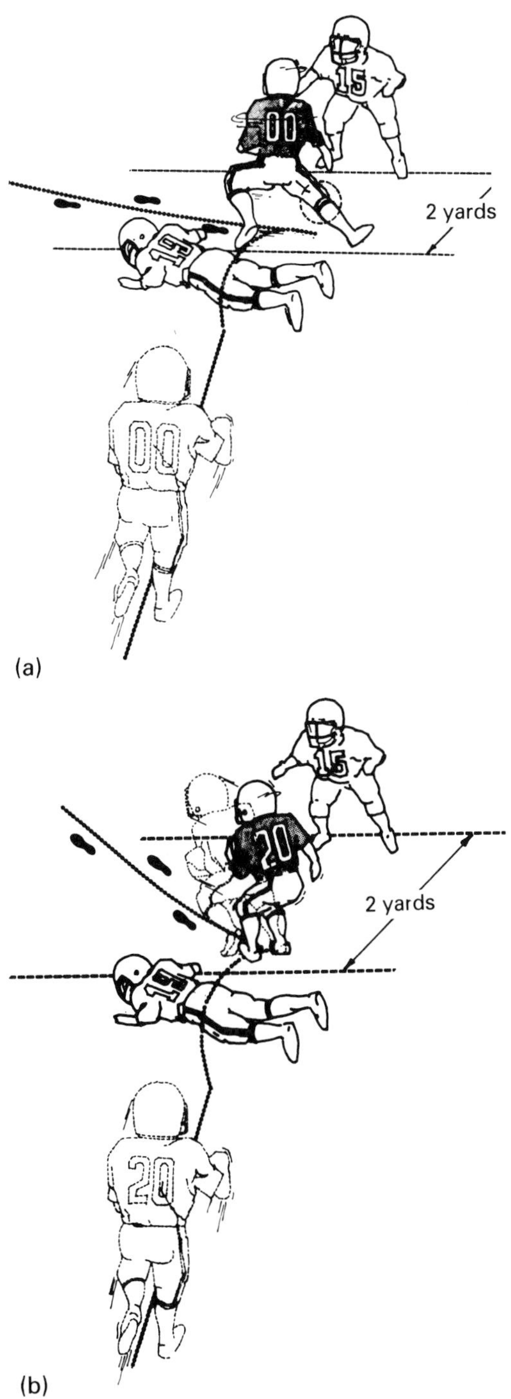

Fig. 11.5 (a) Bad technique: jumping over a downed player. (b) Good technique: jumping over a downed player.

baseball occurs while running the bases. Often the base runner is forced to stop suddenly and reverse direction very quickly. For example, a base runner is told to return to second by the third base coach after rounding second on the way to third. The injury usually occurs when the athlete stops in one step and attempts to push off in the opposite direction to tag up to second base. In this situation, the base runner should decelerate in three small quick steps as his or her centre of gravity is lowered to reverse direction, or utilize the block turn for a quicker turn.

FIELDING THE BALL

Fielding the ball accounts for 33% of ACL injuries in baseball. Most of these injuries are the result of stopping in one step or landing with the leg straight while fielding the ball. Therefore, it is important for fielders to practise the three step stops and bent knee landings as previously described. A good fielder will also check his or her surroundings during the warm-up and between innings for any obstacles, divets, holes or depressions in the terrain in order to avoid a foot contact with these hazards.

Soccer

Many soccer injury-producing situations are the result of running and changing of direction. It is not surprising to find shifting on defence as the most common play situation for ACL tears in soccer (Table 11.5). The defensive player is at risk because of the sudden change of direction by the offensive player. The offensive player has the advantage by controlling the ball and forcing the defender to react. By reacting, the defensive player often uses improper technique when extending or planting the leg to make a directional change. In this situation, the defender should use proper technique by maintaining a good bent knee defensive position. It is also important that the athlete use the inside leg to push off when changing direction. By keeping the knees bent and pushing

Table 11.3 Injury-producing situations for the anterior cruciate ligament in varsity and recreational North American football (n = 154). Offensive, 68 (44%); defensive, 40 (26%); special teams, 18 (12%); drills, 4 (3%); and not applicable, 24 (16%).

					Injury technique						
Injury situation	Total	(%)	Not hit	Hit	PAC	SKL	OSS	TWS	HYP	OTR	Improved player technique
Running with the ball	36	(23)	15	21	9	0	1	4	0	1	ART, TSS, BKL
Plant and fake (no description)	18	(12)	18	0	16	0	2	0	0	0	ART, TSS
Going for a pass	13	(8)	10	3	6	2	0	0	1	1	ART, BKL
Defensive backfield	12	(8)	1	11	1	0	0	0	0	0	ART
Offensive blocking	11	(7)	5	6	3	0	0	0	1	1	ART
Kick off team	9	(6)	4	5	4	0	0	0	0	0	ART, TSS, BKL, BLT
Making a tackle	9	(6)	6	3	3	0	0	1	0	2	ART, TSS, BLT
Kick off return team	7	(5)	4	3	3	0	1	0	0	0	ART, TSS, BKL, BLT
Defensive blocking	7	(5)	0	7	0	0	0	0	0	0	ART, TSS, BLT
Hit (no description)	7	(5)	0	7	0	0	0	0	0	0	
No description	6	(4) 2*	3	1	1	1	1	0	0	2	ART, BKL, TSS
Going for a pass (defence)	5	(3)	5	0	1	3	0	0	0	1	BKL, ART
Clipped	4	(3)	0	4	0	0	0	0	0	0	
Shifting on defence	3	(2)	3	0	3	0	0	0	0	0	ART, TSS, BLT
Punt return	2	(1)	0	2	0	0	0	0	0	0	ART, TSS, BKL, BLT
Lead blocking	2	(1)	1	1	0	0	0	0	0	1	ART, TSS
Trying to stop	2	(1)	1	1	0	0	1	0	0	0	TSS, BLT
Jumping over a downed player	1	(0.5)	1	0	0	1	0	0	0	0	BKL
Total	154		77	75	50	7	6	5	2	9	
%			50	49	32	5	4	3	1	6	

* Not known if hit or not hit.

ART, accelerated rounded turn; BKL, bent knee landing; BLT, block turn; HYP, hyperextended; OSS, one step stop; OTR, other; PAC, plant and cut; SKL, straight knee landing; TSS, three step stop; TWS, twist.

Table 11.4 Injury-producing situations for the anterior cruciate ligament in softball and baseball (n = 64). Hit versus not hit: not hit, 57 (89%); and hit 7 (11%).

Injury situation	Softball (n = 60)	Baseball (n = 4)	Total	Improved player technique
Running base, tried to stop suddenly at base	10	0	10	TSS, BLT, ART
Trying to avoid tag	6	2	8	ART, BLT, TSS
Slid into base	5	1	6	BKL
Hit while running	4	0	4	
Plant while fielding	4	0	4	ART, TSS, BLT
Stop/plant and throw	3	0	3	TSS
Plant to stop and catch fly ball	3	0	3	TSS, ART
Step in hole while fielding	3	0	3	INS
Hit while fielding	3	0	3	
Stepped on a sprinkler head	2	0	2	BKL, INS
Jumping for a ball fielding	2	0	2	BKL, ART
Stretched for the base (hyperextended)	2	0	2	TSS, BLT
Trying to stop (no data as to if fielding or running base)	2	0	2	TSS, ART, BLT
Pushing off base to run	1	0	1	ART
Stealing base	1	0	1	ART, TSS, BLT
Trying to make a tag	1	0	1	ART, TSS
Running base and knee gave out	0	1	1	
Landed off balance after stepping on rough surface between infield and outfield	1	0	1	INS
Injury situation not known	7	0	7	

Injury techniques: plant and cut 20 (31%); one step stop 14 (22%); straight knee landing 6 (9%); twist 2 (3%); hyperextended 4 (6%); and other 11 (17%).
ART, accelerated rounded turn; BKL, bent knee landing; BLT, block turn; INS, inspect field; TSS, three step stop.

off with the inside leg, the risk of ACL injury from quadricep–cruciate interaction force is reduced.

A common injury technique for the soccer defender is trying to stop in one step. Often the defender approaches the offensive player at full speed and will attempt to stop in one step, and usually change direction. This should be discouraged and replaced with a three step deceleration as discussed earlier (see Fig. 11.4b). Other play situations of concern in soccer include the offensive player who stops suddenly on an extended leg to plant and kick the ball. This is also a situation where the three step stop technique with a follow-through step after kicking should be utilized. Landing from a header is a common play in soccer and should be practised using the bent knee landing as described (see Table 11.5).

Volleyball

Volleyball is another sport that involves very little contact. The jumping and landing that occur in volleyball accounts for the majority of all ACL tears in this sport (Table 11.6). Most of the emphasis on injury prevention for the ACL in volleyball is on frontline play at the net. When a player jumps and lands from a spike, block shot or fake, the athlete must land with the knees bent and continue to bend them throughout the landing (see Fig. 11.4b). The athlete is in better position to jump quickly again for a quick tip or block. This technique is consistent with pliometrics commonly used in training.

Another area of concern is reacting to the ball on defence. Care must be taken in keeping the knees bent and pushing off with the inside leg

Table 11.5 Injury-producing situations nor the anterior cruciate ligament in soccer (n = 61). Hit versus not hit: not hit 51 (84%); and hit 10 (16%).

Injury situation	Total	Improved player technique
Shifting on defence	12	ART, TSS, BLT
Running, plant to get open or get ball	11	ART, TSS, BLT
Hit	10	
Plant to kick	7	TSS, BKL
One step stop to reverse or change direction	4	TSS, BLT
Foot stuck on artificial turf	3	
Jumping over a downed player	3	BKL
Tackled low	3	BKL, TSS
Landing from a header	2	BKL
Running for ball, bumped off balance	1	BKL
Dribbling ball, got tangled up with opponent	1	BKL, TSS, BLT
Kicked ball the same time as opponent	1	
Knocked off balance	1	BKL
Slipped in mud	1	
Injury situation not known	1	

Injury techniques: plant and cut 22 (36%); one step stop 8 (13%); straight knee landing 7 (11%); twist 2 (3%); hyperextended 6 (10%); and other 6 (10%).
ART, accelerated rounded turn; BKL, bent knee landing; BLT, block turn; TSS, three step stop.

Table 11.6 Injury-producing situations for the anterior cruciate ligament in volleyball (n = 28). Hit versus not hit: not hit, 28 (100%); and hit 0.

Injury situations	Total	Improved player technique
Spike attempt	10	BKL, TSS
Jumping for the ball	5	BKL, ART, TSS
Block shot attempt	4	BKL
Dig	3	ART, BLT
Landing from a jump	2	BKL
Bump play	1	TSS
Landing on someone's foot	1	BKL
Stop to jump	1	TSS
Injury situation not known	1	

Injury techniques: plant and cut 1 (4%); one step stop 3 (11%); straight knee landing 14 (50%); twist 3 (11%); hyperextended 1 (4%); and other 6 (21%).
ART, accelerated rounded turn; BKL, bent knee landing; BLT, block turn; TSS, three step stop.

when a player is pulled out of position for a pass or during a dig situation (Fig. 11.6).

Conclusion

Feagin and Lambert (1985) suggested that 'too little has been devoted to understanding the mechanism of injury and too much has been devoted to surgical repair' of the ACL. This chapter is intended to better identify and understand the injury-producing situations and associated mechanism techniques and introduce injury-prevention techniques that might be capable of reducing ACL tears.

The coach and athlete can relate better to modification at the play situation level. The purpose of ACL injury prevention is obvious. Athletes involved in any sport that might involve deceleration should be aware of these ideas. The injury-prevention techniques illustrated in this chapter are meant to make previous works done in the field of ACL injury prevention (Abbott & Kress, 1969; Peterson,

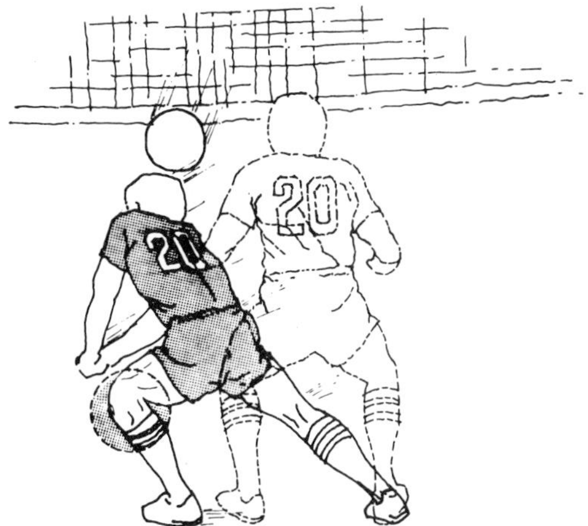

Fig. 11.6 Good technique: good bent knee defensive in reacting.

1970, 1973; Eriksson, 1976) more useful to the coach and athlete. It is our belief that these techniques can be used as building blocks for an effective ACL injury prevention programme.

Ideally, these techniques should be introduced to as many athletes as possible with extra effort placed at reaching the young athlete. The place to start this programme is in the school system as part of the elementary physical education programme. By learning these techniques at an early age, not only will the athlete develop good injury-prevention habits, but many will improve their player performance. The young athlete can apply these techniques as he or she grows and becomes more competitive. The younger and the more often an athlete is exposed to these ideas, the greater the chance of a successful, ACL injury-free career.

Eventually, it will become the responsibility of schools, coaches and parents to convey these skills to athletes of all ages, promoting safe competitive athletic activities.

References

Abbott, H.G. & Kress, J.B. (1969) Preconditioning in the prevention of knee injuries. *Arch. Phys. Med. Rehab.* **50**(6), 326–33.

Butler, D.L., Noyes, F.R. & Grood, E.S. (1980) Ligamentous restraints to anterior-posterior drawer in the human knee. *J. Bone Joint Surg.* **62A**(2), 259–70.

Daniels, D., Biden, E., Malcom, L. *et al.* (1981) *The anterior cruciate–quadriceps interaction.* Presented at the annual meeting of the American Orthopaedic Society of Sports Medicine, South Lake Tahoe, June 1981.

DeLorme, T.L. (1956) *Misconceptions of rehabilitation of the thigh musculature in cruciate injuries.* Presented at the New York Orthopedic Hospital.

Eriksson, E. (1976) Sports injuries of the knee ligaments: their diagnosis, treatment, rehabilitation, and prevention. *Med. Sci. Sports* **8**(3), 133–44.

Feagin, J.A. (1979) The syndrome of the torn anterior cruciate ligament. *Orthop. Clin. N. Am.* **10**(1), 81–90.

Feagin, J.A., Curl, W.W. & Markey, K.L. (1978) Anterior cruciate ligament loss: complications and late results. In *American Academy of Orthopedic Surgeons, Symposium on the Athlete's Knee,* pp. 173–7. CV Mosby, St Louis.

Feagin, J.A. & Lambert, K.L. (1985) Mechanism of injury and pathology of anterior cruciate ligament injuries. *Orthop. Clin. N. Am.* **16**, 41–5.

Fetto, J.F. & Marshall, J.L. (1980) The natural history and diagnosis of anterior cruciate ligament insufficiency. *Clin. Orthop.* **147**, 29–38.

Henning, C.E., Lynch, M.A. & Glick, K.R. (1985) An *in vivo* strain gage study of elongation of the anterior cruciate ligament. *Am. J. Sports Med.* **13**(1), 22–6.

Johnson, R.J., Kettelkamp, D.B., Clark, W. *et al.* (1974) Factors affecting later results after meniscectomy. *J. Bone Joint Surg.* **56A**, 719–29.

Johnson, R.J. & Pope, M.H. (1978) Knee joint stability without reference to ligamentous function. In *Form and Function of the Knee: American Academy of Orthopedic Surgeons, Symposium on Reconstructive Surgery of the Knee*, pp. 14–25. CV Mosby, St Louis.

Kain, C.C., McCarthy, J.A., Arms, S. *et al.* (1988) An *in vivo* analysis of the affect of transcutaneous electrical stimulation of the quadriceps and hamstrings on anterior cruciate ligament deformation. *Am. J. Sports Med.* **16**(2), 147–52.

Lindahl, O. & Movin, A. (1967) The mechanics of extension of the knee joint. *Acta Orthop. Scand.* **38**, 226–34.

Lynch, M.A., Henning, C.E. & Glick, K.R. (1983) Knee joint surface changes long-term follow-up meniscus tear treatment in stable anterior cruciate ligament reconstructions. *Clin. Orthop.* **172**, 148–53.

McDaniel, W.J. & Dameron, T.B. (1983) The untreated anterior cruciate ligament rupture. *Clin. Orthop.* **172**, 158–63.

Marshall, J.L. & Baugher, W.H. (1980) Stability examination of the knee: a simple anatomic approach.

Clin. Orthop. **146**, 78–83.

O'Brien, W. (1989) *Degenerative arthritis of the knee following anterior cruciate ligament injury: a long-term, multicenter, followup study*. Presented at the American Academy of Orthopaedic Surgeons Annual Meeting, Las Vegas, Nevada, February.

Paulos, L., Noyes, F.R. & Grood, E. (1986) Knee rehabilitation after anterior cruciate ligament reconstruction and repair. *Am. J. Sports Med.* **9**(3), 140–9.

Peterson, T.R. (1970) The cross-body block, the major cause of knee injuries. *JAMA* **211**(3), 449–52.

Peterson, T.R. (1973) Blocking at the knee, dangerous and unnecessary. *Phys. Sportsmed.* **1**(2), 46–50.

Renström, P., Arms, S.W., Stanwyck, T.S. *et al.* (1986) Strain within the anterior cruciate ligament during hamstring and quadriceps activity. *Am. J. Sports Med.* **14**(1), 83–7.

Chapter 12

Lower Leg Injuries

SAKARI ORAVA

Lower leg injuries are the most common overuse injuries, but they are seldom seen as acute sports injuries (Orava & Puranen, 1979; Orava, 1980; Pagliano & Jackson, 1989). Acute leg injuries may occur in contact sports, down-hill skiing and in sports demanding maximal power or speed. In the aetiology of acute lower leg injuries, factors include poor or faulty sports technique, poor muscle conditioning, muscle fatigue, breaking the rules, incompetent judges and pure accidents. Chronic or overuse injuries, on the other hand, follow training errors, extreme muscle fatigue, biomechanical faults, poor sports shoes, bad training surfaces, lack of muscle care or too intensive and great training quantities (Friberg, 1982; Viitasalo & Kvist, 1983; McKenzie *et al.*, 1985; Subotnick, 1985; Kujala *et al.*, 1986; Jones *et al.*, 1989; Renström, 1991). There are, in addition to these factors, lots of other reasons for both acute and chronic lower leg injuries. The diagnosis and treatment of them is not always easy and the preventive means are difficult to outline and follow. Plenty of scientific investigations have been performed on this subject, but still there are many uncertain facts which need further studies (Clement *et al.*, 1980; Friden *et al.*, 1983; Komi *et al.*, 1987; Hyvärinen, 1988; Jørgensen & Ekstrand, 1988; Lehto & Järvinen, 1991; Nicol *et al.*, 1991).

Type and frequency of injuries

The type of lower leg injuries in sports has changed with time. For example, the development of down-hill skiing boots changed the pattern of lower leg fractures from typical down-hill injuries to knee ligament injuries, which now represent typical skiing injuries (Johnson & Pope, 1991; Renström, 1991). The vast increase in running and jogging during the last two decades increased the number of leg muscle pains and compartment syndromes (Puranen, 1974; Millar, 1979; Orava & Puranen, 1979; Johnell *et al.*, 1982; Mubarak *et al.*, 1982; Wallensten & Eriksson, 1984; Kmen *et al.*, 1990; Åkermark *et al.*, 1991). The frequency of lower leg injuries in different sports is presented in Table 12.1. A short classification of acute lower leg injuries is presented in Table 12.2. The chronic lower leg injuries can be divided and classified as presented in Table 12.3, with an age distribution in Table 12.4.

The most common overuse injury in athletes according to Orava (1980) was medial tibial syndrome (shin splint syndrome, deep posterior compartment syndrome). Pagliano and Jackson (1989) classified this syndrome as the second in a list of frequency, representing 9.4% of runners' total complaints. About 17% of all overuse injuries of athletes in Finland were localized in the lower leg (Orava & Puranen, 1979; Orava, 1980). Stress fractures of the tibia and fibula are also quite common stress injuries in athletes (Hulkko, 1988; Jones *et al.*, 1989). They often represent diagnostic and therapeutic difficulties (Green *et al.*, 1985; Orava & Hulkko, 1988).

Table 12.1 Division of athletes with lower leg overuse injuries according to sports events. From Orava & Puranen (1979).

	n	%
Track and field:		
Middle/long distance running	219	44.2
Sprinting/hurdling	55	11.1
Jumping/throwing events and decathon	8	1.6
Youth track and field	4	0.8
Jogging	98	19.8
Skiing	45	9.1
Orienteering	36	7.3
Ball events (football, volleyball, baseball, ice hockey, bandy, tennis)	15	3.0
Power events (weightlifting, judo, boxing wrestling)	5	1.0
Gymnastics	3	0.6
Other sports (cycling, skating, ballet dancing, skeet, etc.)	7	1.4
Total	495	100

Acute lower leg injuries

Treatment

In this chapter, the main subject is the sports-related injury panorama. Therefore most severe lower leg injuries can be excluded as uncommon sports injuries and as typical problems of general traumatology.

Muscle injuries of the lower leg in sports can be divided into muscle lacerations, muscle contusions and muscle strains. In strains, disruption of muscle fibres occurs, probably due to muscle strength imbalance of antagonists, which predisposes the weaker muscle to injury. Primary first aid measures including compressive bandage, cold treatment and elevation is the basis of the treatment. Depending on the severity of the muscle strain, active mobilization is started in a few days. By early mobilization and good rehabilitation, the functional state is restored in 2–3 weeks (Millar, 1979; Lehto & Järvinen, 1991). The most common muscle injury in the lower leg is the grade I or II strain of the medial gastrocnemius muscle, so-called 'tennis leg' (Millar, 1979).

Table 12.2 Acute lower leg injuries in sports.

Skin	Wound Laceration Infection Blister
Muscles	Direct muscle injury (contusion, rupture) Indirect muscle injury (strain) Muscle cramps, spasms Acute compartment syndrome: Anterior compartment Lateral (peroneal) compartment Posterior compartment (superficial or calf muscle) exertional acute compartment secondary to other leg injuries
Blood vessels	Venous Arterial
Bones	Periosteal haematoma Tibial or fibular fractures (simple or complicated, closed or open)
Nerves	Contusion and neuroma formation (saphenous nerve, peroneal nerve, sural nerve) Paresis due to intensive use of muscles peroneal nerve (inside anterior muscle compartment)

Contusion of the tibial periosteum may cause painful subperiosteal haematoma or scar and neuroma formation to the superficial branches of the saphenous nerve. Cases with prolonged symptoms can be treated by corticosteroid injections. Direct muscle injury to the anterior compartment of the leg sometimes causes temporary or persistent drop foot by damaging deep peroneal nerve inside the muscle compartment.

Acute muscle compartment syndrome may follow direct trauma of shin bone fractures, too tight cast or bandage and intensive use of muscles (Matsen, 1975; Reneman, 1975; Mubarak, 1981; Kmen *et al.*, 1990). Volkman described, as early as 1881, the contracture of the lower leg muscles as a late result of compartment syndrome (Kmen *et al.*, 1990). Murphy

Table 12.3 Chronic lower leg injuries in sports.

Skin	Blisters, lacerations, abrasions, skin diseases, infections
Muscles	Chronic compartment syndromes: Anterior compartment Lateral (peroneal) compartment Posterior superficial (calf) compartment Medial tibial syndrome (deep posterior compartment, shin splints, traction periostitis of tibial border) Muscle hernias
Blood vessels	Intermittent claudication (atherosclerosis) Aneurysm formation Anomalies
Bones	Stress fracture of tibia (lower third, upper third, anterior midtibia, tibial plateau) Stress fracture of fibula: Distal supramalleolar Middle or upper diaphysis Delayed unions and non-unions (anterior cortex of midtibia)
Nerves	Entrapments: Peroneal nerve (common or deep peroneal nerve, superficial branches) Saphenous nerve Sural nerve Posterior tibial nerve

Table 12.4 Age distribution of athletes with lower leg overuse pains (females 10.5%; and males 89.5%) From Orava & Puranen (1979).

Age (years)	*n*	%
≤9	4	0.8
10–15	27	5.5
16–19	145	29.3
20–29	214	43.3
30–39	74	15.0
40–49	24	4.8
≥50	7	1.4
Total	495	100

explained in 1914 how decreased capillary outflow and pooling of the blood inside a fascial compartment may lead to ischaemia and muscle necrosis (Kmen *et al.*, 1990). Acute compartment syndromes have been described in the anterior, lateral (peroneal) and posterior superficial compartments of the lower leg (Matsen, 1975; Reneman, 1975; Mubarak, 1981; Rorabeck & Fowler, 1988; Puranen, 1991). The diagnosis is done according to clinical symptoms, sensory and motor neurological defects, absence of arterial pulses and by elevated intracompartmental pressure recordings (Mubarak, 1981; Wallensten & Eriksson, 1984). Promptly performed fasciotomy is the only treatment; muscle necrosis and persistent weakness due to neurological deficiencies may follow in a few hours of ischaemia (Kmen *et al.*, 1990).

Prevention

Acute injuries and accidents can be prevented by education and knowledge as well as following the rules. Young athletes should be instructed of rules and made to obey them. The responsibility of the judges in the prevention of injuries is evident. In spite of the fact that the lower leg is usually well protected in contact sports, acute injuries may occur because of improper or missing orthoses and shoes.

Acute indirect muscle injuries can be prevented only by strengthening exercises and elasticity/flexibility training. The avoidance of extreme fatigue may protect athletes from acute muscle compartment syndromes, caused by physical exertion and intensive use of leg muscles.

In different sports, there are plenty of individual and characteristic features, which should be taken into account when trying to keep training as safe and symptom-free as possible (Table 12.5).

Chronic lower leg injuries

Chronic muscle pains in the lower leg are typical in all sports events which require

Table 12.5 Prevention of acute lower leg injuries in sports.

Rules, judges
Education
Equipments, orthoses, supports, braces
Sport fields, halls, areas
Surface, ground
Sport shoes, sport wear
Warm-up
Stretching
Massage, muscle care
General conditioning
Sport performance technique
Avoidance of exhaustive training/competing when poorly conditioned, after training pause or disease
Gradual increase in mileage

running or jumping as the main aerobic training form. The diagnosis is not always easy. However, treatment is an urgent procedure. Muscle hypertrophy, stiffness and increased training often lead to chronic pain syndromes (Slocum, 1967; Puranen, 1974; Goldberg *et al.*, 1975; Mubarak, 1981). Connective tissues changes in the muscles and fascia and increased scarring inside the muscles due to cellular damage from intensive recurrent use of muscles is one aetiological pathway to chronic compartmental pains (Friden *et al.*, 1983; Williams & Goldspink, 1984; Nicol *et al.*, 1991).

Increased pressure inside the fascial compartment is the aetiology for the symptoms in anterior, peroneal and posterior compartments, but the deep posterior compartment pain — medial tibial syndrome — is probably caused by inflammation, fibrosis and fascial thickening near the tibial border from the pull of fascia caused by muscle contractions (Slocum, 1967; Puranen, 1974; Reneman, 1975; Wallensten & Eriksson, 1984). In Fig. 12.1 the fascial compartments of the leg are shown.

Treatment of chronic fascial compartment syndromes

Shin splint syndrome or the medial side pain and of the shin has long been treated by massage, stretching, optimizing the running mileage in a day and by orthotic correction of hyperpronation, which has often been noticed in these athletes (Slocum, 1967; Bates *et al.*, 1979; Eggold, 1981). In spite of conservative treatment, symptoms continue in some athletes. Puranen (1974, 1991) described the fasciotomy of the deep posterior or medial compartment of the leg. Since the early 1970s, surgical treatment has become a routine treatment of chronic symptomatic cases of 'medial tibial stress syndrome' in athletes (Mubarak *et al.*, 1982; Orava *et al.*, 1991). It seems that there are differences between countries and climates in the occurrence of medial tibial pains in athletes. In cold countries, as in Scandinavian countries, relatively more athletes need operative treatment (Orava & Puranen, 1979; Johnell *et al.*, 1982; Åkermark *et al.*, 1990). The fasciotomy is per-

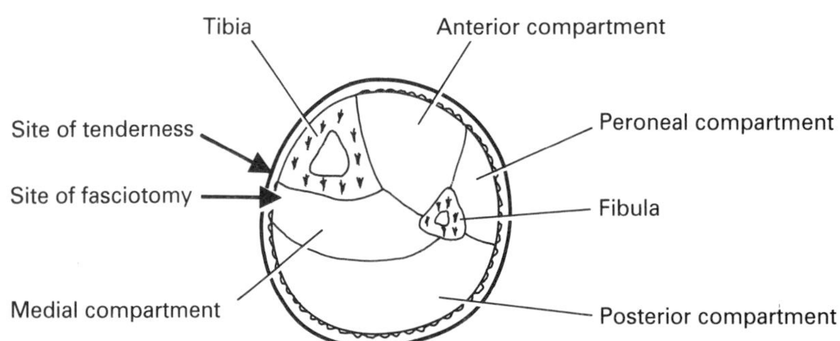

Fig. 12.1 Fascial compartments of the lower leg. Transverse section is from the lower third. The arrows show the site of tenderness and place of fasciotomy in chronic medial tibial syndrome.

formed near the tibial border, near medial malleolus and extends proximally 20–25 cm depending on the site of symptoms, sometimes it can be even longer. The operation is normally performed under sight control through open wound or two wounds. Postoperatively, walking is allowed and good compressive bandages are used for 10 days. Running is usually possible 3 or 4 weeks after the operation.

To decompress the anterior compartment, an open wound of 5–6 cm can be used or the fasciotomy can be performed through a small incision blindly by fasciotomy knife (Matsen, 1975; Reneman, 1975; Orava *et al.*, 1991). If the anterior compartment syndrome develops to a chronic pain, probably either surgery or a clear decrease in running mileage is necessary. By good muscle care and adaptation only can part of the symptoms be eliminated. In Fig. 12.2 the location of medial and anterior syndromes is shown.

Chronic pains located at the peroneal or posterior — calf muscle — compartments can also be treated with the above-mentioned conservative means. Usually they help or give extra time for the athletes to adapt, correct biomechanics, strengthen the weak points and continue training. In certain cases, where sports participation is hampered and which do not react to therapeutic means, fasciotomy may be needed. The surgery in these cases is as effective as in most other fascial compartment pain syndromes (Reneman, 1975; Orava & Puranen, 1979).

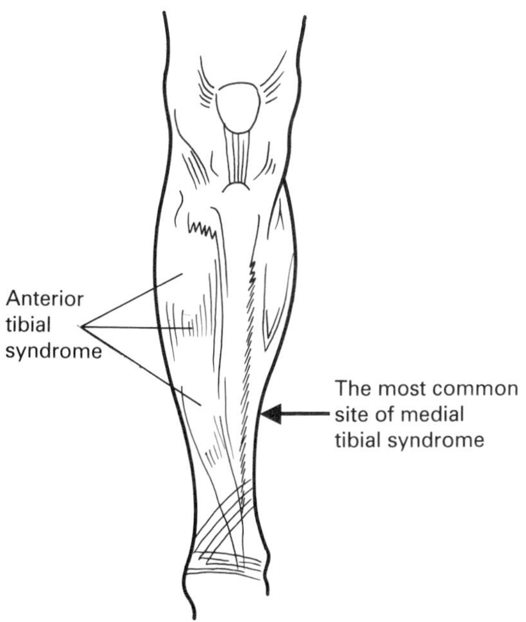

Fig. 12.2 Location of medial and anterior tibial syndromes of the leg. From Orava (1980).

After the surgery, the biomechanical malalignments have to be corrected, good muscle care is needed, running mileage, running surface, training frequency and intensity, etc., have to be considered carefully. Much can be done before the surgery and much should be done after the operation to prevent recurrences and keep the athletes in successful condition.

Prevention of chronic muscle pains and compartment syndromes

The most important biomechanical faults for the development of the medial tibial syndrome (shin splints) are outward rotation of the feet, hyperpronation and poor use of calf muscles (Clement & Taunton, 1980; Segesser & Nigg, 1980; Viitasalo & Kvist, 1983; Pagliano & Jackson, 1989). To correct these malalignments, special orthoses and better sports shoe modifications have been made with success (Bates *et al.*, 1979; Eggold, 1981; Mann, 1982; Subotnick, 1985; Pförringer & Segesser, 1986; Nigg & Morlock, 1987; Hyvärinen, 1988). The so-called 'normal anatomy' variation between individuals is great. Therefore the biomechanical errors are small and difficult to measure (Viitasalo & Kvist, 1983; Komi *et al.*, 1987; Hyvärinen, 1988). To prevent lower leg pains, shoes and orthotic corrective devices have to be tried, if a functional malalignment is detected or even suspected. In future, gait, running and jumping analysis will become more accurate and the meaning of abnormal findings will be understood better. By this development the prevention of lower leg and extremity overuse injuries will become more successful than it is today. Some of the lower leg pains cannot be prevented totally, because modern athletic training includes such vast training quantities that the locomotor system will be on the upper limit of its tolerance. Adaptation will not continue forever. It is also known that some athletes who are prone to overuse syndromes, can still be top level athletes. Table 12.6 shows preventive means.

Treatment of lower leg stress fractures

The total weekly mileage of running, an increased intensity or changes in running training schedule, improper sport shoes, hard road surfaces and faulty biomechanics all influence the appearance of lower leg stress fractures (Clement & Taunton, 1980; McKenzie *et al.*, 1985; Hulkko *et al.*, 1987; Matheson *et al.*, 1987; Hulkko, 1988). In addition to these factors, several others have been mentioned, but still in half of the patients no clear reason is found (Hulkko *et al.*, 1987; Jones *et al.*, 1989). Lower leg length discrepancy (Friberg, 1982), poor shock-absorbing capacity of the heels (Milgrom *et al.*, 1985; Nigg & Morlock, 1987), functionally wrong running style and fatigue of the lower extremity muscles (Mann, 1982; Nicol *et al.*, 1991) are included as possible risk factors. One important phenomenon is that together with the ground reaction (gravity) force, pace and impact twisting of tibia and fibula also occurs (Hulkko, 1988). The muscles of the lower leg thus have two effects: (i) to twist the bones; and (ii) to decrease the impact force during the foot strike in running and jumping. Shoes, orthoses and shock absorbers have been observed to have a positive effect on decreasing the heel and sole contact on the ground during running (Bates *et al.*, 1979; Eggold, 1981; Milgrom *et al.*, 1985; Pförringer & Segesser, 1986; Nigg & Morlock, 1987; Jørgensen & Ekstrand, 1988). It seems that when running on hard surfaces, pure shock absorbers are the most effective in preventing stress fractures, hyperpronation probably does not play as important a role (Clement & Taunton, 1980; Mann, 1982).

Table 12.6 Prevention of chronic lower leg injuries in sports.

Muscle care, massage, physiotherapy, stretching, muscle balance training
General conditioning, muscle strength training
Avoidance of extreme muscle fatigue
Avoidance of extreme dehydration
Proper running and jumping technique
Correction of training errors
Good sport shoes
Orthoses (antipronation soles, arch supports)
Shock absorbers
Good sports wear (according to circumstances)
Gradual increase in mileage

Stress fractures appear during the first few weeks or months following the start of regular physical exercise like running, for example in military recruits and joggers (Hulkko, 1988). In athletes who have regularly trained for years, stress fractures occur later as a consequence of small changes in training, poor adaptation to rising running distances, amenorrhoea due to overtraining in females and of other unknown reasons (Matheson *et al.*, 1987; Hulkko, 1988).

Stress fractures of the lower leg are usually located at the proximal and distal third of the tibia or at the supramalleolar area of the fibula (Hulkko, 1988). More uncommon sites are the fibular shaft and middle tibia. Delayed- and non-unions usually develop at the anterior tibial cortex in the middle part of the bone (Green *et al.*, 1985; Rettig *et al.*, 1988; Orava *et al.*, 1991). These stress fractures are uncommon but represent a clear risk of becoming chronic because of non-union. The diagnosis is usually delayed and the severity is increased. Therefore, complete fractures may occur or surgery is indicated before that to ensure healing and continuation of a sports career. Excision of the non-union area and bone grafting as well as excision and transversal drilling through the anterior cortex both have given good results (Green *et al.*, 1975; Hulkko & Orava, 1988;

Rettig *et al.*, 1988; Orava *et al.*, 1991). However, 6 months have to pass after the surgery before running and jumping exercises can be resumed. By leg orthosis, relative rest (avoiding maximal jumping and running) and early detection, fractures may heal spontaneously. Non-unions of other sites in the lower leg are rare and the treatment of them is similar. By electrical field or magnetic field treatment some fractures have been said to heal faster (Hulkko, 1988). Usually only rest from sports and exercises is needed for 6–8 weeks in tibial stress fractures, and 4 weeks in fibular stress fractures. Stress fracture sites are shown in Fig. 12.3.

Prevention of lower leg stress fractures

Stress fractures are sometimes said to be 'training errors'. Thus the coach has the greatest responsibility for the occurrence of them (Hulkko, 1988). Close monitoring of training amounts, follow-up of the training and avoidance of any sudden increase in mileage are the best prophylactic means. If a stress fracture appears, careful analysis of the exact circumstances must be completed. In athletes involved in abnormally heavy impact, softer shoes or shock absorbers should be used (Milgram *et al.*, 1985). General conditioning and muscle strengthening for the lower leg is also wise. In overtraining situations, metabolic or hormonal changes may affect the skeleton and promote the appearance of stress fractures (Orava, 1980; Hulkko, 1988). The training should be adjusted according to the health state of an athlete. Table 12.7 shows the distribution of chronic leg injuries.

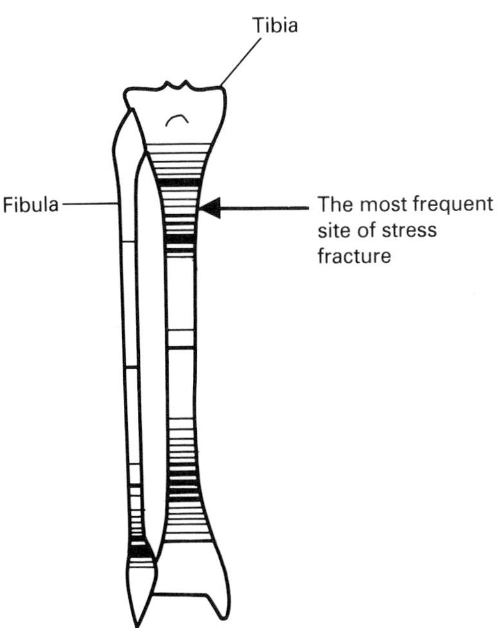

Fig. 12.3 Location of 88 tibial stress fractures and 23 fibular stress fractures in athletes. From Orava (1980).

Nerve injuries of the lower leg

Compressive acute and chronic trauma may cause nerve damage to the peroneal and saphenous nerve. Drop foot or ankle dorsiflexion weakness also follows acute compartment syndrome of the anterior compartment (Kmen *et al.*, 1990). Peroneal paresis, usually temporary, may follow if irritation to the nerve occurs under the tight insertion area of muscles in the fibular neck or from the compression of muscles inside the compartment (Orava, 1980).

Neuroma formation to the branches of the saphenous nerve is possible after direct injury or after chronic irritation by sport shoes, boots, etc. Suralis nerve injury is possible from the pressure of shoes, bandages or other irritation

Table 12.7 Distribution of chronic lower leg injuries in athletes according to diagnosis (%). From Orava (1979).

Medial tibial syndrome	58
Stress fracture of tibia	15
Chronic calf muscle pains	11
Anterior tibial syndrome	6
Stress fracture of fibula	4
Simultaneous pain syndrome in two fascial compartments	3
Other (e.g. diffuse muscle pain (myositis?), peroneal compartment pains, fascial hernias	3
Total	100

on the posterolateral side of the shin and ankle. In the distal anterolateral aspect of the leg, the superficial branches of the peroneal nerve may give pain and distal radiation due to compression or ankle distorsion. Muscle hernia is often associated with superficial peroneal nerve irritation. Posterior tibial nerve is well protected in the leg, but more vulnerable behind the medial malleolus.

In treatment, eliminating the irritative factor is most important. Physiotherapy, corticosteroid injections and even surgery are all needed. In prevention, good care and protection of the lower leg is necessary.

Conclusion

All people engaged in sports training and athletes should develop sound principles in the prevention of acute and overuse injuries. Athletes, who have a history of injuries, should be analysed by experts to find possible risk factors. The evaluation on this aspect is best done at an early age, before the training quantities have risen to high level and before young athletes develop the wrong routines and habits. Muscle care and general conditioning as well as strength training should be made automatic routines. The feedback after injuries is most important; by that procedure only can the athlete and his or her coach learn to create better programmes. Not all injuries can be prevented, but most of them can be treated well. If the postoperative recovery and rehabilitation can serve sporting purposes, then the final result will be the best for all those involved. Experienced coaches, trainers and other sports medical staff are the best prophylaxis against injuries.

References

Åkermark, C., Ljungdahl, M. & Johansson, C. (1991) Long-term result of fasciotomy caused by medial tibial syndrome in athletes. *Scand. J. Sports Med. Sci.* **1**, 59–61.

Bates, B.T., Osternig, L.R., Mason, B. & James, L.S. (1979) Foot orthotic devices modify selected aspects of lower extremity mechanics. *Am. J. Sports Med.* **7**, 338–42.

Clement, D.B. & Taunton, J.E. (1980) A guide to the prevention of running injuries. *Can. Fam. Phys.* **26**, 543–8.

Eggold, J.E. (1981) Orthotics in the prevention of runner's overuse injuries. *Phys. Sportsmed.* **9**, 125–8.

Friberg, O. (1982) Leg length asymmetry in stress fractures. A clinical and radiological study. *J. Sports Med. Phys. Fitness* **22**, 485–8.

Friden, J., Sjöström, M. & Ekblom, B. (1983) Myofibrillar damage following intense eccentric exercise in man. *Int. J. Sports Med.* **4**, 170–6.

Goldberg, A.L., Etlinger, J.D., Goldspink, D.F. & Jablecki, C. (1975) Mechanism of work-induced hypertrophy of skeletal muscle. *Med. Sci. Sports* **7**, 248–61.

Green, N. Rogers, R. & Libscomb, A. (1985) Non-unions of stress fractures of the tibia. *Am. J. Sports Med.* **13**, 171–6.

Hulkko, A. (1988) *Stress fractures in athletes. A clinical study of 368 cases.* Thesis, Acta Universitatis Ouluensis.

Hulkko, A. & Orava, S. (1988) Delayed unions and non-unions of stress fractures in athletes. *Am. J. Sports Med.* **16**, 378–82.

Hulkko, A., Orava, S. & Alen, M. (1987) Stress fractures of the lower leg. *Scand. J. Sports Sci.* **9**, 1–8.

Hyvärinen, T. (1988) *Karhu Ortix. The Shoe System of the Future.* A training manual. Karhu Titan Co., Helsinki, Finland.

Johnell, O., Rausing, A., Wendeberg, B. & Westlin, N. (1982) Morphological bone changes in shin splints. *Clin. Orthop.* **167**, 180–4.

Johnson, R.J. & Pope, M.H. (1991) Epidemiology and prevention of skiing injuries. *Ann. Chirurg. Gynaecol.* **80**, 110–15.

Jones, B.H., Harris, J.M., Vihn, T.N. & Rubin, C. (1989) Exercise induced stress fractures and stress reactions of bone: epidemiology, etiology and classification. *Exerc Sports Sci. Rev.* **11**, 379–422.

Jørgensen, U. & Ekstrand, J. (1988) Significance of heel pad confinement for the shock absorption at heel strike. *Int. J. Sports Med.* **9**, 468–73.

Kmen, A., Schlerka, C. & Puhringer, A. (1990) Akutes, durch muskuläre Überbeanspruchung ausgelöstes Kompartmentsyndrom an der Vorderseite beider Oberschenkel. *Sportver. Sportschad.* **4**, 125–9.

Komi, P.V., Gollhofer, A., Schmidlbleicher, D. & Frick, U. (1987) Interaction between man and shoe in running: considerations for a more comprehensive measurement approach. *Int. J. Sports Med.* **8**, 196–202.

Kujala, U., Kvist, M., Österman, K., Friberg, O.

& Aalto, T. (1986) Factors predisposing army conscripts to knee exertion injuries incurred in a physical training program. *Clin. Orthop.* **210**, 203–12.

Lehto, M.U.K. & Järvinen, M.J. (1991) Muscle injuries, their healing process and treatment. *Ann. Chirurg. Gynaecol* **80**, 102–8.

McKenzie, D.C., Clement, D.B. & Taunton, J.E. (1985) Running shoes, orthotics and injuries. *Sports Med.* **2**, 334–47.

Mann, R.A. (1982) Biomechanical approach to the treatment of foot problems. *Foot Ankle* **2**, 205–12.

Matheson, G.O., Clement, D.B., McKenzie, D.C., Taunton, J.E., Lloyd-Smith, D.R. & McIntyre, J.G. (1987) Stress fractures in athletes: A study of 320 cases. *Am. J. Sports Med.* **15**, 46–58.

Matsen, F.A. (1975) Compartment syndrome: An unified concept. *Clin. Orthop.* **113**, 8–14.

Milgrom, C., Giladi, M., Kashtan, H. *et al.* (1985) A prospective study of the effect of shock-absorbing orthotic device on the incidence of stress fractures in military recruits. *Foot Ankle* **6**, 101–4.

Millar, A.P. (1979) Strains of the posterior calf musculature ('tennis leg'). *Am. J. Sports Med.* **3**, 172–7.

Mubarak, S.J. (1981) Exertional compartment syndromes. In S.J. Mubarak & A.R. Hargens (eds) *Compartment Syndromes and Volkmann's Contracture*, pp. 210–26. WB Saunders, Philadelphia.

Mubarak, S.J., Gould, R.N. & Lee, Y.F. (1982) The medial tibial stress syndrome. *Am. J. Sports Med.* **10**, 201–6.

Nicol, C., Komi, P.V. & Marconnet, P. (1991) Fatigue effects of marathon running on neuromuscular performance: I. Changes in muscle force and stiffness characteristics. *Scand. J. Med. Sci. Sports* **1**, 10–17.

Nigg, B.M. & Morlock, M. (1987) The influence of lateral heel flare of running shoes on pronation and impact forces. *Med. Sci. Sports Exerc.* **19**, 294–302.

Orava, S. (1980) *Exertion injuries due to sports and physical exercise.* Thesis, University of Oulu, Finland.

Orava, S. & Hulkko, A. (1988) Delayed unions and non-unions of stress fractures in athletes. *Am. J. Sports Med.* **16**, 378–81.

Orava, S., Karpakka, J., Hulkko, A., Väänänen, K., Kallinen, M. & Alen, M. (1991) Diagnosis and treatment of stress fractures located at the mid-tibial shaft in athletes. *Int. J. Sports Med.* **12**, 419–22.

Orava, S., Leppilahti, J. & Karpakka, J. (1991) Surgical treatment of overuse injuries in athletes. *Ann. Chirurg. Gynaecol.* **80**, 177–84.

Orava, S. & Puranen, J. (1979) Athletes' leg pains. *Br. J. Sports Med.* **13**, 92–7.

Pagliano, J.F. & Jackson, D.W. (1989) A clinical study of 3500 long distance runners. In *Paavo Nurmi Congress Proceedings*, pp. 191–6. Turku, Finland.

Pförringer, W. & Segesser, B. (1986) Der Sportschuh (The athlete's shoe). *Orthopäde* **15**, 260–3.

Puranen, J. (1974) The medial tibial syndrome. Exercise ischaemia in the medial fascial compartment. *J. Bone Joint Surg.* **56B**, 712–15.

Puranen, J. (1991) The medial tibial syndrome. *Ann. Chirurg. Gynaecol.* **80**, 215–18.

Reneman, R.S. (1975) The anterior and lateral compartment syndromes of the leg due to intensive use of muscles. *Clin. Orthop.* **113**, 69–80.

Renström, P. (1991) Sports traumatology today. A review of common current sports injury problems. *Ann. Chirurg. Gynaecol.* **80**, 81–93.

Rettig, A., Shelbourne, D., McCarroll, J., Bisesi, M. & Watts, J. (1988) The natural history and treatment of delayed union stress fractures of the anterior cortex of the tibia. *Am. J. Sports Med.* **16**, 250–5.

Rorabeck, C. & Fowler, P. (1988) The results of fasciotomy in the management of chronic exertional compartment syndrome. *Am. J. Sports Med.* **16**, 224–7.

Segesser, B. & Nigg, B. (1980) Achillodynie und tibiale Insertiontendinosen (Achilles pain and tibia tendon insertion injuries). *Medizin Sport* **20**, 79–83.

Slocum, D.B. (1967) The shin splint syndrome. Medical aspects and differential diagnosis. *Am. J. Surg.* **114**, 875–81.

Subotnick, S. (1985) The biomechanics of running. Implications for the prevention of foot injuries. *Sports Med.* **2**, 144–53.

Wallensten, R. & Eriksson, E. (1984) Intramuscular pressures in the exercise induced lower leg pain. *Int. J. Sports Med.* **5**, 31–5.

Viitasalo, J. & Kvist, M. (1983) Some biomechanical aspects of the foot and ankle in athletes with and without shin splints. *Am. J. Sports Med.* **11**, 125–30.

Williams, P.E. & Goldspink, C. (1984) Connective tissue changes in immobilized muscle. *J. Anat.* **138**, 343–50.

Chapter 13

Achilles Tendon Injuries

GIANCARLO PUDDU, ANDREA SCALA, GUGLIELMO CERULLO, VITTORIO FRANCO, FOSCO DE PAULIS AND OSVALDO MICHELINI

'Then in answer to him spake Achilles, swift of foot.' (Homer, *Iliad*, I,84)

The Achilles tendon is the thickest and strongest tendon of the human body and it plays a very important role in sport activities. All running and jumping athletes, at professional and recreational levels, are exposed to the risk of injuries to the Achilles tendon (Curwin & Stanish, 1984; Jozsa *et al.*, 1989).

Normal anatomy of the Achilles tendon

The Achilles tendon is common to the gastrocnemius and soleus muscles (Fig. 13.1).

Muscles

The gastrocnemius is a superficial muscle; it has two heads which are connected to the condyles of the femur by strong, flat tendons. The soleus is situated immediately deep to the gastrocnemius; it starts with tendinous fibres from the posterior surfaces of the fibula and tibia with the accessory head to its lower and inner parts usually ending in the Achilles tendon or the calcaneal bone. These two muscles are referred to as calf muscles or triceps surae. Neurophysiological studies on the fibres of the two calf muscles found an 80% prevalence of type I fibres in the soleus, which is characterized by slow and tonic contraction; soleus fibres react by weakening and atrophying which produces prolonged immobilization. The plantaris is a small muscle that arises from the upper part of the posterior aspect of the lateral femoral condyle. Its tendon crosses obliquely between the two muscles of the calf and runs along the medial border of the Achilles tendon, to be inserted with it into the posterior part of the calcaneus. This accessory muscle is present in approximately 93% of people. The insertion of the Achilles tendon on the calcaneal tuberosity is slightly medial to the midline; when the triceps surae contracts the heel is pulled into equinus and inversion.

Achilles tendon

The tenocytes, elongated fibroblastic cells, characterize this highly specialized connective tissue; these cells are separated by collagen fibres which follow the muscle–tendon–bone kinetic chain forces and are gathered in bundles. Primary bundles are the morphofunctional units of tendon tissue; these are collected into larger secondary bundles or fascicles. Fascicles in turn are assembled into tertiary bundles. It is these tertiary bundles which comprise the tendon itself. The tendon, initially fan-shaped, becomes more rounded as it approaches the calcaneus, where it expands slightly to attach to its posterior surface. The two components of the tendon maintain clearly defined characteristics derived from the muscles from which they originate: (i) localization of insertion; (ii) length of contraction

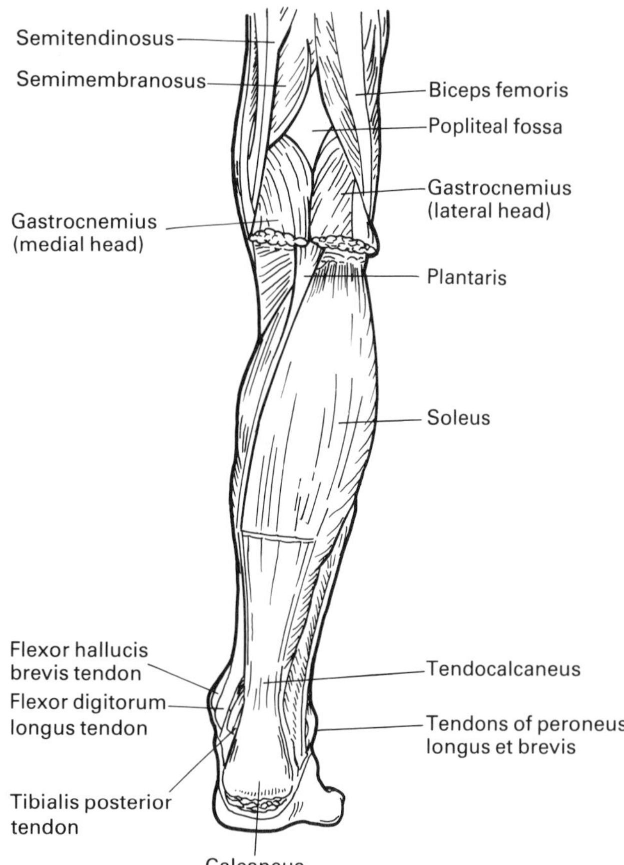

Fig. 13.1 Normal anatomy of the Achilles tendon.

lever; (iii) contraction (slow for the soleus component, fast for the gastrocnemius component); and (iv) innervation.

The tendon is surrounded by loose fibrillar tissue termed the epitendon; this fine sheet continues into the interior of the tendon as the endotendon, to surround the primary and secondary fibre bundles. Between the two layers of aponeurotic covering is the paratendon which contains blood vessels. The epitendon and the paratendon together are often referred to as the peritendon.

Myotendinous junction

The muscle and tendon fibres have numerous interdigitations in this region. The muscle fibres are contained by a basal membrane of the sarcolemma, but the collagen fibres are always separated from the basal membrane.

Osteotendinous junction

As the tendon expands in the bony tissue of the calcaneal tuberosity, the tendon gradually converts to fibrocartilage and stiffens, thus protecting the tendon against oblique traction and abrupt stress. This transition is gradual: the cells lose their elongated shape, become rounded like cartilage cells and form orderly rows containing a variable number of cellular elements. Beyond the area known as the 'blue line' or 'cementing line', the fibrocartilaginous matrix becomes mineralized; the cells keep the same morphological characteristics, while there are hydroxypatite crystals both between and within the collagen fibres. The bony tissue of the underlying stratum does not show any clear separation from the calcified fibrocartilage.

Synovial bursae

The insertion of the Achilles tendon is protected by two synovial bursae: the subcutaneous bursa, between the skin and the tendon, and the retrocalcaneal bursa, between the tendon and the upper part of the calcaneus. The properly defined insertion area on the os calcis is a rough surface situated between the retrocalcaneal bursa and the plantar surface of the calcaneus where the superficial tendinous fibres extend on the posterior part of the fascia plantaris.

Vascularization

The arterial blood supply to the Achilles tendon is provided by branches of the posterior tibial artery and the peroneal artery (Lagergren & Lindholm, 1958). The vascular network that surrounds the tendon is described as follows:

1 A vertical system provided from the peritendon, which is more developed on the anterior aspect of the tendon (mesotendon) and furnishes numerous transversal anastomoses.

2 A descending system arising from the myotendinous junction.

3 An ascending system arising from the osteotendinous junction.

Several authors have demonstrated a zone of reduced vascularity 2–6 cm above the insertion, a site that is commonly involved in rupture (Arner & Lindholm, 1959) and sustains the strain of running.

Innervation

On the medial side, innervation of the Achilles tendon is provided by branches of the tibial nerve. On the lateral side, the sural nerve supplies branches to the Achilles tendon and to the posterior aspect of the lateral malleolus. Inside the tendon, the nerve branches form a network of trunks that run parallel to the main axis of the tendon, anastomosed by branches running transversely and obliquely.

Function

In 1953, Arandes and Viladot recognized this tendon as a portion of the anatomical–functional unit which includes the triceps surae, Achilles tendon, os calcis and fascia plantaris. This muscle–tendon chain plays some role in knee flexion, mostly plantar flexion, and also tends to supinate the foot (Domingo-Pech *et al.*, 1981).

Os calcis appears to be the true os sesamoid of the foot plantar flexor system as the patella is in the extensor apparatus of the knee (Fig. 13.2).

Anatomical anomalies of the Achilles tendon

James *et al.* (1978) assessed the aetiology of running injuries under three categories: (i) training errors; (ii) anatomical factors; and (iii) shoes and surfaces. Achilles tendon injuries also have a multifactorial origin; they often occur as a consequence of anatomical anomalies and biomechanical problems.

The correct diagnosis of these anomalies and the evaluation of their consequences are the keystone of any preventive and/or therapeutic strategy. Subotnick (1979) pointed out that abnormal pronation can cause more symptomatology than any other single foot pathology.

An exaggerated hip anteversion, valgus knee, tibial internal rotation and leg length discrepancies cause secondary hyperpronation of the hindfoot.

Increased pronation is an abnormal state and occurs as a compensatory motion of the subtalar joint secondary to malalignment of the heel–foot or leg–foot deformity. This condition may be due to a forefoot supination, a rearfoot varus, a functional ankle joint equinus, or a

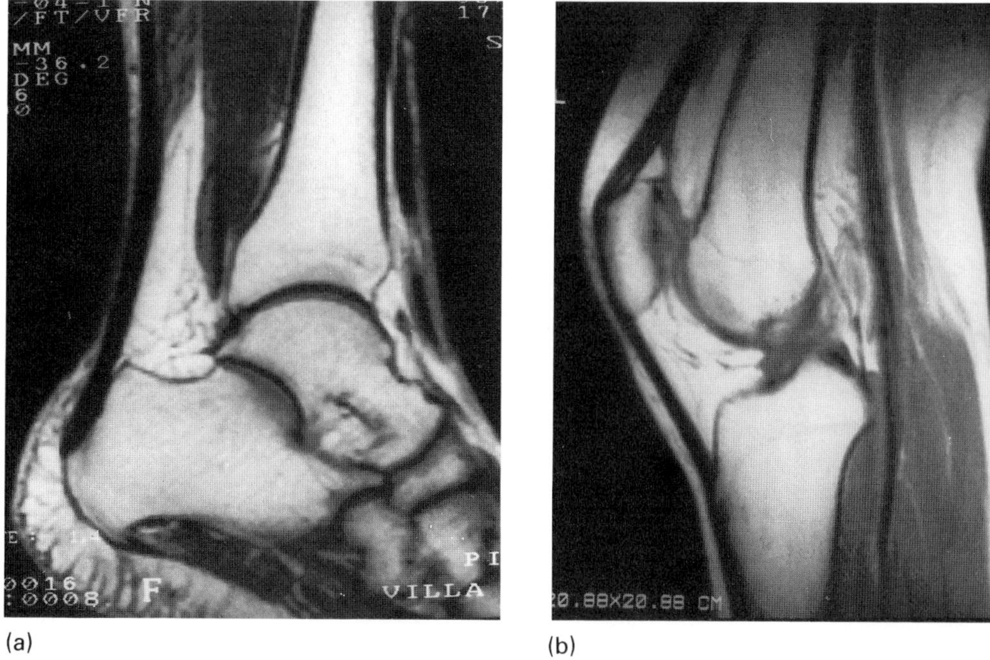

(a) (b)

Fig. 13.2 Magnetic resonance image showing (a) the normal anatomy of the foot plantar flexor system in comparison with (b) the extensor apparatus of the knee.

contracture and tightness of the triceps surae. Overpronation of the foot during running may result in the 'whipping-action' of the tendon (Clement *et al.*, 1984) and increased friction between tendon and peritendon. When examining athletes the following questions must be resolved (Curwin & Stanish, 1984):

1 Where is the pain?
2 When does it occurs?
3 How long does it last?

ASSESSMENT OF ANATOMICAL ANOMALIES

Biomechanical analysis of the forces acting on and within the foot during sport activities, needs high-technology methods of research (Nigg, 1987). However, when these methods are unavailable, or when epidemiological investigation upon a series of athletes is needed, the authors believe that footprint collection can be an acceptable alternative approach to the assessment of anatomical anomalies.

Footprint collection produces information about the longitudinal arch, is a clinically valuable method of classifying feet, and provides a useful guideline for correct diagnosis.

MECHANICAL VARIATIONS

Foot morphology and biomechanics are genetically determined. It is very difficult to decide how to compensate or balance anatomical anomalies, nevertheless the correction of a forefoot varus or valgus, a supinated or hyperpronated hindfoot, a flattened medial arch and a rigid cavus foot, is mandatory. An appropriately prescribed and constructed orthotic device can greatly decrease the likelihood of Achilles tendon injuries (Bates *et al.*, 1979).

Cavus varus — high arched foot (Fig. 13.3). At foot strike, the heel remains in the varus

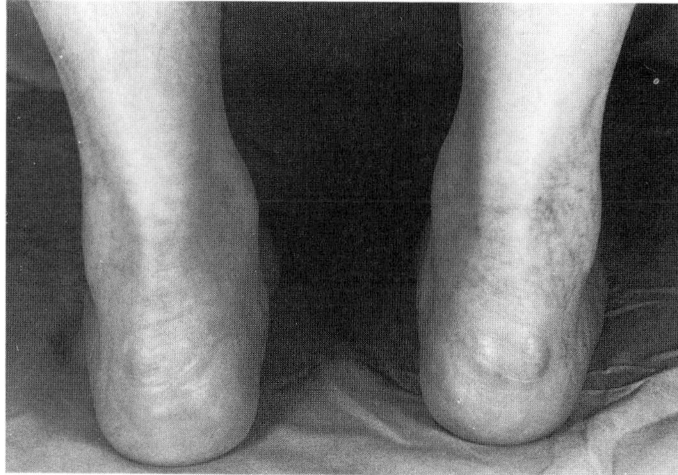

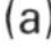

(a)

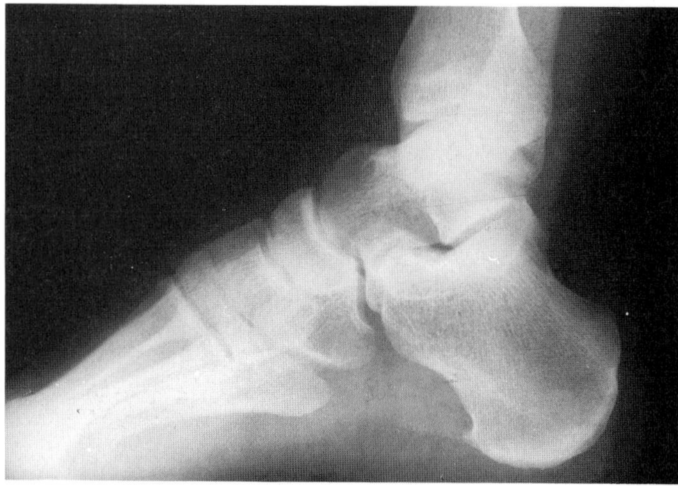

(b)

(c)

Fig. 13.3 (a) Photo and (b) lateral X-ray film of a cavus varus foot; (c) the footprint demonstrates an extremely reduced weight-bearing area connecting the forefoot and rearfoot. In the normal foot a straight line passes through the plantar print of both the second toe and the long axis of the calcaneus. In this case the inward open angle confirms that forefoot and rearfoot are misaligned in a varus position.

position and the longitudinal arch of the foot remains rigid; the stress of loading is thus passed through the lateral side of the foot. Rigidity and lack of shock absorption place the athletes with this type of foot at an increased risk for Achilles tendon injuries.

Pes planus (Fig. 13.4). Individuals with morphology of this type show excessive and prolonged pronation. They suffer from injuries of the Achilles tendon attributable to excessive motion at the subtalar joint. The medial side of the posterior tarsal bones and tendons are also subjected to overload.

Cavus valgus (Fig. 13.5). Muscular contractures,

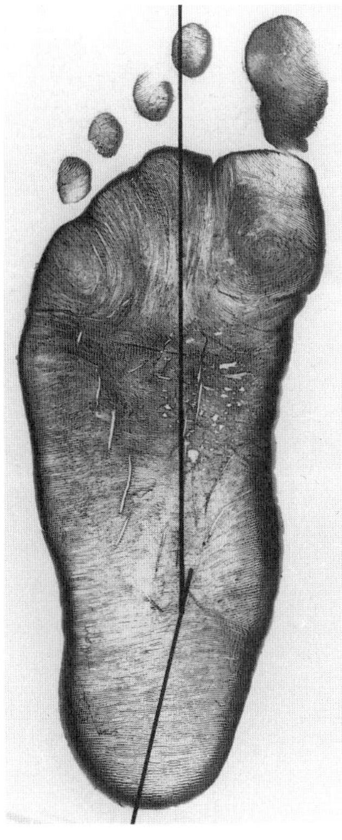

(c)

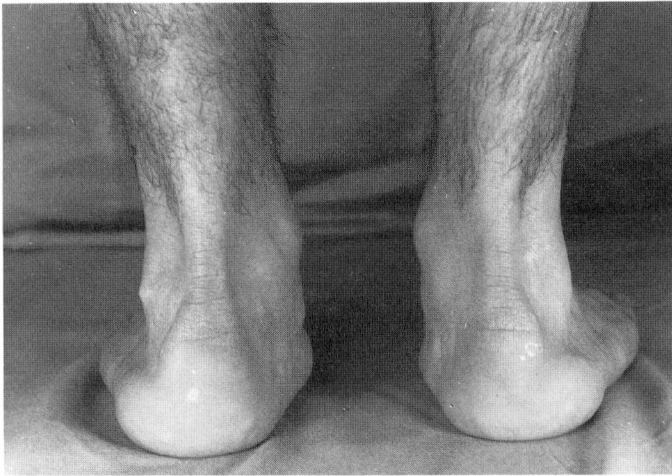

(a)

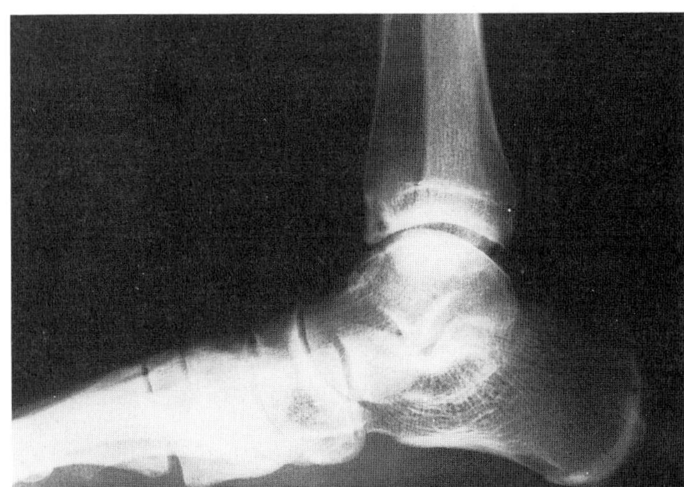

(b)

Fig. 13.4 (a) Photo and (b) X-ray of this type of foot show the collapse of medial tarsal bones; (c) the footprint demonstrates the longitudinal medial arch is abolished and the rearfoot is outwardly oriented.

instability of the subtalar joint and excessive motion of calcaneus with resulting overpronation are the features of this type of foot.

Muscular and myotendinous junction injuries

The triceps surae muscle–Achilles tendon unit is subjected to traumatic injuries (muscular strains and deep muscle contusions) and overuse injuries (peritendinitis).

Traumatic injuries near the myotendinous junction occur more often in young people, and rupture near the distal insertion more often in middle-aged people. Muscular strains are due to indirect force (contraction of the muscle itself), and deep muscle contusions to direct force (Mellion *et al.*, 1990).

Muscular strains are classified as:

First degree: Tear of only a few muscle or tendon fibres, characterized by mild swelling, pain and disability of the calf. The patient is

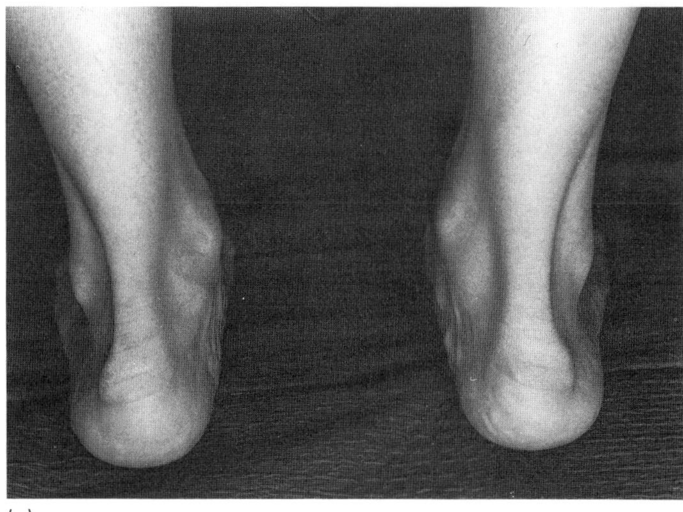

(a)

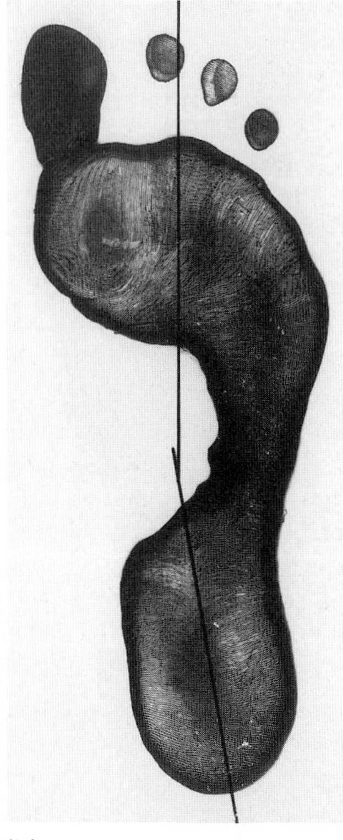

(b)

Fig. 13.5 (a) Photo of a cavus valgus foot: hyperpronated rearfoot and internal displacement of medial tarsal bones; (b) the footprint confirms the valgus (outward) orientation of the rearfoot and the pronounced longitudinal medial arch (cavus) in spite of the medial displacement of tarsal bones and the appearance of flat footedness.

able to produce strong, but painful, muscle contraction.

Second degree: Disruption of a moderate number of muscle or tendon fibres (Fig. 13.6), characterized by pain, swelling, disability and by the patient's weak and painful attempts at muscle contraction.

Third degree: Complete rupture of the muscle–tendon unit. It may be localized to the origin, muscular portion, myotendinous junction,

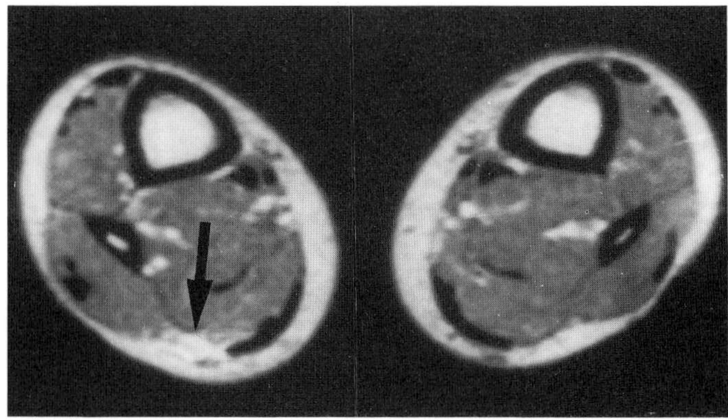

Fig. 13.6 Magnetic resonance image showing the partial rupture laterally of the gastrocnemius muscle (arrow) at level of myotendinous junction.

within the tendon itself or at the tendon insertion. It is characterized by full disability, swelling and pain.

Clinical examination

Muscles are strained more often than tendons in young people; the reverse is true in older people. Physical examination of calf muscles reveals the presence of pain and swelling at the lesion level. The oedematous and inflammatory reaction often impedes palpatory perception of the interruption of the muscular tissue. Muscle function is limited or severely compromised by both pain and tissue disruption. Pain is often diffuse. Ultrasonography, telethermography, computerized tomography (CT) scan and magnetic resonance imaging (MRI) are methods utilized to obtain accurate diagnosis. When a functionally important muscle is ruptured, especially in athletes, early surgical repair is indicated.

Aetiology

The full power of a muscle depends upon the degree of extensibility. Triceps surae tightness increases the risk of muscle ruptures, diseases of the muscle–tendon junction and tendinitis. Strains of the posterior calf musculature are related to overuse of the gastrocnemius muscle (Millar, 1979).

Studies report that males are prone to muscle injuries because of their lack of flexibility, whilst females are prone to muscle injuries because of their lower levels of physical strength and endurance.

Preventive measures

The role of stretching in the prevention of muscle and tendon injury is paramount, and it is widely utilized to increase flexibility, to diminish passive tension after training and performances, and to increase range of motion. Several techniques are recommended to attain the appropriate tension between the triceps surae and muscles of the anterolateral compartment of the leg. The effect on both the muscle–tendon junction and the tendon itself is confirmed by Viidik (1969), who demonstrated a waviness in the collagen fibres of unstretched rabbit Achilles tendon. The contract–relax method of stretching seems to be more physiologically beneficial than both slow static stretch and ballistic stretch.

Treatment

The correct treatment after diagnosis of muscular and myotendinous injuries should be:

1 Pain relief.
2 Passive stretching.
3 Exercise for the antagonists.
4 Exercise for agonists (later).
5 Quadriceps exercise.

Muscular and junctional injuries are precipitated by a stretching manoeuvre, therefore the aim of treatment should be to obtain a scar that is able to tolerate sudden stretches without tearing.

Achilles tendon peritendinitis

The Achilles tendon lacks a true synovial sheath, being surrounded by peritendon. The tendon itself lacks the characteristics of a tissue predisposed to inflammatory processes. However, inflammation may occur in the peritendinous structures (peritendon, paratendon and septae) which are made up of loose connective tissue rich in cells and are well vascularized. Classification of Achilles tendon disease according to Puddu *et al.* (1976) is as follows:

1 Pure peritendinitis — inflamatory process of peritendinous tissue (Fig. 13.7).
2 Tendinosis — degenerative changes of tendon tissue (Fig. 13.8).
3 Peritendinitis with tendinosis — both inflammation of the tendon covering and degeneration of tendon tissue are present (Fig. 13.9).

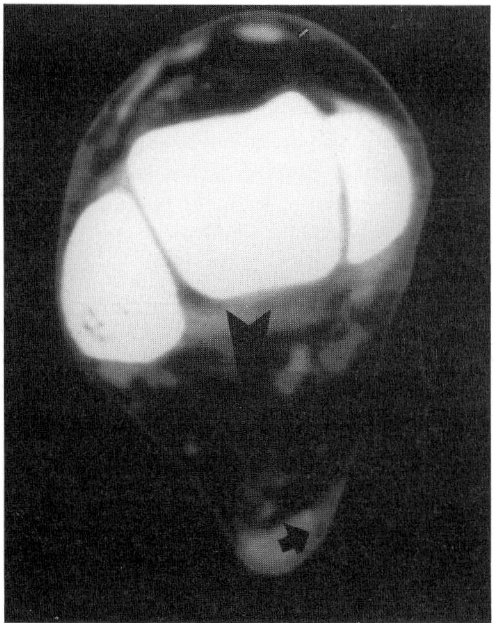

Fig. 13.7 Computerized tomographic scan of peritendinitis of the Achilles tendon (small arrow); the soft tissue and the mesotendon gathered in the Kager triangle are remarkably oedematous (large arrow).

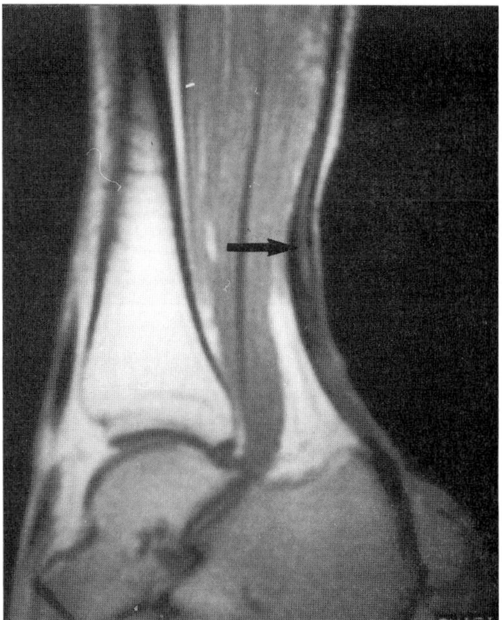

(a)

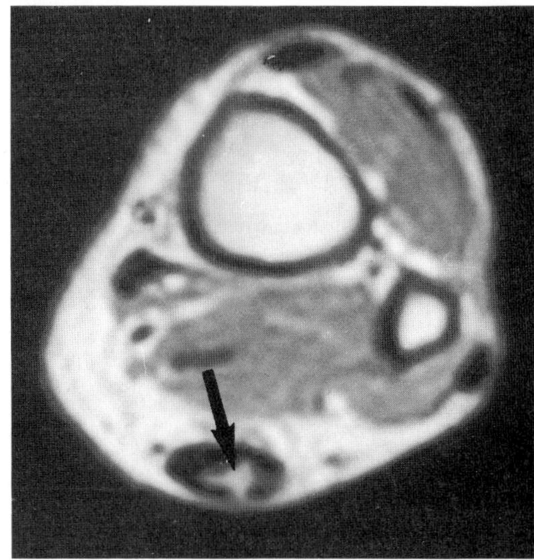

(b)

Fig. 13.8 Magnetic resonance image of a severe case of tendinosis; (a) the sagittal view shows the enlarged and degenerated tendon, the arrow indicates the extension of the non-homogeneous area within the tendon belly that is clearly visible (arrow) in the horizontal view (b).

The pathological changes of tendinosis and peritendinitis with tendinosis create the condition for an impending rupture of the Achilles tendon.

Aetiology

ANATOMICAL FACTORS

Cummins *et al.* (1946) studied the patterns of reciprocal rotation of the Achilles tendon fibres. Based on this work, Christensen (1954) pointed out the peculiar twisting disposition and Barfred (1973) affirmed that the rotation produces areas of stress concentrated in the tendon caused by a 'sawing' action of one part of the tendon as it twists and crosses another. This effect is most marked in the area 2–6 cm above the tendon insertion where rotation is most pronounced.

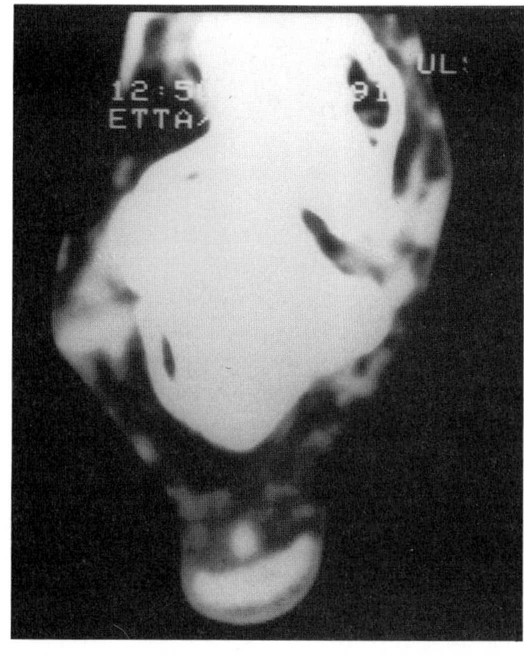

(a)

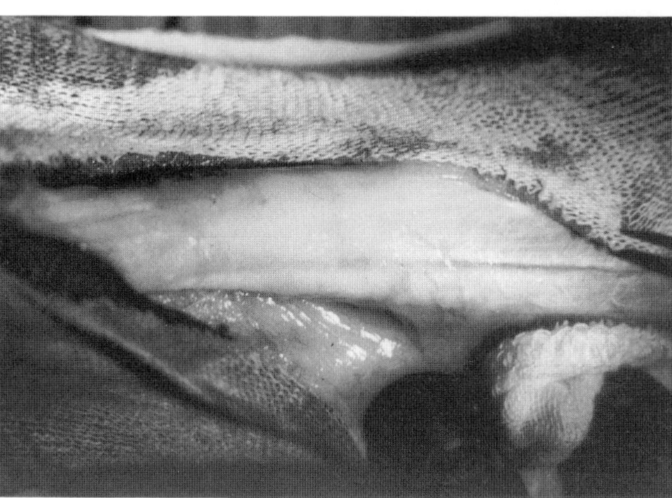

(b)

Fig. 13.9 (a) Computerized tomographic scan showing tendinosis of the Achilles tendon and peritendinitis. (b) The inflammation of the tissues that surround the tendon are revealed by surgical exploration.

BIOMECHANICAL FACTORS

Functional overpronation of the foot is an aetiological factor of primary importance to the Achilles tendon disorders. Pronation generates an obligatory internal tibial rotation which tends to draw the Achilles tendon medially. Clement *et al*. (1984) described this pronation as producing a whipping action in the Achilles tendon. This whipping action may contribute to microtears in the tendon, particularly in its medial aspects, and thus initiate an inflammatory response.

DYSTROPHIC FACTORS

Abnormal tendon structure is considered an aetiological factor of Achilles tendon peritendinitis (Davidson & Taunton, 1987). Factors present may include:

1 Presence of collagen disorders such as rheumatoid disease, ankylosing spondylitis or discoid lupus erythematosus.

2 Hyperuricaemia.

3 Corticosteroid drugs administered for systemic disease or locally injected.

4 Previous trauma, such as previous surgery or scarring around the tendon from laceration or infection.

5 Disuse atrophy.

The physiological senescence process in tendinous tissue seems to play a lesser role in peritendinitis.

MICROTRAUMATIC FACTORS

Sudden modifications in style or quantity of training can produce severe microtrauma in the Achilles tendon. Changes particularly likely to precipitate peritendinitis include (Curwin & Stanish, 1984):

1 Adding hills or sprints to regular training.

2 Running on uneven ground.

3 Changing sports shoes.

4 Changing running surfaces (as when ground freezes).

5 Inadequate emphasis on warm-up and flexibility.

6 Beginning another sport such as basketball, tennis or squash.

7 Sudden increase of mileage.

8 Resumption of training after a long period of inactivity.

Peritendinitis crepitans

This affects the peritendinous covering of tendons without synovial sheets, like the Achilles tendon, and the extensive areas of perimysium at the myotendinous junction. It is typically characterized by crepitation caused by tendon movements or by palpation of the affected area.

PATHOLOGY

The perimysium and the peritendinous tissues are remarkably oedematous and hyperaemic. There is abundant serous exudation and the formations involved are almost always covered by a sheet of fibrin. Histologically, considerable proliferation and dilatation of the capillaries is found at the level of the peritendinous sheets and perimysium, which is itself covered with fibrinous exudate. Thrombosis of the small vessels is always present.

SYMPTOMS

Subjective symptoms are: (i) local pain; (ii) limited function; and (iii) crepitation. Objective signs include diffused local swelling, sometimes with cutaneous hyperaemia. Crepitation is the most typical sign and it is best heard with a stethoscope. It can be induced by provoking muscular contractions or by pressure on the swollen area.

Chronic adhesive peritendinitis

PATHOLOGY

The tendon and peritendon are adherent and appear in a magma of connective tissue. Degeneration of the tendon itself is sometimes evident macroscopically: it loses its natural brightness, becomes chalky, and ulceration and partial tears may be evident. In other cases, changes are evident at histological examination: the most typical findings are the proliferation of capillaries surrounded by fibroblasts at the visceral and parietal peritendon level, and the adhesion between the tendon and the peritendinous structures.

SYMPTOMS

Pain is the basic symptom and it occurs at the Achilles tendon or calf muscles. The pain can be divided into four stages (Walsh *et al.*, 1990):
Stage 1: Pain after activity only; ceases at rest.
Stage 2: Pain during activity; does not restrict performance.
Stage 3: Pain during activity; restricts performance.
Stage 4: Chronic, unremitting pain, even at rest.

Swelling is more or less evident over and around the Achilles tendon. On palpation, the tendon is soft and pain is provoked on the tendon belly, while the myotendinous and osteotendinous junction are painless. Dorsal and plantar flexion movements are painful, especially when exercised against resistance.

DIFFERENTIAL DIAGNOSIS

Partial rupture of the Achilles tendon is a differential diagnosis. Because of the abundance of symptoms that are similar to that of peritendinitis, the diagnosis must be accurate and made only by experienced specialists. Partial ruptures of the Achilles tendon may arise as a consequence of eccentric action due to sport activity (Ljungqvist, 1968).

Peritendinitis is characterized by a thickened and swollen area along the tendon. Partial rupture sometimes shows itself as a small hard nodule (Pagliano, 1987b). Physicians may inject steroids into the area, mistaking symptoms for peritendinitis; this is always a dangerous practice and may occasion a full rupture.

Differential diagnosis must also include: (i) the compression syndromes involving the S1 nerve root; (ii) the congenital 'short' Achilles tendon; (iii) peritendinitis crepitans; and (iv) the insertional tendinopathies. Soft-tissue roentgenogram shows thickening of the tendon shadow; thermography is also a useful diagnostic tool.

When chronic adhesive peritendinitis is associated with tendon degeneration, subcutaneous rupture is the complication to be most feared, especially because it may arise abruptly, often without warning symptoms.

CONSERVATIVE TREATMENT

Suggested treatment is as follows (Clement *et al.*, 1984):
1 A symptomatic reduction in activity level.
2 Attainment of adequate gastrocnemius–soleus strength and flexibility. The authors consider that exercises done to obtain a flexibility of less than 12 times dorsal extension and less than 25 times plantar flexion are inadequate. Athletes lacking ankle flexibility due to tight calf musculature often attempt to gain additional range of dorsiflexion by additional knee flexion thus worsening the muscular contracture.
3 A proper training method after the onset of symptoms. Continued running in the presence of a microtear in the early phases of healing may overload the immature scar. Total rest may also create a scar which is not of sufficient tensile strength. Graded eccentric rehabilitative exercises are superior to total rest during recovery from microtearing of the Achilles tendon.
4 Appropriate installation of corrective orthotic devices. Correction of functional overpronation via a medial rearfoot post minimizes the potential for vascular impairment by reducing or eliminating conflicting internal tibial rotation produced by prolonged pronation (Bates *et al.*, 1979).
5 Well-designed footwear. For maximal rearfoot stability, the shoe must have a firm, well-fitted heel counter and a moderate flared heel. The sole must be flexible under the metatarsal heads to allow the foot to bend easily over the metatarsophalangeal joints. Strain on the Achilles tendon is also increased by an inadequate heel wedge: the heel wedge should be between 12 and 15 mm in all athletic shoes. Additional heel lifts (from 7 to 15 mm in thickness) relieve tension in the Achilles tendon during the symptomatic phase of treatment.
6 Respect for the postsymptomatic phase.

Patients who begin to increase their training levels as soon as they become asymptomatic often experience a total relapse of symptoms.

Conservative treatment may also include the following:

1 Rest; withdrawal from all activities that induce or enhance symptoms; walking with crutches is sometimes necessary in severe cases.
2 Administration of oral and local anti-inflammatory drugs (in peritendinitis crepitans the use of heparin is also advised).
3 Cortisone products administered via the systemic route or locally (avoiding injection into tendon tissue) in order to prevent more adhesions, though not all authors agree with local injection of corticosteroids because of the danger of weakening or rupturing the tendon.
4 Ice massage (effective but temporary relief).
5 Heelcord stretching to stretch the soleus muscle and the Achilles tendon.
6 Ultrasound is largely used but caution must be observed as ultrasonic waves may disturb leucocytes in the inflamed tendon and enhance the inflammatory response.
7 Ionophoresis utilizes non-steroid ions or radicals, such as magnesium salicylate; phonophoresis; and massage to increase local circulation and help to loosen adhesions and reduce stiffness.

The keys to successful conservative treatment are:

1 Respect for the fixed treatment programme.
2 The necessary time is taken for recovery.
3 The gradual and clinically controlled resumption of sports activities.

SURGICAL TREATMENT

Operative treatment should be reserved for those patients in whom conservative treatment has failed and who are motivated with regard to sports (Kvist & Kvist, 1980; Leach *et al.*, 1981; Schepsis & Leach, 1987; Nelen *et al.*, 1989). Surgical procedures include:

1 Extensive tenolysis of the tendon (opening the peritendinous and perimysial sheath).
2 Thorough exploration of the tendon in order to detect signs of peritendinitis or tendinosis.
3 In cases of peritendinitis, the adhesions between the tendon and peritendon are freed; the serous and fibrinous exudates are removed and the hypertrophic paratendon is excised.
4 In cases of *tendinosis*, excision of the degenerated tendon tissue and repair with resorbable suture is performed. Zones having lost their normal luster or nodular thickenings should be split longitudinally.
5 When extensive debridement of the tendon is performed, the tendon is reinforced with turned down tendon flaps.
6 Scarification over the full thickness of the tendon belly (Fig. 13.10). The stimulus to regenerate induced by the incisions makes it possible to replace degenerated tissue with newly formed connective tissue which gradually takes on the structural characteristics of tendon tissue. However, many authors report that this procedure may jeopardize the tendon blood supply.
7 Great care has to be taken not to perform circular exploration of the tendon. The blood supply may be compromised if the fatty tissue of the ventral aspect of the tendon undergoes undue exploration.

POSTOPERATIVE REGIMEN

The regimen suggested by Davidson and Taunton (1987) and Nelen *et al.* (1989) are:

1 2 weeks immobilization in plaster splint or restricted motion brace (early plantar flexion of the ankle is possible).
2 3–4 weeks walking with crutches: non-weight-bearing initially on operated side.
3 6–8 weeks range-of-motion exercises (passive dorsiflexion); stretching exercises (with knee extended as well as flexed); swimming; training while wearing a floating jacket and diving in a swimming pool; stationary bicycling; isometric, isotonic and isokinetic strengthening of the calf muscle; introduction of impact stress (jogging, distance running).

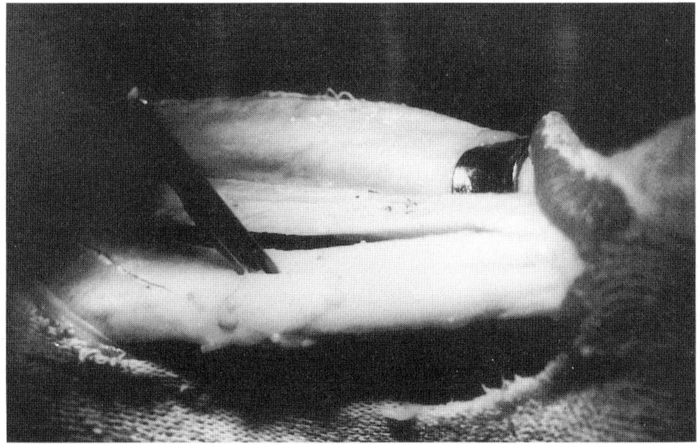

(a)

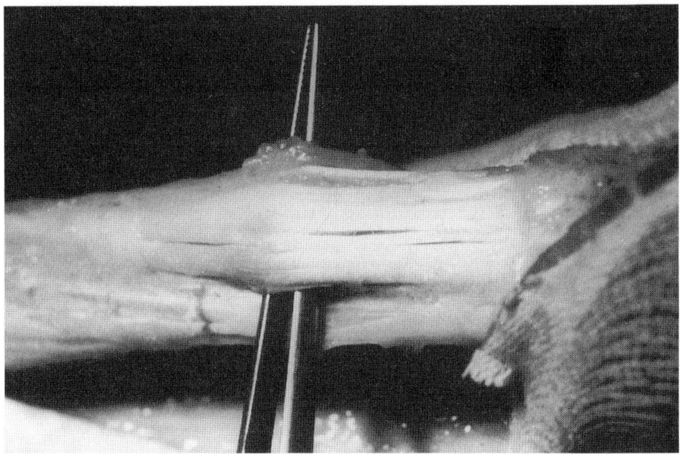

(b)

Fig. 13.10 Surgical treatment of chronic adhesive peritendinitis: (a) extensive tenolysis of the tendon; (b) scarification along the whole length of the tendon.

4 3 months: gradual introduction of high impact stress (sprinting, jumping).
5 4 months: return to competitive sport.

ECCENTRIC EXERCISE PROGRAMME

Curwin and Stanish (1984) pointed out that rest and surgery (which is invariably followed by inactivity) induces muscular atrophy and weakens the tendon structure in athletes. These treatments may relieve symptoms, but recurrence remains as a complication: the athlete may be left with an Achilles tendon too weak for what is demanded of it. A vicious cycle begins, with rest weakening the tendon so that the symptoms recur as soon as activity is resumed. Only in cases of acute peritendinitis, where pain is so intense as to prevent athletic participation, should complete rest be enforced and only until acute symptoms subside. The eccentric exercise programme is a training programme which aims to strengthen the actual tendon tissue and to avoid inactivity.

Example. The eccentric programme for Achilles peritendinitis:

1 Warm-up: moderately vigorous sit-ups, push-ups, and so on.
2 Flexibility exercise for the calf muscle; stretching exercise for the gastrocnemius and soleus.
3 Eccentric exercises: the patient stands on the edge of a step. Body weight is sustained by the forefoot, the heel remaining suspended. The heel is allowed to drop downward with gravity, below the level of the step. Three sets of 10 repetitions are performed. There should be some discomfort in the last 10 of 30 repetitions, but pain should not be present throughout and the level of pain should not be extreme. Ignoring pain means that further damage may occur. Pain is important to judge the severity of tendinitis, for the clinical check on the eccentric programme and to determine the rate of progression of the programme.
4 Progression: increase the speed of the movements or increase resistance:
   (a) to begin, the weight should be supported equally by both feet throughout the exercise session,
   (b) slowly increase the weight, shifting it onto the symptomatic leg,
   (c) gradually, the weight becomes supported by the symptomatic leg only,
   (d) increase speed of dropping, and
   (e) add weight to shoulders.

Achilles tendon rupture

Epidemiology

Epidemiologically, ruptures of the Achilles tendon are showing an increased incidence. Patients who suffer from Achilles tendon rupture are younger than patients with other tendon ruptures (e.g. supraspinatus, long head of biceps brachii) (Turco & Spinella, 1987). Achilles tendon rupture is more frequent in sports in which abrupt or repetitive jumping, cutting and sprinting movements are required (Fig. 13.11).

Aetiology

INFLAMMATION

Two clinical patterns of Achilles tendon rupture are generally observed (Puddu *et al.*, 1976):
1 Tendon rupture preceded by a long history of acute symptoms of peritendinitis.
2 Ruptures suddenly occurring in absence of previous history of Achilles tendon pain. These latter cases are characterized pathologically by the degenerative lesion of tendon tissue ('tendinosis') that presents as rupture in the absence of changes in the peritendon.

Pure tendinosis is the pathological sub-

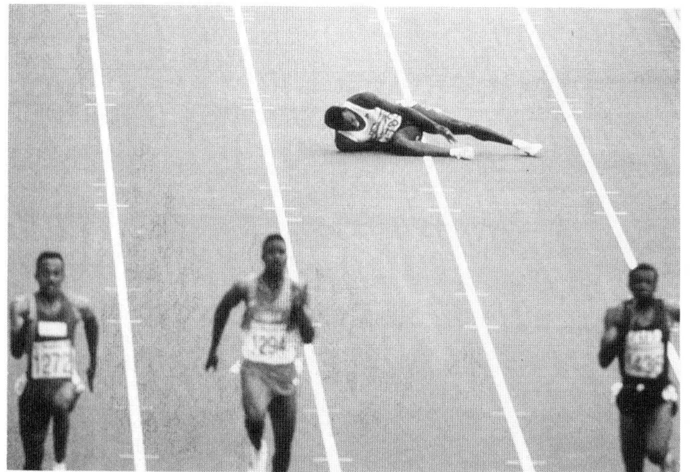

Fig. 13.11 Acute complete Achilles tendon tear occurring during an Olympic 100-m dash. © Vandystadt.

stratum not only for ruptures of the Achilles tendon but for the majority of tendon ruptures (Perugia *et al.*, 1981). As such, it cannot be considered as a special condition leading to predisposition to subcutaneous lesions of the Achilles tendon. The finding of peritendinitis associated with tendinosis may explain the presence of the inflammatory symptoms and reduced mechanical resistance in tendons predisposed to rupture. Peritendinitis by itself does not seems to be an aetiological factor in the genesis of the rupture. The peritendinous inflammation might be an indirect agent, causing changes to the vascular network predisposed to degeneration of the tendon tissue and to rupture (Fox *et al.*, 1975).

IMPAIRED BLOOD SUPPLY

The area of critical blood supply situated 2–6 cm proximal to the insertion of the Achilles tendon is the segment in which ruptures occur (Lagergren & Lindholm, 1958). Arner and Lindholm (1959) studied the histological changes in Achilles tendon rupture and their findings (oedema and disintegration of the tendon tissue, fraying of the collagen bundles, decreased number of cell nuclei) were consistent with an impairment of the blood supply as the causative factor.

ECCENTRIC ACTION

The role of eccentric action as a causative agent of rupture of the Achilles tendon was clearly described by Ljungqvist (1968). All the following examples of Achilles tendon rupture involve eccentric action of the muscle (i.e. the muscle is contracting and lengthening as the tendon is stretched):

1 Pushing off with the weight-bearing foot while simultaneously extending the knee, common in sprinting or running uphill. The calf muscles are maximally contracted.

2 Sudden unexpected dorsal extension of the ankle joint, such as slipping on a stair or stumbling into a hole, where the heel drops suddenly. The calf muscles are moderately contracted but become maximally contracted in reflex due to the sudden stretch.

3 Forced dorsal extension of the ankle, while the foot is plantar flexed, such as jumping or falling. The calf muscles are maximally contracted and sudden movement leads to marked stretching of the muscle and particularly the tendon.

For prevention, the athlete should be well prepared for these motions.

MECHANICAL AETIOLOGY

The mechanical aetiopathogenesis of Achilles tendon rupture is supported by the experimental researches of Barfred (1973) who emphasized the uneven distribution of the stresses in the Achilles tendon fibres on inversion or eversion use of the subtalar joint.

CORTICOSTEROID ADMINISTRATION

This is a well-known and documented aetiopathogenetic mechanism of Achilles tendon rupture. The drug locally injected causes changes within the tendon structure that may lead to rupture. An indirect mechanism of rupture is the premature resumption of athletic activity due to the relief of the symptoms induced by the drug that exposes the impaired tendon to unbearable use.

METABOLIC CONDITIONS

In a series of 42 Achilles tendon ruptures, Beskin *et al.* (1987) reported a surprisingly high incidence of gout (14.3%); another patient in the same series was later diagnosed as having Cushing's disease.

Acute rupture of the Achilles tendon

CLINICAL PATTERN

Patient history is highly suggestive: sudden pain where the injury occurred, just like a direct blow. Sometimes an audible snap is heard. The patient becomes immediately unable to walk or to stand on tiptoe. Weakness, inability to ascend stairs and limping are also observed. The circumstances of the injury are very often the same and some physicians affirm that diagnosis can almost be done without seeing the patient. Nevertheless, the diagnosis is sometimes missed (from 25 to 50% in the largest series). Ankle sprain is most often confused with fresh acute rupture, especially if active plantar flexion is present. Rupture of the medial head of the gastrocnemius is another misdiagnosis. Only later, when there are no signs of improvement, does the patient ask for a second opinion. The physical examination of a fresh rupture reveals: (i) swelling of the calf and Achilles tendon area; (ii) oedema of the perimalleolar lodge; and (iii) a palpable gap in the tendon 2–6 cm above the tendon insertion. The palpation of the gap is painful.

The remaining active plantar flexion may be due to the integrity of the flexor longus hallucis, the flexor longus digitorum and the tibialis posterior. After fresh rupture of the Achilles tendon, dorsal extension of the affected foot with flexed knee results in an exaggerated motion.

On examination, the athlete lies prone with feet out of the bed, the uninjured foot showing equinus position due to the normal tonus of triceps surae, while the affected foot appears to be at 90° to the axis of the leg (Brunet–Guedj sign).

The Thompson test is performed by squeezing the calf muscles ('squeezing test') while the patient lies prone with the knee flexed (Thompson & Doherty, 1962). The plantar flexion of the foot is produced when the Achilles tendon is intact, in tendon disruption the foot does not move.

The 'needle test', described by O'Brien (1984), is performed by inserting a needle at a right angle through the skin of the calf just medial to the midline 10 cm above the superior border of the os calcis. The needle tip should penetrate just within the substance of the Achilles tendon. Motion of the external extremity of the needle in a direction opposite to that of the tendon during passive dorsal extension and plantar flexion of the foot will confirm an intact tendon distal to the level of the needle insertion.

FURTHER INVESTIGATIONS

X-ray examination is useful to exclude ankle and subtalar fractures. In the lateral view the Kager triangle is evident. This is the area observed in the posterior aspect of the distal shaft of the tibia and flexor muscle, with the Achilles tendon profile on the opposite side and the superior aspect of os calcis at the base. In Achilles tendon rupture, changes in this area were thought to be of diagnostic value, but this remains uncertain.

Xeroradiographic examination better shows the Kager triangle and Achilles tendon (Fig. 13.12a). In Achilles tendon rupture, the dimension and radiolucency of the triangle appear to be reduced. The shadow of the Achilles tendon thickens and displaces ventrally, thus reducing the triangle area (Fig. 13.12b). The skin outline forms an obtuse angle of 130–150° with the apex at the point of rupture (Toygar sign). This examination does not produce the definitive diagnosis, especially regarding partial and complete ruptures.

Ultrasonography. Enlargement of the tendon, hypoechogenous aspect of the tendon structure and oedema of the Kager triangle are the signs of fresh rupture (Fig. 13.13). In old lesions, the interruption of the tendon structure is best seen via ultrasonography (Monetti, 1989).

CT scan and MRI. These techniques give more detailed information about the exact level of the lesion, the amount of tendon tissue involved and the extension of the lesion on the sagittal and the horizontal views. MRI has proved to be of great importance in preoperative planning (Keene *et al.*, 1989).

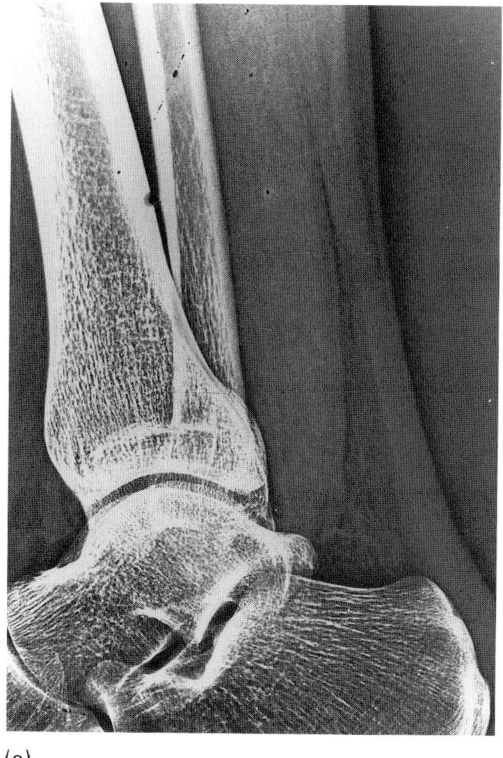

(a)

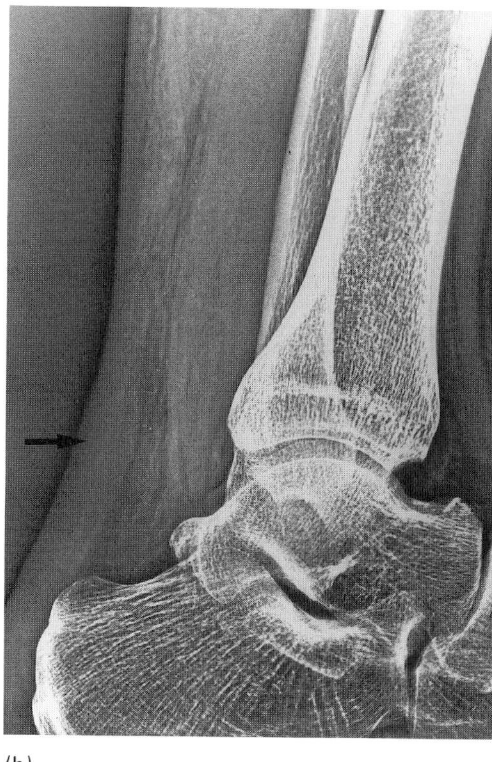

(b)

Fig. 13.12 (a) Xeroradiography of the region of the Achilles tendon. Normally, Kager triangle borders are: (i) anterior margin of Achilles tendon posteriorly; (ii) upper face of os calcis distally; and (iii) muscular masses of the back of the tibia and fibula anteriorly. (b) Kager triangle reduced and deformed in a case of rupture of the Achilles tendon. The arrow indicates the rupture area.

PATHOLOGY

The site of rupture is located 2–6 cm proximally to the insertion on the calcaneal bone. Rupture occurring at the myotendinous junction are usually close to the insertion. Avulsion from the distal insertion are exceptional. The tendon bundles appear completely disarranged at both ends of the disruption; the typical 'horse-tail' feature is not infrequent (Fig. 13.14).

Haematoma, granulation tissue and inflammatory changes are consistent findings. Associated rupture of the plantaris muscle is quite rare.

Old ruptures of the Achilles tendon

A neglected rupture of the Achilles tendon is characterized by the severe retraction of the proximal muscles and separation between the ends. Perugia *et al.* (1981) consider that these changes become fixed and irreversible within 4 weeks.

Old ruptures of the Achilles tendon are lesions at least 4 weeks old. Complete ruptures diagnosed after this limit, and those misdiagnosed and unsuccessfully treated as partial, occur at an average of 25% of all tendon ruptures (Inglis *et al.*, 1976).

CLINICAL PATTERN

Old lesions of the Achilles tendon are characterized by elongation of the Achilles tendon and weakening of the calf muscles. As a consequence of the impaired function, the patient

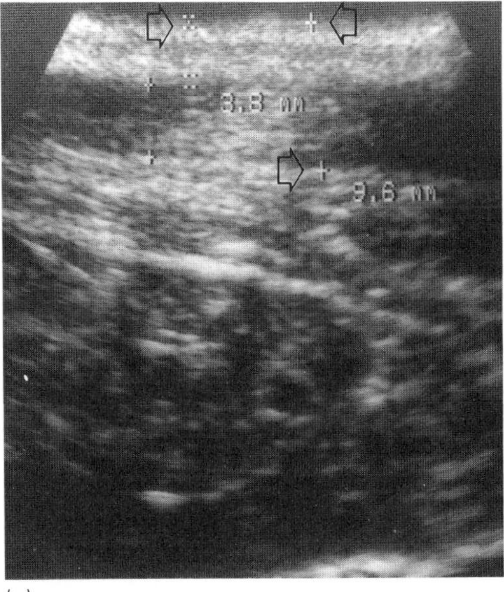

(a)

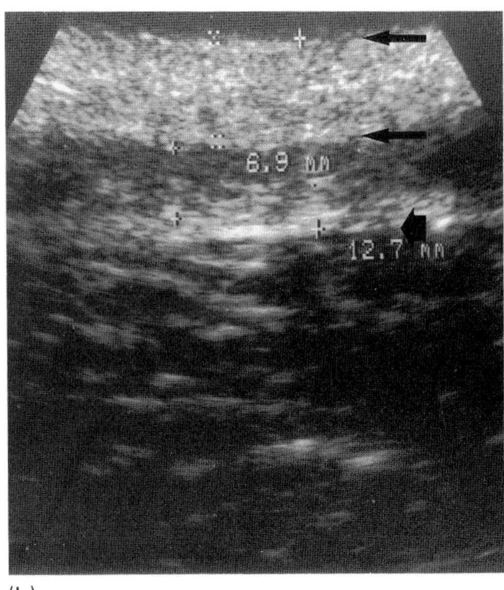

(b)

Fig. 13.13 (a) Ultrasonography of a normal Achilles tendon and (b) in a case of rupture: the tendon is enlarged, hypoecogenic and oedema of the Kager is present.

walks on the heel and lacks the toe-off phase of gait. Standing tiptoe on the affected limb becomes almost impossible. Plantar flexion is reduced, but present. Pain is mild or absent.

PATHOLOGY

Separation between the ends of the tendon measures 5–6 cm. The space is filled by scar tissue, scarcely adhering to the ends; the peritendinous covering appears thickened. The calf muscles are retracted, hypotrophic and fibrotic.

Partial rupture of the Achilles tendon

AETIOLOGY

As previously reported (Puddu *et al.*, 1976),

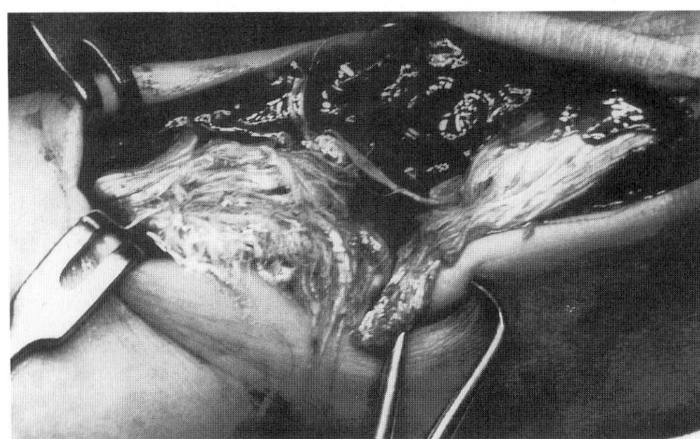

Fig. 13.14 Fresh 'horse-tail' rupture of the Achilles tendon: the disarranged bundles and the degenerative changes at the ends of the tendon are clearly visible.

partial rupture of the Achilles tendon may occur in the course of chronic or recurrent peritendinitis (pure tendinosis and peritendinitis with tendinosis). The role of eccentric contractions must be determined (Ljungqvist, 1968).

CLINICAL PATTERN

Sudden worsening of pain in patients affected by peritendinitis, or sharp pain after an eccentric contraction, followed by asthenia in the calf and limitation of function are presenting symptoms. Hypotrophy of triceps surae is observed very often, but in spite of this finding, the patient is still able to stand and walk on tiptoe. The physical findings are: (i) thickening of the Achilles tendon of variable degrees; (ii) palpatory sensation of a rigid heel cord; and (iii) localized swelling (Pagliano, 1987b).

X-ray examination shows: (i) reduction of the radiolucent Kager triangle area; (ii) blurring of the profile of the tendon; (iii) signs of infiltration of the peritendinous area; and (iv) calcium deposits are sometimes present. Some of these signs are in common with those of peritendinitis thus posing problems in differential diagnosis, especially in cases of partial rupture. CT scan and MRI have proved to be of great help in the assessment of the presence, the extent and the exact nature of the lesion (Fig. 13.15).

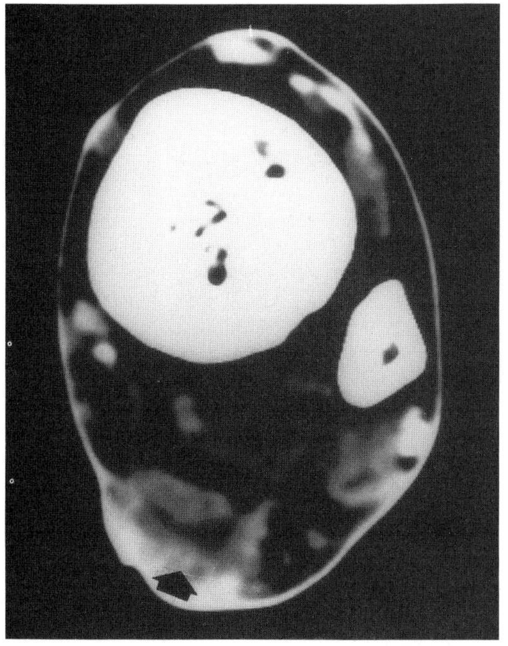

(a)

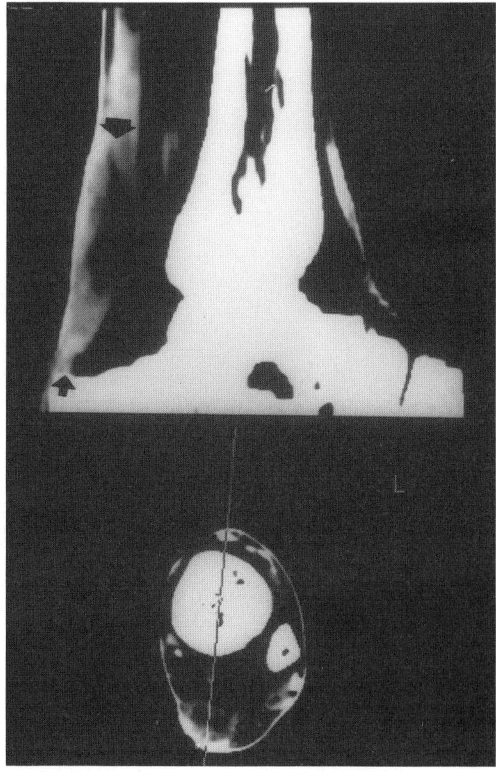

(b)

Fig. 13.15 Computerized tomographic scan of peritendinitis with tendinosis and partial rupture of the tendon: (a) the horizontal view — the arrow indicates the partial rupture in the tendon context; (b) the sagittal view — the extension of the partial rupture is correctly evaluated.

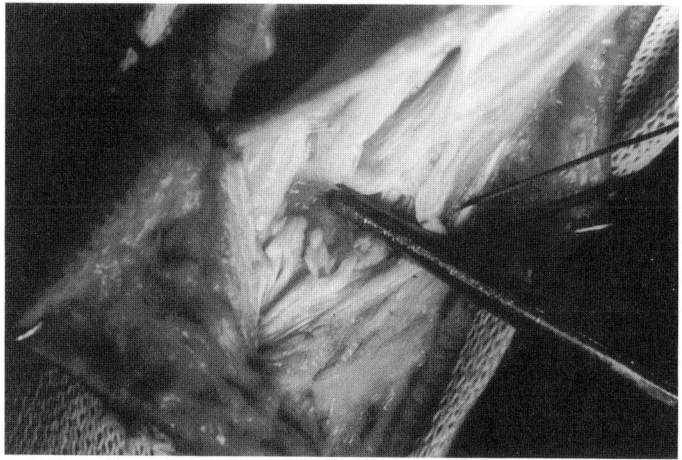

Fig. 13.16 Operative finding in a case of old partial rupture, characterized by fibrotic processes around the ends of the tear.

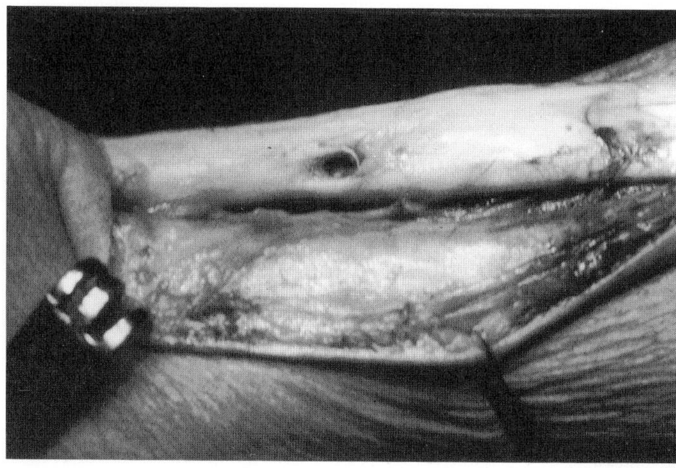

Fig. 13.17 Old partial rupture revealed by a cavity of cystic appearance on the middle third of the tendon.

PATHOLOGY

Fresh ruptures: the main characteristics are: (i) oedema; (ii) haematoma filling the site of the tear; and (iii) inflammatory reaction of the peritendinous tissues around the lesion. The tear may be transverse, oblique or longitudinal, generally with fraying ends.

When the rupture occurs within the tendon parenchyma as a central lesion, extending proximally and distally, the uninjured fibres may conceal the gravity of the lesion.

Old partial lesions are characterized by fibrotic processes around the ends of the tear (Fig. 13.16). The presence of a longitudinal lesion within the tendon, communicating with a cavity of cystic appearance, usually reveals an old partial rupture (Fig. 13.17).

Treatment of complete ruptures

Both conservative and surgical methods are reported to produce satisfactory results. In athletes, surgical treatment seems to fulfil the necessity of early repair and recovery.

CONSERVATIVE TREATMENT

Lea and Smith (1972) list the following elements:

1 Below-knee cast for 8 weeks, the foot in 20° plantar flexion for 4 weeks and in a slight plantar flexion for the remaining 4 weeks. A long-leg cast with knee flexed at 40° is also recommended for the first 4 weeks, in order to attain relaxation of the triceps surae.

2 Removal of the plàster cast and prescription of a heel lift of 2.5 cm for 4 more weeks. Walking (weight-bearing) and physiotherapy are allowed. Movements of the ankle joint are allowed, though strictly avoiding dorsal extension and plantar flexion against resistance.

3 At the beginning of the sixth month, full weight-bearing is allowed with the heel lift. At the end of this period a gradual retraining programme begins.

Advantages

The treatment can be carried out at an outpatient clinic, avoiding hospitalization, the problems inherent in anaesthesia and those related to orthopaedic surgery. Patients with diabetes, peripheral vascular and other recognized conditions of an increased risk for surgical procedures are best treated by non-operative means.

Disadvantages

Recovery of the tendon is obtained at the price of tendon lengthening, with a decrease of the muscular power of the triceps surae. This is only slightly compensated for by hypertrophy of the plantar flexors. Recurrence of the rupture is the most significant complication (10–30%).

SURGICAL TREATMENT

Percutaneous technique

A non-absorbable suture is passed through small cutaneous incisions, first in the proximal stump of the tendon and then to the distal stump. The ankle is held in the equinus position and tension is applied to the suture in a criss-cross manner, bringing the tendon ends together (Ma & Griffith, 1977).

Open techniques

Beskin *et al.* (1987) stress the importance of optimizing local skin conditions before surgical procedures. If control of swelling requires several days or even weeks, this delay is preferred over hasty surgical intervention.

The skin incision is performed on the posteromedial side of the Achilles tendon area. The posterolateral approach is important to avoid damage to the sural nerve (with consequent dysesthesiae) and to the small saphenous vein. Great care should be taken to avoid damaging the anterior tendon sheath and the anterior fatty area, which contains the all-important blood supply of the tendon (Quigley & Sheller, 1980). The peritendinous coverings are sutured only when inflammatory changes are not evident (Saillant *et al.*, 1989).

Methods of surgical repair

These include:

1 End-to-end suture with 'U' or 'X' stitches.

2 Direct repair with Bunnel or modified Kessler suturing of the tendon.

3 Three-tissue bundle technique.

4 Two rectangular flaps of the dorsal surface of the proximal stump of the Achilles tendon are folded and sutured on the distal stump directly, or passed 'U' shaped in the posteroanterior direction. The flaps may be obtained from both stumps.

5 A wide flap of the triceps surae aponeurosis folded down and sutured onto the distal end.

6 Autografts to augment (support) tendons: the plantaris gracilis is the most used. It is attached proximally at the myotendinous junction and then passed in a figure of 8 into the two tendon stumps. It must be noted that the plantaris gracilis muscle is absent in about

15% of the human population. Autograft of the peroneus brevis tendons (Perez-Teuffer, 1972; Turco & Spinella, 1987): the tendon is anchored distally to the stump of the Achilles tendon (in the original technique a transosseous tunnel is made through the calcaneus); the retracted end of the Achilles tendon is pulled distally, and sutured end-to-end and firmly secured to the 'U' shaped transfer of peroneal tendon.

7 Flaps of fascia lata have been used to reinforce an end-to-end suture and to wrap the stump of the tendon.

Surgical repair of partial ruptures

Usually it is possible to perform an accurate end-to-end suture in partial lesions (Denstad & Roass, 1979). When the tear is not recent and when there are fibrous changes, necrotic areas or calcifications build up in peritendinous tissues and excision of the diseased area is necessary. Many surgeons prefer not to perform longitudinal scarifications round the full girth of the intact part of the tendon. When the rupture involves more than 25% of the whole tendon, a flap (or a bundle) of the tendon is taken, folded and sutured to overlap the rupture.

Surgical repair of neglected ruptures

Old lesions are characterized by: (i) severe retraction of the triceps surae; (ii) tendon callus; and (iii) impairment of local blood supply by the oedematous and inflammatory changes. The suggested methods of repair are:

1 Flaps of Achilles tendon obtained from the proximal side of the tendon are folded and sutured to the distal stump. Sometimes it is possible to obtain flaps from both sides of the disrupted tendon.

2 A long strip of aponeurosis of the triceps surae (Bosworth, 1956) is obtained and passed through both stumps and sutured onto itself.

3 Strips or flaps of fascia lata are utilized to unite the two ends or to wrap an end-to-end suture.

4 Plantaris gracilis tendon is transferred using the same procedure described for the fresh ruptures.

5 The transfer of peroneus brevis tendon has proved to be effective in older Achilles tendon ruptures since the peroneal tendon acts as a biological scaffold for the reparative process.

POSTOPERATIVE REGIMEN

1 Immediately following the operation: rest; correct elevation of the affected limb; the knee flexed at 45°; therapy with anti-inflammatory drugs and anticoagulants.

2 5–7 days: below-the-knee plaster splint or restricted motion brace (fixed in slight equinus or square ankle); walking with non-weight-bearing crutches.

3 10–12 days: part-time removal of plaster splint; active dorsiflexion encouraged; neutral or more active dorsiflexion is achieved; walking with non-weight-bearing crutches.

4 6–8 weeks: below-the-knee walking cast in neutral position (there is no general agreement about this procedure); part-time splint or restricted motion braces are preferred since early motion of the operated tendon enhances the formation of collagen with tensile strength properties and anticipates the remodelling phase.

5 End of treatment: removal of the cast; walking with full weight-bearing crutches; active dorsiflexion encouraged.

REHABILITATION PROGRAMME

1 During immobilization, isometric exercises are encouraged.

2 At the removal of the plaster cast and sutures:

(a) electrical stimulations of triceps surae are used,

(b) passive stretching exercises for the heel cord flexibility,

(c) passive dorsal extension of the ankle,

(d) gradual regaining of plantar flexion strength utilizing isometric exercises at first. Only when the problems of swelling, pain

and healing of the surgical scar are solved can isotonic and isokinetic exercises be allowed,
(e) swimming and fin-swimming allow cardiovascular and respiratory conditioning, the maintenance of adequate aerobic qualities and stimulate the tension of the triceps surae–Achilles tendon system in absence of load,
(f) wearing a floating jacket while diving into a swimming pool allows the patient to tread water. This method is very effective in athletes with Achilles tendon injuries because it avoids exaggerated muscular tension and overload impact stresses (the plantar surface of the foot is not used). The movement of the whole body musculature against the water resistance enhances muscle power and cardiac and respiratory conditioning, and
(g) bicycle training is useful for an athlete recovering from an Achilles tendon injury: cardiac and respiratory conditioning are assured as well as increase of muscular power in the absence of impact stresses.

Return to sports

1 After a stop of 3–4 weeks:
(a) training must be resumed at a level of no more than 50% of the previous level,
(b) if pain or muscular tightness does not occur after isometric and isotonic exercises, mild jogging is allowed. Swelling, scar healing or local inflammation must be resolved,
(c) whole days of intensive training must be avoided for 1 month,
(d) slow running is only allowed during warming up, and
(e) care should be taken if athletes compete before optimal condition is regained.
2 After a stop of 6–8 weeks:
(a) training must be resumed at a level of no more than 25% of the previous level, and
(b) the increase in training must not exceed 10% per week.
3 Warming up and stretching: muscular warming up and stretching must be linked to the resumption of impact load stresses. An accurate programme of eccentric exercises is a useful preventive measure against the relapse of injury.
4 Choice of surface: running on regular surfaces is the best way to return to sport activity; surfaces like tarmac or grass absorb the stress due to repeated heel strikes. A smooth surface, even if hard, is preferable to an irregular surface.
5 Choice of shoes: wear only well-fitting shoes, assuring stability, comfort and shock absorption. When sprinting, cutting, jumping and kicking activities are fully reintroduced into training, wearing of sport-specific shoes (football, soccer, field and track athletics, hockey, etc.) is allowed.

Discussion of Achilles tendon ruptures

The surgical repair of Achilles tendon ruptures allows an early resumption of sports activities (Jacobs *et al.*, 1978). The risk of rerupture is currently negligible (1–1.7%). The aim of the operative procedure is to restore the normal length of the tendon. Remarkably, as Turco and Spinella (1987) pointed out, there is experimental evidence and clinical support for a more effective repair when physiological tension is restored to the myotendinous unit at an early stage. Immobilization with the ankle at a right angle is performed to allow the immediate return to normal muscular tone.

The length of the immobilization period is debatable. Beskin *et al.* (1987) compared an early repair group to a late repair group. The average time to weight-bearing was 3.5 weeks in the early repair group, and 5.5 weeks in the late repair group. The time to cast removal averaged 7.2 weeks in the early repair group and 8 weeks in the late repair group. Immobilization of the foot and ankle in an equinus position for more than 14 days counteracts the benefits gained by surgery (P. Renström, personal communication, 1991). The correct tension of the triceps surae–Achilles tendon unit obtained at the time of the surgery, must be maintained by reducing the immobilization period and gradually encouraging active dorsal extension of the foot and ankle. Plantar flexion 0–20° should start after 1–2 weeks. Active motion maintains tension, avoids adherent scars forming between the tendon, peritendon and surrounding tissues and helps in remodelling the tendon.

The use of a heel lift at the end of the immobilization period when full weight-bearing is allowed, is controversial because it causes a delay in restoration of the normal length of the tendon and the tension of the myotendinous unit.

Complications

Nistor (1981) reviewing 2647 cases of Achilles tendon rupture found the incidences of the complications in surgically treated patients as follows: (i) deep infection (1%); (ii) fistula (3%); (iii) skin or tendon necrosis (2%); and (iv) rerupture (2%). Other problems included haematomas, superficial infections, granulomas and skin adhesion in about 5% of operations.

Beskin *et al.* (1987) stress that surgery should only be done when local skin conditions are good. Surgery should be delayed by several days or even weeks, if swelling needs to be controlled.

Inglis *et al.* (1976) studied the influence of surgical experience relative to surgical complications: in the initial series of 130 patients who were operated on 17% suffered from complications. It is interesting to note that in the last 48 patients of the series only two complications were noted and both were wound infections.

Diseases of the calcaneal insertion and bursae

The insertion of the Achilles tendon is protected by two synovial bursae: the subcutaneous bursa is located between the skin and the tendon itself, while the retrocalcaneal bursa lies between the tendon and the posterior aspect of the calcaneus. The subcutaneous and retrocalcaneal bursa may become inflamed and hypertrophied in the following sport-related situations:

1 An overpronated hindfoot during the stance phase of running.
2 A cavus foot.
3 Excessive impact loading due to sport.
4 Poorly constructed shoes.
5 Exaggerated friction of the counter of the shoe on the outside of the heel.

Achilles tendon bursitis appears to be entirely mechanical in origin: pressure on the prominent upper portion of the calcaneus and repetitive abnormal use leads to a chronic inflammation of the bursae (bursitis). As a reaction the bursae and the overlying skin form a painful 'runner's bump'. Haglund (1928) in his classic description of a case of chronic retrocalcaneal bursitis pointed out the role played by the peculiar shape of the calcaneal bone. When the uppermost posterior corner of the calcaneus forms a sharp and prominent angle incongruency arises between shoe and heel: thus the Achilles tendon is pinched between the shoe counter and the prominent corner of the os calcis (Fig. 13.18).

Fowler and Philip (1945) also expressed the opinion that it is the shape of the os calcis itself that determines the condition. They measured the angle between the most posterior and the lowest (plantar) surface of the calcaneus on an X-ray film in the lateral view. They found that in symptomatic patients the angle is larger than 75° while in asymptomatic patients the angle averaged between 44 and 69°. Knobby heel, high-prow heel, hatchet heel and cucumber heel are terms which describe this condition in the literature.

Fiamengo *et al.* (1982) outlined the importance of proper clinical assessment. Features may include: (i) chronic posterior heel pain; (ii) a calcified distal Achilles tendon; (iii) a bony step in the middle of the posterior surface of the calcaneus (Fig. 13.19); and (iv) soft-tissue swelling just proximal to the often 'spurred' insertion of the Achilles tendon. According to Fiamengo *et al.* (1982) in symptomatic cases

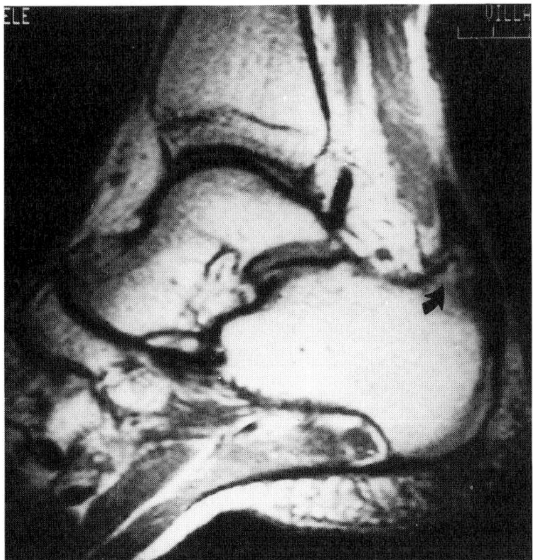

Fig. 13.18 Magnetic resonance image showing the pattern of Haglund's disease: prominent upper posterior angle of the calcaneus, chronic retrocalcaneal bursitis and peritendinitis of the Achilles tendon.

three radiographical signs may become clinically evident: (i) a prominent posterosuperior calcaneal prominence; (ii) a relatively increased horizontal length of the calcaneus; and (iii) the presence of a posterior calcaneal step. These factors would tend to create increased and possibly pathological pressure on the patient's Achilles tendon. The sequence of events may be as follows: (i) repetitive microtrauma or macrotrauma to the tendon causing gross or microscopic collagen fibre disruption, resulting in scar formation; and (ii) decreased vascularity and tendon elasticity. These changes may be revealed by tendon calcification, decreased tendon strength and, eventually, rupture.

CONSERVATIVE TREATMENT AND PREVENTION

Abnormal external pressure in cases of retrocalcaneal bursitis should be alleviated by the following measures:

1 Anti-inflammatory drugs in the early phase of conservative care.

2 Steroid solution injected into the retrocalcaneal bursa, not into the tendon.

3 Physical therapy, including ionophoresis, phonophoresis, transcutaneous electrical nerve stimulation (TENS) or sometimes cycles of X-rays.

4 Reduction of mileage and rest in severe cases.

5 The selection of proper shoes for training and competition is very important for athletes with significant biomechanical abnormalities.

6 Removing or softening the counter of the shoe. According to McKenzie (1987) the heel

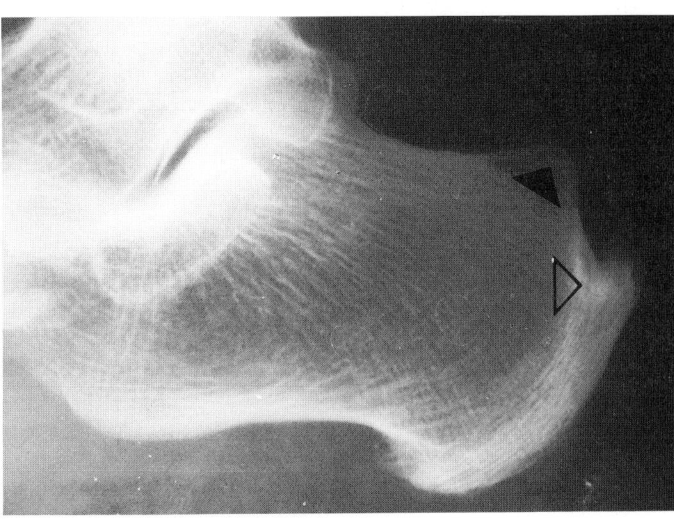

Fig. 13.19 Lateral X-ray film of rearfoot showing a prominent posterosuperior calcaneal border (filled arrow) and a calcaneal bony 'step' (empty arrow).

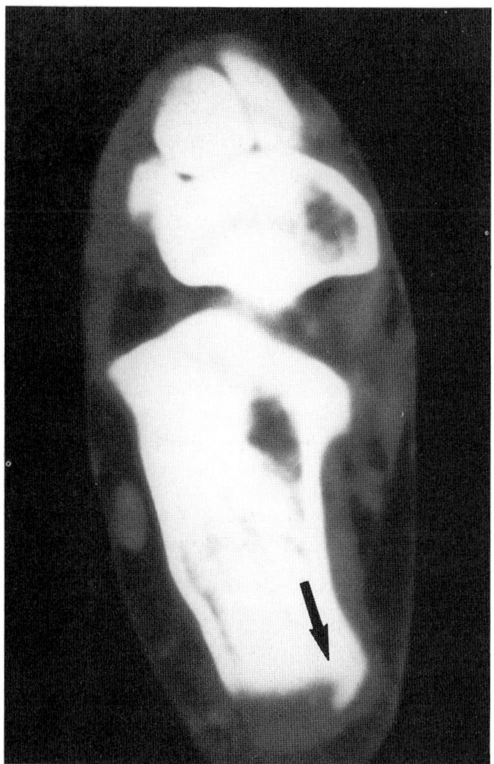

Fig. 13.20 Incomplete bone resection in a case of Haglund's disease resulting in relapse of retrocalcaneal bursitis.

counter should cradle the heel, minimizing rotation and slippage. It should also stabilize the subtalar joint, controlling excessive pronation. For those individuals with overpronation, a rigid heel counter is mandatory, but precautions against exaggerated friction over the bursae must be undertaken.

7 Inserting a heel cup or sponge pad into the shoe to protect the affected area from the irritation.

8 Using socks with soft pads in the heel area.

9 Using a heel wedge is advisable, while the wearing of shoes with a low heel is beneficial in cases of posterior calf musculature tightness. In cases of retrocalcaneal bursitis an elevated heel is advisable because the foot comes easily into neutral position, the equinus of the ankle diminishes and abnormal stress on the osteotendinous junction is less severe.

10 A short leg walking cast from 3 to 4 weeks can be used to allow some degree of training and cardiovascular maintenance.

SURGICAL TREATMENT

In cases resistant to conservative treatment, surgery becomes necessary to prevent further damage. Great care must be taken so that no bony prominences remain to irritate the Achilles tendon (Jones & James, 1984) (Fig. 13.20).

POSTOPERATIVE REGIMEN

Patients who sustain partial ostectomy of the calcaneal bone must follow the same postoperative care and management described for Achilles peritendinitis above.

References

Arandes, A.R. & Viladot, P.A. (1953) Biomechanica del Calcaneo (Biomechanics of the calcaneous). *Med. Clin.* **21**, 5–9.

Arner, O. & Lindholm, A. (1959) Subcutaneous rupture of the Achilles tendon: a study of 92 cases. *Acta Chir. Scand.* **239**(Suppl.), 1–51.

Barfred, T. (1973) Achilles tendon rupture: aetiology and pathogenesis of subcutaneous rupture assessed on the basis of literature and rupture experiments on rats. *Acta Orthop. Scand.* **152**(Suppl.), 1–124.

Basmajian, J.V. (1976) *Primary Anatomy*, 7th edn. William & Wilkins, Baltimore.

Bates, B.T., Osternig, L.R., Mason, B. & James, L.S. (1979) Foot orthotic devices to modify selected aspects of lower extremity mechanics. *Am. J. Sports Med.* **7**(6), 338–42.

Beskin, J.L., Sanders, R.A., Hunter, S.C. & Hughston, J.C. (1987) Surgical repair of Achilles tendon ruptures. *Am. J. Sports Med.* **15**(1), 1–8.

Bosworth, D.M. (1956) Repair of defects in tendo Achillis. *J. Bone Joint Surg.* **38A**, 111.

Christensen, I. (1954) Rupture of the Achilles tendon: analysis of 57 cases. *Acta Chir. Scand.* **106**, 60–70.

Clement, D.B., Taunton, J.E. & Smart, G.W. (1984) Achilles tendinitis and peritendinitis: etiology and treatment. *Am. J. Sports Med.* **12**(3), pp. 179–84.

Cummins, E.J., Anson, B.J., Carr, B.W. & Wright, R.R. (1946) The structure of the calcaneal tendon (of Achilles) in relation to orthopaedic surgery. *Surg. Gynecol. Obstet.* **83**, 107–10.

Curwin, S. & Stanish, W.D. (1984) *Tendinitis: Its Etiology and Treatment*. Collamore Press, Lexington, Toronto.

Davidson, R.G. & Taunton, J.E. (1987) Achilles tendinitis. In R.J. Shepard & J.E. Taunton (eds) *Foot and Ankle in Sport and Exercise*, Vol. 23, pp. 71–9. Karger, Basel.

Denstad, T.F. & Roass, A. (1979) Surgical treatment of partial Achilles tendon rupture. *Am. J. Sports Med.* **7**(1), 15–17.

Domingo-Pech, J., Girvent, F. & Huguet, J. (1981) Anatomia comparada del sistema Aquileo–calcaneo–plantar. *Chir. Piede-Foot Surg.* **5**(1), 1–8.

Fiamengo, S.A., Warren, R.F., Marshall, J.L., Vigorita, V.T. & Hersh, A. (1982) Posterior heel pain associated with a calcaneal step and Achilles tendon calcification. *Clin. Orthop. Rel. Res.* **167**, 203–11.

Fox, J.M., Blazina, M.E., Jobe, F.W. *et al.* (1975) Degeneration and rupture of the Achilles tendon. *Clin. Orthop. Rel. Res.* **107**, 221–4.

Fowler, A. & Philip, J.F. (1945) Abnormality of the calcaneus as a cause of painful heel: its diagnosis and operative treatment. *Br. J. Surg.* **46**, 484–98.

Gray, H. (1975) In C.M. Goss (ed) *Anatomy of the Human Body*, 29th edn, p. 506. Lea & Febiger, Philadelphia.

Haglund, P. (1928) Beitrag zur Klinik der Achilles Sehne (Clinical conditions of the Achilles tendon). *Zeitschr. Orthop. Chir.* **49**, 457.

Hattrup, S.J. & Johnson, K.A. (1985) A review of ruptures of the Achilles tendon. *Foot Ankle* **6**(1), 34–8.

Inglis, A.E., Scott, W.N., Sculco, T.P. & Patterson, A.H. (1976) Ruptures of the tendo Achilles — an objective assessment of surgical and non-surgical treatment. *J. Bone Joint Surg.* **58A**, 990–2.

Jacobs, D., Martens, M., Van Audekerke, R., Mulier, J.C. & Mulier, F.R. (1978) Comparison of conservative and operative treatment of Achilles tendon rupture. *Am. J. Sports Med.* **6**, 107–11.

James, S.L., Bates, B.T. & Osternig, L.R. (1978) Injuries to runners. *Am. J. Sports Med.* **6**(1), 40–50.

Jones, D.C. & James, S.L. (1984) Partial calcaneal ostectomy for retrocalcaneal bursitis. *Am. J. Sports Med.* **12**(1), 72–3.

Jozsa, L., Kvist, M., Balint, B.J. *et al.* (1989) The role of recreational sport activity in Achilles tendon rupture. *Am. J. Sport Med.* **17**(3), 338–43.

Keck, S.W. & Kelly, P.J. (1965) Bursitis of the posterior part of the heel. *J. Bone Joint Surg.* **47A**, 267–73.

Keene, J.S., Lash, E.G., Fisher, D.R. & De Smet, A.A. (1989) Magnetic resonance imaging of Achilles ruptures. *Am. J. Sports Med.* **17**, 333–7.

Kvist, H. & Kvist, M. (1980) The operative treatment of chronic calcaneal paratendonitis. *J. Bone Joint Surg.* **62B**(3), 353–7.

Lagergren, C. & Lindholm, A. (1958) Vascular distribution in the Achilles tendon: An angiographic and microangiographic study. *Acta Chir. Scand.* **116**, 491–5.

Lea, R.B. & Smith, L. (1972) Non surgical treatment of tendo Achillis rupture. *J. Bone Joint Surg.* **54**A, 1398–401.

Leach, R.E., James, S.L. & Wasilewski, S. (1981) Achilles tendinitis. *Am. J. Sports Med.* **9**(2), 93–8.

Ljungqvist, R. (1968) Subcutaneous partial ruptures of the Achilles tendon. *Acta Orthop. Scand.* **113**(Suppl.), 1–86.

Ma, G.W. & Griffith, T.G. (1977) Percutaneous repair of acute closed ruptured Achilles tendon: a new technique. *Clin. Orthop. Rel. Res.* **128**, 247–55.

McKenzie, D.C. (1987) The role of the shoe and orthotics. In R.J. Shepard & J.E. Taunton (eds) *Foot and Ankle in Sport and Exercise*, Vol. 23, pp. 30–8. Karger, Basel.

Mellion, M.B., Walsh, W.M. & Shelton, G.L. (1990) *The Team Physician Handbook*. Hanley & Belfus, Philadelphia and Mosby Yearbook, Chicago.

Millar, A.P. (1979) Strains of the posterior calf musculature ('tennis leg'). *Am. J. Sports Med.* **7**(3), 172–4.

Monetti, G. (1989) *Ecografia Muscolo-Tendinea e dei Tessuti Molli*. SOLEI Edit., Milano, Italia.

Nelen, G., Martens, M. & Burssens, A. (1989) Surgical treatment of chronic Achilles tendinitis. *Am. J. Sport Med.* **17**(6), 754–9.

Nigg, B.M. (1987) Biomechanical analysis of ankle and foot movement. In R.J. Shepard & J.E. Taunton (eds) *Foot and Ankle in Sport and Exercise*, Vol. 23, pp. 22–9. Karger, Basel.

Nistor, L. (1981) Surgical and non-surgical treatment of Achilles tendon rupture; a prospective randomized study. *J. Bone Joint Surg.* **63A**, 394–9.

O'Brien, T.O. (1984) The needle test for complete rupture of the Achilles tendon. *J. Bone Joint Surg.* **66A**, 1099–101.

Pagliano, J. (1987a) Management of the pronated and supinated foot. In R.J. Shephard & J.E. Taunton (eds) *Foot and Ankle in Sport and Exercise*, Vol. 23, pp. 155–60. Karger, Basel.

Pagliano, J. (1987b) Soft tissue injuries of the foot tendinous lesions. In R.J. Shephard & J.E. Taunton (eds) *Foot and Ankle in Sport and Exercise*, Vol. 23, pp. 161–8. Karger, Basel.

Perez-Teuffer, A., Ilizariturri, V.M. & Martinez Del Campo, F. (1972) Rupture traumatiques du tendon d'Achille (Traumatic ruptures of the Achilles tendon). *Revue Chir. Orthop.* **58**(Suppl. 1), 219–23.

Perugia, L., Ippolito, E. & Postacchini, F. (1981) *I*

Tendini Biologia, Patologia, Clinica (Biology, pathology and clinical disorders of tendons). Masson, Milano, Italia.

Puddu, G., Ippolito, E. & Postacchini, F. (1976) A classification of Achilles tendon disease. *Am. J. Sports Med.* **4**, 145–50.

Quigley, T.B. & Sheller, A.P. (1980) Surgical repair of the ruptured Achilles tendon. Analysis of 40 patients treated by the same surgeon. *Am. J. Sports Med.* **8**(4), 244–50.

Saillant, G., Thoreux, P., Benazet, J.P. & Roy-Camille, R. (1989) Pathologie du tendon d'Achille (tendinopathies, ruptures et plaies) (Pathology of Achilles tendons (tendinopathies, ruptures and wounds)). *Encyclopedie Medico-Chirurgicale — Appareil locomoteur*, 14090–A10. Editions Techniques, Paris.

Schepsis, A.A. & Leach, R.E. (1987) Surgical management of Achilles tendinitis. *Am. J. Sports Med.* **15**(4), 308–15.

Stanish, W.D., Ratson, G. & Curwin, S. (1987) Tendinopathies of the foot and ankle. In R.J. Shepard & J.E. Taunton (eds) *Foot and Ankle in Sport and Exercise*, Vol. 23, pp. 80–98. Karger, Basel.

Subotnick, S.I. (1979) *The Running Foot Doctor*. World Publication, California.

Thompson, T.C. & Doherty, J.H. (1962) Spontaneous rupture of Achilles tendon. A new clinical diagnostic test. *J. Trauma* **2**, 126–9.

Turco, V.J. & Spinella, A.J. (1987) Achilles tendon ruptures — peroneus brevis transfer. *Foot Ankle* **7**(4), 253–9.

Viidik, A. (1969) Tensile strength properties of Achilles tendon system in trained and untrained rabbit. *Acta Orthop. Scand.* **40**, 261–72.

Chapter 14

Acute Ankle Injuries

WILLIAM A. GRANA

Injuries of the ankle are common in sports, accounting for 10–15% of all injuries reported (Henry, 1983; Hunter-Griffin, 1990). The reason for this common occurrence is the pivotal role of the ankle in running gait, and the need for a stable ankle as the base of the lower extremity in running and cutting activities (Slocum & James, 1969; Sammarco, 1980; Mann, 1982, 1986). Acute injuries such as fractures and sprains occur most commonly as a result of cutting or side-to-side movement in sports such as basketball, soccer and football. On the other hand, overuse problems such as tendonitis, bursitis and stress fracture occur more commonly in endurance-type activities such as cross-country and the running events in track.

Ankle sprain is by far the most common cause of time loss in sports participation and, as we will see, can also be the cause of chronic pain with long-term disability. Therefore, with the prevalence of ankle injuries which occur in sport, it would seem reasonable to attempt to outline a plan to prevent ankle injury. In order to do this, it is necessary to understand the functional anatomy of the ankle and the implications that this unique anatomy has for injury and prevention of injury.

The purpose of this chapter is to present in a systematic way the functional anatomy of the ankle, common acute injury problems, common overuse problems, and the methods used for treatment and prevention of these problems. As noted above, the ankle is the most commonly injured joint in athletic participation. It is also the most frequently overlooked anatomical area when seriously injured. Casual treatment will result in chronic disability.

Functional anatomy of the ankle

The bony anatomy of the ankle consists of the distal end of the fibula, the lateral malleolus. The tip of the distal end of the tibia is the medial malleolus. The distal end of the tibia forms the tibial plafond, which, with the malleoli, articulates with the dome of the talus. The lateral malleolus is long and rectangular, while the medial malleolus is short and broad. This bony anatomy encourages plantar flexion inversion laxity while the ankle is stable in eversion and dorsiflexion. The tibial plafond is concave for the articular surface of the talus. Together, the malleoli and tibial plafond form the mortise for the tight insertion of the tenon which is the body of the talus. This bony structure provides for an inherently stable joint (Henry, 1983; Wilson, 1990).

There are three main ligamentous complexes which assist in the stability of the ankle: (i) the lateral ligaments; (ii) the deltoid ligament; and (iii) the tibiofibular syndesmosis. Laterally, the anterior and posterior talofibular and calcaneofibular ligaments prevent inversion and anterior drawer of the talus on the tibia and the malleoli. The medial deltoid ligament is a triangular-shaped ligament that has a deep and superficial component. In order for eversion or abduction laxity to occur, both components must be injured. Finally, with abduction or external rotation injury, the tibiofibular syndesmosis may also be stretched or torn, which results in the most severe type of ankle sprain (Henry, 1983; Boytim *et al.*, 1991).

Functionally, the ankle is a hinge joint, however, with plantar flexion, inversion occurs, and with dorsiflexion, eversion and external rotation occurs. As eversion occurs, there is stress placed on the fibula with a tendency to widen the ankle mortise. Therefore, there is bony stability in dorsiflexion as a result of the tight fit of the talus in the tibial plafond. The talus is narrow posteriorly and wider anteriorly. Therefore, it is wedged in position in dorsiflexion, but it is allowed greater excursion in plantar flexion. Of course in sports, cutting activity, particularly involving toe-off, results in an unstable position. Therefore, it is common for ankle injuries to occur with the athlete poised on the ball of the foot ready to move from side to side. The muscular back-up to the unstable plantar flexed position is the weaker anterior compartment and lateral compartment muscles balanced against the much stronger posterior compartment muscles. Therefore, in rehabilitation, efforts should be directed at strengthening the peroneal muscles as well as the tibialis anterior since these are the muscles that produce the stable position of dorsiflexion and eversion (Mann, 1986).

Injuries in sport tend to be of low velocity, and, therefore, the unstable position or plantar flexion, which is common in sport activities, will result in injury to the lateral ligament complex as opposed to fracture which occurs with high-velocity injury. It is only with greater force with the ankle in the stable position of dorsiflexion that more severe injuries such as fractures or injury of the tibiofibular syndesmosis occur. It is also important to remember the 'ring concept' in which the malleoli, tibial plafond and the talus are interconnected by the ligamentous complexes medially, laterally and through the tibiofibular syndesmosis to form a ring. An injury on one side of the ring, such as an injury to the deltoid ligament is often accompanied by an injury on the opposite side of the ring such as fracture of the lateral malleolus with or without injury to the tibiofibular syndesmosis. Always look elsewhere in the ring for further injury. Whether or not the opposite component of the ring injury occurs depends upon the amount of force placed on the ankle.

The primary contribution of the ankle during running is to help the body absorb the impact of the initial ground contact force. These forces are two or three times greater than the vertical forces experienced during walking and the ankle accommodates these forces by rapid dorsiflexion at ground contact. The muscles around the ankle serve to diminish the contact force during running, protecting the articular surfaces of the tibia and talus (Sammarco, 1980; Mann, 1982, 1986).

Acute injuries

In general, fractures are uncommon in sport because of the low velocities generated. Nonetheless, injuries of the ankle that involve the lateral malleolus do occur and must be recognized and treated adequately to prevent residual deformity and disability. The diagnosis of a fracture requires appropriate and adequate radiographic evaluation. Every ankle injury with localized point tenderness over the malleoli or with persistent pain, loss of motion and swelling for more than 48 h should be evaluated by appropriate radiographs. This is the only way that an adequate assessment of the integrity of the ankle mortise can be obtained. The talus must remain in its anatomical relationship to the malleoli and the tibial plafond, and the mortise view is the only way that this is determined. Therefore, a complete set of X-rays must include an anteroposterior (AP), mortise and a lateral view.

A non-displaced lateral malleolus fracture is managed by a brief period of casting or in a functional orthosis until the initial symptoms have subsided. The patient can then move to a hinged ankle orthosis which allows a range of motion but protects against inversion–eversion stress (Wilson, 1990).

On the other hand, if the ankle mortise is disrupted with resultant lateral subluxation of the talus or widening of the medial mortise, then anatomical reduction must be obtained. Usually this will involve open reduction and internal fixation of the lateral malleolus with screw fixation of fractures and a neutralization plate on the lateral aspect of the distal fibula. Open repair of the deltoid ligament may or may not be required depending on the adequacy of the initial reduction of the lateral malleolus, and a transsyndesmotic screw for disruption of the tibiofibular syndesmosis (Wilson, 1990).

About 15% of all acute athletic injury is ankle sprain and 85% of these are the inversion type (Henry, 1983). The vast majority of these injuries are of the lateral ankle ligaments and consist of a double ligament injury involving the anterior talofibular and the calcaneal fibular ligament, one of these two are the anterior talofibular ligament. In a more severe form of injury, the tibiofibular syndesmosis is involved as well. This latter injury requires a longer period of treatment, often twice as long for return to sport (Boytim *et al.*, 1991). The least common sprain is of the deltoid ligament. Virtually all of these injuries can be treated non-operatively with the exception of the tibiofibular syndesmosis injury which has widening of the mortise with separation of the tibiofibular space. This injury requires open reduction and internal fixation with a screw which crosses the syndesmosis. In addition, if the deltoid ligament is torn, this injury may also require open repair, especially when the ligament is folded into the joint (Wilson, 1990; McBryde, 1991).

Most of these ankle sprains are treated non-operatively. The usual course of management involves a period of rest and restriction of activity. This can be done either with appropriate splinting with a preformed air cast or gel cast, or with a commercially available ankle–foot orthosis (AFO). If none of these are available, cast immobilization in a bivalved cast which can be removed for exercise is equally effective. In the less severe injuries, taping or a lace-up ankle stabilizer can be used to provide compression. In addition to the restriction and compression, local icing begins immediately and active range of motion as early as pain will allow. Non-steroidal anti-inflammatories are useful for the control of pain and swelling. Emphasis is on early full range of motion to avoid contracture of the Achilles tendon and subsequent plantar flexion deformity. When the range of motion and normal gait returns, protective immobilization is removed, and the patient uses an air cast or gel cast in a shoe for stability. Emphasis is then on strengthening the peroneal muscles and the anterior compartment muscles. When full strength is obtained by isokinetic testing and calf measurement, running activity is started. As strength returns, agility and coordination activities are begun with balance board mini-trampoline and plyometric exercise (Grana, 1990; McBryde, 1991; Yngve, 1991).

Chronic pain after ankle sprain can result in severe disability (Grana, 1990). As many as 40% of patients with an acute ankle sprain may continue to have pain (Ferkel, 1988). It interferes with athletics or even everyday activity. It is a perplexing diagnostic problem for the clinician and a frustrating problem for the patient. Typically, the patient complains of vague ankle pain. It is often anterior and lateral, frequently involving the sinus tarsi and the area of the anterior talofibular and calcaneal fibular ligaments. Usually, there is a history of an inversion plantar flexion type injury. Often the patient will have had symptoms for several months. The initial injury treatment has consisted of crutch ambulation, non-weight-bearing without compression or immobilization which leaves the foot and ankle in a plantar flexed or equinus position. In addition, no X-ray studies are obtained following the initial injury. As the patient returns to full activity, he or she becomes aware of symptoms such as weakness, fatigue, pain, locking or giving way. Physical examination with reveal crepitation, popping and swelling as well as discoloration.

The differential diagnosis includes the following important diagnostic categories (Grana, 1990):

1 Incomplete rehabilitation. After an ankle sprain, the most common cause of continued chronic pain is incomplete rehabilitation. It is usually manifested by the physical findings of atrophy of the musculature of the calf and foot, and contracture of the Achilles tendon. These patients may also have an appearance of reflex sympathetic dystrophy with skin changes and discoloration as well as dysaesthetic sensations. The most important aspect of the treatment of an ankle sprain is complete rehabilitation of the motion and strength of the muscles about the foot and ankle.

2 Previously undetected trauma.

(a) injury to the syndesmosis ligament can be a continued source of pain. Patients with injury of this ligamentous complex will continue to have pain and prolonged symptoms. Radiographically, heterotopic bone may be seen locally in this area as documentation of this more severe injury,

(b) osteochondral injury of the talus is also a common and unrecognized cause of chronic ankle pain and mechanical complaints. Arthroscopic treatment that includes excision of loose fragments and debridement of the bed of the injury or open reduction internal fixation of an intact fragment may be necessary,

(c) there are a number of different fractures about the foot and ankle that can mimic an ankle sprain. These include fractures of the anterior process of the calcaneus, lateral process of the talus, the lateral aspect of the cuboid, and fractures of the base of the 5th metatarsal,

(d) in children, physeal injury and stress fractures may masquerade as an ankle sprain and produce prolonged symptoms. These can be ruled out with plain X-rays and bone scan with or without a computerized tomography (CT) scan, and

(e) peroneal tendon subluxation can also produce chronic pain. Sometimes it is possible to reproduce the subluxation with the eversion and dorsiflexion of the foot or to produce apprehension when this passive movement is accomplished. The patient localizes pain over the peroneal tendons or actual movement of the tendons can be documented. Reconstruction of the peroneal tendon retinaculum is necessary to correct this problem.

3 Congenital abnormalities. Tarsal coalition or accessory navicular may produce chronic pain following an ankle sprain and mimic some of these other acquired causes of chronic pain after ankle sprain. A careful physical examination and appropriate X-rays will usually rule out these problems.

4 Tumour. Tumours are rare but may occur. The two most common which might produce pain after an ankle sprain are cysts of the talus or cuboid or osteoma of the talus. Either of these benign problems may produce chronic pain either as a result of inherent characteristics of the tumour, or pathological fracture. Careful history and physical examination with appropriate plain radiographs are essential in the evaluation of these chronic problems after ankle sprain. Bone scan, CT scan and magnetic resonance imaging (MRI), when used appropriately are also helpful in the differential diagnosis of these causes of chronic ankle pain. An algorithm of the evaluation and management of chronic ankle pain is included in Fig. 14.1. In most patients, the prevention of the development of such chronic pain syndromes is achievable. For an acute ankle sprain, the key to full rehabilitation is the initiation of a stepwise programme of therapeutic exercise beginning with early range of motion to pain tolerance and then to the restoration of full strength progressing to resistive exercise. The return to sports participation requires training focused on the restoration of function and the careful entry into a well designed graded regimen of activity. Such a treatment programme is most likely to maximize the ankle function and prevent the development of chronic ankle pain.

Tendon rupture

Classically, eccentric loading of the Achilles tendon will result in complete rupture of the

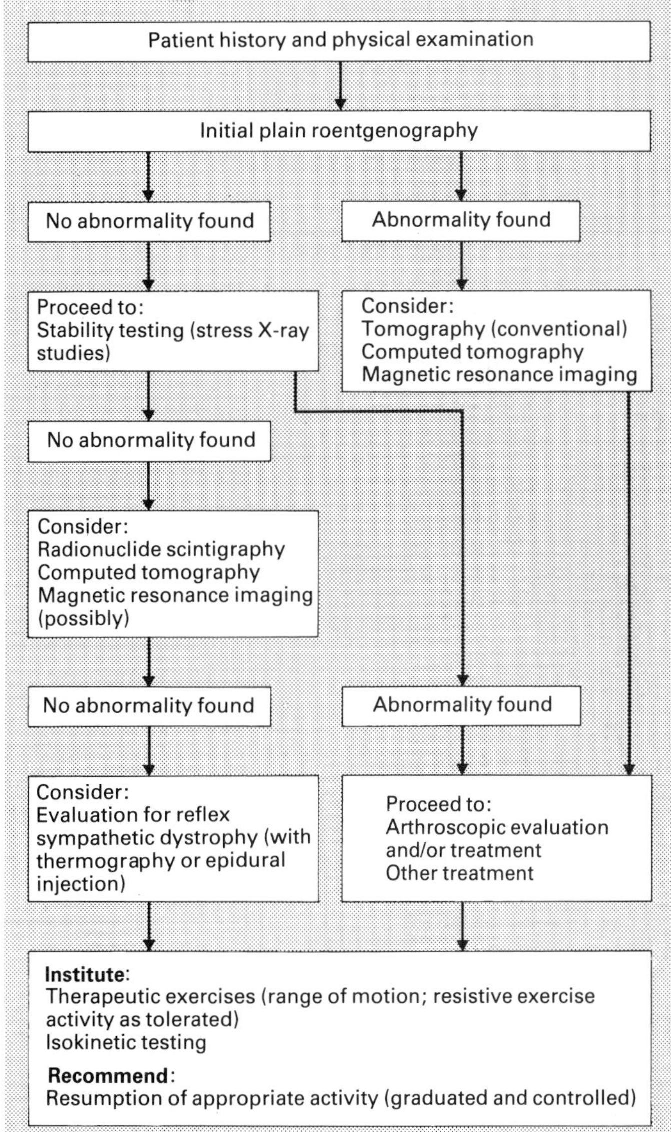

Fig. 14.1 Algorithm for evaluation and management of chronic ankle pain.

tendon. This occurs most commonly in racquet sports or in sprinting in track. The patient perceives a sudden painful pop as if he or she has been kicked hard or hit by an object. Complete rupture is documented by the Thompson's squeeze test. With the patient prone, the knee is flexed to 90° and the affected and unaffected calf is squeezed. The result should be a passive plantar flexion of the foot if the Achilles tendon is intact.

A partial tear is differentiated by a palpable local swelling or even a defect but with an intact passive squeeze test. Partial tear is managed by immobilization for a period of approximately 4 weeks and gravity plantar flexion and non-acinus. Subsequently, the patient begins range of motion activities, calf strengthening exercise and uses a heel wedge. Return to sport is delayed for approximately 4–6 months, depending upon strength and range of motion (Clancy *et al.*, 1976; Schepsis & Leach, 1987; McBryde, 1991).

Complete ruptures require surgical repair when the medical condition of the patient will allow it. In the élite athlete, repair of the ruptured Achilles tendon is mandatory and may require augmentation with plantaris or a portion of the peroneus brevis (McBryde, 1991).

Posterior tibial tendon rupture can occur acutely in the younger athlete but is considered much more likely to produce acute symptoms in the older athlete. The sudden development of flat foot deformity is a sign of posterior tibial tendon rupture. A loss then of plantar flexion inversion strength is diagnostic. Usually the tendon will retrack to the level of the medial malleolus. Early diagnosis allows acute repair followed by a period of immobilization and a delay in return to full activity for a period of approximately 3–5 months (McBryde, 1991).

Overuse problems

Connective tissues are viscoelastic materials that show extreme variance in response to macrotrauma and microstresses. Overuse injury occurs as a consequence of repetitive non-destructive submaximal microstress. The result is a variety of inflammatory and stress reaction problems about the ankle. In addition to the effects of overuse, alignment abnormality such as excessive valgus or varus deformity in the hindfoot may contribute to the impact on the ankle (Stanitski, 1990).

The muscle has a large capacity to respond to imposed demands. The connective tissues, ligament and bone respond at a slower rate. For example, bone takes approximately 2 weeks to respond to a new loading regimen. Muscle strength can increase faster than bone and within 2 weeks of the onset of a training programme, there could be an imbalance of muscle and bone strength as the bone would not yet have responded to the new imposed loading conditions. Therefore, stress fractures may arise as a result of doing too much too soon. Other factors that contribute to overuse or stress reactions include hard training surfaces, improper footwear with inadequate shock-absorbing properties and hormonal factors in women that relate to the onset of puberty or amenorrhoea (Yngve, 1990).

Impingement syndrome

Chronic inflammation about the ankle can result in pain with activity. This may occur anteriorly in association with osteophyte formation at the neck of the talus and the anterior tibia or posteriorly with inflammation in the area of a non-united os trigonum or posterior process of the talus. Plain radiographs and a bone scan that shows diffuse uptake may help in the diagnosis of these problems. Non-operatively, these problems are managed by non-steroidal anti-inflammatory medication, ice and restriction of activity as well as brace support. Arthroscopy is helpful both for diagnosis and management by partial synovectomy. The spurs are removed, and the chronically inflamed synovium is excised (Grana, 1990).

Tendonitis

Chronic tendonitis is a direct result of overuse and can occur in the peroneal tendons, the posterior tibial tendons or the Achilles tendon. The presentation is usually of localized inflammation with pain with the reproduction of symptoms by active contraction of the muscle tendon either involved in manual or passive stretch of the tendon. In addition, there may be localized swelling along the course of the tendon and a palpated or audible sensation of crepitation (Clancy *et al.*, 1976; Schepsis & Leach, 1987; McBryde, 1991).

Management includes rest and restriction or modification of activity, non-steroidal, anti-inflammatory medication, local ice application and appropriate orthotic inserts. For the Achilles tendon, a heel wedge may be useful. For the posterior tibial tendon, an arch support, and for the peroneal tendon, a valgus heel wedge (Clancy *et al.*, 1976; Schepsis & Leach, 1987).

MRI is useful in the evaluation of patients

with chronic tendonitis. Areas of signal abnormality indicate degenerative change within the tendon and a need for operative exploration. Particularly with regard to the Achilles tendon, this is helpful. The area of tendinosis is treated by an excision of hypertrophic degenerative tissue followed by repair and treatment similar to that in the acute rupture. Postoperative treatment is similar to that following the acute repair (Schepsis & Leach, 1987).

Bursitis

A number of bursal sacs exist on the medial and lateral aspects of the ankle, but the most important from a symptom standpoint is the retrocalcaneal bursa. The patient will present with pain anterior to the Achilles tendon and localized swelling. Manual pressure in front of the tendon will reproduce the patient's symptoms. The above management for tendonitis is the treatment of choice (McBryde, 1990). If retrocalcaneal bursitis persists, the area should be explored through an incision medial to the Achilles tendon, bursectomy is carried out and the posterior portion of the angle of the calcaneus is removed with an osteotome (McBryde, 1991; Yngve, 1991).

Stress fracture

About 60% of stress fractures occur over the age of 20, while one-third occur between the ages of 15 and 20, with only 10% occurring below the age of 15 (Yngve, 1990). The ankle *per se* is not a common site of stress fracture, however, fractures of the distal fibula can occur and mimic ankle sprain (Devas & Sweetnam, 1956; Grana, 1990). In addition, vertical stress fractures of the medial malleolus may also occur (Devas & Sweetnam, 1956). The diagnosis is made by localized tenderness and confirmatory radiographs. If the radiographs are negative and symptoms persist, then bone scintigraphy is the evaluation of choice.

Rest is the usual treatment for stress fracture, but in many cases, general conditioning can be maintained during recovery by exercise that does not impact loading or by involvement of other parts of the body. Rarely stress fractures can develop into a complete fracture when they are ignored. In addition, electrical stimulation with use of an orthosis such as an AFO may be useful in the élite athlete to allow a degree of continued physical activity (Yngve, 1990).

Prevention of injuries

Orthotics and taping

The prevention of ankle injuries should focus on the functional anatomy and biomechanics of the ankle joint. We have noted before in this chapter the vulnerability of the plantar flexed in the inverted position. Therefore, anything that can be done to provide stability when the ankle is in the functional position, will help to prevent ankle injury. The vulnerability of the ankle in this position produces the susceptibility to a lateral ankle ligament injury. A variety of braces, shoe inserts and taping techniques are used, though there are very few scientific studies that document the effectiveness of any of these techniques. However, as with bracing of the knee, while there may not be scientific data, subjectively athletes feel that these techniques may help them. The mechanism may be by some proprioceptive input that the braces and taping provides. From experience, certain devices seem to work better in certain situations, and these will be discussed now.

With regard to ankle braces, there are three types that can be listed (Fig. 14.2). The most restrictive type is the ankle–foot orthosis that has a hinge at the ankle joint which very markedly protects against inversion–eversion stress, but which allows flexion–extension of the ankle with some degree of restriction. This can be either purchased off the shelf or can be fabricated by an orthotist. We prefer to use this type of brace following significant injury or fractures as an intermediate form of treatment prior to beginning functional activities and early on when functional activities begin. We also use this postoperatively following ankle ligament reconstruction.

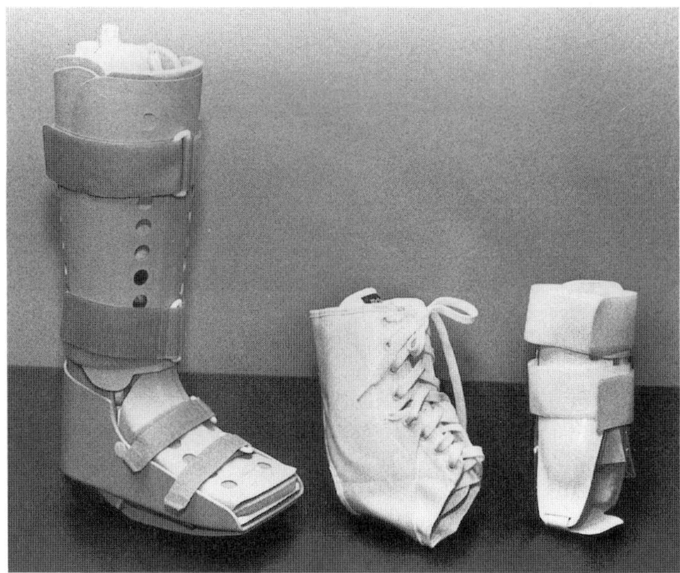

Fig. 14.2 There are several types of orthosis available for protection following ankle sprain. From left to right: (i) an ankle–foot orthosis for protection of the more severe injuries, which can be removed for exercise; (ii) the lace-up ankle stabilizer for return to function; and (iii) a stirrup-type splint which provides intermediate protection and can be removed for exercise.

A second type of brace is the stirrup type that is either padded with an air cell or gel material, and these can also be used in the acute phase following ankle sprain or in intermediate management as the patient is trying to return to activity, and when the patient does return to activity, as a support in place of a soft ankle brace or tape. The disadvantage of this brace is that in certain individuals who have slender ankles, they may twist and not fit as snugly as they should.

The third type of ankle brace is the soft brace, which can vary from a sleeve that fits around the ankle to provide compression, to a lace-up type ankle stabilizer that may have a solid metal or plastic support on the lateral side. These braces can be used for return to activity and also prophylactically and can be used in the place of tape and can be a more cost effective way of providing the same effect. For high schools and small colleges, this type of brace may be a better alternative than the expense of tape and prewrap and the regular services of a trainer.

There are some shoe inserts that are useful for various problems. When the patient has the problem of recurrent ankle sprains, the use of a lace-up type ankle brace in conjunction with a valgus heel wedge, may help to diminish the occurrence of planter flexion–inversion stress. In addition, for the patient who has problems with Achilles and posterior tibial tendonitis, an arch support may help to limit these problems as well. Also, the patient with Achilles tendonitis may find the use of a heel wedge helpful in diminishing the tensile stress on the Achilles tendon. There are a variety of systems available that allow the fabrication of these in the office by a cast technician with appropriate training and experience.

The conventional and traditional method of providing support to the ankle has been ankle taping. A number of studies document the effectiveness of ankle taping, and none have shown conclusively that this modality provides stability to the ankle for a sustained period of time. Tape loosens after a period of 20–30 min after application with exercise and the result is that the instability problems can reoccur. If it is to be used effectively and the patient has a clinical problem, then it is probably preferable to retape at intervals during the competition. Nonetheless, taping can be used effectively to provide compression following acute injury and between rehabilitation sessions when those services are available. Much of the function of taping, however, can be replaced by the newer lace-up type stabilizers.

Ankle rehabilitation

The following is a progression that can be used for the acute rehabilitation of an ankle sprain and with varying degrees of modification for other acute ankle injuries as well. The progression attempts to relieve pain, regain active range of motion, and ultimately full strength.

The key to this ankle rehabilitation progression is daily evaluation. Exercise and activity levels are progressed based upon pain, swelling, ROM and functional ability. The stages below are general guidelines and will vary dependent upon the severity of injury or type of injury and the individual athlete. The last phase of this rehabilitation programme (phase 6) will maintain the level of conditioning established for the athlete.

Phase 1: acute stage

1 Ice: applied 15–20 min every 2 h.
2 Compression: doughnut pad, open basket weave or ACE applied with foot elevated.
3 Crutches: weight-bearing to tolerance.
4 Exercise: passive range of motion (PROM) performed in pain-free range, four times a day, 10–15 min·session^{-1}.

Phase 2: postacute stage

1 Ice: continue ice treatment, may begin contrast bath.
2 Compression: continues as above, may initiate gentle massage or Jobst pump.
3 Crutches: may wean from crutches if pain free.
4 Exercise: PROM continues with progression to active range of motion (AROM). May initiate ankle isometrics.
5 Other: may use other modalities for pain and swelling, i.e. pulsed ultrasound, electrical stimulation. Biking may begin if adequate ROM available.

Phase 3: preactivity stage

Progression now dependent on symptoms.
1 Ice: continue ice if swelling persists, otherwise may decrease to postexercise application.
2 Support: may continue compression dressing or use supportive taping or brace.
3 Exercise: begin tubing/theraband exercise programme. Continue PROM and begin pain-free stretching including the Achilles tendon. Begin ankle proprioceptive neuromuscular facilitation (PNF) patterns. Begin one limb balancing.
4 Other: continue other modalities as needed for pain and swelling.

Phase 4: activity stage

1 Ice: applied post-treatment.
2 Support: supportive brace/taping.
3 Exercise: continue resistive exercises including PNF, tubing/theraband. Stretching programme continues. Begin heel/toe raises, eccentric exercises. Start balance board activities/BAPS (Fig. 14.3).
4 Begin jog–walk programme. May progress to figure of eights and Z cuts starting from slow speed progressing to fast speeds. Plyometrics may begin when tolerated.

Phase 5: return to play/maintenance

1 Ice: continued as needed.
2 Support: supportive brace/taping.
3 Maintenance exercise programme: to continue resistive exercise programme three times per week. Stretching continues daily. Proprioceptive exercise three times per week. Plyometrics three times a week.
4 Athlete should be pain free with no swelling. He or she should be able to perform all sports-specific skills without limitation or pain.

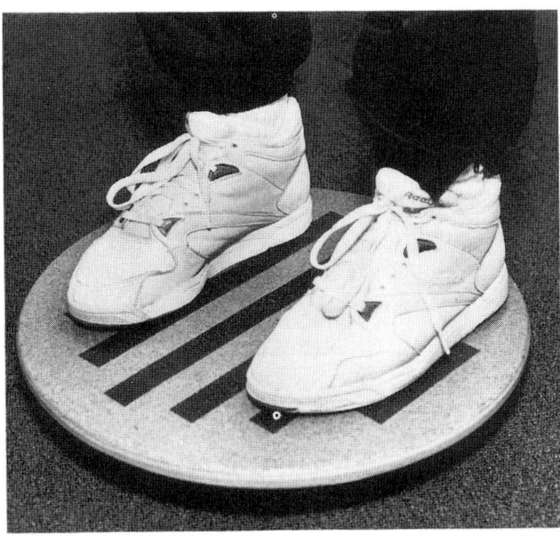

Fig. 14.3 The BAPS board which is used to regain neuromuscular coordination prior to return to function.

Phase 6: maintenance conditioning programme

1 AROM: begin active motion in dorsiflexion, plantarflexion, inversion and eversion. Can also perform alphabet with ankle. Dexterity exercise can include spreading/closing toes, picking up small objects, i.e. marbles, or tracing objects.
2 Resistive exercises: can include ankle tubing/theraband/manual resistance. May start with simple resistance such as pushing towel with foot. Later stage may include ankle weights, sand box, PNF patterns, toe/heel raises and Cybex exercise.
3 Isometrics: includes all ankle motions.
4 Stretching: must be done with pain-free limits and should include Achilles tendon stretching with knee straight/bent positions.
5 Proprioceptive exercises: may begin with single limb balancing (eyes open/closed) and progressing to balance board or BAPS.
6 Plyometrics: start with double leg hop progressing to single limb hop for height and distance. Later stages may include depth jumps and incline board.

Preventive ankle conditioning programme

The prevention of ankle injury includes a specific foot, ankle and calf exercise regimen which is integrated into the patient's general conditioning programme. The ankle programme may be tailored for an individual or be incorporated into a prepractice programme. The ankle programme is performed a minimum of three times a week. A preventive conditioning ankle programme should also include a postural evaluation to evaluate for muscle weakness, laxity, flat or high arch. It is also important to evaluate the playing surface (grass, wood, artificial turf), shoes, and practice conditions.
1 Toe raises/heel raises (40 repetitions).
2 Resistive exercises (40 repetitions):
(a) dorsiflexion,
(b) plantarflexion,
(c) inversion, and
(d) eversion.
3 Balance activities (5 min).
4 Plyometrics (5 min).
5 Stretching (5 min).

Toe/heel raises are done individually or performed as toe/heel walking for 45 m (50 yd). Resistive exercise is performed by theraband programme or manual resistance. Balancing is performed by single limb balancing (eyes open/closed) or use of balance board or BAPS. Plyometric exercise is performed by such activities as single limb hopping, high stepping, incline hopping, skipping or various other plyometric drills. Functional activities such as figure of eights, cutting or other drills are incorporated into the general conditioning programme. Stretching is performed with other stretching exercises. Focus should be on Achilles stretching and hamstring stretching.

Acknowledgments

The above ankle rehabilitation and conditioning programmes were prepared by David Ruhl, RPT, ATC, director of the Oklahoma Center for Athletes.

References

Boytim, M.J., Fischer, D.A. & Neumann, L. (1991) Syndesmotic ankle sprains. *Am. J. Sports Med.* **19**(3), 294–8.

Clancy, W.G., Neidhart, D. & Brand, R.L. (1976) Achilles tendinitis in runners: A report of 5 cases. *Am. J. Sports Med.* **4**, 46–7.

Devas, M.B. & Sweetnam, R. (1956) Stress fractures of the fibula: A review of 50 cases in athletes. *J. Bone Joint Surg.* **38B**, 818–29.

Ferkel, R.D. (1988) *Indications, decision-making, and results of ankle arthroscopy*. Presented at the Arthroscopic Association of North America Continuing Medical Education Course on Arthroscopic Surgery, Palm Desert, California.

Grana, W.A. (1990) Chronic pain persisting after ankle sprain. *J Musculoskeletal Med.* **6**, 35–49.

Henry, J. (1983) Lateral ligament tears of the ankle, 1–6 years follow-up: study of 202 ankles. *Orthop. Rev.* **10**, 31–9.

Hunter-Griffin, L.Y. (1990) Injuries to the leg, ankle, and foot. In J.A. Sullivan & W.A. Grana (ed) *The Pediatric Athlete*, pp. 187–98. American Academy of Orthopaedic Surgeons, Park Ridge, Illinois.

McBryde, A.M. (1991) Disorders of the ankle and foot. In W.A. Grana & A. Kalanek (ed) *Clinical Sports Medicine*, pp. 466–89. WB Saunders, Philadelphia.

Mann, R.A. (1982) Biomechanics of running. In R.A. Mann (ed) *American Academy of Orthopedic Surgeons Symposium on the Foot and Leg in Running Sports*, pp. 30–44. CV Mosby, St Louis.

Mann R.A. (1986) Biomechanics of the foot and ankle. In R.A. Mann (ed) *Surgery of the Foot and Leg in Running Sports*, pp. 1–30. CV Mosby, St Louis.

Sammarco, J. (1980) Biomechanics of the foot. In V.H. Frankel (ed) *Basic Biomechanics of Skeletal Systems*. Lea & Febiger, Philadelphia.

Schepsis, A.A. & Leach, R.E. (1987) Surgical management of Achilles tendinitis. *Am. J. Sports Med.* **15**, 308–15.

Slocum, D.B. & James, S.L. (1969) Classification of running gait. In *American Academy of Orthopedic Surgeons Symposium of Sports Medicine*, pp. 105–10. CV Mosby, St Louis.

Stanitski, C.L. (1990) Repetitive stress and connective tissue. In J.A. Sullivan & W.A. Grana (ed) *The Pediatric Athlete*, pp. 203–10. American Academy of Orthopaedic Surgeons, Park Ridge, Illinois.

Wilson, F.C. (1990) The pathogenesis and treatment of ankle fractures. In W.B. Greene (ed) *American Academy of Orthopaedic Surgeons Instructional Course Lectures*, Vol. 39. CV Mosby, St Louis.

Yngve, D.A. (1990) Stress fractures in the pediatric athlete. In J.A. Sullivan & W.A. Grana (eds) *The Pediatric Athlete*, pp. 203–10. American Academy of Orthopaedic Surgeons, Park Ridge, Illinois.

Yngve, D.A. (1991) Evaluation and management of ankle joint problems in the runner. In W.A. Grana (ed) *Techniques in Orthopaedics: Runner's Injury*, Vol, 5. No. 3, pp. 30–40. Aspen Publishers, Frederick, Maryland.

Chapter 15

Chronic Ankle Injuries

JÓN KARLSSON AND EVA FAXÉN

Lateral sprains of the ankle are the most frequent injuries found during athletic activities. Early diagnosis, functional treatment and rehabilitation are the keys to prevention of chronic ligament insufficiency of the ankle joint. Acute ligament injuries can be divided into grades I, II and III, depending on the damge to the ligamentous and capsular structures and the degree of functional loss. The most vulnerable of the lateral ankle ligaments is the anterior talofibular ligament (ATFL) (Fig. 15.1), which is injured in two-thirds of all ankle ligament injuries, followed by a combined rupture of the ATFL and the calcaneofibular ligament (CFL) in a further 20% of patients. Isolated injuries to the CFL and the deltoid ligament on the medial side are infrequent. Prevention by either coordination training using balance boards or by external support can reduce the number of ligament injuries. Ankle tape and/or functional splinting, proficiently completed by the use of a Air-Stirrup® pneumatic splint are preferred by many athletes. There is hardly any place for primary surgical repair after acute ligament ruptures of the ankle.

The recommended treatment is a rehabilitation programme with functional treatment, i.e. active range-of-motion exercises, coordination training, peroneal strengthening and early weight-bearing. Satisfactory results are reported in 80–90% of athletes after functional treatment. About 10–20% of patients may develop chronic instability in spite of adequate primary treatment.

Ankle joint instability

Ankle joint instability has been defined as either mechanical instability (MI) or functional instability (FI). The MI refers to an objective measurement (e.g. standardized stress radiographs) while FI is an individual description of the athlete's subjective symptoms (e.g. repeated giving way often combined with pain). FI is the most common and serious residual disability after acute lateral ligament ruptures.

The anatomical, biomechanical and pathophysiological factors behind the development of FI are not exactly known, and these factors may vary between different patients. It is, however, clear that FI is a complex syndrome, where mechanical, neurological and muscular factors are at fault, either alone or in combination. The known factors are elongation of the ruptured ligaments, i.e. MI (Staples, 1975; Karlsson *et al.*, 1991a), proprioceptive deficit (Freeman, 1965a,b; Tropp, 1985; Konradsen & Ravn, 1990; Karlsson & Andréasson, 1992; Karlsson *et al.*, 1992), peroneal muscle weakness (Tropp, 1985) and subtalar instability (Zwipp & Tscherne, 1984; Harper, 1991; Schon *et al.*, 1991). Karlsson *et al.* (1991a) have shown a correlation between FI and MI using standardized stress radiographs.

Correlation between FI and isometric peroneal muscle weakness has been shown, using a Cybex II dynamometer (Tropp, 1985). The same author also showed a correlation between FI and decreased postural control, using stabilometric measurements, indicating a proprio-

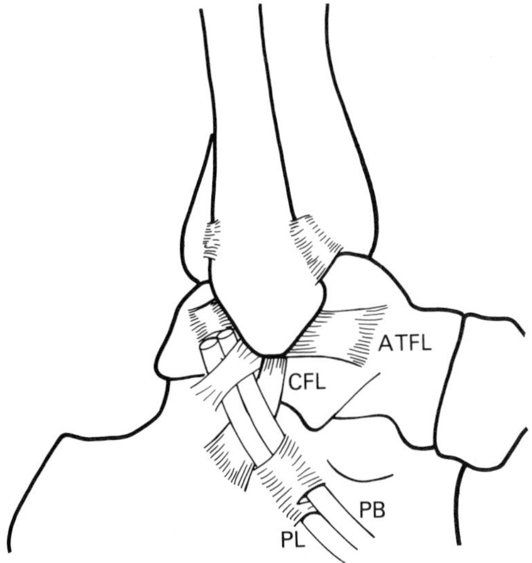

Fig. 15.1 Normal anatomy of the lateral aspect of the ankle. ATFL, anterior talofibular ligament; CFL, calcaneofibular ligament; PB, peroneus brevis tendon; PL, peroneus longus tendon. From Karlsson *et al.* (1989).

ceptive deficit after ligamentous injury. In the above mentioned study there was, however, no constant correlation between FI and MI.

Freeman (1965a,b) found that the majority of his patients had FI after acute ligament ruptures. He found that the proprioceptive deficit was the most important factor behind the development of FI and that MI was less important, and not alone a decisive factor in ankle joint function.

In an electromyograph (EMG) study on the proprioceptive system of the ankle joint, Karlsson and Andréasson (1992) found that the reaction time of the peroneal muscles was significantly slower in mechanically unstable ankles than in stable ones. The same phenomenon has been shown by Konradsen and Ravn (1990). This difference in the reaction time is due to the time that elapses from the start of the inversion movement of the ankle, i.e. start of the ankle sprain, until the mechanoreceptors in the ligaments and the joint capsule are stretched.

It can thus be concluded that FI is caused by a combination of MI and a proprioceptive deficit, i.e. increased reaction time, during quick inversion torque.

Chronic ligament instability

It has been shown that chronic lateral ankle joint instability will develop in 10–20% of patients after acute ligament rupture. This chronic ligament instability, irrespective of FI, MI or a combination of both does not always produce such severe disability that surgical reconstruction is needed. However, surgical reconstruction is often needed for athletes with high demands of stable ankle joints. More than 50 different surgical methods have been described to correct chronic ankle joint instability.

Clinical diagnosis

The diagnosis of chronic ankle joint instability is initially mainly based on a thorough clinical assessment. The clinical evaluation consists of testing the anterior drawer sign and the inversion (supination) test, always comparing results with the contralateral side. Increased anterior movement of the talus upon the tibia in the talocrural joint (positive anterior drawer sign) implies rupture and/or elongation of the anterior talofibular ligament (ATFL). Increased inversion indicates rupture and/or elongation of the calcaneofibular ligament (CFL), or, more commonly, a combination of ATFL and CFL insufficiency.

One must, however, always bear in mind that FI is a complex and composite syndrome where several factors, such as MI, proprioceptive deficit and peroneal muscle weakness, can be at fault, either alone or in combination. Subtalar instability has recently been shown to be one of the factors behind the development of FI (Harper, 1991; Schon *et al.*, 1991). A correlation between chronic ankle instability and prolonged peroneal reaction time has been shown, indicating that a proprioceptive deficit can, at least partly, be responsible for the ankle instability (Konradsen & Ravn, 1990; Karlsson & Andréasson, 1992; Karlsson *et al.*, 1992).

Radiographic diagnosis

Exact knowledge of the mechanical stability of the ankle joint in both the sagittal and the frontal planes gives valuable information in the diagnostic evaluation of chronic FI of the ankle. Roentgenographic measurements of ankle joint stability can be made before deciding upon the treatment of chronic FI. Contrast arthrography, double-contrast arthrography and tendography of the peroneal tendons can give concise information about the extent of ligament damage after acute ruptures, but are nowadays very little used (Broström, 1966; Balduini *et al.*, 1987).

Standardized roentgenographic measurements using stress radiographs should be used in differential diagnostic evaluation and therapeutic assessment. Two radiographic tests are used, the lateral instability test (talar tilt, TT) (Fig. 15.2) and the anterior instability test (anterior talar translation, ATT) (Fig. 15.3) (Lindstrand, 1976; Johansen, 1978; Karlsson, 1989; Karlsson *et al.*, 1991a).

Measurements of ATT and TT have been shown to be reliable with few false positive and negative results (Karlsson *et al.*, 1991a). MI can be defined in patients with unilateral instability as either (i) an ATT $\geq$ 10 mm and a TT $\geq 9°$; or (ii) a Δ ATT $\geq$ 3 mm (i.e. the difference in ATT between the functionally unstable ankle and the contralateral ankle) and/or Δ TT $\geq 3°$. A correlation between FI and MI has been shown (Karlsson *et al.*, 1991a). This correlation is, however, not constant as factors other than MI can also be responsible for the development of FI. Some studies have thus questioned the reliability of stress radiographs, especially the measurements of TT.

Recently, ultrasonography and magnetic resonance imaging (MRI) have been used to delineate injuries to the ankle ligaments. These methods are, however, still little used in clinical practice.

Treatment

NON-SURGICAL TREATMENT

Of all athletes that have sustained acute ligament injuries, probably less than 10% will need stabilizing surgery at a later stage. Before deciding upon surgical treatment in a patient with chronic ligament insufficiency, a well-planned rehabilitation programme based on peroneal muscle strengthening and coordination training should be carried through. Approximately 50% of patients with chronic FI of the ankle will regain satisfactory functional stability after 12 weeks on such a programme (Karlsson *et al.*, 1991b). The goal of the programme is to decrease the muscle weakness of the peroneal muscles, regain normal proprioceptive function around the ankle and to re-establish normal protective reflexes. Those patients most likely to need surgical reconstruction are those with very high-grade MI, measured using standardized stress radiographs.

The recommended rehabilitation programme for patients with chronic FI of the ankle is given in Table 15.1. The estimated rehabilitation time is 12 weeks. Balance and coordination training should be included during the estimated rehabilitation time (Fig. 15.4). The strength training should be both eccentric and concentric. The last weeks of the rehabilitation programme should concentrate on the sports activity (Fig. 15.5).

SURGICAL TREATMENT

Although a variety of different surgical procedures have been described to stabilize the unstable ankle, most of these are minor modifications of: (i) tenodeses; and (ii) anatomical reconstructions.

The most widely used surgical procedures during the past have been the many tenodeses described in the literature. All tenodeses sacrifice some normal tissue around the ankle joint, in most cases either the peroneus brevis or peroneus longus tendons, while some have

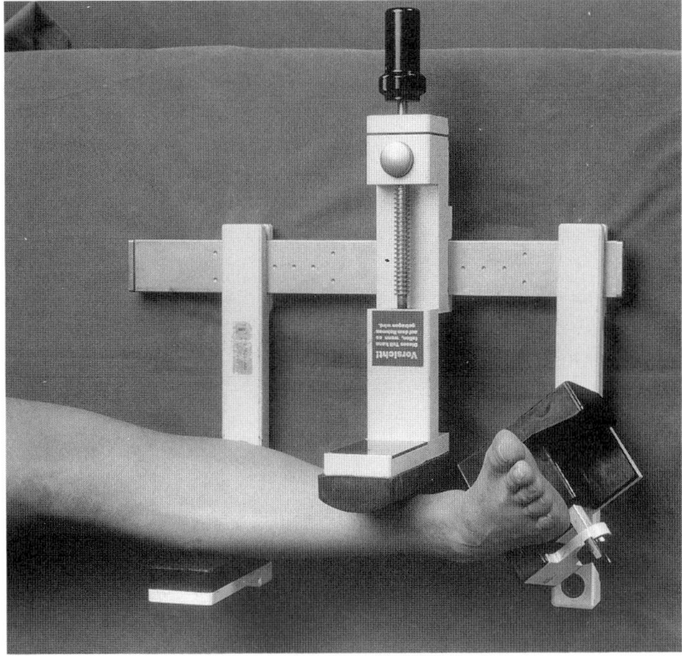

(a)

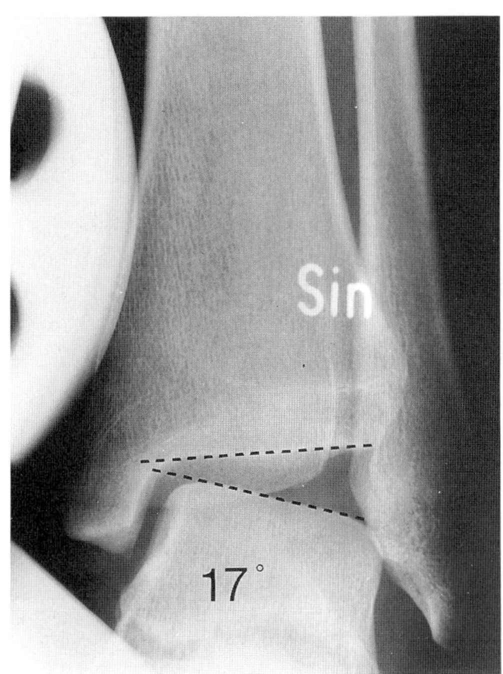

(b)

Fig. 15.2 (a) The talar tilt (TT) is measured with the ankle in 10° of internal rotation and a straight anteroposterior roentgenograph is taken after provocation force (150 N) is applied to the calcaneus for 30 s. (b) The TT is measured in degrees as the angle between the skeletal surfaces of the talus and the tibia after the provocation force has been applied. This figure shows an unstable ankle with a TT of 17°. The mean normal value is 3° (men), 4° (women) and the upper normal value is 9°. From Karlsson *et al.* (1989).

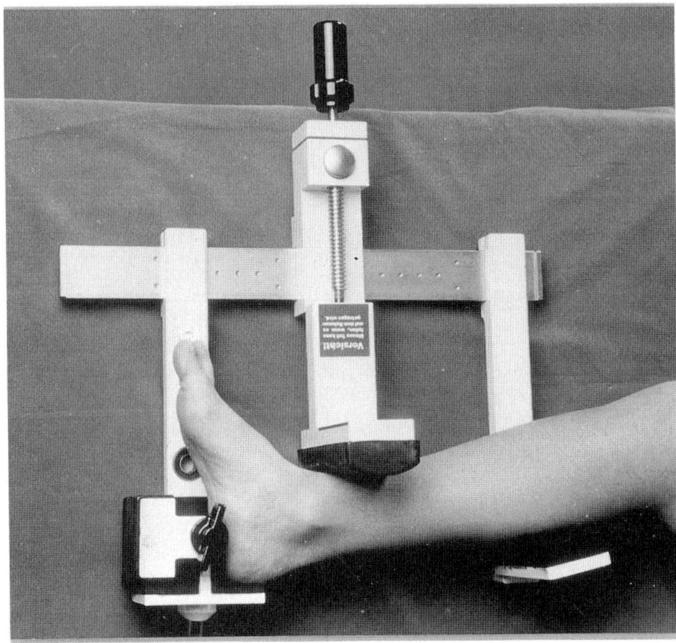

(a)

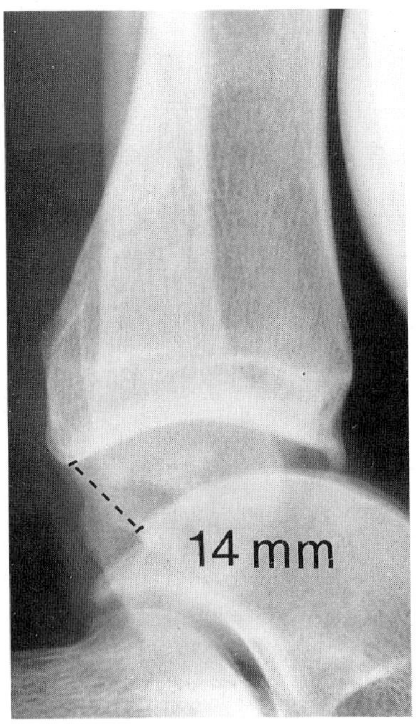

(b)

Fig. 15.3 (a) The anterior talar translation (ATT) is measured with the ankle in 10° of flexion. A horizontal provocation force of 150 N is applied just above the joint line for 30 s. (b) ATT is measured in millimetres as the shortest distance between the skeletal joint surfaces of the talus and the tibia in the posterior part of the ankle joint, after the provocation force has been applied. This figure shows an unstable ankle with an ATT of 14 mm. The mean normal value is 7 mm and the upper normal value is 10 mm. From Karlsson *et al.* (1989).

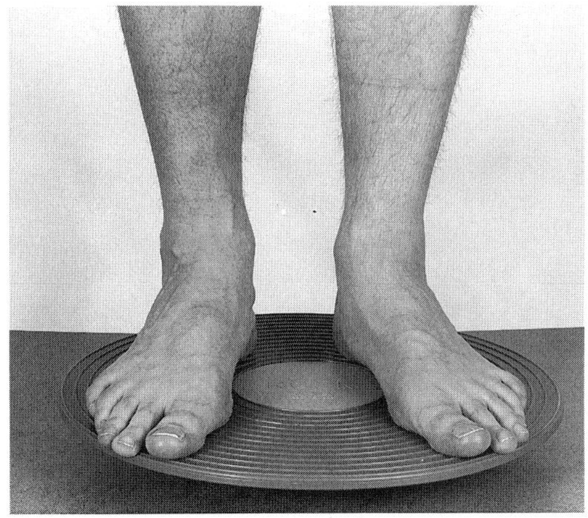

(a)

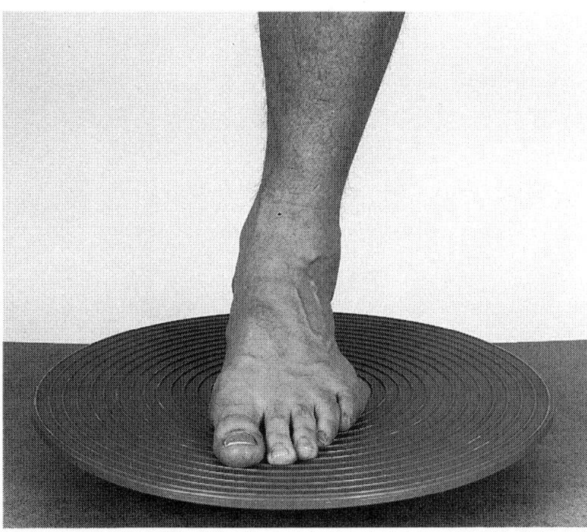

(b)

Fig. 15.4 (a) A balance board is used when training neuromuscular coordination. This training is started by balancing on both feet. (b) As the training progresses, balancing on the injured foot only is an essential part of the rehabilitation programme.

used the plantaris tendon, part of the Achilles tendon or even a free fascia lata graft. None of the tenodeses restore normal anatomy and they always result in altered kinematics and often in limited joint motion and stretching of the reconstructed ligaments, which might cause degenerative changes of the ankle in the long term.

The first report on the reconstruction of the lateral ankle ligaments for chronic lateral instability was made by Nilsonne (1932). He reported on a patient who was successfully treated using peroneus brevis reconstruction, with the transposition of the tendon into a subperiosteal groove behind the lateral malleolus.

The four classic tenodeses (Elmslie, Evans, Watson-Jones and Chrisman–Snook) are all well defined. The Elmslie procedure is, however, hardly used any more. The Evans tenodesis is technically the least demanding of these tenodeses to perform. However, the Evans tenodesis does not biomechanically reconstruct the ATFL or the CFL, but lies in a plane between these two ligaments (Fig. 15.6). Several authors have reported good short-term results after the Evans tenodesis and its modifications (Evans, 1953; Korkala *et al.*, 1991). Varying long-term results have, however, been found. Many patients with satisfactory early results have deteriorated after a few years, resulting in unsatisfactory function in the long run (Karlsson *et al.*, 1988a). Korkala *et al.* (1991) found satisfactory results after 9–12 years in four-fifths of their patients using a modified Evans reconstruction. These authors used the peroneus brevis tendon as a static reconstruction, i.e. a real tenodesis. Karlsson *et al.* (1988a) found less than 50% satisfactory results after a mean follow-up period of 14 years.

The much-used Watson-Jones tenodesis biomechanically reconstructs only the ATFL, not the CFL (Fig. 15.7). This means that patients with insufficiency of the CFL will not benefit from this procedure (Watson-Jones, 1952). Several good short-term results have been reported, but the only long-term follow-up study found in the literature by van der Rijt & Evans (1984) showed disappointing functional results in two-thirds of patients. Late deterioration was common and four-fifths were mechanically unstable when stress radiographs were evaluated.

The Chrisman–Snook tenodesis, which anatomically and biomechanically restores both the ATFL and the CFL, has on the other hand been shown to give satisfactory short- and long-

Table 15.1 Rehabilitation programme for patients with chronic functional instability of the ankle.

Week 1	
Range-of-motion exercises (flexion–extension) for increased blood circulation	3 × 20 repetitions 3 times·day^{-1}
Cycling	
Weeks 2–4	
Isometric contractions in flexion, extension and pronation	Hold the contraction 3 × 10 s; relax 2–6 s between each contraction
Foot exercises: Roll a small ball under the foot back and forth and side to side Wrinkle a towel Pick up marble balls or small rocks	3 min, 2 times·day^{-1}
'Closed-chain' (weight-bearing)	
Balance and coordination training: Toe raises bilaterally Walking on tiptoe alternately with ordinary walking Jog in place Jog on a soft mattress Walk along zig-zag lines, back and forth and from side to side Increase the training by varying the tempo and by turning from 90 to 180° Walk with a surgical tube around the ankle, back and forth and from side to side Stand on one leg Stand on one leg, flex and extend the knee Stand on one leg with the eyes closed for 40 s Increase the balance training by standing on a balance board, first on both feet and thereafter on one foot while flexing and extending the knee at the same time Stand on the balance board on one foot and roll a ball around the balance board with the other foot Use two or three balance boards and try to walk from one to another	3 × 20 repetitions
Endurance and strength training:	
Training with a surgical tube — flexion, extension and pronation	3 × 20 repetitions
Increase the training after a while by shortening the surgical tube	
Stretch gastrocnemius and soleus muscles with straight and flexed knee	2 × 15–20 s

Weeks 5–8	
Increased strength training:	2 × 20 repetitions
Toe raises on one leg	
Step-ups on a box back and forth and from side to side	
Step-ups using two boxes, 1 m apart	
Jog up and down with different steps in between the boxes	
Use a weight-shoe for heavy weight-training of flexion, extension and pronation	
Week 9	
Increased coordination training:	
Walk on uneven surfaces.	
Use different kinds of jumps	
Jog in intervals	
Train with a ball	
Weeks 10–12	
Add to the programme:	
Turnings while jogging	
Starts, stops and rushes	
Cone training	
Slope training	
Sports activity, individual and team training	

term results. Snook *et al.* (1985) reported satisfactory long-term stability in 94% of their patients. It utilizes only half of the peroneus brevis tendon, which leads to less reduction of strength on the lateral aspect of the ankle (Fig. 15.8). This is, however, a technically demanding procedure, primarily modified from the Elmslie tenodesis (Elmslie, 1934). Biomechanical studies with stress provocation have shown better mechanical stability after the Chrisman–Snook reconstruction than after the Evans reconstruction (Chrisman & Snook, 1969). Although this procedure is well defined and has been much used, some problems have been reported, the

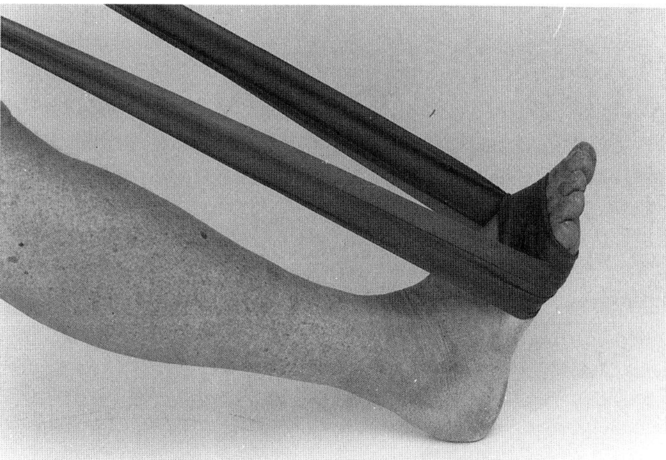

Fig. 15.5 Strength training using a rubber tube.

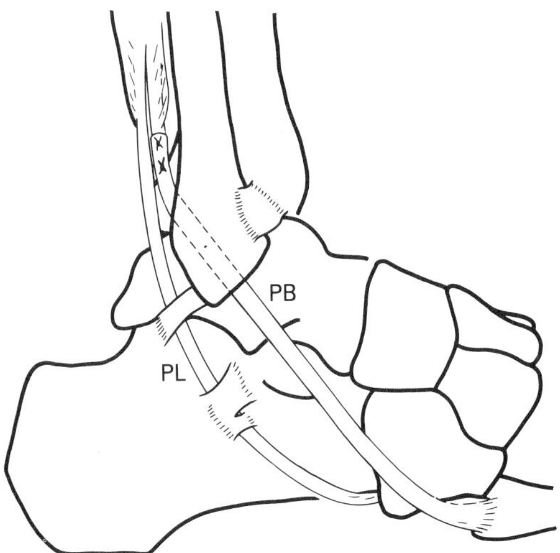

Fig. 15.6 The Evans procedure. The transferred peroneus brevis tendon (PB) lies in a plane between the anterior talofibular ligament and the calcaneofibular ligament. PL, peroneus longus tendon. From Karlsson *et al.* (1989).

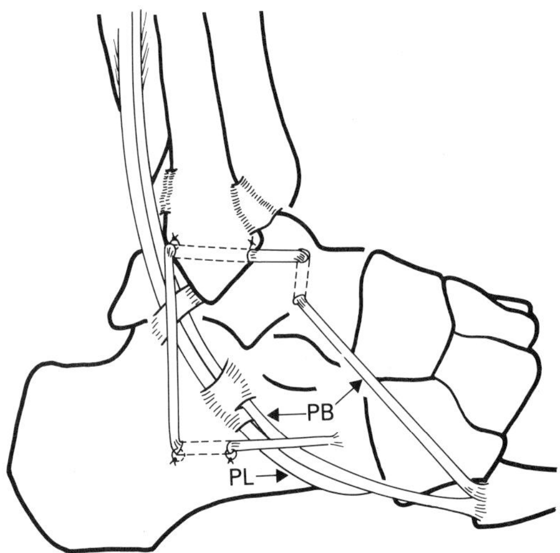

Fig. 15.8 The Chrisman–Snook procedure. Both the anterior talofibular ligament and the calcaneofibular ligament are reconstructed, utilizing only half of the peroneus brevis tendon (PB). PL, peroneus longus tendon. From Karlsson *et al.* (1989).

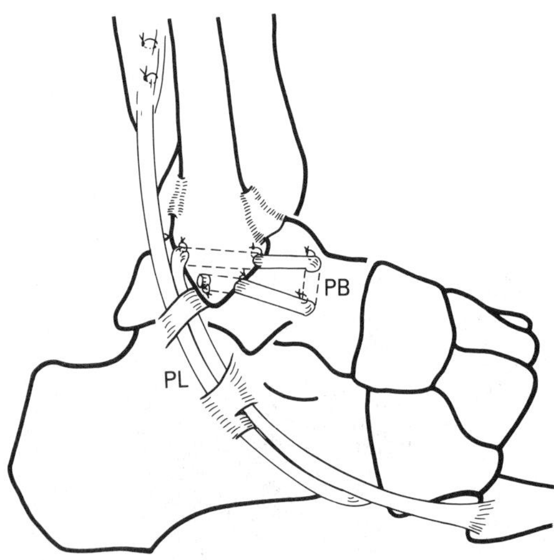

Fig. 15.7 The Watson-Jones procedure. The anterior talofibular ligament, but not the calcaneofibular ligament is reconstructed. PB, peroneus brevis tendon; PL, peroneus longus tendon. From Karlsson *et al.* (1989).

majority of which are related to the long skin incision for harvesting the peroneus brevis tendon. Problems with wound healing, skin sloughs and sural nerve injuries have been described. However, in light of the good functional results after the Chrisman–Snook reconstruction, this procedure is a good alternative to anatomical reconstruction, at least in patients where the latter cannot be performed.

The second method of stabilizing the unstable ankle is anatomical reconstruction, where the tissues of the damaged ligaments are used, thus permitting a reconstruction without sacrificing any normal tissue. Broström (1966) found that dissection of the ruptured and elongated ligamentous ends and direct suture was possible even several years after the primary injury. This is, in fact, the same principle shown by Stener (1962) in his study of inveterated ruptures of the ulnar collateral ligament of the thumb, where many of the ruptured ligament ends were preserved and could be repaired many years after the primary injury.

Several authors have reported satisfactory

functional results after anatomical reconstruction of the lateral ankle ligaments. The surgical technique described by Karlsson *et al.* (1988b, 1989) and Karlsson and Lansinger (1992) is simple and easily performed. The damaged and/or elongated remnants of the ATFL and CFL are transsected, shortened by several millimetres and imbricated. Satisfactory results have been found in approximately 90% of patients, with roentgenographic evidence of satisfactory mechanical stability. Less than satisfactory results were found in patients with generalized hypermobility of the joints, very long-standing ligamentous insufficiency (over 10 years) and in patients who had had previous ligament surgery to the ankle joint. Simultaneous reconstruction of both the ATFL and CFL is recommended, as this gives better results than reconstruction of the ATFL alone. After surgery, the ankle is immobilized in a plaster cast for 6 weeks, allowing weight-bearing (Figs 15.9–15.12).

This method of anatomical reconstruction has been found to be technically simple with very few complications, giving satisfactory functional results both in the short and the long term. Mechanical stability has also been shown to be satisfactory, correlating well with the functional results. It is therefore concluded that anatomical reconstruction should be the primary choice, rather than the more complex tenodeses, in most patients. A positive factor is that normal range of motion is easily regained during the post-operative rehabilitation period after anatomical reconstruction. A loss of motion, which is common after the various tenodeses, is a major drawback for the athlete who is in need of full functional range of motion of the ankle.

Several minor modifications of the anatomical reconstructions have been described. Sjölin *et al.* (1991) described a reinforced anatomical reconstruction, using a periosteal flap from the lateral aspect of the fibula, giving satisfactory short-term results in approximately 85% of patients.

A drawback of anatomical reconstructions is prolonged post-operative immobilization, with 6 weeks in plaster cast. Early controlled range-of-motion (flexion–extension) exercises, e.g. by the use of Air-Stirrup® (Fig. 15.13), can shorten the post-operative disability.

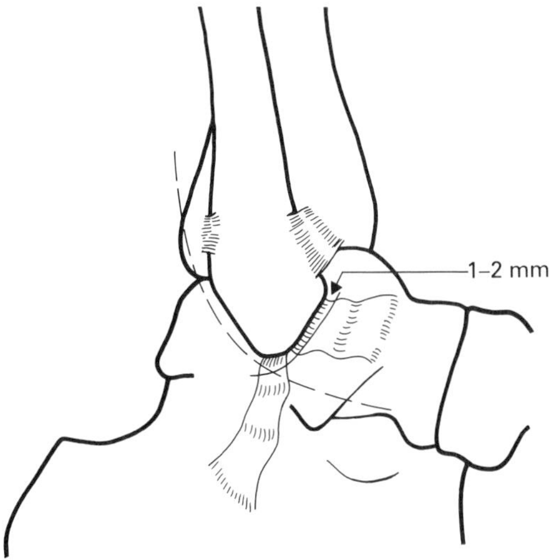

Fig. 15.9 Anatomical reconstruction. The skin incision can be placed either anterior or posterior to the lateral malleolus, but the posterior incision gives better access to the calcaneofibular ligament (CFL) and is therefore preferred. The elongated ligaments, as well as the joint capsule are divided approximately 1–2 mm from the anterior, inferior border of the fibula. Reconstruction of both the anterior talofibular ligament and the CFL is recommended. From Karlsson *et al.* (1989).

The use of fresh frozen allografts to reconstruct the lateral ankle ligaments has lately been reported to give satisfactory results (Horibe *et al.*, 1991). No immunological rejections or complaints of late instability were reported. As no normal tissues are sacrificed this procedure may be considered as an alternative to anatomical reconstructions, especially where the quality of the damaged ligaments is poor.

ARTHROSCOPIC LIGAMENT STABILIZATION

In selected cases, arthroscopic ligament stabil-

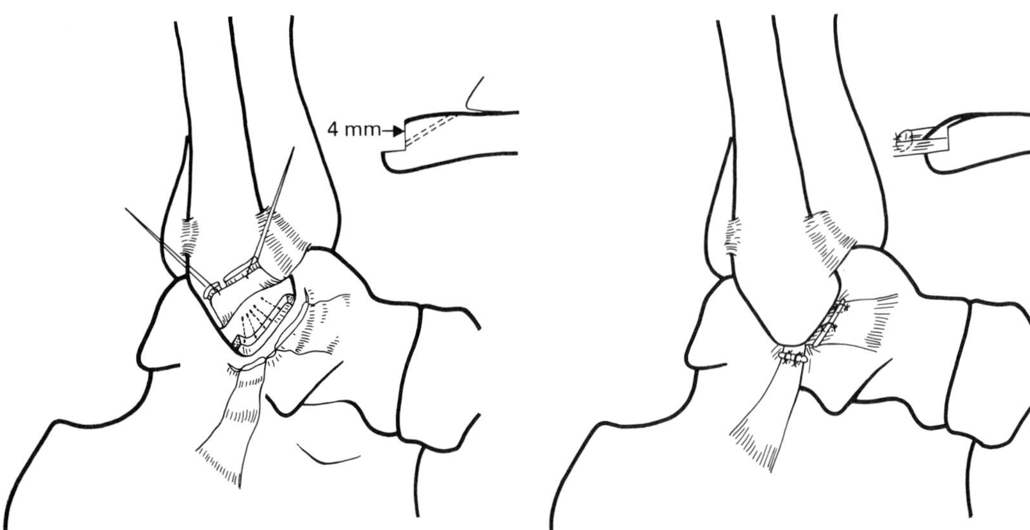

Fig. 15.10 A periosteal flap including the most proximal part of the damaged ligaments is elevated. Thereafter a small bone block, approximately 4 × 4 mm in size, is chiselled away from the anterior, inferior border of the fibula. Drill holes, using a 2.0 mm drill bit are made in the fibula. From Karlsson *et al.* (1989).

Fig. 15.12 The final step of the operation is duplication, using the periosteal flap and the proximal part of the ligaments. From Karlsson *et al.* (1989).

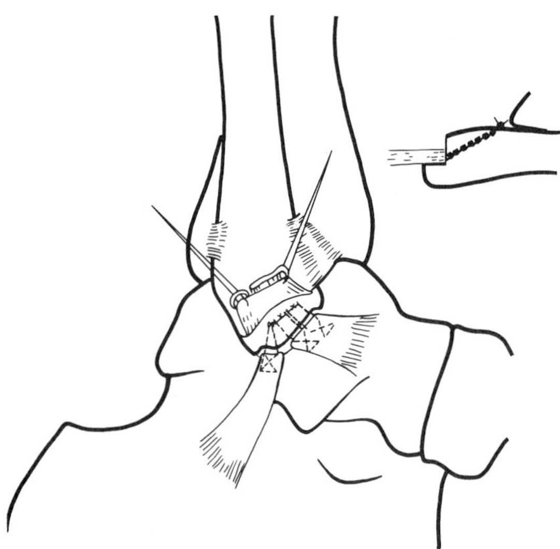

Fig. 15.11 The ligaments are now reconstructed by shortening; thereafter they are tightened. The sutures are drawn through the drill holes in the fibula and tied over bone bridges. From Karlsson *et al.* (1989).

ization may be a valid alternative to open reconstruction. The lateral aspect of the talus is abraded using a shaver. A small-calibre arthroscope is used. The ATFL is shortened and reinserted by the use of a percutaneous staple. Only a few reports on this technique are found in the literature. Hawkins (1987) reported satisfactory clinical results in 23 out of 24 patients after 2–5 years. A special indication for this technique is in children, to avoid damage to the growth plate of the fibula.

A possible drawback of arthroscopic stabilization is that it is only possible to reconstruct the ATFL using the technique. The arthroscopic technique for lateral ankle ligament stabilization is demanding and the procedure should be performed only by surgeons with experience of ankle arthroscopy. Future developments, especially with the development of biodegradable implants might make this procedure more versatile. Further studies are needed to define its role in stabilizing the unstable ankle.

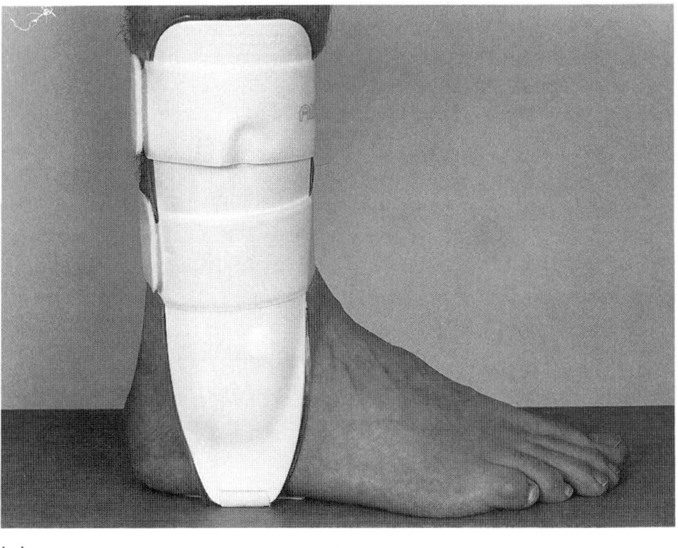

(a)

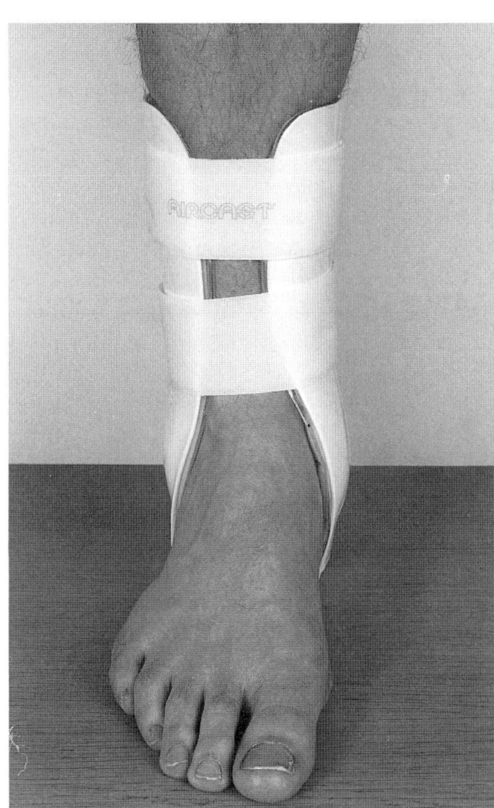

(b)

Fig. 15.13 The Air-Stirrup® can be used to prevent ankle injuries or as a part of the rehabilitation programme after ligament injury. There is an outer shell on each side and the inner lining air bags should be inflated as felt comfortable by the athlete. The two straps around the malleoli can be adjusted by the athlete. The Air-Stirrup® should always be worn over stockings. (a) Lateral view; (b) anterior view.

Prevention

Basically, there are two different methods for the prevention of ligament injuries of the ankle.

1 Coordination training using a balance board. This improves both postural control and functional stability. It has been shown that balance-board training can reduce the incidence of ankle ligament injuries among athletes with a history of previous injury, as well as in those with previously uninjured ankles (Tropp, 1985).

2 External ankle support. This theoretically provides better mechanical stability. Both ankle taping and semirigid braces are used to prevent ankle ligament injuries.

Ankle taping

One of the most commonly used methods of supporting the chronically unstable ankle is external support by the means of ankle tape. Many athletes use ankle tape either temporarily or permanently to deal with their ankle instability. Ankle tape is used directly after injury, during the rehabilitation phase after injury, and prophylactically to prevent the healthy or previously weakened ankle joint from further injury. The mechanisms behind the function of ankle tape is, however, not fully understood. There are three possible theories: (i) reduction of mechanical ankle instability; (ii) limitation of extremes of ankle motion; and (iii) shortening of the reaction time of the peroneal muscles by affecting the proprioceptive function of the ligaments and joint capsule around the ankle joint and the lower leg muscles.

Mechanical instability

The static mechanical instability in the sagittal plane (ATT) and the frontal plane (TT) has, in several studies, been shown to be decreased by the use of ankle tape (Vaes *et al.*, 1984, 1985; Karlsson, 1989). The instability in the frontal plane (TT) is controlled to a greater degree by ankle tape than the sagittal instability. A significant reduction of TT has been shown after ankle taping (Larsen, 1984; Vaes *et al.*, 1984, 1985). The support afforded by ankle tape is, however, generally insufficient to eliminate the TT completely. The greatest degree of protection (decreased MI) is found in ankles with the highest degree of MI. Karlsson and Andréasson (1992) found an insignificant reduction of mechanical ankle instability (both ATT and TT) with ankle tape using standardized stress radiographs.

Limitation of ankle motion

Although ankle tape does not normalize mechanical ankle instability, it significantly affects ankle motion. It has been shown that tape effectively limits the extreme ranges of ankle motion, i.e. partially increases the mechanical stability of the unstable ankle. In spite of the fact that tape becomes looser after exercise, the partial increase in mechanical stability by limiting the extremes of ankle motion is probably a significant factor behind the function of ankle tape.

Functional instability

Ankle tape also works by shortening the reaction time of the peroneus brevis and longus muscles by affecting the proprioceptive function of the ankle ligaments and joint capsule. Ankle tape has been found to have a stimulating effect on the peroneus brevis muscle in mechanically unstable ankles (significant increase of TT) measured with EMG and stop-action films (Glick *et al.*, 1976). The same authors found, however, no effect on the peroneus brevis function in ankles with an insignificant increase of TT. Karlsson and Andréasson (1992) showed a significantly slower reaction time of both peroneus longus and peroneus brevis muscles in mechanically unstable ankles, as compared to stable ones, using EMG measurements of the reaction time. The reaction time of the peroneal muscles was significantly shortened in unstable ankles with ankle tape, as compared to those without. However, these changes were only found in ankles with a significant degree of MI. The reaction time of the peroneal muscles in mechanically stable ankles was not shortened with ankle tape.

INDICATIONS AND USE

Ankle taping may be used in the following situations.

1 Prophylactically to prevent an uninjured ankle from ligament injury.

2 After injury, to prevent an injured or weakened ankle from further injury.

3 During the rehabilitation phase, to bridge the time gap between acute injury and full biological recovery. The tape can be used as a part of the rehabilitation programme. Reduction of the proprioceptive deficit gives increased functional stability.

4 In ankles with chronic ligament instability. Tape is used either temporarily or permanently instead of surgical stabilization of the ankle ligaments, or during a limited period of time before surgery is performed.

Ankle taping can also be used for the following injuries.

1 Lateral ligamentous injuries, i.e. ruptures or insufficiency of the ATFL and/or CFL.

2 Medial ligamentous injuries, i.e. deltoid ligament rupture or insufficiency.

Ankle taping is, however, not recommended after ruptures of the anterior ankle syndesmosis (anterior tibiofibular ligament) or ankle fractures.

Practical use

1 A thorough knowledge and understanding of the anatomy and biomechanics of the ankle joint is necessary. The extent of soft-tissue damage, especially ligament injuries, must be known exactly before a decision is made about the treatment.

2 The skin around the ankle joint should be thoroughly cleaned and shaved to reduce the risk of skin irritation and blisters. Sores and cuts must be protected.

3 Foam tape may be used as an underwrap to prevent skin breaking down. Use of foam tape also facilitates tape removal, but reduces support and stability.

4 Several anchors (1–4) are applied above the malleoli (Fig. 15.14a).

5 Stirrups (5–8) are combined with basketweaves (Fig. 15.14b).

6 The taping is completed with one or two heel-locks, circular anchors proximally and semicircular distally. The heel-lock can be applied both on the medial and the lateral side. When tape is applied on an uninjured ankle the heel-lock is not recommended (Fig. 15.15).

7 Continous taping should not be used as this usually results in unequal pressure on the skin and may impair bloodflow. The tape should be applied in strips, each strip overlapping the preceding one by about one-half to three-quarters and without gaps. The Achilles tendon should always be left without any tape.

8 Tape must never be applied over infected areas.

9 The tape should be removed directly after exercise.

ADVANTAGES AND DISADVANTAGES

Advantages

Tape is highly effective and functional. It partially increases the mechanical stability of the ankle and decreases the range of motion. It is easy to apply and to remove. Complications after the use of tape are few, and none are serious.

Disadvantages

The role of ankle tape is not scientifically proven. Some athletes complain of blisters and/or allergic reactions after the use of tape. The tape loses at least a part of its stabilizing effect after a short period of exercise. The cost is rather high.

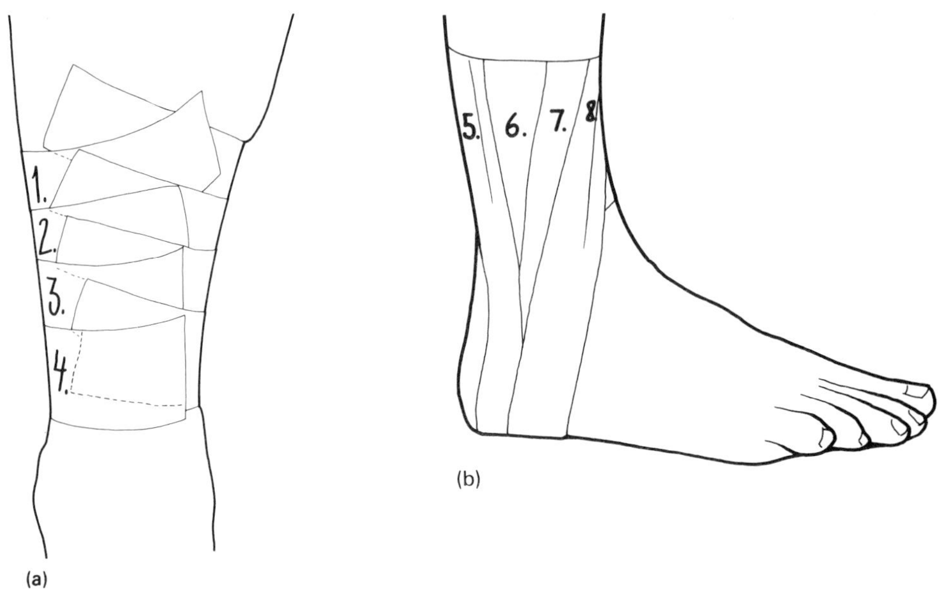

Fig. 15.14 Ankle taping using inelastic tape. (a) Four anchors (1–4) are placed around the lower part of the leg just above the joint line. (b) Four stirrups (5–8) are used to support the lateral aspect of the ankle.

WHY USE ANKLE TAPE?

Ankle support, particularly ankle taping, has been readily adopted by athletes to prevent and treat injuries around the ankle joint. An accurate assessment of the extent of the ankle injury is required before ankle tape is used and it must always be borne in mind that ankle

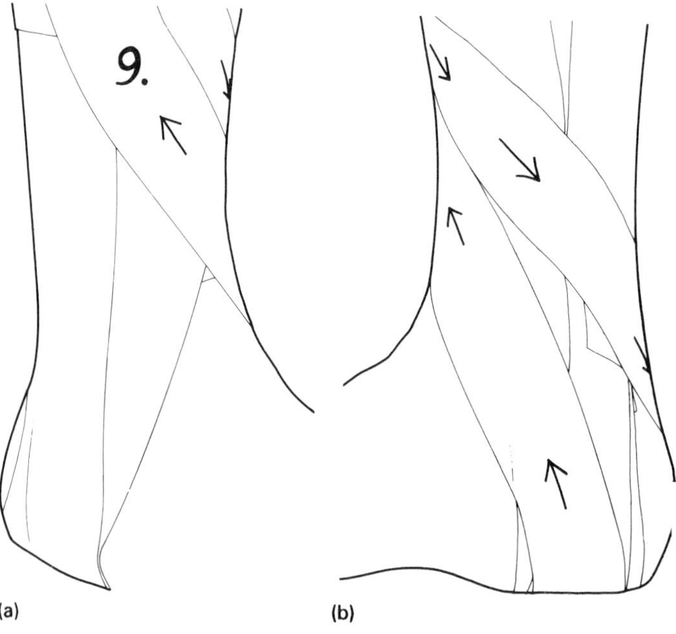

Fig. 15.15 (a) The heel-lock (9) viewed from the lateral side of the ankle. (b) The heel-lock viewed from the medial side of the ankle.

tape is only a substitute for normal soft-tissue function and stability. Tape is most effective in supporting and protecting soft tissues that have been weakened as a result of acute injury or chronic ligamentous insufficiency.

Ankle tape should be used in parallel with a rehabilitation programme, aimed at reduction of inflammation and restoring the normal range of motion, muscular strength and neuromuscular coordination — that is restoring normal functional stability of the ankle.

Several studies have shown that ankle tape is effective in the prevention of ankle ligament injuries (Garrick & Requa, 1973; Glick *et al.*, 1976; Fumich *et al.*, 1981; Larsen, 1984; Tropp, 1985). Prophylactic ankle taping is, however, no more effective than coordination training of the ankle (Tropp, 1985). Freeman *et al.* (1965) have shown that proprioceptive training of the ankle results in increased functional stability and resolution of the de-afferentiation of the ankle receptors.

Although tape is used to a large extent to prevent ankle injuries, it is mostly used as a part of the early rehabilitation programme after acute ligamentous injuries. Ankle tape is also helpful in the prevention of further injuries in athletes who have had previous ankle injuries (Garrick & Requa, 1973).

An obvious drawback in the use of ankle taping is the loss of mechanical support after a short period of exercise, leaving the ankle only partially protected. Rarick *et al.* (1962) showed that approximately 40% of the net supporting mechanical strength was lost after only 10 min of exercise. This is in line with the results of Larsen (1984), who found that after exercise most of the adhesive bandages were loose, the tapes mostly acting as canvas boots. Another drawback is the rather high cost, at least if the tape is used to prevent previously healthy ankles from injury.

Different methods of ankle taping have been described. The inelastic tape is preferred by most athletes and athletic trainers. Four conventional ways of taping are: (i) basketweave; (ii) basketweave and stirrup; (iii) basketweave and heel-lock; and (iv) basketweave with a combination of stirrup and heel-lock. The basketweave combined with a stirrup and heel-lock has been found to the most effective, providing the best mechanical support.

Alternative methods, such as rigid or semi-rigid ankle braces, some of which give good mechanical support, are often cumbersome and are probably little used by athletes.

The most effective and functional alternative to ankle tape is the Air-Stirrup® (Stover, 1980). This is a non-rigid prefabricated shell with an inner lining of air bags, that has been shown to provide protection and reduce the range of ankle motion and TT. The Air-Stirrup® has been used to help bridge the time gap between early tissue healing and full functional recovery (1–12 weeks after injury). It can also be used to treat stable ankle fractures.

In conclusion, ankle tape has been found to be highly effective in protecting the ankle joint from injuries as well as in the rehabilitation phase after acute ligament injuries. The best stabilizing effect is generally obtained in ankles with the highest degree of MI. After exercise, however, the tape is often loose, affording the ankle only limited protection. Tape is a simple and functional method to prevent and treat ligament injuries of the ankle. Whether tape is cost-effective is, however, unknown.

Subtalar instability

Subtalar instability has during the last few years become a better defined clinical entity. The ligamentous support of the subtalar joints consists of three layers, within the sinus tarsi and the canalis tarsi, as well as in the lateral aspect of the subtalar joints. Ligament insufficiency of the subtalar joints is now recognized as one of the important factors behind the development of chronic FI and it is probably more frequent than had been anticipated. The incidence of subtalar instability is, however, still unknown. The diagnostic methods are still not fully developed. There are only a few studies found in the literature on both diagnostic and therapeutic methods, or about the levels of disability associated with subtalar instability.

Chronic instability of the subtalar joints has been corrected either with anatomical reconstruction, where the superficial layer of the extensor retinaculum has been used (Harper, 1991), or by the use of a tenodesis (Schon *et al.*, 1991). The short-term results after both these methods are promising.

Anterior ankle pain

Chronic exertional pain on the anterior aspect of the ankle joint is often seen in athletes, e.g. soccer players and runners. In some cases this pain syndrome is found in combination with chronic instability of the ankle, but often there is only a mild form of MI. The athlete complains of anterior ankle pain during movement (especially extension or hyperextension) and a sense of impingement (locking and catching), i.e. a subjective feeling of FI.

Numerous pathological changes have been reported in patients with anterior ankle pain, such as intra-articular adhesions, meniscoid-type lesions, osteophytes and impingement exostoses (Biedert, 1991; Ferkel *et al.*, 1991; Stone & Guhl 1991). The meniscoid lesion is probably the most frequent of these changes.

Several recent reports have shown satisfactory results after arthroscopic resection of meniscoid lesions for the anterior ankle pain syndrome in the anterolateral gutter of the ankle joint (Stone & Guhl, 1991).

References

Balduini, F.C., Vegso, J.J., Torg, J.S. & Torg, E. (1987) Management and rehabilitation of ligamentous injuries of the ankle. *Sports Med.* **4**, 364–80.

Biedert, R. (1991) Anterior ankle pain in sports medicine: Aetiology and indications for arthroscopy. *Arch. Orth. Trauma Surg.* **110**, 293–7.

Broström, L. (1966) *Sprained ankles. A pathologic, arthrographic and clinical study.* Dissertation, Karolinska Institute, Stockholm.

Chrisman, O.D. & Snook, G.A. (1969) Reconstruction of lateral ligament tears of the ankle. An experimental study and clinical evaluation of seven patients treated by a new modification of the Elmslie procedure. *J. Bone Joint Surg.* **51A**, 904–12.

Elmslie, D.L. (1934) Recurrent subluxation of the ankle joint. *Ann. Surg.* **100**, 364–7.

Evans, D.L. (1953) Recurrent instability of the ankle. A method of surgical treatment. *Proc. Roy. Soc. Med.* **46**, 343–4.

Ferkel, R.D., Karzel, R.P., Del Pizzo, W., Friedman, M.J. & Fischer, S.C. (1991) Arthroscopic treatment of anterolateral impingement of the ankle. *Am. J. Sports Med.* **19**, 440–6.

Freeman, M.A.R. (1965a) Instability of the foot after injuries to the lateral ligament of the ankle. *J. Bone Joint Surg.* **47B**, 669–77.

Freeman, M.A.R. (1965b) Treatment of ruptures of the lateral ligament of the ankle. *J. Bone Joint Surg.* **47B**, 661–8.

Freeman, M.A.R., Dean, M.R.E. & Hanham, I.W.F. (1965) The etiology and prevention of functional instability of the foot. *J. Bone Joint Surg.* **47B**, 678–85.

Fumich, R.M., Ellison, A.E., Guerin, R.K. & Grace, P.D. (1981) The measured effect of taping on combined foot and ankle motion before and after exercise. *Am. J. Sports Med.* **9**, 165–70.

Garrick, J.G. & Requa, R.K. (1973) Role of external support in the prevention of ankle sprains. *Med. Sci. Sports* **5**, 200–3.

Glick, J.M., Gordon, R.B. & Nishimoto, D. (1976) The prevention and treatment of ankle injuries. *Am. J. Sports Med.* **4**, 136–41.

Harper, M.C. (1991) The lateral ligamentous support of the subtalar joint. *Foot Ankle* **11**, 354–8.

Hawkins, R.B. (1987) Arthroscopic stapling repair for chronic lateral instability. *Clin. Podiatr. Med. Surg.* **4**, 875–83.

Horibe, S., Shino, K., Taga, I., Inoue, M. & Ono, K. (1991) Reconstruction of lateral ligaments of the ankle with allogenic tendon grafts. *J. Bone Joint Surg.* **73B**, 802–5.

Johansen, A. (1978) Radiological diagnosis of lateral ligament lesion of the ankle. A comparison between talar tilt and anterior drawer sign. *Acta Orthop. Scand.* **49**, 295–301.

Karlsson, J. (1989) *Chronic lateral instability of the ankle joint. A clinical, radiological and experimental study.* Dissertation, Gothenburg University, Sweden.

Karlsson, J. & Andréasson, G.O. (1992) The effect of external ankle support in chronic lateral ankle joint instability. An electromyographic study. *Am. J. Sports Med.* **20**, 257–61.

Karlsson, J., Bergsten, T., Lansinger, O. & Peterson, L. (1988a) Lateral instability of the ankle treated by the Evans procedure. A long-term clinical and radiological follow-up. *J. Bone Joint Surg.* **70B**, 476–80.

Karlsson, J., Bergsten, T., Lansinger, O. & Peterson, L. (1988b) Reconstruction of the lateral ligaments of the ankle for chronic lateral instability. *J. Bone Joint Surg.* **70A**, 581–8.

Karlsson, J., Bergsten, T., Lansinger, O. & Peterson, L. (1989) Surgical treatment of chronic lateral instability of the ankle joint. A new procedure. *Am. J. Sports Med.* **17**, 268–74.

Karlsson, J., Bergsten, T., Peterson, L. & Zachrisson, B.E. (1991a) Radiographic evaluation of ankle joint stability. *Clin. J. Sports Med.* **1**, 166–75.

Karlsson, J. & Lansinger, O. (1992) Lateral instability of the ankle joint. *Clin. Orthop. Rel. Res.* **276**, 253–61.

Karlsson, J., Lansinger, O. & Faxén, E. (1991b) Conservative treatment of chronic lateral instability of the ankle (Summary in English). *Swedish Med. J.* **88**, 1404–6.

Karlsson, J., Peterson, L., Andréasson, G.O. & Högfors, C. (1992) The unstable ankle: A combined EMG and biomechanical modeling study. *Int. J. Sports Biomech.* **8**, 129–44.

Konradsen, L. & Ravn, J.B. (1990) Ankle instability caused by prolonged peroneal reaction time. *Acta Orthop. Scand.* **61**, 388–90.

Korkala, O., Tanskanen, P., Mäkijärvi, J., Sorvali, T., Ylikovski, M. & Haapala, J. (1991) Long-term results of the Evans procedure for lateral instability of the ankle. *J. Bone Joint Surg.* **73B**, 96–9.

Larsen, E. (1984) Taping the ankle for chronic instability. *Acta Orthop. Scand.* **55**, 551–3.

Lindstrand, A. (1976) *Lateral lesions in sprained ankles*. Dissertation, Lund University, Sweden.

Nilsonne, H. (1932) Making a new ligament in ankle sprain. *J. Bone Joint Surg.* **14**, 380–1.

Rarick, G.L., Bigley, G., Karst, R. & Malina, R.M. (1962) The measurable support of the ankle joint by conventional methods of taping. *J. Bone Joint Surg.* **44A**, 1183–90.

Rijt, A.J. van der & Evans, G.A. (1984) The long-term results of Watson-Jones tenodesis. *J. Bone Joint Surg.* **66B**, 371–5.

Schon, L.C., Clanton, T.O. & Baxter, D.E. (1991) Reconstruction for subtalar instability: A review. *Foot Ankle* **11**, 319–25.

Sjölin, S.U., Dons-Jensen, H. & Simonsen, O. (1991) Reinforced anatomical reconstruction of the anterior talo-fibular ligament in chronic anterolateral instability using a periosteal flap. *Foot Ankle* **12**, 15–18.

Snook, G.A., Chrisman, O.D. & Wilson, T.C. (1985) Long-term results of the Chrisman–Snook operation for reconstruction of the lateral ligaments of the ankle. *J. Bone Joint Surg.* **67A**, 1–7.

Staples, O.S. (1975) Ruptures of the fibular collateral ligaments of the ankle. Result of study of immediate surgical treatment. *J. Bone Joint Surg.* **57A**, 101–7.

Stener, B. (1962) Displacement of the ruptured ulnar collateral ligament of the metacarpo-phalangeal joint of the thumb. A clinical and anatomical study. *J. Bone Joint Surg.* **44B**, 869–79.

Stone, J.W. & Guhl, J.F. (1991) Meniscoid lesions of the ankle. *Clin. Sports Med.* **10**, 661–76.

Stover, C.N. (1980) Air-Stirrup management of ankle injuries in the athlete. *Am. J. Sports Med.* **8**, 360–5.

Tropp, H. (1985) *Functional instability of the ankle joint*. Dissertation, Linköping University, Sweden.

Vaes, P., de Boeck, H., Handelberg, F. & Opdecam, P. (1984) Comparative radiological study of the influence of ankle bandages on ankle stability. *Acta Orthop. Belgique* **50**, 636–44.

Vaes, P., de Boeck, H., Handelberg, F. & Opdecam, P. (1985) Comparative radiologic study of the influence of ankle bandages on ankle stability. *Am. J. Sports Med.* **13**, 46–50.

Watson-Jones, R. (1952) Recurrent forward dislocation of the ankle joint. *J. Bone Joint Surg.* **34B**, 519.

Zwipp, H. & Tscherne, H. (1984) Zur Behandlung der chronischen Rotationsinstabilitet im hinteren unteren Sprunggelenk (On the treatment of chronic rotation instability of the ankle joint). *Unfallheilkunde* **87**, 196–200.

Chapter 16

Foot Injuries

DAVID F. MARTIN

Historically, the foot has been covered in sports by boots, cleats, skates or shoes, and has been easy for the sports medicine specialist to ignore. However, the foot is the contact point for the body and the playing surface. Running, jumping and cutting place great stresses on the foot, which are then distributed up the lower extremity through the leg, knee, thigh, hip, pelvis and, finally, the spine. The foot should be viewed as one part of many that must function as a load receiver and transmitter. During running, the forces applied to the foot approach three times body weight (Lillich & Baxter, 1986) and the foot strikes the ground 480–1200 times$\cdot$km^{-1} (800–2000 times$\cdot$mile^{-1}) (Brody, 1980). A firm understanding of the anatomy and function of the foot and the ability to recognize and correct injury mechanisms in the foot are critical to the sports medicine specialist.

Anatomy of the foot

The anatomy of the foot has evolved as it has changed from a grasping organ to one that allows ambulation with a bipedal gait — an athlete can stand, take off and land on one foot with good stability (Hamilton, 1985; Bordelon, 1989). To accommodate these motions, the bones of the foot function as a series of wedges that can lock and unlock, thereby allowing the foot to be supple on impact while becoming a rigid lever at toe-off.

The foot contains 26 bones (along with a variable number of sesamoids and accessory ossicles) that make up approximately 30 joints. Strong ligamentous and capsular attachments limit motion and contribute to stability. The foot is divided into the hindfoot, the midfoot and the forefoot (Fig. 16.1). The forefoot contains the five toes (five metatarsals, 14 phalanges), which can vary significantly in size and shape and thus contribute to biomechanical problems in some instances. The forefoot articulates with the midfoot at the tarsometatarsal joint of Lisfranc. The midfoot contains the navicular bone, the cuboid bone, and three cuneiform bones, and it articulates with the hindfoot at the midtarsal joint of Chopart. The hindfoot is made up of the talus and the calcaneus, and these two bones control the bulk of foot movement. Each portion of the foot has types of injuries related to its form and function. The metatarsals in the forefoot behave like other long bones; the midfoot is involved in avulsion injuries as the foot is forced to excesses in its range of motion and ligamentous injuries occur. The hindfoot is involved in compressive injuries as it works to absorb forces at heel strike (O'Donoghue, 1970).

The foot is controlled by two muscle systems, the extrinsic system and the intrinsic system (Hamilton, 1985). The extrinsic muscles are located in three compartments of the leg: (i) posterior, mainly plantar flexors and arch supporters; (ii) anterior, mainly dorsiflexors; and (iii) anterolateral mainly evertors and plantar flexors. These muscles function through

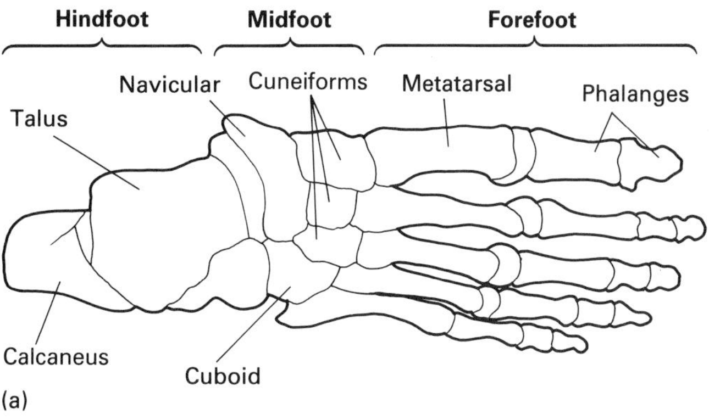

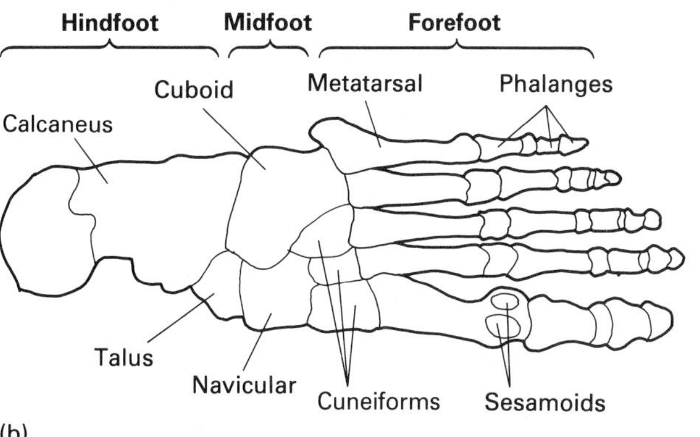

Fig. 16.1 Bony anatomy of the foot: (a) dorsal view; (b) plantar view.

tendons that cross the ankle joint and insert on the foot. These tendons are often injured in overuse injuries. The intrinsic muscles have their origins and insertions in the foot and are primarily concerned with fine motor toe functions (Peterson & Renström, 1986).

The bones of the foot form two arch systems: (i) the transverse arch; and (ii) the longitudinal arch. The transverse arch is formed by the metatarsal bones and the strong ligaments interconnecting them at their bases. This arch is present at rest, but it disappears as the metatarsal heads contact the ground when the foot is weight-bearing. The longitudinal arch (Fig. 16.2) runs from the calcaneus to the metatarsal heads and is supported intrinsically by the plantar calcaneonavicular ligament (spring ligament) and the plantar fascia, which runs from the calcaneus to the proximal phalanges of the toes and acts as a bowstring (Hunter-Griffin, 1991). There is a windlass mechanism that acts to tighten the plantar fascia as the toes are dorsiflexed at toe-off (Fig. 16.3) (Nuber, 1988). The extrinsic support to the longitudinal arch comes from a dynamic sling under the foot formed by tendons of the anterior tibialis, posterior tibialis and peroneus longus muscles. Understanding how the arches are supported is important, because they come under heavy loads as the foot strikes the playing surface.

One other anatomical structure, which is often overlooked when considering the athletic foot, is the fat pad. While the skin overlying the dorsum of the foot and the ankle is only loosely connected to underlying fascia, the skin on the plantar aspect of the foot is firmly anchored to the plantar fascia (Hamilton, 1985). These anchors act to separate the subcutaneous fat into small compartments well suited for weight-bearing (Hunter-Griffin, 1991). The

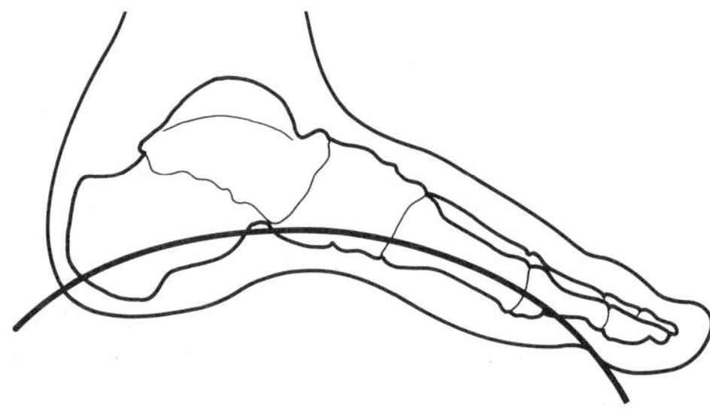

Supports of the longitudinal arch:

Medial	Lateral
Tibialis posterior	Peroneus longus
Flexor digitorium longus	Peroneus brevis
Flexor hallucis longus	Peroneus tertius
Tibialis anterior	Short plantar ligament (calcaneocuboid)
Plantar calcaneo-navicular ligament (spring)	Plantar fascia
Plantar fascia	

Fig. 16.2 The longitudinal arch of the foot.

compartments are larger to permit more shock absorption over the calcaneus and the metatarsal heads. If the vertical fibrous septae are broken down, either due to trauma or surgical incisions, the fat pad loses the ability to absorb forces and calcaneal or metatarsal problems can result (Hamilton, 1985).

Weight-bearing

Weight is distributed equally between the hindfoot and forefoot during stance. This is accomplished through muscle balance: complete muscle relaxation will lead to more weight being borne by the metatarsals (Hamilton, 1985). In normal stance, the 1st metatarsal bears twice the weight of the lateral four metatarsals. Small changes in muscle strength, tone, and coordination can have large effects on the way weight is distributed in the foot.

In evaluating foot injuries, one must also consider other forces: fore and aft shear, medial and lateral shear, and torque. At heel strike, shear is directed forward and medial. This progresses to rearward and lateral directed shear at the toe-off and can approach 20% of body weight (Nuber, 1988). Torque is internally directed at heel strike and this then changes to external torque as the foot flattens, and finally becomes zero at toe-off. The magnitude of these forces can increase up to 50% or more with

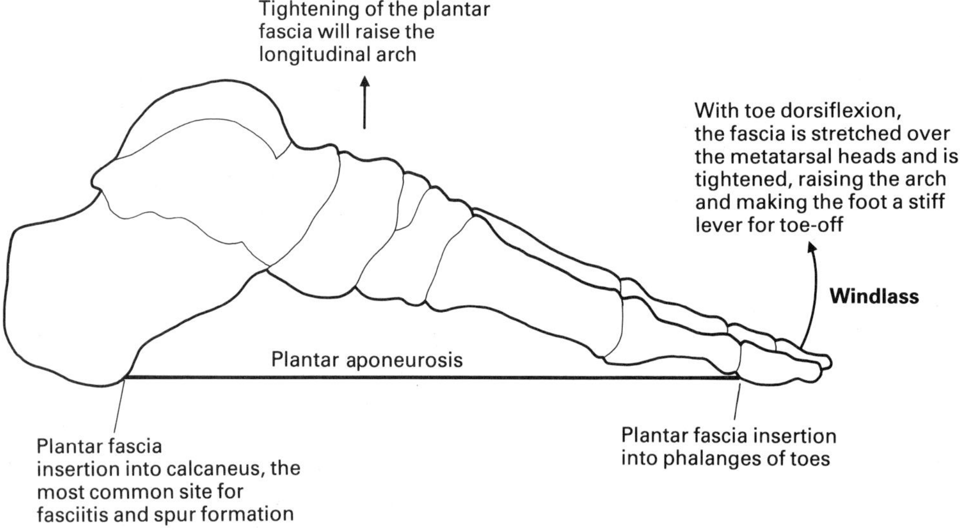

Fig. 16.3 The plantar fascia and the windlass mechanism.

running, cutting and jumping (Mattalino *et al.*, 1989).

Cavanagh (1987) has evaluated forces under the shoes of running athletes and found significant variability, depending on speed, individual and even right or left foot. The sports medicine specialist must therefore individualize therapy and orthotics after thoroughly evaluating an athlete during activity.

Biomechanics and gait

Motion of the foot occurs around two axes: (i) horizontally through the talus where plantar flexion and dorsiflexion of the ankle occur; and (ii) diagonally from the calcaneus forward and upward through the talus where pronation and supination occur (Peterson & Renström, 1986). Pronation and supination occur through the talonavicular and talocalcaneal joints. These subtalar joints are critical to the ability of the foot and ankle to function with the rest of the lower extremity (Mattalino *et al.*, 1989). Internal rotation of the leg leads to eversion of the calcaneus, which results in slight pronation and flattening of the arch at heel strike. External rotation of the leg leads to inversion of the calcaneus, which causes forefoot supination and stabilization of the transverse tarsal joint for stability at toe-off.

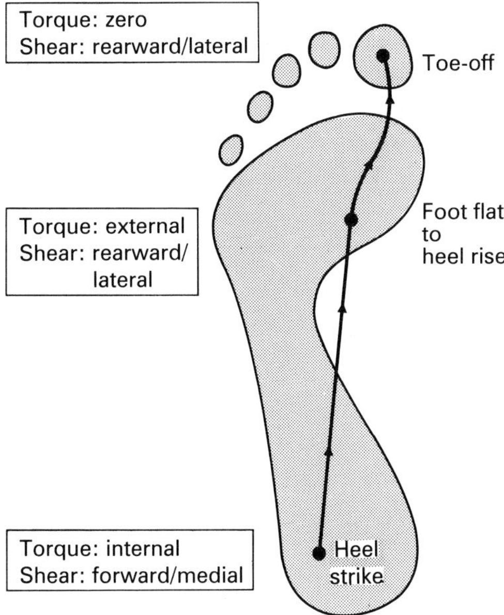

Fig. 16.4 The foot during gait. The load progresses from the lateral heel pad through the forefoot and finally to the great toe as the foot strikes and leaves the ground during gait. The torque between the foot and the ground also varies from internal to external and becomes neutral at toe-off.

The gait cycle (Fig. 16.4) starts with the foot in slight supination prior to the heel strike, which is generally just lateral to the centre of the heel fat pad. At heel strike, the foot pronates as the lower extremity rotates internally and the calcaneus everts — all of which allow the foot to absorb impact and be supple to adapt to the terrain. The foot is pronated for about half of the stance phase. As the longitudinal arch is loaded, the plantar fascia gradually tightens. Concomitantly, the lower extremity externally rotates at midstance and this everts the calcaneus, supinates the forefoot, and locks the transverse tarsal joint, all of which allow the foot to be a rigid lever for toe-off and effective propulsion of the body (Peterson & Renström, 1986; Cavanagh, 1987; Nuber, 1988; Mattalino *et al.*, 1989).

These relationships are dynamic ones; small changes in muscle strength, joint mechanics or foot conformation can alter the entire system. Symptoms and signs can be manifest in the foot, the leg, the thigh or even the lumbosacral spine. The way in which the athletic foot strikes the playing surface can be altered by footwear, orthotics and conditioning techniques; and by correcting aberrations, injuries can be avoided.

Injury risk factors

The foot in the athlete has a complex function — to absorb load from the ground, to bear the weight of the body and, perhaps most importantly, to act as a 'universal' joint to convert the power from thigh–leg musculature into effective locomotion. Locomotion is not enough, however, since most athletic activities require jumping, cutting, acceleration and deceleration. During these activities, numerous risk factors result in abnormal or overload forces and lead to injury. These can be intrinsic (anatomical or biomechanical factors) or extrinsic (shoes, surfaces, training regimens).

Intrinsic factors

Variations in foot anatomy are common; when the variation is significant or the stresses placed on the foot are extraordinary, injury can result.

A flat foot deformity is one in which the foot is held in an excessively pronated position and the heel is generally held in valgus. These are classified as either flexible or rigid and can be due to posterior tibial tendon insufficiency, accessory navicular bones, tight gastrocnemius musculature, genu varum or tarsal coalition (Morgan & Crawford, 1986). The position of pronation causes increased internal rotation of the tibia throughout the stance phase and results in higher loads being placed on the foot, ankle and entire lower extremity. Problems can be seen in the posterior tibialis, the plantar fascia, the forefoot, and additionally, the knee and hip (Lillich & Baxter, 1986; Peterson & Renström, 1986).

A cavus foot, or high arch deformity, is often fixed with limited subtalar motion. Tight calf muscles, varus heel deformity, and clawing of the toes are commonly seen in association with a cavus foot. This deformity decreases the plantar weight-bearing surface and limits shock absorption at heel strike, leading to significant stress on the plantar fascia and the plantar foot pad. Calluses under the heel and metatarsal heads are common, and heel pain with fasciitis/tendinitis can develop quickly (Peterson & Renström, 1986; Hunter-Griffin, 1991).

The weight-bearing surface of the foot can be evaluated using Harris footprints — the foot is placed on an ink pad and then the athlete walks or runs on a foot mat where contact points can be evaluated (Fig. 16.5) (Alexander *et al.*, 1990; Forriol & Pascual, 1990). In addition, the timing and extent of foot position during running and jumping is important, as this can lead to abnormal stresses (Brody, 1980).

Other intrinsic factors that can predispose to injury include forefoot varus or valgus, hallux valgus, Morton's foot (shortened first ray), interdigital cysts and various forms of capsulitis (Lillich & Baxter, 1986). Pads, shoe modifications and orthoses can be used to correct these anatomical abnormalities and avoid the biomechanical imbalances that place undue stresses on the foot and often lead to overuse injury. Proper flexibility and strength balance are also extremely important (Herring & Nelson, 1987).

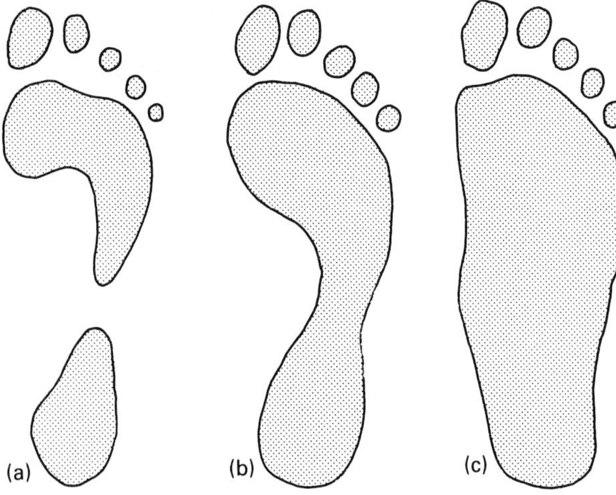

Fig. 16.5 Sample Harris footprints: (a) cavus (high arch) foot; (b) normal foot; (c) planus (flat) foot.

Extrinsic factors

The most important covering of the foot is the shoe. But, in addition to covering the foot, athletic footwear can add support to the foot and ankle and alter mechanics to change foot function (Bordelon, 1989). While footwear for runners has advanced significantly, shoes in other sports have not been as modified and the shoe itself can apply injurious loads to the foot or lack appropriate padding to protect the foot. Obviously, fit and appropriate sock wear are extremely important also, and often are overlooked as the cause of an injury.

The shoe interfaces with the playing surface. This can vary from grass or cinders, where some sliding occurs, to synthetic surfaces (all-weather tracks, artificial turfs, rubber mats), where the shoe–surface interface is more efficient, but friction and torque forces are much greater. In addition, while soft or loose surfaces can result in decreased shear and torque, a surface that is overly soft can allow the foot to absorb too much of the shock and sink more deeply, often leading to tendon and ligament problems (Lillich & Baxter, 1986; Peterson & Renström, 1986).

Uneven terrain, such as crowned roads, also can simulate leg length discrepancies in runners, while hills can lead to tendon imbalances. The sports medicine specialist must take into account the surface an athlete plays *and* practices on when evaluating or attempting to prevent injuries.

An athlete's training regimen is another extrinsic factor that must be evaluated, especially when considering overuse injuries of the foot. Either excessively intense workouts or rapidly changing training regimens can lead to overuse syndromes such as plantar fasciitis, posterior tibial tendinitis or stress fractures. Improper technique, whether in form for runners or in take-off/landing motion for jumpers, can cause undue stresses in the forefoot or the hindfoot (Herring & Nilson, 1987). To avoid injury, technique must be stressed and when overuse does occur, substitute activities to keep the athlete conditioned while decreasing loads on the foot are extremely important.

Evaluation of the injured foot

History

The appropriate history when evaluating an athlete with a foot injury is often overlooked. Symptoms must be described carefully and specifically — those factors that cause worsening of or improvement in symptoms can be important in diagnosis, treatment and prevention. The precipitating events or training regimen, as well as the equipment, playing surfaces and weather conditions, are important. Timing of symptoms as related to gait and ground contact can give the sports medicine specialist clues to the anatomical origin of the problem.

Examination

The athlete with an injured foot must be examined thoroughly, with the entire lower extremity being evaluated in a systematic fashion. Systemic and anatomical abnormalities should be addressed as well as static foot conformation. In addition to anatomical variations in the foot, Achilles tendon tightness, hamstring tightness, genu varus, genu valgus, torsional deformities, leg length discrepancies, hyperlordosis and scoliosis can all contribute to athletic foot injuries (Mattalino *et al.*, 1989). In the foot itself, assessment should include palpation of bony and soft-tissue structures, range of motion testing, stability testing, neurovascular examination and evaluation of muscle strength and flexibility.

Biomechanical assessment

The assessment of foot, ankle and leg mechanics is important in both injury evaluation and prevention. Gait evaluation is easily accomplished in a standard clinical setting, as is evaluation of the athlete's footwear. The wear pattern can give important clues as to the forces being experienced by the injured foot. Pressure distribution can be evaluated with Harris ink footprints or with plain water and footprints on a dry surface (Peterson & Renström, 1986; Alexander *et al.*, 1990) (see Fig. 16.5). More detailed evaluation can be obtained with formal force plate testing and high-speed filming using a treadmill. These tests can often reveal dynamic biomechanical abnormalities that place the athlete's foot under increased pressure.

Radiographic examination

Evaluation of the injured foot should include full roentgenographic studies. Anteroposterior, lateral and oblique plain films of the foot are the minimum. Weight-bearing views are helpful. In addition, special views of the sesamoids and stress views can be important. Technetium bone scanning is an excellent screening examination for overuse and stress injuries.

Foot injuries

While injuries to the foot are much less glamorous and often receive less attention than knee or shoulder injuries, the injured foot can lead to significant disability. In a recent study of over 16000 sports injuries, over 15% were found to involve the foot. Hiking and walking, running, and all types of dance were the sports most commonly involved. Half of the foot injuries reported were overuse injuries (Garrick & Requa, 1988). Clearly, the foot is responsible for significant athletic disability, and with athlete and coach education, many of the overuse injuries can be prevented.

Specific injuries

PLANTAR FASCIITIS

The most common cause of heel pain in athletes is plantar fasciitis. Symptoms of pain, morning stiffness and limping are caused by inflammation resulting from chronic traction on the plantar fascia at its insertion of the calcaneus (Brody, 1980; Torg *et al.*, 1987). Bony spurs of the calcaneus can develop secondary to the traction, but it is most often microtearing and inflammation in the fascia that cause the symptoms and not the heel spur. In mild cases, pain is experienced only before and after workouts and with the first steps taken each morning. More severe cases cause symptoms with every step. Athletes are most tender over the medial aspect of the calcaneus and often exhibit tightness in the Achilles tendon. Treatment starts with heel pads, cups, activity modification, ice, massage and aggressive stretching. Anti-inflammatory medication, phonophoresis and iontophoresis may follow along with taping/strapping.

Corticosteroid injections can decrease inflammation and symptoms. Surgery is rarely necessary, but involves plantar fascia debridement/release and heel spur excision. The differential diagnosis must include plantar fascial arch sprain, tarsal tunnel syndrome, entrapment of the medial calcaneal nerve, retrocalcaneal bursitis, tendinitis of the Achilles insertion, and bruised heel pad. Tarsal coalition must be considered in the overpronated foot that develops plantar fasciitis — increased pronation being a common cause of plantar fasciitis (Kwong *et al.*, 1988).

STRESS FRACTURES

Stress fractures are a common overuse injury of the foot in the athlete and develop from repetitive, cyclical loading at forces lower than those that produce acute fractures (Ting *et al.*, 1988). Competitive, long-distance runners and walkers are at particular risk, as are athletes who suddenly increase the frequency and intensity of their workouts. Complaints centre around pain with activity, the pain being located directly over the involved bone. Point tenderness is the classic sign. Stress fractures can involve the calcaneus, the navicular and the metatarsal bones. If roentgenograms do not reveal a fracture (positive in approximately half of the cases), technetium bone scanning is the test of choice as stress fractures show intense uptake. Treatment involves rest and alternative activities for 6 weeks. If symptoms persist with weight-bearing, crutch walking and immobilization are considered. Certain fractures (the navicular and the 5th metatarsal) may require open reduction and internal fixation. Return to activity is allowed when symptoms resolve — prevention by proper training regimens and correction of biomechanical problems is the key.

FRACTURES AND DISLOCATIONS

Acute trauma to the athlete in collision sports or secondary to falls can lead to fractures or dislocations throughout the foot.

The calcaneus is at risk in falls from heights — the lumbosacral spine then should be evaluated because injuries often occur there in concert with calcaneus fractures. Significant swelling can result, so early elevation is important. With subtalar joint disruption, open reduction with internal fixation to maintain anatomical relationships is being performed more frequently. Because this is best performed early in the course of the injury, appropriate roentgenograms and referral are important in obtaining the best results in this often devastating injury.

Talus fractures occur mainly with twisting-type forces and are associated with problems of blood supply, which place the talus at risk for non-union of the fracture and avascular necrosis (with subsequent collapse). Early anatomical reduction and appropriate fixation/casting to maintain that reduction are critical. Prolonged non-weight-bearing is often necessary.

Metatarsal fractures can occur with twisting or direct trauma to the dorsum of the foot. Careful evaluation of alignment, especially in the lateral plane, is important to maintain good foot function following healing. Fixation is necessary occasionally, especially in fractures of the base of the 5th metatarsal. These often are avulsion injuries involving the peroneus brevis tendon, and healing can be difficult to obtain. Dancers commonly sustain a twisting, oblique fracture of the 5th metatarsal shaft, which can be treated with closed reduction and cast immobilization.

Dislocations occur most frequently at the tarsometatarsal joint, but can be seen at the talonavicular–calcaneocuboid joint or talocalcaneal joint as well, although more infrequently. Anatomical reduction is the treatment of choice, with fixation being used to stabilize the joints if necessary. Early motion is important to avoid stiffness and loss of flexibility, but proper foot conformation must be maintained. The tarsometatarsal joint (Lisfranc's joint) most often requires open treatment with fixation to obtain and maintain anatomical positioning.

HALLUX VALGUS/HALLUX RIGIDUS

The great toe has twice the weight-bearing responsibility of the other toes; therefore, abnormalities and problems at the important metatarsophalangeal joint are magnified. When the metatarsophalangeal joint has a valgus angle greater than 10°, this is called hallux valgus. Insufficiency of the arch, overpronation, muscle imbalance, joint capsule stretching and inappropriate footwear can all lead to hallux valgus. The deformity can lead to an inflamed subcutaneous bursa in the area, a painful bony exostosis, footwear problems and skin breakdown. Shoe modification, padding and strapping are the best initial treatment. Surgery is indicated for pain unresponsive to conservative therapy or for progressive deformity.

Hallux rigidus is characterized by tenderness over the great toe metatarsophalangeal joint and decreased motion, especially in dorsiflexion. This common injury results from repeated stress to this vulnerable joint and significant degenerative changes in the articular surfaces can result. Turf toe, often resulting from stress on artificial surfaces that stresses the joint capsule–ligamentous complex, can also cause symptoms in this area. Ice, elevation, taping and splinting, along with appropriate orthotic treatment, can relieve symptoms. Surgical joint debridement is sometimes necessary.

SESAMOID PROBLEMS

The sesamoid bones can cause symptoms in the athlete, most often due to inflammation (sesamoiditis) or a fracture, while chondromalacia, osteochondritis and stress fractures do occur. The sesamoids are contained in the tendinous insertions of the intrinsic muscles of the great toe, adding joint stability and increasing flexion power while enhancing shock absorption. Inflammation can occur secondary to overuse, acute trauma or biomechanical abnormalities (cavus foot, tight plantar fascia, limited ankle motion). Local tenderness and swelling with occasionally positive roentgenograms are the hallmarks of sesamoid disease. Technetium bone scanning can also be a useful diagnostic tool. Acute fractures should be casted; inflammatory problems are treated most effectively by footwear modification.

Conclusion

The sports medicine specialist should develop a good understanding of foot anatomy and biomechanics — the foot is the body's contact with the playing surface and is the main locomotor in athletics. By gaining insight into injury mechanisms and risks factors, the anatomical and biomechanical knowledge can be applied to prevent many disabling foot injuries.

References

Alexander, I.J., Chao, E.Y.S. & Johnson, K.A. (1990) The assessment of dynamic foot-to-ground contact forces and plantar pressure distribution: a review of the evolution of current techniques and clinical applications. *Foot Ankle* **11**, 152–67.

Bordelon, R.L. (1989) Orthotics, shoes, and braces. *Orthop. Clin. N. Am.* **20**(4), 751–7.

Brody, D.M. (1980) Running injuries: prevention and management. *Clin. Symp.* **32**(4), 1–36.

Cavanagh, P.R. (1987) The biomechanics of lower extremity action in distance running. *Foot Ankle* **7**, 197–217.

Forriol, F. & Pascual, J. (1990) Footprint analysis between three and seventeen years of age. *Foot Ankle* **11**, 101–4.

Garrick, J.G. & Requa, R.K. (1988) The epidemiology of foot and ankle injuries in sports. *Clin. Sports Med.* **7**(1), 29–36.

Hamilton, W.G. (1985) Surgical anatomy of the foot and ankle. *Clin. Symp.* **37**(3), 1–32.

Herring, S.A. & Nilson, K.L. (1987) Introduction to overuse injuries. *Clin. Sports Med.* **6**(2), 225–39.

Hunter-Griffin, L.Y. (1991) *Athletic Training and Sports Medicine*, pp. 425–40. American Academy of Orthopaedic Surgeons, Chicago.

Kwong, P.K., Kay, D., Voner, R.T. & White, M.W. (1988) Plantar fasciitis. Mechanics and pathomechanics of treatment. *Clin. Sports Med.* **7**(1), 119–26.

Lillich, J.S. & Baxter, D.E. (1986) Common forefoot problems in runners. *Foot Ankle* **7**, 145–51.

Mattalino, A.J., Deese Jr, J.M. & Campbell Jr, E.D. (1989) Office evaluation and treatment of lower extremity injuries in the runner. *Clin. Sports Med.* **8**(3), 461–75.

Morgan, R.C. & Crawford, A.H. (1986) Surgical management of tarsal coalition in adolescent athletes. *Foot Ankle* **7**(3), 183–93.

Nicholas, J.A. & Hershman, E.B. (1986) *The Lower Extremity and Spine in Sports Medicine*, pp. 271–600. CV Mosby, St Louis.

Nuber, G.W. (1988) Biomechanics of the foot and ankle during gait. *Clin. Sports Med.* **7**(1), 1–13.

O'Donoghue, D.H. (1970) *Treatment of Injuries to Athletes*. WB Saunders, Philadelphia.

Peterson, L. & Renström, P. (1986) *Sports Injuries: Their Prevention and Treatment*, pp. 353–75. Mosby–Year Book, St Louis.

Resch, S. & Stenstrom, A. (1990) The treatment of tarsometatarsal injuries. *Foot Ankle* **11**, 117–23.

Richardson, E.G. (1987) Injuries to the hallucal sesamoids in the athlete. *Foot Ankle* **7**, 229–44.

Rodgers, M.M. & Cavanagh P.R. (1989) Pressure distribution in Morton's foot structure. *Med. Sci. Sports Exerc.* **21**, 23–8.

Ting, A., King, W., Yocum, L. *et al.* (1988) Stress fractures of the tarsal navicular in long-distance runners. *Clin. Sports Med.* **7**(1), 89–102.

Torg, J.S., Pavlov, H. & Torg, E. (1987) Overuse injuries in sports: the foot. *Clin. Sports Med.* **6**(2), 291–320.

Further reading

Acker, J.H. & Drez Jr, D. (1986) Nonoperative treatment of stress fractures of the proximal shaft of the fifth metatarsal (Jones' fracture). *Foot Ankle* **7**, 152–5.

Adelaar, R.S. (1986) The practical biomechanics of running. *Am. J. Sports Med.* **14**, 497–500.

Ahstrom Jr, J.P. (1988) Spontaneous rupture of the plantar fascia. *Am. J. Sports Med.* **16**, 306–7.

Axe, M.J. & Ray, R.L. (1988) Orthotic treatment of sesamoid pain. *Am. J. Sports Med.* **16**, 411–16.

Clanton, T.O., Butler, J.E. & Eggert, A. (1986) Injuries to the metatarsophalangeal joints in athletes. *Foot Ankle* **7**, 162–76.

Hamilton, W.G. (1988) Foot and ankle injuries in dancers. *Clin. Sports Med.* **7**(1), 143–74.

Hughes, J., Kriss, S. & Klenerman, L. (1987) A clinician's view of foot pressure: a comparison of three different methods of measurement. *Foot Ankle* **7**, 277–84.

Jørgenson, U. (1985) Achillodynia and loss of heel pad shock absorbency. *Am. J. Sports Med.* **13**, 128–32.

Jørgenson, U. & Bojsen-Moller, F. (1989) Shock absorbency of factors in the shoe/heel interaction — with special focus on role of the heel pad. *Foot Ankle* **9**, 294–9.

Kaye, R.A. & Jahss, M.H. (1991) Tibialis posterior: A review of anatomy and biomechanics in relation to support of the medial longitudinal arch. *Foot Ankle* **11**, 244–7.

Kibler, W.B., Goldberg, C. & Chandler, T.J. (1991) Functional biomechanical deficits in running athletes with plantar fasciitis. *Am. J. Sports Med.* **19**, 66–71.

Leach, R.E., Seavey, M.S. & Salter, D.K. (1986) Results of surgery in athletes with plantar fasciitis. *Foot Ankle* **7**, 156–61.

McBryde Jr, A.M. (1991) Disorders of the ankle and foot. In W.A. Grana & A. Kabnah (eds) *Clinical Sports Medicine*, pp. 466–89. WB. Saunders, Philadelphia.

Mann, R.A. (1989) The great toe. *Orthop. Clin. N. Am.* **20**(4), 519–33.

Marshall, P. (1988) The rehabilitation of overuse foot injuries in athletes and dancers. *Clin. Sports Med.* **7**(1), 175–91.

Chapter 17

Dermatology Problems in Sport

WILMA F. BERGFELD AND DIRK M. ELSTON*

A commitment to athletics usually translates into long hours of practice and hard work. Athletes place great demands on their bodies. The skin, despite its marvellous resiliency, sometimes is overwhelmed by these demands. Some skin problems are unique to athletes — some are even unique to a particular sport. Athletes may also experience skin disorders common in the population at large. This chapter will consider the causes of skin disorders of the athlete, as well as the treatment and prevention of these disorders.

Skin disorders in the athlete may be the result of heredity, mechanical forces, environmental factors, allergy, infection, infestation and drugs taken to enhance athletic ability. An appreciation of each of these causes is necessary for accurate diagnosis, treatment and prevention.

Hereditary skin disorders

An hereditary skin disorder may prevent an individual from participating in sports. Often, however, such an individual will continue to participate, and may even excel in sports. Athletes with hereditary skin disease require special care. Particular concern must be directed toward the prevention of skin injury.

Atopic eczema

Atopic dermatitis is characterized by eczematous, itchy skin lesions (Fig. 17.1). Flexures are often involved. Those with atopic dermatitis often have dry, easily irritated skin. Heat and sweating may provoke bouts of intense pruritus. The eczematous skin is often colonized by *Staphylococcus aureus* (Leyden *et al.*, 1974; Hanifer *et al.*, 1986). These individuals may experience repeated episodes of pyoderma.

Obviously, those with severe atopic dermatitis are not likely to participate actively in sports. Milder cases of the disorder are common and do not preclude participation in sports. These individuals are more prone to develop skin problems when they exercise. Flare of eczematous skin lesions, maceration and pyoderma are of particular concern.

Topical corticosteroids remain the mainstay of treatment for atopic dermatitis. Hydrocortisone preparations are mild and generally well tolerated, but they may not be potent enough for many patients with eczema. Mid-strength corticosteroid preparations are more effective than hydrocortisone, and are less likely to produce unwanted side-effects than are the more potent fluorinated corticosteroids. A table of some commonly used mild and mid-strength corticosteroids is included in Table 17.1.

Extremely potent, fluorinated corticosteroids are sometimes needed to manage severe cases of eczema. Caution must be exercised if they are used: cutaneous atrophy and striae may

* The views and opinions expressed in this chapter are those of the authors and are not to be construed as official or reflecting those of the United States Army or the Department of Defense.

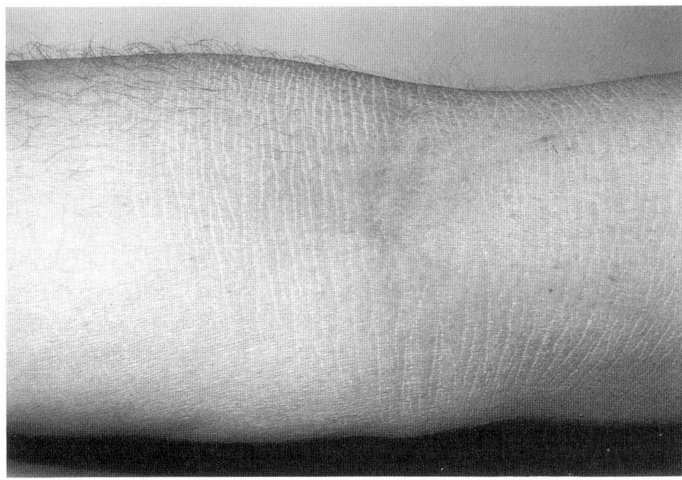

Fig. 17.1 Atopic eczema.

be the result of overuse. Atrophic skin is, of course, prone to mechanical injury, a particular problem in athletes. Overuse of potent topical corticosteroids may also result in cushingoid features and suppression of the adrenohypothalamopituitary axis. In general, the milder corticosteroid preparations are more suitable for long-term treatment. Skin care regimens including soap-free cleansers, skin hydration and emollients are helpful, and decrease the need for corticosteroids.

Secondary staphylococcal infections should be treated appropriately. Treatment of eczema with topical corticosteroids results in healing of eczema and restoration of the skin's normal barrier function. Intact skin is the body's best defence against *Staphylococcus aureus*. It has been demonstrated that treatment of eczematous skin with topical corticosteroids reduces bacterial counts of *Staphylococcus aureus* (Nilsson *et al.*, 1986). This reduces the risk of infection. A new topical antibiotic, mupirocin, may be helpful in some cases of pyoderma (Leyden, 1988). In selected cases, this topical antibiotic may be as effective as oral antibiotics.

Table 17.1 Some commonly used low to mid-strength topical corticosteroids.

Low-strength topical corticosteroids
Hydrocortisone preparations
(Cort-Dome, Hytone, Penecort, Synacort, etc.)
Mild to mid-strength, non-fluorinated corticosteroids
Alclometasone dipropionate (Aclovate)
Betamethasone valerate (Valisone, etc.)
Desonide (DesOwen, Tridesilon)
Hydrocortisone butyrate (Locoid)
Hydrocortisone valerate (Westcort)

Psoriasis

Psoriasis is a common skin condition in which hereditary appears to play a role (Krueger *et al.*, 1984). Psoriasis commonly localizes to sites of cutaneous injury (the Koebner phenomenon). Psoriatic skin lesions typically appear as erythematous papules or plaques covered by a thick, silvery scale (Fig. 17.2). Areas of the body, like the elbows and knees, which are prone to repeated trauma are common sites for psoriatic lesions. The skin of the feet may also be affected by psoriasis. Pustular and hyperkeratotic skin lesions commonly involve the soles. Nails may be thickened and dystrophic. A painful paronychia may accompany severe nail involvement.

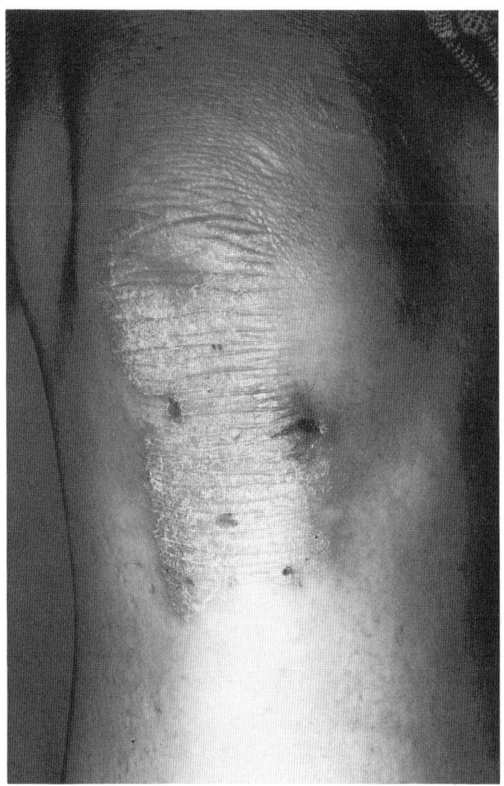

Fig. 17.2 Psoriasis.

Therapy for psoriasis includes the use of topical corticosteroid preparations as well as topical tar and anthralin preparations (Lowe *et al.*, 1984). Oral retinoids (Ellis & Voorhees, 1987), psoralens and ultraviolet A (PUVA) light (Gupta & Anderson, 1987), methotrexate (Roenigk *et al.*, 1988), Azulfidine (Gupta *et al.*, 1990) and cyclosporine (Page *et al.*, 1986) may be useful in more severe cases.

Properly fitted shoes are critical in order to avoid skin injury. Thick, psoriatic nails may predispose to soft-tissue trauma even in the best fitted of shoes. Markedly thickened nails, including those associated with paronychia, may respond to systemic treatments for psoriasis. Psoriatic nails may also be mechanically 'ground down' or chemically dissolved with urea paste. These interventions can help to minimize adjacent soft-tissue trauma.

Lichen planus

Lichen planus is another chronic skin disease which appears to have a genetic component. Characteristic lesions are intensely pruritic, flat-topped, violaceous papules (Fig. 17.3). Flexural surfaces of the wrist and ankle are typically involved. Nails may be involved, with thinning, grooving, splitting or even complete destruction of the nail plate. Treatment of lichen planus generally involves the use of topical and systemic corticosteroids. PUVA (Gonzalez *et al.*, 1984) and antimalarials (Mostofa, 1989) have been used.

Like psoriasis, lichen planus characteristically localizes to areas of trauma. Management must include minimizing further trauma. Protective clothing and properly fitted footwear are essential. Preservation of fingernails and

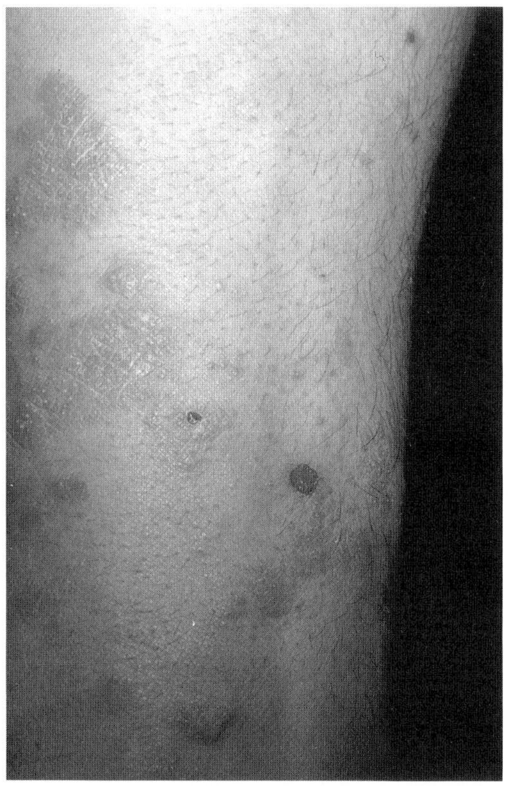

Fig. 17.3 Lichen planus.

toenails by prompt treatment of inflammatory lesions is of critical importance, as loss of nails may result in permanent disability.

Mechanical skin injury

Friction blisters

Friction blisters are common in athletes, and may result in significant disability. A friction blister occurs when the skin is subjected to repeated, rapidly alternating shearing forces. Necrosis of the epidermis occurs below the upper cornified layer (Fitzpatrick, 1987); interstitial fluid gradually fills the resulting cavity. Friction blisters may be large, tense and painful. Secondary infection may cause further disability.

Treatment of friction blisters may include the use of antibiotics to prevent secondary infection. Systemic antibiotics should be effective against *Staphylococcus aureus*. Topical antibiotics such as bacitracin and mupirocin may be helpful.

Tense blisters should be aspirated. The blister roof may be left in place as a natural dressing (Kennedy, 1992). Some synthetic wound dressings may also be helpful in the management of extensive friction blisters. Hydrocolloid dressings, such as Duoderm, are self-adhesive and serve as a physical barrier to further trauma. Hydrocolloid dressings promote rapid re-epithelialization and may reduce the rate of secondary infection (Metz *et al.*, 1985). Thin film, adhesive polyurethane dressings, such as OpSite, have also been used. Caution must be exercised when removing these dressings, as they have been known to strip the new epithelium from the wound. Gel dressings, such as Vigilon feel cool and comforting (Mandy, 1983). They may be refrigerated and used as cool compress and dressing in one. Gram-negative infection may be a problem with gel dressings (Metz *et al.*, 1985).

PREVENTION

Prevention of blisters is obviously the best form of management. Gloves serve as a barrier and absorb most shearing stress. Chalk is commonly used to reduce frictional forces. Proper fitting of footwear is the single most important step in preventing friction blisters of the feet.

Compound tincture of benzoin has been used by some military cadets with the intent of preventing blistering of the feet during training. This practice has been associated with allergic contact dermatitis to allergens in the tincture. An alternative preparation, Mastisol, may be less likely to produce sensitization. Once an individual is sensitized to compound tincture of benzoin, cross-reactions with Mastisol may occur (James *et al.*, 1984).

Friction-induced irritation

Chafing or irritation from repeated frictional forces applied across the skin most commonly involves the thighs and nipples. The result can be extremely debilitating. Chafing of the nipples, described under the name 'joggers nipples' (Levit, 1977) is common in men. Physical barriers, such as braziers, occlusive dressings or 'band-aids' help to prevent chafing. Powders to absorb sweat and reduce friction are useful to reduce thigh chafing. Acute inflammation responds to topical corticosteroids.

Calluses and lichenification

High-intensity frictional forces result in epithelial necrosis and blistering. Low-intensity forces result in epithelial thickening (acanthosis) and thickening of the stratum corneum (hyperkeratosis) (Kennedy, 1992). The result is a broad area of lichenification or a focal callus. This reactive skin thickening generally serves a protective function, serving as a cushion to absorb the shearing forces. Excessive thickening, however, may lead to discomfort. Soft-tissue injury may result from pressure transmitted through a thick callus. Lichenified skin may be pruritic. Scratching produces further lichenification, a vicious cycle referred to as lichen simplex chronicus.

As mentioned above, calluses generally represent a normal protective mechanism. Calluses which do not result in discomfort do not require treatment. Symptomatic calluses may be debrided with a blade or with chemical keratolytics (such as salicylic acid). Gentle debridement can be performed by soaking the callus, then filing it with an emery board or pumice stone (Kennedy, 1992). Recurrence of symptomatic calluses should be prevented. Gloves, chalk and proper fitting of footwear diminish the frictional forces responsible for callus formation.

Lichen simplex chronicus (chronic pruritic lichenification of skin, Fig. 17.4) responds to topical corticosteroids. Barriers that impede scratching and rubbing are also helpful.

Corns

A corn, or clavus, is a compact collection of keratin. Corns develop in areas subjected to extreme pressure. Pressure transmitted through the corn may produce discomfort. Debridement by a blade, chemical keratolytics or filing are effective treatments. The factors that produced the corn must then addressed: footwear must be fitted properly; underlying bony deformity may require surgical correction, ring pads (to distribute pressure) may be helpful (Kennedy, 1992).

Haemorrhage

Splinter nail haemorrhage, calcaneal petechiae (black heel, talon noir) and subungual haematomas are all common in athletes (Kennedy, 1992). These injuries result from shearing stresses applied to capillaries in the superficial dermis.

Splinter haemorrhages and calcaneal petechiae are asymptomatic. The striking black colour of the calcaneal petechiae may cause alarm: the patient may suspect melanoma because of the 'sudden appearance of a black spot'. Simple paring of the stratum corneum will remove the discoloration, and in the process, remove any suspicion that the lesion might represent a melanoma. Painful subungual haematomas should be evacuated. A hot cautery loop applied to the nail plate is effective.

Prevention of traumatic haemorrhage relies on reduction of shearing stress. Gloves, chalk and properly fitted footwear are helpful.

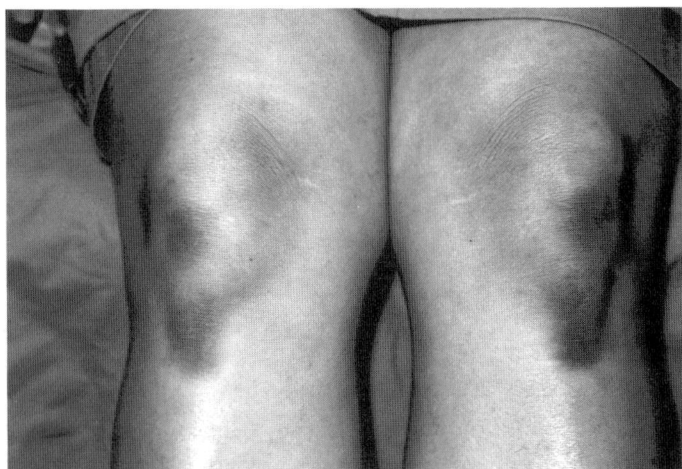

Fig. 17.4 Lichen simplex chronicus.

Piezogenic papules

Piezogenic papules of the feet (piezogenic pedal papules) are the result of pressure-induced fat herniation through defects in the dermis. The papules appear when weight is placed on the foot. They disappear when the foot is not bearing weight (Kennedy, 1992). The papules may be associated with discomfort. Obesity appears to be a predisposing factor.

Environmental skin injury

Maceration

Macerated skin is prone to injury. Maceration softens the protective stratum corneum and produces hydropic degeneration of skin cells. Socks should be changed frequently to avoid maceration. Hydrophobic ointments may be useful in preventing injury from intermittent immersion. Caution must be exercised, as hydrophobic ointments reduce transepidermal water loss and may promote maceration in hot, moist environments (Daniels, 1987).

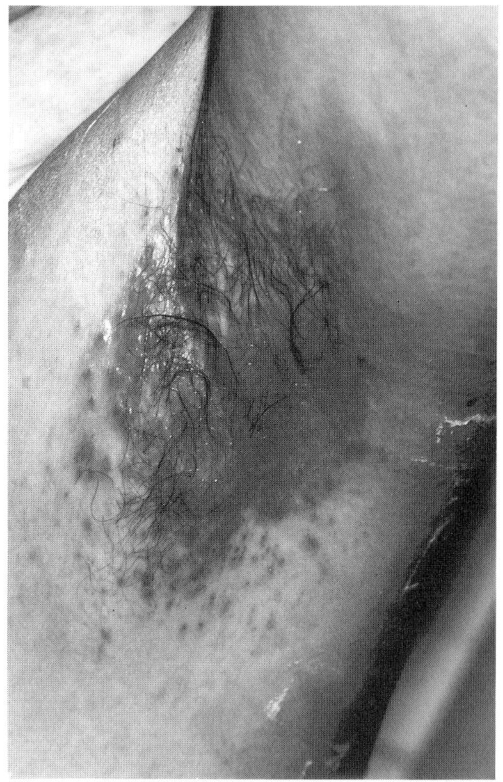

Fig. 17.5 Intertrigo.

Intertrigo

Heat, moisture and occlusion predispose to overgrowth of bacteria and yeast in intertriginous areas. Lesions of intertrigo are characteristically bright red, moist and tender (Fig. 17.5). Treatment of intertrigo includes the use of anti-inflammatory and antifungal agents. Antibacterial/antifungal agents such as phenol and resorcinol have been used in formulas such as Castellani's paint. Zinc oxide ointment has also been used. Weight loss and efforts to avoid maceration of intertriginous areas are helpful in preventing recurrences.

Pernio

Pernio (chilblain) occurs after prolonged exposure to a cold, damp environment. Symptoms of pruritus and burning are generally noted hours after the exposure. Lesions consist of cyanotic subcutaneous nodules. Warm dry clothing offers the best protection — wet shoes, socks or gloves should be changed immediately (Champion, 1992).

Frostbite

Exposure to extreme cold can result in frost bite (Daniels, 1987; Champion, 1992). Frostbite is the result of tissue freezing. It tends to occur on exposed, acral areas of the body. Degrees of frostbite have been described, similar to the classification of thermal burns. First-degree frostbite results in erythema and oedema. Second-degree injuries are characterized by vesicles and bullae. Third-degree frostbite involves the entire thickness of skin. Fourth-degree lesions involve the full thickness of the extremity, and generally become gangrenous.

Repeated freeze–thaw cycles increase tissue injury. The frostbitten area should not be rewarmed *en route* to a medical facility if it is likely to freeze again. Rapid rewarming in a warm water bath should be accomplished after the patient has been evacuated to a warm facility. Analgesia is necessary during and after the rewarming process. Debridement or amputation should not be performed until clear demarcation of the necrotic tissue has occurred.

Warm protective clothing is key to preventing frostbite. Acral areas of the body should be examined regularly for signs of freeze injury. Rapid rewarming is key in preventing progression of superficial freeze injury to frostbite.

Miliara

Miliaria (prickly heat) results from episodes of profuse sweating. The swollen, hydrated stratum corneum may occlude the distal seat duct. Hydrostatic pressure within the duct builds, and results in rupture. If the rupture occurs superficially, a crystalline-appearing accumulation of sweat occurs under the stratum corneum (miliaria crystallina). Deeper rupture of the intraepidermal duct results in red, pruritic papules (miliaria rubra). Very deep rupture of the dermal duct results in deep papular or pustular lesions (miliaria profunda). Widespread miliaria profunda may lead to tropical anhidrotic asthenia. In this condition, occlusion of sweat ducts leads to an inability to cool the body. The result is heat fatigue (Daniels, 1987).

Miliaria crystallina is asymptomatic and does not require treatment. Deeper forms of miliaria may respond to topical corticosteroids. Topical antipruritics, such as camphor and menthol lotion, may provide symptomatic relief.

Extremes of temperature, occlusive clothing, heavy packs (that exert pressure on the sweat duct opening) and possibly staphylococcal colonization of the sweat duct predispose to miliaria (Cage *et al.*, 1987). Prevention of miliaria involves avoidance of heavy, occlusive packs and clothing. Antistaphylococcal agents may be helpful.

Sunburn

Exposure to ultraviolet B (290–320 nm) is responsible for most sunburn reactions. Individuals taking photosensitizing drugs (such as psoralens, tetracycline, thiazides and sulfa) may experience sunburn-like reactions from ultraviolet A light (320–400 nm). Topical exposure to psoralens present in perfumes, limes, celery, and other plants can produce striking patterns of phototoxic sunburn-like reactions (Mitchell & Fisher, 1986). Window glass permits passage of UVA, while blocking UVB. Thus, window glass filtered light is incapable of causing common sunburn reactions, but phototoxic reactions to drugs and psoralens will still occur. At high altitudes, of couse, ultraviolet exposure is more intense.

Sunburn reactions are typically characterized by pain and redness, but in more severe cases, oedema and vesiculation may occur. Phototoxic psoralen reactions as sunburn-like streaks or patches, which typically heal with marked hyperpigmentation.

Prevention of sunburn involves avoidance of prolonged exposure to midday sun, white (reflective) clothing, broad-brimmed hats and the use of chemical sunscreens. Sun protection factor (SPF) is a measure of a sunscreens ability to filter out ultraviolet light in the UVB range. A sunscreen with an SPF value of 15 is recommended for all skin types. Most commercially available sunscreens are not very effective in UVA range. Photoplex is a relatively new sunscreen which has demonstrated efficacy in blocking both UVA and UVB light (Stanfield *et al.*, 1989). In cases of phototoxicity secondary to oral medication, a decision must be made as to whether the drug or sun exposure should be discontinued. Often an alternative, non-photosensitizing drug is available. Individuals who experience phototoxic reactions from topical psoralens must be educated about natural sources of psoralen exposure.

Allergic skin reactions

Allergic contact dermatitis to plants

Allergic contact dermatitis is common in athletes as well as in the population at large. Allergic dermatitis commonly results from contact with the *Rhus* (*toxicodendron*) group of plants (poison ivy, poison oak). These plants are common throughout North America, so those engaged in outdoor sports easily encounter the plants. Allergic plant dermatitis presents with streaks and patches of vesiculation, crusting, oozing and intense pruritus.

Treatment involves the use of topical and systemic corticosteroids. Cool compresses provide relief from itching. Burow's solution compresses are useful for oozing and crusted lesions. Sedating antihistamines, used mostly for their sedative effect, may be helpful at bedtime.

Prevention of allergic plant dermatitis is best accomplished by avoiding the offending plants. Poison ivy is easily recognized by its groupings of three shiny leaves. Topical application of polyamine salts of a linoleic acid dimer may be effective in preventing poison ivy dermatitis (Orchard *et al.*, 1986).

Shoe dermatitis

Rubber allergens contained in rubber adhesives and rubber box toes are the most common causes of shoe dermatitis (Storrs, 1986) (Fig. 17.6). Untreated natural rubber has little tendency to produce contact allergy. Unfortunately, untreated rubber is also inelastic and of limited commercial use. Vulcanization of rubber produces an elastic, resilient (and therefore commercially valuable) product. Rubber accelerators (which accelerate the process of vulcanization) and antioxidants (which prevent deterioration) are the major causes of contact dermatitis to rubber (Taylor, 1986). Two rubber accelerators in particular (mercaptobenzothiazole and tetramethylthiuram disulfide) are commonly implicated in rubber allergy (Storrs, 1986).

Symmetrical involvement of the dorsa of both feet is characteristic of allergic shoe dermatitis. The insteps and toe webspaces are generally spared (Storrs, 1986). This is in contrast to fungal infections of the feet which tend to involve these areas. It would be unusual for fungal infection to produce bilateral involvement of the dorsa of the feet. Allergic reactions to a rubber box toe generally involve the dorsa

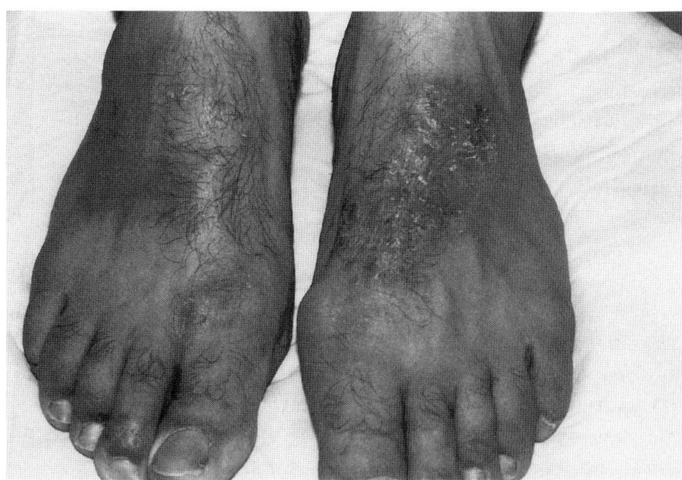

Fig. 17.6 Shoe dermatitis.

of the toes. Both allergic contact dermatitis and fungal infections occasionally cause blistering of the soles. In most cases, a potassium hydroxide (KOH) preparation of the blister roof easily differentiates the two. Fungal hyphae are generally abundant in blistering tinea.

Acute shoe dermatitis is treated with topical or systemic corticosteroids. Prevention, however, is the major therapeutic goal. Patch testing with rubber allergens will identify the offending agent. Shoes free of the allergen can then be purchased. Updated lists of shoe (Adams & Fisher, 1986) and glove (Rich *et al.*, 1991) alternatives for allergic patients appear periodically in the dermatology literature.

Nickel dermatitis

Nickel is ubiquitous in our environment. It is used on belt buckles, snaps, fasteners, chains, earrings, watches, eyeglass frames, coins, keys and whistles (Fisher, 1986). Gold-plated items are first coated with nickel — as the gold wears away, nickel is exposed. Contact dermatitis to nickel commonly occurs on earlobes, under watches and belt snaps, and on the hands. Identification tag chains may produce an eruption of the chest and neck. Occasionally, an eruption simulating Paget's disease of the breast may occur in women who place a coin or key case into a bra cup.

The key to prevention is identification of the allergen. After nickel allergy is confirmed by patch testing, the patient must be educated about sources of nickel. Stainless steel provides an acceptable, hypoallergenic, alternative. Items can be tested for nickel content with dimethylglyoxime test kits. The test is easy to perform and interpret (Fisher, 1986).

Infection

Skin abrasions and cuts, to which athletes are naturally prone, provide portals of entry for infectious agents. The close physical contact inherent to many sports provides further opportunities for transmission of infectious agents.

Bacterial infections

IMPETIGO

Impetigo may present as honey crusted or bullous skin lesions (Fig. 17.7). *Staphylococcus aureus* is responsible for bullous impetigo (Tunnessen, 1985; Swartz & Weinberg, 1987). *Staphylococcus aureus* and *Streptococcus pyogenes* may be involved in honey crusted lesions (Coskey & Coskey, 1987). Individuals with recurrent impetigo may harbour the responsible organisms in the nares. *Staphylococcus* carriers may serve as a source of infection for family members or team mates and are often responsible for outbreaks of food poisoning. Staphylococcal food poisoning often affects large numbers of people at one time, especially in dormitory or training table situations.

Impetigo responds to treatment with sys-

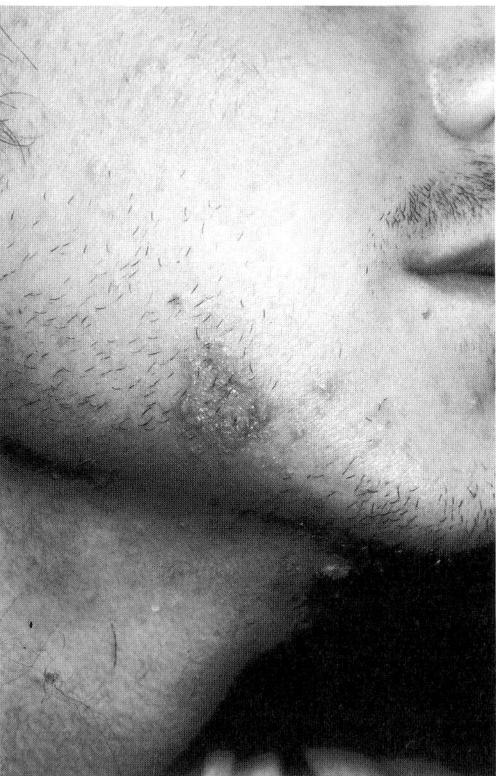

Fig. 17.7 Impetigo.

temic antibiotics. Semisynthetic penicillins, cephalosporins, and the combination of amoxicillin and clavulanic acid are generally effective. Erythromycin has been widely used for the treatment of impetigo. In some years, however, erythromycin-resistant strains of *Staphylococcus aureus* have become common (Feldman & Lynfield, 1987). The topical antibiotic, mupirocin, may be as effective as oral agents in the treatment of impetigo (Medical letter, 1988).

Prevention of impetigo includes efforts to minimize skin injury. Good hygiene is important. Treatment of chronic eczema with topical corticosteroids decreases bacterial counts of *Staphylococcus aureus* (Nilsson *et al.*, 1986). Treatment of *Staphylococcus* carriers has important public health implications, especially in cases of food poisoning. Individuals who have a nasal focus of staphylococcal carriage often respond to combination treatment with a semisynthetic penicillin and rifampin (Feingold & Wagner, 1986).

FOLLICULITIS

Staphylococcus aureus is the organism most commonly implicated in bacterial folliculitis. Lesions begin as erythematous follicular papules, which evolve into pustules. Deep abscess formation may occur. Patients with chronic eczema and nasal *Staphylococcus* carriers are prone to repeated bouts of folliculitis.

Hot tubs and swimming pools may harbour strains of *Pseudomonas aeruginosa*, especially types O-11. Pseudomonas folliculitis resulting from hot tub or swimming pool exposure has been termed 'hot tub dermatitis' (Silverman & Nieland, 1983). Hot tub folliculitis commonly presents with follicular papules and pustules in intertriginous areas and skin covered by the bathing suit.

Drainage is the treatment of choice for a solitary furuncle (Swartz & Weinberg, 1987). Widespread folliculitis responds to antibiotic treatment. Staphylococcal folliculitis responds to the same oral agents used to treat impetigo. Hot tub folliculitis may be self-limited. Oral ciprofloxin is effective.

Prevention of staphylococcal folliculitis includes treatment of chronic eczema (Nilsson *et al.*, 1986), eradication of nasal foci of staphylococcal carriage, and good general hygiene. Prevention of hot tub and swimming pool folliculitis centres on adequate treatment of the water to prevent overgrowth of organisms (Silverman & Nieland, 1983).

PITTED KERATOLYSIS

Pitted keratolysis presents as asymptomatic pitting of the stratum corneum. Generally the sole of the foot is involved. Gram-positive rods have been implicated as pathogens (Zaias, 1982). *Micrococcus sedentarius* may act independently or may act synergistically with Gram-positive rods to produce the disease (Nordstrom *et al.*, 1987). Topical antibiotics and antiperspirants have been effective in treating the disorder.

ERYTHRASMA

Erythrasma presents as reddish brown patches in intertriginous areas. The lesions demonstrate a characteristic coral red fluorescence when examined with midrange ultraviolet A light (a Wood's lamp). The infection is generally asymptomatic. Heat, humidity, obesity, diabetes mellitus and poor hygiene are predisposing factors (Somerville & Lancaster-Smith, 1973). *Corynebacterium minutissimum* is the causative agent (Sarkany *et al.*, 1961).

Erythrasma may respond to oral antibiotics. Topical antibiotics and drying agents have also been used (Swartz & Weinberg, 1987).

Viral infections

WARTS

Warts are a manifestation of skin infection with the human papilloma virus (HPV). Warts commonly occur on the hands, feet and knees (Fig. 17.8). Sites of minor trauma may be prone to inoculation with HPV. The incubation time until a wart becomes clinically evident may be in the order of months. Warts may be filiform,

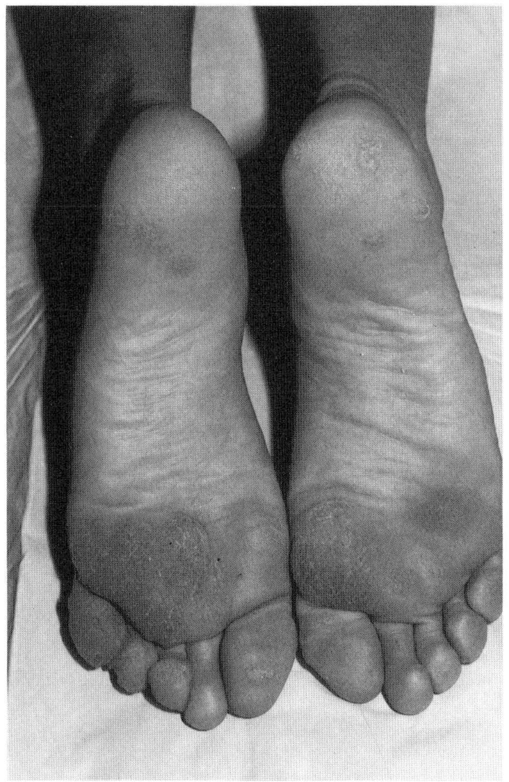

Fig. 17.8 Warts.

with finger-like projections, they may be hyperkeratotic, or they may appear as flat-topped papules. Deep warts on the sole may resemble clavi.

Plantar, and especially, periungual warts may cause pain with ambulation, and may be difficult to eradicate. Some serotypes of HPV have been linked to the development of squamous cell carcinoma (Epstein *et al.*, 1984). HPV DNA sequences have been found in squamous cell carcinoma of a digit (Ostrow *et al.*, 1989).

Cryotherapy with liquid nitrogen is an effective wart treatment. Keratolytic agents, such as salicylic acid are also used. Recalcitrant warts may respond to laser ablation, contact immunotherapy (Nuyler *et al.*, 1988) or intralesional bleomycin (Shumer & O'Keefe, 1983).

Sites of minor trauma may be portals of entry for HPV. Prevention of warts includes minimizing cuts and abrasions of the skin. Shower shoes should be worn to minimize exposure to virus shed from plantar warts. Treatment of warts should begin promptly to minimize spread.

MOLLUSCUM CONTAGIOSUM

Molluscum contagiosum presents as small, skin-coloured to pink, umbilicated papules. Often, multiple members of a family or team are affected. In adults, genital and suprapubic molluscum are typically acquired through sexual contact. An individual with genital or suprapubic molluscum contagiosum should be evaluated for other sexually transmitted disorders.

Individual lesions may be treated with cryotherapy, curettage or applications of cantharidin (a blistering agent). Often, lesions are present in large numbers. Repeated treatment is commonly necessary.

HERPES SIMPLEX

Herpes simplex (HSV) presents as recurrent grouped vesicles on an erythematous base. Paraesthesia or neuralgic pain may be associated with episodes of blistering. The virus may affect any area of skin, with perioral skin being the most common site. The close skin-to-skin contact which occurs in many sports presents an ideal setting for the spread of HSV. Wrestlers, in particular, may be prone to herpes simplex infection. Unusual skin sites are frequently involved because the head, and indeed, the entire body of the wrestler generally become involved in the contest (James, 1984).

Acyclovir can effectively shorten the healing time of HSV lesions. Long-term administration of acyclovir can prevent recurrences. Sunburn and windburn frequently trigger outbreaks of HSV. An effective sunblock can be helpful in preventing recurrences.

Individuals with active lesions should not participate in sports which require close physical contact. Those prone to frequent recurrences may benefit from long-term acyclovir therapy.

Fungal infections

TINEA

Dermatophyte infections are common in athletes, especially tinea pedis (athletes' foot) and tinea cruris (jock itch) (Fig. 17.9). Tinea infections of the feet may present as blistering lesions, or as red and scaly lesions. Toenails may be thick, yellow and dystrophic. Interdigital tinea may lead to bacterial toeweb infection. Tinea cruris presents as an annular erythematous patch with a raised scaly border. The diagnosis is confirmed by demonstration of fungal hyphae in a KOH preparation of scale or a blister roof. KOH examination of a blister roof may be useful in differentiating a blistering tinea from a blistering eczema.

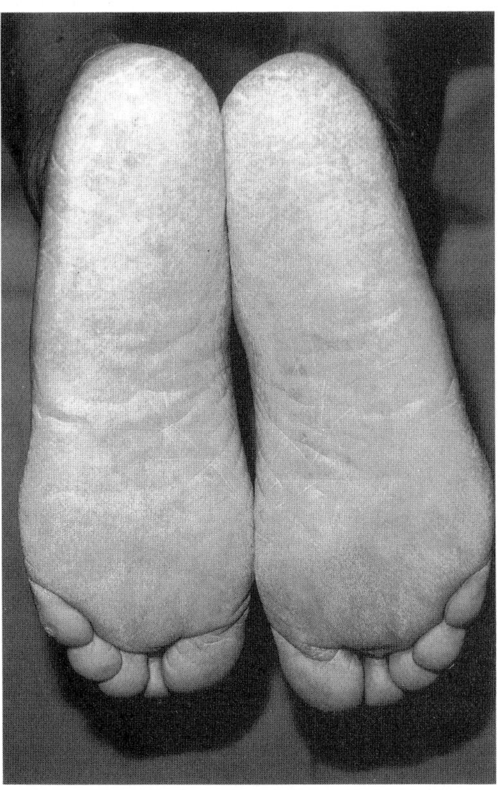

Fig. 17.9 Tinea.

Many topical antifungal agents are available. Some of the newer agents offer such advantages as once daily application and improved nail penetration. Oral agents are generally appropriate for the treatment of fungal nail infections, blistering tinea and other dermatophyte infections not responsive to topical agents. Griseofulvin and ketoconazole are effective oral antifungal agents. Ketoconazole has been associated with hepatotoxic reactions. Itraconazole may be less hepatotoxic, but is not presently available in the USA.

Fungal infections are exceedingly common, and may be difficult to prevent. Shower shoes should be worn in public showers. Blistering and erosive interdigital tinea should be treated promptly to prevent disability and secondary bacterial infection. Often prolonged courses of treatment are necessary. Recurrences are common.

TINEA VERSICOLOR

Tinea versicolor is common in athletes. Lesions may be hypopigmented, hyperpigmented or pink in colour. A fine scale is present over the entire surface of the lesion. Occasionally, the lesions are pruritic, but usually, tinea versicolor is asymptomatic. Heat, humidity and diabetes mellitus are predisposing factors. The lesions may become more prominent in summer when they fail to tan.

Malassezia furfur, the causative fungus is sensitive to many topical antifungal agents, but the lesions are often too widespread for topical treatment with antifungal creams to be cost-effective. Topical selenium sulfide (Selsun and Exsel) is cheap, effective, and suitable for widespread application. Monthly applications of selenium sulfide can prevent recurrences. Oral ketoconazole (Nizoral) has been used for refractory cases.

CANDIDIASIS

Candida albicans infections are common, particularly in women. Maceration, tight-fitting clothes, obesity and diabetes mellitus are predisposing factors. Vaginal yeast infections often complicate antibiotic treatment of bacterial infections. Cutaneous candidiasis is characterized by bright red patches of skin with satellite lesions. Burning and itching are common. KOH preparations and wet mounts confirm the diagnosis.

Topical antifungals provide effective treatment for most cases of candidiasis. Oral ketoconazole is highly active against *Candida*, but griseofulvin is ineffective. Candida paronychia often requires systemic therapy, but topical agents (such as thymol in chloroform or acetone) have also been used.

Efforts to prevent yeast infections should be directed toward the predisposing factors. Skin maceration and tight-fitting clothes should be avoided. Antibiotics should be used judiciously.

Bites, stings and infestation

Bites and stings

Outdoor athletics provide a natural setting for bites and stings. Arthropod bites often cause pruritic or painful skin reactions. Papular, nodular and vesiculobullous lesions may occur. Arthropods may also serve as vectors for infectious disease, including Lyme disease, rocky mountain spotted fever, and viral encephalitis (Kurgansky & Burnett, 1988; Modley & Burnett, 1988).

Bite reactions may require treatment with topical or systemic corticosteroids. Topical antipruritics, such as camphor and menthol lotion may be helpful. Individuals with a history of anaphylactic reactions to stings should carry an epinephrine injector kit (ANA Kit, EPI-PEN). Arthropod-borne infectious disease require appropriate diagnosis and treatment.

Preventive measures include avoidance of perfume and brightly coloured clothing, which attract bees and vespids. Long sleeves and trousers are helpful in preventing bites. Insect repellents, such as diethyltoluamide (DEET) are effective (Medical letter, 1989). Permethrin, an insecticide, may be applied to clothing. It appears particularly effective in the prevention of tick bites (Medical letter, 1989).

Scabies

No segment of the population is immune from scabies infestation. Often large groups of people, especially those living in close quarters, are affected. Affected individuals usually present with intense pruritus. Finger webspaces, areolae and the glans penis are commonly involved. The diagnosis is confirmed by demonstration of an adult mite, eggs or faeces in scrapings from a burrow. In adults, scabies is often transmitted by sexual contact, and may serve as a marker for other sexually transmitted disease.

Permethrin (Elimite), lindane (Kwell) and crotamiton (Eurax) have been used to treat scabies infestation. Permethrin appears to be a highly effective agent, and is less toxic than lindane (Taplin *et al.*, 1986). Care must be exercised to treat all affected areas, especially web spaces and under fingernails. All close physical contacts of an affected individual should be treated.

Scabies infestation may spread to affect many individuals, especially in settings such as barracks, dormitories, hospitals and nursing homes. Prompt diagnosis and treatment are critical in order to prevent spread.

Pediculosis

Humans may be host to body lice, head lice and pubic lice. Pubic lice are often spread through sexual contact. Head lice commonly affect groups of individuals, such as schoolchildren. Prompt diagnosis and treatment, with removal of all nits (eggs), is essential to prevent spread of the infestation. Permethrin (NIX) is a highly effective treatment (Brandenburg *et al.*, 1986). Pyrethrins and piperonyl butoxide (RID, A-200) and malathion may be more effective than lindane (Kwell) against nits (Altschuler & Kenney, 1986).

Cutaneous larva migrans

Canine hookworms, including *Ancylostoma braziliense* and *Uncinaria stenocephala*, cause cutaneous larva migrans, or 'creeping eruption'. Lesions are erythematous, serpiginous, and often intensely pruritic. A given individual may have many lesions. Topical thiabendazole under occlusion is an effective treatment. For widespread infestation, systemic thiabendazole is effective.

The eruption occurs after skin penetration by larval worms, found in soil contaminated by cat or dog faeces. Shaded, moist, sandy areas are ideal for development of the larvae. Prevention of the disorder depends on preventing soil contamination.

Acne

Acne vulgaris and nodulocystic acne are common in athletes. Mechanical factors, such as pressure from a mask or chin strap, may cause striking localization of lesions. Acne may be a sign of excessive androgen production. Women should be questioned about menstrual irregularities, infertility, galactorrhoea, hair thinning (alopecia), hirsutism and more overt signs of virilization such as increasing muscle mass, deepening of the voice or enlargement of the clitoris. Positive findings should prompt investigation for excess androgen production. Ovarian (Marynick *et al.*, 1983) and/or adrenal (Lobo *et al.*, 1981; Baskin, 1987; Siegel *et al.*, 1990) androgen production may be increased. Appropriate laboratory testing may include serum testosterone, free testosterone, dehydroepiandrosterone sulfate (DHEA-S), androstenedione, luteinizing hormone (LH), follicle-stimulating hormone (FSH), prolactin and cortisol. Adult adrenogenital syndrome may be detected by measuring adrenocorticotrophic hormone (ACTH) stimulated production of 17-OH progesterone or by an extended dexamethasone suppression test (Ehrmann & Rosenfield, 1990).

Comedonal acne (black heads and white heads) responds well to topical tretinoin. Individuals using tretinoin should be cautioned about photosensitive reactions. Inflammatory acne may respond to topical benzyl peroxide, topical antibiotics (including erythromycin and clindamycin), tretinoin and oral antibiotics (especially the tetracyclines and erythromycin). High oestrogen oral contraceptives (such as Demulen 1/50) and oral antiandrogens (such as spironolactone) may be useful (Muhlemann *et al.*, 1986; Young *et al.*, 1987). Refractory cases of nodulocystic acne may respond dramatically to the oral retinoid isotretinoin. Isotretinoin has been associated with severe fetal abnormalities. Its use is absolutely contraindicated in women who may become pregnant during (or within 1 month after) treatment.

Prompt intervention can prevent the cutaneous and emotional scarring that can result from disfiguring acne. In individuals with refractory acne, one should consider the possibility that the individual is using anabolic steroids.

Skin disorders caused by performance-enhancing drugs

Anabolic steroids have been used by some athletes in an effort to enhance athletic performance. Skin findings, especially treatment-resistant acne, alopecia and striae, may be signs of anabolic steroid abuse. Identification of illicit steroid use is important to prevent other, potentially serious, side-effects of anabolic steroids.

References

Adams, R.M. & Fisher, A.A. (1986) Contact allergen alternatives: 1986. *J. Am. Acad. Dermatol.* **14**, 951–69.

Altschuler, D.Z. & Kenney, L.R. (1986) Pediculicide

performance, profit, and the public health. *Arch. Dermatol.* **122**, 259–61.

Baskin, H.J. (1987) Screening for late-onset congenital adrenal hyperplasia in hirsutism or amenorrhea. *Arch. Intern. Med.* **147**, 847–8.

Brandenburg, K., Deinard, A.S. & DiNapoli, J. (1986) 1% permethrin cream rinse vs 1% lindane shampoo in treating pediculosis capitis. *Am. J. Dis. Child.* **140**, 894–6.

Cage, G.W., Sato, K. & Schwachman, H. (1987) Eccrine glands. In T.B. Fitzpatrick, A.Z. Eisen, K. Wolff, I.M. Freedberg & K.F. Austen (eds) *Dermatology in General Medicine*, 3rd edn, pp. 691–704. McGraw-Hill, New York.

Champion, R.H. (1992) Reactions to cold. In R.H. Champion, J.L. Burton & F.J.G. Ebling (eds) *Rook's Textbook of Dermatology*, 5th edn, pp. 833–848. Blackwell Scientific Publications, Oxford.

Coskey, R.J. & Coskey, L.A. (1987) Diagnosis and treatment of impetigo. *J. Am. Acad. Dermatol.* **17**, 62–3.

Daniels Jr, F. (1987) Physiologic factors in the skin's reaction to heat and cold. In T.B. Fitzpatrick, A.Z. Eisen, K. Wolff, I.M. Freedberg & K.F. Austen (eds) *Dermatology in General Medicine*, 3rd edn, pp. 1412–24. McGraw-Hill, New York.

Ehrmann, D.A. & Rosenfield, R.L. (1990) Hirsutism — beyond the steroidogenic block. *N. Engl. J. Med.* **323**, 909–11.

Ellis, C.N. & Voorhees, J.J. (1987) Etretinate therapy. *J. Am. Acad. Dermatol.* **16**, 267–91.

Epstein, W.L., Byrstyn, J.C., Edelson, R., Elias, P.M., Lowy, D.R. & Yuspa, S. (1984) Non-melanoma skin cancer, melanosis, warts and viral oncogenesis. *J. Am. Acad. Dermatol.* **11**, 960–70.

Feingold, D.S. & Wagner, R.F. (1986) Antibacterial therapy. *J. Am. Acad. Dermatol.* **14**, 535–48.

Feldman, P. & Lynfield, Y. (1987) Antibiotic choice for pyodermas (letter). *J. Am. Acad. Dermatol.* **17**, 859–60.

Fisher, A.A. (1986) Nickel — The ubiquitous contact allergen. In A.A. Fisher (ed) *Contact Dermatitis*, 3rd edn, pp. 745–61. Lea & Febiger, Philadelphia.

Fitzpatrick, T.B. (1987) Epidermis: Disorders of epidermal and dermoepidermal cohesion — vesicular and bullous disorders. In T.B. Fitzpatrick (ed) *Dermatology in General Medicine*, 3rd edn, p. 547. McGraw-Hill, New York.

Gonzalez, E., Khosrow, M.T. & Freedman, S. (1984) Bilateral comparison of generalized lichen planus treated with psoralens and ultraviolet A. *J. Am. Acad. Dermatol.* **10**, 958–61.

Gupta, A.K. & Anderson, T.F. (1987) Psoralen photochemotherapy. *J. Am. Acad. Dermatol.* **17**, 703–34.

Gupta, A.K., Ellis, C.N., Siegel, M.T. *et al.* (1990) Sulfasalazine improves psoriasis. *Arch. Dermatol.* **126**, 487–93.

Hanifen, J.M., Cooper, K.D. & Roth, H.L. (1986) Atopy and atopic dermatitis (periodic synopsis). *J. Am. Acad. Dermatol.* **14**, 703–6.

James, W.D. (1984) Herpes gladiatorum. *J. Assoc. Milit. Dermatol.* **10**, 4.

James, W.D., White, S.W. & Yanklowitz, B. (1984) Allergic contact dermatitis to compound tincture of benzoin. *J. Am. Acad. Dermatol.* **11**, 847–50.

Kennedy, C.T.C. (1992) Reactions to mechanical and thermal injury. In R.H. Champion, J.L. Burton & F.J.G. Ebling (eds) *Rook's Textbook of Dermatology*, 5th edn, pp. 777–832. Blackwell Scientific Publications, Oxford.

Krueger, G.G., Bergstresser, P.R., Lowe, N.J., Voorhees, J.J. & Weinstein, G.D. (1984) Psoriasis. *J. Am. Acad. Dermatol.* **11**, 937–48.

Kurgansky, D. & Burnett, J.W. (1988) Diptera mosquitoes. *Cutis* **41**, 317–18.

Levit, F. (1977) Joggers' nipples. *N. Engl. J. Med.* **297**, 1127.

Leyden, J.J. (1988) Pyoderma pathophysiology and management. *Arch. Dermatol.* **124**, 753–5.

Leyden, J.J., Marples, R.R. & Kligman, A.M. (1974) *Staphylococcus aureus* in the lesions of atopic dermatitis. *Br. J. Dermatol.* **90**, 525–30.

Lobo, R.A., Wellington, C.P. & Goebelsmann, U.W.E. (1981) Dehydroepiandrosterone sulfate as an indicator of adrenal androgen function. *Obstet. Gynecol.* **57**, 69–73.

Lowe, N.J., Ashton, R.E., Koudsi, H., Verschoore, M. & Schaeffer, H. (1984) Anthralin for psoriasis: Short contact anthralin therapy compared with topical steroid and conventional anthralin. *J. Am. Acad. Dermatol.* **10**, 69–72.

Mandy, S.H. (1983) A new primary wound dressing made of polyethylene oxide gel. *J. Dermatol. Surg. Oncol.* **9**, 153–5.

Marynick, S.P., Chakmakjian, Z.H., McCaffree, D.L. & Hernden Jr, J.H. (1983) Androgen excess in cystic acne. *N. Engl. J. Med.* **308**, 982–6.

Medical letter (1988) Mupirocin — a new topical antibiotic. *Med. Lett.* **30**, 55–6.

Medical letter (1989) Insect repellents. *Med. Lett.* **31**, 45–7.

Metz, P.M., Marshall, D.A. & Eaglestein, W.H. (1985) Occlusive wound dressings to prevent bacterial invasion and wound infection. *J. Am. Acad. Dermatol.* **12**, 662–8.

Mitchell, J.C. & Fisher, A.A. (1986) Dermatitis due to plants and spices. In A.A. Fisher (ed) *Contact Dermatitis*, 3rd edn, pp. 418–53. Lea & Febiger, Philadelphia.

Modley, C.E. & Burnett, J.W. (1988) Tick-borne dermatologic diseases. *Cutis* **41**, 244–5.

Mostofa, W.Z. (1989) Lichen planus of the nail: Treatment with antimalarials. *J. Am. Acad. Dermatol.* **20**, 289–90.

Muhlemann, M.F., Carter, G.D., Cream, J.J. & Wise, P. (1986) Oral spironolactone: An effective treatment for acne vulgaris in women. *Br. J. Dermatol.* **115**, 227–32.

Nilsson, E., Henning, C. & Hjorleifsson, M.L. (1986) Density of the microflora in hand eczema before and after topical treatment with a potent corticosteroid. *J. Am. Acad. Dermatol.* **15**, 192–7.

Nordstrom, K.M., McGinley, K.J., Cuppiello, L., Zechman, J.M. & Leyden, J.J. (1987) Pitted keratolysis: The role of micrococcus sedentarius. *Arch. Dermatol.* **123**, 1320–5.

Nuyler, M.F., Neldner, D., Yarbrough, G.K., Rosio, T.J., Iriondo, M. & Yeary, J. (1988) Contact immunotherapy of resistant warts. *J. Am. Acad. Dermatol.* **19**, 697–83.

Orchard, S., Fellman, J.H. & Storrs, F.J. (1986) Poison ivy/oak dermatitis: Use of polyamine salts of a linoleic acid dimer for topical prophylaxis. *Arch. Dermatol.* **122**, 783–9.

Ostrow, R.S., Shaver, M.K., Turnquist, S. *et al.* (1989) Human papilloma virus-16 DNA in a cutaneous invasive cancer. *Arch. Dermatol.* **125**, 666–9.

Page, E.H., Wexler, D.M. & Guenther, L.C. (1986) Cyclosporine A. *J. Am. Acad. Dermatol.* **14**, 785–91.

Rich, P., Belozer, M.L., Norris, P. & Storrs, F.J. (1991) Allergic contact dermatitis to two antioxidants in latex gloves: 4,4′-thio*bis*(6-*tert*-butyl-*meta*-cresol) (Lowinox 44S36) and butyl hydroxyanisole. Allergen alternatives for glove-allergic patients. *J. Am. Acad. Dermatol.* **24**, 37–43.

Roenigk, H.H., Auerbach, R., Maibach, H.I. & Weinstein, G.D. (1988) Methotrexate in psoriasis: Revised guidelines. *J. Am. Acad. Dermatol.* **19**, 145–56.

Sarkany, I., Taplin, D. & Blank, H. (1961) The etiology and treatment of erythrasma. *J. Invest. Dermatol.* **37**, 283–90.

Shumer, S.M. & O'Keefe, E.J. (1983) Bleomycin for the treatment of recalcitrant warts. *J. Am. Acad. Dermatol.* **9**, 91–6.

Siegel, S.F., Finegold, D.N., Lanes, R. & Lee, P.A. (1990) ACTH stimulation tests and plasma dehydroepiandrosterone sulfite levels in women with hirsutism. *N. Engl. J. Med.* **323**, 849–63.

Silverman, A.R. & Nieland, M.L. (1983) Hot tub dermatitis: a familial outbreak of pseudomonas folliculitis. *J. Am. Acad. Dermatol.* **8**, 153–6.

Sommerville, D.A. & Lancaster-Smith, M. (1973) The aerobic cutaneous microflora of diabetic subjects. *Br. J. Dermatol.* **89**, 395–400.

Stanfield, J.W., Feldt, P.A., Csortan, E.S. & Krochmal, L. (1989) Ultraviolet A sunscreen evaluations in normal subjects. *J. Am. Acad. Dermatol.* **20**, 744–8.

Storrs, F.J. (1986) Dermatitis from clothing and shoes. In A.A. Fisher (ed) *Contact Dermatitis*, 3rd edn, pp. 283–37. Lea & Febiger, Philadelphia.

Swartz, M.N. & Weinberg, A.N. (1987) Infections due to Gram-positive bacteria. In T.B. Fitzpatrick (ed) *Dermatology in General Medicine*, 3rd edn, pp. 2100–21. McGraw-Hill, New York.

Taplin, D., Meinking, T.L. & Porcelain, S.L. (1986) Permethrin 5% dermal cream: a new treatment for scabies. *J. Am. Acad. Dermatol.* **15**, 995–1001.

Taylor, J.S. (1986) Rubber. In A.A. Fisher (ed) *Contact Dermatitis*, 3rd edn, pp. 603–43. Lea & Febiger, Philadelphia.

Tunnessen, W. (1985) Practical aspects of bacterial skin infections in children. *Pediatr. Dermatol.* **2**, 255–65.

Young, R.L., Goldzieher, J.W. & Elkind-Hirsh, K. (1987) The endocrine effects of spironolactone used as an antiandrogen. *Fertil. Steril.* **48**, 223–8.

Zaias, N. (1982) Pitted and ringed keratolysis. *J. Am. Acad. Dermatol.* **7**, 787–91

PART 2

SPORT-SPECIFIC INJURIES: PREVENTION AND CARE

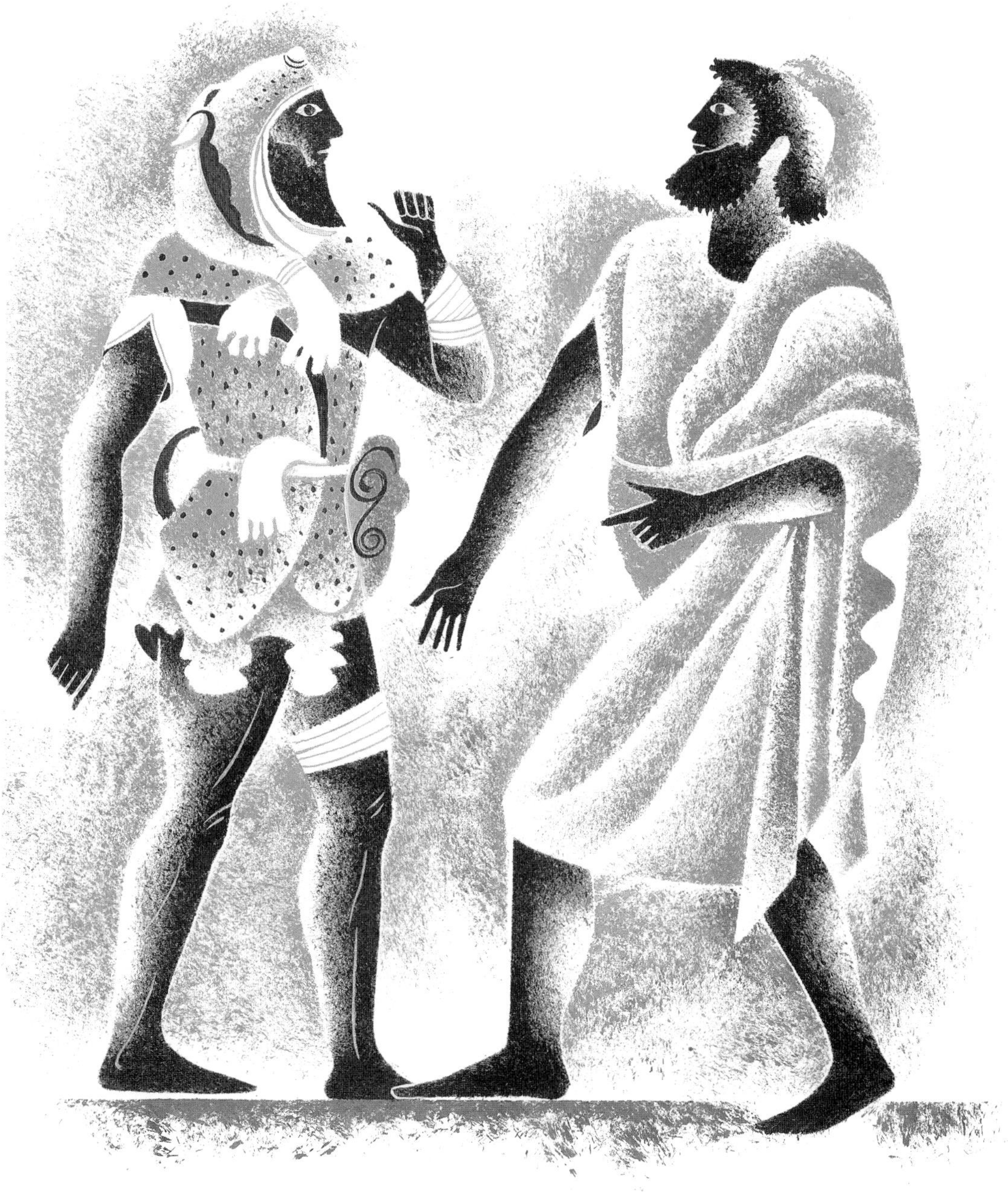

Part 2a

Team Sports

Chapter 18

Injuries in Soccer: Mechanism and Epidemiology

PAOLO AGLIETTI, GIOVANNI ZACCHEROTTI, PIETRO DE BIASE, FRANCO LATELLA AND GIOVANNI SERNI

Soccer injuries are frequent. This can be explained by the high number of participants all over the world (approximately 22 million) and by the specific mechanics of the game which involve kicking, cutting, tackling and prolonged efforts (Fig. 18.1). In Italy, in the season 1989–1990, there were 1419 930 athletes registered in official soccer teams. Among these there were 2746 top professional athletes, 9402 young professionals and 519 117 youth players. In Europe 50–60% of all sport injuries are due to soccer (Franke, 1977).

Many authors have discussed soccer injury epidemiology (Table 18.1). In a study of a professional team during an entire season (McMaster & Walter, 1978) all the players were injured with maximum incidence for strikers and midfielders. The goalkeeper was more at risk according to other studies (Sullivan *et al.*, 1980). Lower extremities are definitely more at risk and include 64–88% of the lesions (Nilsson & Roaas, 1978; Sullivan *et al.*, 1980; Ekstrand & Gillquist, 1982). The most frequent injuries were ankle sprains and muscle strains, but usually the lesions were minor compared to the more severe American football injuries. More than 30% of meniscal tears are produced by sport injuries, and in Europe soccer is responsible for 70% of them (Smillie, 1970). As far as age is concerned, it has been found (Sullivan *et al.*, 1980) that, studying the epidemiology of lesions in a group of 7–19-year-old athletes, the incidence in the entire group was 2.6% but increased to 7.7% when considering only the 14–19-year-old subgroup. Several other authors have found a higher incidence in the older athletes (McMaster & Walter, 1978; Nilsson & Roaas, 1978; Albert, 1983). Nilsson (1978) studying young athletes involved in two 5-day tournaments in Norway, found a higher incidence in the very young athletes but comparing the

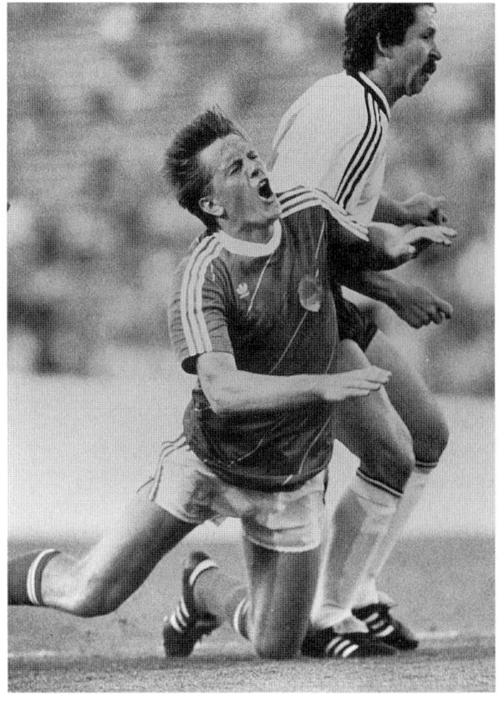

Fig. 18.1 Body contact can cause soccer injuries. © NPP/Los Angeles Times/T. Barnard.

Table 18.1 Soccer injury epidemiology — review of the literature.

Reference	Period	Object	Injury definition	Comments
Albert, 1986	1979–81 outdoor and indoor seasons	56 NASL professionals	Time loss injuries	1.2 injuries·players^{-1}·year^{-1}, 72% lower extremity
McMaster & Walter, 1978	1976–77	15 ASL professionals	Any injury reported	Midfielders and strikers most prone to injuries, ankle and foot most frequently injured site
Nilsson & Roaas, 1978	1975, 1977 two 5-day tournaments	25 000 11–18-year-old players	Any injury reported	Females twice rate of males, 68% lower extremity, injuries in adolescents are less severe and frequent than adults
Sullivan *et al.*, 1980	1979 spring season	1272 7–18-year-old players	Time loss injuries	Females more prone to injuries, youngest players have lower incidence, goalkeepers more injured
Ekstrand *et al.*, 1983a	1980 spring and autumn season	180 amateurs average age 25 years	Time loss injuries	78% lower extremity, 7.6 injuries·1000 h^{-1}, higher incidence during matches
Nielsen & Yde, 1989	1986 outdoor season	123 16–18-year-old players and over 18-year-old players	Time loss injuries	Older youths similar to adults, 84% lower extremity, ankle sprains most common, 28% had symptoms 1 year after end of season

ASL, American Soccer League; NASL, North American Soccer League.

results of the entire group with professional soccer data noted that injuries in youth were less frequent and less severe.

This chapter examines the injuries which occurred in an Italian professional soccer team over a period of 11 years in an effort to study the epidemiology, the mechanisms of injury, the frequency of the various lesions reported, and the importance of factors such as age and role.

A prospective soccer injury study

All the 1018 athletes belonging to an Italian professional soccer team from Florence over a period of 11 years (August 1980 to June 1991) were included in the study. In Italy, the season begins in August with athletic training and ends in June with the end of the various championships. Our study includes 11 complete seasons.

Players were divided into three groups. The first group included the juvenile division composed of 642 young athletes between 13 and 17 years of age. The second group included 186 junior professional athletes 16–20 years old, and finally the third group was composed of 190 top professional athletes competing in the Italian major league (A league). The age ranged from 19 to 37 years.

The players were also divided according to their role in the team. We considered the players registered at the beginning of every season. There were 109 goalkeepers, 352 defenders, 326 midfielders and 231 strikers.

During the observation period, the athletes competed in an average of 50 games (75 h) per year and trained 5 days·week^{-1} for 2 h·day^{-1} (480 h). All the matches and practice took place on grass and equipment was the same for all the players (shoes with cleats, leg protections, etc.).

Lesions were observed and recorded by only two team physicians and reported to the same orthopaedic specialists for subsequent treatment, when necessary. Significant injuries were defined as those involving the absence of athletes for at least one game or one training session.

Results

The total number of injuries observed during the 11-year period was 207 (20%). Forty of these (19%) belonged to the youth, 62 (30%) to the junior professional, and 105 (51%) to the top professional group. The average ages of the three groups at the time of injury were 15, 18 and 26 years respectively. Most of the lesions occurred between 17 and 19 years (Fig. 18.2) and the majority of them, in this age range, belonged to the junior professional group (Fig. 18.3).

Midfielders and strikers had the higher incidence of injuries (22%) compared with the defenders (19%) and goalkeepers (16%). In the top professionals, 80% of the strikers, 58% of the midfielders and 40% of the defenders and goalkeepers were injured. In the young professionals, there was no difference between players, while in the youth group the incidence of injuries by position played was lower and the goalkeeper accounted for most of the lesions (10% of the goalkeepers, while 8% of the midfielders and 4% of the defenders and strikers were injured).

The number of injuries during official games was 112 (54%) and during training 95 (46%). The incidence of lesions was also calculated in relationship to the exposure time. It was 1.4 · 1000 game h^{-1} and 0.2 · 1000 training h^{-1}. During official games, the incidence was 4 · 1000 h^{-1} for the top division, 2.5 · 1000 h^{-1} for the young professionals and 0.4 · 1000 h^{-1} for the youth group. Lesions observed in the top professionals were significantly more frequent than the other two series (55% versus 12%; $P < 0.001$).

About 53% of the injuries occurred in the months of October–November and April–May, that is at the beginning or near the end of the championships (Fig. 18.4). Analysing the three groups of players separately, it was noted

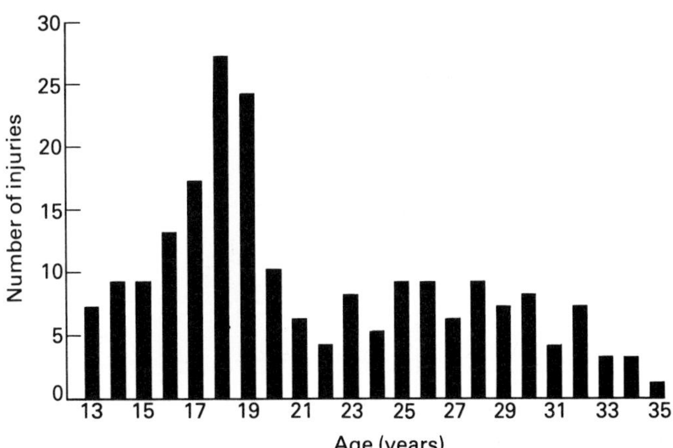

Fig. 18.2 Injuries by age.

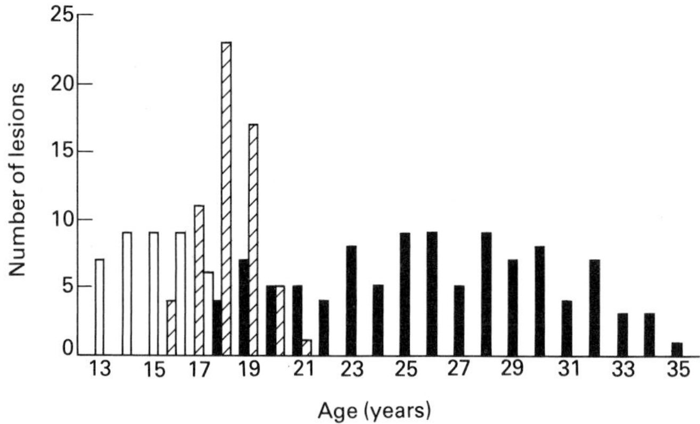

Fig. 18.3 Injuries by age and category: □, youth; ⊠, young professional; ■, top professional.

that the maximum frequency of lesions was reached by the youth group at the end of the championship, by the young professionals at the beginning of the season, while the top professionals had lesions distributed uniformly throughout the season (Fig. 18.5).

The types of injuries recorded are shown in Table 18.2. Lesions were divided in two groups: (i) those involving the muscle–tendon units; and (ii) those involving the osteoarticular units. Osteoarticular lesions represent about two-thirds of all the lesions and comprise mostly joint sprains (52%). The muscle–tendon lesions are mostly composed of muscle strains (78%).

76% of the injuries are localized to the lower extremity, while upper extremity injuries account for 17%, head and face 13%, and torso 3% (Table 18.3). In the lower extremity, the most frequent lesions involved the knee (37%) (Table 18.4) while the ankle accounted for 27%. In the upper extremity, the hand and wrist (28%) were the most frequent lesions, while the shoulder accounted for 16%. Among the head and face injuries, fracture of the nasal bones included a high 58%.

Table 18.5 evaluates the various mechanisms of injury (tackle, running, falling, kicking) for the various positions (goalkeepers, defenders, midfielders and strikers). Contact injuries were

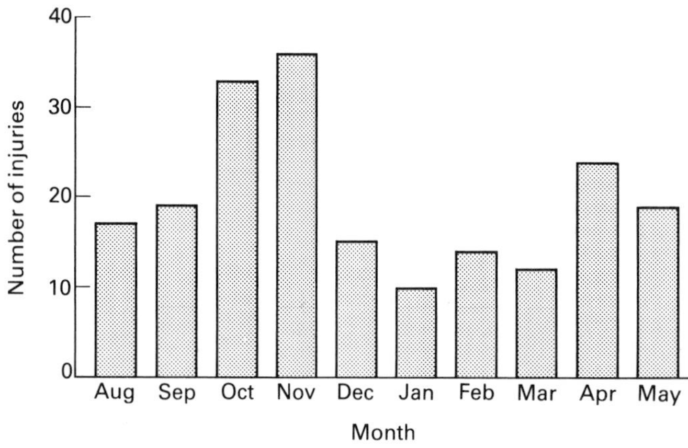

Fig. 18.4 Number of injuries by month.

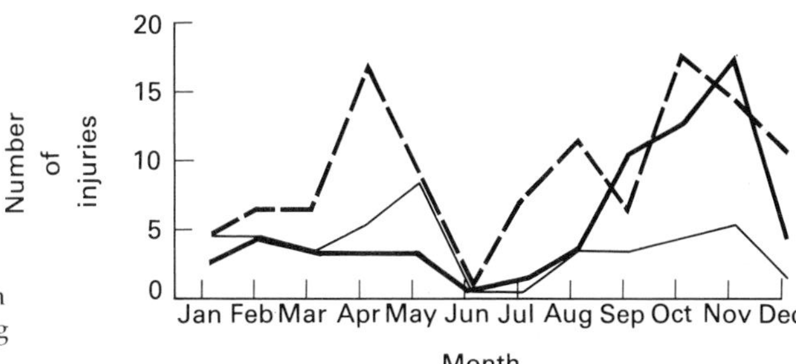

Fig. 18.5 Number of injuries by month and category: ——, youth; **——**, young professional; – – –, top professional.

Table 18.2 Injury type.

Muscle–tendon lesions	
muscle contusions	6 (12%)
muscle strains	40 (78%)
tendinitis	5 (10%)
Total	51 (24.6%)
Osteoarticular lesions	
joint sprains	70 (52%)
dislocations/subluxations	15 (11%)
fractures	50 (37%)
Total	135 (65.2%)
Other	21 (10.2%)

Table 18.3 Anatomical location of injuries.

Upper extremity	
shoulder	11 (16%)
elbow	2 (5%)
wrist and hand	10 (28%)
phalanges	13 (36%)
Total	36 (17%)
Torso	6 (3%)
Lower extremity	
thigh	40 (29%)
knee	51 (37%)
leg	6 (4%)
ankle	37 (27%)
foot	5 (4%)
Total	139 (67%)
Head and face	
face	20 (77%)
head	6 (23%)
Total	26 (13%)

Table 18.4 Knee injuries.

Sprains	
anterior cruciate ligament lesions	17 (47%)
medial collateral ligament lesions	10 (28%)
lateral collateral ligament lesions	2 (5%)
posterior cruciate ligament lesion	1 (3%)
other	6 (17%)
Isolated meniscal lesions	
medial meniscus	7 (78%)
lateral meniscus	2 (22%)
Fractures	
supracondylar	1 (2%)
tibial plateau	1 (2%)
osteochondral fracture	1 (2%)
Total	3 (6%)
Contusions	3 (6%)

the principal mechanisms (79 lesions, 38%). The goalkeepers became injured by contact in 50% of the cases, and this percentage decreased for defenders (42%), midfielders or strikers. Running, falls or kicking injuries are more frequent among midfielders or strikers. Traumatic lesions were more frequent during official competitions (64% of all injuries) than during training (51%, $P = 0.03$).

In the upper extremity, the typical injury was caused by falling on the ground (72%, $P = 0.007$), while for the lower extremity contact injuries represented the major source of fractures and sprains particularly for the knee. In 37% of the cases, knee sprains occurred without contact.

In 47% of all knee sprains, an anterior cruciate ligament lesion was diagnosed, while a lesion of the medial collateral ligament was found in 28% of the cases (see Table 18.4). An anterior cruciate ligament lesion was caused by a contact

Table 18.5 Injury mechanism.

Position	Tackling	Running	Fall	Shooting	Other
Goalkeeper	9 (50%)	1 (5.6%)	—	1 (5.6%)	7 (39%)
Defenders	28 (42%)	16 (24%)	15 (22%)	5 (7.5%)	3 (4.5%)
Midfielders	25 (35%)	21 (29%)	10 (14%)	8 (11%)	8 (11%)
Strikers	17 (34%)	18 (36%)	7 (14%)	7 (14%)	1 (2%)

injury in 81% of the cases, while half of the medial collateral ligament lesions were caused by contact injuries. The posterior cruciate ligament or the lateral collateral ligament were less frequently involved. Half of the isolated meniscal lesions were attributed to a kicking mechanism.

The mechanism of the muscle strains varies according to location. For the rectus anterior, strains usually occur while kicking (86%); for the hamstrings or the gastrocnemius, while sprinting (91%).

Most of the ankle sprains occurred by inversion (70%) and without any contact.

We could not find differences according to the observation year or the various coaches involved.

Mechanism and epidemiology of injuries

A scientific evaluation of epidemiology and mechanisms of injury in soccer is difficult. The literature on the subject includes only a few studies (McMaster & Walter, 1978; Nilsson & Roaas, 1978; Sullivan *et al.*, 1980; Ekstrand & Gillquist, 1982, 1983a,b; Albert, 1983; Ekstrand *et al.*, 1983a,b; Nielsen & Yde, 1989). Keller (1987) stressed the difficulties of finding common denominators to compare the results.

This study used the definition of injury adopted by several authors (Ekstrand & Gillquist, 1982, 1983a,b; Ekstrand *et al.*, 1983a,b; Nielsen & Yde, 1989). An injury is defined as a lesion which prevents the athlete from participating in a game or training session. Injuries occurring during other activities were excluded.

The identification of the frequency of the injuries is a common denominator to all studies. Some authors (Sandelin *et al.*, 1985) have utilized the number of lesions·player^{-1}·year^{-1}. We have adopted the method of Ekstrand and Gillquist (1983a,b) who calculated the frequency of lesions·player^{-1}·exposure time^{-1} (1000 h) as also suggested by Keller *et al.* (1987). The incidence of lesions in our study is lower than that reported by Nielsen and Yde (1989). We have recorded in top professional athletes an incidence of $4 \cdot 1000\ h^{-1}$ for the official matches and $0.5 \cdot 1000\ h^{-1}$ for training sessions, which is less than the $16.9 \cdot 1000\ h^{-1}$ for matches and $7.6 \cdot 1000\ h^{-1}$ in training reported by Ekstrand (1983a).

The incidence of lesions in the youth group is less than the other groups. While the difference between the youth group and top professionals is marked ($0.4 \cdot 1000\ h^{-1}$ versus $4 \cdot 1000\ h^{-1}$), the junior professionals show an incidence closer to the senior athletes ($2.5 \cdot 1000\ h^{-1}$). We can therefore confirm what has been found by other authors (Sullivan *et al.*, 1980; Nielsen & Yde, 1989): that younger players have less injuries than older athletes. This is probably due to the inferior intensity of participation of the youth group compared to the professionals (Nilsson & Roaas, 1978; Keller *et al.*, 1987). The players in the age range 16–19 years, defined in our study as junior professional, show an elevated incidence of lesions similar to the top series.

The lower extremity accounts for most of the lesions, as found by many (Ekstrand & Gillquist, 1982, 1983a,b; Ekstrand *et al.*, 1983a,b; Nielsen & Yde, 1989). The knee in our series is the most frequently involved joint (25% of all lesions). The ankle had lesions in 18% of the cases, about half of that reported by Nielsen (1989). Knee lesions are usually more severe, particularly considering the prolonged absence from playing that they cause. Ankle sprains, however, may cause subsequent reinjuries through a mechanism of chronic instability.

In the knee, in this series of mostly professional athletes, anterior cruciate ligament tears were most frequently caused by contact injuries (81%). Medial collateral ligament lesions occurred equally by contact and non-contact mechanisms, while meniscus tears usually presented after a kick or shooting the ball. We believe that in reality meniscal tears are due to knee sprains but may reveal themselves only after a kick or a shoot. Meniscal injuries can rarely be due to microtrauma (Vecchiet *et al.*, 1990). Lower extremity fractures are rare in soccer and in our study were found in only 5% of players.

Muscle strains of the thigh and calf (Ekstrand & Gillquist, 1982) have been related to poor muscle elasticity. The same authors studied the avoidability of muscle strains in soccer (1983a) and identified a programme of prevention based on adequate training with warm-up and stretching, use of adequate equipment, prophylactic taping of unstable joints, adequate information about the risks during fouls and appropriate rehabilitation. Results were very encouraging with a 75% reduction of injuries in the group prepared with the above-mentioned programme compared to the control group. For preventing hamstring strains, a stretching programme is particularly important. For rectus femoris strains, a warm-up is mandatory during which kicking should be avoided.

Upper extremity lesions are less frequent than lower extremity ones (17%). The hand is vulnerable in soccer players, particularly in goalkeepers. Some authors (Nilsson & Roaas, 1978; Sullivan *et al.*, 1980; Albert, 1983) report a high incidence of hand lesions in the younger group of players. Shoulder dislocation and acromioclavicular dislocation are relatively infrequent and usually occur due to accidental falls.

The mechanism of lesions reported in our study are similar to those described by Nielsen and Yde (1989) who showed 40% of injuries were due to contact and 39% occurred during running. Other authors (Berger-Vachon *et al.*, 1986) showed that in only 17% of the cases is the soccer player injured without contact. In our series, a contact injury was the cause of the lesion in 38% of the cases, and in 27% the lesions occurred during running. The lower incidence of lesions during running can be explained by the conditions of the playing surfaces. Soccer fields can be classified in three types: (i) grass; (ii) synthetic; and (iii) soil. In Italy, only grass fields are used. Xenthalis and Boiardo (1989) noted that European players playing in the USA on synthetic surfaces suffered an unusually high incidence of muscle strains. Changing surfaces accounts for an increase in injury rate (Sullivan *et al.*, 1980; Ekstrand & Gillquist, 1983b; Ekstrand *et al.*, 1983a,b).

The player's position in the team has some significance in determining the injury type. Contact with another player is the most frequent mechanism but the percentage of lesions due to this mechanism decreased progressively starting from the goalkeeper. In the goalkeepers, contact accounted for 50% of the lesions and this decreased to 42% for defenders, and to 35% for midfielders and strikers. For the latter two groups, injuries occurring due to running or kicking became more frequent.

We related the number of players by their position to the incidence of injuries and found that in the top professional group the most frequently injured roles were midfielders and strikers, while in the youth group the goalkeeper sustained a two-fold higher incidence of injury compared with the other positions.

A significant difference has been found between injuries occurring during official matches and during training sessions. The frequency of injuries during the official matches was approximately 10 times higher than during training and this held true for all categories of players. If the exposure time is not considered, then the incidence during matches and training becomes closer (Sullivan *et al.*, 1980; Ekstrand & Gillquist, 1983). Nielsen and Yde (1989) have reported a higher incidence of lesions during matches for older players and the opposite in the youth group.

Conclusion

In conclusion, the incidence of lesions during training is far less than during official matches. Athletes in the juvenile team have a significantly lower incidence of lesions than the top athletes while the junior professionals have an incidence closer to the senior professionals. Severity of lesions increases with age and intensity of participation of players. Lower extremity injuries occur more frequently than upper extremity in general but the youth group showed an increased incidence of upper extremity lesions relative to the other groups. Among the various joints, the knee and the ankle are most frequently involved usually by a twisting injury both due to contact and noncontact mechanisms. Adequate programmes to limit the risks of injury in soccer should include type of training, adequate equipment and education of the rules of the game to decrease fouls.

References

Albert, M. (1983) Descriptive three year data study of outdoor and indoor professional soccer injuries. *Athletic Training* **18**, 218–20.

Berger-Vachon, C., Gabard, G. & Moyen, B. (1986) Soccer accidents in the French Rhone-Alpes Association. *Sports Med.* **3**, 69–77.

Ekstrand, J. & Gillquist, J. (1982) The frequency of muscle tightness and injuries in soccer players. *Am. J. Sports Med.* **10**, 75–8.

Ekstrand, J. & Gillquist, J. (1983a) The avoidability of soccer injuries. *Int. J. Sports Med.* **4**, 124–8.

Ekstrand, J. & Gillquist, J. (1983b) Soccer injury and their mechanism: A prospective study. *Med. Sci. Sports Exerc.* **15**, 267–70.

Ekstrand, J., Gillquist, J. & Liljedahl, S. (1983a) Prevention of soccer injuries. *Am. J. Sports Med.* **11**, 116–20.

Ekstrand, J., Gillquist, J., Möller, M., Öberg, B. & Liljedahl, S. (1983b) Incidence of soccer injuries and their relation to training and team success. *Am. J. Sports Med.* **11**, 63–7.

Franke, K. (1977) *Traumatologie des Sports*. Verlag, Berlin.

Keller, C.S., Noyes, F.R. & Buncher, C.R. (1987) The medical aspects of soccer injury epidemiology. *Am. J. Sports Med.* **15**, 230–7.

McMaster, W.C. & Walter, M. (1978) Injuries in soccer. *Am. J. Sports Med.* **6**, 354–7.

Nielsen, A.B. & Yde, J. (1989) Epidemiology and traumatology of injuries in soccer. *Am. J. Sports Med.* **17**, 803–7.

Nilsson, S. & Roaas, A. (1978) Soccer injuries in adolescents. *Am. J. Sports Med.* **6**, 358–61.

Sandelin, J., Santavirta, S. & Kiviluoto, O. (1985) Acute soccer injuries in Finland in 1980. *Br. J. Sports Med.* **19**, 30–3.

Smillie, I.S. (1970) *Injuries of the Knee Joint*, 4th edn. Churchill Livingstone, Edinburgh.

Sullivan, J.A., Gross, R.H., Grana, W.A. *et al.* (1980) Evaluation of injuries in youth soccer. *Am. J. Sports Med.* **8**, 325–7.

Vecchiet, L., Calligaris, A., Montanari, G., Resina, A. (1990) *Trattato di medicina dello sport applicata al calcio*. Centro di documentazione scientifica, Menarini, 1990.

Xethalis, J.L. & Boiardo, R.A. (1989) Soccer injuries. In J.A. Nicholas & E.B. Hershman (eds). *The Lower Extremity and Spine in Sports Medicine*, Vol. II. CV Mosby, St Louis.

Chapter 19

Injuries in Soccer: Prevention

JAN EKSTRAND

Soccer is the most popular sport in the world, with more than 22 million participants (Pardon, 1977; Ekstrand, 1982). As the popularity of soccer has grown, soccer injuries have become the object of increasing medical interest (Keller *et al.*, 1987). It is estimated that in Europe 50–60% of all sports injuries and 3.5–10% of all hospital-treated injuries are due to soccer (Franke, 1977; Ekstrand, 1982; Keller *et al.*, 1987).

The essence of sports medicine is the prevention of injuries. To prevent injuries occurring in a particular sport, it is necessary to be sport-specific; to analyse the incidence, type and localization of injuries as well as the mechanisms behind the injuries in just that sport (Fig. 19.1). The purpose of this section is to briefly summarize the incidence of soccer injuries and the mechanisms involved, and then discuss various methods of prevention.

Type, localization and incidence of injuries

A fundamental problem associated with an epidemiological assessment of data on sports injuries is the inconsistent manner in which injury is defined and information collected and recorded (Kraus & Burg, 1970; Blyth & Mueller, 1974; Ekstrand, 1982). Current literature on soccer injury epidemiology relies upon a variety of definitions of injury. The meaningful com-

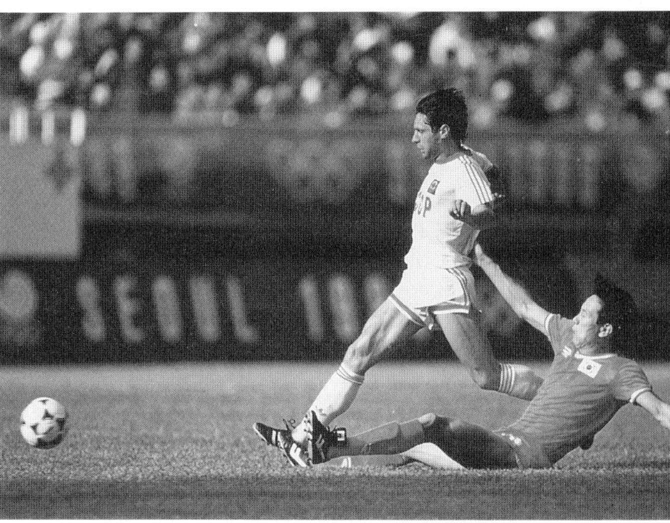

Fig. 19.1 Tackling from behind is a common injury mechanism which should be forbidden. © Allsport/D. Cannon.

parison of data collected in future soccer studies and comparison of soccer injury data with those reported for other sports requires a universal definition of athletic injury (Keller *et al.*, 1987).

It has been suggested (Keller *et al.*, 1987) that only those injuries resulting in lost time from practice or play should be included in the statistics. The duration of restricted athletic performance should also be reported in future studies since this represents a useful measure of the severity of injury (Keller *et al.*, 1987).

Ekstrand and Gillquist (1983b), Brynhildsen *et al.* (1991) and Jørgensen (1984) and others have all used a common definition of injury where injury was defined as any injury occurring during scheduled games or practice and causing the player to miss the next game or practice session. Injuries were classified into three categories according to severity (Table 19.1). The type and localization of injuries from the studies by Ekstrand are shown in Tables 19.1 and 19.2.

Expressed as a percentage of total injuries, lower extremity injuries represent 82–88% for senior male amateur players (Ekstrand, 1982; Jørgensen, 1984), 73% for male professional players (Albert, 1983), 80% for senior female players (Brynhildsen *et al.*, 1991), and 65–68% for youth players (Nilsson & Roaas, 1978; Sullivan, 1980).

To evaluate the real risk for soccer injuries, the exposure factor, i.e. the time the player is at risk, has to be taken into account (Table 19.3).

Table 19.1 Type of injury* (%).

	Total	Minor	Moderate	Major
Sprain	29	16	7	5
Overuse	23	17	5	2
Contusion	20	15	5	0
Strain	18	9	7	2
Fracture	4	1	1	2
Dislocation	2	0	2	0
Other	4	4	0	0
Total	100	62	27	11

* Minor injury, absence from practice for less than 1 week; moderate injury, absence from practice for more than 1 week but less than 1 month; major injury, absence from practice for more than 1 month.

Table 19.2 Localization of injury* (%).

	Total	Minor	Moderate	Major
Foot	12	10	2	0
Ankle	17	11	5	2
Leg	12	6	4	2
Knee	20	11	5	4
Thigh	14	6	5	2
Groin	13	9	3	1
Back	5	4	1	0
Other	7	5	2	0
Total	100	62	27	11

* See Table 19.1 footnote.

Injury mechanisms

The assessment of aetiological factors responsible for soccer injuries is a necessity for injury prevention. The cause of a soccer injury is often multifactorial. Ekstrand and Gillquist (1983a) analysed possible injury mechanisms and the avoidability of soccer injuries by compiling information from a preseason examination and test, a prospective study of injuries, and a training analysis in a Swedish soccer league. The results are summarized in Table 19.4.

Prevention of injuries

Preseason examination

Preseason examination and testing of soccer players are valuable in preventing injury. Incorrect training and individual player factors such as muscle tightness, malalignment, muscle weakness and joint instability are related to many soccer injuries. A preseason examination provides the opportunity to analyse and correct individual factors predisposing to injury. We suggest that a preseason examination should include a physical examination as well as measurement of flexibility and muscle strength.

Table 19.3 Soccer injury exposure rate.

Athlete	No. of injuries·1000 h^{-1}	Reference
Youth		Sullivan *et al.*, 1980
Male	0.5	
Female	1.1	
Youth		Nilsson & Roaas, 1978
Male	1.4	
Female	3.2	
Senior (male)		Ekstrand *et al.*, 1983b
Practice	7.6	
Game	16.9	
Senior (male)	4.1	Jørgensen, 1984
Senior (female)		Brynhildsen *et al.*, 1991
Practice	2.1	
Game	6.5	

Table 19.4 Aetiology of injuries* (%).

Player factors	42	
joint instability		12
muscle tightness		11
inadequate rehabilitation		17
non-training		2
Equipment	17	
shoes		13
shin guards		4
Playing surface	24	
Rules	12	
Other factors	29	

* Combinations of factors were fairly common.

PHYSICAL EXAMINATION

It is recommended that a preseason examination begins with an inquiry about past injuries and an examination to evaluate persistent symptoms from past injuries. Since leg injuries dominate in soccer, the musculoskeletal profile of the lower extremity should be analysed to evaluate persistent symptoms after past injuries. Such an examination includes the following.

Ankle tests

Mechanical instability can be evaluated by the drawer test. If there is mechanical instability, ankle taping is recommended, see below.

Functional instability, i.e. a feeling of 'giving way' and recurrent sprains can be evaluated by stabilometry. Stabilometry is an objective method for the study of postural control where the body sway is measured on a force plate. However, a modified Romberg test can also be used to evaluate functional instability. The player stands on one leg with the other leg raised and flexed at the knee, the arms folded across the chest and the eyes closed (Fig. 19.2). The player should be able to stand for 60 s without putting the raised foot to the ground. Correction movements of the standing leg are allowed. If the player fails to stand for 60 s (three attempts are allowed), he or she is considered to have functional instability and should be recommended ankle disc training (see below).

Test of the knee joint

Measurement of range of movement (ROM)

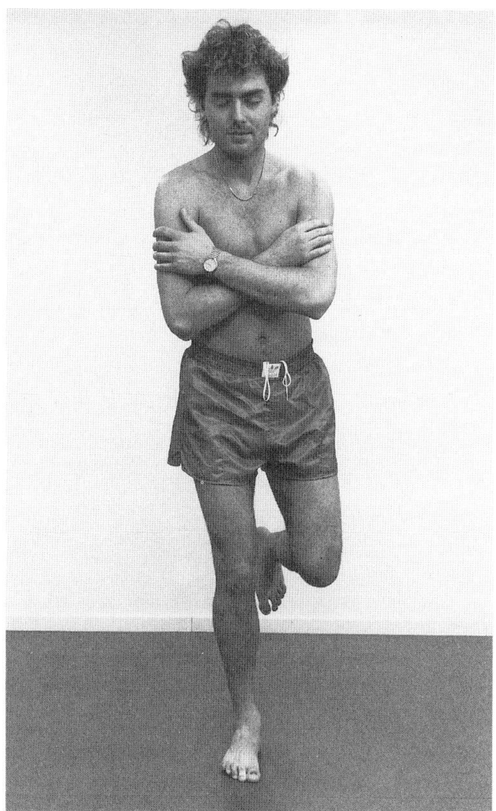

Fig. 19.2 Analysis of functional instability of the ankle joints (modified Romberg test). The player stands on one leg with the other leg raised and flexed at the knee, the arms folded across the chest and the eyes closed.

and clinical instability. The anterior drawer test or Lachmann test used for the evaluation of sagittal stability can be complemented by objective measurement by using a laxity tester.

A player with an insufficient anterior cruciate ligament (ACL) knee is usually unable to continue soccer and should be recommended a reconstruction of the ACL (Ekstrand, 1989b).

Test of the hip joint

Coxarthrosis should be excluded by clinical examination, i.e. analysis of rotation.

Malalignment test

Screening for malalignments or other possible biomechanical risk factors for overuse injuries, should be included in the physical examination. Examples of malalignments include: pes cavus, pes planus, Q angle over 20°, limb length discrepancy, soft heel pads, etc. The use of a mirror-box facilitates the analysis (Fig. 19.3).

MEASUREMENT OF ROM

To disclose muscular tightness of the lower extremity, a preseason examination should include measurement of six movements of the lower extremity: (i) hip flexion with the knee straight; (ii) hip extension; (iii) hip abduction;

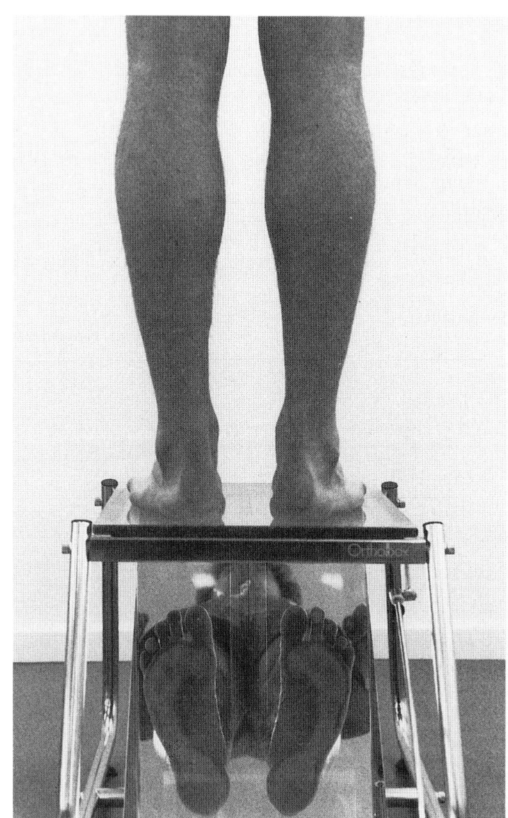

Fig. 19.3 The use of a mirror-box for the screening of malalignments of the lower extremity.

(iv) knee flexion lying prone; (v) ankle dorsiflexion with the knee straight; and (vi) ankle dorsiflexion with the knee bent. In the absence of coxarthrosis, gonarthrosis and neurological disease, these movements are thought to be limited by muscles and ligaments, and to be restricted in the presence of muscular tightness of the hamstrings, iliopsoas, adductors, rectus femoris, gastrocnemius and soleus.

Commonly used clinical methods for ROM measurement have a measurement error of 7–10% (Ekstrand *et al.*, 1982). Ekstrand *et al.* (1982) showed that the accuracy of measurement could be improved (measurement error less than 2%) by the use of goniometers and by secure fixation and marking of anatomical landmarks. Players with muscle tightness are recommended stretching exercises (see below).

MEASUREMENT OF MUSCLE STRENGTH

The maximal muscle strength of the knee extensor (quadriceps) and the knee flexor (hamstrings) muscles can be measured with great accuracy by using an isokinetic dynamometer. In the absence of such devices, muscle strength can be evaluated by using functional tests such as the one leg long jump (Tegner, 1985) or vertical jump (Gauffin, 1991).

Correction of training, warm-up, cool-down and stretching techniques

Soccer players are in general less flexible than non-soccer players of the same age (Ekstrand & Gillquist, 1982). There is a correlation between muscle tightness, strains and tendinitis (Ekstrand & Gillquist, 1983a).

The muscle tightness observed in soccer players is probably correlated to the design of soccer training. In a field study, it was found that the duration of warm-up was adequate but its content was not optimal (Ekstrand *et al.*, 1983b). Since 90% of soccer injuries affect the lower extremities, stretching exercises for the leg muscles (adductors, hamstrings, quadriceps, iliopsoas and triceps surae) should be included in the warm-up and cool-down exercises. Ekstrand *et al.* (1983a) devised a special warm-up programme with contract–relax stretching for the legs combined with a cool-down programme after training. Möller *et al.* (1985) found that this programme increased ROM by 5–20%. Players with muscle tightness detected by ROM measurement at preseason examination, should be recommended individual stretching exercises as well. Other corrections of training design are also valuable in reducing injuries. Shooting at goal before warm-up should be avoided since it increases the risk of muscle strains (Ekstrand, 1982).

Planning of the soccer season is also of importance. Ekstrand *et al.* (1983b) found a correlation between team success and the amount of training which would seem logical, provided the quality of training is adequate. They also found a curved relationship between injuries and training; teams with less than average training showed an increase in the number of injuries with increased training, probably the result of prolonged exposure. It was found, however, that teams with more than average training sustain fewer injuries with increased training, probably a reflection of the well-known fact that well-trained athletes sustain fewer injuries. Another important aspect of the planning of a season is that a high practice to game ratio seems to be beneficial with a tendency towards better performance with fewer injuries.

Ankle taping and ankle disc training

Ankle sprains are common in soccer (Ekstrand, 1982; Tropp, 1985) mostly affecting joints with a previous history of sprain. Several methods for prevention of ankle sprains have been documented (Ekstrand, 1982; Tropp *et al.*, 1985). Based on findings at the preseason examination, it was recommended that players with mechanical instability of the ankle joints are selected for taping or bracing and players with functional instability are selected for ankle disc training.

ANKLE TAPING

Prophylactic taping has become one of the main methods to prevent ankle sprains. The mechanism behind the effect of taping is not fully understood. It is assumed that external support increases ankle stability by reinforcing the ligaments and restricting motions such as extreme inversion (Fumich *et al.*, 1981; Tropp, 1985). A neuromuscular reflex mechanism has also been proposed (Boland & Glick, 1981).

Other questions to be answered are, who should be taped, by whom and by which method? Ekstrand *et al.* (1983a) showed good results by selecting players with mechanical instability for taping, letting the coach, trainer or doctor tape the players before games using a stirrup and horseshoe technique' followed by a figure of eight lock around the heel, and let the players tape themselves before practice sessions using only stirrups and horseshoes. The reasoning behind this procedure was the finding that match injuries are twice as common as practice injuries (Ekstrand, 1982).

ANKLE BRACING

Since ankle taping is expensive and the technique can be difficult to learn, an alternative to ankle taping would be valuable for players with mechanical instability (Tropp *et al.*, 1985). Various functional semirigid ankle braces are available and semirigid supports have been found to be effective in restricting ankle inversion and reducing the risk of ankle sprain (Stover, 1979; Tropp *et al.*, 1985). Some players, however, may complain of discomfort from the use of ankle braces.

ANKLE DISC TRAINING

The most common residual disability after ankle sprain is functional instability. Tropp (1985) found impaired postural control and pronator muscle weakness to be correlated to functional instability. Players with functional instability are predisposed to recurrent ankle sprain (Tropp, 1985). Impaired postural control and pronator muscle weakness as well as the subjective feeling of instability can be improved by coordination training on an ankle disc.

The exercises are performed on an ankle disc, which is a section of a sphere (Fig. 19.4), the supporting leg being straight and the other leg flexed at the knee. The arms should be folded across the chest. The recommended dose and duration of training is 5 min for each leg, 5 days·week^{-1}, for 10 weeks (Tropp, 1985). In players with a history of ankle problems, ankle disc training seems to be the method of choice because it diminishes functional instability and

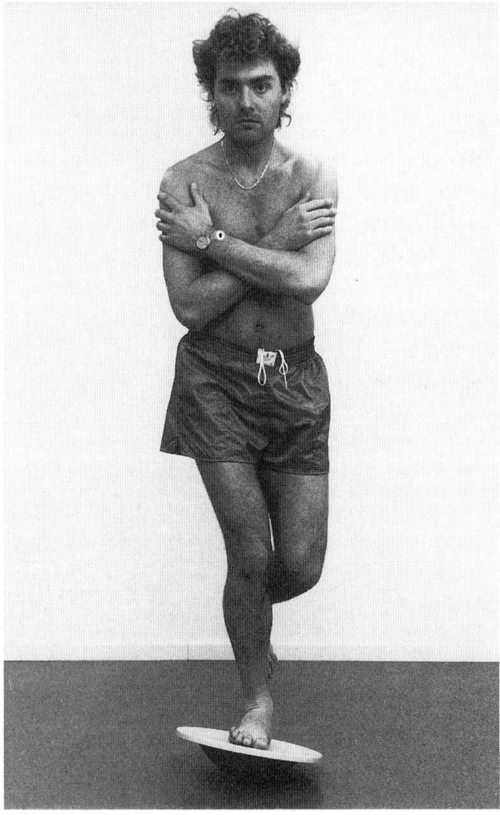

Fig. 19.4 Ankle disc training. The exercise is performed on an ankle disc which is a section of a sphere, the supporting leg being straight and the other leg flexed at the knee. The arms should be folded across the chest.

breaks the vicious circle of recurrent sprain and subsequent atrophy (Tropp, 1985). After an initial sprain, further ankle disc training is indicated even if the player is able to return to soccer play, because of the increased risk of reinjury. This may prevent residual disability and injury predisposition (Tropp, 1985).

Equipment and playing surface

The value of optimum equipment in injury prevention has been stressed (Ekstrand, 1982; Hoerner & Vinger, 1986; Hlobil *et al.*, 1987), Shin guards, shoes and insoles are important in soccer. It has been demonstrated that shock-absorbent, anatomically shaped shin guards, protecting a large area of the lower leg, can prevent injuries to the shin bone in soccer players (Ekstrand, 1982). The variety of soccer shoes available is enormous. When selecting footwear it should be realized that there is interaction between the foot and the shoe and between the shoe and the playing surface (Hlobil *et al.*, 1987; Ekstrand & Nigg, 1989).

High friction between shoe and surface may produce excessive forces on the knees and ankles; too little friction, however, may be the reason for slipping, which affects performance negatively and may cause injuries (Ekstrand & Nigg, 1989) (Fig. 19.5). Frictional resistance must be held within an optimum range.

Furthermore, it is generally assumed that the stiffness properties of the playing surface influence the frequency of injuries. It is assumed that 'hard' surfaces are associated with more injuries than 'soft' and 'well-cushioned' surfaces. The stiffness properties of a surface might have an influence on some chronic overuse injuries which account for about one-third of all soccer injuries (Ekstrand & Nigg, 1989). Overuse injuries can be avoided or reduced by adequate training, gradual adaption to a new surface, by the use of appropriate insoles, by the use if suitable soccer shoes (Jørgensen, 1989), and by adapting the movement to the surface.

Rehabilitation

Incomplete rehabilitation following a sports injury is a causal factor in the recurrence of sports injuries. In a prospective study of soccer players, Ekstrand (1982) found that 17% of the injuries were attributable to inadequate rehabilitation. Rehabilitation following a soccer injury is commonly neglected, yet few injuries sustained by soccer players are so trivial that no form of rehabilitation is unnecessary.

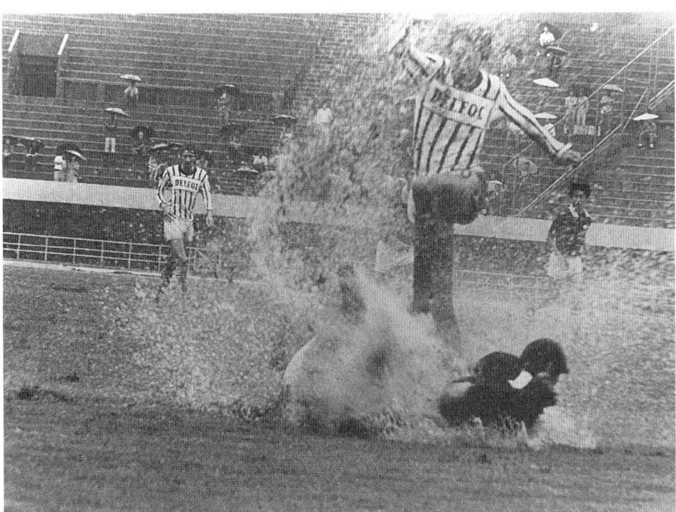

Fig. 19.5 A wet playing surface increases the risk of injury. Courtesy of the CIO archives (K.-J. Lee).

A rehabilitation programme should be sport-specific, gradually increasing the stress on the injured leg, and step by step adaption of the player for return to play. Return to games and practice should be decided by the doctor and physiotherapist, and a full, pain-free ROM, the regaining of coordination and more than 90% of muscle strength should be mandatory. In this way, 'controlled rehabilitation' can reduce the number of soccer injuries (Ekstrand, 1982).

Information and supervision

Many authors regard lack of information regarding the causes of sports injuries as a factor in their occurrence and the provision of information as an important factor in their prevention. In soccer, information should be given to coaches and players about:

1 The importance of disciplined play and the risk of serious own-foul injuries (Ekstrand, 1982).

2 The increased incidence of injury at training camps and how to avoid such injury (Ekstrand, 1982).

3 The importance of the use of protective equipment and other individual protective measures (Hlobil *et al.*, 1987).

Furthermore, supervision by doctors and physiotherapists is an important part of the prophylactic programme.

References

Albert, M. (1983) Descriptive three year data study of outdoor and indoor professional soccer injuries. *Athletic Training* **18**, 218–20.

Blyth, C.S. & Mueller, F.D. (1974) Football injury survey. *Phys. Sports Med.* **9**, 45–52.

Boland, A.J. & Glick, J. (1981) Editorial comment. *Am. J. Sports Med.* **9**, 316–17.

Brynhildsen, J., Ekstrand, J., Jeppsson, A. & Tropp, H. (1990) Previous injuries and persisting symptoms in female soccer players. *Int. J. Sports Med.* **11**, 489–92.

Brynhildsen, J., Tropp, H. & Ekstrand, J. (1993) Injuries in women's soccer — A prospective study. (In press.)

Ekstrand, J. (1982) *Soccer injuries and their prevention*. Linköping University Medical Dissertations, No. 130, Linköping, Sweden.

Ekstrand, J. (1989a) Reconstruction of the anterior cruciate ligament in athletes, using a fascia lata graft: a review with preliminary results of a new concept. *Int. J. Sports Med.* **1**, 225–32.

Ekstrand, J. (1989b) Reconstruction of the anterior cruciate ligament in soccer players. *J. Sci. Football* **2**, 19–27.

Ekstrand, J. & Gillquist, J. (1982) The frequency of muscle tightness and injuries in soccer players. *Am. J. Sports Med.* **10**, 75–8.

Ekstrand, J. & Gillquist, J. (1983a) The avoidability of soccer injuries. *Int. J. Sports Med.* **2**, 124–8.

Ekstrand, J. & Gillquist, J. (1983b) Soccer injuries and their mechanisms: A prospective study. *Med. Sci. Sports Exerc.* **15**, 267–70.

Ekstrand, J., Gillquist, J. & Liljedahl, S.O. (1983a) Prevention of soccer injuries. *Am. J. Sports Med.* **11**, 116–20.

Ekstrand, J., Gillquist, J., Möller, M., Öberg, B. & Liljedahl, S.O. (1983b) Incidence of soccer injuries and their relation to training and team success. *Am. J. Sports Med.* **11**, 63–7.

Ekstrand, J. & Nigg, B. (1989) Surface-related injuries in soccer. *Sports Med.* **8**, 56–62.

Ekstrand, J., Wiktorsson, M., Öberg, B. & Gillquist, J. (1982) Lower extremity goniometric measurements: a study to determine their reliability. *Arch. Phys. Med. Rehab.* **63**, 171–5.

Franke, K. (1977) *Traumatologie des Sports* (Sport Traumatology). VEB Verlag, Volk und Gesundheit, Berlin.

Fumich, R.M., Ellison, A.E., Guerin, G.J. & Grace, P.D. (1981) The measured effect of taping on combined foot and ankle motion before and after exercise. *Am. J. Sports Med.* **9**, 165–70.

Gauffin, H. (1991) *Knee and ankle kinesiology and joint instability*. Linköping University Medical Dissertations, No. 331, Linköping, Sweden.

Hlobil, H., Mechelen, W. van & Kemper, H.C.G. (1987) *How can sports injuries be prevented?* NISGZ Publication No. 25E, Medical Faculty. University of Amsterdam, The Netherlands.

Hoerner, E.F. & Vinger, P.F. (1986) Protective equipment: its value, capabilities and limitations. In P.F. Vinger & E.F. Hoerner (eds) *Sports Injuries*. 2nd edn, pp. 375–6. PSG Publishing, Massachusetts.

Jørgensen, U. (1984) Epidemiology of injuries in typical Scandinavian team sports. *Br. J. Sports Med.* **18**, 59–63.

Jørgensen, U. (1989) *Implications of heel strike — an anatomical, physiological and clinical study with focus on the heel pad*. Linköping University Medical Dissertations, No. 284, Linköping, Sweden.

Keller, C.S., Noyes, F.R. & Buncher, C.R. (1987) The medical aspects of soccer injury epidemiology. *Am. J. Sports Med.* **15**, 105–12.

Kraus, J.F. & Burg, F.D. (1970) Injury reporting and recording. *JAMA* **213**(3), 438–444.

Möller, M., Ekstrand, J., Öberg, B. & Gillquist, J. (1985) Duration of stretching effect on range of motion in lower extremities. *Arch. Phys. Med. Rehab.* **66**, 171–3.

Nilsson, S. & Roaas, A. (1978) Soccer injuries in adolescents. *Am. J. Sports Med.* **6**, 358–61.

Pardon, E.T. (1977) Lower extremities are the site of most soccer injuries. *Phys. Sports Med.* **6**, 43–8.

Stover, G.N. (1979) A functional semi-rigid support system for ankle injuries. *Phys. Sports Med.* **7**, 71–18.

Sullivan, J.A., Gross, R.H. & Grana, W.A. (1980) Evaluation of injuries in youth soccer. *Am. J. Sports Med.* **8**, 325–7.

Tegner, Y. (1985) *Cruciate ligament injuries in the knee. Evaluation and rehabilitation.* Linköping University Medical Dissertations, No. 203, Linköping, Sweden.

Tropp, H. (1985) *Functional instability of the ankle joint.* Linköping University Medical Dissertations, No. 202, Linköping, Sweden.

Tropp, H., Askling, C. & Gillquist, J. (1985) Prevention of ankle sprains. *Am. J. Sports Med.* **13**, 259–62.

Chapter 20

Injuries in Baseball and Softball: A Study of Preventive Measures

DAVID H. JANDA

'Injury is probably the most underrecognized major public health problem facing the nation today, and the study of injury represents unparalleled opportunities for reducing morbidity and mortality and for realizing significant savings in both financial and human terms — all in return for a relatively moderate investment.'

(National Academy of Sciences)

The above statement, now 6 years old, continues to ring hollow in most medical research facilities in North America. All causes of injury have been estimated to kill more than 142 000 Americans each year and cause more than 62 million people to require medical attention annually (National Committee for Injury Prevention and Control, 1989). Injuries are the greatest single killer of people aged 1–44 years and cost the USA approximately $US133.2 billion each year (Rutherford & Miles, 1981). The United States Consumer Product Safety Commission has reported 5 million medically treated injuries associated with 15 of the most popular sports in a 1-year time period (Rutherford & Miles, 1981). In addition, the Consumer Product Safety Commission conducted a study on sports injuries in children between 5 and 14 years of age. The study found more baseball-related fatalities in the 5–14-year-old age group than for any other sport (Rutherford *et al.*, 1984). In a follow-up study, 51 baseball-related deaths of children were documented (Consumer Product Safety Commission, 1983–1989). The most frequent type, 21 cases in total, involved impact of a ball to the child's chest. Of those fatalities, 11 occurred during organized games and the remainder in unorganized recreational play. The Consumer Product Safety Commission has since reported another 11 deaths in children secondary to chest impact from a ball between 1983 to 1990 (Rutherford, 1991). Thus, it is an understatement to say, that sports injuries are an enormous public health problem that continue to use up limited health-care financial resources.

It has been estimated by the National Electronic Injury Surveillance System of the United States Consumer Product Safety Commission that softball and baseball are two of the main sports leading to emergency-room visits in the USA. Between 1983 and 1989, the Consumer Product Safety Commission documented 2 655 404 injuries sustained by individuals playing either softball or baseball (Consumer Product Safety Commission, 1983–1989). Although this figure is an underestimate, because it does not include non-hospitalization visits to the physician, it does indicate the magnitude of the current problem. As the fitness-consciousness level of recreational athletes across the USA has been raised, a large number of individuals play softball and baseball, the most popular team sports in the USA. In fact, it has been estimated by the American Softball Association that 40 million individuals nationally participate in organized softball leagues, playing an estimated 23 million games·year^{-1}. It has also been estimated that 18 million children and young adults are involved in youth baseball, pony league baseball, Babe Ruth baseball and high school baseball. In addition to the participation of individuals at a recreational level, a higher echelon of baseball has developed. This higher echelon consists of individuals playing at the college and professional levels, which include minor and major league baseball. The National Collegiate Athletic Association (NCAA) has 712 teams involved in intercollegiate baseball. In addition, in the professional ranks there are 26 major and 168 minor league teams participating in the highest skill level of baseball.

The cost of a sport-related injury, either recreational, semiprofessional or professional, can be categorized into short- and long-term expenditures. The short-term expenditures include acute medical care costs, time lost from work and expenses related to the injured player's employer concerning replacement or lost production. Long-term expenditures include medical care costs, restriction of future athletic activities, permanent functional impairment and escalating insurance premiums for the injured player, his or her employer, the field owner and the softball or baseball league itself (Janda, 1990). The associated costs of these injuries can be staggering; for financial reasons alone, therefore, prevention is of utmost importance.

Injury prevention is a major public health issue throughout the world. The work place, consumer products and public services are all governed by regulations designed to protect the individual from unnecessary risks. In addition, athletes are also governed by rules and equipment regulations designed to prevent injuries during competition. An athlete's risk of sustaining a sport-related injury is influenced by several factors. High-impact sports, such as American football, place the athlete at an increased risk of musculoskeletal trauma. Governing rules that regulate the games can modify injury patterns. An example has been borne out with restricting pitching times in Little League baseball. Strict enforcement of rules by vigilant officials can foster the safety of the players and greatly reduce the threat of injury (Janda, 1990).

It is difficult to control and regulate adherence to safety rules in recreational athletics, even when games are officiated. As a consequence, passive preventive measures that do not depend on the athlete, referee, level of competition or skill should be incorporated into the sport. Examples of extrinsic or passive preventive measures in sports include using protective eye wear during racquet sports as illustrated by Pashby *et al.* (1982) and head gear during batting.

In the USA, the vast majority, if not the entirety, of physicians' training focuses on treatment and rehabilitation of the injured individual. Little, if any, attention is given to the development of a preventive approach to a problem, let alone an emphasis on the skills needed to evaluate a problem from a preventive approach. This chapter highlights the aetiology of injuries associated with softball and baseball, which has previously been identified as the leading cause of sport-related emergency-room visits in the USA. In addition to highlighting the aetiology of injuries occurring in organized recreational league softball and baseball play, we will focus on previous preventive studies and the methodologies employed which have been instituted in the USA to curb the alarming rate of injuries secondary to softball and baseball.

Treatment of upper and lower extremity traumatic injuries sustained in softball and baseball will not be the focus of this chapter. Many articles have been written in reference to treatment of ankle, knee, shoulder, elbow, wrist and finger injuries (Nichols & Hershman, 1986, 1990). To our knowledge, there have been very few studies on the preventive aspect of these injuries and we would like to focus our attention on those that have been done. If preventive efforts truly have an impact, the need for treatment would be drastically reduced (Janda *et al.*, 1992a).

Aetiology of injuries

Prior to implementation of any preventive measures, the aetiology and distribution of injuries must be ascertained. Softball-related injuries can be grouped into four categories: (i) sliding-related injuries; (ii) collision-related injuries, such as person vs. person, person vs. stationary object (e.g. back stop or fence) and ball vs. person; (iii) falls sustained by the player; and (iv) overuse injuries due to poor conditioning and training or lack of warm-up (such as medial epicondylitis of the elbow, rotator cuff tendinitis and hamstring tendinitis).

In a previous retrospective study conducted by Janda *et al.* (1986) sliding-related injuries were found to comprise 71% of all softball-related injuries sustained in a recreational softball league at the University of Michigan. The majority of the injuries sustained in this retrospective study were to the ankle and foot as the lead extremity impacted the stationary base. Table 20.1 illustrates injury patterns found in recreational baseball caused by a sliding mechanism. In numerous organizations' rule books throughout the USA, it has been stated that the bases may be up to 12.7 cm (5 in) in height and they must be secured to the ground. The standard base used throughout the USA is bolted to a metal post and sunk into the ground and concrete. It takes 4.75 kJ (3500 ft lbs) of force to separate the white portion of the exposed base from its moorings. The common denominators in the sliding-related injuries were found to be poor musculoskeletal conditioning, poor technique, occasional alcohol consumption and, above all, a late decision to slide (Janda *et al.*, 1986). The cost of these traumatic injuries were found to be significant both in the short and long term. The costs consisted of lost wages, restriction of future athletic activities and long-term functional impairment. The unexpected costs of the traumatic events were investigated in order to facilitate and emphasize the discussion of their prevention. The costs of injury

Table 20.1 Sliding-related injuries, 1986–1987.

	Number of injuries	
Type of injury	Stationary bases	Break-away bases
Ankle sprains	18	1
Ankle fractures	6	1
Skin abrasions	5	
Knee, MCL sprain	3	
Knee, ACL tear	2	
Tibia/fibula fractures	1	
Shoulder subluxation	1	
AC joint injury (type 1)	1	
Wrist fractures	1	
Wrist sprains	1	
Foot contusion/sprain	1	
Finger ligament injury (volar plate)	1	
Finger dislocation	1	
Finger fracture	3	
Total	45	2

AC, acromioclavicular; ACL, anterior cruciate ligament; MCL, medial collateral ligament.

to the player, his or her employer and the sponsoring softball organization itself were found to be significant. For example, athletic knee injuries are common, and can pose high morbidity for participants. The average cost for a knee ligament injury treated in a university hospital setting was between $US300 and $US500 (Janda *et al.*, 1988a). If the traumatic knee injury necessitated a reconstruction such as an anterior cruciate ligament reconstruction, this figure rapidly escalated to between $US7000 and $US10 000, again treated in a university hospital setting. It should be noted, these figures did not include the time lost from work and future functional impairments.

In a prospective investigation of slow pitch softball injuries occurring in the military, 25% of the injuries were caused by jamming or collision and 17% were due to falls sustained by the athlete. Wheeler (1984) found that jamming injuries to the upper extremity when struck by a ball are caused by lack of hand–eye coordination and concluded that there did not appear to be any way of preventing these injuries other than practice and good coaching. Further preventive efforts in regard to collisions include improved padding of back stops and immobile objects, such as the outfield walls and dugouts. The most appropriate preventive measure with regard to falls includes meticulous maintenance of playing fields to prevent individuals from stumbling into holes or over roughened areas.

In addition, a multitude of overuse injuries secondary to participation in softball and baseball have been described. The vast majority of these injuries can be attributed to poor conditioning, poor training or lack of an appropriate warm-up period prior to play. This pattern of injuries can affect the upper extremities as well as the lower extremities. One of the more common aetiologies of overuse injuries is related to throwing. Examples include medial epicondylitis of the elbow and rotator cuff tendinitis. The best preventive techniques involve applied commonsense, as well as comprehensive training and conditioning programmes related to all levels of play. In addition, restriction of pitching times and number of pitches has led to a reduction in the number of overuse injuries.

Preventive research

As outlined in the previous section in reference to collision injuries, deformable walls and padded back stops and field maintenance will prevent the majority of injuries secondary to collisions and falls. Better coaching techniques will reduce the number of player versus player collisions. Several measures have been undertaken in the Ann Arbor, Michigan area to prevent sliding-related injuries. In the second and third phases of a study by Janda *et al.* (1988a, 1990) various options were tried in order to prevent sliding-related injuries from occurring. It was found that making sliding illegal was impractical, since giving up sliding was unacceptable to the participants. Instructional courses were then offered; however, few of the recreational athletes attended. Recessed bases, such as a home plate, are a viable alternative; however, umpires objected because poor visualization made safe versus out calls an overwhelming problem. These solutions did not deal with the problem of indecision in the mind of the base runner, poor musculoskeletal conditioning, occasional alcohol consumption and a desire to impress one's team mates and fans. Considering these factors, it was felt an altered base design, such as a quick-release or break-away base, would provide a practical, reliable and cost-effective means of reducing sliding injuries. Because most injuries occur during rapid deceleration against a stationary base, quick-release bases were chosen to modify this mechanism of injury (Janda *et al.*, 1990).

Break-away bases were placed on half the softball fields at the University of Michigan. The break-away bases used were the Rogers Break-Away Base (Rogers Sports Corporation, Elizabethtown, Pennsylvania) (Fig. 20.1). Each set of three bases costs $US400 (1993 prices), which is twice the cost of a standard set of stationary bases. It should be noted that each set of break-away bases lasted four times as long as the standard stationary bases previously used at the university. The Rogers break-away system consists of a rubber mat which is flush with the in-field surface and is anchored into the ground by a buried metal post similar to that used with standard stationary bases. Rubber grommets arise from a rubber mat which attaches to anchoring sockets on the under surface of the break-away portion of the base. This particular system is available in four models (youth, teen, adult and professional), each differing in the amount of force needed to cause the base to break away and in the consistency of the top portion of the base (i.e. the youth model is less rigidly held and breaks away more easily than the teen, adult or professional models). The adult model, which we used, required 0.95 kJ (700 ft lbs) of force for the break-away portion of the base to release, or 20% of the force necessary for a stationary base to disassemble. Base sliding injuries that occurred on the study fields were documented by field supervisors and follow-up was performed by one of the authors. In addition, local hospital emergency rooms, the student health service and private practice orthopaedic surgeons were requested to keep logs of patients if they were injured on the study fields; these patients were also seen in follow-up by the authors.

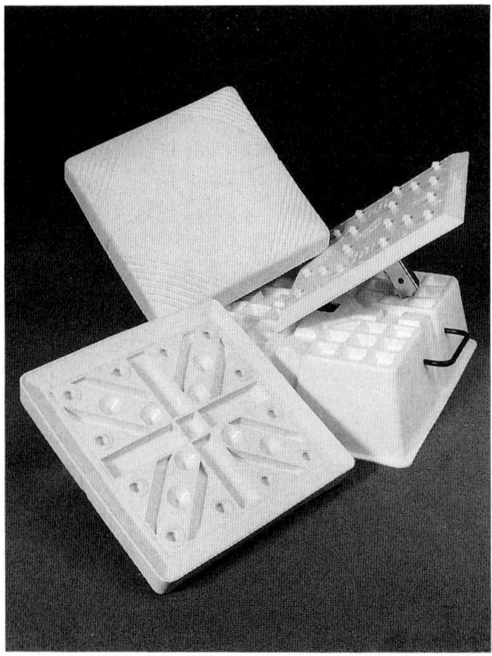

Fig. 20.1 The Roger's Break-Away Base utilized in preventive studies in Ann Arbor, Michigan.

In the second phase of the study (Janda *et al.*, 1988a), 633 games were played on break-away base fields and 627 games were played on stationary base diamonds in the Ann Arbor summer league. The players ranged in age from 18 to 55 years and included college students, labourers, executives and physicians. Teams were assigned to one of four leagues based on skill level and previous experience. Women participated in a co-ed league. Teams were assigned to playing fields on a random and rotating basis. All fields were maintained in the same manner and all experienced the same weather conditions. During the two seasons, a total of 45 sliding injuries occurred on the stationary base fields, while only two sliding injuries occurred on the break-away base fields, a 96% reduction in injuries. This difference was statistically significant ($P < 0.001$). Of the 45 injuries sustained by players sliding into stationary bases, 43 involved the lead foot or hand. The distribution of ankle injuries sustained on the stationary base fields is shown in Table 20.1. Ankle injuries predominated, accounting for 24 of the 45 total injuries.

The total medical charges for these 45 players was approximately $US55 000 ($US1223 per injury). Two other players were injured when they tripped over the stationary bases as they ran around the diamond. One of these players sustained an ankle fracture and the other a scaphoid fracture. However, these injuries were not included in the analysis, as they did not occur as a result of sliding, and we were unsure whether break-away bases could have prevented these injuries from occurring. Two isolated injuries occurred on the break-away bases; a nondisplaced medial malleolar ankle fracture and an ankle sprain. The total medical charges for these two players was approximately $US700 ($US350 per injury). It should be noted that in these two sliding injuries, the bases did not break away.

The director of field supervisors was interviewed 2–3 times each month during the study concerning experiences with the break-away bases. The field supervisors felt that softball play was not significantly delayed with the use of break-away bases, even though sliding players broke away the bases up to six times during each game. Properly seated break-away bases did not detach during routine base running. The umpires did not have any difficulty with judgement calls (safe versus out) when the bases released. For continuation of play circumstances, when the break-away portion of the base did break away, the rubber mat that was flush with the in-field service was considered the base when determining if the runner was safe or out.

Finally, in the third phase of the study, a follow-up 1035 games were played on fields that had all been switched over to break-away bases (Janda *et al.*, 1990). The same surveillance system was utilized. Two injuries occurred during the study period. Each player sustained an ankle sprain that was treated with protected weight-bearing. The total medical costs for these injuries was $US400. One player sustained a lateral collateral ligament ankle sprain to his left foot which was not his lead leg. This injury was sustained as the player caught his cleat on the ground; he never reached the base. The second injured player sustained a deltoid ligament sprain to her lead foot while sliding into the base.

These prospective studies support the concept that modifying the bases can alter the frequency of sliding injuries. An analysis of the injury rates reveals that one injury occurred in every 13.9 games (7.2%) on stationary base fields, while on the break-away base fields, one injury occurred every 316.5 games (0.3%) in phase 2, and every 517.5 games (0.19%) in phase 3. In other words, for each sliding injury on the break-away base fields there were more than 23 sliding injuries on the stationary base fields. It should be noted, even with break-away bases, injuries still occur. Most are the result of judgement errors by the runner. Improper sliding technique, poor timing, inadequate physical conditioning and alcohol consumption contribute to sliding injuries at the recreational level of play. Break-away bases, however, can modify the outcome when these factors are involved.

In a follow-up study, 19 teams within the NCAA and professional minor league baseball utilized break-away bases for two consecutive seasons. 498 games were played on stationary bases and ten sliding-related injuries were documented. Of the ten injuries, three injuries were sustained to the knee and seven injuries to the ankle. The same teams played 486 games on break-away bases with two sliding-related injuries. Therefore, one injury was documented every 243 games on break-away bases, which translates into 0.41 injuries every 100 games on break-away bases. In regard to the stationary base injuries, one injury occurred every 49.8 games which translates into 2.01 injuries every 100 games. Therefore, an 80% reduction ($P <$ 0.05) was noted in the high-performance baseball population utilizing break-away bases (Janda *et al.*, 1993).

The quick release feature of the break-away base utilized in these studies decreases the impact load generated against the athlete's limb and subsequent trauma inflicted upon it. Sliding players come in all sizes and approach the base from all angles, so that no one preventive system can be completely foolproof. The forces generated by the trajectory athlete against the ground or other players may still be more than sufficient to result in severe injuries to the musculoskeletal system. An actuarial analysis by the Section of Epidemiology and Injury at the Center for Disease Control in Atlanta, Georgia, has estimated (based on phase 2 of the study conducted by Janda and colleagues and data from the Consumer's Power

Safety Commission) that by changing from stationary to break-away bases across USA, approximately 1.7 million injuries·$year^{-1}$ would be prevented and over $US2 billion in medical care costs·$year^{-1}$ could be saved (Janda *et al.*, 1988b).

As previously mentioned, more baseball-related fatalities occur in the USA between the ages of 5 and 14 years of age than for any other sport. The most common mechanism is impact of a baseball into a child's chest. Currently, various manufacturers have developed protective chest gear that could attenuate the forces being delivered to the chest by a baseball impact. In addition, softer baseballs have been developed for similar reasons. However, many products that claim to prevent injuries have not been independently tested, evaluated or certified.

In a study by Viano *et al.* (1992), an animal model was utilized to investigate the fatal blunt impact of baseballs to the upper torso. In that investigation, pigs subjected to midsternal blunt chest trauma by a baseball accelerated to 42.8 m·s^{-1} (95 mph) developed fatal arrhythmias including ventricular fibrillation, ventricular tachycardia and asystole. These arrhythmias are identical to the on-field events which have occurred to children after being struck by a baseball. A sharp drop-off in cardiac arrhythmias causing death was found at lower projectile speeds and survival was related to the use of ventilatory support. It was the purpose of a follow-up study to investigate the usefulness of a second experimental model, namely the biomechanical Hybrid III crash dummy, for the purpose of independently testing protective equipment in low-mass, high-velocity chest impacts from baseballs. A second purpose of the study was to determine the characteristics of impacts produced to the chest area of the crash dummy by various types of 'protective' baseballs used in combination with various chest protectors. In this study, the standard hard ball was used as a test control to compare the impact characteristics of various softer core baseballs (Janda *et al.*, 1992b).

The internal deflection and viscous response values obtained from the Hybrid III dummy showed minimal reduction in response when chest protectors were used compared to the unprotected dummy. Using a generic closed cell foam chest protector impacted by a standard hard baseball, the impact force increased between 6 and 43%, and the momentum delivered increased between 10 and 15%. When a softer core baseball was used with generic closed cell foam protection, the force measured increased between 15 and 58%, and the momentum delivered increased between 14 and 18%. Impact tests using the standard hardball and the softer core baseball on the unprotected chest showed minimal differences in the viscous response measured. Closed cell foam protectors, including ABS plastic hard shell-covered generic closed cell foam, had only a marginal effect in reducing levels of chest viscous response. This study concluded that the different types of softer core baseballs utilized in this study had no appreciable protective effect and in some cases may exacerbate the impact force of a baseball to the chest. In addition, chest protectors and the various types of chest protector materials studied had minimal protective effects and may also exacerbate the impact force to the chest. Therefore, to date, no effective preventive approach has been developed to eliminate or reduce chest injuries from baseball impact in the paediatric population (Janda *et al.*, 1992b).

In a recently published study focusing on head impacts with both standard hard baseballs and softer core baseballs, Hybrid III crash systems were utilized. The authors found that at 95 km·h^{-1} (60 mph) the risk of head injury with a hard ball was 20% and between 12 and 16% with a softer core ball. The study concluded that, in reference to head impacts, softer baseballs do decrease the risk of injury, but not to the extent claimed by the manufacturers (Viano *et al.*, 1993).

Implementation of preventive research

On the one hand, research directed towards documenting the efficacy of preventive measures in sports seems to be logical, straightforward and relatively simple. Unfortunately, this is not the case at present. Even with well-substantiated studies, the enforcement of protective rules and utilization of protective equipment continues to be shunned by the athletic community at large. Tradition has been one of the major obstructions to introducing new rules or equipment to prevent injuries. Implementing equipment changes such as break-away bases may offend the traditionalist and undermine traditional aspects of the sport. In addition, other obstacles such as ignorance or lack of recognition of safety measures can delay or block instituting preventive measures. Unfortunately, the general public may be misled in regard to prevention, if unethical promotion of products by the business community is allowed. Furthermore, implementation of some protective equipment may be expensive and resisted by communities, schools and organizations, since they must absorb the additional cost without benefiting directly from reduced insurance premiums (Janda, 1992).

It is of paramount importance that citizens, organizations, and most importantly, physicians, researchers and other health-care professionals maintain persistent pressure on all organized sports groups, school leagues, city leagues, professional and college sports to consider and promote improved equipment, safer techniques and preventive measures. The cornerstone to diminished injuries consists of a safer environment for the recreational softball and baseball player to participate in. A safer environment consists of well-maintained fields and facilities, padded walls and back stops, a good stretching programme prior to commencement of play, a comprehensive conditioning and techniques programme, a reduction or cessation in alcohol consumption and the utilization of break-away or quick-release bases.

References

Consumer Product Safety Commission (1983–1989) *Product Summary Reports*. National Electronic Injury Surveillance System, Washington, DC.

Janda, D.H. (1992) Prevention has everything to do with sports medicine. *Clin. J. Sports Med.* **2**, 159–60.

Janda, D.H., Hankin, F.M. & Wojtys, E.M. (1986) Softball injuries, cost, cause and prevention. *Am. Fam. Phys.* **33**, 143–4.

Janda, D.H., Maguire, R., Mackesy, D., Hawkins, R.J., Fowler, P. & Boyd, J. (1993) Sliding injuries in college and professional baseball. *Clin. J. Sports Med.* **3**, 78–81.

Janda, D.H., Viano, D.C., Andrzejak, D.V. & Hensinger, R.N. (1992b) An analysis of preventive methods for baseball-induced chest impact injuries. *Clin. J. Sports Med.* **2**, 172–9.

Janda, D.H., Wojtys, E.M., Hankin, F.M. & Benedict, M. (1988a) Softball sliding injuries. A prospective study comparing standard and modified bases. *JAMA* **259**, 1848–50.

Janda, D.H., Wojtys, E.M., Hankin, F.M. & Benedict, M. (1988b) Softball sliding injuries — Michigan 1986–1987. *Morbidity and Mortality Weekly Report* **37**, 169–70.

Janda, D.H., Wojtys, E.M., Hakin, F.M., Benedict, M.E. & Hensinger, R.N. (1990) A three phase analysis of the prevention of recreational softball injuries. *Am. J. Sports Med.* **18**, 632–5.

Janda, D.H., Wold, D.E. & Hensinger, R.N. (1992a) Softball injuries — Aetiology and prevention. *Sports Med.* **13**(4), 285–91.

National Academy of Sciences (1988) In *Injury Control*, p. 7. National Academy Press, Washington, DC.

National Committee for Injury Prevention and Control (1989) Injury prevention: Meeting the challenge. *Am. J. Prevent. Med.* **3**(Suppl.), 1.

Nichols, J.A. & Hershman, E.B. (1986) *The Lower Extremity and Spine in Sports Medicine*. CV Mosby, Toronto.

Nichols, J.A. & Hershman, E.B. (1990) *The Upper Extremity in Sports Medicine*. CV Mosby, Toronto.

Pashby, T.J., Bishop, P.J. & Easterbrook, W.M. (1982) Eye injuries in Canadian racquet sports. *Can. Fam. Phys.* **28**, 967–71.

Rutherford, G.E. (1991) *National Summit Presentation*, September 1991. National Youth Sports Coaches Association, Orlando, Florida.

Rutherford, G.E., Kennedy, J. & McGhee, L. (1984) *Hazard Analysis; Baseball and Softball Related Injuries*. United States Consumer Product Safety Commission, Washington, DC.

Rutherford, G.E. & Miles, R. (1981) *Overview of Sports Related Injuries*. United States Consumer Product

Safety Commission, Washington, DC.
Viano, D.C., Andrzejak, D.V., McCleary, J. & Janda, D.H. (1993) An analysis of baseball head impacts — hard baseballs vs. softer core baseballs. *Clin. J. Sports Med.* (in press).
Viano, D.C., Andrzejak, D.V., Polley, T.Z. & King, A.I. (1992) Mechanism of fatal chest injury by baseball impact: Development of an experimental model. *Clin. J. Sports Med.* **2**, 166–71.
Wheeler, B.R. (1984) Slow-pitch softball injuries. *Am. J. Sports Med.* **12**, 237–40.

Chapter 21

Injuries in Basketball

JEFF MINKOFF, BARRY G. SIMONSON, ORRIN H. SHERMAN AND GREGG CAVALIERE

Basketball differs from other sports in that it originated in the USA and then disseminated to other countries. It also, with few exceptions, demonstrates an apparently different anthropometry than other sports; its élite participants being extremely tall as a rule (well over 2 m) and thin. Its anthropometry may have a bearing upon the nature of the more commonly observed afflictions among basketball players. The majority of injuries are derived from contact in one form or another. About 75% of injury occurrences in the National Collegiate Athletic Association (NCAA) were attributable to contact with another player, playing surface, backboard, rim or board posts, while 25% were independent of any contact (1990). Included in the latter group are many significant injuries which derive from the repetitive performance of the complex and ballistic movements that characterize the sport.

A report from the US Consumer Product Safety Commission indicated that just under 0.5 million people were seen in emergency rooms for injuries sustained in non-recreational basketball in 1989 (Chandy & Grana, 1985). The frequency of injuries sustained by élite competitors, with which this report is primarily concerned, is even greater than that observed in the recreational population. There are some basic differences between professional and amateur (collegiate, Olympic and high school) basketball that enhance the exposure of professionals to injury. One is the length of the game, professional games being 48 min versus 40 min for college and 32 min for high-school games (Hollander & Sachare, 1989). Practices are more frequent, intense and of longer duration in the professional ranks. National Basketball Association (NBA) professionals play many more games per season (80 versus 30 for collegians). The 24-s clock accelerates the speed of the professional game and they play more years than high-school/collegiate players, thus incurring extra wear and tear. Not infrequently, amateur players with apparent physical tolerance for basketball, succumb to injuries and overuse afflictions when subjected to the more intense, protracted schedules of the professional game.

Interestingly, NBA players with 2–7 years experience average 1.8 injuries·player^{-1}·year^{-1}, whereas players with an NBA experience of 10–15 years average 2.6 injuries·player^{-1}·year^{-1}. Rookies averaged 1 injury·player^{-1}·year^{-1} (NBTA, 1989). These figures do not account for exposure (minutes played), position, occurrences in the same player in a given year, or other important variables. Nevertheless, the trend would suggest that the longer a player is in the league the more likely he or she is to sustain an injury. Rookies may have lower incidences by virtue of less accrued or degenerative damage and a reduced exposure time.

The basketball court and injury

Few injuries are directly attributable to the basketball court *per se*. The dimensions of the court are of little import other than as it relates to the amount of running done per game (see stress fractures). The backboards are suspended by cushioned poles into which players may impact on occasion. The backboards (often plexiglass) can shatter, but without a known production of injuries. The basket rims are an unheralded source of injury for players who dunk the ball (see hand and wrist injuries).

A single season incidence of injuries ascribable to the rim and backboard in the NBA (1990) was a mere 0.2%. This is probably a lower than actual incidence, many of the injuries not being evident at the time of impact. To reduce such injuries, break-away rims were initiated into the NBA in the mid-1980s.

Playing surface

The floor of the court is a recognized source of injury. Floor surface materials range from asphalt to parquet wood floors. Injuries sustained as a result of direct contact with the floor (especially of knees, elbows, hands and wrists) are evident at the time of occurrence. More subtle and more speculative in derivation are injuries of attrition and overuse, such as stress fracture, to which floor resilience may be a contributor of some measure in a game of incessant running and jumping.

The human body and its tissues resonate in a frequency of range known to bioengineers. This has led to an ability to construct athletic playing surfaces with resonating frequency ranges harmonious to those of human tissues.

McMahon and Green (1979) demonstrated that an enhanced performance and fewer injuries resulted among runners using a running track tuned to the elastic characteristics of the human body. Shorten (1987) has likened the muscle–tendon unit to an elastic spring, and the body to a type of mass spring, both manifesting natural frequencies of vibration. When the forces acting upon the body are at the same frequency, the result is a resonance which maximizes performance and minimizes harmful effects. The playing surface participates in these mechanics, and should be structured to accommodate to the resonant frequency of the body with respect to that activity (Shorten, 1987).

Under the auspices of the Maple Flooring Manufacturers Association (MFMA), the Drucker Research Company undertook to resolve the controversy that existed regarding the potential contribution to injury by maple wood versus synthetic floorings (MFMA, 1988). Studies of 50 secondary schools and colleges housing both floor types or having made a transition from one to the other were studied. Results of this study demonstrated that injuries were much more likely to occur on synthetic surfaces than on maple floors (63 versus 37% respectively) when basketball (45% of all injuries) as well as other sports were considered. The higher incidence of synthetic surface injuries was observed as well in the NCAA–ISS report for 1989–1990, but not nearly with the same disparity shown here. In the NCAA (1989–1990), players sustained injuries at a rate of $5.07 \cdot 1000$ exposures^{-1} on wood and at a rate of 5.47 on composite surfaces.

To date, no effort has been made to create basketball floors in compliance with the resonance frequencies of the human body.

Injuries: epidemiology and general trends

The epidemiology of disabilities produced by basketball at the élite level may be determined from several sources (Abdenour *et al.*, 1979; DeLee *et al.*, 1983; Giladi *et al.*, 1987). What is described below is largely extrapolated from three primary sources: the National Basketball Trainers Association (NBTA) annual injury report for 1989–1990 (1990), the NCAA annual injury report for 1989–1990 (1990), and the multi-year, single franchise study (Henry *et al.*, 1982).

In recent years, the NBA trainers collectively determined to record all injuries for each professional team and to submit their recordings to a central authority for computer analysis. This has come to be known as the NBTA Injury Reporting System.

In 1982, an injury surveillance system (ISS) was developed for the NCAA providing reports predicated upon a minimal sampling of participating colleges within each division (I, II and III). Hence, injuries and their patterns are expressed as a rate (e.g. projected number or incidence per 1000 participations). More specifically, injuries are expressed as a function of exposure, whereby each game or practice constitutes an exposure (but without regard to duration of the event or the individual's participation time). Furthermore, to qualify as an injury worthy of reporting, the injury must be sustained as a consequence of intercollegiate participation, must require trainer or physician attention, and must result in restricted participation for at least 1 day after the incident.

NBA and NCAA general statistics

In the NBA, approximately 40% of players are guards, 40% are forwards and 20% are centres. The preponderance of players are between 23 and 28 years of age (65%), but some are younger than 20 or older than 40 years of age. Player height peaks are most evident between 1.9 and 2.1 m (6 ft 3 in and 6 ft 11 in) (75% of all players). Player weight peaks are evident between 77 and 113 kg (170 and 250 lb) (about 95% of all players). About 70% of NBA players wear high-top sneakers and about 10% wear three-quarter height sneakers (NBTA, 1990).

In the NBA the number of injuries sustained in games was more than double the number of those sustained in practices for a single season. This resulted in an average of more than 2 injuries per player and accounted for an average of seven practices and games missed for each injury (NBTA, 1990). Henry *et al.* (1982) also observed a nearly 2:1 ratio for injuries sustained in games versus practices. In the NBA, practices are somewhat more frequent than games, but apparently (on the basis of the division of injuries) games are more intense. Indeed, Henry *et al.* (1982) state that contrary to earlier contentions, basketball is a contact sport. They cite statistics presented at the 1980 meeting of NBA physicians which revealed an average of 48 fouls and 15 considered acts of violence in games played during the previous season. Nevertheless, they concede that the incidence of 'severe' injury in basketball is quite low.

ISS statistics for the 1989–1990 NCAA men's basketball season reveal that injuries were sustained primarily in practices. However, there were almost five times the number of practices as there were games. Hence, the rate of injuries in games was almost twice that of practices (9.36–4.28 · 1000 exposures^{-1} respectively) (NCAA, 1990).

In terms of injury demographics in the NBA, almost twice as many injuries occurred at home as on the road (NBTA, 1990), potentially reflecting a greater intensity of play by the home player. Similarly in the NCAA, the incidence of injuries due to game exposures was 50% greater at home than on the road (NCAA, 1990).

In the NBA, the ratio or injuries varied little in each of the final three-quarters, but was substantially less in the first quarter (NBTA, 1990). This may represent a lesser level of intensity at the outset of the game or a less susceptible 'starting five'. It is noteworthy that the NBTA report accounts for a single year and many teams in the NBA. Interestingly, the study by Henry *et al.* (1982) of a single NBA franchise spanning 7 years corroborates a substantially lower incidence of first period injuries.

The NCAA ISS reports that injuries in the second half of games were more than 50% greater than those sustained in the first half and that injuries in the second half of practices were nearly 50% more plentiful as those sustained in the first half (NCAA, 1990). These findings would seem to imply that an insufficient quantity of fitness (cardiovascular and/or muscular) and a progression of injury inductive fatigue are significant factors in the ranks of college basketball. The alternative consideration is that an increased intensity in the second half of games and practices is responsible, but this is a less likely contention.

More than 80% of NBA injuries are acute, 14% are chronic, and 2–3% are reinjuries. Almost 65% of NBA injuries occurred in the lower extremities (NBTA, 1990).

Projections in the NCAA reveal an injury rate of a little more than $5 \cdot 1000$ exposures^{-1}, 80% of which represent new injuries, and 20% of which represent recurrences or complications of previous injuries (NCAA, 1990).

An analysis of injuries sustained by body part in the NCAA revealed the same lower extremity bias observed among basketball players in the NBA (Apple, 1988; NBTA, 1990), the combine physicals, (DeBenedette, 1991), and women's professional basketball players (Zelisko *et al.*, 1982). Injuries to the ankles predominated with a projected occurrence of $1.64 \cdot 1000$ exposures^{-1}, or about 30% of the occurrence of all qualifying injuries (NCAA, 1990). Injuries to the knee and the groin area were the next most frequent, together representing about 18% of the total (NCAA, 1990). Chandy and Grana (1985) surveyed injuries in 130 Oklahoma secondary schools over a 3-year period and found that female basketball players had a higher injury rate ($35.9 \cdot 1000$ athletes^{-1}) than male players ($26.3 \cdot 1000$ athletes^{-1}). In addition, females had more severe injuries and more knee surgeries.

In the multi-year study of a single NBA team by Henry *et al.* (1982) only 6% of all games missed could not be accounted for by an injury to or about a lower extremity joint. The study reaffirms the above listed assertions of others, that the most commonly observed injuries were those of the knees and ankles. In fact, injuries of these joints accounted for 84% of all player games missed over a 7-year period (66% knees, 18% ankles). The majority of knee afflictions were listed as patellar tendinitis, while the majority of ankle injuries were diagnosed as lateral ligament sprains.

Apart from the lower extremities, occurrence rates for injuries of the groups constituted by the lower back, the hand and wrist, and the head, eyes and nose, each represented about 7% of the total (Henry *et al.*, 1982).

Nearly 80% of NBA injuries are comprised of sprains (28%), strains (21%), contusions (18%) and tendinitis (12%). The rank order of athletically related injury sites is demonstrated in Fig. 21.1 (NBTA, 1990).

In the study by Henry *et al.* (1982), lower extremity injuries apart from those of the knees and ankles, accounted for about 14% of all injuries. More importantly, nearly three-quarters of these were accounted for by thigh

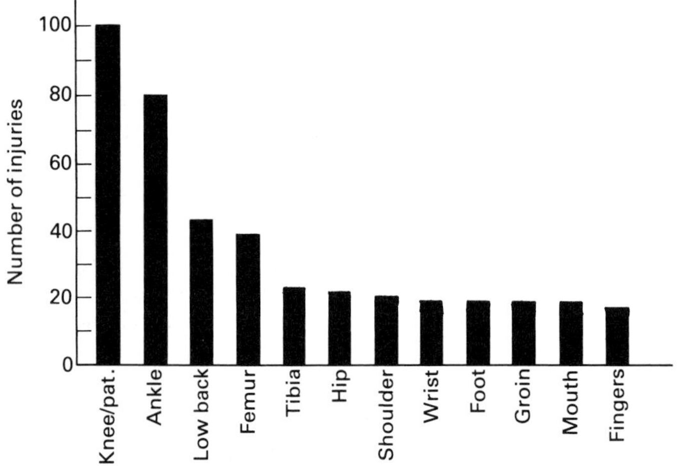

Fig. 21.1 Rank order of National Basketball Association (NBA) injuries 1989–1990. Adapted from NBTA annual injury report (1990).

contusions, which raises the issue of whether hip and thigh padding should be initiated as a prophylactic measure. Contusions of the lower extremities and back alone constituted nearly 20% of all injuries reported in the study.

Back and hip injuries represented 11.5% of all injuries in the study by Henry *et al.* (1989). The majority of these injuries were contusions. Several lumbosacral sprains were reported in this study. In a 5-year period with an NBA team, the present authors have witnessed several disc herniations, one advanced spinal stenosis, and numerous lumbosacral sprains which have accounted for several operations and many player days missed.

With respect to upper extremity injuries, Henry *et al.* (1982) reported that injuries of the shoulder girdle, most of which were contusions and strains, constituted a meagre 3% of injuries, and were responsible for only 1% of games missed. Elbow injuries, comprised primarily of hyperextensions and contusions, represented only 2% of injuries. Injuries of the wrist, hand and fingers accounted for 15% of injuries, a figure which underscores the susceptibility of exposed acral parts to injury. Injuries of the fingers *per se* represented 75% of these distal injuries, the vast majority (90%) of which were accounted for by contusions and sprains of the proximal interphalangeal (PIP) and metacarpophalangeal (MCP) joints (Henry *et al.*, 1982).

Finally, Henry *et al.* (1982) reported that the incidence of head and facial injuries was 12%, but that these injuries rarely resulted in missed player days. Nearly 80% were due to contusions and lacerations; 16% were due to facial fractures (mostly nasal and zygomatic). Flying elbows and fists are responsible for oral injuries as well. In this regard, mouth protectors are important preventive devices. 38 of the 40 oral injuries reported in the NCAA in the 1989–1990 season were in players who wore no mouth guard (NCAA, 1990).

As in the NBA, the most common injury types in NCAA basketball were sprains and strains. They represented about 40 and 20% respectively of the total projected injury rate. Contusions, fractures and overuse injuries were the next most frequent types (NBTA, 1990, NCAA, 1990). Among injuries in the NBA, fractures cost an average of 17 player days missed while strains resulted in an average loss of 9 days; and overuse injuries in an average loss of 4 days (NBTA, 1990). Almost 80% of the injuries reported in the NCAA (1989–1990) prevented a return to play for less than 1 week (NCAA, 1990).

In the NBA, correlations between position played and injury incidence reveals no position which is preselected for a general occurrence of injury. This is not true, however, for specific types of injuries as for example, cruciate tears or stress fractures (Lombardo, 1990). In the NCAA, forwards were injured about 40% more often than guards, who in turn, were injured about 65% more often than centres (NCAA, 1990). The reasons for the occurrence differential between the NBA and the NCAA is not clear. For their NBA team, Henry *et al.* (1982) noted that forwards sustained more injuries on the average ($9.8 \cdot \text{player}^{-1}$) than did guards ($8.3 \cdot \text{player}^{-1}$). The former sustained a higher proportion of upper extremity injuries, and the latter a higher proportion of lower extremity injuries.

On the whole, the statistical data provided by the NCAA's ISS and the NBTA's injury reporting system are of interest and value. Unfortunately, these systems have not regression correlated the multiple variables for which data is reported. Hence, there is only limited insight provided toward a comprehension of specific trends and associations.

Career-threatening injuries

As already indicated, injuries in competitive élite basketball players are reasonably abundant. The vast majority are comprised of 'commonplace' strains, sprains and contusions. Naturally, injuries which threaten the termination of a career are less abundant, but are of particular concern. Most notable among the latter injuries has been a complete rupture of the anterior cruciate ligament (ACL) with resulting instability of the knee.

ACL sprains

The number of ACL (partial or complete) ruptures in the 7-year period spanning 1983–1990 was 30 (Lombardo, 1990). This represents an average incidence of a little more than four per season, and constitutes less than 1% of all reported injuries. The distribution of ACL ruptures was as follows: 50% in forwards, 30% in centres and 20% in guards (Lombardo, 1990).

Ruptures of the ACL are usually easy to diagnose. In contact sports, such as American football, ruptures are often sustained as a result of direct contact to the knee by an opponent. Many, however, are sustained due to cutting motions which impart great stresses to the knee joint. ACL ruptures in basketball players are almost always sustained in the absence of direct contact. Rapid pivots, landing off-balance from a jump, and sudden decelerations of various forms are mechanisms which can result in rupture. The player will have heard and/or felt a pop. Pain and/or a sense of knee instability are common immediate sequelae. The development of a haemarthrosis normally ensues within hours. Examination in the absence of severe guarding will reveal a positive Lachman test (anterior displacement of the tibia at 30% of flexion), often a positive anterior drawer test (anterior tibial displacement at 90% of knee flexion), and not infrequently a positive pivot shift test to detect anterior rotational displacement of the lateral tibial plateau.

When a diagnosis of a cruciate ligament rupture exists, and when the history and physical examination are equivocal, and plain X-rays fail to substantiate the presence of instability (a bone fragment avulsed by the ligament or capsule), further diagnostic pursuits are in order. Computerized ligament testing devices (knee arthrometers) can overcome guarding and subjectivity in analysing tibiofemoral displacements. Many varieties are available. In addition, magnetic resonance imaging (MRI) is highly diagnostic of major disruptions, but more equivocal when only a portion of the ligament is ruptured. Absence of the ligament shadow or altered morphology in the form of a sag, attenuation or irregularity of contour, or bright signal replacing the normally dark band of signal void representing the ligament, are all diagnostic of ACL rupture (Fig. 21.2). MRI offers the additional advantages of demonstrating lesions of the menisci and of chondral and osteochondral fractures with a high degree of accuracy and sensitivity. There is almost never a need to consider an examination under anaesthesia or a diagnostic arthroscopy to establish the diagnosis.

Once the diagnosis has been established, a decision must be made with respect to treatment. Short-term and long-term considerations must be weighed. Whereas in gliding sports such as ice hockey, élite performance in the face of anterior knee instability (with a ligament brace) is not infrequently possible, in a running, cutting and jumping sport such as basketball, a severe curtailment of performance ability and a promise of a progressive degenerative disorder of the knee is the rule rather than the exception. If the instability is not overly severe, strengthening and use of a ligament brace may allow a continuation of play until a progression of instability and knee damage preclude reasonable performance. In almost every instance today, knee ligament repair and/or reconstruction is the best treatment choice. While such procedures offer no assurance of success and no chance for 'normality', they offer the best opportunity for achieving the most optimally functioning knee and the only real chance for longevity of performance.

In a 1991 article (Demak, 1991), it is contended that seven élite NBA players sustained and were operated upon for complete ruptures of the ACL in the past three seasons, and that an effective performance return has been the rule rather than the exception. Improved reconstructive techniques and more efficacious postoperative rehabilitation programmes have contributed

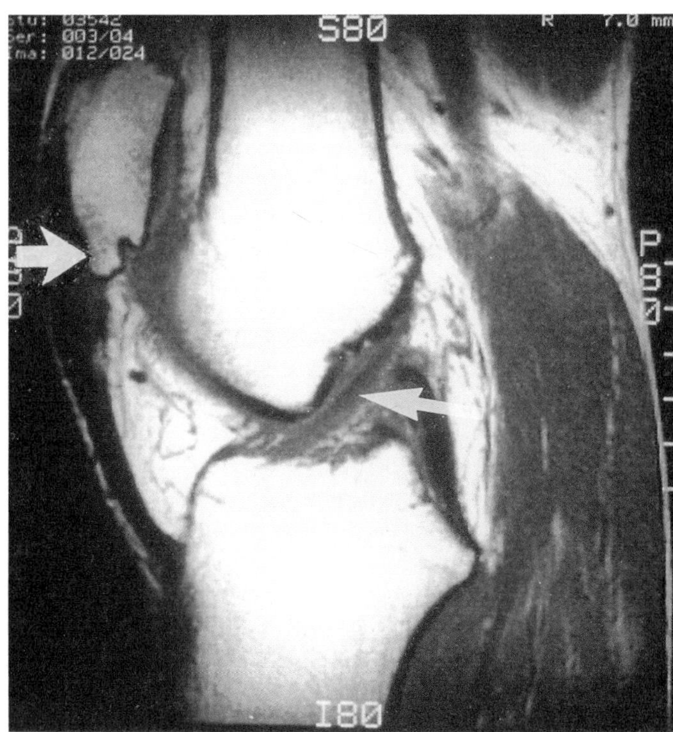

Fig. 21.2 Magnetic resonance imaging. Sagittal image of the knee of a National Basketball Association player with inferior patellar pole pain, recurrent effusions and mild tibiofemoral instability. Note the large inferior pole osteophyte (thick arrow) and the sagging, though homogeneous anterior cruciate ligament (thin arrow).

measurably to this more recent trend. Hence, the present issues regarding the ruptured ACL are not so much those regarding an ability to return to play but are those of longevity of performance, ability and the potential for arthritic degeneration. Some physicians interviewed indicated that a number of NBA players are functioning well with partial tears and have not undergone surgery. Among physicians interviewed, the most popular operative procedure was an arthroscopically assisted bone–patellar tendon–bone substitution for the ACL. After such a procedure, players are generally restrained from play for no less than a year, and until completion of a slowly evolving progression of motion, strength and agility formats, which pit therapeutic acceleration against fear of disrupting the implanted substitute.

Stress fractures

With the possible exception of ruptured cruciate ligaments, few basketball injuries are more dreaded than stress fractures. It is not that the annual incidence is dramatic. In fact, the incidence of stress fractures in the NBA during the 1989–1990 season was only 0.6% (NBTA, 1990). In a single NCAA basketball year with 92 participating colleges, and just under 150 000 exposures, stress fractures were observed at a rate of 0.07 · 1000 exposures^{-1} (NCAA, 1990). In the NBA, of course, the intensity of play is greater, the games are longer, and the number of games is greater, thereby representing a greater exposure from several vantage points.

Anyway, it is not so much the incidence as the potential severity of stress fractures, in terms of time missed, career implications and treatment options, that constitute their perils. Like cruciate ligament ruptures, stress fractures have resulted in career terminations in some élite and professional basketball players. Furthermore, among NBA players there is at least a 50% chance that at least 6 months of playing time will be lost when a stress fracture has been sustained (Haas, 1988).

An evaluation of stress fractures in any athletic population is difficult. The definition of a stress fracture, mechanism of production, and therefore, the incidence of occurrence are not matters of universal accord. The terms 'overuse', 'fatigue', 'spontaneous' and 'insufficiency' have been used in the literature as facsimiles of 'stress' and as modifiers of the word 'fracture' (Frankel, 1975; Walter & Wolf, 1977; Stanitskie *et al.*, 1978; Jackson & Strizak, 1982).

Haas (1988) cautioned that it is virtually impossible to differentiate between acute fractures and the so-called stress fractures. Jackson and Strizak (1982), Frankel (1975), Stanitski *et al.* (1978), and Taunton *et al.* (1981) are among those who debate the role of the muscles, which may provide too much force by one view, or inadequate force (and energy absorption) by another view, as mechanisms of producing stress fracture. Markey (1987) argued that in the presence of certain stresses the normal homeostasis of bone remodelling is adversely affected, a theory which was also promulgated by Taunton *et al.* (1981). In any case, it would appear that the 'certain stresses' alluded to above are comprised of combinations of exercise frequency, intensity and duration (Kavanaugh *et al.*, 1978; McBryde, 1985). This is commensurate with distance runners having the highest incidence of stress fractures (Cavanagh & Robinson, 1989). Matheson *et al.* (1987). Orava *et al.* (1978) and Taunton *et al.* (1981), relate the following range of distribution of reported stress fractures for all athletes: (i) tibia 49–54%; (ii) fibula 7–14%; (iii) femur 6–7%; (iv) metatarsals 9–18%; and (v) tarsals <1–25.3%.

This distribution is dramatically different from that noted in NBA players by Haas (1988). Haas reported 44 fractures in 36 players over a period of about 5 years, an incidence of about 3% among basketball players for that time period. Only 13% occurred in the tibia, 9% in the fibula, only 2% in the femur and over 75% of the fractures occurred in the foot. In fact, over 50% occurred in the 5th metatarsal alone and 20% occurred in the navicular. Of 86 élite college players evaluated at the annual NBA, predraft physicals in 1990, 8% were reported as having had a stress fracture of the foot sometime during their playing career. This represented 70% of all reported lower extremity fractures in this group (J.A. Hefferson, personal communication).

The distribution of stress fractures in élite basketball players, with an overwhelming concentration in the foot, is different than that observed in other sports. One is left to ponder whether this peculiarity is due to the nature of the game or due to any predisposing structuring among its participants.

It is evident that as a group, basketball players are anthropologically unique. With rare exceptions they are stereotypically tall and lean. It could be speculated that the size and structure of basketball players may play a critical role in the production of disabling lower extremity stress fractures.

Interestingly, Haas (1988) reported a disproportionate incidence of stress fractures among guards, the shortest and lightest of the players. Cavanagh and Robinson (1989) observed that guards run more than other players, averaging between 3.2 and 4.8 km (2 and 3 mile) per professional game.

Relevant sport-specific and anthropometric factors in basketball were studied by Cavanagh and Robinson (1989) in an attempt to deduce correlations between these factors and the potential for stress fractures. They used cinematographic techniques, and Hughes (1985) used biomechanical analyses to explain predisposing factors in the creation of stress fractures of the feet.

To aid their study, Cavanagh and Robinson (1989) studied players from five teams, measuring their body dimensions and the morphology, kinetics and kinematics of the feet of the players during a variety of simulated game movements. They determined that there are 13 essential movement patterns in basketball:

1 Running.
2 Cutting.
3 Lay-up take-off.
4 Lay-up landing.
5 Starting.
6 Stopping.
7 Jump shot take-off.
8 Jump shot landing.
9 Vertical jump take-off.
10 Vertical jump landing (Fig. 21.3).
11 Shuffling (Fig. 21.3).
12 Maximum vertical jump take-off.
13 Maximum vertical jump landing.

These studies revealed that professional basketball players have proportionately increased thigh and shank lengths, and shoulder and hip widths than is anticipated for the average male height. Of perhaps greater interest, since stress fractures are most common in the feet, is that the players had smaller feet than extrapolations from a population of recreationally active males; nevertheless, the heel to metatarsophalangeal (MTP) joint length was greater, and hence it was the phalanges which were relatively shortened.

Biomechanics is an important contributor. Cavanagh and Robinson (1989) cite Taunton *et al.* (1981) who noted that varus alignment in runners predisposed to stress fractures. They also cite Valiant and Cavanagh (1987), who observed that peak ground reaction forces in landing from a jump varied between one-fifth and four times body weight depending on whether landing occurred on the forefoot or flatfooted.

Cavanagh and Robinson (1989) studied ground reaction forces for each of the above 13 manoeuvres. Using force plates, jump landings from lay-ups and jump shots produced vertical forces up to seven and five times body weight respectively, far exceeding those recorded for runners. Forces for other basketball movements were also high compared to related movements in other sports.

The kinematic studies of Cavanagh and Robinson (1989) also hinted at alarming factors predisposing to injury in basketball players. In the knee, lay-up and vertical jump take-off required about 70° of knee flexion, and lay-up landings, starts and stops demonstrated knee flexion velocities of $500-600°\cdot s^{-1}$ versus less than $400°\cdot s^{-1}$ in running. Jump take-off knee extension velocities exceeded $600°\cdot s^{-1}$ versus less than $300°\cdot s^{-1}$ in running. In fact, jump shot take-offs produced the widest range of knee and ankle motion, and knee extension and ankle plantar flexion velocities. Many other potentially pertinent kinematic results were noted. Studies of pressure distribution upon the sole

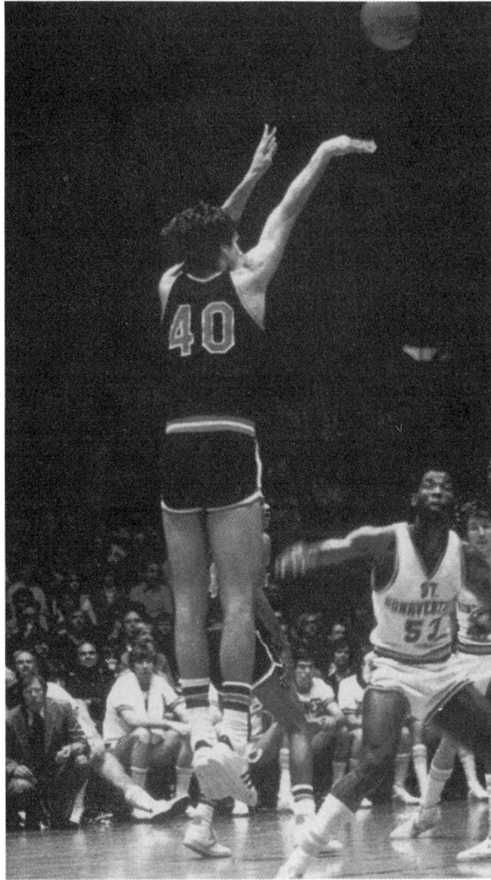

Fig. 21.3 Typical basketball movements. Player shooting the ball is 'descending from a vertical jump' while the defending player in white is posed to spring off his right leg and is 'shuffling'. Courtesy of Paul Bereswell.

of the foot revealed interesting patterns but none which specifically explain the incidence of stress fractures to the 5th metatarsal.

Gross and Nelson (1988) evaluated 11 recreational basketball players in an effort to determine if various forms of surface cushioning effectively reduced the shock of landing from jumps. The surfaces included the cast aluminum force plate, tartan rubber (as used in gymnasium floors) and one duromer of a foam used in running shoe soles. Attenuations produced by these surfaces were insignificant relative to the peak forces attributable to the natural kinematics of landing.

While stress fractures have been alleged to manifest typical patterns of symptom evolution, including prodromal pain occurring first after, and later, during activity (Walter & Wolf, 1977; Taunton *et al.*, 1981; McBryde, 1985; Markey, 1987), such warnings are not always present. Recalcitrance and recurrence patterns of stress fractures among professional basketball players have raised discussions among NBA team physicians as to whether aggressive primary treatments, including bone grafting and internal fixation, should be considered for the majority. Certainly the most feared stress fracture is that which occurs in the tibia and to which has been called 'the dreaded black hole', an anterior cortical stress fracture of the midtibia (Fig. 21.4). It is feared because of its persistence, recalcitrance to union and propensity for refracture.

As suggested above, stress fractures occupy a section in this chapter more by virtue of their recalcitrance to union and the protraction of disability for which they are notorious, than by virtue of their frequency of occurrence. Orava and Hulkko (1988) studied 369 stress fractures in competitive athletes and runners and reported an alarming 10% rate of delayed- or non-union.

On the basis of a review of 369 stress fractures in athletically active competitors, Orava and Hulkko (1988) identified the midtibia, 5th metatarsal, tarsal navicular and great toe sesamoids as preselected sites for delayed- or non-unions in the lower extremities. Also in this series of 369 stress fractures, more than half of the 37 cases with tardy or absent pro-

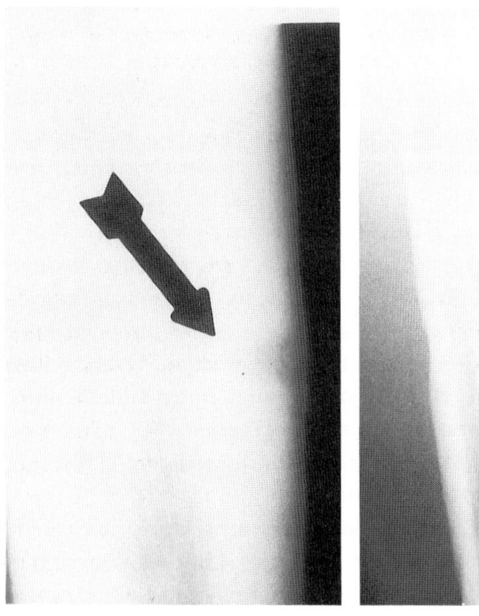
(a)

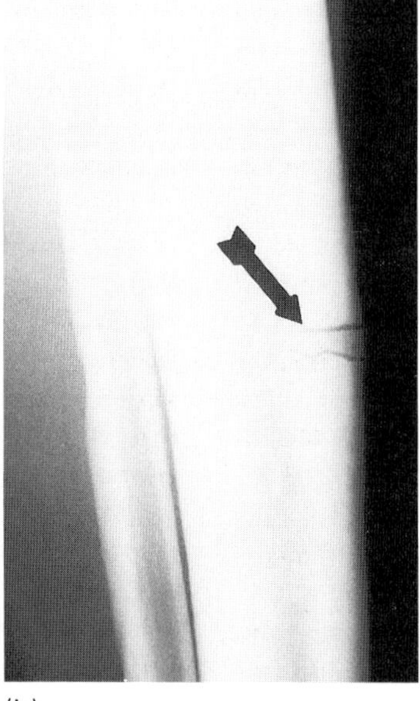
(b)

Fig. 21.4 Radiographs demonstrating progressive phases of the dreaded anterior tibial cortical stress fracture.

gression toward union required surgery, of which a return to full activity required 3–6 months postsurgery.

Probably the most controversial stress fractures dealt with by basketball physicians are those of the tibia and the 5th metatarsal. Information pertaining to these fractures is plentiful but falls short of providing adequate answers to questions of pathogenesis, prevention and management.

Stress fractures of the tibia

Devas (1958) was among the pioneers in recognizing the possible presence of tibial stress fractures as causes of tibial pain in active individuals. As early as the 1950s, he appreciated that the syndrome of 'shin soreness' consequent to running often represents a unicortical stress fracture of the tibia. In reviewing 16 tibial stress fractures diagnosed personally and 78 reported in the literature in a 'prefitness era', it was evident that virtually all such fractures occurred as a result of running, walking with loads (army recruits), and ballet in individuals between 14 and 30 years of age.

With respect to physical findings, Devas (1958) observed that tenderness is present from the outset (most often at the medial border of the tibia) but that thickening of the tissues over the site of infraction is not consistently observed until a later stage. The production of tibial pain by 'springing' the tibia (i.e. bending it over a fulcrum) is highly suggestive of stress fracture even if radiographs are non-diagnostic. In cases of the more commonly observed fracture of the posteromedial cortex, radiographs reveal proximal and lateral propagation of the fracture line. Commonly, oblique views will demonstrate evidence of new bone formation before any views demonstrate a fracture lucency (Fig. 21.5). Blank (1987) reported on five transverse tibial stress fractures, four of which were anterior, and three of which were associated with basketball; of these latter three, two were proximal (one anterior and one posteromedial).

Frequently, evidence of stress fracture is lacking on plain radiographs for weeks to months subsequent to the onset of symptoms, therefore scintimetry and other nuclear bone imaging techniques have become the definitive tests for the detection of stress fractures once their presence was suspected (Devas, 1958). The interpretations of such tests can nevertheless be misleading (Fig. 21.6).

The 1977 study of Prather *et al.* helped establish the importance of scintimetry as a diagnostic standard for the detection of suspected stress fractures. Subsequently, Holder (1982) reinforced its value for this purpose. Prather *et al.* (1977) evaluated 42 patients, virtually all males, between 17 and 35 years of age who presented with signs and symptoms suggestive of stress fracture. 50% were determined as having a stress fracture by scintimetry; 50% had negative roentgenograms at the time of scan.

The average time between symptom onset and the performance of a bone scan was just over 15 days in the study by Prather *et al.* (1977). Of equal interest was that the average delay between a positive bone scan and a positive plain X-ray was only 10.5 days.

MRI can detect the presence of stress as well as other fractures, while demonstrating morphology not demonstrable by the much more invasive nuclear techniques. Lee and Yao (1988) reported on five patients with stress fractures examined by MRI within a month of symptom onset. Early plain radiographs failed to reveal evidence of a fracture in each case. In all five cases, a low signal band representing the fracture was seen to extend various depths into the marrow from the site of cortical origin (see Fig. 21.13). T2 imaging, when performed within 2 weeks of symptom onset, may reveal juxtacortical areas of high signal, and when performed within 3 weeks of symptom onset, may demonstrate bright signal within the marrow cavity (Lee & Yao, 1988).

Tibial stress fractures derive from excessive or 'overloading' activities performed with persistence. Athletes and military trainees have

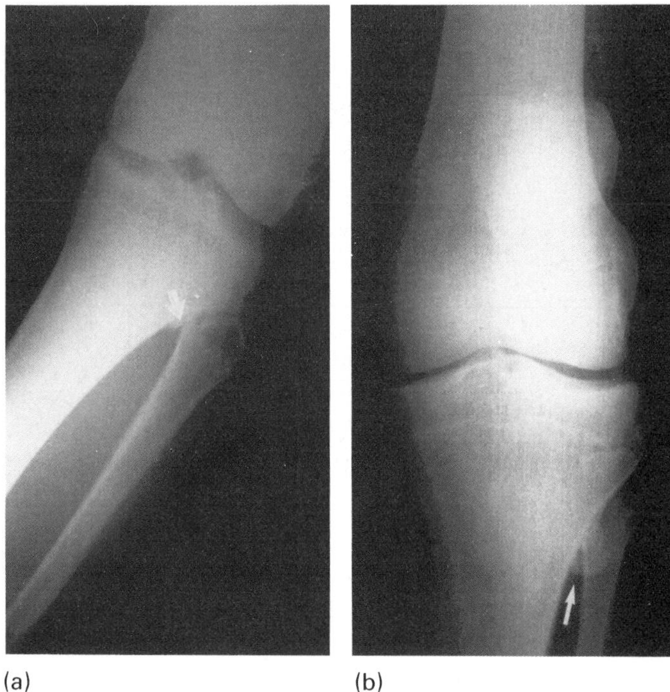

Fig. 21.5 Anteroposterior radiographs of two National Basketball Association players with ossifying responses in the proximal region of the tibiofibular membrane (arrows). (b) Player with symptoms of a peroneal neuropathy confirmed by nerve conduction studies and treated successfully by neurolyses and excision of the calcified mass. The precise aetiology of these responses is unknown.

been the prototypic victims by virtue of the running, jumping and load-bearing inherent in their daily formats.

Daffner *et al.* (1982) reported the tibial stress fracture to be the most common type among runners. Of all stress fractures, those of the tibia were found to be the most common ones in the Israeli Army (Giladi *et al.*, 1985, 1987; Milgrom *et al.*, 1988), and among the more common ones in the American Army (Protzman & Griffis, 1977). Common to the military groups is the use of extensive running and walking as part of a training programme. Scully and Besterman (1982) reported a reduced incidence of the tibial stress fracture as a result of eliminating hard surface running. Assuming the role of percussive stresses in the aetiology of tibial stress fractures, Milgrom *et al.* (1988) studied the effect of shock-absorbing boot orthotics on the incidence of occurrence, and noted no significant effect.

One factor which may influence or predispose to the occurrence of tibial stress is race. Prather *et al.* (1977) found a single Black patient with a stress fracture among the 21 stress fractures discovered; this was significant in light of the fact that more than one-quarter of the population from which the patients were drawn were Black. Prather *et al.* cite the study of Provost and Morris (1969) as providing additional evidence of a low incidence of stress fractures in Black patients. Nevertheless, American basketball suffers no lack of stress fractures among its Black players.

Few studies report the influence of gender upon predisposition to tibial stress fractures. Protzman and Griffis (1977) reported on the incidence of stress fractures among new cadets at the USA Military Academy. Both male and female cadets were subjected to exhaustive daily training sessions over an 8-week period, including a progression of running, marches with packs, calisthenics and field training. There were 12 stress fractures among 1228 males and 10 among 102 females, representing 10 : 1 female to male incidence of fractures. The tibia

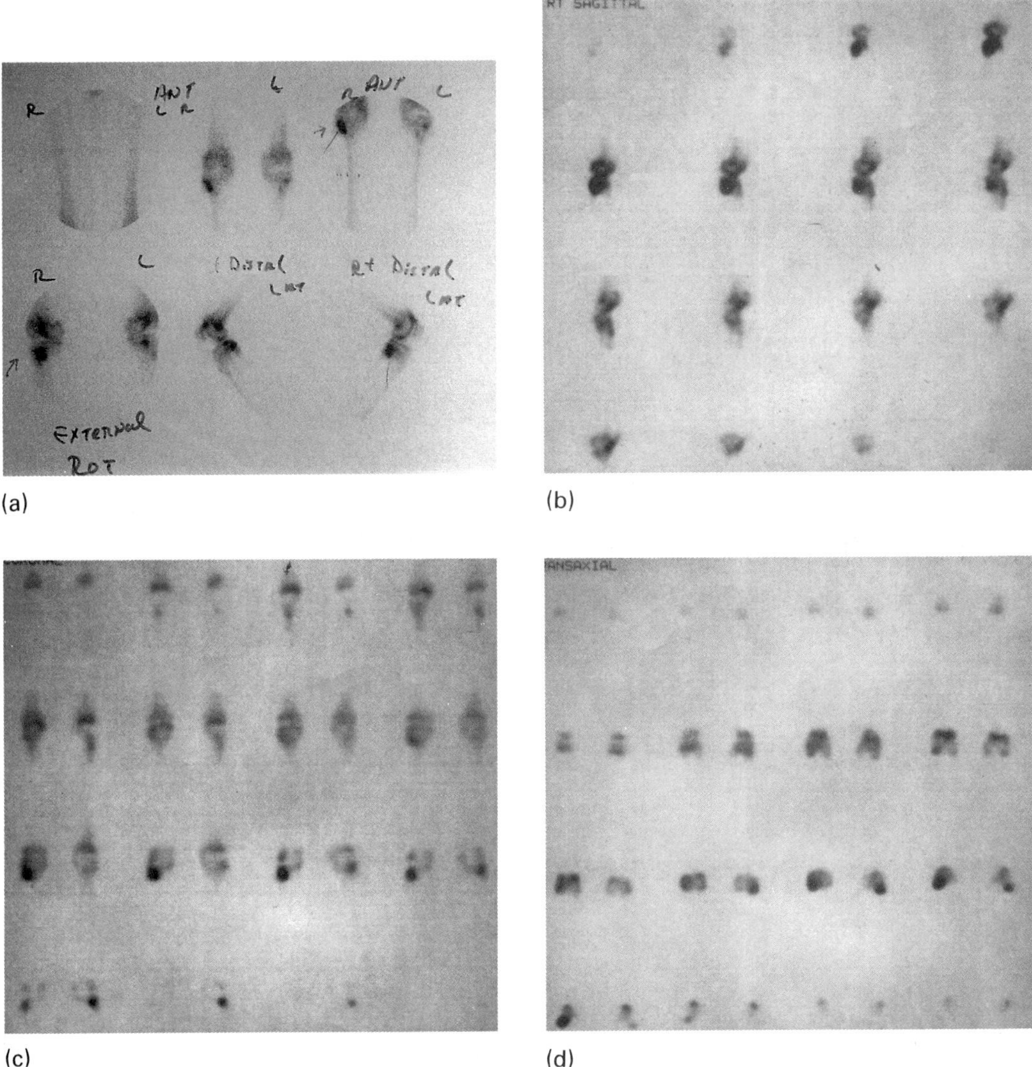

Fig. 21.6 (a) Standard technetium bone scan of the knee of a National Basketball Association player with complaints of pain near the fibular head. The scan was interpreted as having demonstrated a stress fracture of the proximal end of the fibula. (b–d) Sagittal, coronal, and transaxial SPECT (single photon emission computerized tomography) scan images of the knee of the same player 2 months later. Images demonstrate the presence of a process in the proximal portion of the tibiofibular membrane. A stress fracture was ruled out.

was the bone most frequently involved. This study may have little relevance to the gender risk of sports in which the female is not burdened with force levels conceived to substantially stress males.

A number of more sophisticated bioengineering studies have been undertaken to gain insight into kinematic and anthropometric factors of influence.

Milgrom *et al*. (1988) studied nearly 300 Israeli infantry recruits in whom the incidence of tibial stress fracture was inordinately high, approximately 20%. These workers measured the cortical and whole bone widths of the tibia in multiple planes, at their narrowest points. They found that the mediolateral width of the tibia correlated significantly with the incidence of tibial stress fractures, and conversely, that recruits with wider tibiae had a lower incidence of tibial stress fracture. They found that the area moment of inertia where the anteroposterior (AP) width of the tibia was narrowest had the greatest statistical relationship to the incidence of stress fractures in this study where almost every fracture was in the medial aspect of the midportion of the diaphysis. For fractures in this location, the bending strength of the bone about the AP axis seems to be a critical factor. In a related study, Giladi *et al.* (1987) indicated that the ratio of tibial width to the height of the subject added nothing to the significance of the study.

It is axiomatic that mechanical stresses influence the physiology and remodelling of bone, and in a like manner, that they play a key role in the production of stress fractures. Lanyon *et al.* (1975) hypothesized that a measurement of bone deformation occurring with certain activities might provide some understanding of the nature of those stresses which influence bone response. These workers implanted a rosette strain gauge on the anteromedial cortex of the tibial midshaft of a young active male of average dimensions and recorded bone deformation occurring during phases of walking and running gait. Use of a single subject and of a single discrete bone locus for the taking of measurements preclude validation of any conclusions drawn from the results. Nevertheless, it is interesting to note that the largest deformations occurred in running, and the second largest in the pre-toe-off stance phase of walking. The wearing of shoes reduced these peak deformations (Lanyon *et al.*, 1975). It may be presumed that cyclic bone deformations do occur with activity; whether these derive from the pull of the muscles attaching to the bone, from inadequacies in the shape or structure of the bone, or from other factors, and whether and how they may correlate to the production of stress fractures is not yet known.

Of what significance are the sites along the tibia at which stress fractures occur? Devas (1958) observed that the most common site for tibial stress fractures is the posteromedial cortex at the junction of the middle and lower thirds of the bone. However, beneath this general observation a pattern of specificity by which site and activity type could be correlated was recognized. Devas noted that stress fractures in 'athletes' and in recruits were observed in the proximal third of the bone. He cited Burrows' (1956) observation that all tibial stress fractures in ballet dancers were in the middle third of the bone, as was the fracture in the only ballet dancer in his personal series (Devas, 1958).

Such implications of specificity would imply additional correlations between specific sports or movement patterns and the character and spectrum of stress responses they induce. Furthermore, recognizing the stress response patterns produced by given specific activities might lead to formulated hypotheses of mechanisms of production and experimental designs to prove them.

Of the 81 tibial stress fractures discovered by Milgrom *et al.* (1988) among 286 army recruits, 88% occurred in the middle third of the tibia and 100% involved the medial cortex. The theme of specificity of activity as a correlate to specificity of stress fracture type is perhaps best demonstrated by the reports of Symeonides (1980) and Mutoh *et al.* (1980) relative to the proximal end of the fibulae.

Mutoh *et al.* (1980) reported 10 cases of stress fracture of the proximal end of the fibula due to squat jumping. In the same year, Symeonides (1980) reported a 40% incidence of proximal fibular stress fractures in military recruits subjected to a programme of squat jumps. The author contends, though without proof, that specific muscular activities produce particular types of stress fractures.

The site of a tibial stress fracture has a bearing upon prognosis with respect to a proclivity for union, length of disability, and other behavioural issues.

Green *et al.* (1985) reported that posteromedial cortical stress fractures of the proximal third of the tibia are common and usually heal without incident. They asserted that anterior cortical fractures of the middle third of the tibia are much less common and often fail to unite without difficulty (see Fig. 21.4).

Five of six anterior cortical middle third stress fractures reported by Green *et al.* (1985) went on to an acute complete fracture, three having denied symptoms prior to the completion of fracture.

As already indicated, theories concerning the aetiology of stress fractures are numerous. Most authors have implicated repetitive compressive loading. Green *et al.* (1985) indicated that anterior cortical stress fractures of the middle portion of the tibia result from tensile forces, a factor which may relate to the propensity for non-union demonstrated by these fractures.

Green *et al.*, referring to anterior cortical stress fractures, suggested casting for several months, followed by absence of union should be treated by excision of the fibrous union and bone grafting (1985).

In 1971, Friedenberg reported that 'fatigue' fractures of the tibial diaphysis are uncommon, and once diagnosed, rarely present a problem in treatment. However, he reported two cases of stress fracture of the anterior cortex of the middle portion of the tibia, both in teenagers, and both resistant to union. Persistence of symptoms and a cortical defect for more than 6 months resulted in biopsies in each case. Histopathology revealed compact bone with empty lacunae, sparse granulation tissue and no osteogenesis. It was reckoned that tensile loading was responsible for delaying or preventing union.

Brahms *et al.* (1980) discussed an anterior cortical diaphyseal tibial stress fracture in a professional football player who presented with a painless lump. He played uneventfully for two seasons before the site of the stress fracture converted to a complete, comminuted fracture without direct trauma. The authors presumed that reduced muscle strength (and a consequent reduction in energy absorption) aided and abetted tensile forces encouraging the anterior cortical fracture.

As the years and the literature progressed, it became increasingly apparent that the anterior cortical diaphyseal stress fracture of the tibia ('the dreaded black line') carried the stigmata of delayed union, non-union, refracture and a propensity for progressing to a complete fracture.

Rettig *et al.* (1988) reported eight cases of anterior cortical stress fractures of the tibia, all of which were in competitive basketball players. According to Rettig *et al.*, the typical radiographic appearance of the anterior cortical stress fracture of the tibia is best appreciated on the lateral view (see Fig. 21.4), and is characterized by a V-shaped defect, open anteriorly and variably surrounded by reactive cortical bone.

Discrete anterolateral tenderness and a palpable fibrous mass are the characteristic features on physical examination (Rettig *et al.*, 1988). Rettig *et al.* reported an average disability time (from symptom onset to return to full activity) of just over 1 year with a maximum of 19 months. One player who had healed his fracture, subsequently played in the NBA for 30 asymptomatic months before sustaining a similar fracture at a different cortical location. The majority of patients in the series of Rettig *et al.* were treated by a combination of rest, immobilization and pulsed electromagnetic stimulation (PEMS) for an average duration of 7.5 months.

Rettig *et al.* (1988) offer the possibility that increased anterior bowing of the tibia may be a predisposing cause for the tension failure to which the anterior cortical stress fracture is attributed. However, they offer no tibial angular measurements as proof.

In a recent and exceptional review of tibial stress fractures, Beals and Cook (1991) report on 15 anterior stress fractures of the midtibia to be added to the mere 36 reported cases accounted for in the pre-existing literature. Hence, the authors were able to analyse 51 such fractures in 46 patients. Of the 51 fractures, 20 (about 39%) were clearly associated with participation in basketball.

Beals and Cook summarize treatment options (Table 21.1) and the case histories of each of the 51 reported fractures. Of eight patients allowed to perform with their fractures, five ultimately fractured completely. Of those treated with rest or casting, only 38% could return to full activity without refracture after a period of 1–14 months. Of only eight patients treated with electrical stimulation and rest, six could return to full activity after an average of more than a year and two required additional treatment. Only four of 10 cases treated by excision were able to return to full activity. When grafting was added, success was minimally better. Of six cases treated by excision and drilling with or without grafting, all were able to return to full activity at an average of less than 10 months. Of all cases, only one was treated by primary intramedullary nailing; the fracture eventually united despite technical difficulties. It is not known whether anterior bowing was present at the time of nailing. Among complete fractures, unsatisfactory results were virtually guaranteed by closed treatment forms.

As bottom lines, Beals and Cook (1991) conclude that most anterior midtibia stress will heal with rest for a protracted time, but that a desire for expediency requires invasive treatment. They suggest that excision and drilling (with or without grafting) is the most successful procedure based upon their review of the literature. However, a review of their data reveals that of the mere six cases so treated, only one was a basketball player despite basketball being the sport most frequently associated with this fracture.

Table 21.1 Treatments for anterior midtibial stress fractures. From Beals & Cook (1991).

Incomplete fractures
Observation
Relative rest (activity modification/cast)
Electrical stimulation (and rest)
Excision and/or graft and/or drilling
Graft (with or without excision)
Internal fixation (plate or rod and/or graft)
Complete fractures
Closed methods (e.g. cast)
Electrical stimulation
Graft without external fixation
External fixation (plate or rod) with or without graft

Most tibial stress fractures reported have been in active individuals between 15 and 25 years of age. The importance of age is not addressed in the literature. Though targeted at non-stress isolated tibial fractures, the study by Teitz *et al.* (1980) is of interest and possible relevance to the tibial stress fracture. They studied middle and lower third tibial fractures (not of the stress variety) with an intact fibula. One-quarter of patients over 20 years of age developed a delayed or non-union. Fresh cadaver studies revealed that a tibiofibular length discrepancy results from the tibial fracture, promoting delays in union, and that the compliance of the fibular and soft tissues as an aid to length adjustment is reduced in patients over 20 years of age. Hence, in this older group, the fibula may add to the tensile forces distracting the fracture.

Iatrogenic fracture of the fibula has not been reported as a treatment for incomplete stress fractures of the tibial shaft. Professional basketball players are over 20 years of age and the compliance of their tibiofibular membranes are often compromised by calcifying or ossifying processes.

DIFFERENTIAL DIAGNOSES OF TIBIAL STRESS FRACTURES

Stress fractures of the anterior tibial cortex are the most revered, but not the only afflictions of athletes to be considered when anterior tibial pain is the presenting complaint. The lower leg segment, approximately spanning the diaphyseal length of the tibia, is subject to several common types of pain-producing afflictions in basketball players. Differential diagnoses of tibial stress fractures include anterior (and/or lateral) compartment syndromes and shin splint syndromes. Each provides a threat of protracted disability.

Compartment syndromes result when the fascial container of a muscle compartment is not sufficiently compliant to allow an increase in muscle volume with exercise without a compromise in blood flow and an excessive rise in tissue pressure. Such syndromes are most frequently observed in the anterior and lateral compartments of the leg, either as an acute or as a chronic syndrome.

Veith *et al*. (1980) studied 11 anterior compartment syndromes in seven patients, none of which were provoked by an acute trauma. The syndromes were characterized by exercise-induced tightness in the compartment muscles, dorsiflexor weakness and dorsal paraesthesias of the foot, manifestations reproducible by repetitions of resisted dorsiflexion. Fascial hernias were a commonly associated finding. Average resting compartment pressures (18 mmHg) were more than 50% greater than the average pressures of controls (11 mmHg).

Nkele *et al*. (1988) established definitive pressure parameters for the diagnosis of anterior compartment syndromes. Their studies suggested that regardless of the patient's age, the diagnosis is established when the resting compartment pressure exceeds 12 mmHg, when exercise induces compartment pain, and when with exercise, the elevated pressure does not return to the pre-exercise level within 5 min.

Measuring pressures is the only proof of the presence of the condition and surgery is the only definitive treatment if activity modifications fail to bring about resolution. There is no preventive measure known for the competitive basketball player who is obligated to a programme of continuous training and play. Once the condition is recognized, especially in cases of acute compartment syndromes, early fasciotomy can prevent necrosis of the compartment muscles, or even a Volkmann's ischaemic contracture.

In discussing a series of 61 cases of anterior and/or lateral compartment syndromes of the chronic variety, Reneman (1975) indicated that objective findings were inconsistent. Compartment tautness in conjunction with cramp-like postexercise discomfort were common features. Perhaps most alerting, however, was the presence of fascial defects in nearly 60% of cases.

Reneman suggested that compartment pressure measurements and phlebography were the most valuable diagnostic aids for the anterior compartment, but more difficult to interpret with respect to disorders of the lateral compartment (1975). He also determined that the incremental change in compartment pressure between that at rest and that at 6 min after exercise (δ P6) was a more reliable index of disease than absolute pressure levels and that a δ P6 greater than 15 cmH_2O suggested a need for surgical decompression. Phlebograms performed sequentially were considered to be abnormal when the anterior tibial veins failed to fill within 2–4 min after exercise.

Styf (1988) agreed that the diagnosis of exercise-induced anterior leg pain is difficult because of the many possible causes and the few specific signs. He evaluated nearly 100 presentations of anterior leg pain in a young population, the majority of which were thought to represent anterior compartment syndromes. All patients were studied by physical examination, compartment pressure measurements, electromyography and radiography. Nearly 50% of the subjects had periosteal symptoms with no pathology demonstrated by objective testing as would be the case with shin splints. About one-quarter of the patients satisfied criteria for an anterior compartment syndrome. Of great interest and pertinence to basketball players was the finding of superficial peroneal nerve compression in nearly 15% of the patients. Of course, such compression may accompany a proximal fibular stress fracture, ossifying responses in the proximal portion of the tibiofibular membrane, and lateral compartment syndromes. Mimics are uncommonly encountered, they have presented problems in élite basketball players with a sufficient frequency that the present authors have dealt with protracted disabilities from these entities in at least three players during a 10-year experience with professional basketball teams (see Figs 21.5 & 21.6).

The report of Goodman (1980) is of interest in light of the fact that ankle sprains are the most frequent injuries among basketball players at all levels of play. Goodman presented a case of lateral compartment syndrome as a result of an inversion ankle sprain. The syndrome was accompanied by peroneal nerve conduction delays below the popliteal fossa, and by a lateral compartment pressure elevation to 70 mmHg (versus less than 15 mmHg in the uninvolved leg). Goodman makes the point that the combination of abnormal electrophysiology and elevated compartment pressure (versus neurapraxia alone) warrants compartment decompression and debridement. He would recommend that testing for myoglobinuria be added to the tests performed by Styf (1988), since its presence is suggestive of myonecrosis.

It may be concluded that compartment syndromes are observed periodically in athletes, and that their presentation of signs and symptoms is often nebulous. Acute compartment syndromes are rarely observed, and when present, justify expedient fasciotomy. Chronic compartment syndromes are more common. Their presence is established by the performance of a reliable method of compartment manometry in pre-exercise and postexercise states. Lateral, rather than medial, compartment syndromes have been more frequently observed in basketball players by the authors, often in conjunction with ossifying processes between the tibia and fibula. Manometry reliability for the lateral compartment is more controversial than for the anterior compartment.

Electrodiagnostic testing and testing for myoglobinuria are worth considering to rule out neural damage and muscle necrosis when these entities are suspected. There are no known methods of preventing these syndromes apart from non-participation.

Shin splints must be included in the differential of tibial pain syndromes. Andrish and Work (1990) indicate that the differential diagnosis of shin splints includes the tibial stress syndrome, tibial stress fracture, periostitis and compartment syndromes. It is known, fortunately, that shin splints are not a dangerous entity as are some of its differential diagnoses. Unfortunately, and despite its frequency of occurrence, the specific pathology of this entity remains unproven. Its presence is suspected when tibial pain is focused at the posteromedial face of the tibia near the junction of its middle and lower thirds; that it is most often induced by running and jumping activities, and particularly in the wake of having initiated a new intensity of activity after a lay-off; the only certain means of reducing the symptoms is by avoidance of running and jumping for a variable period. Relative to basketball, this means that shin splints are most often experienced during training camp, after a period of deconditioning between seasons, and that the consequence is likely to be a period of disability during which training must be curtailed. Though commonly recommended, strengthening and stretching exercises, the use of cushioned athletic shoes, and various physical therapy modalities may modify symptoms, but do not consistently succeed in producing relief. Probably the best preventive measure is the maintenance of a high level of conditioning all the year round so that no dramatic alteration of activity intensity is experienced. It is vital to distinguish shin splints from a tibial stress fracture.

Lilletvedt *et al.* (1979) evaluated a group of female athletes with existing, or once existing shin splints, and compared them to a group that had never experienced shin splints. They found significant structural differences between the two groups. Those afflicted tended to have greater external rotation of the extended hip, increased ankle dorsiflexion with the knee flexed, and abnormalities in the tilts of the hindfoot joints. The implication is that the only alterable variable (other than activity moderation) relates to the foot. Orthotics may be of help in this regard.

The relevance of medial shin pain ('medial tibial syndrome') in relation to stress fractures and shin splints is not clear. Orava and Puranen (1979) determined that the medial stress syndrome was the most common entity among 465 shin pain presentations due to overuse in runners. In the absence of a positive bone scan, the authors considered release of the fascia about the posterior tibial group of muscles to be the treatment of choice. Seemingly the identical condition was termed fibro-ostosis of the crural fascia by Matsuzaki (1979), who claimed that it could be distinguished from stress fracture by an absence of radiographic findings and a dramatic response to injection of steroid.

Wallenstein (1983) suggests that shin splints, medial tibial syndrome and periostitis, are different names for the same entity.

According to E. Kramer (personal communication), head of the section of nuclear imaging at New York University Medical Center, only two entities among the differential diagnoses of anterior tibial syndromes are appreciated by nuclear diagnosticians. They are tibial stress fractures, which produce a focal response on bone scan at the fracture site, and shin splints, which produce a diffuse response of uptake about the medial and posterior border of the middle portion of the tibia. Furthermore, the natural history of progression of scan positivity in relation to length or intensity of symptoms has not been reported. The medial tibial syndrome, as it is called, is an entity nominally unfamiliar to American radiologists.

Jones' fracture

Among metatarsal fractures in the NBA, the Jones' fracture of the 5th metatarsal has been the most frequent and worrisome. Jones sustained the fracture which bears his name in 1896, and later (1902) described its characteristics. Carp (1927), Morrison (1937) and Key and Conwell (1946) each discussed its propensity for delayed or non-union (Kavanaugh *et al.*, 1978). Nevertheless, the distinction between the malevolent Jones' fracture and the innocuous avulsion fracture of the base of the 5th metatarsal was often forgotten.

In more modern literature, anatomical descriptions by Stewart (1960), and later by Dameron (1975), refocused orthopaedists to the specific attributes of the Jones' diaphyseal fracture, included among which are delayed union and a tendency to refracture.

A second confusion relates to a possible distinction between the Jones' fracture as an immediate consequence of an identifiable trauma versus as a consequence of repetitive and summating microtrauma (a so-called 'stress fracture'). The distinction relates not only to the mode of onset (including the characteristics of the initial X-rays), and to the subjects who sustain these fractures (athletes versus non-athletes), but more particularly to the prognosis and treatment attached to each.

Seitz and Grantham (1985) reported a series of Jones' fractures in non-athletes. In 74% of the 53 patients, fracture onset could be ascribed to an acute inversion injury, and in all but four cases, to a definitive traumatic episode. All cases received non-operative treatment in the form of casts or compression dressings and weight-bearing delays of days to weeks. Only two delayed unions were experienced in this group of non-athletes. Clearly the behaviour trend of the fracture in this group differs from that in the competitive athlete; the issue is why. Perhaps most striking in the series reported by Seitz and Grantham was the prevalence of acute traumatic onsets and, therefore, the presence of fresh, sharp fracture surfaces; whereas in athletes there is often a symptom and/or radiological prodrome antedating discovery of the fracture, at which time the fracture line is already widened or demonstrates evidence of intramedullary sclerosis; these factors resist a normal progression of union. Of course, other factors, such as bone mineral content, bone dimensions and the stresses imparted by ligament and tendon attachments to the bone, may prejudice the behaviour pattern of these fractures in athletes versus non-athletes.

Kavanaugh *et al.* (1978) reviewed their experience with 23 fractures in 22 patients, almost all of which were between 15 and 25 years of age. Incredibly, about 50% of fractures demonstrated delayed union and nearly 50% suffered refractures. Basketball was the sport most commonly associated with the fractures in this series; three of 10 basketball players were forced to miss an entire season while awaiting union. In conjunction with the length of disability, 75% of delayed unions were ultimately internally fixed at almost 9 months after injury.

Anatomical dissections by Kavanaugh *et al.* (1978) confirmed the observations of Jones. The fracture occurs about 0.5 cm distal to the insertion of the peroneus brevis and at or near the articulation between metatarsals 4 and 5; the latter is firmly bound by strong ligaments.

Kavanaugh *et al.* recommend intramedullary screw fixation as the treatment of choice in athletes and in instances of delayed union and recurrent fracture (1978). In their series, non-operative treatment, regardless of a participation in sports, resulted in a 66.7% incidence of delayed union.

Two-fifths of the patients in the series reported by Kavanaugh *et al.* (1978) reported a minimum prodrome of 2 weeks. Two-thirds of the initial X-rays of patients reported by Zelko *et al.* (1979) demonstrated periosteal reaction. While in the above cited series, a statistical correlation relating length of prodrome and stage of radiographic fracture progression to prognosis was not specifically determined, the reader is left with little doubt that the 'stress' type of Jones' fracture in young athletes is most likely to result in a complicated progression of healing, or in refracture. Torg *et al.* (1984) emphasize the radiographic distinction between stages of the Jones' fractures. They indicate that three categories exist:

1 Acute fractures with sharp borders and an absence of periosteal and endosteal response.
2 Fractures manifesting delayed union, characterized by periosteal and endosteal response (sclerosis) and widening of the fracture line.
3 Non-unions with complete obliteration of the medullary canal by sclerotic bone.

The series by DeLee *et al.* (1983) is the only one found by the authors in which every case reported (n = 10) was of the stress fracture variety, and in which all subjects were athletes. The authors defined their criteria for qualification as a stress fracture as follows:

1 Prodromal symptoms over the lateral aspect of the bone prior to any episode precipitating the seeking of medical attention.
2 X-ray evidence of a 'stress' phenomenon in the bone: radiolucent line, periosteal reaction, heaping up of callus and intramedullary sclerosis.

The report is fortunate in that it demonstrated uncomplicated union at an average of 7.5 weeks in all cases when intramedullary fixation was used (DeLee, 1983). It is unfortunate that there are no controls (no non-athletes, non-operative treatments or acute fracture onsets) by which to sort out the meaning of results reported in previous studies. Refracture in this athletic group was not witnessed after an average post-operative follow-up period of 14.5 months. Kavanaugh *et al.* (1978) were disheartened by refracture in several of their cases (6–12 months after injury, and after union appeared to be solid) and by jeopardy to professional careers imposed by protracted disability in five athletes. These authors concluded that immediate screw fixation of the fracture was the best treatment option for athletes. Both Kavanaugh *et al.* (1978) and DeLee *et al.* (1983) achieved good results with this technique followed by non-weight-bearing for 1–2 weeks, and then progressive weight-bearing and functional rehabilitation.

It would appear that for athletes, and especially those with 'stress' Jones' fractures, internal fixation with an intramedullary screw is the answer to a difficult problem. Whether this is so in the professional basketball player remains to be proven. Larkin and Brage (1991) indicate that screw breakage and painful hardware have been reported in the literature.

A number of other issues remained unresolved. What types of screws are ideal and why? When and should the screw be removed? What is the role of bone grafting, and is it an important consideration when severe sclerosis is seen at the fracture site? Is sclerosis mistaken for union? What is the import (*re* treatment form and prognosis) of complete fracture, especially when displacement is present?

F. Thompson (personal communication) indicates two axioms with respect to the Jones' fracture. The first is that a failure to achieve an anatomical reduction when the fracture is complete can shift or create pathological stresses to adjacent skeletal structures. The second is that the large diameter screws commonly (and appropriately) used to internally fix the Jones' fracture must be removed after apparent union to allow the internal architecture of the bone to strengthen without being stress shielded. These concepts are demonstrated in the case of one basketball player who sustained several Jones' type fractures of one foot (Fig. 21.7); his fracture was ultimately internally fixed with a medullary screw, and after apparent union, eventually recurred. The fracture was then bone grafted and unified, but due to a shift of weight-bearing, a stress fracture developed in the adjacent 4th metatarsal; this healed and recurred. Surmising the abnormal shift of forces to the 4th ray by the entire sequence of events and by the progression of exquisite tenderness under the 4th metatarsal head, Thompson performed a dorsal angulation osteotomy of the neck of the 4th metatarsal (personal communication). The player subsequently played at least two seasons in the NBA without foot symptoms. There are obviously additional answers to be sought with respect to the Jones' fracture.

Eye injuries

Eye injuries are considered in this chapter because of their potential severity and their ability to produce permanent, vision-threatening disabilities. Fortunately, their frequency is small.

The annual eye injury projection for the 1989–1990 NCAA year was only $0.1 \cdot 1000$ exposures^{-1} or about 2% of the total (NCAA, 1990). Nevertheless, eye injuries in basketball can be quite severe. While the NCAA and NBA report relatively few injuries, Jones (1989) cites the 1982 National Electronic ISS, indicating that basketball accounted for about 25% of all reported eye injuries sustained in sports, primarily in the 15–24-year age group. He cites Vinger (1985), proclaiming that the preponderance of ocular injuries sustained in basketball are due to blunt trauma from the fingers and elbows of other players (Jones, 1989). Jones cites Karlson and Klein (1986) as having found that about 75% of basketball eye injuries were caused by this mechanism (Jones, 1989). Several authors have reported optic nerve avulsions in basketball (Jones, 1989). Eye protection should be seriously considered. It was the recommendation of Jones (Benton, 1969) that all basketball players wear polycarbonate eye protectors. Its impact resistance is unsurpassed by currently competitive products, but has a nuisance liability in that it scratches easily.

Sudden death syndrome

Sudden death in young athletes has been a shocking and media-publicized event with an unwelcome frequency. Chillag (1991), citing Kuller *et al.* (1967), defines 'sudden cardiac death' as that which occurs within 24 h of the onset of the fatal event. Physically larger athletes have seemed to be the most frequent victims. In a comprehensive study of 29 such deaths among athletes by Maron *et al.* (1980), 11 of the individuals were competitive basketball players. In more than 96% of cases, death was essentially instantaneous and in about 80% it

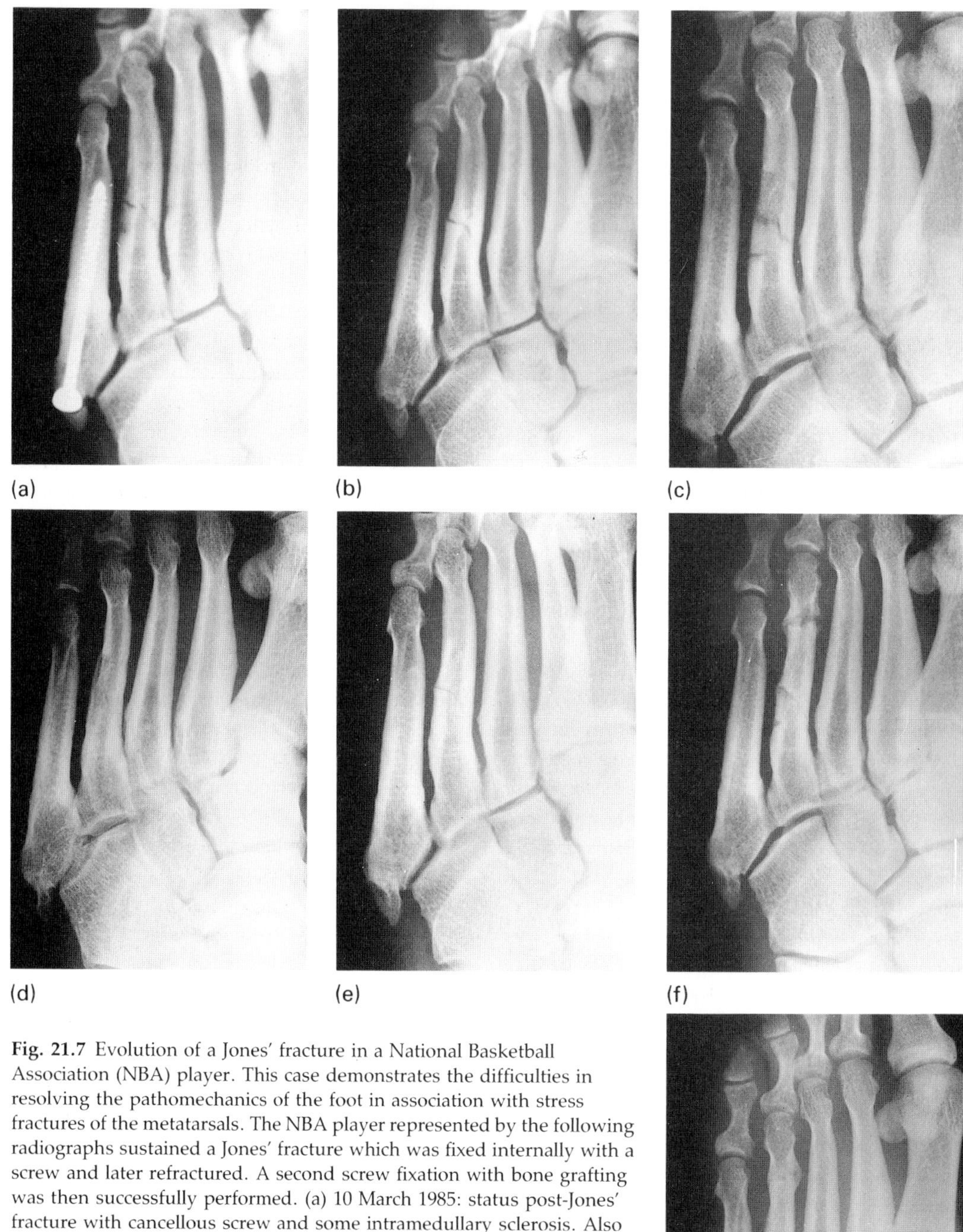

Fig. 21.7 Evolution of a Jones' fracture in a National Basketball Association (NBA) player. This case demonstrates the difficulties in resolving the pathomechanics of the foot in association with stress fractures of the metatarsals. The NBA player represented by the following radiographs sustained a Jones' fracture which was fixed internally with a screw and later refractured. A second screw fixation with bone grafting was then successfully performed. (a) 10 March 1985: status post-Jones' fracture with cancellous screw and some intramedullary sclerosis. Also noted is an oblique diaphyseal stress fracture of the 4th metatarsal. (b) 2 January 1986, screw has been removed from 5th metatarsal. There is a recurrent diaphyseal fracture in the 4th metatarsal. (c) 18 February 1986: no change in 5th metatarsal. There has been a progression of fracture lines in the 4th metatarsal. (d) 16 June 1986: after a period of cast immobilization, the 4th metatarsal fracture appears to be healed. (e) 20 November 1986: recurrence of stress fracture of the diaphysis of the 4th metatarsal. (f) 9 April 1987: presuming the recurring fracture to be due to a postural abnormality of the 4th ray, a distal, dorsal angulation osteotomy was performed. (g) No recurrence of difficulty has since been evidenced.

(g)

occurred during or just after athletic exertion. Necropsy findings revealed that 78% of these athletes had unequivocal predisposing cardiovascular disease, preponderantly of a congenital variety (86%) (Maron *et al.*, 1980).

Perhaps the most alarming statistic offered by Maron *et al.* (1980) in the context of injuries and their prevention, is that 21 of the 29 decedents had been asymptomatic. The remaining eight athletes had transient symptoms which included one or more of the following: syncope, presyncope, chest pain, fatigue and palpitations. Evaluations in those with suspected or demonstrated disease led to diagnoses which included a 'normal athletic heart', Wolff–Parkinson–White syndrome, Marfan's syndrome, hyperlipoproteinaemia and hypertrophic cardiomyopathy (HCM). No pursuit of diagnostics or therapeutics had been sufficient to obviate sudden death (Maron *et al.*, 1980).

The obvious question which derives from these statistics is: what constitutes an appropriate athletic screening? Of seven athletes suspected of disease while alive, five had normal electrocardiograms (ECGs) and one had an abnormal angiogram; but it would probably have required a good quality echocardiogram to establish the correct diagnosis (HCM). The sad fact is that the majority of cases of sudden death would have been properly identified as being at risk by a thorough personal and family history, physical examination, ECG and echocardiogram (Maron *et al.*, 1980).

Epstein and Maron (1986) list the following disorders as the most common causes of sudden death in athletes under 35 years of age:

1 HCM

2 Idiopathic left ventricular hypertrophy.

3 Aortic rupture (cystic medial necrosis).

4 Coronary artery disease.

5 Congenital coronary abnormalities.

They list less common causes as:

1 Valvular aortic stenosis.

2 Prolonged QT syndrome.

3 Primary cardiac electrophysiological abnormalities.

4 Cardiac sarcoidosis.

5 Myocarditis.

Certainly, HCM, the hallmark of which is left ventricular hypertrophy without dilation, is the most common and important cause of sudden death in young athletes. HCM was present in about half of the 29 cases reported by Maron *et al.* (1980). These authors indicated that substantiation of the diagnosis requires at least one of the following features:

1 Asymmetrical septal hypertrophy (determined by measurements). Epstein and Maron (1986) indicate that the upper limits of the thickness of the ventricular septum is about 12 mm. Thicknesses of 13–14 mm, for example, may alert the physician to the presence of HCM, but may merely represent what has been eponymically termed 'the normal athletic heart'.

2 Marked disorganization of cardiac muscle cells in the ventricular septum.

3 Clinical and/or echocardiographic evidence of HCM in at least one close family member.

Physical examination has a poor sensitivity for detecting HCM (Epstein & Maron, 1986). Chest X-rays are useful when cardiac enlargement is present. A history of syncope or a family history of HCM or sudden death in a first-degree relative should particularly alert the physician to the possibility of cardiomyopathy. While 90% of those who succumb to HCM demonstrate abnormal ECGs, they are not specific for the disease. Only M-mode and two-dimensional echocardiography of the athlete (and first-degree relatives) have a great likelihood of detecting this often autosomally dominant condition (Epstein & Maron, 1986).

Chillag (1991) states that his experience reveals that anomalous coronary artery disease and HCM each account for 20% of exercise-induced deaths in athletes under 30 years of age. While Chillag concedes that echocardiography is the only usable test to screen for asymptomatic congenital heart disease, he indicates that it is imperfect in the detection of anomalous coronary disease and HCM.

Aortic rupture secondary to cystic medial necrosis (e.g. Marfan's syndrome) also demonstrates a variance in the sensitivity of available diagnostic tests. Chest X-rays may reveal aortic dilation and auscultatory ejection sounds may herald the condition, but neither is reliably sensitive. The greatest sensitivities in detection derive from M-mode and two-dimensional echocardiography and from root contrast angiography.

Congenital and acquired coronary artery disease may require invasive studies (radionucleotide stress testing or coronary angiography) for adequate diagnostic sensitivity, but still with a disturbing yield of false positive results.

Aortic stenosis is usually easily detected by auscultatory physical examination by virtue of the characteristic murmur.

Table 21.2 summarizes the efficacies of the various diagnostic modalities for conditions known to have produced sudden death in athletes.

Approximately 0.005% of asymptomatic aspiring athletes may succumb to the sudden death syndrome. In terms of screening for such an event, about 200 athletes would have to be screened to find one with potentially fatal cardiovascular disease (Epstein & Maron, 1986). Tests such as echocardiography have been considered to be too costly for community screening projects. The NBA has been willing and supportive of such tests for their draftees. In two consecutive years of screening élite college players expected to be drafted by professional (NBA) teams, (a total of slightly less than 180 players), no echocardiograms (M-mode or two-dimensional) were considered sufficiently abnormal to preclude participation in the sport (J.A. Hefferson, personal communication).

In the 1990 NBA combined physicals, a single case of aortic dilatation was detected (with a possible implication of Marfanoid cystic medial necrosis). In the 1991 combined physicals, about 10% of players demonstrated ECG abnormalities during Bruce protocol stress testing; stress echocardiography of these players revealed no significant abnormalities (J.A. Hefferson, personal communication). In a population of middle-aged men, potentially fatal silent cardiac disease is estimated to be present in about 3% (Epstein & Maron, 1986).

Table 21.2 Possible community-initiated screening strategies for identifying the athlete at risk of sudden death. Adapted from Epstein & Maron (1986).

Screening battery	Will detect	Will miss
History, auscultation	All AS, 25% of all HCM, some CMN	75% of HCM, all CAD/CAA, most CMN
History, auscultation, chest X-ray film	All AS, 30% of all HCM, many CMN	70% of HCM, all CAD/CAA, many CMN
History, auscultation, chest X-ray film, 12-lead ECG	All AS, most HCM at risk of SD	Many CMN, virtually all CAD/CAA
History, auscultation, chest X-ray film, 12-lead ECG, echocardiography (M-mode)	All AS, most HCM, most CMN	Virtually all CAD/CAA
History, auscultation, chest X-ray film, 12-lead ECG, echocardiography (M-mode), exercise ECG	All AS, most HCM, most CMN, ~20% of CAD/CAA at risk of SD	~80% of CAD/CAA at risk of SD

AS, aortic stenosis; CAA, coronary artery anomalies; CAD, coronary artery disease; CMN, cystic medial necrosis; ECG, electrocardiogram; HCM, hypertrophic cardiomyopathy; SD, sudden death.

Cocaine

At least among college and professional basketball players in the USA, sudden death syndromes are not exclusively in the domain of congenital and/or hereditary cardiac abnormalities. Cocaine has been an all too frequent cause of sudden death syndrome in these groups.

Cocaine was first used medically in 1884 as a local anaesthetic (Cantwell & Rose, 1986). Its well known and compelling addictions have been made legendary.

Cocaine enhances catecholamine response (Lombardo, 1986). It will impair the athlete by accelerating mental processes, with euphoria and a sense of increased ability, or perhaps, with paranoia (Cantwell & Rose, 1986). A list of mental and physical responses known to occur with cocaine use are listed in Table 21.3.

Organs with sympathetic innervation (e.g. the heart) are particularly influenced by cocaine. The drug can induce coronary vasospasm (in a young athlete without arteriosclerosis) or severe arrhythmias, either of which can result in death (sudden or delayed) by various pathways. The vasospasm or arrhythmia can result in myocardial infarction directly, or produce stasis of flow with coronary thrombosis, thereby resulting in infarction or stroke (Cantwell & Rose, 1986). Pasternack *et al.* (1988) indicate that in addition to these liabilities, cocaine in very high doses can have a direct toxic effect on heart muscle to produce cardiac failure and sudden death.

Table 21.3 Signs and symptoms of cocaine abuse. Adapted from Cantwell & Rose (1986) and Lombardo (1986).

Psychomental	*Cardiovascular*
Tremulousness	Tachycardia
Agitation	Ectopic beats
Restlessness	Coronary spasm
Paranoia	Stroke
Hallucinations	Hypertension
Delusions	Ventricular arrhythmia
	Myocardial infarction
Other	
Hyperthermia	
Epistaxis	

Lombardo (1986) points out that athletes are targets of cocaine distributors by virtue of their presence, influence upon children and finances (if a professional). Many of these athletes are so talented that the influence of the drug is not appreciated in watching their performance. The initial clues revealing the presence of a problem in an athlete are an altered (more 'hyper') personality and tardiness (especially to team meetings and events). Both cardiac abnormalities and substance abuse can lead to impaired performance, often in conjunction with fatigue (or

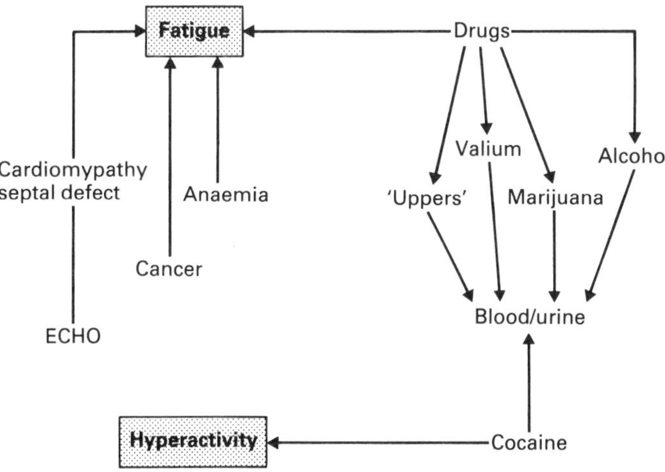

Fig. 21.8 Poor performance is not always due to inadequate training and/or skills. Fatigue and/or hyperactivity are not infrequently manifestations of problems characterized in this schematic. A current concern is the human immunodeficiency positive athlete who may also manifest fatigue as a primary symptom. ECHO, echocardiogram.

hyperactivity in some cases of cocaine abuse) (Fig. 21.8).

Mandatory drug testing is not always allowable at all levels of basketball as it is for Olympic competition. All Olympic participants are automatically tested. Analysis of the urine is the usual method of corroborating cocaine use. The drug is usually detectable for about 3 days after use. Those who are habitually addicted will not usually abstain for that number of days.

Other injuries

Ankle sprains

It has already been acknowledged that ankle sprains are the most frequent lower extremity injury in basketball at all levels of competition. Garrick (1987) studied injuries sustained by students (n = 3049) in four high schools over a 2-year period. Ankle sprains were the single most common group of injuries among male and female basketball players, representing between 40 and 50% of all injuries sustained in the sport. In a separate study of 8029 ankle injuries recorded in a sports medicine practice from participants in 12 sports, basketball players demonstrated the highest proportion of ankle sprains versus other injuries.

Zelisko *et al.* (1982) acknowledged the increased popularity of women's basketball in recent decades. They compared men's and women's professional basketball injuries and discovered the injury rate in women to be $51 \cdot 1000$ exposures^{-1} versus $32 \cdot 1000$ exposures^{-1} in men. The women's rate was 60% higher. However, the most commonly injured area for both groups was the ankle, approximating 20% of all injuries for each group. Even in the absence of overt injury to the ankles, the wear and tear of basketball is often evident in the subjacent tissues (Fig. 21.9).

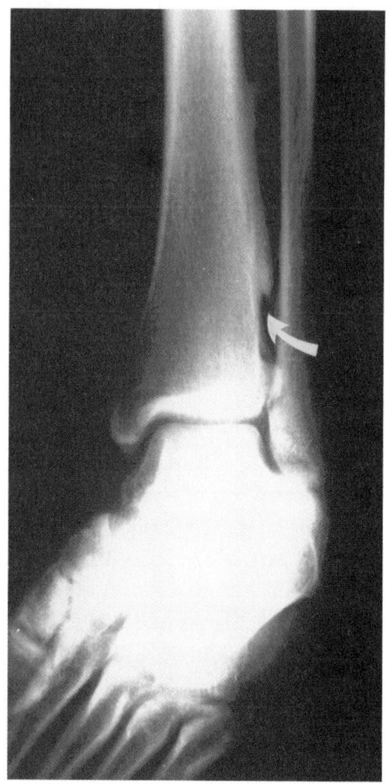

Fig. 21.9 Radiography of the ankle of a National Basketball Association player devoid of any symptoms. Note the notching effect of the distal end of the lateral aspect of the tibia created by the proximal ossifying response in the tibiofibular membrane from repeated microtrauma.

LATERAL LIGAMENTS

The ligament complexes about the ankle are demonstrated in Fig. 21.10. The present discussion is essentially limited to the lateral ligament complex, since it is by far the most frequently injured.

Most lateral sprains occur by the mechanism of plantar flexion and inversion, as in landing from a jump with an inverted foot. The usual sequence of lateral complex failure proceeds

Fig. 21.10 (*Opposite*) (a) Ligaments of the ankle: (i) anterior view, (ii) posterior view. (b) Deltoid ligament (primary stabilizer of the ankle joint): (i) superficial portion; (ii) deep portion. (c) Ligaments of the ankle and foot: (i) lateral view, (ii) medial view. From Reckling *et al.* (1990).

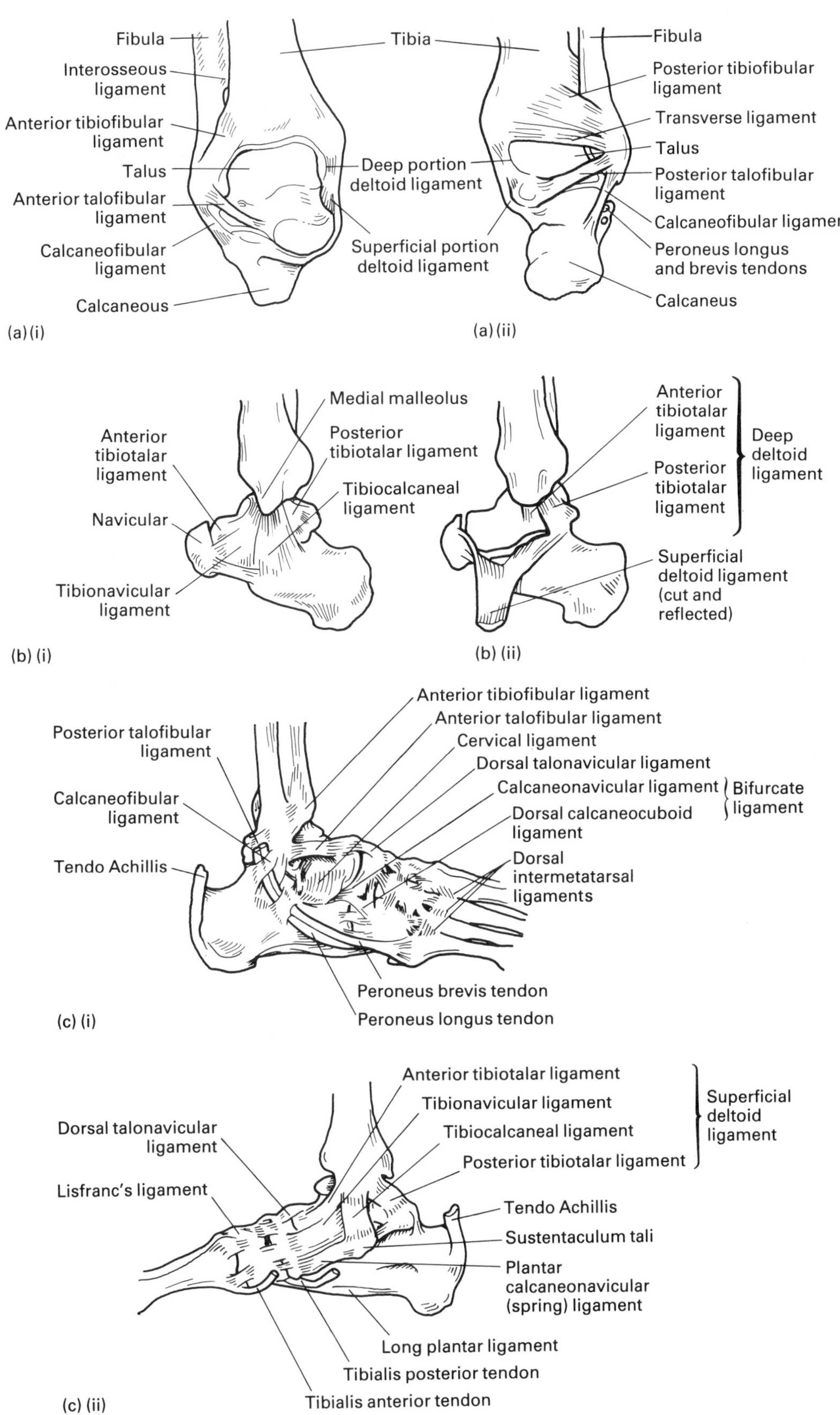
Fibula
Interosseous ligament
Anterior tibiofibular ligament
Talus
Anterior talofibular ligament
Calcaneofibular ligament
Calcaneous
Tibia
Deep portion deltoid ligament
Superficial portion deltoid ligament
(a) (i)
Fibula
Posterior tibiofibular ligament
Transverse ligament
Talus
Posterior talofibular ligament
Calcaneofibular ligament
Peroneus longus and brevis tendons
Calcaneus
(a) (ii)
Medial malleolus
Anterior tibiotalar ligament
Posterior tibiotalar ligament
Tibiocalcaneal ligament
Navicular
Tibionavicular ligament
(b) (i)
Anterior tibiotalar ligament
Posterior tibiotalar ligament
Deep deltoid ligament
Superficial deltoid ligament (cut and reflected)
(b) (ii)
Anterior tibiofibular ligament
Anterior talofibular ligament
Cervical ligament
Dorsal talonavicular ligament
Calcaneonavicular ligament
Bifurcate ligament
Dorsal calcaneocuboid ligament
Dorsal intermetatarsal ligaments
Posterior talofibular ligament
Calcaneofibular ligament
Tendo Achillis
Peroneus brevis tendon
Peroneus longus tendon
(c) (i)
Anterior tibiotalar ligament
Tibionavicular ligament
Tibiocalcaneal ligament
Posterior tibiotalar ligament
Superficial deltoid ligament
Dorsal talonavicular ligament
Lisfranc's ligament
Tendo Achillis
Sustentaculum tali
Plantar calcaneonavicular (spring) ligament
Long plantar ligament
Tibialis posterior tendon
Tibialis anterior tendon
(c) (ii)

from the anterior talofibular ligament to the lateral calcaneofibular ligament, and then finally to the posterior talofibular ligament (Larkin & Brage, 1991).

The anterior talofibular is the single most frequently injured ligament. It is the broadest, but weakest of the lateral ankle ligaments (Larkin & Brage, 1991). The fact that it is intra-articular is of significance in interpreting its rupture by arthrography. The calcaneofibular is the only lateral ligament to span the talocalcaneal as well as tibiotalar articulations; it helps inhibit inversion in plantar flexion as well as dorsiflexion. It is not infrequently torn in severe sprains, but always in addition to the anterior talofibular ligament (Larkin & Brage, 1991). The fact that the calcaneofibular ligament is extracapsular and forms the floor of the peroneal tendon sheaths is vital to the interpretation of its disruption by arthrography. The strong posterior talofibular ligament is rarely torn (Larkin & Brage, 1991).

Jaskulka *et al.* (1988) reported the frequency of lesions discovered at surgery in 268 ankles with fresh ruptures of the lateral ligament complex:

1 Anterior talofibular ligament only: 18.3%.

2 Combined rupture of the anterior talofibular and calcaneofibular ligaments: 75%.

3 Combined rupture of all three lateral ligaments: 6%.

These percentages apply to a young population (average 25.8 years) in which nearly 25% of the injuries were sustained in sports activities.

EVALUATING ANKLE SPRAINS

The evaluation of the 'apparent sprain' serves more than one purpose. A critical purpose is to ascertain whether the severity of injury warrants consideration of a surgical repair. A certain quantity of diagnostic study is indicated to determine the presence of differential diagnoses which may warrant surgery (e.g. osteochondral fractures of the talus, tibiofibular dissociations) and to formulate prognostic information for the future.

The described mechanism of injury, and the locations and severity of pain may provide clues about the specific structures involved and the extent of damage. Physical examination will reveal loci of tenderness, the range of motion, the presence of effusion and the state of stability. The presence of an effusion or haemoarthrosis may add to the pain response, reduce the range of motion, and inhibit an adequate stability evaluation. Aspiration and an injection of local anaesthetic may relieve pain and thereby facilitate further diagnostic evaluation and expedite the initiation of physical therapy for the development of motion and strength.

Ray *et al.* (1991) indicate that the 'anterior drawer' is the easiest stability test to perform. Larkin and Brage (1991) cite Castaing and Delplace (1972) as having indicated on the basis of cadaver studies that anterior translations of 8–10 mm imply disruption of the anterior talofibular ligament while excursions of 10–15 mm imply disruption of additional lateral complex ligaments. The variability of inversion stress testing results reduces its value to some degree (Larkin & Brage, 1991). Talar tilts up to 25° have been considered to be normal (Larkin & Brage, 1991). They also indicate that most authors would agree that a talar tilt in excess of 20° or one which is 10° greater than that of the uninvolved ankle is consistent with ruptures of both the anterior talofibular and the calcaneofibular ligaments.

Anterior drawer and inversion testing are both performed with the foot plantar flexed to maximally elicit the existing laxity. Inversion stress testing is performed with the talus internally rotated (15–20°) as well as plantar flexed (Larkin & Brage, 1991). Both anterior and inversion stress tests are applied by grasping the heel to direct an anterior force for the former and to avoid a bias due to forefoot movement in evaluating the latter. Laxity of the involved and uninvolved ankles should be compared. Stress testing is most accurately performed upon a relaxed ankle using a mechanized stress applicator in conjunction with X-ray documentation of the extent of displacement. Stress testing devices help to regulate the quantity of applied force and to assure the plane of motion in which displacement is to be measured. To ensure testing upon a relaxed ankle, the use of local anaesthetic may be necessary, general anaesthesia is an extreme measure. Clark *et al.* (1965) reported the use of high lateral popliteal nerve blocks, in preference to peroneal or sural blocks, to gain relaxation of the ankle for stress radiography.

Routine radiographs, including AP, lateral and mortise views of the ankle should be performed to rule out the presence of fractures prior to the performance of any stress testing (Ray *et al.*, 1991).

Ray *et al.* (1991) indicate that arthrography and tenosynoviography are not practical in the evaluation of acute sprains, though they have been used to document the magnitude of damage. Larkin and Brage (1991) state that arthrography is rarely indicated and offers little information in the 'acute' setting. However, arthrography is only of value in the acute setting; if arthrography is not performed within several days of the acute sprain, areas of potential contrast leakage may become sealed.

Fussell and Godley (1973) studied acute ankle sprains by arthrography in 29 athletic individuals, 40% of whom sustained their injuries in basketball. The uninvolved ankles of the subjects were studied as controls. These authors claim that arthrograms are not only accurate in distinguishing between tears of the anterolateral structures, syndesmoses and medial joint capsule, but in quantitating the magnitude of disruption (of the anterolateral complex). In this regard, they contend that anterolateral extravasation of contrast more than 5.5 cm above the distal tip of the fibula indicates a severe (and possibly surgical) disruption of the lateral complexes. Yet, in reviewing their tables of subjects and results, it is interesting to note that there was a very low correlation between cases with a positive anterior drawer and those with an extravasation height of 5.5 cm or more. Furthermore, the heights of the subjects in this study are not provided to help evaluate the possible significance of extravasation due to height in a population of basketball players well over 2 m (6 ft 10 in) in height.

Sauser *et al.* (1983) undertook a study of the comparative values of stress radiography and arthrography in quantifying instabilities resulting from acute inversion sprains of the ankle. 55 patients with acute inversion sprains were subjected to stress radiography of the injured and uninjured ankle, followed by arthrography of the injured one. A critical point reiterated by the authors is that any validation of stress testing results requires the use of a mechanical device which reproducibly applies designated forces in designated planes (the Telos apparatus in this case).

The arthrographic technique used by Sauser *et al.* (1983) was a facsimile of that reported by Broström (1966). Absence of extravasation about the lateral malleolus or communicating with the peroneal tendon sheath was presumed evidence of normality. Extravasation about the lateral malleolus was interpreted as evidence of a tear of the anterior talofibular ligament; and communication with the peroneal sheaths was presumed to indicate an associated tear of the calcaneofibular ligament (with which the peroneal sheaths are contiguous).

The stress test results of the study by Sauser *et al.* (1983) are presented in Table 21.4. The authors conclude that stress radiography, even when a sophisticated testing apparatus is used, is diagnostically less accurate than arthrography (within 72 h of injury). If any stress test is of value, it is the inversion stress test. Sauser *et al.* (1983) determined that a 10° or greater tilt provides a 99% certainty of lateral ligament injury.

Forward and internal rotatory glide of the talus (the 'anterior drawer sign' of the ankle) was demonstrated by Dehne (1933) by a combination of *in vitro* and *in vivo* studies (Broström, 1966). Broström indicated that this was the most common sign of ligamentous insufficiency in evaluating the results of treatment for sprains and, as indicated above, Ray *et al.* (1991) pro-

Table 21.4 Stress test results. Adapted from Sauser *et al.* (1983).

Test	Torn ligaments	Displacements/tilts	
		Range	Average
Anterior drawer	None	2–10 mm	5.1 mm
	ATFL	3–10 mm	6.3 mm
	ATFL + CFL	4–15 mm	7.2 mm
Inversion stress	None	0–13°	2.6°
	ATFL	0–18°	8.0°
	ATFL + CFL	0–20°	8.8°

ATFL, anterior talofibular ligament; CFL, calcaneofibular ligament.

claimed it to be the easiest sign or test to demonstrate. Nevertheless, Sauser *et al.* (1983) indicated that anterior stress displacements bear no statistical significance as predictors of lateral complex disruption. Arthrography predicted ligamentous disruption in about 85% of the acute sprains studied, possibly because incomplete disruptions were present in the remaining 15%.

In 1962, Anderson *et al.* sponsored the performance of primary repair of acutely torn ligaments only when both the anterior talofibular and calcaneofibular ligaments are torn (Clark *et al.*, 1965). Disciples of this recommendation are obligated to demonstrate disruption of both ligaments before proceeding with a surgical repair. Evans and Frenyo (1979) review the disadvantages of stress testing and arthrography, but particularly from the perspective of distinguishing ruptures of the individual ligaments of the lateral complex. As a general objection to inversion stress testing they reiterate the wide variation of 'normal tilts' and side-to-side differences that may be interpreted as normal; Bonnin (1944), Laurin *et al.* (1968) and Cox and Hewes (1979) indicated a range of normal up to 25°, while Rubin and Witten (1960) indicated that normal side-to-side differences can be as much as 19°. With respect to determining which ligaments are torn, Leonard (1949) indicated that an excessive talar tilt in the plantar flexed ankle relates to a ruptured anterior talofibular ligament, and when present in a plantigrade ankle, additional rupture of the calcaneofibular ligament is implied (Evans & Frenyo, 1979). The anterior drawer stress test does not distinguish between isolated and combined ligament ruptures.

By contrast, arthrography is effective in discerning acute ruptures of the anterior talofibular ligament. Since this ligament is intracapsular, contrast escapes through the capsule representing an easily visible sign. In attempting to discern ruptures of the calcaneofibular ligament, however, one encounters too many false negative studies. This conclusion of Fordyce and Horn (1972) and of Staples (1975) is explicable on the basis of the likelihood that contrast will often more easily escape through the capsular rent created by the always associated anterior talofibular ligament, rather than into the peroneal tendon sheath with which the extracapsular calcaneofibular ligament is intimately associated (Evans & Frenyo, 1979). Black *et al.* (1978) suggested that peroneal tenography can overcome this inability to distinguish separate ruptures of the calcaneofibular ligament (Evans & Frenyo, 1979). Contrast injected into the peroneal tendon sheath enters the ankle joint when this ligament is ruptured. The accuracy of the technique was corroborated at surgery by Evans and Frenyo (1979).

The study of Johnson and Markoff (1983) goes a long way toward explaining the interpretations of ankle stress testing reported in the literature. These workers used fresh-frozen cadaver tibiotalar joints and studied displacement curves relative to AP force, inversion–eversion movement and internal–external rotary torque.

When the anterior talofibular ligament was sectioned, AP laxity increased most dramatically in dorsiflexion, an average of 4.3 mm. The greatest increases in inversion were noted in plantar flexion and averaged 5.2°. Increases in rotational laxity were also maximum in plantar flexion, averaging 10.8°. Johnson and Markoff (1983) make the point that the increases in talar excursion after anterior tibiofibular sectioning are often too small to be readily detected by stress testing, even when symptoms are present.

The small average increase in displacement is consistent with the conclusion of Sauser *et al.* (1983) that anterior stress testing is unreliable, and particularly if measurements are recorded in a neutral or plantar flexed position. Segregated recordings of varus and/or talar rotary displacements are difficult to accomplish in live subjects as is the demonstration of a predominance of one versus the other (which is clearly a function of foot position during testing). Since varus and internal rotation are often coupled motions (as in typical sprains), displacements exceeding norms should be more easily demonstrable in the presence of a rupture of the lateral complex. This contention is also consistent with the greater reliability of 'varus' stress testing as an indication of lateral instability (Sauser *et al.*, 1983) despite the aforementioned wide variability of a normal range of varus tilting. Regardless of its disputed merits, stress radiography, apart from symptoms and physical examination, is the only objective measure of ligament disruption after 1 week (and the loss of reliability of arthrography due to sealing of sites of contrast leakage).

Factors other than testing technique may relate to the presence or persistence of instability in the absence of negative or equivocal stress test evaluation. Sammarco and diRaimondo (1988) indicated their belief that there are forms of subtalar instability which do not derive from calcaneofibular incompetence (though they do not identify the causes). Furthermore, the authors cite two studies which evaluated 750 and 75 ankles respectively. In the former, more anterior than 'normal' position of the calcaneofibular ligament was noted in more than 20%, and in the latter, the angular orientation of the ligament (relative to the long axis of the fibula) was noted to be quite variable. How and if these findings relate to instability stress test results is not known. Sammarco and diRaimondo indicated that 20% of the patients for whom they indicated surgery for persistent instability symptoms had greater than a 20% anterior subluxatability of the talus with the ankle in a plantigrade position. They also cautioned that two of 43 patients had a tarsal coalition.

Neither stress testing nor arthrography is necessarily indicated if a non-operative approach to treatment has been predetermined. On the other hand, when surgical intervention is a prospective treatment, both arthrography and stress testing are worthwhile diagnostics, regardless of which may be a more sensitive indicator of the nature and quantity of ligamentous disruption.

HISTORY OF TREATMENT

Watson-Jones (1941) established plaster immobilization as a treatment of choice for ankle sprains, at least until Anderson and LeCocq (1954) reported success with acute surgical repairs (Clark *et al.*, 1965). Thereafter, controversy regarding the best treatment for ankle ligament rupture has prevailed to the present.

Perhaps no author demonstrated greater wisdom and science in treating ankle sprains than Broström (1966). Though a quarter of a century old, his wisdom is as pertinent today as it was at the time of its writing. Broström recognized three possible treatment formats for the acute sprain: cast immobilization (6–12 weeks), surgical repair and early mobilization. In assessing the efficacy of the various methods, he cites studies which used physical examination and talar tilt (stress X-rays) as benchmarks for determining the presence of instability. Guttner (1941) reported roughly a 20% incidence of instability amongst nearly 100 ankles examined 1–2 years after plaster immobilization for an acute sprain (Broström, 1966). Leonard (1959) treated two groups of sprained ankles. The stable sprains (n = 24) were treated by novocaine and mobilization and the unstable sprains (n = 23) were treated by casting. More than a third of the former group, and none of the latter group had persistent symptoms (Broström, 1966). Bosien *et al.* (1955) reported symptoms in one-third, and physical evidence of instability in nearly two-thirds of more than 100 ankles examined a few years after non-immobilizing, non-surgical treatment; however, they claimed that none had radiographic evidence of instability (Broström, 1966). Pock-Steen (1958) determined that results of plaster treatment for sprains were not improved by more than 4 weeks of immobilization (Broström, 1966). Ruth (1961) indicated superior results in surgically repaired ankles, while two-thirds of a group of plaster-treated ankles were unstable despite good function and an absence of symptoms at a 2-year follow-up (Broström, 1966). Caro *et al.* (1964) randomly selected sprained ankles for treatment with hydrocortisone injection, strapping or plaster immobilization. The hydrocortisone treatment produced the best results and plaster immobilization produced the worst (Broström, 1966). Freeman (1965) reported residual symptoms in 25–58% of ankles evaluated 1 year after treatment with ankle strapping and mobilization, plaster immobilization, or surgery and then immobilization.

While the above-cited studies are not quite comparable with respect to evaluative criteria and treatment methodology, it is quite clear that a treatment of choice had not been definitively established by the mid-1960s. As recently as 1979, Evans and Frenyo pointed out that an ongoing controversy persisted with respect to the treatment of choice for acutely injured unstable ankles among athletes. Evans and Frenyo (1979) cite proponents of early motion and function (McMaster, 1943; Freeman, 1965; Jackson *et al.*, 1974), proponents of plaster immobilization (Leonard, 1949; Chirls, 1973; Gross & MacIntosh, 1973), and those partial to surgery (Ruth, 1961; Broström 1966; Niethard, 1974; Staples, 1975). Essential issues emanating from the results of the studies cited are germane to today's élite game, where periods of disability are all important. Is it better to mobilize and rehabilitate quickly and perhaps risk a residual instability and persistent symptoms (not usually preclusive of play), or to accept a protracted early treatment disability (from surgery or plaster), hoping that it will avert later difficulties? How much should the quantitatively documented severity (by stress tests, arthrography and arthrosocopy) of sprain influence the selection of a treatment?

Even a relatively modern study of treatment for acute sprains (Jaskulka *et al.*, 1988) reiterates that there remains '. . . some controversy, even when diagnosis has been established, as to what constitutes the optimal therapeutic method'.

Jaskulka *et al.* (1988) treated 268 acute sprains by surgery and 6 weeks of plaster immobilization. Despite only a rare initiation of physical therapy, the authors' claim that 94.4% of patients returned to all activities, including sports, at an average of less than 10 weeks. Frankly, such results, especially in the absence of a major rehabilitation programme, are difficult to believe, unless the sports to which the subject returned were those which require a minimum of running or jumping.

Criteria of objective instability used by Jaskulka *et al.* (1988) were based on stress radiography, whereby a talar tilt and/or an anterior displacement exceeding that of the uninjured side by 5° and/or 5 mm respectively constituted justification for surgical repair and/or evidence of post-treatment instability.

Jaskulka *et al.* (1988) reported surgical repairs to be superior to other treatments for acute ankle sprains. Using a combination of stress radiography and subjective complaints they claimed 80% good results. This statistic is not too far removed form the 20% incidence of instability symptoms reported for non-surgical treatment by Broström (1966) (see below).

Clark *et al.* (1965) reported a comparison of surgically and walking plaster-treated ankles of military men. The criteria for inclusion in the study were clinical evidence of a severe sprain and at least 3° or more of talar tilt on the involved side on stress testing using regional anaesthesia. Stress testing revealed better stability among the surgically repaired ankles, but no observable functional differences between the surgically and plaster-treated groups. Furthermore, those treated by plaster (ambulatory) returned to duty at an average of 8 weeks while those treated surgically returned at an average of 12 weeks. Clark *et al.* (1965) determined that with the longer early disability, morbidity risk and lack of obvious functional superiority amongst surgically treated patients, surgical repair should be reserved for those young athletes with extremely severe lateral complex tears.

Pertinent to the issue of length of disability, Broström (1966) studied multiple groups of patients with sprained ankles treated by a variety of protocols. It was determined that strapping and mobilization produced the shortest disability, plaster a moderate one, and surgery a longer one (i.e. weeks for non-athletes to return to work). However, specific symptoms of ankle instability were reported by only 3% of surgically treated patients, but by nearly 20% of those treated non-operatively. In a related finding, the anterior drawer sign was found in about 5% of surgically repaired ankles, but in about 30% of non-surgically treated ankles (Broström, 1966). Perceptively, Broström reasoned that the large percentage of patients with a residual anterior drawer sign, but with no symptoms, could be explained by a controlling quantity of strength in the ankle controlling musculature.

On the basis of his study, Broström concluded unequivocally that suture repair of acutely ruptured ligaments followed by plaster immobilization (3 weeks) resulted in the highest percentage of stable ankles and the lowest percentage of residual symptoms (3%). This conclusion contrasted significantly with a 20% incidence of symptomatic instability afforded by non-surgical treatments.

Nevertheless, Broström does not recommend acute surgical repair routinely. Reasons to defer surgical repair are listed in Table 21.5.

MINIMIZING THE PERIOD OF DISABILITY

Whether the treatment of the acute sprain or the recurrent sprain is early mobilization, plaster immobilization or surgery, rehabilitation is the expedient factor in minimizing the period of disability. Modalities are often helpful in reducing swelling and pain so that active motion can be initiated. Resistance exercises in dorsiflexion, plantar flexion, eversion and inversion are progressed as rapidly as tolerated without sponsoring pain or swelling (Fig. 21.11). Strengthening of the ankle is supplemented by strengthening of the entire lower

Table 21.5 Reasons to defer ankle ligament surgery.

While one-fifth of ankles treated non-operatively manifest symptoms of instability:
- (i) the symptoms are usually not disabling, even for athletics
- (ii) ankle supports and strengthening can reasonably control most ankles

'Downside' risks of surgery in élite athletes are to be feared more than most instabilities:
- infection
- scar discomfort
- neuroma formation
- postoperative osteoarthritis

Late surgical repairs and/or reconstructions may be performed in the eventuality of persistent disabling symptoms of instability

Disability time after surgery is protracted

When the most 'optimal' functioning ankle is not a 'necessity' for performance, surgery can be deferred

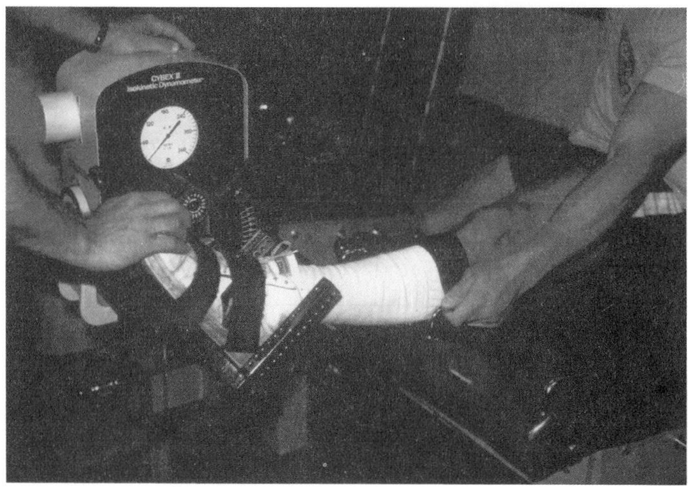

Fig. 21.11 Rehabilitation of an ankle using a Cybex II isokinetic dynamometer in a concentric plantar flexion–dorsiflexion mode. Eversion and inversion strengthening can also be performed with such machinery. Eccentric and other strengthening modes should also be performed for prophylactic and rehabilitative purposes.

extremity, using both joint isolation as well as closed chain machines. Aerobic formats, such as exercycling, can often be initiated early on, and then progressed toward stairmaster, kinetron, trampoline and treadmill training. Ultimately, agility drills, including the BAPS board, and sport-specific training techniques are progressed with circumspection.

Often, it is worthwhile taping, strapping, or bracing the ankle for added support and protection during the rehabilitative programme.

Once the rehabilitation programme is initiated, even in basketball, it is uncommon for a player not to return to play within a period of 2–6 weeks. On occasion, the disability time seems inexplicably protracted. In this regard, the study by Nitz *et al.* (1985) is of particular relevance. While case reports, such as those of Hyslop (1941) and Nobel (1966), have described isolated instances of peroneal nerve injury following ankle sprains, the frequency and magnitude of nerve injuries associated with ankle sprains were only appreciated after the study of Nitz *et al.* (1985). Based upon the laboratory derived classification of Dias (1979), Nitz *et al.* studied 30 grade II (lateral complex and deltoid ligament disruption) and 36 grade III (grade II plus anterior tibiofibular ligament disruption) sprains in an athletic population; they performed EMG and nerve conduction studies and evaluated the progression of functional return and symptom alteration with time. Electrical studies performed at 2 weeks postinjury revealed denervation potential in the peroneal and tibial nerve distributions of a moderate number of subjects with grade II sprains (17 and 10% respectively), but normal distal latencies and conduction velocities. Abnormal findings in those with grade III sprains were more numerous and of greater magnitude. Denervation potentials for the peroneal and tibial nerves were noted in more than 80% of cases, some also demonstrating increased distal latencies. Conduction delays, and sensory disturbances were absent by retesting at 3 months postinjury. It was hypothesized that the mechanism of injury to the peroneal and tibial nerves was traction at the bifurcation of the sciatic nerve caused by inversion of the ankle. Cadaver experiments revealed that sectioning of the ankle ligaments in conjunction with inversion stress result in a 5–8 mm excursion of the sciatic, peroneal and tibial nerves near the knee. Liu *et al.* (1948) demonstrated that as little as 6% elongation can result in traction nerve injuries (Nitz *et al.*, 1985).

Delayed functional recovery, persistent instability, popliteal tenderness and atrophic changes within the leg after severe sprains, may at least in part be due to neurological sequelae. In the presence of severe sprains or tardy recoveries, and especially when rupture of the anterior tibiofibular ligament is suspected, the performance of electrical diagnostic studies should be considered. Positive findings may stimulate consideration of epineural haematomas and compartment syndromes as differential diagnosis.

PROPHYLAXIS

The best preventives are assurance of 'support'. Support may be extrinsic (braces, tape, wraps), or intrinsic (strength of the ankle-controlling musculature).

The frequency of ankle sprains in sports has been an inducement to finding means of preventing both primary and repeated occurrences. Nearly 60 years ago, Belik (1934) indicated that taping ankles was a most effective protector against ankle injuries (Rarick *et al.*, 1962). 12 years later, Quigley *et al.* (1946) advocated the use of ankle taping as a prophylaxis against sprain (Rovere *et al.*, 1988). After reviewing the existing literature prior to 1979, Emerick (1979) concluded with weak conviction that taped ankles may be more resistant to being sprained.

If ankle taping serves a prophylactic function, by what means is this accomplished? Restriction of the extent and force of inversion at which a sprain is likely to occur has been one contention. Abdenour *et al.* (1979) compared taped and untaped ankle motion and torque development in seven young males. They determined that among all ranges of ankle function, not only motion, but torque production was impaired for inversion movements alone. It was presumed by the authors that this impairment serves a protective function.

Rarick *et al.* (1962) studied the effectiveness of ankle taping in inhibiting ankle motions predisposing to sprains. They studied subjects taped by each of four methods and used a cable tensiometer to measure restraint to the direction of motion being studied. They conceded that strappings of all types were effective in providing support restricting passive motion of the ankle. However, effectiveness of taping diminished substantially after only 10 min of exercise (up to 40% of the pre-exercise level). The point made by Rarick *et al.* is not that tape is ineffective, but that it is less effective during athletics than presumed by many physicians and trainers. For whatever it is worth, these authors indicated that the greatest support was provided by a basket weave with the combination stirrup and heel lock (Fig. 21.12).

Laughman *et al.* (1980) used three-dimensional electrogoniometry to study the effects of taping in inhibiting the motions that result in lateral ankle sprains. They tested 20 subjects with no known history of disability by having them exercise on a level surface and on a 10° slope. The exercise level was minor by athletic criteria. 'Sprain' motions were reduced an average of 27% by taping prior to exercise, and by an average of 19% after exercise. The authors claim that the effectiveness of taping is due in part to the more dorsiflexed position of the taped ankle during function.

In a given year (1989–1990) in the NBA, ankle sprains resulted in an average of 4.15 player days missed. Players whose ankles were taped had about the same average loss of days as those with untaped ankles. This does not imply that taped ankles fail to prevent sprains in some individuals, but merely that when sprains occur in taped ankles, there is no reduction in the resulting disability time when compared to that resulting from sprains of untaped ankles (NBTA, 1990).

The effectiveness of taping may be related to other factors which influence the support and placement of the foot during athletic participation.

Garrick and Requa (1977) studied the effects of taping versus non-taping in recreational basketball players. They found a nearly five-fold rate of injury in untaped players wearing high tops and nearly a two-fold rate of injury in untaped players wearing low tops.

Rovere *et al.* (1988) studied football players in an effort to determine the relative efficacies of

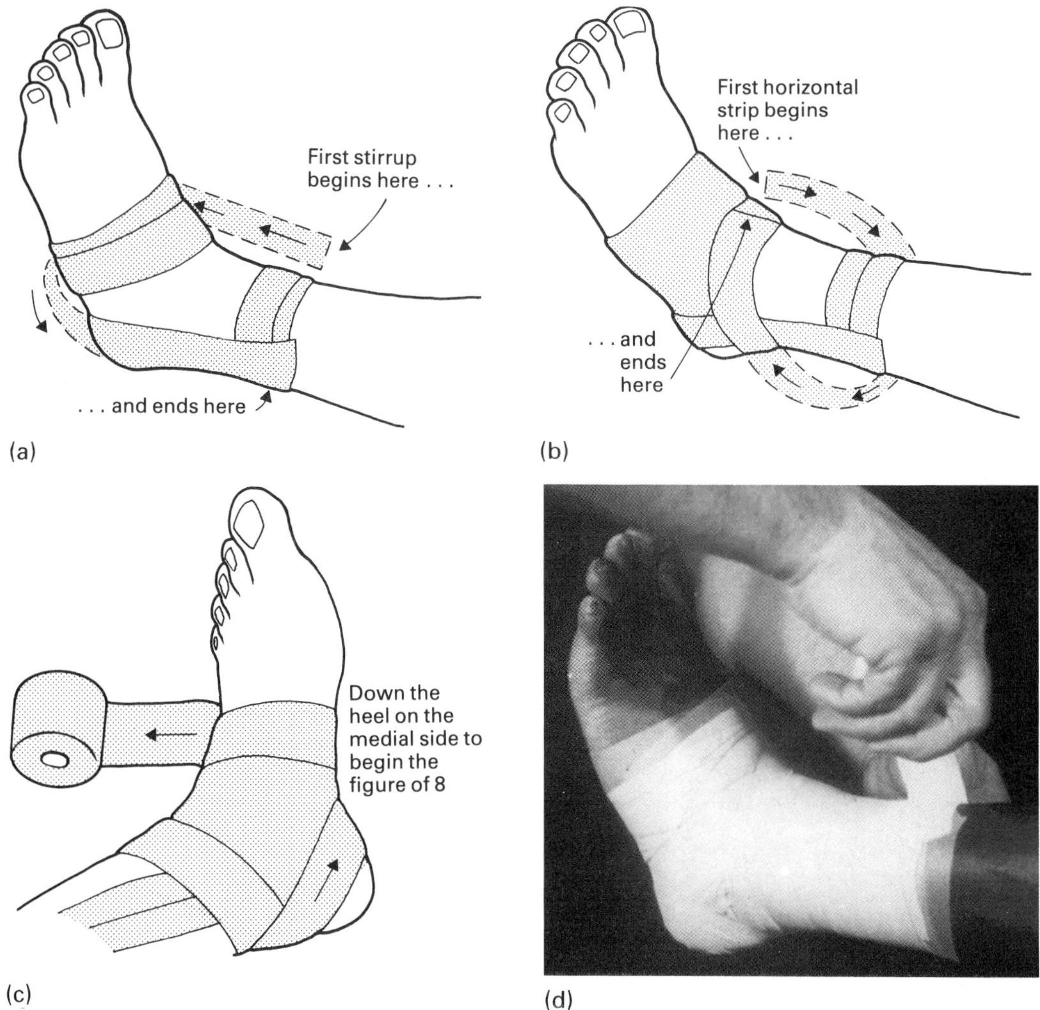

Fig. 21.12 Ankle taping. (a) Demonstration of application of 'stirrups' to initiate common taping of an ankle. (b) Horizontal tape strips are used to anchor the stirrups. (c) Figure of eight 'heel locks' increase the security of tape fixation. (d) Appearance of completed ankle taping. The protective taping liner material shows through at the top and bottom of the taping. Courtesy of Johnson & Johnson, New Brunswick, New Jersey.

ankle taping and an ankle stabilizer with laces. Over a several year period, 297 players sustained 224 ankle injures with 24 reinjuries. It was found that the ankle lacer reduced the risk of injury to 50% of that provided by taping. All reinjuries but one occurred in those wearing tape. The fewest injuries of all occurred in those using laced stabilizers and wearing low-top shoes. The study is not necessarily a blot on the efficacy of taping since there were no controls in the form of subjects wearing no support.

In a study by Hughes and Stetts (1983), 29 subjects had one ankle taped and the opposite ankle splinted by a thermoplastic material. Motion was evaluated by a Leighton flexometer which revealed an equal effectiveness by taping and splinting in restricting inversion movement after 20 min of a prescribed exercise routine. The reusable thermoplastic stabilizer was considered to be a more economical selection for repeated usage.

Of 353 reported ankle injuries among NCAA players in a given year, approximately one-third of players were wearing tape, other wrappings, or braces, while about two-thirds wore no protective device (NCAA, 1990).

From the studies of Garrick and Requa (1977), Rovere *et al.* (1988) and Hughes and Stetts (1983), the following may be deduced. First, that tape would appear to have prophylactic value, but that more formal braces (e.g. lacers and thermoplastics) may have greater prophylactic capacity, are more economical (reusable), and are less apt to lose their restraining ability as a function of time in activity. Second, that low top (versus high top) shoes seem to enhance the preventive effectiveness of ankle supports. The reason is not clear, but improved proprioceptive ability may be among the reasons. Freeman (1965) hypothesized the importance of proprioception as a protective mechanism for the unstable ankle. The hypothesis implies that injury, instability and surgery can interfere with proprioceptive protection and that its return may take some time. Tropp *et al.* (1985) studied the predisposition to ankle sprains among soccer players. Test groups were created whereby controls were pitted against those wearing a specially designed ankle orthosis and others training on a balance disk (similar to the now popular BAPS board). The ankle orthosis and the balance disc each substantially reduced the incidence of sprain among those with a previous history of sprain.

Balance and agility training may, in a sense, qualify as muscle 'strengthening' techniques. Whether they do or not, strengthening, which may be defined in numerous ways, is a major prophylactic asset. In 1934, Belik recognized that strengthening of the ankle-controlling musculature is an effective preventive (Rovere *et al.*, 1988). In 1966, Broström suggested that sufficient ankle muscle strength could subdue symptoms of instability. There is little doubt, that a weak ankle (or extremity for that matter) predisposes to sprain, especially in an individual with previous incidences. A continuum of strengthening exercises for all ankle musculature throughout the season is undoubtedly the best prevention against sprains (see Fig. 21.11).

Knee disabilities (other than ACL)

Diagnostic tests are often required in the evaluation of basketball injuries. It must be recognized in interpreting the results of these tests that élite college and professional athletes have been subjected to repetitive trauma on an almost constant basis. The consequence is the production of overuse pathology which may be detectable by special testing and yet play no active role in causing the symptoms for which the testing is done. In this regard Selesnick *et al.* (1990) performed routine MRIs on 26 asymptomatic knees in 13 professional basketball players. Some quantity of medial meniscus abnormality was present in 20 knees and none of the 26 knees was interpreted by the radiologist as normal. In a 10-year experience with professional basketball, the senior author (J.M.) has performed a single meniscectomy. It can be surmised that meniscal abnormalities, though common in élite basketball players, infrequently require surgical attention.

HYPEREXTENSION INJURIES

The kinematics of basketball movements (elucidated earlier), with excessive knee ranges of motion and angular velocities on jump take-offs and landings, subject players to hyperextension injuries of the knee, especially if the knee is contacted anteriorly by an opponent at the same time. Cruciate ligament injuries may be a result, but uncommonly. Nevertheless, most players develop an effusion and immediate disability, and a return to play is usually permitted when symptoms abate. Today, MRI has elucidated the pathology and confused the treatment plan. Figure 21.13 demonstrates sagittal MRI images representing the knees of two professional players who had

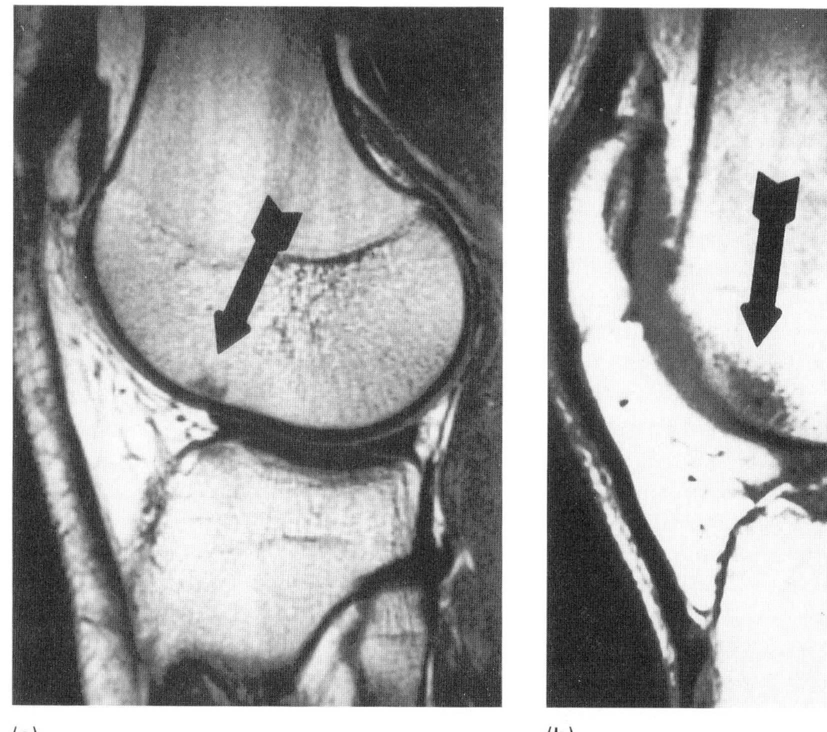

(a) (b)

Fig. 21.13 Magnetic resonance imaging (MRI). Sagittal images of the knees of two National Basketball Association basketball players injured during the same season. Both players sustained hyperextension injuries and underwent MRI evaluation within hours. The arrows indicate the presence of a bone bruise where the distal end of the femur impacted upon the adjacent joint structures. Resolution ordinarily takes several weeks.

sustained hyperextension injuries in the same season. The marrow signal alteration noted in the anterior portions of the femora of these players are considered 'bone bruises', attributable to bleeding within the marrow cavity. Radiographers suggest that such bruising usually resolves after several weeks and that failure of activity curtailment during the recovery period may result in damage to the articular surfaces (M. Rafii, personal communication).

When hyperextension injuries occur, and especially when they produce an effusion and disability, evaluation for capsuloligamentous disruptions and intra-articular fractures is necessary. The simplest way to make a determination of the presence of these entities when physical examination is equivocal is with an MRI. If MRI is not readily available, then a consideration of arthroscopy is justifiable, especially if the force or consequences of the episode seemed substantial. If no ruptured ligament, torn meniscus or intra-articular fracture is discovered, or if an MRI reveals only a 'bone bruise', the player must be withheld from participation for at least 2–3 weeks as physical therapy is progressed from modalities and range of motion through progressive resistance exercises, agility and cardiovascular retraining, limited practice and then full practice. It may be necessary to utilize a ligament brace which blocks hyperextension to allay apprehension and to protect the knee. Obviously, the discovery of a ligament disorder, torn cartilage or fracture dictates the specific treatments appropriate to each entity.

PATELLAR MECHANISM AFFLICTIONS

While patellar mechanism problems are not commonly responsible for the loss of a great number of player days missed, patellar mechanism problems are extremely common. Even when their disability is not apparently significant, players may be forced to compromise their level of performance or the number of minutes played per game. In most instances there is a structural predisposition to the development of symptoms which is instigated by the intensity of basketball. Many players thus afflicted fail to enter the season adequately strengthened from a summer programme; and even if an intraseasonal diligence of resistive exercises is adopted, the player may still not 'catch up' sufficiently, or in time to overcome the inflammatory response initiated during training camp and the season's beginning.

It is a given that the patellofemoral mechanism is among the most complex and least understood in the body. Its disorders, to which have been ascribed the nebulously defined diagnoses of chondromalacia, maltracking, malalignment and instability, are among the more commonly seen ones in sports medicine practices comprised of young athletes.

Parapatellar disorders, such as patellar tendinitis and retinacular inflammation are common, even among élite athletes, especially those participating in sports requiring repetitive percussion and/or decelerations of the eccentric loading type. Basketball is a prime example.

Eighty-six players were examined in the 1990 'combined physicals' which serve to screen top college players expected to be drafted by the NBA. Injuries recorded during these physicals represent those which occurred to any significant degree during each player's high school and/or college career. Patella-related problems were the most numerous among all recorded injuries and diagnoses. They included: chondromalacia with maltracking and/or alta, status postpatellectomy, patellar tendinitis, patellar fracture and ruptured patellar tendon. Yet, despite the range and apparent severity of some of the entities listed, no player manifested a degree of disability preclusive of play (J.A. Hefferson, personal communication).

Despite the frequent presence of patellar laxity and alta among élite basketball players, patellar tendinitis is frequently the only symptomatic (versus instability or retropatellar pain) component. Patellar tendinitis, like Osgood–Schlatter disease and Sinding-Larson–Johansson syndrome, is part of a continuum of chronologically related 'traction' lesions within the patellofemoral apparatus. Its most common symptomatic focus at the élite level is at the distal pole of the patella. The presenting symptoms, focal pain and swelling, are a result of the player's having participated in activities characterized by eccentric and impulsion loading of the extensor mechanism.

Pathologically, the entity represents a partial tear of the patellar tendon just distal to the inferior pole. Plain radiography is usually unremarkable in cases of less than several months duration, but in more chronic cases, fibrocartilaginous metaplasia within the tendon may produce radiographic opacification in the region, contiguous with the inferior pole (Blazina *et al.*, 1975; Martens *et al.*, 1982; Crenshaw, 1987; Ray *et al.*, 1991) (Fig. 21.14).

Options for treatment are dependent upon the severity, chronicity and expediency of the case in point. Moderation of activity (reduced impulsion-type activities) is often necessary for the abatement of the inflammatory stimulus. Physiotherapeutic modalities (ice, ultrasound, iontophoresis, electrotherapy) and nonsteroidal anti-inflammatory drugs (NSAIDs) are soothing and may accelerate the reduction of inflammation. Steroidal injections should be avoided when possible; they may result in direct degeneration of tendon or produce indirect damage. The latter is accomplished by masking symptoms while ignoring the cause. Nevertheless, steroid injections are used all too often. A frequent tell-tale sign in the USA, where Black people pervade the élite ranks, is a blanching of the black skin just over the patellar tendon, consequent to the depigmenting action of steroidal medication.

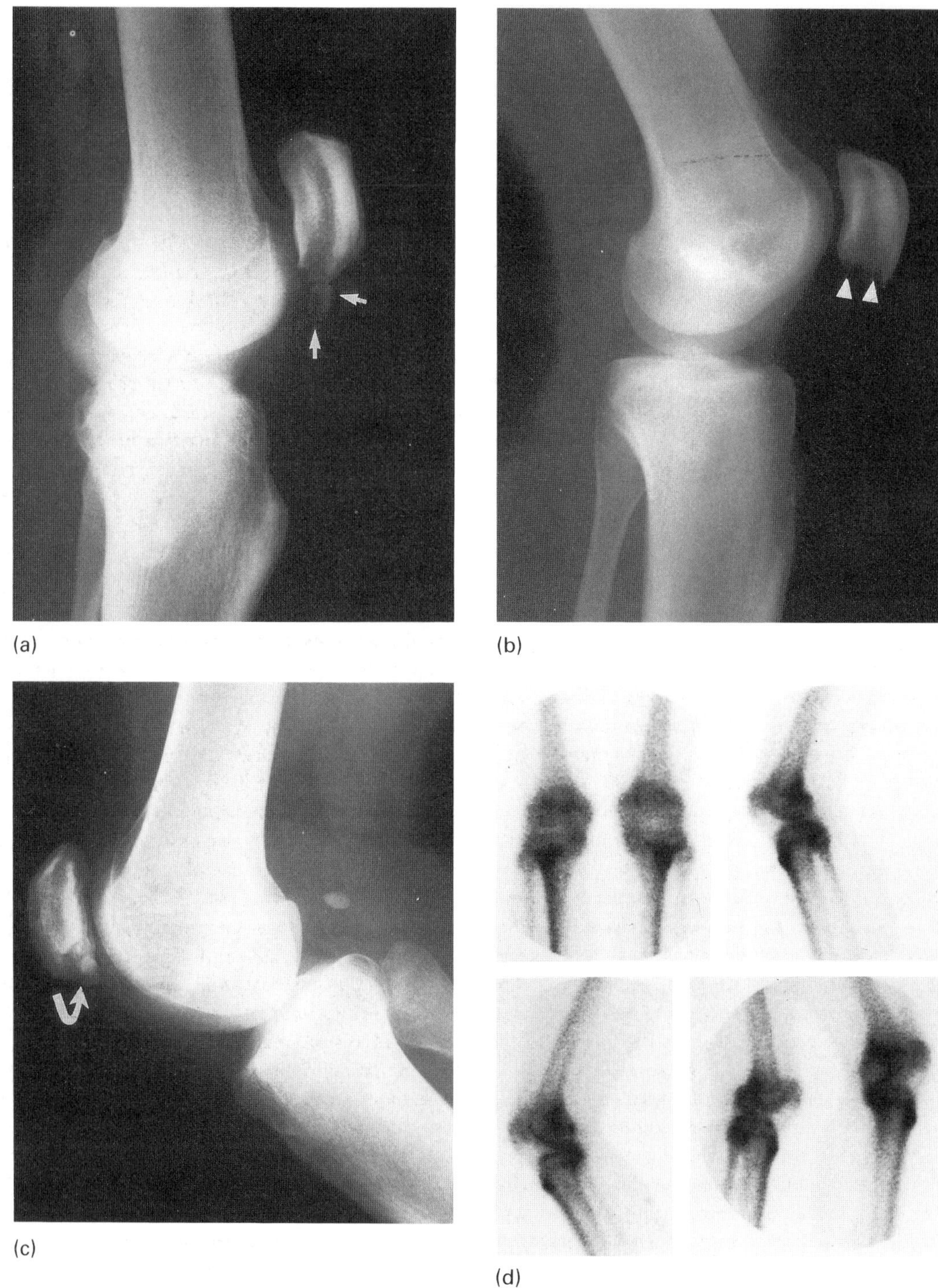
(a)
(b)
(c)
(d)

Apart from the application of modalities, physical therapy must include a strengthening and stretching programme for all groups of the entire lower extremity. Respecting that strengthening may provoke the symptoms, each exercise, load and arc of movement subtended by the load must be titrated to tolerance. The speed of performance, repetition patterns, frequency and other factors must be titrated (and progressed) to avoid provocation. Eccentric strengthening of the quadriceps mechanism must be included in the regimen to help make the extensor mechanism more resistant and better able to absorb the energy of impulsion activities. Quadriceps stretching is also vitally important in alleviating the traction effects upon the inflamed tendon. Frequent stretching produces a stress relaxation in the long, two-joint extensor apparatus, improving glide, facilitating contraction and reducing the likelihood of tendon fibre avulsion from the patella.

In some cases, patellar restraining braces are helpful. They may reduce pain by supporting the mechanism and by diffusing the forces which might otherwise be more focused at the site of inflammation.

Recalcitrant cases may need surgical intervention, though such invasive treatment is uncommonly necessary. Surgery aims to accomplish the excision of necrotic and degenerated tendon tissue and of any calcified metaplastic tissues within the tendon substance.

Martens *et al.* (1982) reviewed 90 athletes (mostly volleyball and soccer players) after no less than 2 years. Nearly half of the cases had indentifiable instigating or associated pathologies such as chondromalacia patella or patellar hypermobility. Elongation of the distal pole of the patella and ossification within the patella tendon were each noted in about 7% of cases.

The classification of disease staging used by Martens *et al.* (1982) is an adaptation of that of Blazina *et al.* (1975) (Table 21.6). Surgery, performed primarily on stage II and III cases after 6 months to 2 years of symptoms, consisted only of patellar tendon debridement without drilling or excision of the lower pole of the patella. Mucoid degeneration and fibrenoid necrosis were consistent histopathological findings as were areas of fibroelastic regenerative proliferation. Significant relief of symptoms at follow-up was documented in about 90% of those operated upon.

The nature of any abnormal tissue which comprises the tendon is a function of the duration of the condition. A common temporal progression pattern is outlined in Table 21.7.

Postoperatively, passive motion, quadriceps and hamstring stretching are initiated immediately. Once a full range of motion is achieved, a slow progression of resistive exercises is begun.

Table 21.6 Classification of disease staging. Adapted from Martens *et al.* (1982).

Stage	Classification
I	Pain only after sports
II	Pain early in activity, then disappearing, then later reappearing
III	Constant pain at rest/during activity and unable to do sports
IV	Complete rupture

Fig. 21.14 (*Opposite*) Patellar tendinitis — lower pole. (a) Lateral radiograph of a knee of a National Basketball Association (NBA) player demonstrating ossification of the proximal end of the tendon (arrows). Symptoms are mild in this case. (b) Lateral radiograph of a knee of an NBA player with acute tendinitis. Resorption of bone is noted at the distal pole of the patella (arrow heads). (c) Lateral radiograph of a recreational basketball player with inferior pole disruption (arrow). He is presently asymptomatic. As an adolescent he had avulsed his patellar tendon from the distal pole in conjunction with treatment for leukaemia which has been arrested for 10 years. (d) Three-phase bone scan demonstrating the knee of a 20-year-old college basketball player with chronic patellar tendinitis. Increased uptake is noted at the tubercle in each image.

Table 21.7 Temporal pathological sequence of patellar tendinitis. Adapted from Evarts (1983).

Time (months)	Pathology
3–4	Degenerated collagenous tissue
6–12	Haemorrhage and cyst formation
>12	Gritty (and/or calcified) metaplastic cartilage

Ultimately, agility, proprioceptive and pleiometric activities are progressed toward a return to athletic function. The foregoing sequence is usually accomplished over a period of 3–4 months.

It must be reiterated that alta patellae, lax patellae, patellar mechanisms with excessive dynamic Q angles, and various malalignments are among the underlying structural aberrations which may participate in the production of a manifested patellar tendinitis or chondromalacia syndrome. The relative severity of these contributing components may determine a consideration for treatments beyond those necessary for tendinitis alone, such as patellar mechanism realignment. The stereotypically tall, élite basketball player often manifests alta and other of the components listed above. Their commonly elongated tendons are subjected to whipping and jerking by the rotatory and jumping movements of basketball. Still, the senior author (J.M.) has had occasion to surgically intervene in only two cases of recalcitrant patellar tendinitis in a 10-year experience with professional basketball players.

CONSTITUENTS OF PATELLAR DISORDERS

The confusingly related entities of chondromalacia, patellar instability and patellar malalignment are among the banes of the orthopaedic surgeon. The orthopaedic literature has dealt with each of these entities as if they were primary and (often) isolated pathologies. This has been particularly true of chondromalacia patella, a commonly found, but uncommonly symptomatic entity among élite basketball players. Chondromalacia, the literal meaning of which is 'softened cartilage' has inappropriately become an eponym for all manner of anterior knee symptoms. Hayes *et al.* (1990) stated that patellofemoral contact pressures have been implicated in the pathogenesis of patellar articular degeneration. In many instances such degeneration is a consequence of direct trauma (as in striking the knee against the floor of the court or the knee of an opponent) or of patellar instability or maltracking. Fulkerson and Shea (1990) correctly indicate that correlations between articular cartilage degeneration (with crepitus) and patellar pain are inconsistent. When chondromalacic manifestations impede function, anti-inflammatory and physiotherapeutic measures, as indicated for tendinitis, are in order. Patellar restraining braces may help allay symptoms by stabilizing patellar glide. Bracing is sometimes a detriment, the compression increasing the sensation of disturbing crepitation or pain.

Maltracking of the patella is an especially difficult subject to comprehend and discuss. The intricacies of its dynamics have yet to be reasonably elucidated. Instability may result in maltracking due to the severity of laxity (medial, lateral or both), and/or due to muscle weakness, and/or due to dysplasias of the bony or soft tissue components of the extensor mechanism.

Whether the issue is chondromalacia, instability or maltracking, there are few absolute parameters which define the limits of normal versus abnormal with respect to treatment. Attempts to define and/or distinguish these entities by radiographic indices have been numerous, but not altogether gratifying. For a comprehensive review of the values and limitations of radiographic criteria used in the evaluation of these entities, the reader is referred to the review by Minkoff and Fein (1989) (in which European readers will appreciate a relative absence of evaluative parameters using lateral views, a popular European method of evaluation).

The indiscriminate use and interchange of descriptive terms implying the presence of a patellar disorder has added measurably to the confusion on the subject. 'Maltracking' is not 'instability' but may be due to the latter. 'Malalignment' may produce 'maltracking'; either may produce 'chondromalacia' or be affiliated with 'instability', but need not be. 'Patellar tendinitis' may be produced by repetitive overuse of the extensor mechanism, but it may also be an accompaniment of and partially induced by 'malalignment' and/or 'instability'. Similarly, the term 'subluxation' is frequently misused. It is used by most to imply that the patella has an ability to partially dislocate from the trochlea; it is used by others in referring to a fixed partial dislocation of the patella. In the former instance it should be said that the patella is 'subluxable', while in the latter it should be stated that the patella is permanently 'subluxed' (i.e. manifests a fixed malalignment).

As indicated, major surgical procedures for patellar mechanism abnormalities are rarely needed. There is no need to review the various procedures here. For the élite competitive athlete, temporal considerations may dictate the treatment option selected. Such an individual afflicted in the midst of the season, or approaching a critical event, can most often be restored to a competitive level by the immediate initiation of physical therapy to reconstitute motion, strength and agility (as long as no loose fracture fragment is present). Year round maintenance of strength (by resistive exercises, not play) and flexibility is the best preventive measure.

The possible importance of patella mechanism orientation (and anthropometry) as a derivative of injuries in basketball is pointed out by the study of Shambaugh *et al.* (1991). 45 players in a community basketball league were evaluated for Q angle, leg girth, foot and ankle posture, leg length inequality and the amount of weight born by each extremity (i.e. weight-bearing difference). Using regression analytical techniques for the eight variables studied, Shambaugh *et al.* discovered a 91% prediction of injury when only the left Q angle and the difference in the amount of weight borne by each lower extremity were considered. The reason for the 'left' Q angle being significant is not clear. The concept is interesting but the players were not élite, not necessarily of 'typical' basketball stature, and the numbers of variables and injury types may have been insufficient to permit reasonable conclusions.

Achilles tendinitis

Achilles tendinitis is a common affliction among basketball players, whose activities combine the activities known to induce the affliction, mainly running and jumping. According to Leach *et al.* (1991), the onset of Achilles tendinitis in basketball players is usually acute and consequent to the dramatic forces of jumping, accelerations and decelerations. Often, there is a partial tear of the substance of the tendon (Fig. 21.15). The acute episode often results in a chronic affliction as disruption, inflammatory response and fibrous repair are cyclically stimulated by continued activity.

When pathology is acute and/or localized, the presentation is often one of focal pain overlying an area of fusiform swelling at the supramalleolar level of the tendon (Leach *et al.*, 1991). As additional damage accrues from the stress of activity, inflammatory and cicatricial response produce a diffuse thickening of tendon with erythema, heat, and swelling, and an inhibition of active and passive dorsiflexion of the ankle (Leach *et al.*, 1991).

Pathology may involve the tendon proper and/or its sheath (Achilles tenovaginitis). Inflammation of the retrocalcaneal bursa may occur in conjunction with tendinitis or independently in relation to a prominent posterior calcaneal angle (Leach *et al.*, 1991). Enlargement and thickening of the Achilles mechanism may produce secondary inflammation by virtue of compression by the back of the sneaker (Ray *et al.*, 1991).

The diagnosis of Achilles tendinitis is not

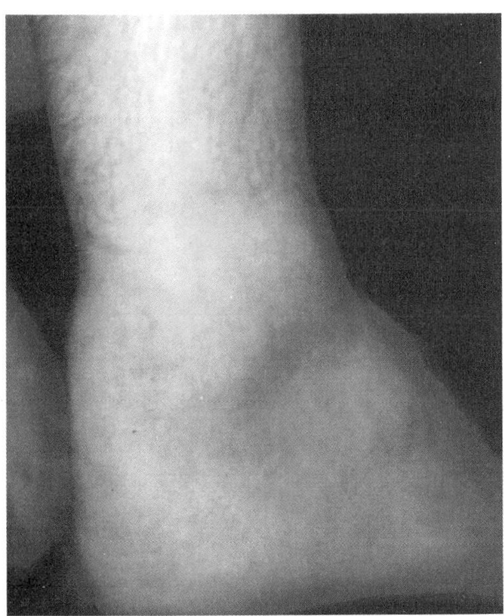

Fig. 21.15 Extreme swelling of the posterior aspect of the ankle. The differential diagnosis includes a range from acute and severe Achilles tendinitis to partial or complete rupture of the Achilles tendon.

difficult. What is difficult is the rendering of a temporal prognosis with respect to length of disability, and more importantly, the delineation of a magnitude, distribution and severity of pathology (particularly in chronic cases). Plain X-rays are usually valueless. On occasion, an area of degeneration within the tendon may be marked by calcific opacities. The most discerning diagnostic modality is MRI by which regions of inflammation and degeneration are characterized by increased signal intensity. Partial or complete tendon disruptions are also discernible by MRI. Bright signal in the region of the retrocalcaneal bursa signifies the presence of fluid (i.e. bursitis).

When symptoms are acute (Fig. 21.16), the most important treatment is a reduction of activity (running and jumping). During the period of relative rest (e.g. the period of acute pain and tenderness), NSAIDs may be used to accelerate the abatement of acute symptoms. These should be discontinued once activity has been reinitiated to avoid masking a response to damage. Modalities such as ultrasound, iontophoresis and whirlpool baths, may also serve to reduce inflammatory manifestations. These may be continued once activity has been reinitiated. Range of motion should be encouraged from the outset to avert a progression of contracture inhibitory to dorsiflexion. As soon as tolerated, posterior ankle and hamstring stretching should be initiated, as well as progressive resistance exercises for all groups of

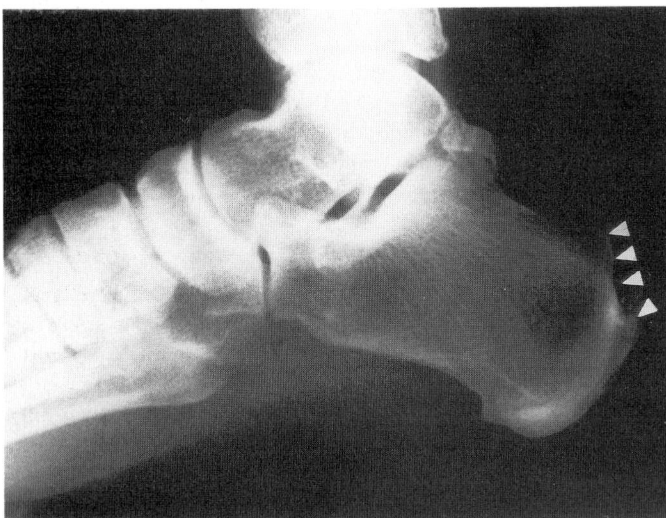

Fig. 21.16 Chronic Achilles tendinitis with pain concentrated at attachment of tendon to os calcis (arrow heads). Note the bony excrescence at this site, where the maximum tenderness exists.

the ankle. Eccentric strengthening modes must be progressed as must the loads and speeds of performance. The rest of the extremity must be strengthened concurrently. Non-percussive aerobics (e.g. cycling, swimming) should be initiated at the outset and progressed to intermediate forms (e.g. stairmaster, trampoline, kinetron) in an effort to maintain conditioning toward a return to basketball *per se*.

On returning to activity a slight heel lift can help relieve symptoms. Orthotics may dramatically alter symptoms if the pathology is not too chronic nor too severe. The reasons are speculative.

In most instances tendinitis comes under control with time, rest and physical therapy. On occasion, manifestations progress or remain recalcitrant. Even at their relative young age, élite basketball players may sustain an acute rupture of the Achilles tendon (encountered once in a 10-year professional experience by the authors). The best treatment in such cases is surgical repair with an expectation of disability lasting about a year, some ultimate loss of function (even if minor) and a predisposition to rerupture.

When chronic Achilles tendinitis precludes effective performance by an élite player, surgical intervention must be considered. Tenovaginectomy and debridement of necrotic areas within the tendon are the options determined by existing pathology. MRI may help determine whether to consider filleting the tendon to excise degenerative tissue. Though immobilization is not necessary, recovery is protracted (many months). Fortunately, this is rarely necessary in players who have complied with conservative treatment regimens.

In 1976, Puddu *et al.* attempted a clarification of the existing classification of Achilles tendon disease processes on the basis of histopathology observed at surgical exploration (Puddu *et al.*, 1976). Whereas the standard nomenclature of athletic injuries (of the American Medical Association), had considered Achilles tendon disorders to be contained within the categories of tenosynovitis, tendinitis and rupture, Puddu *et al.* offer 'more precise' classification:

1 Pure peritendinitis.
2 Peritendinitis with tendinosis (rupture).
3 Tendinosis (rupture).

In 'peritendinitis', only the coverings and penetrating vascular septae are involved; they are thickened and adherent to the tendon, and demonstrate histological evidence of capillary and inflammatory cell proliferations which entirely spare the tendon itself. When, on the other hand, the tendon manifests thickening, softening, yellowing, and/or fibrillations with a secondary vascular invasion from the peritendinous tissue, there exists a 'tendinosis' in addition to peritendinitis. This combination of pathologies is most likely the cause of prodromal symptoms which not infrequently precede tendon rupture. Tendinosis alone is often asymptomatic and can result in ruptures without a prodrome.

The point made by Puddu *et al.* (1976) is that tenolysis is often gratifying when only peritendinitis is present. However, when a tendon with areas of fibrillation and necrosis coexist, tenovaginectomy alone will not resolve the problem. The tendon must be explored through longitudinal excisions to extricate the necrotic areas and to stimulate the ingrowth of a population of new mesendymal cells (Puddu *et al.*, 1976).

When retrocalcaneal bursitis is persistent and disabling, steroid injection into the bursa may be of value. If the bursitis is unresponsive, surgical excision of the bursa becomes a consideration. Leach *et al.* (1991) indicate that when the posterior angle of the calcaneous is resected with the bursa, patients do better.

From the standpoint of prevention, it is vital to restrict activity and to initiate treatment as soon as symptoms of significance are registered so that a progression of disease and damage is averted. Players with flat feet are best fitted with orthotics before the fact. Maintenance of strengthening and stretching of all segments of the lower extremities throughout training and the season are vital.

Hand and wrist injuries

Injuries to the hands and wrists are quite common in basketball. Among 86 players evaluated during the 1990 combined physicals, the injuries recorded are seen in Table 21.8.

Among NBA injuries reported for the 1989–1990 season (NBTA, 1990) the hand accounted for 5.5% and the wrist for 3.25% of the total. In the NCAA, single season hand and wrist injuries occurred at a rate of 0.38 · 1000 exposures^{-1} (NCAA, 1990).

Common mechanisms by which hand and wrist injuries are sustained in basketball include:

1 Contact with the floor.
2 Contact with the ball.
3 Contact with other players.
4 Contact with the basket rim.
5 Ballistic wrist movements (as in dunking or 'rim-rocking').

Items 1–3 are not preventable without altering the basic format of the game. Injuries due to the rim may have been reduced by 'breakaway' rims. Many players capable of dunking and rim-rocking refrain from these actions to avert injury. Malreceptions of the ball and player contact often result in mallet fingers, sprains or fracture–dislocations of the fingers. The little finger is often predilected by virtue of its mobility and acral position (Fig. 21.17).

Direct contact with hard surfaces, such as the floor or rim, may produce metacarpal fractures and fractures or sprains of the carpus. Contact of the volar aspect of the wrist or ballistic volar flexion movements of the wrist in performing these activities can impose acute or attritional injuries upon the carpus and its ligaments. Scapholunate sprains are the most deserving representatives of the eponym 'rim-rocker's wrist' (Fig. 21.18). These sprains are not always acute or dramatic. In fact, there may be long periods of quiescence between the time of injury and the appearance of noteworthy signs or symptoms. Often, no specific injury is recollected. Flare-ups of pain and swelling may wax and wane or may appear and persist.

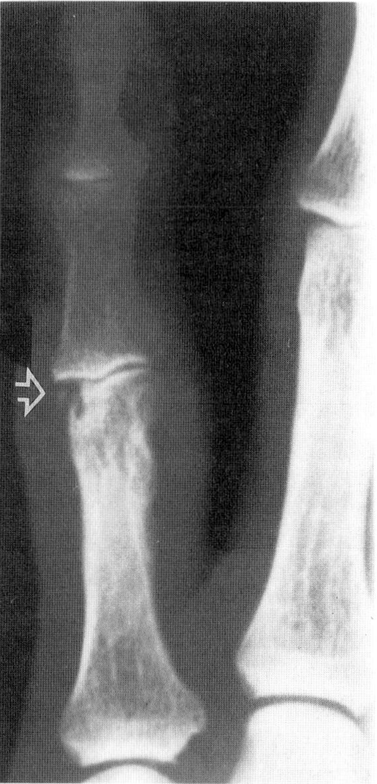

Fig. 21.17 Little finger injuries are all too common, producing fractures and sprains of each of the joints. This radiograph demonstrates the residua of a proximal interphalangeal joint dislocation, capsular disruption and bone avulsion (arrow). Chronic recurrent instability was the ultimate result. Fusion may be necessary.

Table 21.8 Hand and wrist injuries: 1990 combined physicals. Data from J.A. Hefferson (personal communication).

Hand	
Finger fractures	11
Finger dislocations/sprains	10
Mallet finger	1
Metacarpal fractures	2
Wrist	
Sprains	2
Non-specific fractures	3
Healed scaphoid fractures	2
Scaphoid non-unions	2

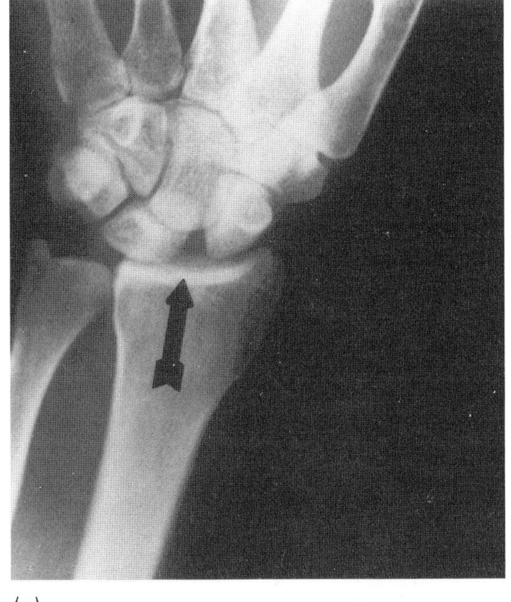

(a)

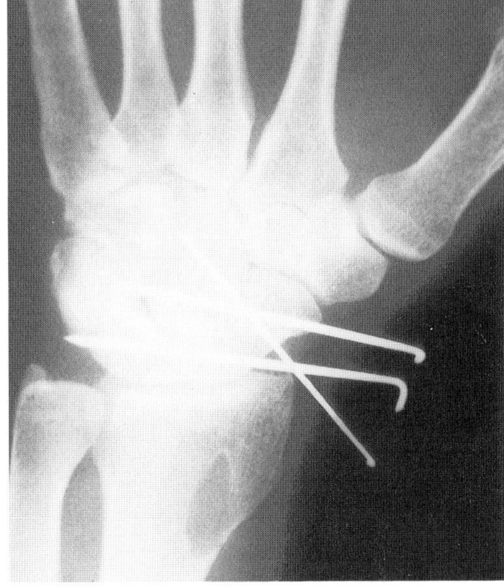

(b)

(c)

Fig. 21.18 Carpal ligament rupture and separation of the navicular and lunate demonstrated by the arrow (a). Reduction and internal fixation uniting navicular to capitate (b). Postoperative result demonstrating capitate–navicular union (c).

Conclusion

Basketball is a contact sport in which injuries are sustained by contact as well as non-contact mechanisms. Many overuse injuries are witnessed as a result of basketball, including the tendinidites and stress fractures. The most dreaded entities are knee ligament ruptures, stress fractures, sudden death syndromes and substance abuse. The most frequent injury producing missed player days is the sprained ankle.

The spectrum of injuries and disabilities associated with basketball is great. Only selected afflictions have been chosen for discussion in this chapter. While many injuries are not preventable unless the intensity of the game is altered, many can be avoided or minimized by maintaining a year round vigil of extremity strengthening and stretching and of cardiovascular fitness. There is some evidence to suggest that strappings or bracing of the ankle can reduce the incidence of the most common injury, the ankle sprain.

References

Abdenour, T.E., Seville, W.A., White, R.C. *et al.* (1979) Effect of ankle taping upon torque and range of motion. *Athletic Training* **4**, 227–8.

Anderson, K.J. & LeCocq, J.F. (1954) Operative treatment of the fibula collateral ligament of the ankle. *J. Bone Joint Surg.* **36A**, 825–7.

Anderson, K.J., LeCocq, J.F. & Clayton, M.L. (1962) Athletic injury of the fibula collateral ligament of the ankle. *Clin. Orthop.* **23**, 146–9.

Andrish, J. & Work, J.A. (1990) How I manage shin splints. *Phys. Sportsmed.* **18**(12), 113–14.

Apple Jr, D.F. (1988) Basketball injuries: An overview. *Phys. Sportsmed.* **16**(12), 64–74.

Beals, R.K. & Cook, R.D. (1991) Stress fractures of the anterior tibial diaphysis. *Orthopedics* **14**(8), 869–75.

Belik, S.E. (1934) *The New Trainer's Bible.* Atsco Press, New York.

Benton, W. (1969) *Encyclopedia Britannica*, Vol. 3, pp. 247–54. Chicago.

Black, H.M., Brand, R.L. & Eichelberger, M.R. (1978) An improved technique for the evaluation of ligamentous injury in severe ankle sprains. *Am. J. Sports Med.* **6**, 276–82.

Blank, S. (1987) Transverse tibial stress fractures. *Am. J. Sports Med.* **15**(6), 597–602.

Blazina, M.E., Kerlan, R.K., Jobe, F.W. *et al.* (1975) Jumper's knee. *Orthop. Clin. N. Am.* **4**, 665–9.

Bonnin, J.G. (1944) The hypermobile ankle. *Proc. Roy. Soc. Med.* **37**, 282–6.

Bosien, W.R., Staples, O.S. & Russel, S.W. (1955) Residual disability following acute ankle sprains. *J. Bone Joint Surg.* **37A**, 1237–43.

Brahms, M.A., Fumich, R.M. & Ippolito, V.D. (1980) Atypical stress fracture of tibial in professional athlete. *Am. J. Sports Med.* **8**, 131–2.

Broström, L. (1966) Sprained ankles; V. Treatment and prognosis in recent ligament ruptures. *Acta Chir. Scand.* **132**, 537–50.

Burrows, H.J. (1956) Fatigue infraction of the middle tibia in ballet dancers. *J. Bone Joint Surg.* **38B**, 83.

Cantwell, J.D. & Rose, F.D. (1986) Cocaine and cardiovascular events. *Phys. Sportsmed.* **14**(11), 77–82.

Caro, D., Craft, I.L., Howells, J.B. & Shaw, P.C. (1964) Diagnosis and treatment of injury of lateral ligament of the ankle joint. *Lancet* **ii**, 720–3.

Carp, L. (1927) Fracture of the fifth metatarsal, with special reference to delayed union. *Arr. Surg.* **86**, 308–20.

Castaing, J. & Delplace, J. (1972) Interet de l'etude de la stabilite dans le plan sagittal pour le diagnostique de gravite. Recherche radiographique du tiroir astragalien anterieur. *Rev. Chir. Orthop.* **58**(51), 1665–700.

Cavanagh, P.R. & Robinson, J.R. (1989) *A biomechanical perspective on stress fractures in NBA players. A final report to the National Basketball Association.* Research partially supported by and submitted to the NBA.

Chandy, T.A. & Grana, W.A. (1985) Secondary school athletic injuries in boys and girls. A three year comparison. *Phys. Sportsmed.* **13**(3), 106–11.

Chillag, S.A. (1991) Is exercise-related sudden death preventable? *Your Patient Fitness* **4**(2), 12–15.

Chirls, M. (1973) Inversion injuries of the ankle. *J. Med. Soc. New Jersey* **70**, 751–3.

Clark, B.L., Derby, A.C. & Power, C.R.I. (1965) Injuries of the lateral ligament of the ankle: conservative vs. operative repair. *Can. J. Surg.* **5**, 358–63.

Cox, J. & Hewes, T.F. (1979) Normal talar tilt angle. *Clin. Orthop.* **140**, 37–41.

Crenshaw, A.N. (ed) (1987) *Campbell's Operative Orthopedics*, 7th edn. CV Mosby, St Louis.

Daffner, R.H., Martinez, S.M. & Gehweiler, J.A. (1982) Stress fractures in runners. *JAMA* **247**(7), 1039–41.

Dameron Jr, T.B. (1975) Fractures and anatomical variations of the proximal portion of the fifth metatarsal. *J. Bone Joint Surg.* **57A**, 788–92.

DeBenedette, V. (1991) Bad breaks in basketball: Unforgettable injuries. *Phys. Sportmed.* **19**(3), 135–9.

Dehne, E. (1933) Die Klinik der frischen und habituellen Adduktionssupinationsdistorsion des Fusses (Clinical picture of healthy and recurrent abduction supination sprains of the ankle). *Deut. Z. Chir.* **242**, 40–61.

DeLee, J.C., Evans, P.J. & Julian, J.D. (1983) Stress fracture of the fifth metatarsal. *Am. J. Sports Med.* **11**(5), 349–53.

Demak, R. (1991) One false move. *Sports Illustrated* **29 April**, 52–8.

Devas, M.B. (1958) Stress fractures of the tibia in

athletes or 'shin splints'. *J. Bone Joint Surg.* **40B**, 227–39.

Dias, L.S. (1979) The lateral ankle sprain: An experimental study. *J Trauma* **19**, 266–9.

Emerick, C.E. (1979) Ankle taping: prevention of injury or waste of time? *Athletic Training* **14**, 149–50.

Epstein, S.E. & Maron, B.J. (1986) Sudden death and the competitive athlete: perspectives on preparticipation screening studies. *J. Am. Coll. Cardiol.* **7**(1), 220–30.

Evans, G.A. & Frenyo, S.D. (1979) The stress-tenogram in the diagnosis of ruptures of the lateral ligament of the ankle. *J. Bone Joint Surg.* **61B**(3), 347–51.

Evarts, C.M. (ed) (1983) *Surgery of the Musculoskeletal System*, pp. 145–74. Churchill Livingstone, New York.

Fordyce, A.J.W. & Horn, C.V. (1972) Arthrography in recent injuries of the ligaments of the ankle. *J. Bone Joint Surg.* **54B**, 116–21.

Frankel, V.H. (1975) Biomechanics can Tibia Frackuren en van Vermoeidheidsfractured. *Gen. Sports* **2**, 30–3.

Freeman, M.A.R. (1965) Instability of the foot after injuries to the lateral ligament of the ankle. *J. Bone Joint Surg.* **47B**, 669–77.

Friedenberg, Z.B. (1971) Fatigue fractures of the tibia, *Clin. Orthop. Rel. Res.* **76**, 111–15.

Fulkerson, J.P. & Shea, K.P. (1990) Mechanical basis for patellofemoral pain and cartilage breakdown: articular cartilage and knee joint function. J.W. Ewing (ed) *Basic Science and Arthroscopy*, pp. 93–102. Raven Press, New York.

Fussell, M.E. & Godley, D.R. (1972) Ankle arthrography in acute sprains. *Clin. Orthop. Rel. Res.* **93**, 278–90.

Garrick, J.G. (1987) Epidemiology of foot and ankle injuries. *Med. Sport Sci.* **23**, 991–7.

Garrick, J.G. & Requa, R.K. (1977) The frequency of injury and epidemiology of ankle sprains. *Am. J. Sports Med.* **5**, 241–2.

Giladi, M., Ahronson, Z., Stein, M. *et al.* (1985) Unusual distribution and onset of stress fractures in soldiers. *Clin. Orthop. Rel. Res.* **192**, 142–5.

Giladi, M., Milgrom, C., Simkin, A. *et al.* (1987) Stress fractures and tibial bone width. *J. Bone Joint Surg.* **69B**(2), 326–9.

Goodman, M.J. (1980) Isolated lateral compartment syndrome. *J. Bone Joint Surg.* **62A**, 834–45.

Green, N.E., Rogers, R.A. & Lipscomb, A.B. (1985) Nonunions of stress fractures of the tibia. *Am. J. Sports Med.* **13**(3), 171–6.

Gross, A.E. & MacIntosh, D.L. (1973) Injury to the lateral ligament of the ankle: A clinical study. *Can. J. Surg.* **16**, 115–17.

Gross, T.S. & Nelson, R.C. (1988) The shock attenuation role of the ankle during landing from a vertical jump. *Med. Sci Sports Exerc.* **20**(5), 506–14.

Guttner, L. (1941) Erkennung und Behandlung des Banderrisses am Ausseren Knochel mit Teilverrenkung des Sprungbeines im Sinne der Supination (Subluxatio supinatoria pedis). *Arch. Orthop. Unfallchirurg.* **41**, 287–98.

Haas, S.S. (1988) *Lower extremity injuries in the NBA 1983–1987*. Presented to the NBA Physicians in Palm Beach, Florida, September, 1988.

Hayes, W.G., Huberti, H.H., Lewallen, D.G. *et al.* (1990) Patellofemoral contact pressures and the effects of surgical reconstructive procedures; articular cartilage and knee joint function. In J.W. Ewing (ed) *Basic Science and Arthroscopy*, pp. 57–77. Raven Press, New York.

Henry, J.H., Lareau, B. & Neigut, D. (1982) The injury rate in professional basketball. *Am. J. Sports Med.* **10**(1), 16–18.

Holder, L.E. (1982) Current concepts review: Radionuclide bone-imaging in the evaluation of bone pain. *J. Bone Joint Surg.* **64A**, 1391–6.

Hollander, Z. & Sachare, A. (eds) (1989) *The Official NBA Basketball Encyclopedia*. Villard Books, New York.

Hughes, L.Y. (1985) Biomechanical analysis of the foot and ankle for predisposition to developing stress fractures. *J. Orthop. Sports Phys. Ther.* **7**, 96–101.

Hughes, L.Y. & Stetts, D.M. (1983) A comparison of ankle taping and a semirigid support. *Phys. Sports Med.* **11**(4), 99–103.

Hyslop, G.H. (1941) Injuries to the deep and superficial peroneal nerves complicating ankle sprain. *Am. J. Surg.* **51**, 436–8.

Jackson, D.W., Ashley, R.L. & Powell, J.W. (1974) Ankle sprains in young athletes. *Clin. Orth. Rel. Res.* **101**, 201–15.

Jackson, D.W. & Strizak, A.M. (1982) Stress fractures in runners excluding the foot. In R.P. Mack (ed) *The Foot and Leg in Running Sports*. C.V. Mosby, St Louis.

Jaskulka, R., Fischer, G. & Schedl, R. (1988) Injuries of the lateral ligaments of the ankle joint: operative treatment and long-term results. *Arch. Orthop. Trauma Surg.* **107**, 217–21.

Johnson, E.E. & Markolf, K.L. (1983) The contribution of the anterior talofibular ligament to ankle laxity. *J. Bone Joint Surg.* **65A**, 81–8.

Jones, N.P. (1989) Eye injury in sports. *Sports Med.* **7**, 163–81.

Jones, R. (1902) Fracture of the base of the fifth metatarsal by indirect violence. *Ann. Surg.* **35**, 699.

Karlson, T.A. & Klein, B.E. (1986) The incidence of acute hospital treated eye injuries. *Arch. Ophthal.*

104, 1473–6.

Kavanaugh, J.H., Brower, T.D. & Mann, R.V. (1978) The Jones' fracture revisited. *J. Bone Joint Surg.* **60A**(6), 776–82.

Key, J.A. & Conwell, H.E. (1946) *The Management of Fractures, Dislocations and Sprains*, 4th edn. CV Mosby, St Louis.

Lanyon, J.E., Hampson, W.G.J., Goodship, A.E. & Shah, J.S. (1975) Bone deformation recorded *in vivo* from strain gauges attached to the human tibial shift. *Acta Orthop. Scand.* **46**, 256–9.

Larkin, J. & Brage, M. (1991) Ankle, hindfoot, and midfoot injuries. In B. Reider (ed) *Sports Medicine, The School-Age Athlete*, pp. 365–405. WB Saunders, Philadelphia.

Laughman, R.K., Carr, T.A., Chao, E.Y. *et al.* (1980) Three-dimensional kinematics of the taped ankle before and after exercise. *Am. J. Sports Med.* **8**(6), 425–31.

Laurin, C.A. (1968) Talar and subtalar tilt: An experimental investigation. *Can. J. Surg.* **11**(3), 270–9.

Leach, R.E., Schepsis, A.A. & Takai H. (1981) Achilles tendinitis. *Phys. Sportsmed.* **19**(8), 87–92.

Lee, J.K. & Yao, L. (1988) Stress fractures: MR imaging. *Radiology* **169**, 217–20.

Leonard, M.H. (1949) Injuries of the lateral ligaments of the ankle. *J. Bone Joint Surg.* **31A**, 373–7.

Leonard, M.H. (1959) Strains and sprains of the ankle. *Am. J. Orthop.* **1**, 227–38.

Lilletvedt, J., Kreighbaum, E. & Phillips, R.L. (1979) Analysis of selected alignment factors related to shin splint syndrome. *J. Am. Podiatr. Assoc.* **69**, 211–17.

Liu, C.T., Benda, C.E. & Lewey, F.H. (1948) Tensile strength of human nerves. *Arch. Neurol. Psychiat.* **59**, 322–36.

Lombardo, J.A. (1986) Stimulants and athletic performance (Part 2): cocaine and nicotine. *Phys. Sportsmed.* **14**(12), 85–90.

Lombardo, S.J. (1990) Communication to NBA Physicians, 15 December.

McBryde, A.M. (1985) Stress fractures in runners. *Clin. Sports Med.* **4**(4), 737–52.

McMahon, T.A. & Green, P.R. (1979) The influence of track compliance on running. *J. Biomech.* **12**, 893–904.

McMaster, P.E. (1943) Treatment of ankle sprain. *JAMA* **122**, 659–60.

Markey, K.L. (1987) Stress fractures. *Clin. Sportsmed.* **6**(2), 405–25.

Maron, B.J., Roberts W.C., McAllister, H.A. *et al.* (1980) Sudden death in young athletes. *Circulation* **62**(2), 218–30.

Martens, M., Wouters, P., Burssens, A. & Mulier, J.C. (1982) Patellar tendinitis: pathology and results of treatment. *Acta Orthop. Scand.* **53**, 445–50.

Matheson, G.O., Clement, D.B., McKenzie, D.C., Taunton, J.E., Lloyd-Smith, D.R. & Macintyre, J.G. (1987) Stress fractures in athletes: a study of 320 cases. *Am. J. Sports Med.* **15**(1), 46–58.

Matsuzaki, A. (1979) Painful condition of legs of runners. *Orthop. Traumatol Surg.* **22**, 479–85.

MFMA (1988) *Incidence of Injury Study: Maple Flooring vs. Synthetic.* Maple Flooring Manufactures Association.

Milgrom, C., Giladi, M., Simkin, A. *et al.* (1988) An analysis of the biomechanical mechanism of tibial stress fractures among Israeli infantry recruits. *Clin. Orthop. Rel. Res.* **231**, 216–21.

Minkoff, J. & Fein, L. (1989) The role of radiography in the evaluation and treatment of common anarthrotic disorders of the patellofemoral joint. *Clin. Sports Med.* **8**(2), 203–66.

Morrison, G.M. (1937) Fractures of the bones of the feet. *Am. J. Surg.* **38**, 721–6.

Mutoh, Y., Yoshiro, S. & Sugiura, Y. (1980) Stress fractures of the fibula due to the so-called rabbit jump. *Orthop. Traumatol Surg.* **23**, 332–8.

NBTA (1990) *Injury Report, 1989–90.* National Basketball Trainers Association.

NCAA (1990) *1989–90, Basketball.* National Collegiate Athletics Association injury surveillance statistics.

Niethard, F.U. (1974) Die Stabilitat des Sprunggelenkes nach Ruptur des lateralan Bandapparates (Stability of the ankle joint after a tear of the lateral ligament). *Arch. Orthop. Unfallchirurg.* **80**, 53–61.

Nitz, A.J., Dobner, J.J. & Kersey, D. (1985) Nerve injury and grade II and III ankle sprains. *Am. J. Sports Med.* **13**, 177–82.

Nkele, C., Aindow, J. & Grant, L. (1988) Study of pressure of the normal anterior tibial compartment in different age groups using the slit-cather method. *J. Bone Joint Surg.* **70A**, 98–101.

Nobel, W. (1966) Peroneal palsy due to hematoma in the common peroneal nerve sheath after distal torsional fractures and ankle sprains. *J. Bone Joint Surg.* **48A**, 1484–95.

Orava, S. & Hulkko, A. (1988) Delayed unions and non-unions of stress fractures in athletes. *Am. J. Sports Med.* **16**(4), 378–82.

Orava, S. & Puranen, J. (1979) Athletes' leg pains. *Br. J. Sports Med.* **13**, 92–7.

Orava, S., Puranen, J. & Ala-Ketola, L. (1978) Stress fractures caused by physical exercise. *Acta Orthop. Scand.* **49**(1), 19–27.

Pasternack, P.F., Colvin, S.B. & Baumann, F.G. (1988) Cocaine-induced angina pectoris and acute myocardial infarction in patients younger than forty years. *Am. J. Cardiol.* 1 March.

Pock-Steen, O.Ch. (1958) Distorsio pedis (Ankle sprains). *Ugeskr. Laeg.* **120**, 561–8.

Prather, J.L., Nusynowitz, M.L., Snowdy, H.A. *et al.* (1977) Scintigraphic findings in stress fractures. *J. Bone Joint Surg.* **59A**(7), 869–74.

Protzman, R.R. & Griffis, C.G. (1977) Stress fractures in men and women undergoing military training. *J. Bone Joint Surg.* **59A**(6), 825.

Provost, R.A. & Morris, J.M. (1969) Fatigue fracture of the femoral shaft. *J. Bone Joint Surg.* **51A**, 487–98.

Puddu, G., Ippolito, E. & Postacchini, F. (1976) A classification of Achilles tendon disease. *Am. J. Sports Med.* **4**(4), 145–50.

Quigley, T.B., Cox, J. & Murphy, J. (1946) Protective wrapping for the ankle. *JAMA* **132**, 924.

Rarick, G.L., Bigley, G., Karst, R. & Malina, R.M. (1962) The measurable support of the ankle joint by conventional methods of taping. *J. Bone Joint Surg.* **44A**(6), 1183–90.

Ray, J.M., McCombs, W. & Sternes, R.A. (1991) Basketball and volleyball injuries. In B. Reider (ed) *Sports Medicine The School-Age Athlete*, pp. 365–405. WB Saunders, Philadelphia.

Reckling, F.W., Reckling, J.B. & Mohn, M.P. (1990) *Orthopaedic Anatomy and Surgical Approaches*. Mosby-Year Book, St Louis.

Reneman, R.S. (1975) The anterior and the lateral compartmental syndrome of the leg due to intensive use of muscles. *Clin. Orthop. Rel. Res.* **113**, 69–79.

Rettig, A.C., Shelbourne, K.D., McCarroll, J.R. *et al.* (1988) The natural history and treatment of delayed union stress fractures of the anterior cortex of the tibia. *Am. J. Sports Med.* **16**(3), 250–5.

Rovere, G.D., Clarke, T.J., Yates, C.S. & Burley, K. (1988) Retrospective comparison of taping and ankle stabilizers in preventing ankle injuries. *Am. J. Sports Med.* **16**(3), 228–33.

Rubin, G. & Witten, M. (1960) The talar tilt angle and the fibular collateral ligaments of the ankle. *J. Bone Joint Surg.* **42A**, 321–6.

Ruth, C.J. (1961) The surgical treatment of injuries of the fibular collateral ligaments. *J. Bone Joint Surg.* **43A**, 229–39.

Sammarco, G.J. & DiRaimondo, C.V. (1988) Surgical treatment of lateral ankle instability syndrome. *Am. J. Sports Med.* **16**(5), 501–11.

Sauser, D.D., Nelson, R.C., Lavine, M.H. & Wu, C.W. (1983) Acute injuries of the lateral ligaments of the ankle: comparison of stress radiography and arthrography. *Radiology* **148**, 653–7.

Scully, T.J. & Besterman, G. (1982) Stress fracture — A preventable training injury. *Milit. Med.* **147**, 285–7.

Seitz Jr, W.H. & Grantham, S.A. (1985) The Jones' fracture in the nonathlete. *Foot Ankle* **6**, 97–100.

Selesnick, F.H., Arena, D. & Bush, J.J. (1990) *The competitive basketball player's knee: prospective clinical and MRI scan analysis*. Presented to the Association of NBA Physicians, Boca Raton, Florida, September.

Shambaugh, J.P., Klein, A. & Herbert, J.H. (1991) Structural measures as predictors of injury in basketball. *Med. Sci. Sports Exerc.* **23**(5), 522–7.

Shorten, M.R. (1987) Muscle elasticity and human performance. *Med. Sport Sci.* **25**, 1–18.

Stanitski, C.L., McMaster, J.H. & Scranton, P.E. (1978) On the nature of stress fractures. *Am. J. Sports Med.* **6**(6), 391–6.

Staples, O.S. (1975) Ruptures of the fibular collateral ligaments of the ankle. Result of immediate surgical treatment. *J. Bone Joint Surg.* **57A**, 101–7.

Stewart, I.M. (1990) Jones' fracture: fracture of the base of fifth metatarsal. *Clin. Orthop.* **16**, 190–8.

Styf, J. (1988) Diagnosis of exercise-induced pain in the anterior aspect of the lower leg. *Am. J. Sports Med.* **16**, 165–9.

Symeonides, P.P. (1980) High stress fractures of the fibula. *J. Bone Joint Surg.* **62B**, 192–3.

Taunton, J.E., Clement, D.B. & Webber, D.B. (1981) Lower extremity stress fractures in athletes. *Phys. Sportsmed.* **9**, 77–86.

Teitz, C.C., Carter, D.R. & Frankel, V.H. (1980) Problems associated with tibial fractures with intact fibulas. *J. Bone Joint Surg.* **62A**, 770–6.

Torg, J.S., Baldkini, F.C., Zelko, R.R. *et al.* (1984) Fractures of the base of the fifth metatarsal distal to the tuberosity. *J. Bone Joint Surg.* **66A**, 209–14.

Tropp, H., Askling, C. & Gillquist, J. (1985) Prevention of ankle sprains. *Am. J. Sports Med.* **13**(4), 259–61.

Valiant, G.A. & Cavanagh, P.R. (1987) A study of landing from a jump: implications for the design of a basketball shoe. In D.A. Winter, R.W. Norman, R.P. Wells, K.C. Hayes & A.E. Patta (eds) *Biomechanics-XB*, pp. 117–22. Human Kinetics, Illinois.

Veith, R.G., Matsen, F.A. & Newell, S.G. (1980) Recurrent anterior compartmental syndromes. *Phys. Sportsmed.* **8**, 80–8.

Vinger, P.F. (1985) The eye in sports medicine. *Clin. Ophthal.* **5**, 12–15.

Wallenstein, R. (1983) Results of fasciotomy in patients with medial-tibial syndrome or chronic anterior compartment syndrome. *J. Bone Joint Surg.* **65A**(9), 1252–5.

Walter, N.E. & Wolf, M.D. (1977) Stress fractures in young athletes. *Am. J. Sports Med.* **5**(4), 165–9.

Watson-Jones, R. (1941) *Fractures and Other Bone and Joint Injuries*, 2nd edn. E & S Livingstone, Edinburgh.

Zelisko, J.A., Noble, H.B. & Porter, M. (1982) A comparison of men's and women's professional basketball injuries. *Am. J. Sports Med.* **10**(5), 297–9.

Zelko, R.R., Torg, J.S. & Rachun, A. (1979) Proximal diaphyseal fractures of the fifth metatarsal — treatment of the fractures and their complications in athletes. *Am. J. Sports Med.* **7**, 95–101.

Chapter 22

Injuries in Team Handball

ÅKE ANDRÉN-SANDBERG

In recent years, a number of surveys have shown that increased physical activity is conducive to good health (Fentem & Bassey, 1979). However, all physical activity, and especially sports, are associated with injuries. Therefore, it is of utmost importance to minimize the injuries in sports to get a positive balance of increase in health versus injuries.

Handball is sometimes called team handball in order not to confuse it with the individually and recreationally played handball in northern America which uses racquets, not hands. Handball is a rather tough game most commonly played indoors (Fig. 22.1). Each team has 12 players (including two goalkeepers), with seven individuals playing in the court at each time. A match is 60 min long. The world and Olympic champions have so far come from Germany, Sweden and eastern Europe, but handball is also played in China, Japan, northern Africa and Cuba. In sports medicine, handball is known to have problems with both number and severity of injuries (Fig. 22.2).

Injury incidence

The injury rate in a particular sport, however, varies under different circumstances. During one decade, we have investigated the injury incidence in handball in different settings, from world élite championships to childrens tournaments. The aim of the studies has been to gather data, thus providing possibilities for prevention. The following is a summary of

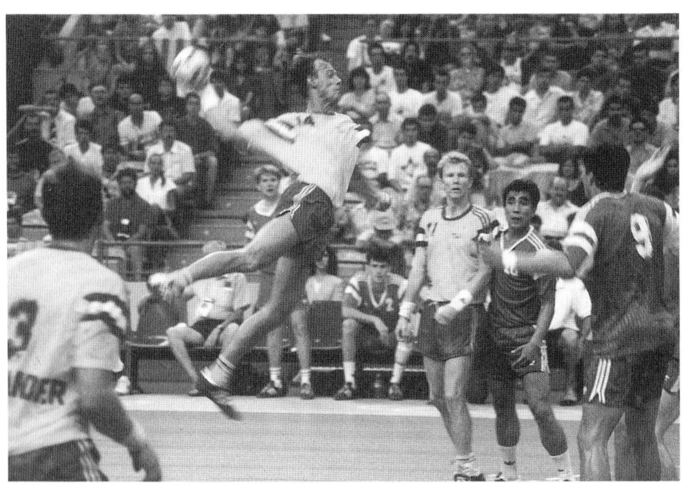

Fig. 22.1 Team handball is a sport which includes many activities which can induce trauma. Courtesy of Dr P.A.F.H. Renström.

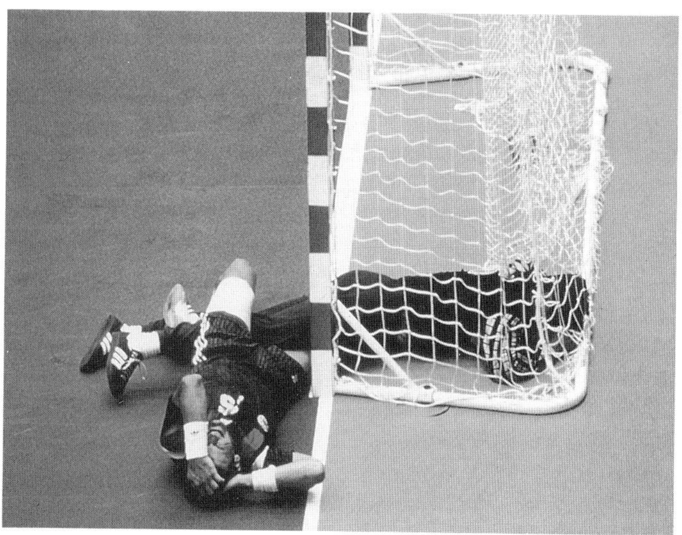

Fig. 22.2 Collisions between the goalkeeper and players, although not common, can result in serious injury. © Vandystadt.

some of the findings.

During two consecutive world championships, the risks of being injured was calculated. In both tournaments there were 12 teams playing, and the injuries which occurred during the tournament were reported by the team doctor through a special protocol. The injury was reported if the player concerned could not play the next match due to the injury.

There were 79 injuries reported during 44 matches, giving an injury rate of 0.9 injuries·match^{-1}·team^{-1} or 0.13 injuries·h^{-1}·player^{-1} (goalkeepers included). The types of injuries are given in Table 22.1.

During 12 consecutive years, the Swedish first handball league were covered for all major injuries. The team doctors or the coaches were interviewed at least once a year for injuries, with special regard to injuries requiring surgery. Only injuries leading to an interruption of practice and playing for at least 14 days were reported, leaving most overuse injuries outside of the study parameters. Included in surgery is arthroscopy and closed reduction of fractures, but not superficial incisions of haematomas or suturing of simple wounds (Table 22.2).

Statistically, there were nine injuries of this severity per team per year, giving an average of

Table 22.1 Team doctors reported injuries in two consecutive world championships in handball.

Site of injury	Injury not requiring immobilization	Injury requiring immobilization or more extensive treatment
Head, neck	2	—
Trunk	2	—
Shoulder	3	2
Arm	1	—
Hand	5	5
Hip, groin	1	—
Thigh	2	—
Knee	21	8
Leg below knee	10	17

Table 22.2 Team doctors or coaches reported injuries during 12 consecutive years in all 12 teams in the first league. Number of injuries are given, with number of injuries leading to surgery in brackets (only one note is given per injury for surgery, even if one injury did require repeated operations).

Site of injury	Fractures, torn ligaments	Contusions, distorsions	Overuse injuries
Head, neck	31 (11)	—	—
Trunk	2	21	69
Shoulder	18 (8)	8	17
Arm	20 (16)	3	12
Hand	111 (26)	13	4
Hip, groin	—	8 (2)	3 (1)
Thigh	—	1	31
Knee	172 (153)	211	69
Leg below knee	202 (39)	259	22

one injury every second year per player. Of the 256 injuries treated with surgery, 60% affected the knees.

During two consecutive years, the élite handball players in 10 teams in Sweden were covered for injuries by an agreement of the team doctors. The registration of injuries was performed prospectively, after a thorough preseason investigation of each player. All injuries requiring interruption of at least one planned practice or match were reported. 87% of the injuries were acute, the other 13% were of overuse type (Table 22.3). 68% of the injuries occurred during matches.

In a study of injuries of intercompany (recreational) handball, 313 matches of 2 × 18 min duration were looked at. A doctor was present at the side of the arena during play and registered the injuries immediately after investigation.

In total, 77 injuries were registered; 20 of them resulted in incapacity to play for at least 1 week. Thus, there was 1 injury $\cdot$ 2.4 h^{-1} of playing, and a risk of 2.9% of sustaining any injury for each player per played hour, and less then 1% risk of sustaining an injury resulting in incapacity to play of at least 1 week. Of the 20 more severe injuries, 16 resulted in incapacity for at least 3 weeks and eight injuries for at least 6 weeks. Of them, five were located in the knee and in four cases an operation was performed (Andrén-Sandberg *et al.*, 1981).

Table 22.3 Team doctors reported injuries during 2 consecutive years in 10 teams in Swedish élite handball.

	Handball given up for		
Site of injury	1–7 days	1–3 weeks	>3 weeks
Head, neck	2	—	1
Trunk	5	1	13
Shoulder	17	9	22
Arm	21	30	18
Hand	78	21	7
Hip, groin	8	2	23
Thigh	2	1	2
Knee	48	37	72
Leg below knee	63	41	26
Total	244	142	184

Injuries in junior league handball were investigated during a 3-day junior handball tournament, 'Lundaspelen', held in Lund yearly. The 7320 participants were boys and girls between 10 and 18 years old. The older ones had in most instances practised at handball regularly for several years, while the younger ones had trained regularly for less than 2 years. In the lower age groups, handball is more technical, and less tough than in the higher age groups, but as elimination rules apply in a cup tournament the level of commitment was high and the potential injury risk was considered great.

During the 3 years under investigation, the same doctor was available for the treatment of injuries, on call and with special visiting hours once a day. The history and the findings on physical examination made by the doctor were prospectively registered. At all nearby centres with casualty and emergency service (one hospital and three clinics), all patients 18 years or younger with injuries sustained during the tournament days in 1980 were asked whether they had been injured while participating in the handball tournament. The case records were examined and compared with the tournament doctor's case sheet (Andrén-Sandberg & Lindstrand, 1982). The results are presented in Table 22.4.

Considerations for prevention and care

In the registration of sports injuries, it is often unclear which injuries have and have not been considered and how large was the population concerned. We attempted to determine the validity of a survey of sports injuries and to calculate the injury risk in handball in one of the studies (Andrén-Sandberg & Lindstrand, 1982). In the other studies, there was only a calculation of the actual risks, as the populations were more easily identified.

Level of competition

The injury rate can be expressed in various ways: for example, with respect to the number of teams in the tournament, the number of players, the number of players on the court at the same time, per played unit of time, or per 'effective' number of players and unit of time (e.g. per 1000 players per hour). When compared with other sports or activities, injuries are best expressed in proportion to the unit of time played by each individual player. One should, however, take into account the fact that different participating situations involve different risks for injury, probably due to various levels of commitment on the part of the players; a cup tournament with honour and prizes at stake is presumably associated with a greater degree of intensity than an ordinary league or friendly match. It has also been clearly shown in all our studies that there is a higher injury rate in playing a match than while training, so that the injury rate during the tournament was

Table 22.4 Injuries, total and grade III (requiring immobilization or more extensive treatment), treated by the tournament doctor classified according to age and gender, both in absolute terms and in relation to the number of players and played match time during the entire tournament.

Categories of players (age in years)	Number of injuries	Number of players	Injuries·1000 players^{-1}	Number of hours	Injuries·100 h^{-1}	Number of injuries grade III	Injuries grade III·100 h^{-1}
Males							
17–18	11	648	17.0	70.5	15.6	5	7.1
15–16	8	912	8.8	97.0	8.2	3	3.1
13–14	3	1032	2.9	73.3	4.1	2	2.7
11–12	2	948	2.1	67.0	3.0	1	1.5
<11	1	600	1.7	39.0	2.6	0	—
Females							
17–18	6	384	15.6	52.5	11.4	1	1.9
15–16	5	744	6.7	84.5	5.9	1	1.3
13–14	2	1020	2.0	78.0	2.6	1	1.3
11–12	2	696	2.9	48.7	4.1	0	—
<11	1	336	3.0	32.9	3.1	0	—

higher when compared with the rate for the entire year. Also, intercompany playing had a lower yield of injuries than more competitive and serious playing.

Age

It is also apparent from our surveys that despite the rather small number of registered injuries, there is a clear tendency for the higher age groups to sustain more injuries than the lower. This can partly be explained by the intensity of the game; strength and speed of the game being greater; and the older players being bigger and generally playing at a faster pace. The pattern of increased injuries despite better training is a constant feature of other team games in Sweden: the higher divisions in all sports having more injuries than the lower.

A notable result of our survey is that the younger children do not seem to sustain any appreciable injuries even though they play intensively. There is thus no reason to advise against, or not to recommend this sport for children and youngsters on the basis of the injury risk. However, the pattern of injuries is somewhat different in children than in adults. This, together with different motivation for playing, makes the work of prevention different in the young players.

Type of trauma

The most important experiences, from a sports medicine point of view, is the high incidence of severe injury to the knee. Work in progress at Lund University is an analysis of knee injuries caught on video (most matches are taped on video to be analysed by the coaches and players after the match). In a series of 13 severe injuries, at arthroscopy found to be ruptures of the cruciate ligaments with or without collateral ligaments and meniscus ruptures, the violence in 11 cases was small or moderate. In 11 of 13 cases, the ball-holding player jumped up (never more than about 60% of their maximum capacity) and simulated a shot (no one actually shot). In the air, the player received a small lateral push against the body (the push was not allowed according to the rules, but it was insignificant enough not to be punished by the referee). While the player concentrated on the ball and the players, he 'forgot' his sense of balance, and obviously did not react properly. When returning to the floor, the leg was unprepared for the lateral shift of the gravitational centre of the body and the heavy player (about 82–90 kg or 180–200 lb) produced a valgus or varus force centred on the knee, resulting in the injury. It was always the leg leaving the floor last during the jump that received the injury. From these preliminary results, it can be anticipated that information on the mechanisms of injury given to the players, aiming at their sense of fair play, is important. The referees must also be more aware of the risks of even small pushes on jumping players.

Role of the referee

During the studied period, on both a national and an international level, the referees had started to act much harder on catching the hand of a player free to shoot. This has obviously reduced the number of acute shoulder injuries, which was almost exclusively confined to the earlier time periods of the longitudinal studies.

Shoes and surface

Ankle injuries are still very frequent and although they more seldom require surgery, the players miss both training and matches. This may in part be due to the modern sport shoes. There are several theories of how best to construct the shoe of the players. Too little friction obviously results in more stumbles, but too much friction also gives a higher frequency of stumbling. Also, the low cutting of the shoe results in greater acceleration, but a higher cutting, or even a shoe giving protection over the ankle, results in a lower risk of sprains to the ankle. The possibilities of better training of both strength and coordination of the ankle has yet to be investigated.

The injury pattern is remarkably constant for older handball players in all our studies; injuries to the lower extremities dominating in élite handball, with serious knee injuries being quite frequent. Similar relationships have been shown for female top-level handball (data not shown). It is obvious that a certain injury rate cannot be given for one sport; it is different between different settings. It is highest when played at top levels, and lowest among young participants. If there were a more specific pattern, there would be greater possibilities for more specific prevention. However, the evaluation of the prophylactic activity has yet to be done.

Conclusion

In summary, injuries in handball can be prevented by carrying out a general training programme aiming at good flexibility and strength, by a specific programme including concentric and eccentric jumping and throwing activities, by wearing adequate shoes, by having good and well-educated referees, and by continuous research.

References

Andrén-Sandberg, Å., Berg, P.L., Bergsten, H. *et al.* (1981) Low risk of injuries in inter-company handball. Knee injuries giving most severe injuries. *Läkartidningen* **78**, 4444–5.

Andrén-Sandberg, Å. & Lindstrand, A. (1982) Injuries sustained in junior league handball. A prospective study of validity in the registration of sports injuries. *Scand. J. Soc. Med.* **3**, 101–4.

Fentem, P.H. & Bassey, E.J. (1979) *The Case for Exercise.* Sports Council Research Working Papers, London.

Chapter 23

Injuries in Volleyball

JAMES WATKINS

Over the past two decades, volleyball has evolved from a recreational activity into a highly competitive, highly skilled sport with Olympic and, in some countries, professional status (Schafle *et al.*, 1990). The International Volleyball Federation (FIVB) represents about 150 million players in approximately 170 countries; consequently, in terms of participation, it is one of the most popular sports in the world (Ferretti *et al.*, 1990).

Volleyball is a dynamic sport involving rapid and forceful movements of the body as a whole, both horizontally and vertically, and of the arm and hand when spiking the ball. Because of the large forces involved in such movements, it is inevitable that injuries occur. Whereas the incidence of injuries which occur in some sports, such as tennis, gymnastics and swimming, have been well documented over a fairly long period (Richardson, 1983), there are few studies of injuries resulting from participation in volleyball (Schafle *et al.*, 1990). Comparison of the results of existing studies is difficult because of differences in research design and the variables investigated. However, most studies show a fairly high incidence of injuries to knees, ankles and fingers (Table 23.1).

A number of injury risk factors for volleyball have been identified including jumping, landing, hand contact with ball during spiking, hand contact with ball during blocking, hardness of playing surface, shock absorbency of shoes, collision with fellow team member or opponent, and level of physical conditioning (Ferretti *et al.*, 1984, 1992; Schafle *et al.*, 1990). In a longitudinal study of sport-related injuries in schoolchildren, Backx *et al.* (1991) showed that, in general, sports involving a high risk of injury were characterized by: (i) contact versus non-contact; (ii) high jump rate versus low jump rate; and (iii) indoor versus outdoor location. Whereas volleyball is not a contact sport in the normal sense, collision with a team member or opposing team member, especially on landing following a block jump, is a significant cause of injury in volleyball (Hell & Schonle, 1985; Schafle *et al.*, 1990; Watkins & Green, 1992). Jumping (in spiking and blocking) and landing is a major feature of volleyball; élite performers average 150 maximum effort vertical jumps per match (Schafle *et al.*, 1990). Volleyball can be played indoors or outdoors. Indoor surfaces are usually quite hard which tends to increase the likelihood of injury compared to softer surfaces (Ferretti *et al.*, 1984; Neri, 1991; Watkins & Green, 1992). Consequently, in relation to the three criteria identified by Backx *et al.* (1991), volleyball is a high-risk sport. The major injury risk factors in volleyball are discussed in the section on injury prevention later in this chapter.

Effects of loading on the body

Mechanical load and the musculoskeletal system

The musculoskeletal system, which is also

Table 23.1 Location of injuries by body part.

Study	Level of performance	Total number of injuries	Shoulder (%)	Hand and wrist (%)	Finger (%)	Knee (%)	Ankle (%)	Foot (%)	Back (%)
Watkins & Green (1992)	Good/élite	46	2		22	30	26	9	17
Schafle *et al.* (1990)	Good	154	8	10†		11	18	6	24‡
Lohmann *et al.* (1988)	Good	242		18	41	10	26	8	
Schmidt-Olsen & Jørgensen (1987)	Élite	69	10		29	8	25*		
Yde & Buhl-Nielsen (1988)	Good	33			33		25		
Gerberich *et al.* (1987)	Mixed	106				59	22		
Hell & Schonle (1985)	Élite	214		2	22	8	53	2	3
Byra & McCabe (1981)	Mixed	53	23		22	20	28*		

* These figures include both ankle and foot.
† This figure includes wrist, hand and fingers.
‡ This figure includes neck and back injuries.

referred to as the locomotor system, enables the body to counteract the effects of body weight and bring about desirable movements of the body. By coordinated activity between the various muscle groups, the forces generated by the muscles are transmitted via the bones and joints to enable the individual to maintain an upright body position and/or bring about voluntary controlled movements of the body for the purpose of transporting the body (such as walking, running and jumping) and manipulating objects (such as spiking a volleyball). Consequently, the musculoskeletal system is constantly subjected to mechanical loading, i.e. forces. The amount of mechanical loading, i.e. the magnitude and frequency of forces acting on the musculoskeletal system, depends upon the intensity of physical activity; the greater the intensity of physical activity the higher the loading tends to be. The components of the musculoskeletal system continually adapt their size, shape and structure to withstand the mechanical loading imposed by the activities of everyday life.

Biopositive and bionegative effects of mechanical loading

The response of the musculoskeletal system to mechanical loading can be biopositive or bionegative (Nigg *et al.*, 1984). Bionegative effects can result from either too much load or too little load. Too much load is likely to result in injury — that is structural tissue damage involving one or more components of the musculoskeletal system resulting in functional impairment (for example muscle tears, tendon and ligament strains or bone fractures). Too little load is likely to lead to, for example, atrophy in muscles, tendons and ligaments. Biopositive effects include the effects of training, such as increased strength in muscles, tendons and ligaments. Biopositive effects result from medium-range loading, i.e. not too much and not too little (Fig. 23.1).

Adaptation and injury

In relation to physical training, the principle of overload is well established. In order to develop muscle strength, muscular endurance and cardiorespiratory endurance, it is necessary to stress the systems of the body concerned to a higher level than that to which they are normally subjected, i.e. to increase their functional capabilities the musculoskeletal and cardiorespiratory systems must be overloaded. Like all well-designed mechanical systems, the musculoskeletal system has a safety margin in terms of overload. Whereas moderate overload will result in biopositive effects in terms of increased functional capacity, excessive overload will result in bionegative effects, i.e. injury to musculoskeletal components.

It should be appreciated that during physical training, the musculoskeletal system is subjected to considerable mechanical loading and that hard training sessions are likely to result in microtrauma (small amounts of tissue damage) to musculoskeletal components, es-

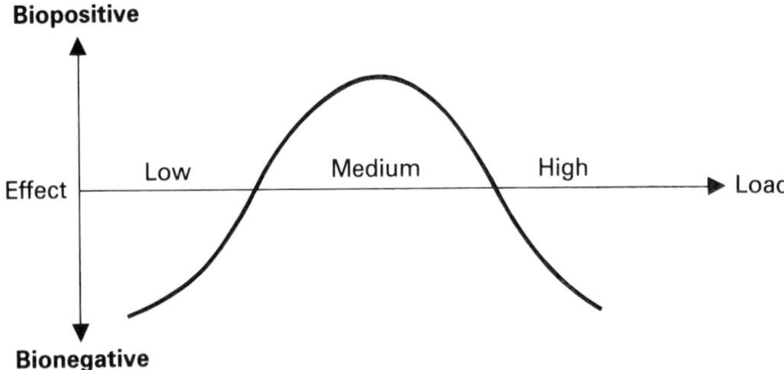

Fig. 23.1 Effects of loading on the musculoskeletal system. Adapted from Nigg *et al.* (1981).

pecially muscles and tendons, and the local capillary and connective tissue networks. Given adequate rest the tissues will not only heal, but also adapt (remodel) their structures over time in order to more readily withstand the stress of mechanical loading imposed during training and competition. However, when rest periods are inadequate the fatigue process (rate at which microtrauma occurs) outpaces the remodelling process such that microtrauma gradually accumulate and eventually result in what is termed a chronic or overuse injury (Williams, 1993) (Fig. 23.2).

Jumper's knee is a good example of an overuse injury which occurs as a result of participation in volleyball. The syndrome is characterized by pain at the insertion of either the quadriceps tendon at the upper pole of the patella, or of the patellar tendon at the lower pole of the patella or at the tibial tuberosity (Fig. 23.3) (Ferretti *et al.*, 1990). As described in Table 23.2, the third and final stage in the development of jumper's knee is characterized by fairly persistent pain which is usually severe enough to prevent participation in sports. Continuing to train and/or play at this stage, despite the pain, is likely to result in complete rupture of the patellar tendon (Ferretti *et al.*, 1990).

This type of injury is referred to an acute injury, i.e. an injury which occurs suddenly and is severe enough in terms of pain and/or functional disablement to prevent further participation, at least temporarily. The severity of acute injuries ranges from minor, such as a minor muscle tear, to very severe, such as a complete rupture of a muscle, tendon or ligament, or a complete bone fracture (Peterson & Renström, 1986). However, as Ferretti *et al.* (1990) point out, many acute injuries, especially in tendons, ligaments and bone, are often the sudden end result of progressive degeneration of the structure concerned. Acute injuries, due to their disabling effect, tend to bring about enforced rest, thereby allowing the healing and remodelling processes to occur unhindered by the stress of continued activity. It is the enforced rest, allied to appropriate treatment and rehabilitation procedures, which often leads to a better recovery from acute injuries than from chronic injuries. Ferretti *et al.* (1990) suggest that negligence of players, in terms of continuing to train or play with a chronic injury or following a minor injury such as a minor muscle tear or minor ankle sprain, significantly increases the severity and long-term prognosis of most injuries.

Load capacity

Each of the musculoskeletal components has a certain load capacity or strength (Nigg *et al.*, 1984). In accordance with the principle of biopositive and bionegative response to loading discussed earlier, the load capacity of a particular musculoskeletal component will vary depending upon the magnitude and frequency of loading imposed on it by everyday life. For an athlete, everyday life is likely to involve a substantial amount of physical training. Properly structured training will result in an increase in the load capacity of the various components of the musculoskeletal system. The increased load capacity is likely to have two main benefits: (i) reduced risk of injury (components will

Table 23.2 Classification of jumper's knee according to symptoms. Adapted from Blazina *et al.* (1973) and Roels *et al.* (1978).

Stage 1	Pain after practice or after a game
Stage 2	Pain at the beginning of activity which disappears after warm-up and reappears after completion of activity
Stage 3	Pain present before, during and after activity such that the individual is unable to participate

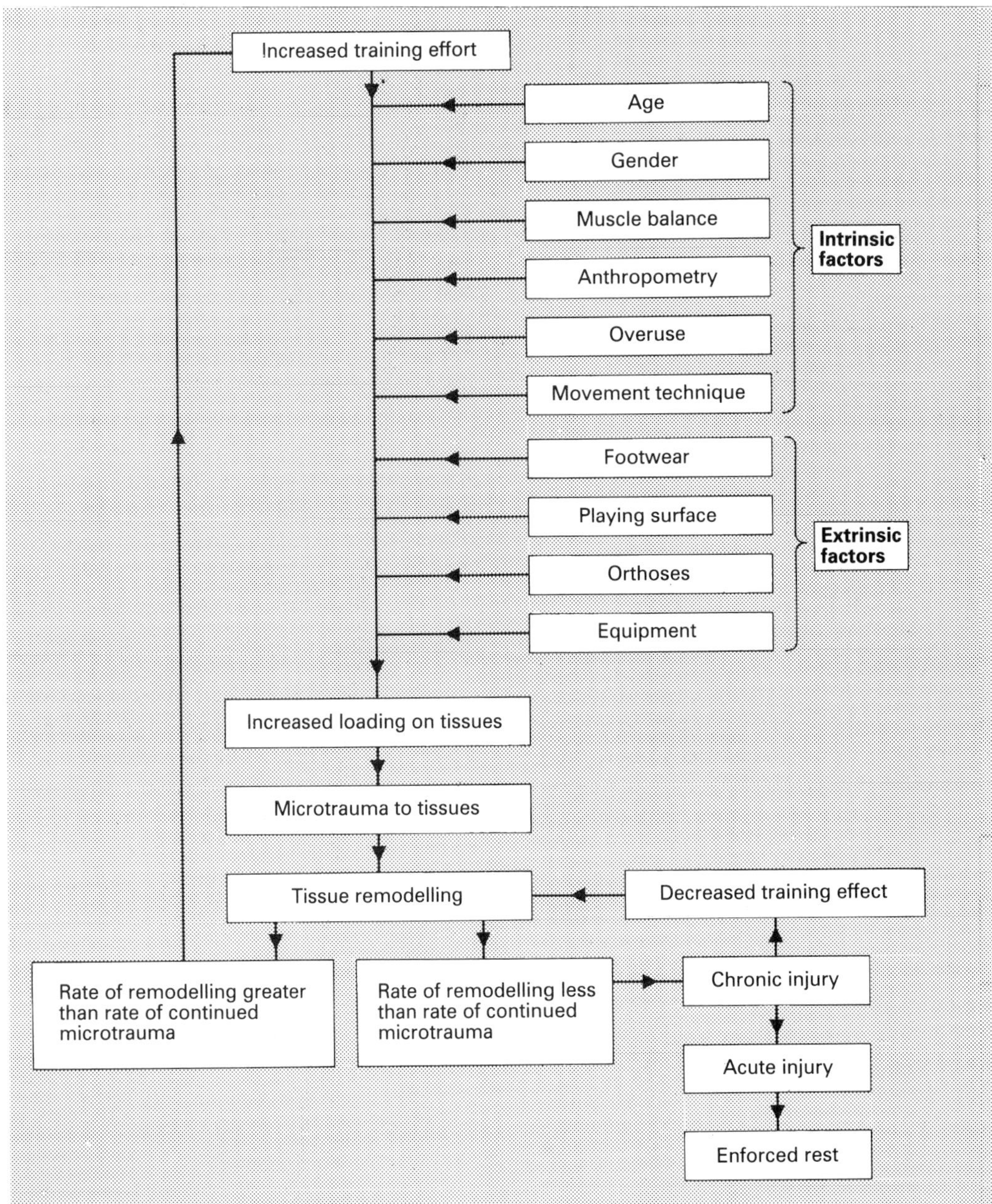

Fig. 23.2 Model of development of injury in relation to intrinsic and extrinsic risk factors. Adapted from Williams (1993).

be able to tolerate greater loads than before training), and (ii) increased functional capacity of the musculoskeletal system as a whole (especially in terms of speed and power).

Active (non-impact) and passive (impact) loading

Exceeding the load capacity of a particular

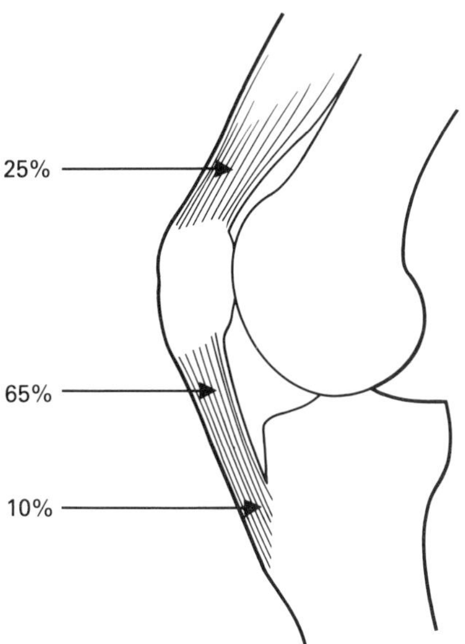

Fig. 23.3 Location of pain in jumper's knee. Adapted from Ferretti *et al.* (1990).

component of the musculoskeletal system will result in injury. Whether or not a particular load exceeds the loading capacity of a component depends upon both the magnitude of loading and the rate of loading.

In order to move the body quickly in a horizontal direction, as in a sprint start, or vertically, as in a vertical jump, it is necessary for the individual to push hard against the support surface; the more powerful the push or drive, the greater the speed of movement generated. Put another way, the coordinated action of the muscles (internal forces) enables the individual to generate a force between foot and floor (external ground reaction force) which drives the body in the desired direction. In these circumstances, where the magnitude and direction of the external force is controlled by the active muscles, the force produced is referred to as an active load or non-impact load (Nigg *et al.*, 1981). By definition, the rate of loading (rate of development of the force) of an active load is controlled by the muscles such that harmful high rates of loading are avoided. In contrast, there are many situations when external forces act, albeit briefly, on the body outside the control of the muscles due to the latency (response time) of the muscular system. Muscles take approximately 30 ms to respond to the stimulus of an external load. During this brief period, high rates of loading may occur which are likely to result in injury. External loads which are not under the control of the muscles are called passive loads or impact loads (Nigg *et al.*, 1981).

The body is subjected to passive loading during, for example, heel strike in running and heel strike following the pre-jump prior to a spike jump in volleyball. Figure 23.4 shows the force–time curves of the vertical component of the ground reaction force for two élite male volleyball players during take-off in a spike jump (Watkins *et al.*, 1988). The movement of the body during the ground contact period, i.e. the period corresponding to that of the force–time curves, is shown, more-or-less, by the middle three figures of the picture sequence. The first and last pictures are included in order to show the full spiking action. The force–time curves show peak impact forces of approximately 5.0 and 2.8 times body weight for subjects 1 and 2 respectively. The magnitudes of these forces are fairly low in terms of the capacity of the body to withstand external loading (Nigg, 1985). However, it is also clear from the force–time curves that the rate of loading is very high in both cases, i.e. in the region of 160–170 times body weight·s^{-1}. Such high rates of loading tend to generate shock waves which propagate throughout the musculoskeletal system (Valiant, 1990). Repetition of such loading over a prolonged period tends to cause progressive damage to certain parts of the musculoskeletal system, especially articular cartilage and subchondral bone (Radin, 1987).

Prevention of injuries

Increased training effort results in increased loading on the musculoskeletal system. However, the degree and location of the increase in

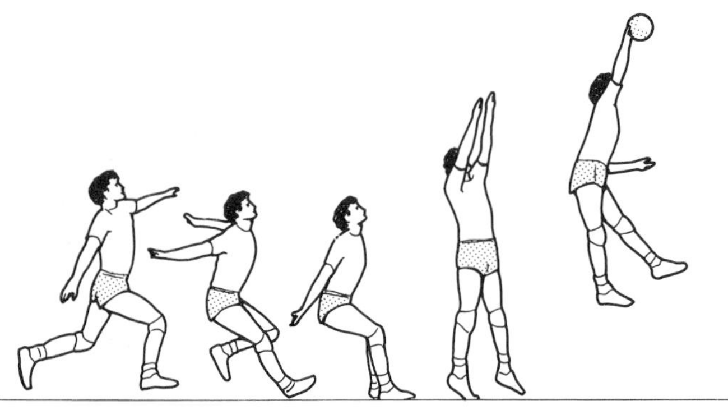

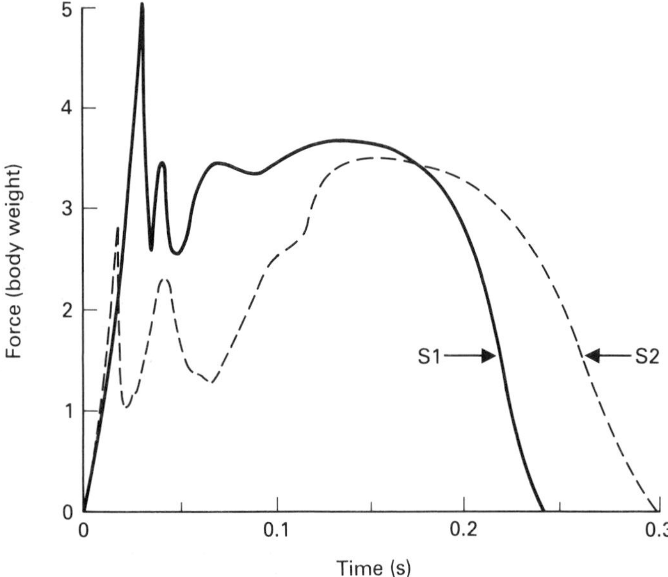

Fig. 23.4 Force–time curves of the vertical component of ground reaction force for two élite male volleyball players (S1, S2) during take-off in a spike jump.

loading will depend to a considerable extent upon the influence of a number of intrinsic and extrinsic risk factors. Figure 23.2 shows a model of the development of injury in relation to the main intrinsic and extrinsic risk factors. Intrinsic factors refer to those personal characteristics, including age, gender and anthropometry, which distinguish individuals from each other. Included in this category are level of physical conditioning and individual styles of movement. Extrinsic factors refer to environmental characteristics such as footwear and playing surface. All forms of orthosis are included in this category.

Age and gender

With regard to age, there are two major areas of interest concerning injuries to the musculoskeletal system, that is injuries which occur prior to maturity and injuries which occur after maturity. Compared to adults, skeletally immature athletes have more pliable bone, softer cartilage and their ligaments are stronger than associated centres of bony growth (Micheli, 1983). Consequently, loading that would cause a ligament or tendon tear in an adult may cause an epiphyseal or apophyseal fracture in an immature athlete. Unless properly diagnosed and treated, such damage to epiphyseal and/or apophyseal regions may result in abnormal bone growth (Peterson & Renström, 1986).

Knee injuries and knee pain are the most common orthopaedic complaints in children and adolescents (Kannus *et al.*, 1988). This finding is particularly pertinent to volleyball since participation in the sport results in considerable stress on knee joints in general and on the knee extensor mechanism in particular. Osgood–Schlatter disease (inflammation and pain at the insertion of the patellar tendon to the tibial tuberosity) is a frequent complaint of young athletes, especially those involved in volleyball and other sports which involve a high rate of jumping and landing (Peterson & Renström, 1986). Just as rupture of the patellar tendon may follow the final stage of chronic jumper's knee in an adult (Ferretti *et al.*, 1990), avulsion of the tibial tuberosity may follow chronic Osgood–Schlatter disease in an immature athlete (Fig. 23.5). Unless properly treated, avulsion of the tibial tuberosity may result in patella alta which, in turn, may result in disorders of the patellofemoral joint (Kujala *et al.*, 1989). Anderson (1991) provides a good overview of knee injuries in young athletes.

With regard to the effect of gender on the incidence of injury, there does not appear to be much information on volleyball players. However, the information which is available would suggest that women are more prone to injury in volleyball than men. Schafle *et al.* (1990) reported a higher injury rate in females than males in a national volleyball tournament. Ferretti *et al.* (1992) reported 52 cases of serious knee ligament injuries in volleyball players over a 10-year period (1979–89). The most frequent cause of injury (92%) was landing from a jump in the attack zone. Forty-two of the cases (81% of the total) were women, whereas the percentage of women in the population group (Italian Volleyball Federation) was only 61%. No satisfactory explanation could be given concerning the disproportionate number of injuries in females.

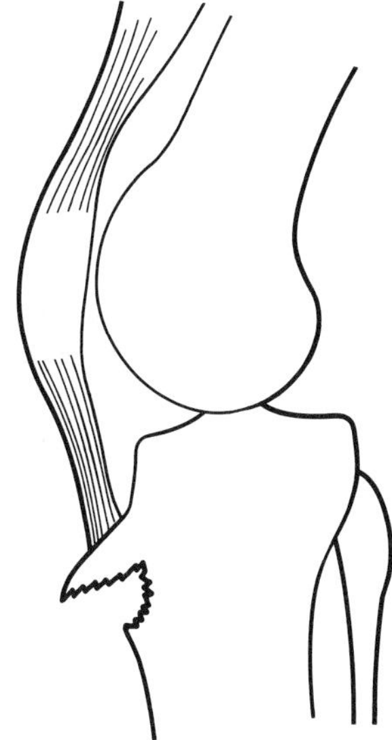

Fig. 23.5 Avulsion of the tibial tuberosity in an immature athlete.

Muscle balance, anthropometry and overuse

The intrinsic and extrinsic injury risk factors shown in Fig. 23.2 interact with each other to a certain extent. This is particularly the case concerning muscle balance, anthropometry and overuse. Normal joint movement involves a high degree of coordination between the members of the various antagonistic pairs of muscles which control joint movement. The coordination between the opposing groups in each antagonistic pair is largely dependent upon a functional balance between the groups in terms of strength and extensibility. A strength imbalance between the groups may occur if one group is trained more than the other; for example, overemphasis on strengthening the quadriceps relative to the hamstrings is likely to result in a strength imbalance between the two groups (Grace, 1985). In a similar way, highly repetitive and exclusive movement patterns, such as running or jumping and landing, are likely to reduce extensibility of the muscle groups concerned (Bach *et al.*, 1985). Strength imbalances combined with reduced extensibility are likely to result in muscle imbalances which predispose the athlete to injury (Grace, 1985).

Muscle imbalance is manifested in a number of ways, in particular: (i) imbalances between left and right sides of the body (Knapik *et al.*, 1991); (ii) imbalances between opposing groups within antagonistic pairs of muscles (Bach *et al.*, 1985); and (iii) imbalances between muscle groups of different joints which work together to bring about particular movements, for example, imbalance between the hip extensors, knee extensors and ankle plantar flexors in jumping and landing (Sommer, 1988). There appear to be few reported studies of muscle imbalance in volleyball players. However, one study by Sommer (1988) involving volleyball and basketball players illustrates the likely effect of muscle imbalance between the leg extensor muscle groups. The study examined the effect of fatigue on the movement of the hips, knees and ankles in jumping and landing. The results showed that as fatigue increased there was an increasing tendency for the knee joints to be forced into abduction during the powerful phases of leg extension (jumping) and leg flexion (landing). Sommer suggested that this was due to imbalances in strength and flexibility of the muscles controlling the hip joints, in particular the gluteal muscles, and that the effects of the imbalance became more pronounced as fatigue increased.

The likely effect of knee abduction during intense activity of the knee extensor muscles would be: (i) lateral tracking of the patella; (ii) strain on the medial ligaments and other medial supporting structures; and (iii) asymmetric loading on the quadriceps tendon and patellar tendon, especially at their insertions on the patella. Lateral tracking would be likely to result in patellar chondromalacia or patellar chondropathy, and asymmetric loading on the quadriceps tendon and patellar tendon would be likely to result in the classic symptoms of jumper's knee, i.e. inflammation and pain at the upper and lower poles of the patella.

The tendency for abductor loading to occur at the knee during jumping and landing would be increased not only by muscle fatigue linked to muscle imbalance, but also by adverse anatomical alignments, such as genu valgum, rearfoot valgus, forefoot varum and instability in related joints, such as excessive pronation in the ankle. With regard to anatomical alignment, there is a larger medial angle between the upper leg and lower leg in the frontal plane in females than in males, i.e. the lateral valgus angle at the knee is smaller in females than males. This may result in a greater tendency for knee abduction to occur during jumping and landing in females than in males, especially as fatigue increases. This may account, at least in part, for the disproportionately higher incidence of serious knee ligament injuries in females reported by Ferretti *et al.* (1992).

Overuse will result in injury whether or not muscle imbalances and adverse anatomical alignments are contributory factors. However, lack of muscular strength and endurance will result in earlier fatigue which, in turn, may lead to overuse. Ferretti *et al.* (1984) reported a clear positive relationship between frequency of play and the incidence of jumper's knee in volleyball players play (Fig. 23.6).

Movement technique

In sports, the movement pattern used by an individual during the performance of a particular movement or sequence of movements is usually referred to as the individual's technique. Good technique is a movement pattern which is not only very effective in terms of the desired outcome, such as spiking a volleyball, but one which also minimizes the load on the musculoskeletal system. Poor technique, due to inappropriate distribution of load throughout the musculoskeletal system, is likely to excessively overload certain muscles and joints resulting in injury. In the absence of other predisposing factors, excessive overloading is the result of: (i) inappropriate use of the various muscle groups which could contribute to a movement; and (ii) abnormal joint movements.

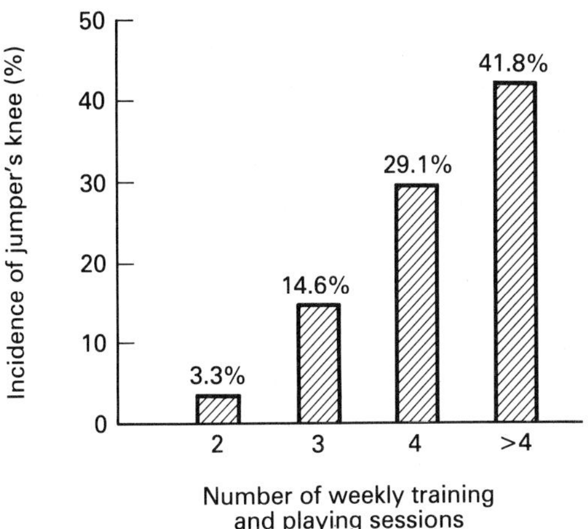

Fig. 23.6 Incidence of jumper's knee in relation to frequency of play. Adapted from Ferretti *et al.* (1984)

INAPPROPRIATE USE OF MUSCLE GROUPS

In the volleyball spiking action the objective is to hit the ball downwards into the opponent's court. The speed of the ball on leaving the hand depends upon the size of the force applied to the ball and the contact time between hand and ball. In order to apply a large force to the ball, the hand must be moving as quickly as possible on impact with the ball. With good technique, hand speed is generated mainly by the large hip flexor and trunk flexor muscles, with little movement of the shoulder of the hitting arm (Fig. 23.7a & b). Using the large hip flexor and trunk flexor muscles minimizes the load on the shoulder and arm muscles and enables the arm to exert control over the hand movement prior to ball contact. Lack of involvement of the hip and trunk muscles is usually compensated by excessive shoulder movement involving intense activity of the shoulder muscles (Fig. 23.7c & d). This is likely to excessively overload the shoulder muscles and supporting structures resulting in injury to, for example, the rotator cuff muscles (Brunet *et al.*, 1982). In turn, damage to the rotator cuff may result in sub-acromial bursitis (Reilly & Nicholas, 1987).

ABNORMAL JOINT MOVEMENTS

Overhead movements of the arms which occur in spiking, swimming and many racquet games, are brought about by movements in three joints: the shoulder, acromioclavicular and sternoclavicular joints. When range of movement in the acromioclavicular and/or sternoclavicular joints is restricted, the shoulder joint must be hyperabducted in order to achieve the overhead position. In doing so the supporting structures of the shoulder are likely to impinge upon the acromion process and associated ligaments resulting in a range of painful disorders such as shoulder-impingement Syndrome (Duda, 1985).

Footwear and playing surfaces

Different types of footwear have been shown to affect both the magnitude and rate of impact loading (Williams, 1993). In general, the results of studies concerning the effect of footwear on impact loading indicate that soft-soled shoes tend to reduce both the magnitude and rate of impact loading compared to harder-soled shoes. This effect is illustrated in Fig. 23.8 which shows the force–time curves of the vertical component of the ground reaction force of a runner running at 5 $m \cdot s^{-1}$ while wearing a soft-soled shoe and then a hard-soled shoe (Nigg *et al.*, 1981). It is clear that both the magnitude and rate of loading of the impact force are lower for the soft-soled shoe. In contrast, it can be seen that the active phase of the ground contact period is very similar for both types of shoe.

Just as softer-soled shoes tend to reduce the magnitude and rate of impact loading compared to harder-soled shoes, softer playing surfaces tend to reduce the magnitude and rate of impact loading compared to harder surfaces. Both Ferretti *et al.* (1984) and Watkins and Green (1992) found a clear positive relationship between the hardness of the playing surface and the incidence of jumper's knee in volleyball players (Fig. 23.9). In a study of knee injuries in

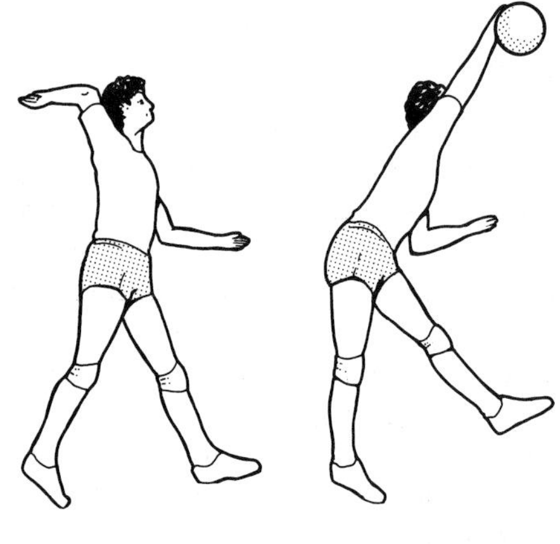

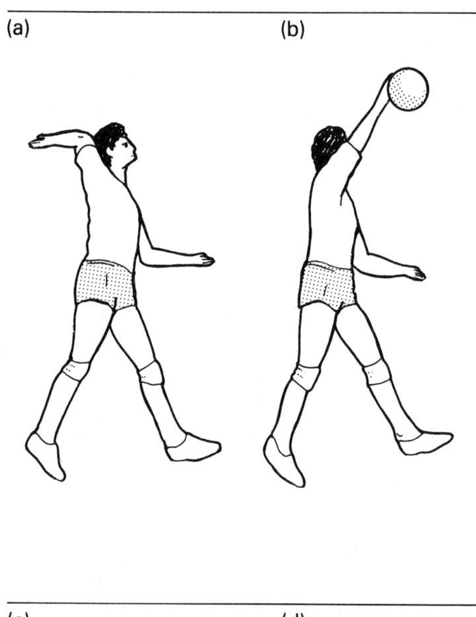

Fig. 23.7 Spiking actions: (a–b) good technique with emphasis on hip and trunk flexion; (c–d) poor technique with emphasis on shoulder extension.

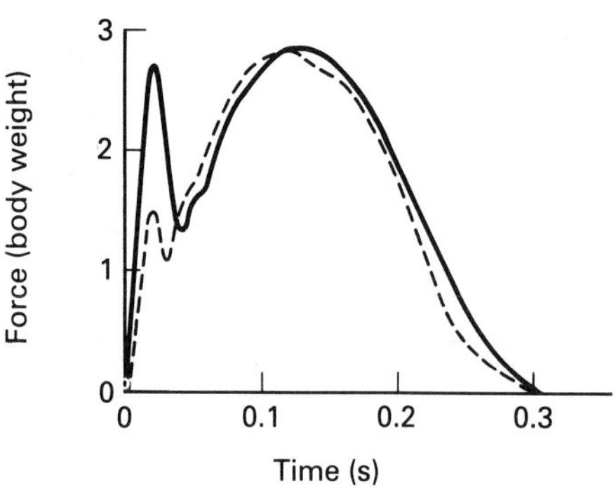

Fig. 23.8 Effect of hard-soled (———) and soft-soled (– – –) shoes on the vertical component of the ground reaction force while running at 5 m·s^{-1}. Adapted from Nigg *et al.* (1981).

tennis players, Nigg and Segesser (1988) found that the incidence of injury was greater on hard courts than on softer surfaces such as grass.

Orthoses

An orthosis is any form of external appliance which is used to: (i) prevent a high rate of passive loading, and/or (ii) protect a joint or joint complex from injury by helping to prevent or restrict the extent of abnormal movement which may occur during physical activity.

PREVENTION OF IMPACT LOADING

In volleyball, orthoses in this group include shock-absorbing shoe insoles, elbow pads and knee pads. Shock-absorbing shoe insoles, i.e. insoles which reduce the magnitude and/or rate of passive loading, have been shown to reduce the risk of knee and ankle injuries when running on hard surfaces (Rooser *et al.*, 1988). The use of such insoles would seem to be a reasonable injury prevention measure for volleyball players. There seems to be little reported information on the use of such insoles by volleyball players, but in a survey of injuries to National League players, Watkins and Green (1992) found that only 10% of players used shock-absorbing insoles.

With regard to elbow pads and knee pads, there seems to be little reported information concerning their use by volleyball players. However, there is considerable anecdotal evidence that knee pads are widely used at all levels of performance. In contrast, elbow pads seem to be used much less frequently. By the

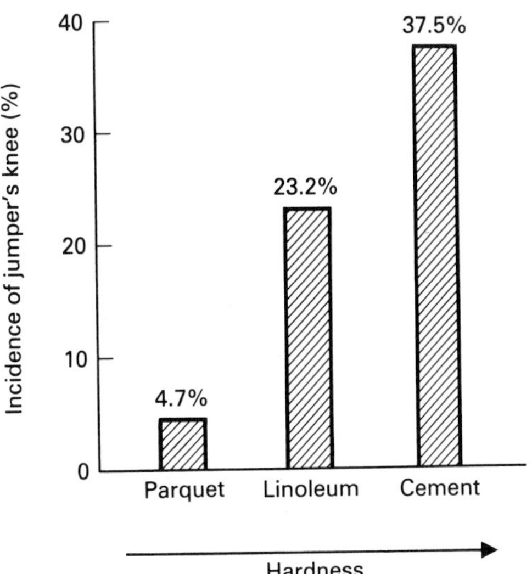

Fig. 23.9 Incidence of jumper's knee in relation to hardness of playing surface. From Ferretti *et al.* (1984)

nature of the game, especially when diving across court in order to retrieve a ball, players often hit the playing surface with their hands, elbows, hips or knees. In such circumstances, the use of elbow pads and knee pads can help to prevent injury to the body in general and the elbows and knees in particular. The use of elbow pads and knee pads is particularly important in the prevention of haemobursitis (bleeding into bursa following impact loading) of the olecranon bursae and the prepatellar bursae (Peterson & Renström, 1986). Knee pads also help to prevent haemobursitis of the superficial and deep infrapatellar bursae (Roland *et al.*, 1992). Most knee pads consist of a cushioned pad attached to an elasticated sleeve; the pad is positioned over the anterior aspect of the knee and is held on to the knee by the elasticated sleeve. In some designs the cushioned pad extends laterally and medially, thereby helping to protect the lateral and medial aspects of the knee as well as the anterior aspect. Elbow pads have a similar design to knee pads; the cushioned pad is located over the posterior aspect of the elbow.

PREVENTION OF ABNORMAL JOINT MOVEMENTS

Orthoses in this group range from well-established taping and strapping (bandaging) methods to, for example, semirigid knee braces (Zachazewski & Geissler, 1992). In sports, the value of this type of orthosis depends upon the extent to which the orthosis is able to prevent damage to the joint-supporting structures (by restricting range of motion in abnormal directions) while simultaneously allowing normal joint movements and unrestricted motor performance.

With regard to tape, the general finding is that it provides initial support, but quickly stretches or loosens in some other way so that its effectiveness is quickly and significantly reduced (Gross *et al.*, 1987; Anderson *et al.*, 1992). With regard to the effectiveness of

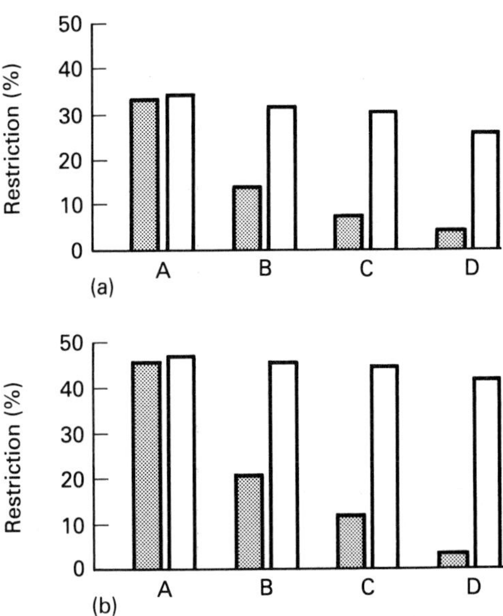

Fig. 23.10 Effect of tape (▩) and semirigid orthosis (□) on percent restriction of (a) eversion range of motion and (b) inversion range of motion before, during and after exercise. Adapted from Greene & Hillman (1990). A, after application of support but before exercise; B, after 20 min of exercise; C, after 60 min of exercise; D, after 180 min of exercise.

lace-on fabric and semirigid orthoses, there have been a number of studies concerning knee braces in various sports (Zachazewski & Geissler, 1992), but few, if any, concerning volleyball. There have, however, been a number of studies concerning the effectiveness of various forms of ankle supports for volleyball players. In one of the most recent and interesting studies, Greene and Hillman (1990) compared the effectiveness of adhesive tape and a semirigid orthosis in providing inversion–eversion range-of-motion restriction before, during and after a 3-h volleyball practice session. The effect of each form of support on the subjects' vertical jump performance was also assessed. Passive inversion–eversion range of motion was measured on an ankle stability test instrument during five testing sessions: (i) before application of support; (ii) after application of support but before exercise; (iii) after 20 min of exercise; (iv) after 60 min of exercise; and (v) after 180 min of exercise. The results of the study are shown in Fig. 23.10.

Both types of support were more or less equally effective in restricting eversion (tape 33.6%, orthosis 34.7%) and inversion (tape 45.8%, orthosis 47.1%) before exercise. The taped ankles showed a large decrease in percent restriction after only 20 min of exercise for both eversion (from 33.6% to 13.7%) and inversion (from 45.8% to 20.5%). Percent restriction provided by the tape showed a further decrease after 60 min of exercise for both eversion (from 13.7% to 7.5%) and inversion (from 20.5% to 11.7%) and further decreases over the next 2 h. At the end of the 3-h practice session the percent restriction provided by the tape was only 4.0% for eversion and 3.0% for inversion. In contrast, the percent restriction provided by the semirigid orthosis decreased only slightly over the first hour of exercise for both eversion (from 34.7% to 30.2%) and inversion (from 47.1% to 44.4%) with further slight decreases over the next 2 h. At the end of the session the orthosis still provided 25.9% and 41.5% restriction for eversion and inversion range of motion respectively compared to only 4.0% and 3.0% restriction provided by the tape. With regard to motor performance, neither form of support affected the subjects' vertical jumping ability.

Since inversion ankle sprains are the most common form of ankle injury in sports (Rijke *et al.*, 1988) and account for many ankle injuries in volleyball, the results of the Greene and Hillman (1990) study are particularly important concerning the ability of the orthosis to restrict inversion. If percent restriction is a reliable indicator of a support system's protective value, the ability of this particular orthosis to provide significant inversion range-of-motion restriction throughout 3 h of exercise suggests that it may be effective in the prevention of acute ligamentous sprains and in providing support for players with chronic lateral ankle instabilities. Whereas the Greene and Hillman study involved a semirigid orthosis, lace-on fabric ankle supports have been shown to reduce the incidence of ankle injury among football players (Rovere *et al.*, 1988).

There would appear to be little information on the use of ankle, knee and other supports by volleyball players. The information which is available would suggest that supports other than taping are not widely used (Schafle *et al.*, 1990; Watkins & Green, 1992).

Immediate treatment and rehabilitation

Immediate treatment

It is widely accepted that the best form of immediate treatment for acute muscle and joint injuries is rest, ice, compression and elevation (RICE) (Peterson & Renström, 1986). The purpose of RICE treatment is to restrict the flow of blood into the injured area while the body's healing mechanisms carry out the process of closing-off the torn blood vessels. In this way the size of the haematoma (blood pool in the injured area) is kept to a minimum. The first stage of tissue repair involves removing the haematoma and, consequently, the smaller the haematoma, the more quickly tissue repair can begin.

The extent to which RICE treatment is used

for volleyball injuries is not clear; there seems to be very few studies of volleyball injuries which refer to the use of RICE treatment. Schafle *et al.* (1990) reported that lots of ice was used during a national volleyball tournament and that it was quite common to see players icing knees and shoulders after matches. In a survey of injuries in National League male volleyball players, Watkins and Green (1992) found that two or more of the four elements of RICE treatment were used in 15% of injuries. Since all of the injuries resulted in pain and/or other symptoms which prevented the players from training or playing for 3 or more consecutive days, the use of RICE treatment in only 15% of cases was surprising. It was also surprising to find that in 28% of cases the players resumed training or playing within a few minutes of injury. In 78% of cases players sought further treatment (medical or paramedical) some hours or days after the injury. It is reasonable to assume that this figure could have been much lower had all the players concerned received immediate RICE treatment, with no further activity.

Rehabilitation

Thorough coverage of the principles of rehabilitation and rehabilitation modalities is beyond the scope of this chapter and the interested reader is referred to Peterson and Renström (1986) and Purdam *et al.* (1992). There are four main stages in the rehabilitation process and the stages overlap with each other as functional capacity is gradually restored.

1 Restoration of joint flexibility.

2 Restoration of muscle strength and muscular endurance.

3 Restoration of proprioception.

4 Restoration of motor ability.

Tippett (1990) provides good guidelines and exercises for all four stages, including a special section on functional progression for volleyball.

Conclusion

Volleyball is a high-risk sport, especially concerning injury to the knee and ankle. Care should be taken by coaches and therapists to ensure that: (i) progression in training is at an appropriate rate to prevent overuse; (ii) the influence of intrinsic and extrinsic injury risk factors are minimized; (iii) RICE treatment is administered when appropriate; and (iv) the rehabilitation process is allowed to progress at an appropriate rate through the four major stages (see above).

References

Anderson, K., Wojyts, E.M. & Lambert, P.V. (1992) A biomechanical evaluation of taping in reducing knee joint translation and rotation. *Am. J. Sports Med.* **20**(4), 416–21.

Anderson, S.J. (1991) Acute knee injuries in young athletes. *Phys. Sportsmed.* **19**(11), 69–76.

Bach, D.K., Green, D.S., Jensen, G.M. & Savinar, E. (1985) A comparison of muscular tightness in runners and non-runners and the relationship of muscular tightness to low back pain in runners. *J. Orthop. Sports Phys. Ther.* **6**(6), 315–23.

Backx, F.J.G., Beijer, H.J.M., Bol, E. & Erich, W.B.M. (1991) Injuries in high-risk persons and high-risk sports: A longitudinal study of 1818 schoolchildren. *Am. J. Sports Med.* **19**(2), 124–30.

Blazina, M.E., Karlan, R.K. & Jobe, F.W. (1973) Jumper's knee. *Orthop. Clin. N. Am.* **4**, 665–73.

Brunet, M.E., Haddad, R.J. & Porsche, E.B. (1982) Rotater cuff impingement syndrome in sports. *Phys. Sportsmed.* **10**(2), 86–97.

Byra, M. & McCabe, J. (1981) Incidence of volleyball injuries. *Volleyball Tech. J.* **7**, 55–7.

Duda, M. (1985) Prevention and treatment of throwing arm injuries. *Phys. Sportsmed.* **13**(6), 181–6.

Ferretti, A., Papandrea, P. & Conteduca, F. (1990) Knee injuries in volleyball. *Sports Med.* **10**(2), 132–8.

Ferretti, A., Papandrea, P., Conteduca, F. & Mariani, P.P. (1992) Knee ligament injuries in volleyball players. *Am. J. Sports Med.* **20**(2), 203–7.

Ferretti, A., Puddu, G., Mariani, P.P. & Neri, M. (1984) Jumper's knee: An epidemiological study of volleyball players. *Phys. Sportsmed.* **12**, 97–106.

Gerberich, S.G., Luhmann, S., Finke, C., Priest, J.D. & Beard, B.J. (1987) Analysis of severe injuries associated with volleyball activities. *Phys. Sportsmed.* **15**(8), 75–9.

Grace, T.G. (1985) Muscle imbalance and extremity injury: A perplexing relationship. *Sports Med.* **2**, 77–82.

Greene, T.A. & Hillman, S.K. (1990) Comparison of support provided by a semi-rigid orthosis and adhesive ankle taping before, during and after exercise. *Am. J. Sports Med.* **18**(5), 498–506.

Gross, M.T., Bradshaw, M.K. & Ventry, L.C. (1987) Comparison of support provided by ankle taping and semi-rigid orthosis. *J. Orthop. Sports Phys. Ther.* **9**, 33–9.

Hell, H. & Schonle, C. (1985) Ursachen und Prophylaxe typicher Volleyballverletzungen (Causes and prevention of typical volleyball injuries). *Zeitschr. Orth. Grenz* **123**, 72–5.

Kannus, P., Nittymaki, S. & Jarvinen, M. (1988) Athletic overuse injuries in children; a 30 month prospective follow-up study at an outpatient sports clinic. *Clin. Paediatr.* **27**(7), 333–7.

Knapik, J.J., Bauman, C.L. & Jones, B.H. (1991) Preseason strength and flexibility imbalances associated with athletic injuries in female collegiate athletes. *Am. J. Sports Med.* **19**(1), 76–81.

Kujala, U.M., Aalto, T., Ostermann, K. & Dahlstrom, S. (1989) The effect of volleyball playing on the knee extensor mechanism. *Am. J. Sports Med.* **17**(6), 766–9.

Lohmann, M., Holmich, P. & Overbaek-Pedersen, A. (1988) *Danish EHLASS Project*. Herlev Hospital, Copenhagen.

Micheli, L.J. (1983) Overuse injuries in children's sports; the growth factor. *Orthop. Clin. N. Am.* **14**(2), 337–60.

Neri, M. (1991) An epidemiological study of jumper's knee in volleyball players. *J. Sports Traum. Rel. Res.* **13**(2), 95–101.

Nigg, B. (1985) Biomechanics, load analysis and sports injuries. *Sports Med.* **2**, 367–79.

Nigg, B.M., Denoth, J., Kerr, B., Luethi, S., Smith, D. & Stacoff, A. (1984) Load, sports shoes and playing surfaces. In E.C. Frederick (ed) *Sports Shoes and Playing Surfaces*, pp. 1–23. Human Kinetics, Champaign, Illinois.

Nigg, B.M., Denoth, J. & Neukomm, P.A. (1981) Quantifying the load on the human body: Problems and some possible solutions. In A. Morecki, K. Fidelus, K. Kedzior & I. Wit (eds) *Biomechanics VIIB*, pp. 88–99. University Park Press, Baltimore.

Peterson, L. & Renström, P. (1986) *Sports Injuries: Their Treatment and Prevention*. Martin Dunitz, London.

Purdam, C.R., Fricker, P.A. & Cooper, B. (1992) Principles of treatment and rehabilitation. In J. Bloomfield, P.A. Fricker & K.D. Fitch (eds) *Textbook of Science and Medicine in Sport*, pp. 218–34. Blackwell Scientific Publications, Melbourne.

Radin, E.L. (1987) Osteoarthritis; what is known about prevention. *Clin. Orthop. Rel. Res.* **222**, 60–4.

Reilly, J.P. & Nicholas, J.A. (1987) The chemically inflamed bursa. *Clin. Sports Med.* **6**(2), 345–70.

Richardson, A.B. (1983) Overuse syndromes in baseball, tennis, gymnastics and swimming. *Clin. Sports Med.* **2**, 379–90.

Rijke, A.M., Jones, B. & Vierhout, P.A. (1988) Injury to the lateral ankle ligaments of athletes. *Am. J. Sports Med.* **16**, 256–9.

Roels, J., Martins, M., Mulier, J.C. & Burssens, A. (1978) Patellar tendinitis (jumper's knee). *Am. J. Sports Med.* **6**, 362–8.

Roland, G.C., Beagley, M.J. & Cawley, P.W. (1992) Conservative treatment of inflamed knee bursae. *Phys. Sportsmed.* **20**(2), 67–76.

Rooser, B., Ekbladh, R., Roels, J. & Lidgren, L. (1988) The shock absorbing effect of soles and insoles. *Internat. Orthop.* **12**, 335–8.

Rovere, G.D., Clarke, T.J. & Yates, C.S. (1988) Retrospective comparison of taping and ankle stabilisers in preventing ankle injuries. *Am. J. Sports Med.* **16**, 228–33.

Schafle, M.D., Requa, R.K., Patton, W.L. & Garrick, J.G. (1990) Injuries in the 1987 National Amateur Volleyball tournament. *Am. J. Sports Med.* **18**(6), 624–30.

Schmidt-Olsen, S. & Jørgensen, U. (1987) Patterns of injuries in Danish elite volleyball. *Ugeskr. Laeger* **149**, 473–4.

Sommer, H.M. (1988) Patellar chondropathy and apicitis, muscle imbalances of the lower extremities in competitive sports. *Sports Med.* **5**, 386–94.

Tippett, S.R. (1990) *Coaches Guide to Sport Rehabilitation*. Leisure Press, Champaign, Illinois.

Valiant, G.A. (1990) Transmission and attenuation of heelstrike accelerations. In P.R. Cavanagh (ed) *Biomechanics of Distance Running*, pp. 225–48. Human Kinetics, Champaign, Illinois.

Watkins, J. & Green, B.N. (1992) Volleyball injuries: A survey of injuries in Scottish National League male players. *Br. J. Sports Med.* **26**(2), 135–7.

Watkins, J., Nicol, A.C. & Nicol, S.M. (1988) Impulse characteristics of the ground reaction force in spike jumping. In: A.E. Goodship & L.E. Lanyon (eds) *European Society of Biomechanics: Bristol 1988*, pp. 27–8. Butterworth Scientific, Sevenoaks.

Williams, K.R. (1993) Biomechanics of distance running. In M.D. Grabiner (ed) *Current Issues in Biomechanics*, pp. 3–32. Human Kinetics, Champaign, Illinois.

Yde, J. & Buhl-Nielsen, A. (1988) Epidemiological and traumatological analysis of injuries in a Danish volleyball club. *Ugeskr. Laeger* **150**, 1022–3.

Zachazewski, J.E. & Geissler, G. (1992) When to prescribe a knee brace. *Phys. Sportsmed.* **20**(1), 91–9.

Chapter 24

Injuries in Ice Hockey

PETER DALY, TIMOTHY FOSTER AND BERTRAM ZARINS

The study of injuries in ice hockey has become mandatory because of the fast pace and high impact forces that are inherent to the sport. Ice hockey involves rapid acceleration and deceleration forces that occur within the unyielding confines of rigid boards upon the ice skating surface. Because impact injuries are frequently sustained from hockey sticks, pucks and skate blades, physicians have become involved in the treatment of injuries and are looking for ways to prevent ice-hockey injuries. Orthopaedic surgeons, neurosurgeons and ophthalmologists have dedicated talents and time toward the treatment of ice-hockey injuries. Improved methods of reporting injuries and studying epidemiology have helped establish a basis for preventing injuries. In this chapter we will discuss the risks of injury to hockey players, data on physiology and epidemiology, specific injury types, and finally, ways to prevent injuries.

Injury potential

One of the main factors that predisposes hockey players to serious injury is the high velocity that is achieved while skating. Sim and Chao documented skating velocities of approximately 48 km·h^{-1} (30 mile·h^{-1}) in senior amateur players and 32 km·h^{-1} (20 mile·h^{-1}) in young players (age 12 years) (1978). Utilizing high speed cinematography, they recorded sliding speeds of approximately 24 km·h^{-1} (15 mile·h^{-1}). The skill of a player is often dependent upon the ability to obtain high skating speeds quickly and to manoeuvre without slowing; therefore, collisions with the rigid goal posts, boards or other players often result in significant injuries to the extremities, viscera, head and neck.

The hockey puck is another significant source of injury. The puck acts as a high-velocity missile, reaching velocities of up to 192 km·h^{-1} (120 mile·h^{-1}) in professional players, 144 km·h^{-1} (90 mile·h^{-1}) in senior recreational hockey players, and more than 80 km·h^{-1} (50 mile·h^{-1}) in young hockey players (Daly *et al.*, 1990). The puck is made of hard rubber that is frozen for use. A puck weighs approximately 170 g (6 oz), and when travelling at the aforementioned velocities can impart significant impact forces. Sim and Chao studied the maximal impact forces that a puck imparts at its terminal velocity (1978). The force attained by the puck was 567 kg (1250 lb). Bishop (1976) and Norman *et al.* (1980) have studied the impact of the puck and its effect upon hockey equipment. They estimated that face masks deformed when the puck reached speeds of 80 km·h^{-1} (50 mile·h^{-1}) and that actual face-to-mask contact occurred when the puck travelled at speeds of 96 km·h^{-1} (60 mile·h^{-1}). Because players younger than 14 years old generally do not impart puck velocities of greater than 80 km·h^{-1} (50 mile·h^{-1}), it would appear that face masks worn by players in these age groups would be sufficiently protective.

However, players older than 14 years often

hit the puck with sufficient force to generate velocities greater than 96 km·h^{-1} (60 mile·h^{-1}); therefore, when a puck hits the face mask of a player in this age group injury can occur (Sim & Chao, 1978). Information derived from these biomechanical studies has lead to safety standards for hockey helmets and face masks (Fig. 24.1). The Canadian Standard Association subsequently raised the standards for face masks, requiring that they be made of heavier material than in the past and be mounted further away from the face. This raises the theoretical concern that with a heavier mask there may be an increased mass moment of inertia of the head and, therefore, an increased potential for cervical spine injuries. Bishop *et al.* (1983), however, did not believe this increased weight significantly contributed to excessive neck flexion when the head was impacted.

Another cause for injury in ice hockey that has been studied is the velocity achieved by the hockey stick (Sim & Chao, 1978). The angular velocity of the hockey stick has been measured to be between 20 and 40 rad·s^{-1} (100–200 km·h^{-1}) assuming a 1.4 m distance from the centre of rotation of the stick to the point of puck contact). This is clinically important because Pashby (1977, 1979) and Pashby *et al.* (1975) have documented that a blow from the hockey stick is the most common cause of eye injury. Sane *et al.* (1988) found that maxillofacial and dental injuries were most frequently caused by being hit with the stick.

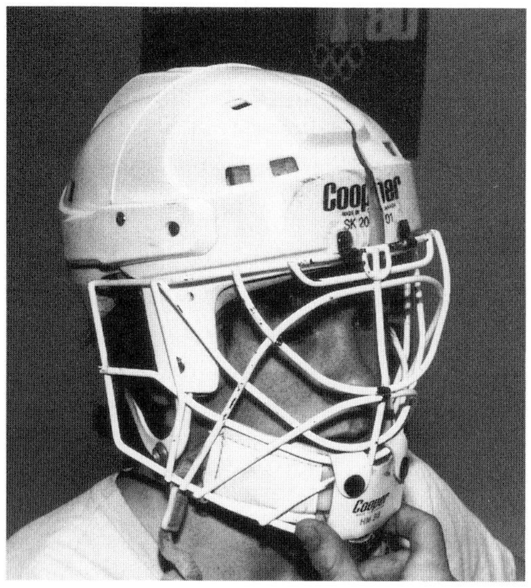

Fig. 24.1 This USA Olympic hockey player sustained a direct blow to his head cracking the helmet. This illustrates the significant forces involved in hockey and the protective effect of the helmet and face mask.

The sharp blades of the skates can injure hockey players in a different manner than the afore-mentioned blunt injuries. Boot-top lacerations of the extensor tendons of the foot and ankle have been reported, as have lacerations to the major blood vessels of the neck (Bull, 1985).

Adopting and enforcing rules to ensure fair play are important to keep the injury rate low. Fighting has no place in sports and should not be permitted in hockey (Fig. 24.2).

Indirect forces that are generated in non-contact injuries usually affect the muscles and tendons. One biomechanical study measured the forces generated during push-off in skating; using a force plate, Sim and Chao measured vertical reaction forces of between 1.5 and 2.5 times the player's body weight (1978). Posterior directed push-off force of the skate blade against the force plate peaked at approximately 668 N (150 lb) but depended on the skating style of the individual. Lateral forces were small reaching up to 353 N (80 lb); vertical twisting moments between the skate and surface ranged from 4.5 to 9 N·m^{-2} (40 to 80 lbf·in^{-2}). Thus, tremendous forces have to be generated by the hip muscles to achieve a quick skating start. Lorentzon *et al.* (1988a) demonstrated the clinical significance of these forces in a prospective study of Swedish élite hockey players, noting that the groin was the most common site of muscle strains.

The stamina and endurance of an athlete are important factors in preventing injury. Studying the physiology and peak performance in ice-hockey players has improved our understanding of the stresses involved in this sport.

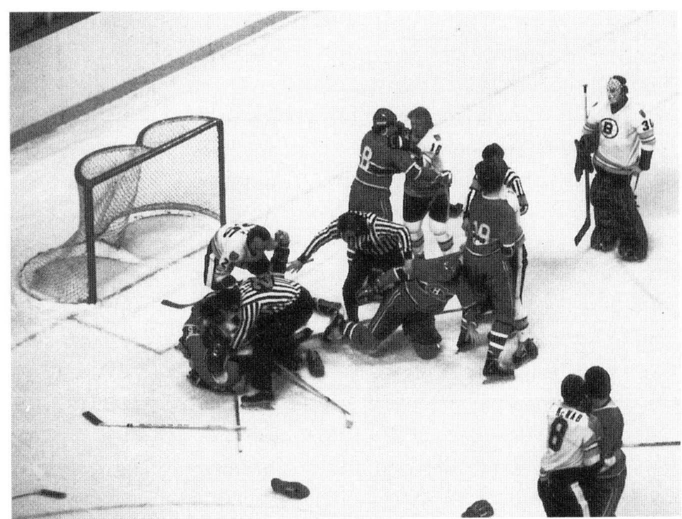

Fig. 24.2 Fighting is a shameful part of ice hockey and should not be tolerated. The shedding of gloves and other protective equipment during fights only worsens the potential of injury to the player.

Houston and Green (1976) studied Canadian junior A and college hockey players and found that the player's skills rather than size were determinants of success. Defencemen were slightly taller and heavier than the forwards because of the nature of their respective positions. The percentage of body fat of all players averaged 10%.

The cardiovascular system of ice-hockey players functions at a high level of performance (Mitin & Gladyseva, 1972; Houston *et al.*, 1973; Houston & Green, 1976). Hockey players have been measured to have a mean aerobic capacity of 55 $ml \cdot kg^{-1} \cdot min^{-1}$. This value is not as high as other endurance athletes such as long-distance runners, whose aerobic capacity averaged 79 $ml \cdot kg^{-1} \cdot min^{-1}$ (Ferguson *et al.*, 1969). Hockey, however, involves rapid changes in acceleration and deceleration that are different from the continuously paced effort of long-distance runners; therefore, anaerobic parameters may more accurately reflect performance of hockey players than aerobic parameters (Sim & Chao, 1978). Minkoff (1982) found no correlation between cardiovascular testing results and the performance of professional ice-hockey players. Nonetheless, optimization of energy delivery systems via adequate aerobic and anaerobic training programmes is important to fully realize the potential of individual hockey athletes.

To determine the effectiveness of the aerobic and anaerobic energy delivery systems in ice-hockey players, Green *et al.* (1976) analysed the time–motion and physiological parameters of play. They estimated that forwards played 14–21 shifts per game with each shift on the ice averaging 85 s. Because of stoppages of play, the average continuing playing time per shift was 39 s. The average velocity was 227 $m \cdot min^{-1}$ (8.5 $mile \cdot h^{-1}$). Telemetry was utilized to monitor pulse rates; the average pulse was 170 $beat \cdot min^{-1}$ This correlates to 80% of a player's maximal aerobic capacity. Ferguson *et al.* (1969) measured the maximal oxygen uptake during ice skating and found that hockey players working at an energy expenditure of 80% of the maximal oxygen consumption would reach an estimated average velocity of 400 $m \cdot min^{-1}$ (14.9 $mile \cdot h^{-1}$). This is higher than the velocity of 227 $m \cdot min^{-1}$ that was measured in the time–motion study by Green *et al.* (1976). Ferguson emphasized that although skating velocity reflects work intensity, other aspects of play include acceleration, change of direction, shooting and checking. These additional demands add significantly to the energy expended during competition.

Epidemiological analysis

Study of the patterns of injury are important so that efforts can be made to prevent injury. Injury patterns at varying levels of competition have been studied in several countries. However, one cannot compare these different studies directly. Injury reporting is non-uniform, and definitions of injury vary as do the numbers of players who constitute a group at risk for injury. Protective equipment that is worn and the players' ages and skill levels are also important variables that affect the statistics that are generated. Hayes (1972, 1975) prospectively studied nine American and 21 Canadian college hockey teams during the 1970–1971 season and etimated an incidence of 1.17 injuries·team^{-1}·game^{-1}. He noted that non-goalkeepers were most frequently injured and that most injuries were accidental (85%). Only 15% of injuries were caused by a player incurring or deserving a penalty. Most injuries (81%) kept the player out of competition for less than 2 days, and only 1% of injuries prevented a player from returning to hockey the same season. The shortcoming of these studies was that a detailed analysis of the circumstances surrounding the injuries were not recorded. True injury rates cannot be estimated since the population at risk (the denominator, or total number of players) was not known.

Harnof and Napravnik (1973) published a retrospective study in which they reviewed all injuries that required medical treatment for more than 14 days to 65 881 hockey players in Czechoslovakia during the 1967–1968 season. Reports of injuries that kept a player out for less than 14 days were obtained from a collective insurance system; minor injuries were, therefore, not reported. This definition of injury introduces the variables of severity of injury, individual recovery rates and the difficulty in defining what constitutes a 'treatment'. This injury definition also assumes there was an equal response of different players to treatment. The overall rate of injury calculated from this study was 29.6 · 1000 players^{-1}·year^{-1}. 45% of injuries occurred during practice or training and 55% occurred during games. The actual exposure of each player was unknown, since the participation by all players was not equal (Sim *et al.*, 1987). The most common mechanism of injury was collision with either a puck or stick (54%), collision with the boards (17%), or collision with other players (16%). Injuries were categorized primarily by the tissues involved rather than the anatomical sites. For example, skin was involved in 37% of injuries, joints in 34%, and bones in 15%.

In 1973, Biener and Muller published a retrospective study gathered from insurance reports during a 5-year period of hockey in Switzerland. The limitations of the study are similar to that of Hornof and Napravnick since it was retrospective and included only injuries that were reported to a health insurance company. They found that 2680 hockey injuries were reported over the 5-year period, 70% of which occurred during actual competition and 30% during practice. The most common cause of injury was the hockey stick (25%), followed by collisions with opposing players (17%), the puck (17%) and the skate (5%) (Table 24.1). The most common sites of injury were the head or face (42%) followed by the legs (21%) and the arm (11%). Although contusions and muscle strains were the most common types of injury, there were also 230 fractures, usually involving the nose and clavicle (Table 24.2).

In 1976, Sutherland published an excellent epidemiological study of ice-hockey injuries. This was a prospective study that established a denominator that could be used to calculate

Table 24.1 Mechanisms of ice-hockey injuries. With permission from Daly *et al.* (1990).

Mechanism	Biener & Muller, 1973 (%)	Lorentzon *et al.*, 1988a (%)
Stick	25	11.8
Puck	17	14.5
Collison	17	57.9
Skate	5	2.6
Miscellaneous	36	13.2

Table 24.2 Anatomical sites of ice-hockey injuries. With permission from Daly *et al.* (1990).

Site	Hornof & Napravnik, 1973 (%)	Biener & Muller, 1973 (%)	Sutherland, 1976 (%)	Lorentzon *et al.*, 1988a (%)
Head	37.1	42	7.0	4.8
Scalp and face			45.9	23.3
Eye			2.6	
Shoulder	21.9	18	8.6	5.6
Hand			2.1	10.5
Thigh (groin)	35.7	21	18.4	15.3
Knee			11.6	17.0
Trunk				
Miscellaneous (back, ribs, foot, ankle)	5.3	19	3.8	23.3

injury rates. He studied a cross-section of all age groups ranging from 5 years old to adults during one season of hockey. A total of 707 minor league and junior amateur players (11–14 years old), 207 high-school players (15–18 years old), 25 on a college team (19–21 years old), and 17 on a professional team were studied. With knowledge of the number of players involved and the number of games and practices in which they participated, Sutherland was able to provide reliable data on the injury rates. At the youngest age level, an injury rate of $1 \cdot 100\ h^{-1}$ of playing time was calculated (17 injuries among 707 players). At the high-school level, the hours played per injury occurrence was 16 (41 injuries among 207 players). At the college level the hours played per injury was 11 (62 injuries among 25 players). At the professional level, there was an injury every 7 h played (51 injuries among 17 players). Thus the number of injuries per player per year ranged from 0.02 for youth hockey players to 3 for professional hockey players. One drawback of the study was that information on differences in playing style and equipment were not assessed and, therefore, the aetiology of different injury rates could not be elucidated (Sim *et al.*, 1987). Nonetheless, Sutherland's prospective study gave validity to the observation that injury rates increase with age and level of play.

Another important study completed in a prospective fashion was that by Lorentzon *et al.* (1988a). From 1980 to 1985 Lorentzon personally attended all practice and game sessions of one Swedish élite hockey team. He recorded the injuries as they occurred and defined an injury as an accident that caused a player to miss the next practice or game. Injuries were classified as minor if the absence was less than 7 days, moderate if the absence was 8–30 days, or major if the absence was greater than 30 days. Of 95 total injuries, 73% were minor, 19% were moderate and 8% were major. Most injuries occurred during games (76%). The injury rate in hours of playing time per injury were 12.7 during games and 714.3 during practice. This rate is similar to Sutherland's rate in college hockey players of 11 h of playing time per injury. 20% of injuries were due to overuse or from indirect forces, and 80% were caused by direct impact, such as collisions. The most common severe injury noted was a complete tear of the medial collateral ligament of the knee. Jørgensen & Schmidt-Olsen (1986) also found this to be the most common severe injury among hockey players.

Because the reporting by Lorentzon *et al.* was prospective and data was personally obtained by a trained clinician, the results are likely to be reliable. Facial lacerations and other minor injuries, however, that did not result in absence from practice or play were not included in the rate of injury calculations. Lorentzon *et al.*

(1988b) also studied injury rates in international ice-hockey players. They found these rates to be nearly identical to those of Swedish élite players despite their expectation of finding a higher rate because of the increased intensity of play at the international level.

Important epidemiological reports were published by Pashby, an ophthalmologist in Toronto who studied eye injuries in Canadian hockey (1977, 1979; Pashby *et al.*, 1975). The importance of his studies was that the effect of introducing new rules and equipment upon injury rates was measured. Utilizing questionnaires sent to members of the Canadian Ophthalmologic Society, 478 eye injuries to hockey players were identified during the 1972–1973 season. The most common injury was to soft tissues (43%). Hyphema accounted for 19% of the injuries. The cause of the injury was usually the stick (74%) followed by the puck. This work (Pashby *et al.*, 1975) helped establish the rules governing the use of a stick and instituted a penalty for high sticking. Partially as a result of this study, use of a helmet with a face mask became required in the 1976–1977 season (Sim *et al.*, 1987). A subsequent study by Pashby (1979) in the 1976–1977 season showed that the number of reported eye injuries had decreased from 253 (1974–1975 season) to 90 (1976–1977 season). The findings proved that the use of face masks could decrease the frequency and severity of eye injury in ice hockey.

In Pashby's third study in 1979, he noted a further decrease in the number of reported eye injuries to 42 injuries during the 1978–1979 season. However, 90% of the eye injuries were sustained by players older than age 16 years. Thus, since the exposure to injury among older players should not have increased during this period, one can assume that the higher rate of eye injuries in older players was due to lower compliance of wearing face protection. The older players did not use face protection early in their hockey careers, and were, therefore, less likely to do so later during informal senior men's leagues.

As a result of the work by Pashby in Canada and Vinger (1977) in the USA, amateur hockey players in North America must now wear face protection by order of the Canadian Amateur Hockey Association and the American Amateur Hockey Association of the USA.

Injury types

Head injuries

Severe head and neck injuries (excluding facial and eye injuries) are less common than other injuries in ice hockey. However, they are important because they can have a devastating effect upon brain and spinal cord function because of the high velocity at impact. Both Benoit *et al.* (1982) and Fekete (1968) reported hockey players who died from head injuries sustained during minor league games. In Benoit's study, two of the hockey players killed were teenagers who had inadequate helmet protection; there was poor coverage of the temporal region, poor shock absorption of the helmet, and inadequate inner padding. They advocated improved helmet design as had been done for motorcyclists and football players.

The types of head injuries that occur in hockey vary from mild concussions that require no treatment to epidural haematomas that are neurosurgical emergencies. In a grade I concussion, a player is momentarily stunned but does not lose consciousness nor have a headache or amnesia. Usually, the player may return to competition immediately.

A concussion is classified as grade II if the player is confused and has post-traumatic amnesia (inability to recall events that occurred just after the injury). A grade III concussion is characterized by post-traumatic amnesia and retrograde amnesia (lack of recall for events prior to the injury). Players with a grade II or III concussion should be held out from play and observed to be sure there is no progression of symptoms. If all symptoms clear within 24 h, the athlete may return to play (Sim *et al.*, 1989). If a player is unconscious for more than 10 s, this is a grade IV concussion. This injury carries the potential for a significant central nervous system injury. These players should not be allowed to participate in activities that carry the risk of trauma to the head for at least 3 days. Any player who has a persistent headache or any focal neurological deficit, such as a sensory or motor change, should be evaluated immediately by a neurological specialist. Imaging studies such as computed tomography of the cranium are useful. The player may need to be hospitalized and monitored closely.

A comprehensive study of head injuries in hockey players was performed by Nagobads during the 1970–1971 Amateur Hockey Association season in the USA (1971). Nagobads identified 79 injuries: 41 were caused by sticks, 25 by pucks and 13 by collisions with boards or goal posts. A majority of the head injuries were lacerations (56%), 15% were concussions, 15% fractures about the head or face, and 10% contusions. 90% of the players who were injured wore helmets. Nagobads, however, felt that the helmet failed to provide protection in 41% of the injuries. He concluded that the helmets used were inadequate in providing appropriate protection. Nagobads' report combined with reports of head injuries resulting in deaths of hockey players (Fekete, 1968; Benoit *et al.*, 1982) helped provide impetus for further research into helmet design as well as certification standards.

Neck injuries

To protect the head from injury, helmets became more protective and heavier. The increased weight of the helmet and the tendency for a player to abandon caution because the head was protected may have contributed to an increasing frequency of cervical spine injuries (Tator & Edmonds, 1984). They noted an increase in the number of admissions of hockey players to a spinal cord injury treatment centre. Information was gained by surveying Canadian neurosurgeons. To evaluate the question of whether or not using a helmet changes the loading of the head and neck region and predisposes a player to sustain a cervical spine injury, Smith *et al.* (1985) evaluated how head dynamics change when the helmet is worn. In a biomechanical model, they could detect no difference between the dynamics of a head that wore a helmet compared to one that did not. Smith *et al.* (1985) could find no evidence to show an increased risk of cervical spine injury by the addition of a helmet. It is possible that the increase in the number of cervical spine injuries during the 1980 season noted by Tator and Edmonds (1984) was due to incomplete reporting prior to 1980. Helmets were introduced prior to the 1980 season and there was no concomitant increase in the number of cervical spine injuries immediately after the introduction of helmets.

Serious cervical spine injuries, such as subluxations or dislocations, can occur in ice hockey. Proper positioning of injured players and removal of them from the ice are important to remember. In general, one should not remove the helmet or move the head or neck. The face mask can be cut away using a bolt cutter. When lifting or moving the patient onto or off a backboard, mild traction to the neck should be applied. The neck should be immobilized using sandbags or rolled towels. The need to control the patient's airway can complicate management of a cervical spine injury. Pulling the jaw forward without moving the neck itself is often all that is needed to prevent the tongue from displacing posteriorly over the player's airway.

A neck injury can primarily cause shoulder pain ('shoulder burners'). The injury may occur from a direct contusion of the lateral aspect of the cervical spine causing a neurapraxia of the cervical nerve roots or upper trunk of the brachial plexus. The player typically has a burning sensation about the neck and shoulder region and weakness in the muscles that are innervated by C5 and C6 nerve roots. These muscles include the deltoid, biceps, infraspinatus and teres minor. The motor deficit often disappears rapidly, but return to full activity must be delayed until all neurological signs are absent and radiological evaluation of the cervical spine has been completed. Congenital narrowing of the space available for the spinal cord in the cervical region has also been reported and can be assessed by measurements from the lateral cervical spine X-ray (Torg & Pavlov, 1987).

Possible measures to prevent neck injuries include isometric and isokinetic strengthening exercises of the paravertebral and shoulder girdle muscles. Preseason flexibility programmes are also helpful to assure that the neck, shoulders and upper back are adequately supple prior to participation.

Eye and facial injuries

Eye injuries in hockey players have been extensively studied by Pashby (1977, 1979) and Pashby *et al.* (1975). Periorbital lacerations, hyphema and iris damage are the most common injuries and are usually due to trauma inflicted by the hockey stick or puck. A player with hyphema or iris injury should be evaluated for a coexisting fracture of the bony floor of the orbit. The use of face protectors has definitely decreased the number of eye injuries (Fig. 24.3). Since the majority of eye injuries are caused by blows from a hockey stick, continued enforcement of the high sticking rule will hopefully lead to a further decline in these injuries.

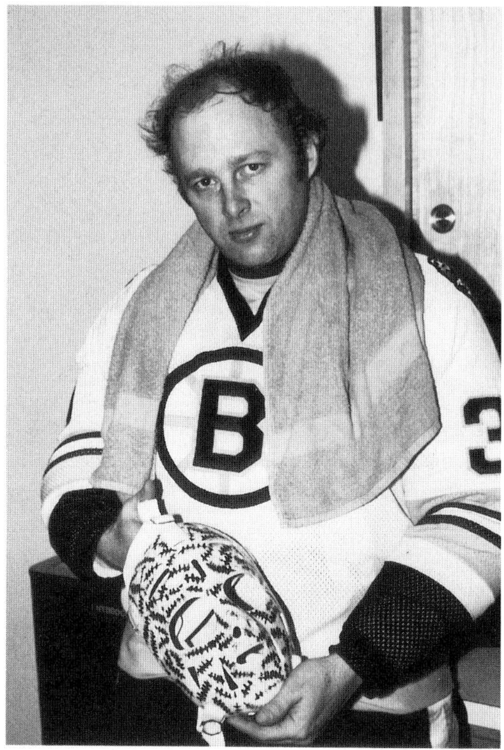

Fig. 24.3 Gerry Cheevers was one of the early professional goalkeepers to wear a face mask. He has marked his face mask at the site of puck contact documenting the protective effect of the face mask.

Dental and maxillofacial injuries are also frequent in ice hockey. Sane *et al.* (1988) studied these injuries in Finnish hockey players from 1979 to 1985. They found that 85% of facial injuries involved the teeth. The most common cause was a blow from the hockey stick and the second most common was injury from the puck. Fractures of the crown (enamel portion of the tooth) were the most common dental injury. Fractures of the maxilla and mandible were rare and accounted for only 7% of all dental injuries in their series. Sane *et al.* (1988) documented a significant decrease in the incidence of dental injuries following the mandatory introduction of a full cage face mask. This drop in the number of injuries also translated into a significant decrease in the cost of care for these athletes. If a player does not use a face mask, a mouth guard should be worn (Fig. 24.4).

Other common facial injuries have been lacerations. Wilson *et al.* (1977) noted that by the time hockey players reached college age, 95% had sustained facial trauma requiring medical attention. Their study, however, was completed in 1975 before the mandatory use of face masks existed. Lorentzon *et al.* (1988a) found that 86% of the facial lacerations occurred to players who were not wearing face visors and that only 14% occurred to those who were wearing visors. They also found that the frequency of facial lacerations was greater in the unprotected part in which area the face visor did not reach ($P < 0.05$). Facial fractures can

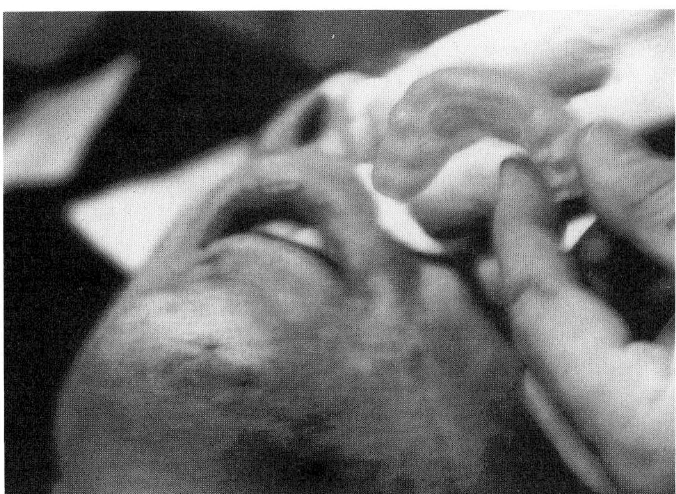

Fig. 24.4 This player received a blow to the face causing a large laceration. The intraoral mouth guard shown here prevented injury to the teeth.

also occur; however, use of face masks and chin guards appears to have reduced the number of these injuries, particularly in goaltenders.

Upper extremity injuries

Shoulder injuries are extremely common in hockey players, particularly at the college and professional levels where the aggressive player receives and delivers frequent direct blows to the shoulder during checking. The most common shoulder injury is acromioclavicular (AC) separation. A study peformed at the Massachusetts General Hospital of college and professional players (B. Zarins, personal communication) confirmed that AC joint injuries were most common, followed by anterior shoulder dislocation. A mild AC sprain (grade I) causes pain but the player can often finish the game. More severe AC joint injuries (grades II and III) typically cause the player to miss from 2 to 6 weeks of competition but usually do not require surgery. A completely displaced distal clavicle in which the distal clavicle is button-holed through a rent in the deltotrapezial fascia usually needs to be repaired surgically. A posteriorly displaced distal clavicle tends to cause persistent pain and should also be treated with surgical correction. Norfray *et al.* (1977) evaluated 77 professional hockey players and found that 45% had symptomatology referrable to the AC joint as well as radiographic abnormalities at the AC joint and distal clavicle. These abnormalities included osteolysis of the distal clavicle and callous from united and un-united distal clavicle fractures.

Shoulder dislocations, while not as common as AC joint injuries, represent a serious injury. Hovelius (1978) reported an 8% incidence of shoulder dislocations in Swedish hockey players. A primary dislocation in a young athlete usually leads to repetitive subluxations or dislocations. Several studies have documented recurrent instability rates from 27 to 94%. Simmonet and Cofield (1984) documented an 82% redislocation rate in athletes and a 30% redislocation rate among non-athletes. Rowe and Sakellarides (1961) reported a 94% redislocation rate among athletes under the age of 20 years. The management of an initial shoulder dislocation in a young hockey player has been debated. There is little correlation between the duration of immobilization following a first-time dislocation and the incidence of recurrence. Immobilizing the shoulder for approximately 3 weeks followed by a supervised rehabilitation programme may lessen the likelihood of recurrence. The incidence of recurrence is directly related to the age of the athlete at the time the first dislocation is sustained (Rowe & Sakellarides, 1961; Hovelius, 1978).

Overuse injuries affect the shoulder of hockey players who can develop rotator cuff tendinitis from repetitive shooting. The phases of the shooting includes a wind-up phase, cocking phase and acceleration phase followed by deceleration and follow-through phases. Inflammation of the supraspinatus tendon can occur. The external rotators can also be involved due to excessive eccentric contraction during the deceleration phase of the shooting motion. Moderate to severe cases of tendinitis often require a period of rest followed by physiotherapy for strengthening the rotator cuff. Full thickness rotator cuff tears can occur and have been documented by Lorentzen *et al.* (1988a).

Soft-tissue injuries about the elbow are common in hockey players. Olecranon bursitis frequently occurs and is usually the result of repetitive hits into the boards or ice. This injury can be prevented by using adequate protective elbow pads. Occasionally, surgical excision and debridement of the bursa is required.

If a player sustains a laceration to the olecranon, the bursa should be mostly excised and the area thoroughly irrigated before closing the wound. Oral antibiotics should be given and the elbow should be splinted in extension for approximately 1 week. If the laceration is simply sutured and the player returned to normal use of the elbow, the incidence of infection is prohibitively high.

Tendinitis at the lateral epicondyle of the elbow at the origin of the wrist extensors is another frequent overuse disorder. The extensor carpi radialis brevis tendon is most frequently involved. Repetitive dorsiflexion of the wrist in shooting predisposes to this injury. Medial epicondylitis is also common and is caused by repetitive use of the wrist shot. Management includes anti-inflammatory medications and counterforce straps around the forearm. Recalcitrant cases often require cortisone injections, and physiotherapy to strengthen the wrist extensors. Rarely, surgery is required if conservative measures fail over several months and the athlete is sufficiently impaired.

Injuries involving the hand and wrist are common in competitive ice hockey. Lorentzon *et al.* (1988a) reported that 20% of injuries requiring more than 1 week's absence from play were due to wrist and hand injuries. Rupture of the ulnar collateral ligament of the thumb metacarpophalangeal joint ('gamekeeper's thumb') typically occurs when the player falls with the hockey stick in the hand and sustains an abduction force to the thumb (Cooney, 1984; Lorentzon *et al.*, 1988a). Partial tears of this important ligament can be treated with splinting or taping of the thumb to prevent excessive abduction motion. Surgery, however, is recommended for complete ruptures of the ligament because interposition of the soft tissues can prevent the ligament from healing in its normal position. Tendon injuries to the hand are not common in hockey players. Nonetheless, avulsion of the flexor digitorum profundus tendon from the distal phalanx, particularly in the ring and little fingers, have occurred and often necessitate surgery. Rupture of the profundus tendon may occur during fighting when the player grabs the opponent's jersey.

The most significant fracture about the hand and wrist occurs in the scaphoid. This is the most frequently fractured carpal bone and may require an extended time to heal. Most scaphoid fractures heal within 3 months. Immobilization in a thumb spica cast and anatomical reduction of the fracture fragments are important to prevent non-union and arthrosis. Metacarpal and thumb fractures occur and often require the player to miss games. Dislocations of the interphalangeal joint of the thumb are common in all levels of hockey competition. Gloves normally protect the hand from injury but when removed while fighting, significant injuries can occur. Extensor tendon lacerations at the metacarpophalangeal joint may be the result of a bite wound sustained when a player strikes the opposing player's tooth during a fight. These are dangerous wounds since contamination by oral bacteria can cause serious infections. The wound should be left open and antibiotics should be given.

Abdominal injuries

Injury to the abdominal viscera is not uncommon in contact sports. Tenderness in the left upper quadrant of the abdomen must be investigated thoroughly because of the risk of a splenic rupture or subcapsular haematoma. A computerized tomography scan of the abdomen can be used to rule out significant splenic trauma. Splenic enlargement due to infectious mononucleosis is sometimes seen in high-school and college players. An inflamed spleen is more susceptible to rupture than a normal one; therefore, players who have mononucleosis should avoid contact sports until the splenomegaly has resolved. Flank contusions can result in renal injury. Urinalysis should be performed to diagnose haematuria. Repeat urinalysis and further urogenital imaging studies may be required to completely rule out a urinary tract injury. Adequate kidney padding or flank vests can help protect against these kidney injuries.

Low back injuries

Acute injuries to the lower back are not common in ice hockey; however, repetitive stress due to playing in a position of forward flexion may result in acute low back pain and lumbar muscle spasm. Common causes are intervertebral disc disease and spondylolysis. When low back pain is persistent and does not respond to the usual physical therapy modalities, radiographs and a technetium three-phase bone scan are helpful to assess the integrity of the lamina and pars interarticularis (Sim *et al.*, 1989). Magnetic resonance imaging can be used to diagnose disc disruption. Prophylactic back and abdominal muscle strengthening exercises help prevent recurrent disability in players who have spondylolysis.

Lower extremity injuries

Soft-tissue injuries are much more common than bone injuries in the lower extremity of ice-hockey players. Thigh contusions may occur as the result of direct trauma from hitting the knees of opposing players. The swelling that occurs in a contused thigh is due to an intramuscular haematoma. Swelling and discomfort prevent a full range of knee motion. The severity of thigh contusions is based upon the degree of knee flexion when the patient is prone. A thigh contusion is classified as grade I when the knee has greater than 90° of motion. In a grade II injury, the knee flexes between 45 and 90°. If knee flexion is restricted to less than 45°, the player has a grade III contusion. A player should not return to participation until a full range of motion is regained. The initial treatment of thigh contusions is important in preventing the formation of a haematoma. Immediate compressive dressing with the knee flexed as much as possible along with cold application, rest and crutches are important. The serious risk is the potential of a thigh haematoma to form bone, a condition known as myositis ossificans (Fig. 24.5). In myositis ossificans, bone forms within the muscle in an abortive attempt at healing. Gradual resorption of this ectopic bone occurs; however, it takes several months for the initial formative phase to complete and many years to resorb. The activity of the bone formation process can be monitored with serial technetium bone scans. The average time from injury for a player who develops myositis ossificans to return to play is 6 months. Late surgical excision of the area of myositis ossificans can be performed, but it is important to delay surgery until all bone formation has ceased as documented by bone scan.

Muscle strains in the adductor muscles of the groin are a common occurrence due to the thrust of the hip adductor muscles required in the skating stride. Sim and Chao (1978) estimated hip joint forces to be as high as 2.5 times body weight during push-off of the skate blade. Thus, adductor muscle strains or 'groin pulls'

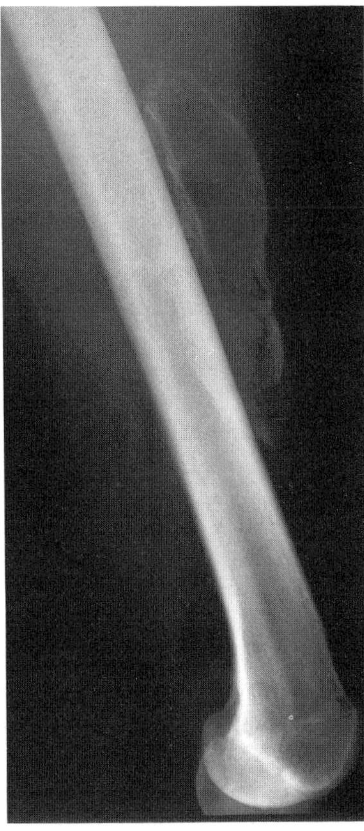

Fig. 24.5 Lateral radiographs of the thigh showing a large area of myositis ossificans in the quadriceps muscles. This player sustained blunt trauma to the anterior thigh from a knee during a check. The disability from myositis ossificans lasts a minimum of 6 months. A player should not return to play until full range of knee motion has been regained and has no pain in the thigh.

not unexpectedly can limit the athlete's playing ability. Lorentzon *et al.* (1988b) found that hip adductor muscle strains accounted for more than 10% of the injuries in their series. Osteitis pubis, an inflammatory process at the symphasis pubis with symmetrical resorption of bone at the medial pubis, can also be considered in the differential diagnosis of groin discomfort in hockey players. Inguinal hernias and stress fractures of the hip or pelvis are also considerations. Treatment of muscle strains in the groin typically involves cold application and anti-inflammatory agents. Use of local injection of steroids may sometimes assist. Stretching and strengthening of hip flexor and adductor muscles along with assessment of proper skating technique are important in preventing further injuries.

A common chronic condition is pain at the insertion of the rectus abdominus into the pubis in the inguinal area. The pain can migrate into the upper groin area as well. This lower abdominal–upper groin pain is one of the most common causes of disability in hockey players. Recently, surgeons have been performing herniorrhaphy operations for this condition with good results. The exact pathology has not been identified, but exploring and repairing the external inguinal ring has been successful.

Ice-hockey players skate with their knees in a semiflexed position making the knee vulnerable to injury. When a player sustains a blow to the lateral aspect of the knee, a valgus external rotation stress occurs and the medial collateral and anterior cruciate ligaments are at risk for injury. An isolated tear of the medial collateral ligament can be treated non-operatively but only after ruling out injuries to other important structures such as the cruciate ligaments and menisci. Injury to the anterior cruciate ligament is usually accompanied by a pop and immediate knee swelling. Fortunately, because the player's foot is usually not fixed to the ground at the time of impact in ice hockey, injuries to the anterior cruciate ligament are less common in ice-hockey players than football players. When a tear of the anterior cruciate ligament occurs, however, recurrent instability of the knee can result; the player is at risk of sustaining meniscus tears and damage to the articular surfaces. Return to competitive play in ice hockey is usually possible with bracing and rehabilitation. Recurrent instability requires surgical correction but functional instability in ice-hockey players due to loss of the anterior cruciate ligament is less likely than in sports that require pivoting motions. The effectiveness of knee braces in preventing knee injuries is controversial. The brace, however, may be useful in a patient who has instability by providing proprioceptive feedback and external support.

The treatment of recurrent instability due to loss of the anterior cruciate ligament most commonly involves replacing the torn ligament with autogenous tissue. The middle third of the patellar tendon (bone–tendon–bone autograft) is a good graft and can be implanted utilizing an arthroscopically assisted technique. Postoperatively, the patient can begin immediate full weight-bearing on the leg using crutches in a brace locked in full extension if stable fixation of the graft has been achieved. Range of motion exercises are begun on the second postoperative day and are performed several times daily when out of the brace.

Meniscus repair or excision can be performed as an arthroscopically assisted or open procedure. If the meniscus tear is located in the peripheral third of the meniscus, then repair is often possible. Magnetic resonance imaging is an expensive but excellent non-invasive technique that allows visualization of the menisci and ligaments of the knee.

Patellofemoral problems are common in hockey players especially softening and fibrillation of the patellar articular cartilage (chondromalacia patella). Persistent pain in the extensor mechanism with this condition can cause significant disability. Occasionally, symptoms from chondromalacia can be improved by arthroscopic debridement. Patellar fractures can also occur, such as from hitting the boards with a flexed knee (Fig. 24.6). If completely non-displaced, the fracture can be treated non-operatively. Otherwise, surgical intervention can be required to achieve anatomical reduction. Early motion, and even continuous passive motion in severe cases, are important in the postoperative phases.

Foot and ankle injuries occur in ice hockey especially from being hit by a puck. The stiffness of the skate boot helps to protect the ankle from frequent sprains. Direct trauma through the skate does occur and fractures of the talus, navicula, and metatarsals may result (Fig. 24.7).

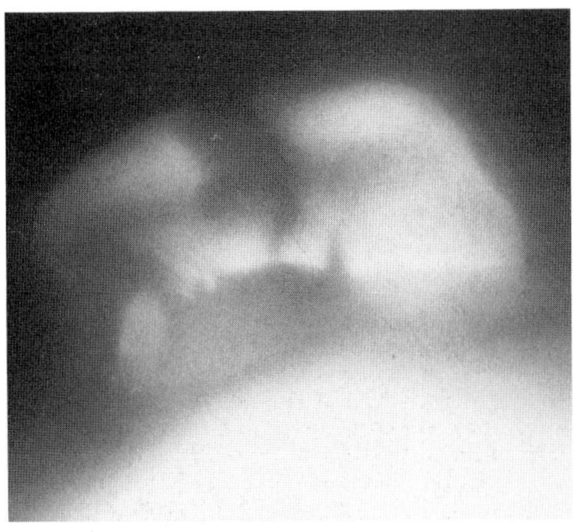

Fig. 24.6 Lateral tomograph of a professional hockey player's fractured patella. He hit the boards with a flexed knee causing a severely comminuted patella fracture. The importance of adequate protective padding is obvious.

These fractures can be difficult to diagnose on plain radiograms. Tomography or computerized tomography are sometimes needed to diagnose occult fractures, especially medially for the navicula. Lacerations of the ankle caused by sharp skate blade have been reported to cause tendon and vessel lacerations at the level of the ankle (Hovelius & Palmgren, 1979). Extensor tendon lacerations at the level of the ankle can be missed unless appropriate care is utilized when examining lacerations over the front of the ankle.

Injury prevention

An important way to prevent injuries in ice hockey is to have an adequate training programme. This should occur both in the preseason and during active competition. Off-ice conditioning exercises, such as bicycling and rollerblading, are activities that specifically strengthen the skating muscles. Physiological testing can be helpful to assess conditioning levels. Cycle ergometry for measurement of maximal oxygen volume (aerobic capacity) and 30-s maximal power tests (anaerobic ca-

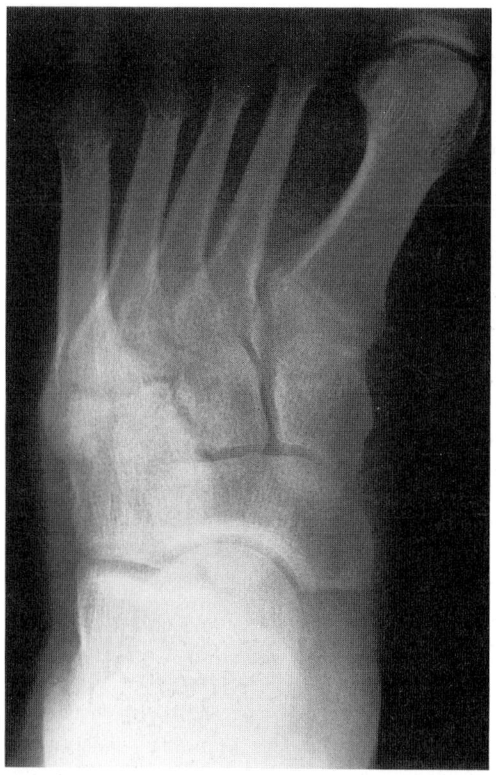

(a)

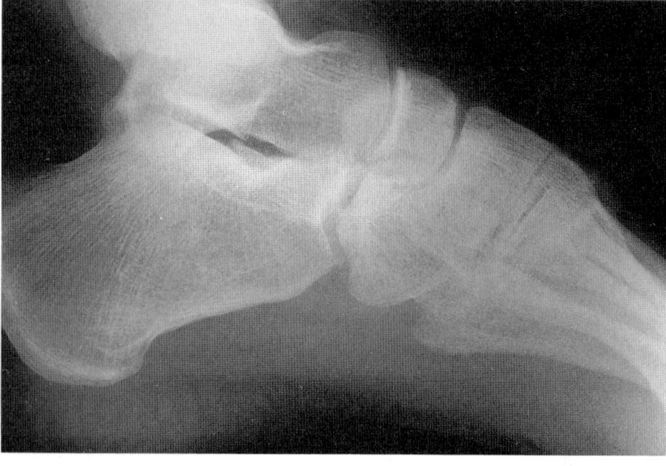

(b)

Fig. 24.7 Anteroposterior (a) and lateral (b) radiographs of a foot of a hockey player who was hit by a puck on the medial side of the midfoot while blocking a shot. No fractures were identified on these views.

pacity) allow assessment of training levels (Sim *et al.*, 1989). Preseason and postseason examinations help to identify injuries and training deficiencies to assist in designing proper rehabilitation schedules.

Protective equipment is an obvious form of injury prophylaxis in ice hockey. Adequate padding over the hip and pelvis, knee and leg, upper extremity, head and face are essential for preventing many of the injuries discussed here.

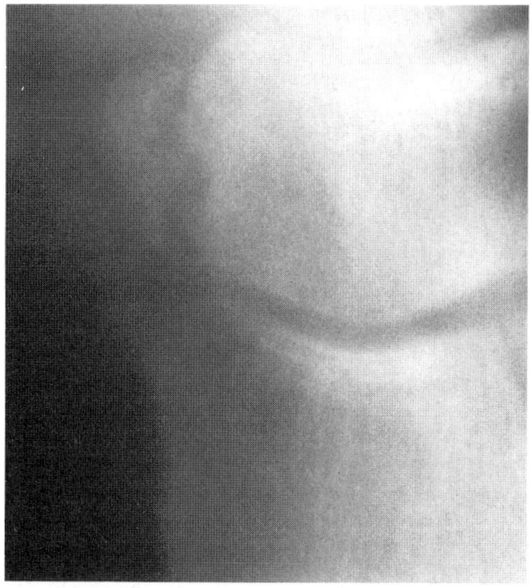

(c)

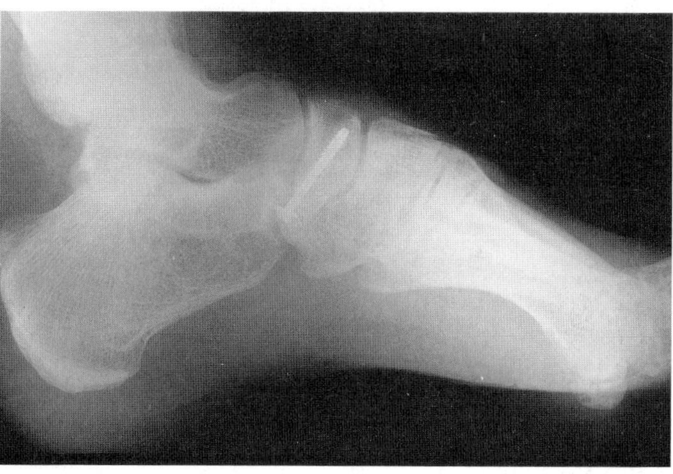

(d)

Fig. 24.7 (*Continued*) Because of persistent pain, an antero-posterior tomograph (c) was obtained showing a fracture of the tarsal navicular. Delayed union of the fracture was treated by internal fixation using a compression screw (d). The fracture has healed and there is no long-term disability. This is not a rare injury.

Protective equipment has become mandatory at most levels of play. The American Amateur Hockey Association of the United States has established guidelines that mandate the use of face and mouth protection. Helmets have reduced the incidence of closed head injuries. The importance of studying injury patterns and applying epidemiological principles to ice-hockey injuries have certainly enhanced the development of adequate protective wear for hockey players (Editorial, 1969; Vinger, 1977; Pashby, 1979).

Further results of analysing injury patterns in hockey have been the establishment of appropriate rules and the enforcement of such rules. Lorentzon *et al.* (1988a) documented that 39% of injuries were caused by plays involving penalties. Appropriate officiating helps decrease the incidence of high sticking and elbowing violations that cause facial injuries. Penalties for cross-checking are particularly important: a player who is checked from behind near the boards may sustain a cervical spine injury and quadriplegia if forced into the boards head down. This situation occurs with offensive forechecking. Further curtailment of fighting is also needed to decrease the incidence of hand, wrist and facial injuries.

Conclusion

Acceptance of ice-hockey injuries as an integral part of the game is no longer tolerated. Epidemiological studies have helped define injury patterns, helped design protective equipment, promulgated improved rules and given impetus to the enforcement of fair play. The increased awareness of injuries and the improved reporting by health-care personnel have also improved the safety of ice hockey. Continued interest in treating the musculoskeletal manifestations of trauma and overuse injuries in these athletes will result in continued improvements in the prevention, identification and treatment of injuries in ice hockey.

References

Benoit, B.G., Russell, N.A., Richard, M.T. *et al.* (1982) Epidural hematoma: report of seven cases with delayed evolution of symptoms. *Can. J. Neurol. Sci.* **9**, 321–4.

Biener, K. & Muller, P. (1973) Les accidents du hockey sur glace (Ice-hockey accidents). *Cash. Med.* **14**, 959–62.

Bishop, P.J. (1976) Head protection in sports with particular application to ice hockey. *Ergonomics* **19**, 451–64.

Bishop, P.J., Norman, R.W., Wells, R., Ranney, D. & Skleryk, B. (1983) Changes in the centre of mass and movement of a inertia of headform induced by hockey helmet and face shield. *Can. J. Appl. Sports Sci.* **8**, 19–25.

Bull, C. (1985) Hockey injuries. In R.C. Snyder, J.C. Kennedy & M.L. Plant (eds) *Sports Injuries: Mechanisms, Prevention and Treatment*, pp. 90–113. Williams & Wilkins, Baltimore.

Cooney III, W.P. (1984) Sports injuries to the upper extremity: How to recognize and deal with some common problems. *Postgrad. Med.* **76**, 45–50.

Daly, P.J., Sim, F.H. & Simonet, W.T. (1990) Ice hockey injuries; a review. *Sports Med.* **10**(3), 122–31.

Editorial (1969) Ice hockey can be safer. *JAMA* **207**, 1706.

Fekete J.F. (1968) Severe brain injury and death following minor hockey accidents: the effectiveness of the 'safety helmets' of amateur hockey players. *Can. Med. Assoc. J.* **99**, 1234–9.

Ferguson, R.J., Marcotte, G.G. & Montpetit, R.R. (1969) A maximal oxygen uptake test during ice skating. *Med. Sci. Sports* **1**, 207–11.

Green, H., Bishop, P., Houston, M. *et al.* (1976) Time–motion and physiological assessments of ice hockey performance. *J. Appl. Physiol.* **40**, 149–53.

Hayes, D. (1972) *The nature, incidence, location and causes of injury in intercollegiate ice hockey*. Thesis, University of Waterloo, Ontario, Canada.

Hayes, D. (1975) Hockey injuries: How, why, where and when? *Phys. Sportsmed.* **3**(1), 61–5.

Hornof, Z. & Napravnik, C. (1973) Analysis of various accident rate factors in ice hockey. *Med. Sci. Sports* **5**, 283–6.

Houston, M.E. & Green, H.J. (1976) Physiological and anthropometric characteristics of élite Canadian ice hockey players. *J. Sports Med. Phys. Fitness* **16**, 123–8.

Houston, M.E., Green, H.J. & Norman, B. (1973) Anthropometric and physiologic characteristics of ice hockey players (Abstract). *Med. Sci. Sport* **5**, 65.

Hovelius, L. (1978) Shoulder dislocation in Swedish ice hockey players. *Am. J. Sports Med.* **6**, 373–7.

Hovelius, L. & Palmgren, H. (1979) Laceration of tibial tendons and vessels in ice hockey players. *Am. J. Sports Med.* **7**, 297–8.

Jørgensen, U. & Schmidt-Olsen, S. (1986) The epidemiology of ice hockey injuries. *Br. J. Sports Med.* **20**(1), 7–9.

Lorentzon, R., Wedren, H. & Pietila, T. (1988a) Incidence, nature, and causes of ice hockey injuries: a three-year prospective study of a Swedish élite ice hockey team. *Am. J. Sports Med.* **16**, 392–6.

Lorentzon, R., Wedren, H., Pietila, T. & Gustavsson, B. (1988b) Injuries in international ice hockey: a prospective, comparative study of injury incidence and injury types in international and Swedish élite hockey. *Am. J. Sports Med.* **16**, 389–91.

Mitin, V.V. & Gladyseva, A.A. (1972) Proportions of body, power and mobility of hockey players (in Russian). *Teoriya Prak. Fizicheskii Kulturi* **36**, 23–26.

Minkoff, J. (1982) Evaluating parameters of a professional hockey team. *Am. J. Sports Med.* **10**, 285–92.

Nagobads, G. (1971) *Amateur Hockey Association of the United States — Head Injuries Study*. Reprinted by Youth Hockey Coaches Association.

Norfray, J.F., Tremaine, M.J., Groves, H.C. & Bachman, D.C. (1977) The clavicle in hockey. *Am. J. Sports Med.* **5**, 275–80.

Norman, R.W., Bishop, P.J. & Pierrynowski, M.R. (1980) Puck impact response of ice hockey face

masks. *Can. J. Appl. Sports Sci.* **5**, 208–14.
Pashby, T.J. (1977) Eye injuries in Canadian hockey. Phase II. *Can. Med. Assoc. J.* **117**, 671–2, 677–8.
Pashby, T.J. (1978) Eye injuries in Canadian hockey. Phase III. Older players now most at risk. *Can. Med. Assoc. J.* **121**, 643–4.
Pashby, T.J., Pashby, R.C., Chisholm, L.D.J. & Crawford, J.S. (1975) Eye injuries in Canadian hockey. *Can. Med. Assoc. J.* **113**, 663–6, 674.
Rovere, G.D., Gristina, A.G., Stolzer, W.A. & Garver, E.M. (1975) Treatment of 'gamekeeper's thumb' in hockey players. *J. Sports Med.* **3**, 147–51.
Rowe, C.R. & Sakellarides, H.T. (1961) Factors related to recurrences of anterior dislocations of the shoulder. *Clin. Orthop.* **20**, 40.
Sane, J., Ylipaavalniemi, P. & Leppanen, H. (1988) Maxillofacial and dental ice hockey injuries. *Med. Sci. Sports Exerc.* **20**, 202–7.
Sim, F.H. & Chao, E.Y. (1978) Injury potential in modern ice hockey. *Am. J. Sports Med.* **6**, 378–84.
Sim, F.H., Simonet, W.T., Melton III, L.J. & Lehn, T.A. (1987) Ice hockey injuries. *Am. J. Sports Med.* **15**, 30–40.
Sim, F.H., Simonet, W.T. & Scott, S.G. (1989) Ice hockey injuries: causes, treatment and prevention. *J. Musculoskeletal Med.* **6**(3), 15–44.
Simonet, W.T. & Cofield, R.H. (1984) Prognosis in anterior shoulder dislocation. *Am. J. Sports Med.* **12**, 19–24.
Smith, A.W., Bishop, P.J. & Wells, R.P. (1985) Alterations in head dynamics with the addition of a hockey helmet and face shield under inertial loading. *Can. J. Appl. Sports Sci.* **10**, 68–74.
Sutherland, G.W. (1976) Fire on ice. *Am. J. Sports Med.* **4**, 264–9.
Tator, C.H. & Edmonds, V.E. (1984) National survey of spinal injuries in hockey players. *Can. Med. Assoc. J.* **130**, 875–80.
Torg, J.S. & Pavlov, H. (1987) Cervical spinal stenosis with cord neurapraxia and transient quadriplegia. *Clin. Sports Med.* **6**(1), 115–33.
Vinger, P.F. (1977) 'Too great' a risk spurred hockey mass development. *Phys. Sportsmed.* **5**, 70–3.
Wilson, K., Cram, B. & Rontal, M. (1977) Facial injuries in hockey players. *Minn. Med.* **60**, 13–19.

Chapter 25

Injuries in Rugby

MYLES R.J. COOLICAN AND THOMAS K.F. TAYLOR

Rugby, a body contact sport played around the globe, is the world's most popular football code after soccer. The speed, frequency of collisions and lack of external protective equipment collectively make Rugby a game destined to produce a variety of injuries ranging from the trivial to the catastrophic. Hence, injury is an accepted and probable risk for those who play the game. It is the purpose of this chapter to examine the musculoskeletal injuries which occur in Rugby with particular emphasis on their prevention.

The prevention of injuries to Rugby players is a responsibility shared by all who are involved in the sport. The administrators and their medical advisors have a responsibility to regularly gather data on both the incidence and the range of injuries seen and then to adjust the rules of play accordingly. Coaches have a dual role. Obviously technique is important but they also have the responsibility of instilling in all players the ethics of fair play and good sporting behaviour. This is particularly important for juniors and schoolchildren. Lastly, the players themselves have a duty of care to their opponents, to themselves and, an important point, to schoolchildren whose behaviour on a Rugby field will be greatly influenced by the example set before them.

In Rugby, there is more than ample opportunity for aggressive, even violent, play and this increases the likelihood of injury. It is self-evident that in a body contact game aggression breeds aggression, and, similarly, violence engenders violence. Thus, the stage is set for injury. The phrase 'controlled violence' is often used by the media to report incidents in Rugby matches. However, all too frequently this fragile control is lost by the players and a free-for-all brawl erupts, much to the enjoyment of spectators and the media. It is a sad commentary that these events make good copy.

In the 1980s, there were many major changes in sport generally, and in most Western societies there is a widening compass of sporting activities. New games are being introduced and existing ones are being modified and diversified. These events reflect certain ill-defined, but nevertheless definite cultural trends, and the links (theoretical or otherwise) between sport (physical activity) and so-called good health. Governments are now laying considerable emphasis on preventative health programmes. They provide substantial funding for selected games, institutes and academies of sport on the basis that sport is a positive move towards better health. Success in the ultimate arena, the Olympic games, is seen as a decidedly positive index of a country's international standing — a symbol of its youth and its future. It is remarkable how these images are divorced from reality in the ingenious international marketing of all forms of sport. The hero status of the world champion is carefully exploited and so often with political or quasi-political implications.

There is another quite complementary aspect of this complex matter. Sport today is far removed from what it was once accepted to be. It is, no doubt, a giant entertainment industry. No longer is it simply something which is a good thing for young people to do — the embodiment and enactment of leadership, teamwork, camaraderie, fair play, the pleasure of participation and the honour of representation. Admittedly, it is almost impossible to define exactly what these things mean, but they are generally understood. While it is true that these elements are still present in sport they are, now, far less relevant, or as accepted as they once were. Today, the financial rewards for a top athlete are potentially huge, and he or she can hold public acclamation to hero (gladiator) status. In the 1990s, the behaviour on the sporting field of top performers particularly in professional sport, is so often the antithesis of what good sporting behaviour is really all about. Such behaviour cannot be unexpected when one considers the enormous financial implications of the difference between winning and losing in some sports. Society now permits unsporting behaviour where once it would simply not have been allowed. Aggressive, if not violent, play is condoned. The pattern of sporting behaviour affects young people, and as is always the case, they tend to style their approach to any game on those who are most successful at it. Once patterns of sporting behaviour and attitude are established they are difficult, and perhaps impossible, to change.

Rugby is an amateur game but in these times the fine line between this status and that of the professional in all sports is, unquestionably, becoming increasingly blurred. Thus, the above comments on the ethos of sport apply in greater or lesser part to Rugby.

A brief history of Rugby

The modern game of Rugby has evolved over 2000 years from the wild mêlées of ancient Britain to its present form. Obviously the injuries produced are related to the way in which the game is played and, as such, a brief history of the game's evolution is pertinent.

The origins of football are obscure but, it is known that all codes stem from the cited mêlées. The origin of these mêlées is debated but they were likely derived from a Roman game called *Harpastum*. Football evolved between Roman times and the beginning of the nineteenth century, from wild brawls involving hundreds of men in a mêlée spread over several miles, to a version similar to modern football with play within defined boundaries by teams of equal size. The rules and mode of play varied, depending to a large extent on the region. It was in schools that football flourished but no two schools seem to have had the same rules. For example, at Westminster School in London, tackling was impossible, due to the surrounding cobble-stones. A game similar to modern day soccer was played here. At Rugby School, in the English Midlands, surrounded by grasslands, a more vigorous game was played which ultimately evolved into present-day Rugby.

Varying types of games were played until 1860 when the Football Association was formed and rules were promulgated. Soccer had thereby begun. Rugby was similarly put on a formal basis in 1871 with the establishment of the Rugby Football Union. Thus, Rugby did not directly evolve from soccer, but rather both stemmed from a common ancestor.

Preparation

Once, football was viewed as a means of keeping fit between cricket seasons. Indeed, a game called Australian Rules, one quite different from Rugby, was introduced into Australia in 1859 for such purposes. In modern Rugby, high levels of physical fitness are required in order to play the game and to minimize injury. For most team positions, this means aerobic conditioning and maintenance of flexibility, plus specific muscle strengthening exercises.

Cardiovascular fitness

It is said that the first recorded case of sudden death following athletic endeavour was that of

Pheidippides in 490 BC. He ran from Marathon to Athens in order to warn of the imminent Spartan invasion. Whilst the cause of Pheidippides's death is not known, in all probability it was a catastrophic cardiac event. The commonest cause of sudden death in sports is pre-existing cardiac disease, and sudden death in athletes is largely a preventable tragedy and one which may be minimized by a thorough preparticipation examination.

In a study of 29 cases of sudden death in athletes of less than 30 years of age, Maron *et al.* (1980) found that 28 (96%) had a structural cause. These included 19 (65%) with hypertrophic cardiomyopathy, five (17%) with coronary artery anomalies, three (10%) with coronary artery disease, two (7%) with a dissecting aneurysm and one with mitral valve prolapse. Other similar studies (Virmani *et al.*, 1982; Waller, 1985) have confirmed the high incidence of detectable abnormalities in athletes who have died suddenly. Notably, only seven of the 29 cases of Maron *et al.* were symptomatic prior to death.

A detailed medical examination is required before an American professional footballer is allowed to commence training. Whilst this vigorous screening programme is not paralleled for Rugby, it is considered to have merits. Therefore, it is germane to set down what is desirable in a pretraining assessment.

A thorough, preliminary history plus a physical examination will minimize the possibility of sudden death. A history of rheumatic fever, hypertension, heart murmur, diabetes, plus chest pain, syncope and a family history of coronary heart disease should be sought. Physical examination should include an assessment of body habitus (Marfan's syndrome), blood pressure, pulses, heart sounds and murmurs. Further investigation may be indicated in those with suspect findings on physical examination. Which special tests are performed is controversial and usually depends on the time and money available. A 12-lead electrocardiogram (ECG) is a good screening test with other tests being performed as indicated by the history and physical findings (Robinson, 1989). Occasionally, a cardiology referral is necessary. In general, players with conditions which place them at higher risk of sudden death are advised not to play Rugby.

Most trainers and coaches begin the season with a prescription heavily based on aerobic exercise but one which leaves some time for work on strength, speed and skills relevant to each player. Cardiorespiratory adaptation to training ('getting fit') occurs both centrally and peripherally. Central mechanisms include both an increase in stroke volume with a capacity for higher cardiac output, and a decrease in the resting myocardial oxygen demand and heart rate. The heart becomes larger and stronger and blood volume increases. Peripherally, an increase in blood flow to muscle is noted, as well as an increase in the arteriovenous oxygen difference, indicating that oxygen is being more efficiently removed from haemoglobin. Below maximum exercise level less lactic acid is produced. More mitochondria appear in muscle, so improving the body's ability to oxidize both fat and carbohydrates. Myoglobin levels are higher and there is an increase in capillary density. Maximal breathing volumes increase during exhaustive exercise. These changes occur gradually but do allow a player to improve exercise tolerance and consequently, to exercise harder at subsequent training sessions (Cox, 1991).

Avoiding 'burn-out' (overtraining) is important and a 24–48 h recovery time between training times improves aerobic fitness and reduces the risk of musculotendinous overload and of stress fractures.

Flexibility

Flexibility remains one of the first lines of defence against injury for the Rugby player. Flexibility is the ability to move a joint or joints easily through a full range of motion. Another way of describing flexibility is the ease with which a joint moves. Flexibility increases to young adulthood and then decreases with age.

It increases with heat, and decreases with cold, and this is largely due to the effect of heat on the extensibility of skeletal muscles. Muscles with greater extensibility are less likely to be overextended during vigorous exercise (Anderson & Burke, 1991). Stretching after exercise will decrease the postexercise muscle soreness which can occur after strenuous play. Most conditioners of Rugby teams utilize a stretching programme prior to training and playing which includes quadriceps, hamstring and calf stretches as well as spinal and shoulder stretching. The stretch is maintained for at least 30 s and bouncing is avoided.

Strength training

Milo, the ancient Greek Olympic wrestler, is said to have been the first to utilize the principle of 'progressive resistance exercise'. Milo carried a baby calf each day until it was fully grown. His accommodation to the demands of the burden he carried demonstrates the ability of skeletal muscle to respond to training. The major principles of strength training in the Rugby player are overload and specificity.

Overload occurs when the demand on a given muscle is greater than is usual. The load may be increased progressively by either increasing the resistance, or the number of repetitions (Di Nubile, 1991). Each team position places varying demands on the musculoskeletal system and it is important to develop strength and endurance in the areas required. Discussion of the exercise programmes for each player position is beyond the scope of this chapter but some general comments are pertinent.

Players in the front row concentrate their strength training on trunk exercises, particularly the cervical spine, whereas the second row requires strength and endurance in the lower limbs plus explosive power for line-out jumping. An exercise programme directed at the quadriceps and calf muscles is appropriate. All forwards need to maintain an upper body strength programme. This is of less value to backs who need to work on strength and endurance in the lower limbs. Some backs will do upper body work, particularly if an increase in bulk is needed. In general, strength is best achieved with higher weights and lower repetitions whereas endurance is improved by utilizing lower weights with higher repetitions.

Warm-up

Warming-up prior to training or to playing a match can be achieved by any activity which increases the core body temperature. Most Rugby coaches utilize a combination of graduated running, stretching and skills rehearsal in approximately a 30-min period prior to a match. The results of a good warm-up include:

1 Increased muscle temperature with improvement in flexibility, and hence a reduced chance of injury.

2 Increased blood temperature which reduces the affinity of the haemoglobin molecules to oxygen, thereby making oxygen more available to working muscles.

When warm-up is combined with a stretching programme, optimal prematch preparation is achieved. It is of interest to record that one of the authors (M.R.J.C.), when serving as a team physician to a representative Rugby side in Australia noted that, in general, Rugby teams from the Northern hemisphere do not leave the locker room between dressing for a match and running on to the field. This may well be related to the ambient temperature during the Rugby season in the Northern hemisphere.

Prevention and treatment of infection

The environment of the Rugby player can be a hazardous place and attention to detail by all involved in team management is required to minimize injury and illness in each player. One of the authors once played in a team which on one occasion had five players unavailable because of infected grazes, one of whom was admitted to hospital with staphylococcal septicaemia. The source was ultimately traced to 'blood and bone' fertilizer being used by the groundsmen. Biological fertilizers such as blood and bone, and various manures which have the potential to carry bacteria, have a place on Rugby fields only in the off-season. All grazes in Rugby players can become contaminated wounds and are well treated with povidone-iodine ointment. If possible they should be kept covered while playing. Tetanus prophylaxis is imperative for all players.

The close contact of Rugby players makes possible the transmission of communicable diseases. The occasional bleeding wound raises the question of transmission of blood-borne diseases, particularly hepatitis and acquired immune deficiency syndrome (AIDS). All Rugby players should be immunized against hepatitis B and should have antibody titres checked periodically. The International Rugby Board is to be commended for its recent alteration to the rules which allows temporary replacement of a player with a bleeding wound. If this can be controlled, the player may subsequently return to the field of play.

Impetigo is a highly communicable staphylococcal infection which has been known to decimate front rows in touring teams. Failure to shave on match day adds to the possibility of transmission as bristly faces scratch one another at scrummage, creating a portal of entry for bacteria in addition to upsetting the concentration of the opponents. Similarly, the herpes simplex type 1 virus may be transmitted by close contact between players at scrummage. In addition there is the risk of players developing herpes keratoconjunctivitis and systemic herpes simplex, cases of which have been documented by White and Grant-Kels (1984). In the USA, wrestlers with herpes simplex are excluded from competition and there is good reason for the International Rugby Board to act similarly. At present Rugby has no specific rules regarding the participation of players with infectious diseases. The responsibility in these matters rests with the player, the coach and the team physician.

Communal bathing after Rugby matches remains relatively common, particularly in the UK. In the past this was considered good for team spirit and the beginning of postmatch celebrations. These circumstances carry a possible risk of transmission of herpes simplex, impetigo, fungal infections and scabies. Many players carry open wounds to the bath and these are portals of entry for common bacteria as well as the more sinister viruses. Torre *et al.* (1990) have documented a case of HIV-1 seroconversion in Rugby when a player collided with an opponent who was an intravenous drug abuser and HIV-1 positive. Both players received facial lacerations with seroconversion noted 2 months later in a player who had no other known exposure to HIV-1. For these reasons, showering after Rugby rather than communal bathing is recommended.

Coaching and refereeing

The Rugby coach has a responsibility to impart to the team the knowledge of the laws of the game, the skills and techniques of safe play and, most important, a sense of the spirit of fair play. The process begins at school level where the role set by senior school players and State and national representative teams in setting a good example cannot be overstated. Whilst the matter of correct technique belongs more in the coaching manuals, some points on fair play are made, particularly where absence of fair play can produce injury.

Of all the modes of play, it is the tackle and subsequent ruck or maul, which produce the greatest number of injuries. These include fractures of both upper and lower limb bones and facial bones, soft tissue injuries and lacerations and, rarely, injuries to the spine. Whilst Rugby remains a body contact sport, the risk of injury from tackling, albeit low, will remain. The subsequent ruck or maul can at times revert to the wild mêlées of ancient Britain. At senior level and above, a player lying on or near the ball, caught in the opposite side of the ruck, is considered fair game by the opponents. The resultant trampling is painful and many injuries result. It may lead, at worst, to an escalation of violence or, more commonly, later retaliation until the match resembles a brawl with repeated fisticuffs and a high level of frustration amongst the players, the referee and the spectators.

The key to minimizing lacerations, trampling injuries and violent outbursts in this mode of play is astute refereeing. Spectators do not enjoy a match where every tackle is rapidly followed by a scrum because, after all, second and third phase play are by far the most exciting. The experienced referee should sense what is happening in the early stages of the game and know when to 'shorten the whistle' and when to let play proceed in the anticipation of early second phase play with a lesser chance of trampling injury.

Poor refereeing may also lead to injury, particularly if players see the referee as favouring their opponents and so decide to take justice into their own hands. Infringements, particularly at line-out, allow one player an advantage over the other and subsequent possession of the ball. Illegal strategies include stepping on the toes of an opponent who is trying to jump, using the opponent's shoulder to push off when jumping and deliberate elbowing when an opponent is in the air. The experienced referee will keep the players well apart at line-out and quickly, correctively and decisively, penalize offenders.

Deliberate collapsing of a scrum is a ploy which is sometimes used to gain an advantage. For example, when one team with a more powerful set of forwards is likely to score a push-over try, the opponents may attempt to prevent the try by deliberately collapsing the scrum. This is dangerous play and carries a significant risk of spinal cord injury. It is now common practice for referees to award a penalty try in this situation.

All Rugby bodies affiliated with the International Rugby Board utilize a judiciary committee to deal with players who have been sent from the field. Clubs are also able to cite opponents to appear before the judiciary when foul play has occurred undetected by the referee or the touch judges. The decision of such committees receives close media attention and, as such, the attitude of the whole code to foul play is embodied in the decisions and suspensions which are handed down. Judiciary committees come under pressure to suspend players for long periods when the injury produced by foul play is significant, and to be somewhat more lenient when the injury is trivial. An example is trampling on an opponent's head in a ruck, when that player is on the ground away from the ball. Here the injuries so produced vary from insignificant to major. The possibilities include extensive avulsion of scalp flaps, lacerations to the face, eye and mouth, partial avulsion of an ear, concussion and faciomaxillary fractures. A mechanism is now in place to discipline players who engage in deliberate foul play. Guilty verdicts with a long suspension affects the players and their families, the team and its coach and the club. The opprobrium of suspension is not to be lightly cast aside.

Equipment

One of the hallmarks of Rugby is the absence of protective clothing worn by players. The standard equipment is a Rugby jersey, athletic support, shorts, socks and Rugby boots. The player also takes little onto the field which could be used as an offensive weapon in the way American footballers use their shoulder pads and helmets. The laws of Rugby are quite specific about the use of such equipment. Rugby law books in the UK and in Australasia simply state that the use of anything containing metal or hard plastic is illegal. In the law books issued by the USA Rugby Football Union, two pages are devoted to listing equipment which is banned. This equipment is very familiar to American footballers. It includes wrestling-type ear muffs, knee pads, forearm guards, casts of any material for the protection of existing bony or soft tissue injuries, shoulder pads and helmets.

Some Rugby players, particularly forwards, wear protective head gear consisting of a soft leather or canvas strapping, including a cover for the ears with a strap under the chin. This is permitted but may lead to chafing and it is not unknown for opposition players to pull the straps and dislodge the head gear or even cause extreme respiratory difficulty. Most players achieve the same level of ear protection by winding elastic or self-adhesive tape around their head immediately above the eyes and below the equator of the skull. Protection from lacerations in the area covered by the tape is achieved, but plastering the ear to the skull gives no protection against an occasional subperichondrial haematoma which leads to cartilage necrosis and the familiar, thickened, collapsed 'cauliflower ear'.

All dental authorities recommend the use of a mouth guard to protect the upper teeth. The mobility of the mandible reduces the likelihood of the lower teeth being damaged. Only adolescents with orthodontic braces are advised to use both upper and lower mouth guards to protect the buccal mucosa. The support provided by a mouth guard certainly improves the chance of the tooth surviving a direct blow. A mouth guard also helps in finding a totally avulsed tooth which can then be cleansed and reinserted into its socket. The compliance with mouth guard use is variable. Chapman in 1989 reported that although 95% of the 1987 USA World Cup Rugby team believed a mouth guard was beneficial, only 50% used one. The 1984 Australian side fared a little better with an 80% utilization rate. Common complaints include partial respiratory obstruction and local discomfort, both of which can be minimized by the use of a professionally fitted guard.

Rugby in the Southern hemisphere is frequently played on hard fast grounds which, in part, explains the world-wide differences in the way the code is played. Hard grounds result in frequent grazes, particularly of the elbows and knees. Elbow grazes can be minimized by the use of longer sleeved jerseys. Knee grazes are accepted as part of the game by most backs but their severity can be reduced by an elastic guard or by the application of petroleum jelly before the game and again at half-time. All grazes should be thoroughly cleansed after a match and rubbed with povidone-iodine ointment to minimize infection.

Ankle injuries, as in all forms of football, are common in Rugby. The prevention of the common anterior talofibular sprain is multifactorial. Ground staff should prepare a playing surface which is free from potholes and depressions. The value of taping is debatable but it is recommended for all players with a history of earlier ankle sprain. The mainstay of prevention of subsequent ankle injuries is an intense, graduated ankle rehabilitation programme.

Attention to footwear is important. Higher cut boots may offer protection to the ankle but it is certain that they reduce the possibility of having the boot accidentally pulled off during a match. Studs (cleats) improve traction. There are set rules on stud dimensions. Longer studs are necessary on wet days, particularly in the tight five. One of the authors (M.R.J.C.) has treated a Rugby player whose anterior cruciate ligament tore because he had failed to revert to dry weather studs. The foot was planted and could not twist with the body. The use of appropriate studs is strongly advised.

In 1983, the International Rugby Board introduced compulsory inspection of boots and, in particular, of studs, prior to a match. The Board became concerned about cuts and lacerations occurring from both sharp studs and the outer margins of the plastic sole used on some boots. When abraded against dry, hard ground throughout a season, stud margins can become razor-sharp and dangerous. This is particularly so for the outer studs in players who run with pronated feet (Fig. 25.1). A weekly inspection of boots helps to prevent possible wounds. A single, leading stud is barred.

Subperiosteal haematoma and lacerations to the subcutaneous border of the tibia are common in front rowers and tend to occur at scrummage when the opposition hooker strikes for the ball. Shin pads of the type commonly worn inside the socks by soccer players give good protection from these injuries and are

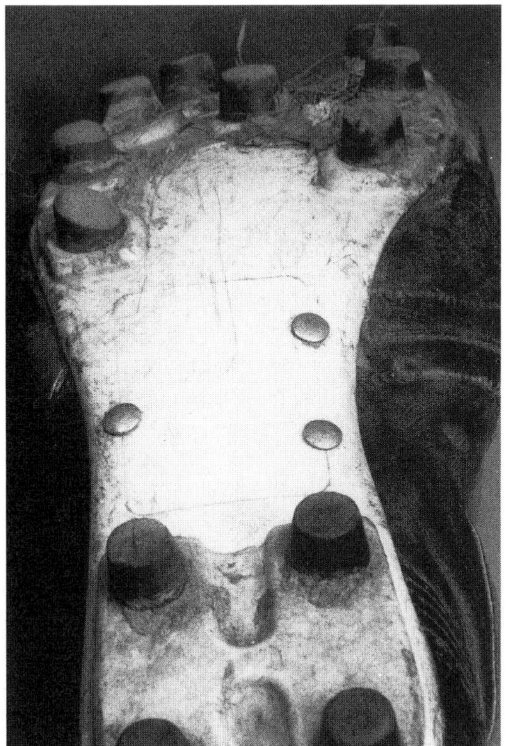

Fig. 25.1 A Rugby boot from a player who ran with pronated feet causing asymmetrical wear of the outside studs. The sharp margin may lacerate an opponent. Regular inspection of boots is important in prevention.

recommended for all front rowers. They are also recommended for any player recovering from a soft-tissue injury along the subcutaneous border of the tibia.

Management of common Rugby injuries

The principal role of the team medical officer in Rugby is to deal with the musculoskeletal injuries produced by the game. Prevention, the major thrust of this chapter, is achieved by sound preparation, good coaching in both attitude and technique and by the use of permitted protective equipment. The players' health comes before any short-term objective of the coach and that of the team. An important role of the team physician is to advise when it is safe to return to play and also advise in the prevention of recurrence of injury. Whilst the management of all injuries seen in Rugby is beyond the scope of this work, some of the more common problems encountered are discussed below.

Facial lacerations

Myers (1980) showed the head and neck to be the most common area affected by lacerations in Rugby (Fig. 25.2). Infection is rare and can be minimized by cleansing the wound and by immediate closure using interrupted sutures. Unless extensive, and provided the bleeding is

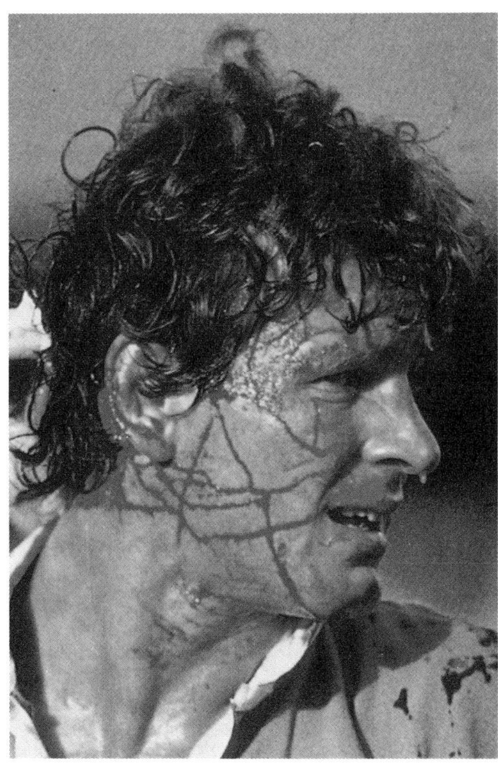

Fig. 25.2 This Rugby player has been forced to leave the field because of a bleeding scalp wound. The International Rugby Board rule changes in 1990 now allow temporary replacement whilst the bleeding is controlled.

controlled, the player may return to the field and turn out the following week with the removal of sutures after the subsequent match. Protective covering is recommended if possible.

Closed head injuries

The International Rugby Board has made specific recommendations on the management of concussion and return to play. Any concussion as defined by a period of unconsciousness should be treated as a potentially serious head injury. The player is removed from the field and does not return to play until given a clearance after thorough neurological examination.

Digital fractures

Fractures and dislocations of the digital phalanges are commonly seen in Rugby as a result of twisting or, occasionally, stomping. The players usually request that the digit be 'buddy' taped for the immediate resumption of play. Close examination to exclude malrotation at the fracture site is necessary. Radiographs are indicated if malalignment is suspected. Failure to correct this results in long-term deformity, particularly if an articular surface is incongruous. The authors recommend hand surgery referral for displaced digital fractures, particularly those involving a joint.

Closed tendon injuries

Closed tendon avulsions, namely the insertion of flexor digitorum profundus and the central slip of the extensor hood are commonly missed as acute injuries. However, the diagnosis of both is easily made by a careful examination. Early referral to a hand surgeon is advised to prevent the deformity and disability which may later result from these injuries.

Acromioclavicular joint injuries

Lack of shoulder pads and other protective equipment around the shoulder in a running collision sport predisposes Rugby players to injure the ligaments which support the acromioclavicular joint. This most often occurs in tackles and falls. Non-operative management with physiotherapy and measures to decrease pain and swelling are appropriate with most acromioclavicular joint injuries. Radiographs are necessary to exclude a type II fracture of the outer end of the clavicle which can closely mimic subluxation or dislocation of the adjacent joint. Many Rugby locker rooms contain players, particularly back rowers, with bilateral grade 3 acromioclavicular separations but who have little or no disability and continue to play at a high level of competition.

Dislocation of the shoulder

Acute anterior dislocation of the shoulder is commonly seen in Rugby players, usually after a tackle. Recurrent subluxation or dislocation is the usual outcome and reconstructive surgery is often required. The authors obtain radiographs of the shoulder for a player's first-time dislocation, but otherwise they recommend prompt relocation of the shoulder either on the field or in the locker room, with subsequent orthopaedic referral. A neurovascular check is mandatory. Posterior dislocation is extremely rare in Rugby particularly as the American football tactic of using the ulnar border of the forearm in blocking is illegal.

Costal cartilage injuries

The junction between costal cartilages and ribs is a notorious area for injury in Rugby, and notably so for front rowers. A direct blow to the costochondral junctional area is the mechanism of injury, often in a pile up or tackle. These are particularly painful injuries. Failure to take adequate time out of playing and training often leads to persistence of symptoms for weeks or even months. Not infrequently symptoms do not subside until the off-season. Anti-inflammatory and pain-relieving medication may help, but generally it is safe for the player to return to competition when local tenderness has settled.

Knee ligament injuries

Isolated injury to the medial collateral ligament is probably the commonest knee ligament injury seen in Rugby. This injury may be combined with a lateral meniscal tear but is rarely associated with a medial meniscal tear.

The authors manage isolated medial knee ligament injuries non-operatively utilizing a limited motion brace, anti-inflammatory medication and an exercise regime to strengthen both the quadriceps and hamstring muscles. Most return to training 3–6 weeks after injury with progression of activity depending upon resolution of pain and local tenderness.

Anterior cruciate ligament tear remains a major problem in Rugby and frequently curtails a player's career, although less so today than in previous years. The injury is almost always indirect and occurs as a player changes direction at speed. Occasionally, it is part of a valgus injury when the knee is torn asunder, but this is less common in Rugby than in American football, as blocking in Rugby is illegal. The authors recommend early clinical evaluation of the knee with radiographs and, if necessary, examination under anaesthetic. The preferred method of treatment is arthroscopic substitution of the injured anterior cruciate with a bone–tendon–bone preparation of middle third autologous patellar tendon.

The correct timing of return to Rugby after anterior cruciate ligament reconstruction is by no means universally agreed upon. However, biomechanical studies in animal models of grafted anterior cruciates show no increase in the force to failure of grafts between 1 and 2 years after surgery (Clancy *et al.*, 1981), and so there is no good reason to keep the player out of the game for more than 12 months. The authors current protocol allows for a graduated return to training at 3 months with sprinting, pivoting and all sudden starts and stops being avoided until 6 months postsurgery. This is sooner than the time at which animal studies suggest the graft has 'plateaued' in strength but parallels the return to full function in the quadriceps and hamstrings.

Meniscal tears are commonly seen in Rugby players and are arthroscopically repaired if this is feasible. The implication of repair, particularly the time out of playing, are discussed prior to surgery. Most Rugby players expect to return to play 2 weeks after arthroscopic knee surgery and must be warned that meniscal repair is followed by 6 weeks limited flexion with return to Rugby at 8–10 weeks. When the long-term risks and arthritis are discussed, few, if any, opt for meniscectomy.

Ankle ligament sprains

Anterior talofibular ligament sprains remain the most common ligament injury seen in Rugby. Early treatment is with ice, elevation, rest and a compressive support with early protected motion. The authors warn players with ankle ligament injuries of the adverse effects of standing for prolonged periods drinking alcohol at after match functions.

Most players with anterior talofibular ligament sprains can usually return to play at approximately 3 weeks after injury, although those with recurrent minor injuries may be able to return earlier. A graduated physiotherapy programme is employed for most sprains. This concentrates on peroneal exercises and the use of a wobble-board. The authors have used the liposuction technique described by Dowden *et al.* (1990) to remove a large haematoma which can accompany these injuries. This simple manoeuvre can considerably shorten the rehabilitation time. The player returns to the game when comfortable sprinting is possible.

Fractures

The management of long bone fractures in a Rugby player is largely carried out along conventional lines and little variation is required. A major exception is a fracture of the shaft of the radius and/or the ulna, where we recommend intramedullary fixation (contoured Rush nails) rather than the conventional dynamic compression plate. The major problem with plates is the differential coefficient of elasticity at the bone–metal interface which may lead to a fracture at the end of the plate should a player return to the game with the fixation *in situ*.

When a plate is removed, the screw holes are sites of possible refracture until cortical reconstitution occurs. This is helped by normal use of the limb. Accordingly, the remodelling process must be followed by careful radiographic evaluations before the patient is permitted to return to competitive play.

Return to play

The decision to allow a player to return to training and playing after injury or surgery can be difficult, and depends upon several factors. Arthroscopic surgery of the knee, particularly partial meniscectomy, no longer has the long rehabilitation period that once was required after open surgery. An arthroscopy portal heals within 1–2 weeks and players frequently, and unrealistically, expect to return to the field after this time. At this stage post-surgery, the knee is often irritable with a small effusion and a degree of synovitis. The atrophy of quadriceps and hamstrings which occurs with disuse takes some time to reverse and premature return to play often results in a larger effusion and a painful, swollen knee. Patellofemoral pain may then ensue and the player, despite resolution of meniscal symptoms, may remain symptomatic for many weeks. The key to early, maximal recovery is adequate rehabilitation with a graduated return to training so that quadriceps endurance is sufficient to protect the joint throughout a game.

In general, capsular and ligament sprains heal in a consistent time period, approximately 3–6 weeks, and return is permitted when range of motion of the joint is restored and muscle strength and endurance is near normal. Muscle and tendon strains are much more variable in healing time. Quadriceps, hamstring and calf muscle strains are particularly prone to recurrence, especially in back row forwards and backs. The authors do not inject local anaesthetic agents into muscles or around tendons, so allowing players to return to play.

Spinal disorders and contraindications to participation

In the question of prevention of injury, the presence of pre-existing conditions should be considered; also to be considered are those circumstances where a specific injury, or simply just playing, leads to the detection of spinal pathology. The latter is a not uncommon event.

Spondylolisthesis

In our view, asymptomatic spondylolisthesis, even with a slip of up to 25%, does not constitute a contraindication to play Rugby. Not infrequently, a Rugby player will first present after a transient episode of low back pain following a game (Fig. 25.3). Subsequently, when the player is without symptoms, the question of returning to the game is raised. Providing that a full range of spinal motion (for that patient) has been regained, and that there are no other abnormal physical signs, playing is permitted. If pain recurs, then withdrawal is advisable, but not absolutely so. In two decades of giving such advice to Rugby players, no adverse effects have occurred through this approach. The presence of protracted root symptoms in spondylolisthesis, although uncommon in younger age groups having smaller slips, is viewed as a contraindication to continued participation. Patients with slips greater than 25%, particularly if in the rapid growth phase, are advised on general grounds not to play Rugby, though we suspect it would probably be quite safe to do so.

The natural history of spondylolisthesis is

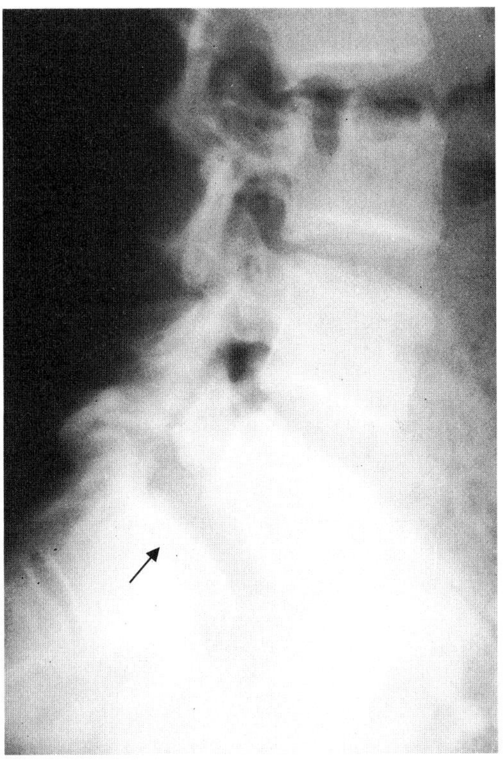

Fig. 25.3 Lateral radiograph of the lumbar spine in a 16-year-old male, which demonstrates an L5–S1 spondylolisthesis. There is an approximately 20–25% slip with the pars defects clearly shown (arrow). This pathology, in the absence of symptoms, is not considered to be a contraindication to playing Rugby.

quite unpredictable. For example, an episode or two of short-lived back pain, with a later, complete recovery and no further difficulty in adult life, is by no means uncommon. Clearly, each player must be managed on an individual basis. The assessment of the keen Rugby player with spondylolisthesis who admits to chronic, though not severe, low back pain is far from easy. Young players who, for one reason or another, are desperate to play, are rarely communicative and tend to understate their symptoms. Frequently, Rugby is the very essence of their being. Furthermore, they are anxious not to be viewed by their peers as being either incapacitated, or just not up to the mark.

Restriction of lumbar spinal motion is a reliable indicator of symptomatic spondylolisthesis but firm pressure which produces tenderness at the level of the slip is even more so. If there is no tenderness on examination, it is most unlikely that the slip is the cause of the patient's symptoms. Hamstring tightness is not a reliable indicator, and it shows poor correlation with either the presence, or absence, of pain.

Unilateral and bilateral stress fractures in the pars interarticularis at all levels in the lumbar spine are not often seen as a complication of conventional Rugby training unless the training programme entails strenuous and repetitive weightlifting and similar activities. Such fractures are usually managed by rest, then a gradual return to training with maximum protection of the lumbar spine under guidance is permitted. If this pathology is suspected a bone scan is helpful. A positive scan confirms the diagnosis. Long-standing lesions, which usually have well-defined cortical margins, do not show increased uptake. Each case must be managed on an individual basis. Stress fractures of this type are common in weightlifters. They also occur in fast bowlers in cricket, gymnasts, trampolinists and ballet dancers. Repetitive rotatory and other forces acting on the lumbar spine in these activities are clearly implicated in the mechanism of fracture in the dense cortical bone of the pars interarticularis which fails in tension.

Scheuermann's disease (osteochondrosis)

This condition is relatively common in Australia and it is far more prevalent here than in North America. It is one of the more common causes of back pain in the teenage years besides presentation as a spinal deformity. Various sports may precipitate symptoms and in Rugby, notably forward play.

The spinal distribution of Scheuermann's disease is variable in the extent of the changes at a given spinal level and the number of levels involved. Classically, the disorder affects the thoracic spine with concomitant arcuate kyphosis with little, if any, pain. Then the problem is primarily, though not invariably, a cosmetic one.

Our attitude to patients with Scheuermann's disease playing Rugby is, in general terms, much the same as it is for spondylolisthesis. If pain is precipitated by playing, and it quickly resolves with rest, then the patients are allowed to return to the game on the proviso that if symptoms recur, they should consider sports other than Rugby. This advice equally applies to those with a degree of thoracic kyphosis not sufficient to warrant brace treatment. Only patients with extensive and severe lumbar involvement are strongly advised against playing Rugby (Fig. 25.4). Players who have recurrent back pain from specific injuries, or from simply playing, usually decide of their own accord, to give up the game. We have yet to see a patient with this condition who has become permanently incapacitated by back pain from playing Rugby.

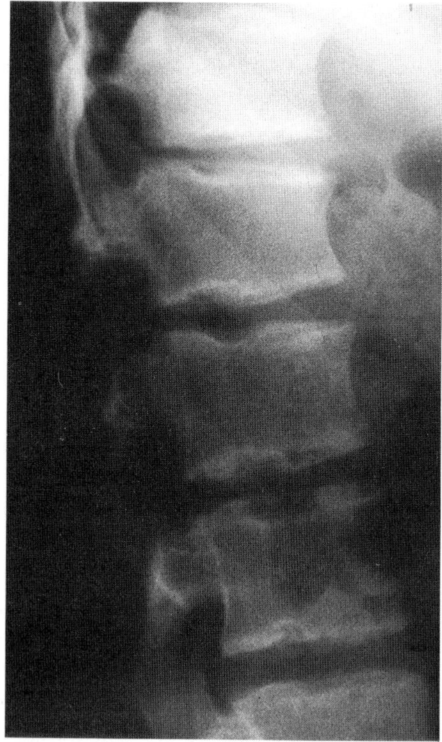

Fig. 25.4 Lateral radiograph of the lumbar spine of an 18-year-old male showing severe osteochondrosis at all levels of the lumbar spine. Patients with such extensive spinal involvement are advised against participation in Rugby.

Lumbar intervertebral disc degeneration and prolapse (herniation)

Low back pain and sciatica as a result of disc prolapse is a common clinical disorder in most Western societies, and footballers are equally subject to these problems as are those who do not play these games. Similar comments apply to low back pain from disc degeneration but without overt prolapse. There is, however, no evidence that trauma (injury) is an aetiological factor in the pathogenesis of prolapse *per se* or of disc degeneration. Rather, an injury or unusual strain acts as a precipitating factor in a structure already weakened by degenerative (degradative) change. Recurrent low back pain often leads to a Rugby player (front row forwards in particular) giving up the game, and this is usually the player's own decision and not an action based on medical advice. Simply, it is the recurrent pain and disability which forces the player to retire. We have never observed major neurological consequences as a result of Rugby in players with proven lumbar disc prolapse. The player who has sufficient symptoms to warrant lumbar discectomy is advised on general grounds to stop playing.

Disorders of the cervical spine

Because of the importance of cervical spine injuries in Rugby, the detection of pre-existing pathology and the return to playing after recent injury are matters which need to be considered. We see no clear place for mandatory screening programmes, including X-ray examination, but players should be aware that if they have had symptoms referable to the cervical spine then they should seek appropriate advice before taking up the game, especially if they plan to play in the forward pack. Similarly, players should seek clearance from their doctors before commencing full training and play after a recent injury. It should be noted that Rugby players do not wear protective head gear or a full-face helmet as worn in American football and which offer a measure of protection to the cervical spine.

Contraindications to participation

The following are considered absolute contraindications to playing Rugby:

1 Os odontoideum, odontoid hypoplasia and agenesis with C1–C2 instability.

2 Congenital abnormalities of the craniocervical junction with restricted neck motion (Fig. 25.5).

3 Congenital vertebral fusion of two or more vertebrae, with or without limitation of neck motion (Fig. 25.6).

4 A one- or two-level surgical fusion for trauma is similar to its congenital counterpart (*vide supra*). Our data suggests that the adjacent intervertebral discs are subject to increased stress and are prone to early degenerative disorder. Such events may well be hastened by a long football career and the activities in forward play.

5 Proven acute cervical disc prolapse with radicular symptoms.

6 Proven instability at one or more interspaces following injury (with or without a bony component). Whilst instability is far from easy to define in precise terms, the criteria put forward by White *et al.* (1975) provide reasonable guidelines. These authors define clinical instability as more than 3.5 mm of translatory displacement at an interspace on a standard lateral radiograph and when the angle subtended by the end-plates at a given interspace is more than 11° at either adjacent interspace. This is a matter which is far from settled.

Relative contraindications which are open to wide interpretation include the following:

1 Healed facet and lateral mass fractures.

2 Healed non-displaced odontoid fractures.

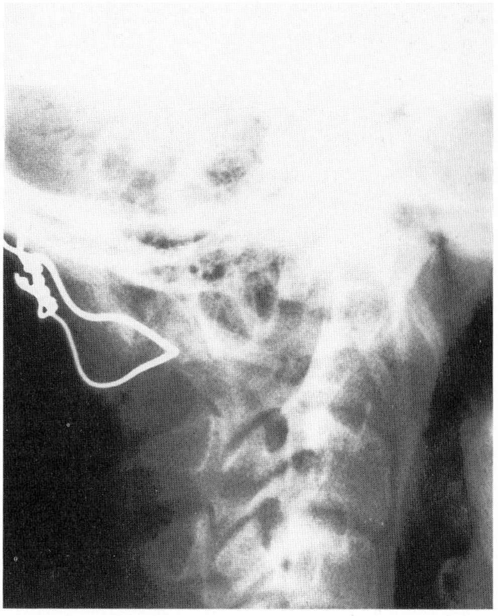

Fig. 25.5 Lateral radiograph of the cervical spine of a 16-year-old male following C2 to the skull fusion. The operation was performed for pain and symptoms suggestive of embarrassment of the midbrain, including dizziness on head movement. A congenital fusion of C1 and C2 is present with hypoplasia of the occipitocervical articulations and absence of the anterior arch of C1. After operation he had only 50% of rotation in both directions. Despite strong advice to the contrary, he returned to Rugby and amateur boxing.

3 Healed Jefferson fractures.

4 Previous wedge compression fractures with no demonstrable instability.

Uncomplicated, healed minor laminar and spinous process fractures do not constitute a contraindication to playing Rugby.

Developmental narrowing of the cervical spine has been linked with transient loss of spinal cord function. Narrowing (stenosis) at one or more cervical levels is considered to be present when the canal to body ratio is 0.8 or less (Torg *et al.*, 1986). However, the relevance of this finding to a given player is far from clear. Players who sustain transient loss of spinal cord function or impairment of such, and in whom complete recovery occurred (as is

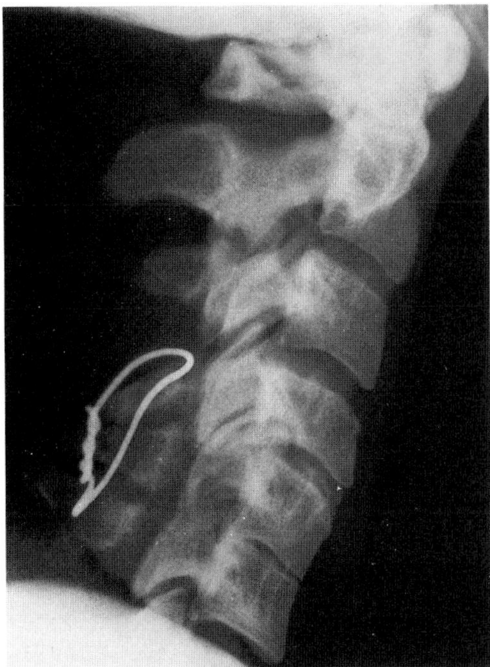

Fig. 25.6 Lateral radiograph of the cervical spine in a 26-year-old male showing a bifacetal dislocation of C4 on C5. There is a congenital fusion of C5 and C6. This patient had an incomplete cord lesion sustained at scrum engagement. Had this anomaly been detected previously, he would have been advised against playing Rugby, let alone in the hooker position.

usual), do not have subsequent loss of spinal cord function even with continued contact activities. Hence, presence of stenosis does not predispose a player to permanent neurological injury. However, it seems prudent to advise players against continuing in the sport if they have been shown to have stenosis and have experienced an episode of cervical cord neurapraxia.

Cervical spine injuries

Almost exclusively, these are unifacetal or bifacetal subluxations or dislocations. They occur primarily at the C4–C5 and C5–C6 levels. Sudden axial loading such as at the moment of scrum engagement, is the principal mechanism of injury (Taylor & Coolican, 1987). Experimental data support this aetiological concept (Bauze & Adran, 1978) and the cervical spine has low intrinsic stability. These injuries occur when a player is caught 'off guard'. Strong cervical musculature does not protect the spine in such instances (Taylor & Coolican, 1988). Burst fractures are rare indeed and have only been seen as a result of impact when a player in full flight at high speed, is tackled.

The alarming increase in spinal cord injuries which occurred in amateur and professional (League) Rugby in the late 1970s and early 1980s led the present authors to undertake the first comprehensive study of spinal cord injuries in Australian footballers. Until then, there were many misconceptions as to how these injuries were produced. It was widely thought, though incorrectly so, that scrum collapse was the major factor in injury production and in Rugby Union some measures had been taken to improve scrum stability. In simple terms, an appropriate study had not been carried out. Pin-pointing risk factors is essential for any effective preventative programme.

There are six spinal cord injury units in Australia and it has long been accepted there that patients with spinal cord injury are best managed in these facilities. Early transfer to the units is standard practice. In a retrospective study covering the years 1960–1985 the authors identified 37 Rugby Union players who had sustained spinal cord injury in play. The following factors were identified with clear implication for some of them being relevant in injury production.

Player positions

Scrum injuries are all but exclusively limited to the front row with the hooker being injured twice as often as the props. The injuries sustained by the tight head props were more severe than in those who played in the loose head position, and further, the latter made more complete recoveries. In approximately 20% of the cases studied, the injured front row forward was in a position not usually held, and moreover, two-thirds of these injuries were in scrummage. Hence, playing out of position in a Rugby scrum is to be avoided, and only those skilled in scrummage technique should play in the front row.

Phase of play

Only 2% of the injured players were hurt in open play. Tackles accounted for 22% and in three-quarters of these cases it was the ball carrier who was injured. Rucks and mauls produced 14% of the injuries and scrums, 62%.

Scrummage

The scrum injuries were analysed in detail. The mechanism of injury for adults and schoolboys is given in Table 25.1. 65% of the injuries occurred at engagement. In 1988, the alterations to law 20 on scrummage, were introduced into Australia by the International Rugby Football Board. In promulgating the rule change, the Board stated that it had been introduced 'to minimize the force of impact on engagement of the front rows, which has been identified as the point of most serious injury in scrums in recent years. This is considered to be a vital safety measure'. However, scrum injuries could all but be eliminated if the two front rows were to pack separately (Fig. 25.7) and then, in succession, the second and back rows added. This move would effectively 'depower' the scrum and avoid the forceful 16-player engagements (Fig. 25.8) which have been shown to be the major cause of spinal cord injury at scrummage. However, in view of the perception of the scrum being a vital part of Rugby, this suggestion has not been welcomed in Australia. In

Table 25.1 Mechanism of scrum injury, Rugby Union and Rugby League 1960–1985.

	Adults		Schoolboys	
Mechanism	Rugby Union	Rugby League	Rugby Union	Rugby League
Engagement	4	2	11	7
Collapse	2	1	2	2
Push after collapse	1	–	2	1
'Popped'	1	–	–	–
Late push after props released bind	–	1	–	–
Totals	8	4	15	10

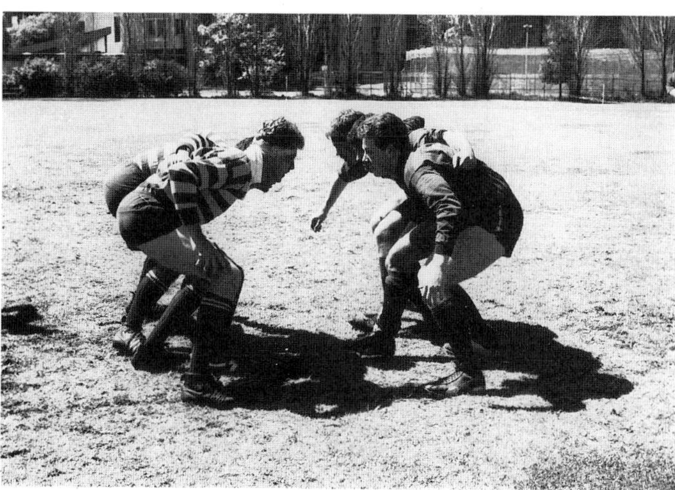

Fig. 25.7 The authors' proposal to prevent spinal cord injury occurring at scrum engagement — a scrum where opposing front rowers engage with the other forwards added in succession.

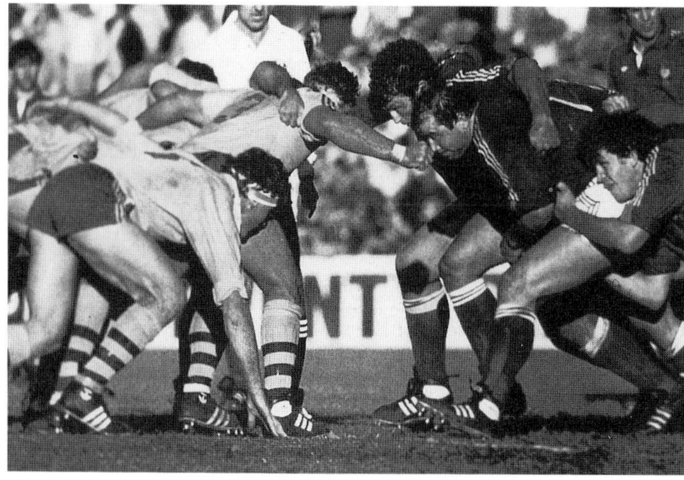

Fig. 25.8 Scrum engagement involves both expression of great force and a resultant high potential for injury.

New Zealand, steps were taken in 1985 to make scrummage safer and, following these rule changes, there was a sharp fall in the incidence of spinal cord injuries. In 1988, Burry and Calcinai reported that on the basis of existing figures nine spinal cord injuries could have occurred in the preceding 3 years, but only one did.

Neck exercise programmes

No evidence has yet been presented to indicate that neck-strengthening exercises prevent these scrum injuries. Rather such programmes, although commendable, have diverted attention from the real issue of the mechanisms of injury as described. It is of note that there were no players under 14 years of age in the series. Until the latter part of the teenage years, players simply do not have enough strength for power scrummage in its various forms. Further, the mobility of the cervical spine in young schoolchildren is, in itself, a protective factor (Taylor & Coolican, 1988).

Management: transport of suspected spinal injuries

It is now well-established that in cervical dislocations with spinal cord injury, the neurological deficit may be increased by injudicious handling during transport from the scene of the accident. In particular, turning the head from one side to the other should be avoided because, with unstable dislocations, this may well further embarrass the injured spinal cord.

If it is suspected that a player who is down has suffered a cervical spine injury, extreme care is needed in removing the player from the field of play. Referees are well-educated on the methods of lifting and stretcher-bearing. Medical officers and voluntary ambulance staff are present at most games in Australia, particularly those with a high profile.

A player who is face down and in whom a cervical spine injury is suspected, should first be returned to the supine position with the cervical spine in neutral. Control of the head and cervical spine is achieved by cradling the skull and neck with the forearms while three other persons gently rotate the torso and lower limbs. A lifting frame (Jordan frame) is ideal for removing the injured player from the field. This frame is based on transverse connecting slats which are passed under the injured player and then connected to a rectangular metal frame. If a frame or similar device is not available, one person (preferably trained in first aid) should hold the head and neck as described above and three persons on each side of the injured player should pass their hands under the torso and lower limbs grasping those of three others opposite to them. This is a safe way for a controlled lift to be made for taking the player off the field.

Medicolegal aspects of Rugby injuries

In view of the financial rewards of professional football, it is easy to understand how a player unable to compete for some months or even an entire season because of an injury inflicted (purposefully or otherwise) by an opponent might resort to legal action. Clearly, the same principal applies to an amateur player who cannot work because of injury so sustained. Now, with video recordings of incidents between teams, this material is later available as evidence, albeit incomplete. Violence is one thing, but in legal terms, inciting to violence with subsequent retaliation is quite another. Hence, visual records of an incident which led to a player apparently intentionally injuring an opponent, is only one aspect of a very complex matter. In the 1991 Rugby League season in Australia, a player successfully sued an opponent for a broken jaw. Unless a watching brief of this evolving situation is maintained, the future of the games is in some jeopardy.

Understandably, administrators of professional Rugby League have become acutely aware of the possibilities associated with these events and they have far-reaching implications for the sport, given the nature of precedents in legal proceedings. Administrators are also anxious to protect players from injuries in games already beset by musculoskeletal injuries. The continued participation by the players is integral to the success of the club, the representative team and the coach. Increased penalties for illegal and foul play are gradually being introduced and these can only be of benefit. They represent, in one form or another, effective preventative measures.

As a result of changes in the laws of the games which are described elsewhere in this chapter, a considerable responsibility now lies with the referees to ensure that the codes are played under existing rules. For example, a referee who did not enforce the rules of scrummage might well be held culpable by a court if a player suffered a spinal cord injury in a scrum engagement where the lines now set down for players under 19 years of age were not followed.

Similar close scrutiny of the actions of team medical officers will doubtlessly come before the courts. The authors consider that the prime concern of the team physician is the continued good health of the players, and any review of the team physician's work should reveal this.

The use of local anaesthetic agents to permit a player to participate in Rugby remains controversial. The International Rugby Board has issued an edict banning the use of local anaesthetic injections to allow a player to participate in Rugby. On the other hand, the International Olympic Committee, the United States Olympic Committee and the National Collegiate Athletic Association (USA) permit the use of such agents to allow an athlete to participate provided:

1 Xylocaine, procaine or carbocaine are used.

2 Adrenaline (epinephrine) or other vasoconstrictive agents are not added.

3 The injection is local or topically applied. Intravenous administration is not permitted.

4 The use is medically justified and the injection specifically permits the athlete to continue the competition without potential risk to health.

5 The medical officials supervising the sporting occasion are notified.

No doubt this issue is a complex one but it can be reduced to a question of medical ethics. The team physician's most important role is to protect the short-term and long-term health of the players under his or her jurisdiction. Occasions often arise where a player suffers an injury which would cause pain, but participation (with the aid of injection) would not prejudice the long-term healing of the injury. Common examples of this set of circumstances include minor fractures of the digits, grade I acromioclavicular joint separations and ligament sprains around the hand. We consider it justifiable to use an injection of local anaesthetic in these situations to allow a player to take to the field, particularly in a touring team when a substitute for the player carrying the minor injury is not readily available. However, repeated injections over several weeks is not in the player's best interests, nor, do we feel, is the injection of local anaesthetic agents into muscle strains or around inflamed tendons.

Conclusion

Rugby remains one of the world's most popular body contact football codes, but participation is not without risk. The likelihood of injury can be diminished by a sensible approach to the game. Aerobic fitness is all important and needs to be approached in a graduated manner after an adequate preparticipation examination.

Various infections can face the football player. The common ones such as impetigo and herpes simplex are easily avoided by an isolation policy. Vaccination against hepatitis B is mandatory and the present restriction of players with bleeding wounds participating in a game is a sound way of minimizing the chance of transfer of the human immunodeficiency virus (HIV).

The attitude of players is paramount in the prevention of injury. There is no doubt that all manner of violence can occur on a Rugby field and a sensible approach by the coach, and a good example set by senior players, will minimize unnecessary roughness which may result in injury.

The rules of Rugby allow minimum equipment to protect the player from injury. Recommended is the use of protective headwear particularly for forwards, as well as a mouth guard and long sleeves to prevent grazes. There is little evidence that neck exercise programmes in any way prevent spinal cord injuries. The International Rugby Board has made several rule changes to minimize the impact on the cervical spine at scrum engagement and it is the authors' impression that these rule changes have reduced the incidence of cervical spine injury since their introduction. Continued review of the data is paramount.

The authors regard congenital cervical spine problems, including fusion and os odontoideum, as absolute contraindications to playing Rugby. Likewise, instability of the spine, any surgical fusion or proven cervical disc prolapse with radicular pain all remain absolute contraindications.

Participation in Rugby remains a great pleasure for thousands worldwide. It is character-building and embodies camaraderie, team spirit and fair play. It is not without risk of serious injury, but simple precautions keep these to a minimum.

References

Anderson, B. & Burke, F.R. (1991) Scientific medical and practical aspects of stretching. *Clin. Sports Med.* **10**, 63–86.

Bauze, R.J. & Adran, G.M. (1978) Experimental production of forward dislocations in the human spine. *J. Bone Joint Surg.* **60B**, 239–45.

Burry, H.C. & Calcinai, C.J. (1988) The need to make Rugby safer. *Br. Med. J.* **296**, 149–50.

Chapman, P.J. (1989) Players attitudes to mouthguards and prevalence of orofacial injuries in the 1987 US Rugby Football Team. *Am. J. Sports Med.* **17**(5), 690–1.

Clancy, W.G., Narechania, R.L., Rosenberg, T.B., Gmeiner, J.G., Wisnefske, B. & Large, T.A. (1981) Anterior and posterior cruciate ligament reconstruction in rhesus monkeys. *J. Bone Joint Surg.* **63A**, 1278–84.

Cox, M.H. (1991) Exercise training programmes and cardiorespiratory adaptation. *Clin. Sports Med.* **10**, 19–32.

Dowden, R.V., Bergfeld, J.A. & Lucas, A.R. (1990) Aspiration of haematomas with liposuction apparatus. *J. Bone Joint Surg.* **72A**, 1534–5.

Maron, B.J., William, M.D., Roberts, C. *et al.* (1980) Sudden death in young athletes. *Circulation* **62**, 218–29.

Myers, P.T. (1980) Injuries presenting from Rugby Union Football. *Med. J. Australia* **2**, 178–80.

Nubile Di, N.A. (1991) Strength training. *Clin. Sport Med.* **10**, 33–62.

Robinson, J.B. (1989) Pre-participation exam — heart disease and sports participation. In J.A. Bergfeld & J.A. Lombardo (eds) *Proceedings of the Cleveland*

Clinic Foundation Sports Medicine Fellow Conferences, Vol. 1, pp. 406–30. Cleveland Clinic Foundation, Cleveland.

Taylor, T.K.F. & Coolican, M.R.J. (1987) Spinal cord injuries in Australian footballers 1960–1985. *Med. J. Australia* **147**, 112–18.

Taylor, T.K.F. & Coolican, M.R.J. (1988) Rugby must be safer: preventive programmes and rule changes. *Med. J. Australia* **149**, 224.

Torg, J.F., Pavlov, H., Genuario, S.E. *et al.* (1986) Neurapraxia of the cervical spinal cord with transient quadriplegia. *J. Bone Joint Surg.* **68A**, 1354–70.

Torre, D., Sampietro, C., Ferraro, G., Zeroli, C. & Speranza, F. (1990) Transmission of HIV-1 infection via sports injury. *Lancet* **335**, 1105.

Virmani, R., Robinowitz, M. & McAllister, H.A. (1982) Non traumatic death in joggers. A series of 30 patients at autopsy *Am. J. Med.* **72**, 874–89.

Waller, B.F. (1985) Exercise related sudden death in young and old conditioned subjects. In N.K. Wenger (ed) *Exercise and the Heart*, pp. 7–73. FA Davis, Philadelphia.

White, A.A., Johnson, R.M. & Punjabi, M.M. (1975) Biomechanical analysis of clinical instability in the cervical spine. *Clin. Orthop.* **109**, 85–96.

White, W.B. & Grant-Kels, J.M. (1984) Transmission of herpes simplex virus type 1 infection in Rugby players. *JAMA* **252**(4), 533–5.

Chapter 26

Injuries in School Physical Education Classes

FRANK J.G. BACKX

In most Western countries, school-aged children get 1 or 2 h of physical education (PE) classes a week. Although it is questionable if this number of PE classes contribute substantially to the physical development and health of a young individual (Jüngst, 1991), it is presumed to be beneficial in the short and long term.

In Europe, sports activities are not explicitly incorporated into the school system as much as in the USA. On the one hand, this has resulted in PE classes being less competitive whereas, on the other hand, club sports activities in Europe have increased, accompanied by more sports injuries (Backx *et al.*, 1989).

PE at school, in which all school-aged children participate, is aimed at an all-round physical conditioning by a diversity of movements. However, the participation in PE classes diminishes as one grows older (Calvert, 1979). Nowadays, not all secondary schools offer PE at every grade level, although this trend seems to be independent of the increased number of injuries during PE classes. Data concerning injuries in PE classes are mostly implemented in large epidemiological studies. Consequently, little specific information is available.

This chapter makes focuses on the epidemiology and prevention of injuries sustained in PE.

Incidence rates

In general, the numbers involved in sports participation and consequently the numbers of sports injuries in young people have increased considerably in the last two decades. Nowadays, it is evident that although the number of schoolchildren is declining in most European countries, there is still an increase in sports accidents (Rummele, 1987). Unfortunately, data concerning injuries incurred in PE lessons are scarce at present. Only a few studies on sports injuries in children and adolescents have outlined the frequency and types of injuries in PE lessons. Analogous to studies performed outside the school system, these studies suffer from a lack of comparability because of:

1 A lack of uniform definitions of sports injury.
2 Limited reliability of collected data.
3 Insufficient information on the population at risk (Tursz & Crost, 1986).
4 Insufficient information on the sports exposure time.

Furthermore, these investigations vary enormously in extent and depth. The scope of data gathered depends strongly on the methods of data acquisition, particularly on the locus of measurement.

Overall in literature, studies on children and adolescents have been rarely population-based; some were registrations in out-patient clinics or in casualty departments (Hammer *et al.*, 1981; Sahlin, 1990) and other registrations were based on reports of PE teachers (Medved & Pavisic-Medved, 1973; Backx *et al.*, 1989). Probably the number of injuries that occur in PE classes is much higher, because many schools do not maintain good records in this area (Calvert, 1979). Another problem arises when pupils themselves have to fill in a registration form. Retrospective studies, in particular, introduce a recall bias resulting in under- or over-recording.

As a result of several differences in the definitions of injury, locus of measurement and content of the PE classes, it is not surprising that incidence rates according to injuries in PE classes vary between 0.75 (Pospiech, 1981) and $11.7 \cdot 100$ schoolchildren^{-1}·year^{-1} (Backx *et al.*, 1991).

Obviously, diagnosis by medical staff or assessment by PE teachers and school-aged children themselves can affect results on sports injuries considerably. It is clear that the medical system is aware of only a small and distorted segment of the total injury problem. In this context, reference is made to the well-known 'iceberg' phenomenon. Therefore, the population approach to injury is preferable, as it allows considerable insight into the rate of occurrence, the causes of injury and the identification of high-risk groups (Walter *et al.*, 1985). The disadvantage of this approach is the registration of a majority of less severe injuries.

The very wide variety of activities undertaken during PE classes is another concern. Because each kind of sports activity has its own characteristics, one has to deal with important differences in sport-specific risk factors.

Risk of injury

It is interesting to compare the risk of getting injured during PE classes with the risk during organized and non-organized sports.

Tursz and Crost (1986) stated that the frequency of accidents in out-of-school sports in France was much higher than for those in PE classes. This is in line with data from a population-based study in The Netherlands (Backx *et al.*, 1989), where sports injuries also were more likely to occur during competition games at sports clubs than in PE classes and non-organized sports activities (Table 26.1) (risk ratio, 1.75). The injuries sustained in organized sports matches led to more absence from PE classes and to medical consultation (risk ratios for both, 1.50). A comparison of year incidence rates per 1000 young athletes in organized sports in relation to physical education is given in Table 26.2.

The finding that the risk of injury in PE classes and non-organized sports is low relative to the number of exposure hours can be explained mainly by the lower intensity of the

Table 26.1 Observed versus expected* numbers of injuries (risk ratios) according to the nature of sports participation. From Backx *et al.* (1989).

		Risk ratio			
			Injuries followed by non-attendance of		
Nature of sport	No. of school children	All injuries	PE classes	School	Injuries with medical consultation
PE	7468	0.63	0.97	1.05	0.66
Club training†	6458	1.04	0.99	0.76	1.05
Club match†	4439	1.75	1.50	1.11	1.50
Non-organized sports	4762	0.81	0.95	1.14	1.01
Total	23127	1	1	1	1

* Expected numbers are based on the injury rate, i.e. all injuries occurred in the total study population.
† Pupils with two or three memberships respectively are counted for two or three persons, respectively.
PE, physical education.

Table 26.2 Incidence rates in organized sports* and physical education (per 1000 young athletes a year). From Backx *et al.* (1991).

Basketball	998
Handball	814
Korfball	809
Volleyball	548
Field hockey	528
Soccer	492
Club gymnastics	399
Martial arts	388
Baseball	387
Track and field	295
Badminton	204
Table tennis	193
Tennis	147
Horse-riding	134
Swimming	123
Physical education	117
Ice skating	79
Ballet	73
Dance	0

* Only types of sport with more than 15 participants.

physical exertion involved. Additionally, activities during PE lessons are mostly adapted to the abilities of the pupils (Rummele, 1987), which is in contrast to the common management of team sports.

PE lessons containing activities like gymnastics (specifically trampolining) and ball games (especially basketball) provoked most damage (Zaricznyj *et al.*, 1980; Hammer *et al.*, 1981). Rummele (1987) registered the number of sports accidents occurring in German schools. He found that three areas (ball games, apparatus gymnastics and athletics) accounted for 88% of all sports accidents. In comparison with the preceding 10 years, accidents from ball games had increased tremendously while the accidents arising from gymnastics and track and field sports had remained relatively constant. This trend has also been seen in other countries (Backx *et al.*, 1991).

Location of injury

Comparisons to medically treated home, school and road accidents reveals that medically treated sports accidents have the highest rate (43%) of upper limb injuries (Tursz & Crost, 1986). Naturally, the location of the injuries on the body depends substantially on the activities taught in the PE classes.

Figure 26.1 summarizes the reported injuries by body area. The distribution of injuries related to body area and to category of sports activity revealed that PE classes gave rise to relatively more upper extremity injuries (Backx *et al.*, 1991).

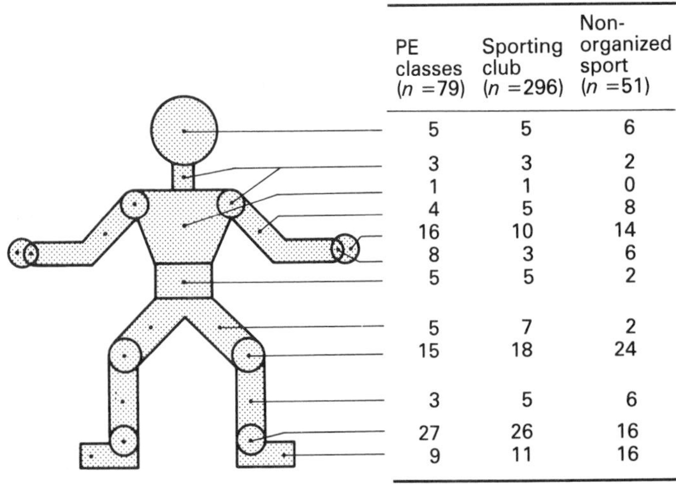

PE classes (*n* =79)	Sporting club (*n* =296)	Non-organized sport (*n* =51)
5	5	6
3	3	2
1	1	0
4	5	8
16	10	14
8	3	6
5	5	2
5	7	2
15	18	24
3	5	6
27	26	16
9	11	16

Fig. 26.1 Correlation (in %) of sports activity category and anatomical region of injury (399 injuries involving 426 anatomical regions). From Backx *et al.* (1991).

Based on the popularity of ball games in schools, the ball is considered to be an important factor in sustaining a finger injury. Finger injuries are dominant amongst younger children, while ankle joint injuries occur more in older pupils (Rummele, 1987). This is in accordance with an injury registration system in an Austrian hospital in which hand and finger injuries were most frequently treated (Schmidt & Höllwarth, 1989).

Type of injury

The distribution of injury types in relation to PE classes shows no uniform pattern, which is caused primarily by the difference in injury definition, the locus of measurement and type of activity.

In studies using a broad injury definition, the fracture rate is low and most injuries are light contusions and sprains (Backx *et al.*, 1989). Measurements in hospital have shown a rather different picture. Depending on the type of sport, the fracture rate varies between 15 and 60% of the acute sports traumas (Schmidt & Höllwarth, 1989; Sahlin, 1990).

Significantly more fractures or dislocations occurred in PE classes in comparison with out-of-school sports. Nearly all of these fractures were located at the upper limb. Also sprains, especially involving the ankle, often occur although less frequently than during organized sports (Backx *et al.*, 1991).

Besides acute macrotrauma, the importance of microtrauma and overuse injuries in children is still growing. The latter type of injury will not be described in this context, because the direct influence of PE classes on the origin of overuse injuries is still unknown. Furthermore, it is also important to investigate the influence of biological growth on injury rates.

Severity of injuries

It is obvious that a high incidence rate of sports injuries is no indicator of injury severity. Therefore, van Mechelen *et al.* (1987) have distinguished six factors of importance in describing the severity of injuries.

Nature of sports injury

Very serious sports accidents in young people, e.g. brain or spinal cord damage or lesions of the heart, leading to invalidity or death, are exceptional (Tursz & Crost, 1986). This corresponds with Nathorst Westfelt (1982) who registered only a few injuries, ranging from life-threatening to fatal, according to the abbreviated injury scale (AIS) severity codes 4, 5 and 6, which is commonly used in traffic accidents. Most of the injuries sustained in PE classes can be categorized as AIS 1 and 2. Sprains were the most common type of injury and the ankle was the most injured body area (Austin *et al.*, 1980).

Nature and duration of treatment

From an epidemiological point of view, only 25% of all injuries registered called for medical attention from a general practitioner or a medical specialist. Pupils who were injured in PE classes had to consult a doctor more frequently compared with other sports activities (Backx *et al.*, 1991).

Watson (1986) observed that 13% of injured Irish schoolchildren in his study spent 1 or more days in a hospital. In two other studies concerning macrotrauma requiring medical care, the hospitalization rate was 10–11%. There is no consensus concerning to the influence of age and gender on hospital admission (Zaricznyj *et al.*, 1980; Tursz & Crost, 1986).

The type and duration of treatment in the case of injuries in school-aged children has not been analysed thoroughly, although there are indications that the claim on health-care professionals seems to be less than in adults.

Time lost from sport

The actual number of days lost until the athlete returns to sports activity is often reported as a measure of injury severity (Noyes *et al.*, 1988). Although van Mechelen *et al.* (1987) stated that the length of sports absenteeism gives the most precise indication of the consequences of a sports injury to an athlete, it is questionable with regard to school-aged children. Bias can easily develop, induced by factors such as an individual's pain tolerance, type of treatment, parents and coach. The time-loss definition of injury is not useful in studies including non-organized sports.

Work absenteeism

In the case of youngsters, injury severity in terms of work absenteeism must be transformed into school absenteeism. Defining the severity of an injury by the amount of time lost in school is highly subjective. It is a useful though unreliable parameter.

In general, most injuries were neither severe nor long-lasting and resulted in little loss of time from PE classes or school. Pupils who were injured in PE classes had more time lost from PE and total schooldays in comparison with those injured in club sports (Backx *et al.*, 1991).

Permanent damage

Until this moment there was no solid data available about the residual and long-term effects of injuries sustained in PE lessons. Zaricznyj *et al.* (1980) recorded in schoolchildren participating in sports and PE that 1.2% of the injuries (such as a compression fracture of the spine or ruptured spleen) became permanent. Actually, it is rather difficult to predict correctly whether or not effects will be permanent.

Costs

Severity in terms of costs have to be included in the direct costs resulting from (para)medical treatment and also the indirect social costs (i.e. sick leave) to the injured pupil and his or her family and school (Watson, 1986). The financial costs stemming from sports injuries in youth are not explored as a single category. The calculations known are roughly derived from figures concerning adults.

Aetiology of injuries

Usually the most important factors affecting sports injuries are divided in two main categories: (i) internal; and (ii) external factors. It is clear that injuries are mostly caused by a combination of factors (van Mechelen *et al.*, 1987). Generally, it seems that internal factors, such as physical build, physical fitness, skills and joint stability are much more important than external factors such as the referee, the opponent or sports material.

It is noticeable that specific information on aetiology and, consequently, injury prevention concerning school-aged children is rarely available. Most of the relevant investigations do mention the causes, primarily informed by the subject or reconstructed by the coach or physician. For example, retrospective data from a population-based study revealed that most reported causes of sports injuries were falling/stumbling (24%), mis-step/twist (22%) and kick/push (18%) induced by the injured person rather than by other pupils (Backx *et al.*, 1991). It is important that in the near future more observational studies are carried out; the findings can then be transferred into preventive measures.

Prevention of injuries

If the benefits of life-long sports participation, based on the potential benefits on health, are to be realized, injury prevention is a must. One of the strategies in the battle against injuries is aimed at behaviour modification of the participants in sports (Kok & Bouter, 1990). Health education as a tool in realizing behavioural change can be implemented in school curricula and, consequently, given by well-educated teachers in PE or biology (Backx, 1991).

The need for the PE teacher to become involved in the field of sports injury prevention may vary from one country to another, depending on the number of other professional groups working in the same area (Table 26.3). The PE teacher can help educate school-aged children in practical and theoretical aspects of injury prevention. This kind of information will also be helpful in out-of-school sports activities (Hess, 1987). Although the effects of health education in this specific area still have to be proven, there are strong indications that in the short term it can be beneficial in reducing the number of sports injuries. The effects in the long run are only speculative.

In The Netherlands, a controlled experimental study has been performed in which special lessons in PE and biology were given in injury prevention. The practical topics instructed in PE classes included warming up, stretching exercises, cooling down, exercises for ankle stabilization and general coordination, and techniques of correct falling. Those practical items were supported by theoretical information given by teachers in biology. Additional education took place concerning adequate sporting shoes, protective materials and first aid in sports. Because the results of this health education programme were very encouraging, it seems to be worthwhile to start with the implementation of this kind of health education into school curricula on a more regular basis (Backx, 1991). It will also be necessary to set up postacademic courses for the teachers in order to optimize their role in the prevention of sports injuries.

Table 26.3 The involvement of the physical education teacher depends on the following aspects. From Watson (1987).

Supervision of qualified coaches
Screening of physical defects
Medical supervision
Qualification in sports medicine and injury prevention
Public awareness

References

Austin, G.J., Rogers, K.D. & Reese, G. (1980) Injuries in high school physical education classes. *Am. J. Dis. Child.* **134**, 456–8.

Backx, F.J.G. (1991) *Sports injuries in youth; etiology and prevention.* Thesis, Janus Jongbloed Research Center on Sports and Health, Utrecht, The Netherlands.

Backx, F.J.G., Beijer, H.J.M., Bol, E. & Erich, W.B.M. (1991) Injuries in high-risk persons and high-risk sports. A longitudinal study of 1,818 school children. *Am. J. Sports Med.* **19**, 124–30.

Backx, F.J.G., Erich, W.B.M., Kemper, A.B.A. & Verbeek, A.L.M. (1989) Sports injuries in school-aged children; an epidemiologic study. *Am. J. Sports Med.* **17**, 234–40.

Calvert Jr, R. (1979) *Athletic injuries and deaths in secondary schools and Colleges, 1975–1976.* National Center for Education Statistics, Washington.

Hammer, A., Schwartzbach, A.L. & Paulev, P.E. (1981) Children injured during physical education lessons. *J. Sports Med.* **21**, 423–31.

Hess, H. (1987) Präventivmassnahmen im Breitenssport und Leistungssport aus orthopädischer Sicht (Preventive orthopaedic measures in recreational and competitive sport). *Off. Gesundh. Wes.* **49**, 496–500.

Jüngst, B.K. (1991) Schulsport; Traume und Wirklichkeit (School sports; myths and reality). *Deut. Z. Sportmed.* **42**, 87.

Kok, G.J. & Bouter, L.M. (1990) On the importance of planned health education. Prevention of ski injury as an example. *Am. J. Sports Med.* **18**, 600–5.

Mechelen, W. van, Hlobil H. & Kemper, H.C.G. (1987) *How can sports injuries be prevented?* National Institute for Sports Health Care, Oosterbeek, The Netherlands.

Medved, R. & Pavisic-Medved, V. (1973) Causes of injuries during the practical classes on physical education in schools. *J. Sports Med. Phys. Fitness* **13**, 32–41.

Nathorst Westfelt, J.A.R. (1982) Environmental factors in childhood accidents. A prospective study in Götenborg, Sweden. *Acta Paediatr. Scand.* **291**(Suppl.), 6–61.

Noyes, F.R., Lindenfeld, T.N. & Marshall, M.T. (1988) What determines an athletic injury? Who determines an injury? *Am. J. Sports Med.* **16**(Suppl. 1), 65–9.

Pospiech, R. (1981) Analyze von 1000 Unfällen beim Schulsport (Analysis of 1000 accidents in school sports). *Med. Sport* **21**, 78–82.

Rummele, E. (1987) Sports injuries in the Federal Republic of Germany, Part two. In C.R. van der Togt, A.B.A. Kemper & M. Koornneef (eds) *Council of Europe: Sport for All; Sports Injuries and their Prevention*, pp. 37–49. Proceedings of the 2nd meeting, Oosterbeek. National Institute for Sports Health Care, The Netherlands.

Sahlin, Y. (1990) Sport accidents in childhood. *Br. J. Sports Med.* **24**, 40–4.

Schmidt, B. & Höllwarth, M.E. (1989) Sportunfälle im Kindes und Jugendalter (Sports accidents in children and adolescents). *Z Kinderchir.* **44**, 357–62.

Stanitski, C.L. (1989) Common injuries in preadolescent and adolescent athletes; recommendations for prevention. *Sports Med.* **6**, 32–41.

Tursz, A. & Crost, M. (1986) Sports-related injuries in children. A study of their characteristics, frequency and severity, with comparison to other types of accidental injuries. *Am. J. Sports Med.* **14**, 294–9.

Walter, S.D., Sutton, J.R., McIntosh, J.M. *et al.* (1985) The aetiology of sports injuries: a review of methodologies. *Sports Med.* **2**, 47–58.

Watson, A.W.S. (1986) *Sports Injuries in Irish Second-level Schools During the School Years 1984–1985*. Department of Education, Dublin.

Watson, A.W.S. (1987) The role of the physical educator in the prevention of sports injuries. In C.R. van der Togt, A.B.A. Kemper & M. Koornneef (eds) *Council of Europe: Sport for All; Sports Injuries and their Prevention.* Proceedings of the 2nd meeting, Oosterbeek. National Institute for Sports Health Care, The Netherlands.

Zaricznyj, B., Shattuck, L.J.M., Mast, T.A., Robertson, R.V. & D'Elia, G. (1980) Sports-related injuries in school-aged children. *Am. J. Sports Med.* **8**, 318–24.

Part 2b

Individual Sports

Chapter 27

Injuries in Running

WILLEM VAN MECHELEN

The popularity of running as a form of exercise and recreation has grown rapidly since the 1970s, first in North America and later, from the beginning of the 1980s, in Europe. One of the reasons for this worldwide trend is the low cost involved: all that is needed is a tracksuit and a pair of running shoes. Reasons for jogging are health/fitness, pleasure/relaxation and competition/personal performance (Clough *et al.*, 1989; Ooijendijk & Van Agt, 1990). More and more people are taking part in such major events as the New York, Los Angeles, Amsterdam or London marathon. In Switzerland, the number of regular joggers has increased 100% over the period between 1978 and 1984, constituting 8% of the total population (Marti *et al.*, 1988). According to Walter *et al.* (1989) the number of Canadians jogging or running doubled from 15% in 1976 to 31% in 1983. Jacobs and Berson (1986) state that the USA counts 30 million runners of all levels, of whom 10 million run regularly and about 800 000 to 1 million enter races. In The Netherlands in 1978, 8% of the Dutch adult population was engaged in running, while in 1984 this number had increased to 17% (Manders & Kropman, 1982, 1987). This 1984 figure meets the results of a telephone survey covering 1000 respondents which was carried out between mid-July and mid-August 1985 by the Amsterdam Market Research Institute Inter/View and which indicated that there are around 2 450 000 joggers in The Netherlands (on a total population of around 14 million). Of this total, around 2 million run at least once a week. It would thus appear that running is the major national sport in The Netherlands.

Running is widely considered to have a preventive effect on cardiovascular problems (Hartung, 1980; Eichner, 1983; Powell & Paffenbarger, 1985). There are benefits associated with the three main risk factors in cardiovascular disease, namely obesity, hypertension and smoking (Koplan *et al.*, 1982; Eichner, 1983): as a group runners smoke less, have a lower percentage of body fat and are less likely to have high blood pressure.

Running is not only a sport in its own right but is also a major element in many other sporting activities, and as a result the typical injuries associated with running are also common in other sports.

Most runners and joggers are not members of any sports association and thus do not appear in any membership records. The fact that their activity does not take place in any organized framework notwithstanding, many of those concerned practice their sport intensively, devoting several hours a week to it. Distances of over 90 km·week^{-1} are far from exceptional (Hølmich *et al.*, 1989).

The purpose of this chapter is to describe preventive measures with respect to running injuries. Prescribing prevention can only be done on the basis of knowledge of the aetiology of running injuries. Much of the existing information is presented as a result of the analysis of case series or common sense. As explained

Table 27.1 Person incidence rates (%) of running injuries based on studies with an incidence time period of 1 year.

Reference	Injury definition (all self-reported)	Numbers; F/M; age (years)	Runners	Design	Yearly incidence rate (%)*
Koplan *et al.*, 1982	Training reduction, medical treatment, medication	693; M; average age 33 730; F; average age 29	Recreative entrants road race >9.5 km·week^{-1}	Retrospective cohort questionnaire	All injuries M, 37% F, 38% Medical consultation: M, 13% F, 17%
Blair *et al.*, 1987	Training reduction >7 days	438; M & F; average age 44	Members fitness club, average 40 km·week^{-1}	Retrospective cohort questionnaire	24%
Lysholm & Wiklander, 1987	Training reduction >7 days	19 sprinters; M & F; average age 21; 13 middle-distance runners; M & F; average age 19; 28 long-distance runners; M & F; average age 35	Competitive athletes	Prospective cohort with: log-analysis, medical injury evaluation, baseline questionnaire	Sprinters, 68% Middle-distance, 77% Long distance, 57%
Ijzerman & van Galen, 1987	Training reduction, medical treatment	757, M; 50, F; age 15–70	Half and full marathon runners average 70 km·week^{-1}	Retrospective cohort questionnaire	56% training reduction 38% medically treated
Marti *et al.*, 1988	Training reduction	4335; M; age 17–64	Entrants 16-km road race average 24 km·week^{-1}	Retrospective cohort questionnaire	45.8%
Hølmich *et al.*, 1989	Training stop	1310; M; average age 34	Marathon entrants 75% of participants training more than 30 km·week^{-1}	Retrospective cohort questionnaire	31% training stop

Clough *et al.*, 1989	Subjective (self-defined)	489 marathon finishers; M; average age 33; 440 marathon drop outs; M; average age 31	Marathon finishers; average 1959 km·year^{-1}; 440 marathon drop outs; average 1212 km·year^{-1}	Retrospective cohort questionnaire	41% marathon finishers 49% marathon drop outs
Macera *et al.*, 1989	Training reduction, medical treatment, medication	485; M; average age 42 98; F; average age 36	Entrants to road races; M, average 39 km·week^{-1}; F, average 37 km·week^{-1}	Prospective cohort with baseline questionnaire, log-analysis	M, 52% (48% retrospective) F, 49% (49% retrospective)
Walter *et al.*, 1989	Training reduction, medical treatment, medication	985; M; age 14–50+ 303; F; age 14–50+	Entrants to road races; M, average 49 km·week^{-1}; F, average 35 km·week^{-1}	Prospective cohort with baseline questionnaire, 4, 8, 12-month telephone questionnaire, baseline check-up LE	M, 49% F, 46% (49% retrospective whole population)
Ooijendijk & Van Agt, 1990	Training reduction, medical treatment	256, M; 60, F; average age 39	Entrants to road races average 30 km·week^{-1}	Retrospective cohort questionnaire	27% training reduction 24% medical treated

* Person incidence rates.
F, female; LE, lower extremity; M, male.

by Walter *et al.* (1985) the methodology of case series, however, does not allow any conclusions on the causes of running injuries. However, epidemiological studies may allow these kind of conclusions. Therefore this review of the literature is predominantly based on the outcome of epidemiological studies.

Incidence of running injuries

There is no unanimity in the literature regarding the incidence of running injuries. Different incidence figures are presented: person incidence rates (number of injured runners·100 runners^{-1}), injury incidence rates (number of injuries·100 runners^{-1}), and incidence per exposure (number of injuries·1000 h^{-1} of running). Differences in definitions, in runner characteristics and in research design may influence injury incidence, as well as differences in the time period of data collection. This should be kept in mind when the incidences of various studies on running injuries are compared.

In Table 27.1, yearly incidence rates are presented from studies with a data collection time period of 1 year. All the studies referred to in this table are cohort studies, either prospective or retrospective. The incidence rate varies from 24 to 77%. If one restricts oneself only to studies in which samples of more than 500 subjects were used the yearly incidence rate varies from 37 to 56%.

One can speculate about the fact that studies, based on a time period of data collection not equivalent to a full year, do not provide representative yearly incidence rates since running participation does not necessarily need to be of the same intensity during 12 months of the year. For instance Lysholm and Wiklander (1987) registered a significantly higher incidence rate during spring and summer and Walter *et al.* (1989) calculated that running whole year round was significantly related to a higher incidence rate. In contrast, Ijzerman and van Galen (1987) found that the time of year did not influence the chance of sustaining a running injury. It was found by van Galen and Diederiks (1990) that 85% of the runners in their study were running whole year round.

In Table 27.2, incidence rates are presented from four studies with a time period of data collection not equivalent to 1 year. Two of these studies are cohort studies with incidence rates varying from 17.5 to 46.5%. The other two studies concern trials in which the running load was programmed by the study and therefore, as will be discussed later, largely influenced by the study design. The incidence rates in these two studies varied from 0 to 67%.

With all limitations in mind to summarize the data as presented in Tables 27.1 and 27.2 it seems that for the 'average' recreational runner, who is steadily training and who participates in a long-distance run every now and then, the overall yearly incidence rate for running injuries is about 37–56%. Depending on the specificity of the group of runners concerned (competitive athletes, boys and girls) and on different circumstances these rates may vary.

In Table 27.3, incidences for running injuries expressed per 1000 h of running are presented. The studies of van Galen & Diederiks (1990) and van Mechelen (1992) are more or less comparable with regard to running characteristics and present incidences varying from 3.6 to 5.5 injuries·1000 h^{-1} of running. For competitive athletes, this incidence figure varies from 2.5 to 5.8 injuries·1000 h^{-1} of running depending on the specialization of the athlete. In the study of Bovens *et al.* (1989), in which running performance was largely inflicted by the study itself, the incidence varied from 12.1 to 7 injuries·1000 h^{-1} running depending on the weekly running distance. This study also clearly demonstrated that with increasing exposure the incidence·1000 h^{-1} of running decreases, whereas the incidence rate (%) increases as a result of the cumulative effect of increased exposure (compare Bovens *et al.* in Tables 27.2 and 27.3). This phenomenon was also demonstrated by Marti *et al.* (1988).

If it comes to the risk of running compared to that of other sports, it is known from Switzerland that running injuries are 2–2.5 times less

Table 27.2 Incidence rates (%) of running injuries based on studies with an incidence time period other than 1 year.

Reference	Injury definition (all self-reported)	Numbers; F/M; age (years)	Runners	Design, time period	Incidence rate (%)
Pollock *et al.*, 1977*	Training stop >7 days	2 groups of male inmates: 87 M, 70 M; age 20–35	3 times·week^{-1} (15, 30 or 45 min) 30 min (1, 3 or 5 times·week^{-1})	Prospective randomized trial with baseline physiological assessment, time period: 20 weeks	22%, 24%, 54% 0%, 12%, 39%
Jacobs & Berson, 1986†	Training reduction, training stop	355; M; average age 34 96; F; average age 32	Entrants to a 10-km race, M & F, average 61 km·week^{-1}	Retrospective cohort questionnaire, time period: 2 years	46.5%
Watson & DiMartino, 1987†	Training ≥ two sessions, training reduction, missed meet	257 boys & girls; average age 16	Members of high school track teams, average training 10 h·week^{-1}	Prospective cohort with medical evaluation of injury, registration of training and performance, time period: 1 season (77 days)	17.5%
Bovens *et al.*, 1989†	Training reduction	58; M; average age 35 15; F; average age 34	Recreative runners training to compete in a marathon average km·week^{-1}: 24, 35, 44 (training phase dependent)	Prospective trial with log analysis, baseline medical check-up, supervised training, time period: 18 months	58%, 60%, 67% depending on training phase

* Injury incidence rates.
† Person incidence rates.
F, female; M, male.

Table 27.3 Incidence of running injuries·1000 h^{-1} of running (time period as indicated).

Reference	Injury definition (all self-reported)	Numbers; F/M; age (years)	Runners	Design, time period	Incidence·1000 h^{-1} of running
Lysholm & Wiklander, 1987	Training reduction >7 days	19 sprinters; M & F; average age 21; 13 middle-distance runners; M & F; average age 19; 28 long distance runners; M & F; average age 35	Competitive athletes	Prospective cohort with log-analysis, medical injury evaluation, baseline questionnaire	Sprinters 5.8 Middle-distance 5.6 Long-distance 2.5
Bovens *et al.*, 1989	Training reduction	58; M; average age 35 15; F; average age 34	Recreative runners training to compete in a marathon average km·week^{-1}: 24, 35, 44 (training phase dependent)	Prospective trial with log-analysis, baseline medical check-up, supervised training, time period: 18 months	12.1, 10, 7 depending on training phase
Van Galen & Diederiks, 1990	Any self-defined injury in relation to sports, medical treatment	257, M; 139, F; average age 33 (drawn from a random population sample of 66 804 persons)	Recreational joggers, average 2.9 h·week^{-1}	Retrospective population study: questionnaire by telephone, time period: 4 weeks	3.6 (all injuries) 1.6 (medically treated)
Van Mechelen, 1992	Training stop, medical treatment, work time loss, pain or stiffness >10 days	421 M split into two groups: 210 experimental subjects, 211 control subjects; average age both groups 40	Recreational runners: average distance: 25 km·week^{-1} average frequency: 2.7 times·week^{-1} (runners matched for age, mileage and knowledge on prevention of injuries)	Prospective intervention trial on effect of warm-up, cool-down and stretch, log-analysis, medical injury evaluation, baseline questionnaire, time period: 16 weeks	All injuries: control group 4.9 experimental group 5.5

F, female; M, male.

frequent than injuries from all other sports and about six times less frequent than ski injuries (Marti *et al.*, 1988). In The Netherlands in the van Galen and Diederiks (1990) study the overall Dutch sports injury incidence was estimated to be 3.3 injuries·1000 h^{-1} of sports, running/jogging, jointly with squash and motor sports, ranking 14th with an incidence of 3.6 (95% confidence limits (CL); 2.7–4.8) injuries·1000 h^{-1}.

Severity of running injuries

Medical diagnosis

Only three of the studies mentioned in Tables 27.1–27.3, give more or less detailed information on the medical diagnosis of the registered injuries (Table 27.4). In competitive athletes, tendinitis was the most frequent registered injury (Lysholm & Wiklander, 1987), in boys and girls periostitis/stress fracture (Watson & DiMartino, 1987) and in an 'average' jogging population strain and tendinitis (Marti *et al.*, 1988).

In order to gain more insight into the most frequent diagnosis of medically treated running injuries it is useful to mention the results of Clement *et al.* (1981), who carried out a retrospective clinical survey of 1650 runners, 987 men and 663 women. These runners had sought medical help in connection with a running injury over a 2-year period. In all 1819 injuries had been sustained; the frequency of the 10 commonest diagnosis of injury — accounting between them for 69% of all injuries — is shown in Table 27.5. In the study of Clement *et al.* (1981) all injuries involved the knee, the leg or the foot. Most of the running injuries are associated with overuse (Mirkin, 1975; Clement *et al.*, 1981; Eggold, 1981; Andrews, 1983; Dressendorfer & Wade, 1983; Lehman, 1984; Stanish, 1984) — understandably, since running involves the constant repetition of the same movements. Marti *et al.* (1988), Ooijendijk and Van Agt (1990) and van Mechelen (1992) found in their respective studies about 75% of all injuries to be of an overuse nature, whereas Ijzerman and van Galen (1987) registered 54% overuse injuries (Table 27.6).

Due to the overuse character of running injuries these injuries tend to recur (Walter *et al.*, 1989). Data from the epidemiological studies on the recurrence of injuries however are inconsistent, with figures varying from 21 to 70% (Table 27.7). This large range is probably strongly affected by differences in the definition of a recurrent injury and by differences in research methodology. Walter *et al.* (1989) also mentioned that with respect to the recurrence of injuries there are major differences with respect to the affected part of the body: rates of

Table 27.4 Distribution of running injuries according to medical diagnosis (%).

	Lysholm & Wiklander, 1987 (n = 55)	Watson & DiMartino, 1987 (n = 41)	Marti *et al.*, 1988 (n = 877)
Tendinitis	33	10	17
Inflammation (other than tendinitis)	4	15	—
Strain	15	15	18
Chondromalacia	11	5	—
Periostitis/stress fracture	15	22	12
Sprain	11	17	14
Other	9	17	39

Table 27.5 Frequency of the 10 commonest medically treated injuries sustained by 987 male and 663 women runners. After Clement *et al.* (1981).

	Males		Females		Total	
	%	*n*	%	*n*	%	*n*
Patellar pain syndrome*	24.3	262	27.9	206	25.8	468
Tibial stress syndrome†	10.7	115	16.8	124	13.2	239
Inflammation Achilles tendon	7.9	85	3.2	24	6.0	109
Fasciitis plantaris‡	5.3	57	3.9	28	4.7	85
Inflammation patellar tendon	5.6	60	2.8	21	4.5	81
Iliotibial friction syndrome§	4.6	50	3.8	28	4.3	78
Metatarsal stress syndrome	3.3	36	3.0	22	3.2	58
Tibial stress fracture	2.4	26	2.8	21	2.6	47
Tendinitis m. tibialis posterior	1.9	21	3.2	14	2.5	45
Tendinitis m. peroneus	2.0	22	1.6	12	1.9	34
Total	68.0	735	69.0	510	68.7	1244

* Patellar pain syndrome (chondromalacia patellae) is a disorder of the kneecap.
† Tibial stress syndrome (shin splints) is caused by strain on the points of attachment of the foot flexors.
‡ Fasciitis plantaris is a disorder of the sole of the foot.
§ Iliotibial friction syndrome is pain on the outer side of the knee.

Table 27.6 Distribution of overuse and acute running injuries (%).

	Ijzerman & van Galen, 1987 (n = 644)	Marti *et al.*, 1988 (n = 877)	Ooijendijk & Van Agt, 1990 (n = 64)	Van Mechelen *et al.*, 1991 (n = 44)
Overuse injuries	54	73	73	75
Acute injuries	46	27	27	25

Table 27.7 Distribution of recurrent and new running injuries (%).

	Marti *et al.*, 1988 (n = 1994)	Macera *et al.*, 1989 (n = 300)	Walter *et al.*, 1989 (n = 620)	Van Mechelen *et al.*, 1991 (n = 44)
Recurrent injury	21	70	46	30
New injury	79	30	54	70

new injuries ranged from 29% for back injuries to 73% for shin injuries.

Localization of injury

Most of the authors of the cited epidemiological studies have mentioned an injury distribution by part of the body affected. In Table 27.8 a summary of these results is given. In the majority of the studies the knee is the most frequently injured part of the body: around 25% of all injuries. In general one can say that running injuries are located from the knee downwards in about 70–80% of all injuries.

Table 27.8 Anatomical distribution of running injuries (%).

	Jacobs & Berson, 1986 (n = 210)	Blair & Kohl, 1987 (n = 105)	Ijzerman & Van Galen, 1987* (n = 644)	Lysholm & Wiklander, 1987 (n = 55)	Watson & DiMartino, 1987 (n = 41)	Marti *et al.*, 1988† (n = 877)	Bovens *et al.*, 1989‡ (n = 34)	Macera *et al.*, 1989 (n = 300)	Walter *et al.*, 1989† (n = 747)	Ooijendijk & Van Agt, 1990 (n = 64)	Van Mechelen, 1992 (n = 44)
Knee	21	31	20	13	20	28	25	24	27	42	25
Foot	5	15	8	13	2	13	6	22	16	8	14
Ankle	12	15	9	11	17	15	12	—	15	20	2
Lower leg (incl. Achilles tendon)	12	11	31	18	2	24	32	—	6	16	21
Shin	10	11	—	15	20	6	—	—	6	—	7
Upper leg	7	10	13	18	15	5	6	—	7	3	14
Back	—	5	6	5	10	3	5	—	11	8	2
Hip/pelvis/ groin	—	2	6	7	3	6	11	—	9	3	14
Other	33	—	6	—	11	—	3	64	4	—	—

* Only injuries leading to training reduction.
† Only injuries resulting in full training stop.
‡ Only medically treated injuries.

Social consequences of running injuries

The severity of sports injuries can also be judged by its social consequences, e.g. sporting time lost, medical treatment and/or absence from work. Table 27.9 gives a summary of social consequences of running injuries as assessed in 10 epidemiological studies.

From these studies it can be concluded that running injuries lead to a reduction of training or training stop in about 30–90% of all injuries, about 20–70% of all injuries lead to medical consultation or medical treatment and 0–5% result in absence from work. Again it should be mentioned that these figures must be judged with precaution, bearing in mind the particularities of the studies involved.

Marti *et al.* (1988) gave the most extensive description in this respect: 44% of 1994 running injuries resulted in a full training stop with an average duration of 4.8 weeks, 31% lead to medical consultation with an average number of 3.8 consultations and 5% to absence from work with an average duration of 10.1 days. Clough *et al.* (1989) found significant differences between marathon finishers and drop outs with respect to the length of full training stop: 35% of all injured marathon finishers suffered from a training stop lasting 4 weeks or more opposed to 65% of all injured marathon drop outs. Hølmich *et al.* (1989) found in a retrospective cohort study (time period of data collection: 1 year) that the percentage of injured runners suffering a full training stop as a result of a running injury increased with the distance covered per week: 23% of all runners running

Table 27.9 Social consequences of running injuries.

Reference	Social consequences of injury
Koplan *et al.*, 1982 (n = 256 M, n = 277 F)	Medical consultation M, 13%; F, 17%
Jacobs & Berson, 1986 (n = 210)	66% full training stop, 70% medical consultation
Ijzerman & van Galen, 1987 (n = 807)	56% training reduction, 38% medical treatment
Watson & Di Martino, 1987 (n = 41)	27% medical consultation
Marti *et al.*, 1988 (n = 1994)	44% full training stop (av. duration: 4.8 weeks), 31% medical consultation (av. no. 3.8), 5% absence from work (av. no. of days 10.1)
Bovens *et al.*, 1989 (n = 174)	20% medical treatment
Clough *et al.*, 1989 (n = 198 & 214)	Full training stop marathon drop outs, 89%; finishers, 65%
Hølmich *et al.*, 1989 (n = 1310)	31% full training stop, 1% absence from work
Macera *et al.*, 1989 (n = 300)	29% medical consultation, 21% medication without medical consultation
Ooijendijk & Van Agt, 1990 (n = 163)	27% training reduction, 24% medical treatment
Van Mechelen, 1992 (n = 44)	43% training stop, 0% absence from work

av., average; F, female; M, male.

0–30 km·week^{-1} were prevented from running as a result of a running injury gradually increasing to 53% of all runners running more than 120 km·week^{-1}. Up to this moment there are no studies known in which the direct and/or indirect cost of running injuries are calculated.

Causes of musculoskeletal running injuries

Running injuries are of a diverse nature and vary as outlined by Powell *et al.* (1986) from metabolic abnormalities such as anaemia, amenorrhoea, hypothermia and hyperthermia to extrinsic hazards such as dog bites and traffic collisions (Fig. 27.1). However, the discussion on the causes of running injuries will be limited to musculoskeletal injuries which constitute the most running injuries.

Table 27.10 presents information on risk factors significantly and not significantly related to running injuries. Almost all of the cited authors have, in order to distinguish relevant factors, in their studies compared injured and non-injured runners by using univariate statistical techniques. However, many of the factors which are identified in this way may interact or be interrelated. For instance in the Ijzerman and van Galen (1987) study after univariate analysis many factors were found to be significantly ($P < 0.05$) associated with running injuries. A key factor in their analysis was membership of an athletic club which 'pooled' a number of other significant factors such as more malalignment disorders, no participation in other sports, higher weekly running distance, higher running speed, more running on a hard surface, frequent change of running shoes, running more marathons per year, high motivation to compete, etc. A second example of interrelation comes from the study by van Mechelen (1992) who found intercorrelation coefficients between weekly running distance, weekly running time and weekly running frequency varying from 0.81 to 0.97. In order to cope with problems associated with interrelation and interaction of risk factors some authors (Ijzerman & van Galen, 1987; Marti *et al.*, 1988; Macera *et al.*, 1989; Walter *et al.*, 1989; van Mechelen, 1992) have, in addition to univariate analysis, also used multivariate statistical techniques, such as discriminant analysis and step-wise logistical regression (Dixon *et al.*, 1990) leading to a clearer sight on the relative importance of risk factors. Using a review by Powell *et al.* (1986) on the causes of running injuries as a starting point the risk factors will be discussed below.

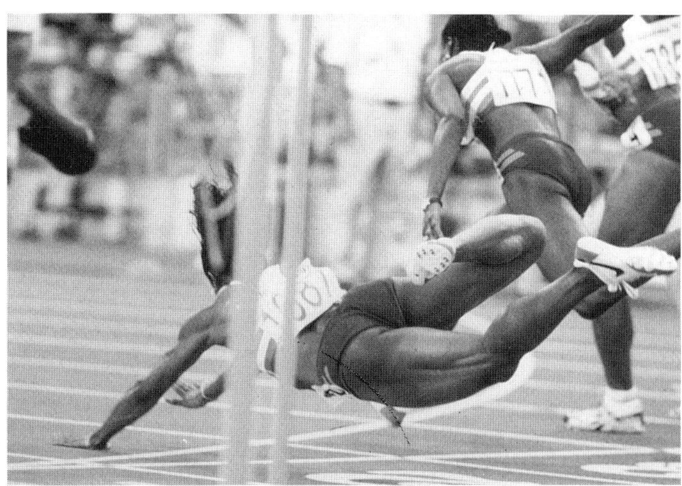

Fig. 27.1 Unexpected running injuries can result from a simple fall. © Vandystadt.

Table 27.10 Summary of the univariate relationship between factors and running injuries, based on the findings of the listed epidemiological studies.

Reference	Factors significantly related to running injuries	Factors not significantly related to running injuries
Pollock *et al.*, 1977*	Running frequency, running duration	
Koplan *et al.*, 1982	Weekly distance	Age, BMI, speed, running experience
Jacobs & Berson, 1986	Weekly distance, number of runs·week^{-1}, running speed, number of races·year^{-1}, stretching, no participation in other sports	Age, gender, duration of run, marital status, education, occupation, running marathons, income, running experience, running surface, ground contact (rear foot vs. mid-distance), running intervals, running sprints, hills
Blair *et al.*, 1987	BMI, weekly distance	Time and place of running, frequency of stretching, age
Ijzerman & van Galen, 1987	Club members,† high motivation score,† stretching exercise,† running according to training scheme,† training with others,† younger age,† malalignment,† training distance, irregular training,† marathon running, best time half marathon,† frequent change of shoes, weekly distance, weekly massage, running speed†	Training speed, gender, body weight, running experience, other sports, time of year, hard surface
Lysholm & Wiklander, 1987	Monthly distance, time of year (spring/summer), training fault (excessive distance, sudden change of training routine), malalignment (?)	Gender
Watson & DiMartino, 1987	Performance level	Exposure time·week^{-1}
Marti *et al.*, 1988	Weekly distance, running speed, previous running injury,† using in-shoe orthoses, running experience, competitive running,† age, BMI < 19.5 and $26 \leq$ BMI ≤ 28	Running frequency, shoe brand, hard running surface, overweight, regular practice of other sports
Bovens *et al.*, 1989	Weekly distance, running one side of the road (?)	
Macera *et al.*, 1989	*Men*: previous injury,† running experience <3 years, running 6–7 times·week^{-1}, running $\geq$32 km·week^{-1}, running $\geq$64 km·week^{-1}, running 1 marathon·year^{-1} *Women*: running 1 marathon·year^{-1}, running on concrete,† running 48–64 km·week^{-1}	Age,† BMI,† running in the dark, hills, running in the morning, stretch before running

Table 27.10 *Continued.*

Reference	Factors significantly related to running injuries	Factors not significantly related to running injuries
Walter *et al.*, 1989	Competitive running, running >64 km·week^{-1}, running >2 days·week^{-1}, running 12 months·year^{-1}, longest run·week^{-1} >8 km, (sometimes) stretching, body height, previous injury,† no warm-up, owning >2 pairs of shoes, training speed	Age, gender, running experience, frequency of race competition, amount of other non-sport activity during the day, BMI, body weight, running surface, running hills, use of cool-down, use of 'hard' training days, performing other sports, smoking status, femoral neck anteversion, pelvic obliquity, knee/patella alignment, rear foot varus, pes cavus/planus, somatotype, shoe characteristics (wedge, sole, etc.)
Van Mechelen, 1992†	Running frequency·week^{-1}, running time·week^{-1}, low attitude score towards cool-down, age,‡ running frequency,‡ low attitude score towards measures on the prevention of running injuries,‡ high attitude score towards cool-down	Knowledge and attitude towards the prevention of running injuries, knowledge and attitude towards warming up and stretching exercises, knowledge of cool-down, running time·week^{-1}, running distance·week^{-1}, running speed

* Controlled experimental trial.
† Remains significant after multivariate analysis.
‡ Only significant after multivariate analysis.
BMI, body mass index.

Characteristics of runners

AGE

In the somewhat comparable studies with regard to study population of Koplan *et al.* (1982), Blair *et al.* (1987), Jacobs and Berson (1986), Macera *et al.* (1989) and Walter *et al.* (1989) age proved to be not significantly related with running injuries. In the study of Ijzerman and van Galen there was a significant but low correlation (0.1) between running injuries and age, runners at a younger age sustaining more injuries than older runners. Younger age also contributed in this study significantly to the prediction of injury after discriminant analysis. However, the meaning of this finding was questioned by the authors by the fact that younger runners train at a higher speed, also running more kilometers per training session than older runners. In the study of Marti *et al.* (1988) after age-stratification a significant decrease of running injuries was found with an increase of age. It was speculated by Marti *et al.* that this finding could be due to a 'healthy runner effect' by which only those runners remaining free of injuries continue to run. Since Marti *et al.* also found, after stratification for length of jogging career, a decrease of injuries with an increase of years of running it was also speculated that this finding could be due to a possible long-term adaptive process of the musculoskeletal system. However, after multiple logistical regression, age was not confirmed as an independent risk factor. Finally, van Mechelen (1992) found age to be an independent risk factor after multiple step-wise logistical regression (odds ratio for runners older than 40 years: 1.05–95% CL, 1.01–1.1).

In conclusion, in the majority of studies, age was not associated with running injuries or it was speculated that the association was biased by factors such as running experience, weekly running distance or running speed. In only one study after multivariate analysis did age prove to be a statistically significant risk factor for running injuries, the odds ratio being, however, relatively low.

GENDER

Powell *et al.* (1986) concluded that 'gender *per se* does not seem to be an important risk factor for running injuries'. This seems to be confirmed by the fact that none of the four epidemiological studies had enough female subjects to take this factor into account (Jacobs & Berson, 1986; Ijzerman & van Galen, 1987; Lysholm & Wiklander, 1987; Walter *et al.*, 1989).

ANTHROPOMETRICS

One may speculate that larger and/or overweight individuals sustain a greater chance of running injuries as a result of greater forces on bones, joints or connective tissue. On the other hand, one may assume that at least in larger people these greater forces will be balanced by stronger muscles, larger bone surface areas, etc.

In only two studies was the relation between body weight and running injuries evaluated; Ijzerman and van Galen (1987) and Walter *et al.* (1989) did not find a significant association between body weight and running injuries.

Body height was only evaluated in one study (Walter *et al.*, 1989) showing after age-adjusted univariate logistical regression that taller men were at greater risk of injury then shorter men, an effect that remained even when height was adjusted for weight.

The association between body mass index (BMI), defined as w/h^2 (w, weight in kg; h, height in m^2) and running injuries was evaluated in five studies. Koplan *et al.* (1982) found BMI to be not independently related to running injuries. A similar finding was reported by Macera *et al.* (1989) and Walter *et al.* (1989). In contrast to these findings Blair *et al.* (1987) found a significant, but low, correlation of 0.1 between running, BMI and running injuries. However, Marti *et al.* (1988) found runners with a BMI smaller than 19.5 and runners with a BMI greater than 27 to be at greater risk of running injuries, although overweight, defined as BMI 26–28, did not prove to be a risk factor in this study. It should be noted though that overweight amongst runners is a rare finding. In the study of Marti *et al.* (1988) only 79 out of 4358 runners had a BMI greater than 27. In a study by Hølmich *et al.* (1989) only 8% out of a total of 1426 non-élite marathon runners had a BMI greater than 25. From these studies it seems that with some precaution it can be concluded that BMI is not related to running injuries, while perhaps taller runners are at greater risk.

MALALIGNMENT

In the literature, many alignment defects are mentioned as giving rise to overuse running injuries such as (i) difference in limb length (Subotnick, 1985); (ii) femoral anteversion (Stanish, 1984); (iii) knee anomalies, such as knock-knees or bow-legs and too large or too small patella (Gudas, 1980; Clement *et al.*, 1981; Andrews, 1983); (iv) foot anomalies, such as varus and valgus of the heel or rearfoot, flat feet and high arches (Doxey, 1985; McKenzie *et al.*, 1985; Renström & Johnson, 1985).

In 1986, Powell *et al.* noted that no epidemiological study had evaluated the effect of malalignment as a risk factor for running injuries. Since then, two epidemiological studies have mentioned malalignment to be significantly associated with running injuries. Lysholm and Wiklander (1987) found, in an attempt to retrospectively analyse the causes of prospectively registered running injuries, that in 40% of the cases malalignment was at least one of the factors causing the injury. Malalignment in this study included 'foot insufficiency, lower extremity muscle stiffness, genu varum and high Q angle'. In their retrospective study by questionnaire Ijzerman and van Galen (1987) included questions on asymmetry of the lower extremity as assessed during previous medical check-ups. After univariate analysis they found a significant correlation of 0.14 between asymmetry and medically treated injuries. This remained significant after multivariate analysis. Walter *et al.* (1989) is the only epidemiological study in which at baseline a physical assessment of the lower extremity was included. None of the measured variables (femoral neck anteversion, pelvic obliquity, knee and patella alignment and rearfoot valgus) was significantly associated with running injuries. From these scarce and contradictory results the importance of malalignment as a cause of running injuries is still not made clear. However, as stated by Powell *et al.* (1986) 'the hypothesis that structural abnormalities are a risk factor for running injuries is too reasonable to deny ... [and] ... careful, abnormality-specific studies should be a top priority for future research'.

MUSCULAR IMBALANCE AND RESTRICTED RANGE OF MOTION

Running strengthens the muscles at the back of the thigh and leg (the hamstrings and calf muscles) relatively more than those at the front (Mirkin, 1975; Clement *et al.*, 1984; Subotnick, 1985), and the resulting imbalance supposedly facilitates the occurrence of various types of overuse injuries. A weak vastus medialis is thought to be a causal factor in damage to the patellar cartilage (Stanish, 1984). It is also speculated that overuse injuries may result from a lack of flexibility, the physiological shortening of the muscle through tiredness, insufficient muscular strength and endurance, a strength imbalance between the left and right hamstrings, an imbalance between the hamstrings and the quadriceps, asymmetrical contraction of the hamstrings and too early a resumption of sporting activity following an injury (van Mechelen *et al.*, 1987). In a case-control study in which subjects were matched for age and weekly running distance van Mechelen (1992) found a significant restriction of range of motion of the hip joint of injured runners in comparison to non-injured runners. Because of the retrospective nature of this study however, it is not possible to attribute this finding to running. No other epidemiological studies mention this factor. More research is needed.

RUNNING EXPERIENCE

Running experience is thought to be a factor associated with running injuries, the inexperienced runner being more susceptible to running injuries (Powell *et al.*, 1986) (Fig. 27.2). This factor did not prove to be significantly associated with running injuries in the studies of Koplan *et al.* (1982), Blair *et al.* (1987), Ijzerman and van Galen (1987) and Walter *et al.* (1989).

Marti *et al.* (1988) found in an age-specific analysis among men of similar age a positive association between years of jogging and decreased incidence of running injuries. In the study by Macera *et al.* (1988) after univariate analysis it was found for men that running regularly for less than 3 years was significantly associated with running injuries of the lower extremity. This association remained after multivariate logistical regression: runners with less than 3 years of running experience had an odds ratio of 2.2 (95% CL, 1.5–3.3).

These findings suggest that at least for men, running experience, resulting in a better adaptation to running on the biomechanical and/or tissue level, may lead to less injuries, although bias as a result of a 'healthy runner effect' should be taken into consideration (Marti *et al.*, 1988).

PREVIOUS INJURY

According to Powell *et al.* (1986) persons with a previous injury may be more likely to become

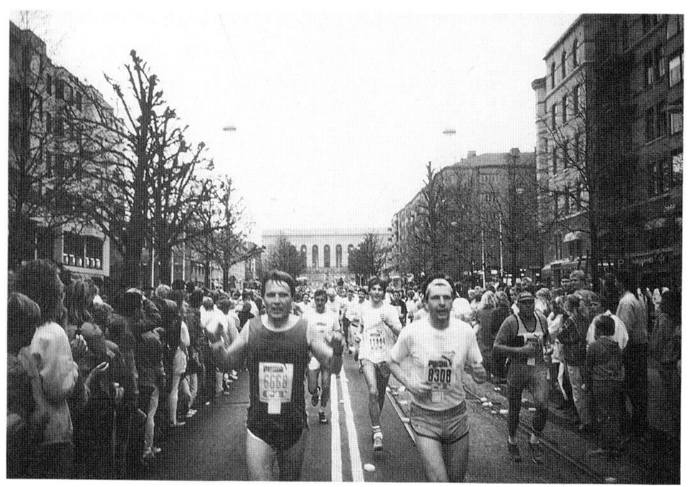

Fig. 27.2 The increasing popularity of the half marathon encourages inexperienced and untrained people to run long distances. Courtesy of Dr P.A.F.H. Renström.

injured again because (i) the original cause may remain; (ii) the repaired tissue may function less well or be less protective than the original tissue; or (iii) the injury may not have healed completely.

In three epidemiological studies previous injury, defined as 'a positive history of running injury in the 12 months prior to the start of the study', was associated with running injuries. Marti *et al.* (1988) found in univariate analysis, after adjustment for differences in weekly running distance a 65% increased risk of injury for runners with a history of previous injury. This remained after multivariate analysis. Macera *et al.* (1989) found for men a history of previous injury to contribute significantly to injury after univariate age-adjusted logistical regression (odds ratio of 2.7; 95% CL, 1.9–3.9). After multivariate analysis, the odds ratio remained the same. Walter *et al.* (1989) found after univariate age-adjusted logistical regression for men a significant odds ratio for previous injury of 1.7 (95% CL, 1.2–3.5) and for women of 2.4 (95% CL, 1.3–4.1). After multiple logistical regression in which age and gender were featured, previous injury proved to be one of the two strongest predictors for running injury with an odds ratio of 1.5. From the findings of these three studies it can be concluded that previous injury as defined above is an important independent risk factor for running injuries, although the mechanisms still needs clarification.

PARTICIPATION IN OTHER SPORTS

It is speculated that runners participating in other sports sustain less running injuries than runners who do not. Reasons for this phenomenon may be that runners who run more miles per week have less time for participating in other sports, as well as that runners who spend more time in other sports use different muscle groups and in this way decrease their risk of overuse injuries associated with running (Jacobs & Berson, 1986).

Jacobs and Berson (1986) found injured runners significantly not participating in other sports in comparison with non-injured runners. However, Ijzerman and van Galen (1987) found no relationship between participation in other sports at least once a week and running injuries. Also Marti *et al.* (1988) found that regular practice of other sports was not associated with reduced running injury risk. Finally, Walter *et al.* (1989) found that participation in other sports was essentially not associated with the risk of running injury. Similar risks were found in runners who reported to be active in a large variety of forms of activity. Only ice skating and dancing showed a significant relation to running injuries with about one-third less risk of injury. In this study also, the risk of injury was studied according to the usual proportion of time spent sitting, standing or walking during the day; no significant relationship could be established.

From these findings it seems reasonable to conclude that participation in other sports is not an independent risk factor. However, this point needs further studying.

PSYCHOLOGICAL AND BEHAVIOURAL FACTORS

Notwithstanding the presence of any evidence in relation to running, Powell *et al.* (1986) presumed psychological factors to be related to running injuries. Ijzerman and van Galen (1987) found that the injury incidence was significantly related to a motivation score. The higher the motivation score, the larger the incidence for medically treated injuries. They speculated that more motivated runners ignore first signs of injury more than less motivated runners therefore having a higher injury incidence. After multivariate analysis, motivation still contributed significantly to the risk of sustaining a running injury. Both Marti *et al.* (1988) and Walter *et al.* (1989) found competitive running, in contrast to running for fitness or recreation, to be significantly associated with running injuries. In the Marti *et al.* study, this association proved to be independent after multivariate analysis.

Van Mechelen (1992) measured overall and specific attitudes towards the prevention of running injuries. After multiple step-wise logistical regression it was found that a low overall attitude score and a high attitude score with respect to cool-down significantly contributed to the risk of running injury.

It can be concluded that psychological and behavioural factors seem important and need further future investigation.

Characteristics of running

WEEKLY RUNNING DISTANCE, FREQUENCY AND TIME

Almost all of the cited authors state weekly running distance as the most important risk factor for running injuries. In a randomized trial, Pollock *et al.* (1977) found weekly running frequency and duration of running to be related to running injuries. Both increasing duration and increasing frequency produced more injuries. Koplan *et al.* (1982) found an almost straight relationship between increasing weekly distance and running injury incidence for both men and women. Jacobs and Berson (1986) found weekly distance to be significantly associated with running injury. The same was confirmed in epidemiological studies of Blair *et al.* (1987), Ijzerman and van Galen (1987), Marti *et al.* (1988), Macera *et al.* (1989), Walter *et al.* (1989) and Bovens *et al.* (1989). Lysholm and Wiklander (1987) found running injuries to be significantly associated with monthly running distance. Only one epidemiological study did not confirm the relation between exposure time and injuries (Watson & DiMartino, 1987). In this study, exposure time was defined as 'time spent training and competing on a weekly basis'. No difference in exposure time was found between injured and non-injured athletes. However, the population in this study was different from the above-mentioned studies in terms of age and participation in athletic events.

It should be mentioned, however, that despite the fact that the absolute risk of running injury increases with increasing weekly distance the relative risk (risk·exposure time^{-1}) decreases as was shown by Marti *et al.* (1988), Walter *et al.* (1989) and Bovens *et al.* (1989).

In terms of prevention, one can speculate about the effect of dividing total weekly distance over several shorter sessions if running injuries are related to weekly distance. In some studies a significant relationship between running frequency (Jacobs & Berson, 1986; Macera *et al.*, 1989; Walter *et al.*, 1989; van Mechelen, 1992) and running injuries was found, although this relation was not confirmed by Marti *et al.* (1988). Marti *et al.* (1988) examined in their study a subgroup running the same weekly distance in two, three or four weekly sessions. No significant differences appeared in the incidence of running-related injuries. In the study of Jacobs and Berson (1986) duration of running was not associated with increased running injury incidence. With respect to the abovementioned variables, it should be borne in mind that these variables are strongly interrelated.

In conclusion it can be stated that weekly running distance is a strong determinant of running injuries. The role of running frequency and weekly running time remains unclear.

TRAINING SPEED AND OTHER INDICATORS OF PERFORMANCE LEVEL

Training speed was not associated with increased risk of running injuries in the studies of Koplan *et al.* (1982), Ijzerman and van Galen (1987), Walter *et al.* (1989) and van Mechelen (1992). In the study of Jacobs and Berson (1986), however, training speed was significantly associated with an increased risk of running injuries, as in a subpopulation of younger runners in the study of Ijzerman and van Galen (1987). Apart from training speed, level of speed, level of performance can for instance also be operationalized by participating in marathon running, fastest time run on a certain distance, running whole year round, running at least 8 km once a week, etc.

Watson and DiMartino (1987) found performance level based on a percentile ranking of the best season performance to be significantly associated with injury. Ijzerman and van Galen (1987) found marathon running and the best time on a half marathon to be significantly associated with an increase in injury risk. Marti *et al.* (1988) found the best time on a 16-km run to be significantly associated with running injury. Macera *et al.* (1989) found running of at least one marathon a year to be significantly associated with injury risk. Walter *et al.* (1989) found running the whole year round and running at least 8 km once a week to be significantly associated with running injury. Frequency of race competition was not associated with running injury in this study.

From these findings the relation between running speed/level of running performance and injury risk remains unclear.

STABILITY OF RUNNING HABITS

A sudden change in weekly running distance or training habits is supposed to be a cause of running injuries, because of lacking capacity of tissue to adapt to these kinds of sudden changes (Powell *et al.*, 1986). Training errors such as running too often, too fast or for too long are major causes of injury in both beginners (Franklin *et al.*, 1979; Kowal, 1980) and experienced runners. Any sudden increase in the weekly distance (Koplan *et al.*, 1982) or any change to a specific form of training (such as interval training or hill training) without a gradual build-up is regarded as a training error (Andrews, 1983; Clement *et al.*, 1984).

Lysholm and Wiklander (1986) found training errors (e.g. sudden change in training routine) to be associated with running injury in about 60% of all injuries. Ijzerman and van Galen (1987) found a low, but significant correlation (0.08) between irregular training and running injuries. On the other hand in this study also a significant difference was found in injury incidence between runners training according to a training scheme set out by a trainer (incidence rate, 53%) and runners running without such a scheme (incidence rate, 35%). In the study of Walter *et al.* (1989) no association was found between 'the use of hard training days' and running injuries.

Running sprints or intervals was not related to running injuries in the study of Jacobs and Berson (1986). In the same study, 33% of the injured runners had changed either their technique or running shoes prior to their injury.

WARM-UP, STRETCHING EXERCISES AND COOL-DOWN

Lack or improper use of warm-up, stretching exercises and cool-down is thought to be a risk factor with regard to running injuries (van Mechelen *et al.*, 1987).

Jacobs and Berson (1986), as well as Ijzerman and van Galen (1987) found injured runners to have stretched significantly more before running than non-injured runners. It was discussed by Jacobs and Berson that certain stretching exercises such as the hurdler stretch can lead to injury of medial collateral ligament and to the medial meniscus. Both studies put forward that runners who are injured stretch because of their injury. Walter *et al.* (1989) found runners who 'sometimes' stretch to be significantly at risk of injury in contrast to runners who 'always, usually or never stretch' leaving this finding unexplained. Blair *et al.* (1987) found frequency of stretching to be unassociated with running injuries. Macera *et al.* (1989) found stretching before running to be not associated with running injury.

With regard to warming up, Walter *et al.* (1989) found runners who say they never warm up to run a significantly smaller risk of running injury in comparison to runners who say they 'always, usually or sometimes' use warm-up. In the same study, regular use of cool-down was not related to running injuries at all.

Finally, van Mechelen (1992) was not able to detect any preventive effect in terms of a reduction of running injury incidence from a standardized programme of warm-up, stretching exercises and cool-down in a randomized trial, in which runners were matched for age, weekly distance and knowledge on the prevention of running injuries.

Characteristics of running environment

SHOES

Running is a cyclical movement comprising two phases, one in which one foot is in contact with the ground (support phase) and one in which both feet are off the ground (air-borne phase). In the course of the ground-contact phase, the weight of the body is absorbed by the foot and then lifted as the next stride begins. Two types of landing are distinguished, namely on the heel (rearfoot strikers, 80% of all runners) and on the front part of the foot (mid-foot and forefoot strikers, 20% of all runners); types of landing intermediate between the two may also occur, depending on speed. With respect to type of landing, Jacobs and Berson (1986) did not find any difference in injury incidence in relation to the part of the foot first contacting the ground. The forces involved in landing may be as great as 2–5 times body weight (McKenzie *et al.*, 1985; Subotnick, 1985). A runner with a stride of 1.5 m makes contact with the ground about 670 times$\cdot$km^{-1}, and if we assume a body weight of 70 kg and an average force on landing of 2.5 times body weight this implies that each leg is subject to a force of around 60 t$\cdot$km^{-1}. These shocks are absorbed by the thigh and particularly leg muscles, and by the movement of the foot with pronation (taking the load on the inner edge of the sole of the foot) playing an important part.

It seems evident that a training shoe providing cushioning, support and stability can play an important role in shock absorption and thereby injury prevention. Ijzerman and van Galen (1987) found a significant correlation of 0.1 between the regular change of shoes and medically treated running injuries. A possible explanation for this phenomenon is the fact that injured runners try to solve their problem by changing shoes. Marti *et al.* (1988) found in their study no difference in injury incidence between runners preferring one of the three most popular running shoes (Adidas, Nike, Puma). Runners having no preference for any brand of shoes whatsoever sustained significantly fewer injuries than runners who had a preference for a specific brand. From this finding the conclusion was drawn that no particular shoe has a preventive advantage over other brand names. Runners wearing inexpensive shoes (less than 60 Swiss Francs) did not sustain more injuries, whereas runners wearing expensive shoes (more than 140 Swiss Francs) sustained significantly more injuries. A likely explanation put forward by Marti *et al.* (1988) is that injury-prone runners or high mileage runners choose to wear expensive shoes. It is said that the use of orthotic devices is capable of correcting minimal alignment abnormalities, in this way creating normal running conditions. Marti *et al.* (1988) found the use of in-shoe orthotics to be significantly related with both a positive history of previous injury and with running-related injuries during the period of study. Selection bias with injury-prone runners favouring orthotics was considered as an explanation.

Walter *et al.* (1989) found owning two pairs of shoes to be significantly related with a 50% increase in injury risk. However, in this study shoe characteristics (presence of varus wedge, waffle sole, wear pattern and personal shoe repair) were not related with injury risk. The effect of owning more shoes was said to reflect greater levels of training of such runners.

Although the role of running shoes in running injury prevention remains unclear, the importance of shock absorbance by running shoes does not seem to be denied by the cited epidemiological studies. In addition to this it should be realized in accordance with Cook *et al.* (1990) that the shock-absorbing qualities of wet running shoes is reduced and that all running shoes lose between 30 and 50% of their shock-absorbing characteristics after as much as 400 km of running.

RUNNING SURFACES AND HILL RUNNING

Running on too hard a surface causes mechanical shocks and may overload joints, tendons, etc. (Clement & Taunton, 1981), while too soft a surface quickly tires the muscles and it is thought that it may thereby give rise to injury (Gudas, 1980). Surface irregularities — potholes, the roots of trees, pavement edges and so on — may cause acute injury to the ankle and knee. In the case of running on public roads, problems may arise not only through the hardness of the surface but also through its camber, which places a different loading on the legs and can thus give rise to overuse injuries of various types, e.g. short leg syndrome (Gudas, 1980).

Jacobs and Berson (1986) did not find a correlation between running surface and running injury, but this finding was probably biased by the fact that the majority of the runners in their study were running on concrete and asphalt. The same was found by Ijzerman and van Galen (1987) who added bias as a result of a 'healthy runner effect' (all runners run on hard surfaces and even those who remain uninjured are still running on hard surfaces) as a possible explanation. Marti *et al.* (1988) were not able to prove an advantage or disadvantage from the usual running surface (predominantly hard, predominantly natural or combined). Walter *et al.* (1989) found no significant relation between injuries and frequency of running on asphalt, concrete, grass or dirt.

Macera *et al.* (1989) found, after both univariate and multivariate analysis in women a significant difference in injury risk for running on a concrete surface (odds ratio 5.6; 95% CL, 1.1–29.3). This relation was not found in men. Bovens *et al.* (1989) found injuries of the lower leg and Achilles tendon to be significantly more localized on the left-hand side. This was explained by the unequal load of the leg caused by the surface of the street, which is a little convex in order to drain rain.

From these findings it seems as if, at least in men, different running surfaces as such do not largely influence running injury risk, although it should be kept in mind that bias probably plays an important role.

Hill running is associated with increased injury risk (Clement *et al.*, 1981). Jacobs and Berson (1986), Macera *et al.* (1989) and Walter *et al.* (1989) did not find any relation between hill running and increased injury risk.

TIME OF DAY AND YEAR

It has been suggested that persons who run in the morning are more likely to be injured than those who run at other times of the day (Powell *et al.*, 1986), although this finding was not confirmed by Blair *et al.* (1987), Jacobs and Berson (1986), Macera *et al.* (1989) and Walter *et al.* (1989), who all found no association between time of day and increased injury risk.

Powell *et al.* (1986) suggested that due to climatical circumstances, such as snow or rain, roads may be slippery thereby causing falls leading to more injuries during winter and autumn. In only one study was climate taken into consideration: Ijzerman and van Galen (1987) found no relation between running injuries and time of year, although according to them this finding could be biased by unequal exposure throughout the year. Walter *et al.* (1989) found running whole year round to significantly enlarge the risk of running injury. This may either reflect climatical influence or differences in exposure.

Other health risks associated with running

In addition to the orthopaedic complications already discussed, three other categories of risk are mentioned in the literature, namely sudden death associated with running, heat illness and traffic accidents. However, as mentioned by Powell *et al.* (1986) with respect to traffic accidents, all of the reported findings are based on analysis of numerator data (case reports and case studies) without information on the population at risk. Without the denominator or estimates of them, the risks of the various categories cannot be compared. Also it is not possible to establish risk factors reliably. This makes recommendation of research-based preventive measures difficult. For this reason the other health-related risks associated with running will only be discussed very briefly.

The risk of a fatal heart attack is enhanced in runners with pre-existing cardiovascular problems (Eichner, 1983), but for those in good health the risk from running is no greater than from ordinary day-to-day activities (Koplan, 1979).

Running generates a great deal of heat (Hughson, 1981), and in warm weather, especially when relative humidity is high, the result can be a build-up of heat in the body. Sunshine and an inadequate intake of liquid exacerbate the problem (Fig. 27.3). Older people, children and the overweight runner are at particular risk.

Runners making use of public roads are exposed to the danger of traffic accidents, especially in conditions of poor visibility (Williams, 1981).

Preventive measures

Based on the available data it seems clear that

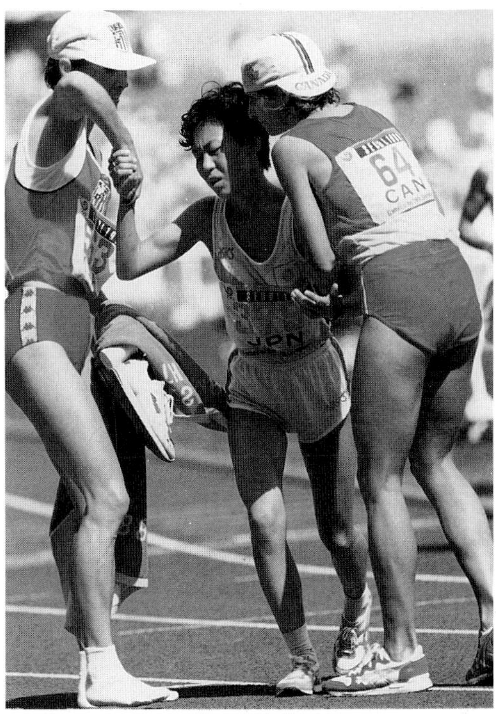

Fig. 27.3 Runners suffering from exhaustion and/or inadequate fluid intake need immediate treatment. Courtesy of the IOC archives.

previous injury, lack of running experience, running to compete, excessive weekly running distance and performing warm-up and stretching exercises are associated with running injuries. The association between running injuries and factors such as body height, malalignment, muscular imbalance, restricted range of motion, running frequency, level of performance, stability of running pattern, shoes and in-shoe orthoses and running on one side of the road remains unclear or is backed by contradictory or scarce research findings. Factors such as age, gender, BMI, running hills, running on hard surfaces, participation in other sports, time of the year and time of the day seem not to be associated with running injuries. The fact that information on some factors is contradictory or scarce and that other factors do not seem to be related to running injuries does not necessarily mean that these factors are of no importance at all. It should be kept in mind, as stated by Walter *et al.* (1989), that this merely reflects that in epidemiological research the range of effects of these factors are probably not important within the range of the majority of runners, but they can undoubtedly be causative for some individual injuries.

Measures aimed at preventing running injuries must be geared to the aetiological factors involved (Clement & Taunton, 1981). However, the causes of running injuries are so multifactorial and diverse that any specific single measure proposed would probably be of help to only a small minority of runners (Marti *et al.*, 1988).

The implications of the risk factors discussed in this chapter speak, in terms of preventive measures, for themselves and will, apart from brief indications with regard to the factors undoubtedly related with running injuries, not be further discussed.

Complete rehabilitation

Dealing with the risk factor 'previous injury', complete rehabilitation and early recognition of symptoms of overuse injuries seem very important. Without going into the precise nature of a rehabilitation programme, some authors state that it can prevent the recurrence of injuries to the postural and movement system (Hayes, 1974; Proctor, 1980; Stulberg, 1980; Davies, 1981; Ekstrand, 1982; Harvey, 1982; Thompson *et al.*, 1982; Runyan, 1983; Lysens *et al.*, 1984; Watson, 1984).

Rehabilitation is a way of preventing an injured athlete recovering 'incompletely' and thus restarting his or her sporting activities at the preinjury level too soon. A rehabilitation programme cannot be regarded as having been completed until (Proctor, 1980; Ekstrand, 1982):

1 The athlete is free from pain.

2 Muscle strength has returned to about the preinjury level.

3 Articulatory mobility has recovered.

In cases of articulatory instability the purpose of rehabilitation is to strengthen the muscles around the unstable joint, compensating for the instability and thus reducing the risk of repeated injury to a ligament or tendon (Runyan, 1983). The author is not aware of any results of research into the effects of a rehabilitation programme with respect to running, although it has been demonstrated that a whole package of measures including 'controlled rehabilitation' can reduce the number of sports injuries in soccer (Ekstrand, 1982). With regard to early recognition of overuse injuries a runner should be taught to respect 'the language of the body' and reduce or temporarily stop, rather then to continue or increase, running when suffering from pain or stiffness of joints and tendons as a result of running.

Warm-up and stretching exercises

According to the literature (van Mechelen *et al.*, 1987; Safran *et al.*, 1989) warm-up and stretching are essential to the prevention of musculoskeletal injuries. However, warm-up and stretching are associated with a higher injury risk in runners. As indicated before, this finding is probably biased by the fact that runners, once injured, start paying attention to the use of warm-up and stretching exercises. In a true experiment in runners, no injury reduction was found as a result of a standardized programme of warm-up, stretching and cool-down, though this finding can perhaps be explained by the fact that the majority of runners in the control group also performed warm-up and stretching exercises quite similar to the experimental group (van Mechelen, 1992).

It is also known that the majority of recreational runners (80–90%) perform a warm-up or stretching exercises one way or the other (Ooijendijk & Van Agt, 1990).

Despite all these findings it still makes sense to promote warm-up and stretching exercises as preventive measures. Safran *et al.* (1989) formulated the following: 'Warm-up should be performed to raise body and muscle temperature — to cause some sweating but not so intense as to cause fatigue. Warm-up reduces the muscle viscosity to promote smoother contractions, causes systematic enhancement of contraction and relaxes muscle neurally. When warm-up is combined with stretching, the elasticity of muscle is temporarily increased requiring greater force and degree of lengthening to tear muscle. Stretching should always be performed after warm-up.' And, 'Stretching regularly will produce enhanced flexibility and also cause a load–stress relaxation. The stretch should be slow, relaxed and graceful — either passive, static or contact-relax, but not ballistic. The stretch position is assumed gently and slowly until muscle tightness, not till pain is felt'.

Health education

Lack of running experience and running to compete are risk factors which are probably hard to deal with in terms of prevention other than through health education by which the runners are made aware of the importance of these factors. It should be stressed that health education will only be effective if it is put forward as a planned strategy (Kok & Bouter, 1990). With regard to lack of running experience, some general training guidelines were formulated by van Mechelen *et al.* (1987). Training should be built up gradually; running speeds should be such that the runner can continue to speak without shortness of breath; the untrained should start their training gradually, e.g. on alternate days; and in group training, each individual should have his or her own training programme (this is helped by a division into groups of more or less equal performance).

Excessive weekly distance can only be dealt with by reducing running itself. However, this does not seem to be an acceptable measure for joggers who are determined to run. At the level of the individual runner the question 'How much is too much?' can only be answered by trial and error. Perhaps this factor may also be made accessible by health educational intervention. Ijzerman and van Galen (1987) state that reducing participation in long-distance runs (marathons) should be one of the aims of health education.

The experiment of van Mechelen (1992) did show a significant improvement in knowledge with respect to warming up as a preventive measure, which can be pointed out as a favourable finding in terms of health education (Kok & Bouter, 1990).

References

Andrews, J.R. (1983) Overuse syndromes of the lower extremity. *Clin. Sports Med.* **2**(1), 137–48.

Blair, S.E., Kohl, H.W. & Goodyear, N.N. (1987) Rates and risks for running and exercise injuries: Studies in three populations. *Res. Q. Exerc. Sport* **58**(3), 221–8.

Bovens, A.M.P., Janssen, G.M.E., Vermeer, H.G.W., Hoeberigs, J.H., Janssen, M.P.E. & Verstappen, P.T.S. (1989) Occurrence of running injuries in adults following a supervised training program. *Int. J. Sports Med.* **10**, S186–90.

Clement, D.B. & Taunton, J.E. (1981) A guide to the prevention of running injuries. *Australia Fam. Phys.* **10**, 156–64.

Clement, D.B., Taunton, J.E., Smart, G.W. & McNicol, K.L. (1981) A survey of overuse running injuries. *Phys. Sportsmed.* **9**, 47–58.

Clement, D.B., Taunton, J.E. & Smart, G.W. (1984)

Achilles tendinitis and peritendinitis: Etiology and treatment. *Am. J. Sportsmed.* **12**(3), 179–84.

Clough, I.J., Dutch, S., Maugham, R.J. & Shepherd, J. (1987) Pre-race drop-out in marathon runners: Reasons for withdrawal and future plans. *Br. J. Sports Med.* **21**(4), 148–9.

Clough, P.J., Shepherd, J. & Maugham, R.J. (1989) Marathon finishers and pre-race drop-outs. *Br. J. Sports Med.* **23**(2), 97–101.

Cook, S.D., Brinker, M.R. & Mahlon, P. (1990) Running shoes. Their relation to running injuries. *Sports Med.* **10**(1), 1–8.

Davies, J.E. (1981) Injuries and physical stress. *J. Biosoc. Sci.* **7**(Suppl.), 151–7.

Dixon, W.J., Brown, M.B., Engelman, L. & Jennerich, R.I. (1990) *BMDP Statistical Software Manual*, Vol. 2. University of California Press, Berkeley.

Doxey, G.E. (1985) Management of the metatarsalgia with foot orthotics. *J. Orthop. Sports Phys. Ther.* **6**(6), 324–33.

Dressendorfer, R.H. & Wade, C.E. (1983) The muscular overuse syndrome in long-distance runners. *Phys. Sports Med.* **11**(11), 116–30.

Eggold, J.F. (1981) Orthotics in the prevention of runners' overuse injuries. *Phys. Sports Med.* **9**(3), 125–31.

Eichner, E.R. (1983) Exercise and heart disease. Epidemiology of the 'exercise hypothesis'. *Am. J. Med.* **75**, 1008–23.

Ekstrand, J. (1982) *Soccer injuries and their prevention.* Linkoping University Medical Dissertation No. 130, Linkoping, Sweden.

Franklin, B.A., Lussier, L. & Buskirk, E. (1979) Injury rates in women joggers. *Phys. Sports Med.* **7**, 105–12.

Galen, W. van & Diederiks, J. (1990) *Sportblessures Breed Uitgemeten* (A Population Study on Sport Injuries). De Vrieseborch, Haarlem, The Netherlands.

Gudas, C.J. (1980) Patterns of lower-extremity injury in 224 runners. *Compr. Ther.* **6**(9), 50–9.

Hartung, G.H. (1980) Jogging — the potential for prevention of heart disease. *Compr. Ther.* **6**(9), 28–32.

Harvey, J. (1982) The preparticipation examination of the child athlete. *Clin. Sports Med.* **1**(3), 353–69.

Hayes, D. (1974) Risk factors in sport; human factors. **16**(5), 454–8.

Hess, G.P., Capiello, W.L., Poole, R.M. & Hunter, S.C. (1989) Prevention and treatment of overuse tendon injuries. *Sports Med.* **8**(6), 371–84.

Hølmich, P., Christensen, S.W., Darre, E., Johnsen, F. & Hartog, T. (1989) Non-élite marathon runners: health, training and injuries. *Br. J. Sports Med.* **23**(3), 177–8.

Hughson, R. (1981) Canadian association of sports sciences position paper on protection from exertional heat injuries. *Can. J. Appl. Sport Sci.* **6**, 99–100.

Ijzerman, J.C. & Galen, W.C.C. van (1987) *Blessures bij lange afstandlopers* (Injuries in Long Distance Runners). Royal Dutch Athletic Association (KNAU), The Netherlands.

Jacobs, S.J. & Berson, B.L. (1986) Injuries to runners: a study of entrants to a 10 000 meter race. *Am. J. Sports Med.* **14**(2), 151–5.

Kok, G. & Bouter, L.M. (1990) On the importance of planned health education: Prevention of ski injury as an example. *Am. J. Sports Med.* **18**, 6.

Koplan, J.P. (1979) Cardiovascular death while running. *JAMA* **242**, 2578–9.

Koplan, J.P., Powell, K.E., Sikes, R.K., Shirley, R.W. & Campbell, G.C. (1982) An epidemiological study of the benefits and risks of running. *JAMA* **248**(32), 3118–21.

Kowal, D.M. (1980) Nature and causes of injuries in women resulting from an endurance training program. *Am. J. Sports Med.* **8**, 265–9.

Lehman, W.L. (1984) Overuse syndromes in runners. *Am. Fam. Phys.* **29**, 157–61.

Lysens, R., Lefevre, J. & Ostyn, M. (1984) The predictability of sports injuries. A preliminary report. *Int. J. Sports Med.* **5**(Suppl.), 153–5.

Lysholm, J. & Wiklander, J. (1987) Injuries in runners. *Am. J. Sports Med.* **15**(2), 168–71.

Macera, C.A., Pate, R.R., Powell, K.E., Jackson, K.L., Kendrick, J.S. & Craven, T.E. (1984) Predicting lower-extremity injuries among habitual runners. *Arch. Intern. Med.* **149**, 2565–8.

McKenzie, D.C., Clement, D.B. & Taunton, J.E. (1985) Running shoes, orthotics and injuries. *Sports Med.* **2**, 334–47.

Manders, Th. & Kropman, J. (1982) *Sportbeoefening: Drempeles en stimulansen* (Determinants of Sports Participation). Institute for Applied Social Sciences, University of Nijmegen, The Netherlands.

Manders, Th. & Kropman, J. (1987) *Sport Ontwikkelingen en kosten* (Sports: Trends and Costs). Institute for Applied Social Sciences, University of Nijmegen, The Netherlands.

Marti, B., Vader, J.P., Minder, C.E. & Abelin, T. (1988) On the epidemiology of running injuries. *Am. J. Sports Med.* **16**(3), 285–94.

Mechelen, W. van (1992) *Aetiology and prevention of running injuries.* Thesis, Vrije Universiteit, Amsterdam.

Mechelen, W. van, Hlobil, H. & Kemper, H.C.G. (1987) *How can Sports Injuries be Prevented?* NISGZ Publication No. 25E, Papendal, The Netherlands.

Mirkin, G. (1976) The prevention and treatment of running injuries. *J. Am. Podiatr. Assoc.* **66**, 880–4.

Ooijendijk, W.T.M. & Agt, L. Van (1990) Preventie

van hardloopblessures (The prevention of running injuries). *Gen. Sport* **23**(4), 146–51.

Pollock, M.L., Gettman, L.R., Milesis, L.A., Bak, M.D., Durstine, L. & Johnson, R.B. (1977) Effects of frequency and duration of training on attrition and incidence of injury. *Med. Sci. Sport* **9**(1), 31–6.

Powell, K.E., Kohl, H.W., Caspersen, C.J. & Blair, S.A. (1986) An epidemiological perspective on the causes of running injuries. *Phys. Sports Med.* **14**(6), 100–14.

Powell, K.E. & Paffenbarger, R.S. (1985) Workshop on epidemiologic and public health aspects of physical activity and exercise, a summary. *Publ. Health Rep.* **100**, 118–26.

Proctor, A. (1980) The medical responsibilities of the athletic trainer. *N. Carolina Med. J.* **41**, 519–20.

Renström, P. & Johnson, R.J. (1985) Overuse injuries in sports, a review. *Sports Med.* **2**, 316–33.

Runyan, D.K. (1983) The preparticipation examination of the young athlete. Defining the essentials. *Clin. Pediatr.* **22**, 674–9.

Safran, M.R., Seaber, A.V. & Garrett, W.E. (1989) Warm-up and muscular injury prevention (an update). *Sports Med.* **8**(4), 239–49.

Stanish, W.D. (1984) Overuse injuries in athletes: A perspective. *Med. Sci. Sports Exerc.* **16**, 1–7.

Stulberg, S.D. (1980) Sports injuries and arthritis. *Compr. Ther.* **6**, 8–11.

Subotnick, S.I. (1985) The biomechanics of running, implications for the prevention of foot injuries. *Sports Med.* **2**, 144–53.

Thompson, J.R., Andrish, J.T. & Bergfeld, J.A. (1982) A prospective study of a preparticipation sports examinations of 2670 young athletes: methods and results. *Clev. Clin. Q.* **49**, 225–33.

Walter, S.D., Hart, L.E., McIntosh, J.M. & Sutton, J.R. (1989) The Ontario cohort study of running-related injuries. *Arch. Intern. Med.* **149**, 2561–4.

Watson, A.W.S. (1984) Sports injuries during one academic year in 6799 Irish schoolchildren. *Am. J. Sports Med.* **12**, 65–71.

Watson, M.D. & DiMartino, P.P. (1987) Incidence of injuries in high school track and field athletes and its relation to performance ability. *Am. J. Sports Med.* **15**(3), 251–4.

Williams, A.F. (1981) When motor vehicles hit joggers: an analysis of 60 cases. *Publ. Health Rep.* **96**, 448–51.

Chapter 28

Injuries in Throwing Sports

JOE P. BRAMHALL, DOROTHY F. SCARPINATO AND JAMES R. ANDREWS

Understanding the management of the throwing athlete's arm has been difficult and controversial. With the technological advancements in arthroscopy and the convergence of ideas from the traditional shoulder surgeons and the sports medicine physicians, a better understanding of the pathology and treatment is evolving.

The most important aspect of diagnosis in the throwing athlete is the history and physical examination. The exact mechanism of injury, the activity that reproduces symptoms, the location and duration of pain and aggravating factors are a necessary part of history taking. The physical examination cannot be overemphasized. Identifying areas of tenderness, limitations of range of motion and other physical findings such as rotator cuff dysfunction and capsular laxity can be elicited.

The initial management in the majority of throwing injuries is conservative. With active rest and a well-designed rehabilitation programme, the athlete will often recover and return to competition. In certain instances, the diagnosis cannot be ascertained by physical examination thus ancillary tests such as computerized tomographic (CT) arthrogram, magnetic resonance imaging (MRI) or isokinetic testing are necessary. In some instances, arthroscopy becomes important in providing information leading to the appropriate diagnosis and treatment. Surgical treatment, should be as conservative as possible. Operative arthroscopy, has its role especially after conservative treatment fails. In other more severe cases, open operative intervention has a place in the treatment armamentarium.

Prevention of injuries

Injuries to the upper extremity caused by the throwing motion in sports are preventable by employing proper body mechanics and maintaining good conditioning. Proper pitching or throwing mechanics are of primary importance in avoiding injury from repetitive microtrauma due to the overhand throwing motion. Poor throwing mechanics are often developed at an early age. Once these faulty throwing mechanics are established, they become set kinematics for the individual (Anderson & Ciocek, 1989).

The stresses placed on the throwing arm emphasize the importance of proper pitching mechanics to avoid chronic overuse injuries. Evaluating pitching mechanics by the use of high speed three-dimensional videography is helpful in detecting improper biomechanics. The throwing motion that is biomechanically sound decreases the chance of injury and promotes increased longevity of competition for the athlete. A shoulder performing at or near its physiological limitations without proper throwing mechanics, conditioning or warm-up, will eventually break down from overuse (Derscheid, 1988; Feiring & Derscheid, 1989).

Phases of throwing

The pitching motion has been divided into five phases: (i) wind-up; (ii) cocking; (iii) acceleration; (iv) deceleration; and (v) follow-through. The motion and the position for the entire body during the different phases of throwing must be considered when evaluating pitching mechanics.

Wind-up. The wind-up is a smooth preparation phase of throwing in which no excessive strain is placed on the pitcher's shoulder or elbow. In this phase, kinetic energy is stored and the body is placed in a position so that the entire body contributes to the throw. The wind-up begins with a two-legged stance and terminates at the top of the leg kick with the ipsilateral leg planted when the ball is removed from the glove. The body is ready to begin a forward motion (Fig. 28.1).

Cocking. The cocking phase positions the throwing arm for delivery of the ball. The opposite leg is extended forward and planted directly toward the plate or in a slightly closed position. A right-handed pitcher would ideally stride toward the plate or to the right of the midline. The trunk rotates toward and faces the plate. The arm is positioned with the humerus horizontal and the elbow flexed approximately 90° (Fig. 28.2). The humerus is externally rotated to approximately 160°. There is very little forward motion of the ball during this phase so that at the end of the cocking phase the shoulder has advanced to eccentrically load both the humeral adductors, the pectoralis major and the subscapularis, and the internal rotators, the latissimus dorsi and teres major muscles. The development of this extrinsic loading is a smooth, well-controlled phase.

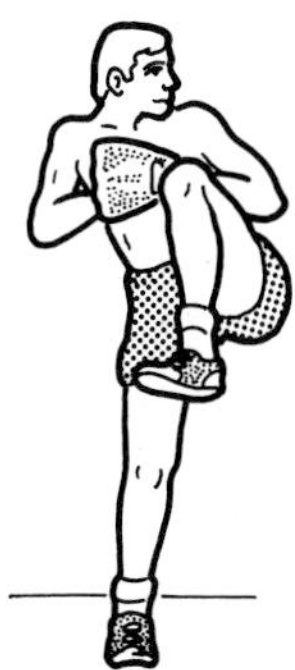

Fig. 28.1 The balanced body position.

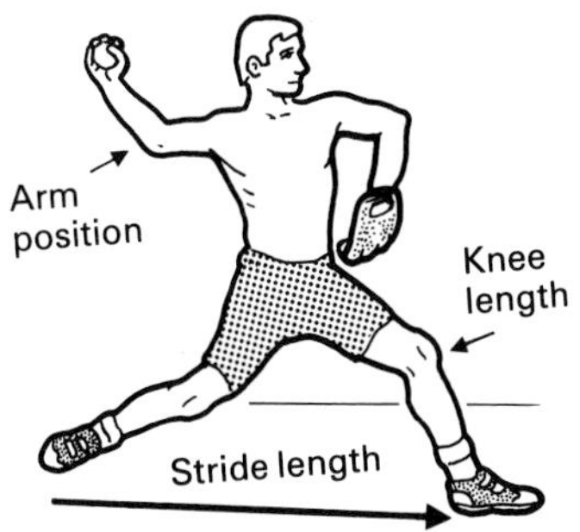

Fig. 28.2 Body position during foot contact.

Acceleration. The acceleration phase spans from the end of the cocking phase, when the velocity of the ball is zero, to the point of ball release (Fig. 28.3). As the trunk is rotated anteriorly during the cocking phase, the anterior motion of the shoulder is stopped to allow a transfer of this anterior momentum from the trunk to the arm to provide acceleration of the ball. As this extrinsic load is applied to the arm, the anterior muscles, the pectoralis and subscapularis also contract to add intrinsic acceleration to the arm. During the first half of the acceleration phase the humerus is accelerated anteriorly. The internal rotator muscles, the latissimus dorsi and the teres major, also contract to initiate internal rotation of the humerus. The first half of acceleration is a smooth, well-controlled phase, but as the rate of humeral adduction increases, the torque on the elbow joint needed to accelerate the forearm is very high (Bradley & Tibone, 1991).

In the second half of the acceleration phase, the rate of humeral adduction is decreased by the firing of the teres minor, infraspinatus and supraspinatus muscles (Bradley & Tibone,

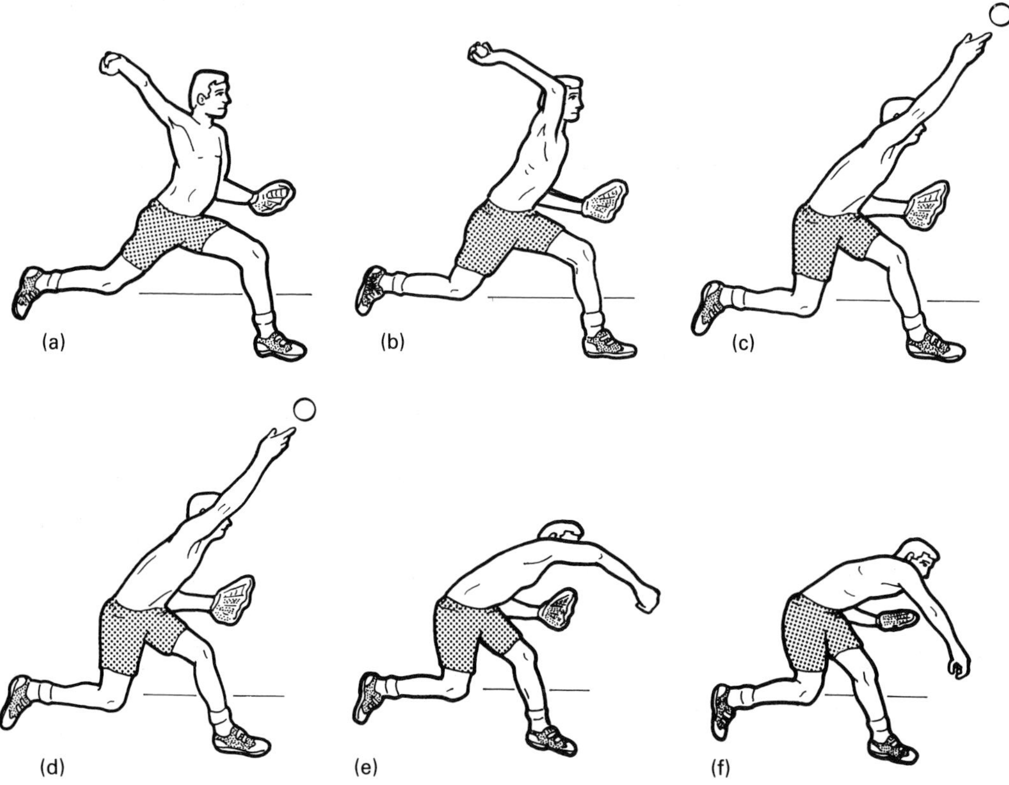

Fig. 28.3 Body positions during delivery (a–c) and release (d–e): (a) delivery phase, (b) maximum external rotation, (c) release of ball, and (d–f) follow through.

1991). This deceleration of the humerus allows the momentum to be transferred to the forearm and increases the rate of internal rotation of the humerus further accelerating the ball. The centrifugal force imposed on the ball and forearm extends the elbow joint. The rate of elbow extension is controlled by the antagonistic action of the elbow flexors. It is the combination of this high acceleration torque on the elbow, as well as the rapid rate of extension of the elbow that causes high shear forces to be imposed on the articular surfaces. The end of the acceleration phase occurs just before ball release. At this point, the external rotators such as the posterior deltoid and teres minor are beginning to contract to stop the arm. This allows a transfer of momentum to the hand and the ball, and the ball is released. The phase between stopping the acceleration of the arm and complete extension of the wrist with subsequent ball release is called the release point. This marks the beginning of the deceleration phase.

Deceleration. The deceleration phase lasts from point of ball release to the end of the humeral internal rotation. This is the most violent phase in the throwing mechanism. All the muscles of the shoulder are contracting violently during this phase (Bradley & Tibone, 1991). The acceleration phase of throwing has created an outward distraction force on the arm that is equal to the body weight. This force must be opposed to maintain stability of the glenohumeral joint. In addition to opposing this outward force, the muscles of the shoulder must decelerate the rotatory motions of the arm. Deceleration forces are much higher but of a much shorter duration than the acceleration forces. In addition, the elbow extension velocity must be decelerated to prevent hyperextension injuries. However, if elbow extension is decelerated too rapidly, the high flexion forces can cause overstress problems with the biceps tendon.

Follow-through. During the follow-through phase, the body moves forward with the arm to create a smooth transition of arm deceleration and reduction of the shoulder distraction force. This phase also allows balance to be regained. A smooth, full follow-through is associated with fewer deceleration injuries to the throwing arm.

Preseason and year-round conditioning

In order to maintain the level of performance at which today's athletes compete, an off-season programme that stresses conditioning, strength and flexibility is necessary (Feiring & Derscheid, 1989). Maintenance programmes should stress flexibility and strength (Derscheid, 1988) and include a good throwing programme.

Professional level pitchers will demonstrate increased flexibility in external rotation of the throwing shoulder (Bradley & Tibone, 1991). This allows for a more fluid delivery and generation of increased arm speed. Strength of the shoulder during the pitching motion provides for dynamic stability and prevents fatigue of the shoulder musculature. Balance must exist between the anterior and posterior muscles of the shoulder.

In assessing rehabilitation potential, frequently, posterior capsular tightness causing a decrease in internal rotation will be noted. Subtle signs of secondary impingement and scapular winging are occasionally found. It is now recognized that a tight posterior capsule in the throwing athlete must be eliminated to allow for appropriate posterior translation of the humerus (Silliman & Hawkins, 1991). Capsular tightness preventing normal posterior translation of 6–10 mm at the extreme of external rotation, may result in impingement secondary to anterior subluxation.

Considerable information exists in the literature that describes the theoretical and practical benefits of preseason conditioning. In theory, a clear relationship exists between preseason conditioning and injury prevention. Less clear is evidence that shows that preseason conditioning has a causal effect on the prevention of injuries on the field. The reason for this disparity between laboratory and field research is the difficulty in controlling for events on the field that affect the valid interpretation of data (Derscheid, 1988; Feiring & Derscheid, 1989). General and specific training will help prevent athletic injuries that might occur during the season. To maximize this benefit, the exercise programme must simulate as closely as possible the sport for which the athlete is training (Feiring & Derscheid, 1989).

The preseason evaluation is an important aspect of the evaluation of the high-performance athlete. It gives an indication of the condition of the athlete and should detect deficiencies that may lead to injury. For instance, it is assumed that with a bilateral comparison that no more than a 10% difference in muscle function is acceptable (Davies, 1984; Åstrand, 1987). More than a 10% difference indicates a muscle that is predisposed to injury, and strength conditioning is recommended to bring it to the acceptable level (Davies, 1984).

In conditioning for a sport, one of the most critical aspects of that training is sports specificity (Feiring & Derscheid, 1989). Specific training techniques should create the muscle function needed to prevent injuries during a specific activity. As previously stated, cardiovascular, flexibility and resistance exercises should all be constructed to meet the specific demands of the sport.

A complete preseason and maintenance programme should stress three major areas: (i) cardiovascular endurance; (ii) flexibility; and

(iii) strength. Each area has a specific role in preventing injury.

Cardiovascular exercise has multiple benefits. The increased aerobic endurance provided by cardiovascular exercise improves muscle conditioning which prevents injury by preventing muscular fatigue. The fact that fatigue of the muscles stabilizing a joint leads to injury of that joint is true in any sport but is especially important in injuries of the throwing shoulder. Cardiovascular conditioning may have a role in joint injury prevention due to the elimination of extra stress placed across the joint by the mass effect of the fat, which has no joint stabilizing properties (Fleck & Falkel, 1986).

The relationship of flexibility to injury prevention and improved performance has become more clearly defined. Improved flexibility increases the muscle–tendon unit's efficiency of action by accommodating the stress imposed on it and dissipating impact shock (Fleck & Falkel, 1986).

Resistance training is the exercise of choice with strength programmes. There are many positive effects of resistance training to the structural integrity of the joint. If the muscle–tendon unit and its corresponding joint are stressed in a constructive manner, the structural integrity of this complex is improved (Åstrand, 1987). Many researchers believe that connective tissue is the key element in improving the structure and function of the muscle–tendon complex. Resistance training has been shown to increase the thickness, weight and strength of tendon and ligaments (Fleck & Falkel, 1986).

Resistance and flexibility training of the muscle–tendon unit increases the dynamic stability of the joint to support the passive protection of the ligaments. This protection has been advocated for the knee, ankle, elbow and shoulder.

Warm-up procedures increase the intramuscular temperature so that the load at which muscle fails is increased (Åstrand, 1987). Isokinetic training is recommended for resistance training because of its specificity of training effect (Ellenbecker *et al.*, 1988). Conditioning intensity should be increased based on performance level (Derscheid, 1988). At higher levels of athletic performance there is an increased risk of injury.

Mechanism of injury

Shoulder injuries

ANTERIOR IMPINGEMENT

During the throwing motion, the humeral head and its overlying biceps tendon/rotator cuff must pass rapidly under the coracoacromial arch composed of the anterior acromion and the coracoacromial ligament. Impingement of these structures by the coracoacromial arch may occur by several mechanisms. First, increase in the size of the structures passing underneath the arch may lead to impingement. This can occur either by hypertrophy of the muscle–tendinous cuff or by inflammation of the cuff. Second, decreased space available underneath the arch secondary to osteophyte formation of the acromion and fibrosis of the subacromial space may lead to impingement. Third, weakness or incompetence of the rotator cuff allows the humerus to ride up and impinge against the coracoacromial arch with motion of the shoulder.

POSTERIOR TENSION INJURIES

As described, the deceleration phase of throwing is the most violent in the entire throwing mechanism. The muscles about the shoulder must contract to oppose the outward distraction force of the arm, which can approach approximately body weight to maintain stability of the glenohumeral joint. These forces must also decelerate the rotatory motions of the arm. These deceleration torques are nearly twice as great as the acceleration torque on the arm. It is in this phase of throwing that the decelerating rotator cuff muscles may fail under tension and cause the posterior tension failure rotator cuff tears.

AVULSION INJURIES

Avulsion of the anterosuperior labrum at the insertion of the biceps tendon is a well-described lesion in the throwing shoulder of pitchers. It is during the violent deceleration phase that the biceps tendon is actively contracting to oppose extension of the elbow. This eccentric contraction of the biceps, to decelerate the elbow is transmitted to its proximal attachment. As the humerus is rapidly internally rotated, additional forces are placed on the biceps tendon between its position in the bicipital groove and its attachment to the glenoid tubercle. It is the combination of these two forces that can result in avulsion of the anterosuperior labrum at the site of the biceps insertion.

ANTERIOR LAXITY

As with the posterior tension injuries, repetitive injuries leading to anterior laxity occur during the deceleration phase of throwing. As the muscles about the shoulder contract to oppose the outward distraction and internal rotation of the humerus, anterior translation of the humerus on the glenoid occurs. This anterior translation results in repetitive microtrauma to the anterior labrum and capsular structures. This repetitive microtrauma to the anterior structures results in anterior labral tears and capsular laxity.

Elbow injuries

MEDIAL TENSION INJURIES

Medial tension injuries occur during the acceleration phase of throwing. During this phase, there is a transfer of anterior momentum from the anteriorly rotating trunk into the shoulder and arm. Additional momentum is supplied by the anterior muscles, pectoralis major and subscapularis, contracting to increase the acceleration of the humerus in an anterior direction. At this time, there is also a significant contribution by the shoulder internal rotators, subscapularis, latissimus dorsi and the teres major, which are all contracting to start the internal rotation of the humerus. It is at this point in the acceleration phase that tremendous forces are generated in the humerus. The forearm, hand and the ball are essentially left behind the anteriorly rotating trunk and humerus. This results in extreme valgus stress at the elbow producing significant tensile forces across the medial side of the elbow joint.

LATERAL COMPRESSION INJURIES

During the acceleration phase of throwing, the lateral side of the elbow also experiences abnormal forces. Extreme compression forces result between the radial head and capitellum when the elbow is subjected to this valgus moment. It is at this phase that the lateral compression injuries occur.

POSTERIOR COMPRESSION INJURIES

As the forearm and ball are accelerated, significant centrifugal forces are generated and an extension force across the elbow occurs that subjects the posterior aspect of the elbow to compression and shear injuries. This results in impingement in the posteromedial olecranon fossa with subsequent osteophyte formation of the posterior and posteromedial aspect of the olecranon and chondromalacia of the olecranon fossa.

Evaluation of specific lesions

Primary impingement

Primary impingement can be defined as compressive cuff disease caused directly by the shape of the acromion, such as a type III hooked acromion (Bigliani *et al.*, 1986), or an os acromiale. It can also be caused by prominence of the acromioclavicular joint or occasionally by hypertrophy of the coracoacromial ligament.

Compressive cuff disease results in an outside-in type of rotator cuff tear.

Throwing and serving motions that require using the arm in a fully flexed, adducted and internally rotated position are likely to produce impingement symptoms. This is reproducible on physical examination by forceful forward flexion — a positive impingement sign (Hawkins & Kennedy, 1980). Pain relief by injecting 1% lignocaine into the subacromial space helps confirm the diagnosis. Most patients respond to a conservative programme of relative rest, non-steroidal anti-inflammatory medication, and progressive rotator cuff strengthening and stretching exercises (Andrews & Angelo, 1991).

If the athlete's symptoms are not relieved by non-operative measures, surgical treatment may be warranted. Arthroscopy of the subacromial space may reveal bursitis that can be easily debrided with a motorized resector. If impingement of the rotator cuff by the acromion or the coracoacromial arch complex is visible, an acromioplasty and coracoacromial ligament resection is performed to decompress the subacromial space. Approximately 8 mm of the anterior acromion is removed extending medially to the acromioclavicular joint. If there is partial tearing of the superior surface of the rotator cuff, this is debrided to healthy, bleeding tissue. At this time, the humeral head is rotated to assess the adequacy of the amount of space available between the acromion and the rotator cuff.

Arthroscopic decompression of the subacromial space has minimal morbidity because the insertion of the deltoid is not violated (Jobe & Glousman, 1991). It also allows for early rehabilitation, which in turn allows for earlier return to competition (Fig. 28.4).

Secondary impingement

Impingement may be secondary to another underlying problem, such as glenohumeral instability (Jobe & Glousman, 1991). The correct diagnosis is mandatory, as treatment includes alleviating the primary problem. The patient may present only with a complaint of pain; therefore, a thorough history and physical examination must be performed. Emphasis should be placed on comparing range of motion and anterior/posterior translation of the humeral head to the opposite shoulder. Generalized ligamentous laxity should be noted. A special test that is helpful is the Lachman test of the shoulder. With the patient supine and the shoulder abducted 90°, an anterior force is applied to the humeral head to assess the tension and end-point of the anterior capsule.

If anterior laxity is evident, treatment options in this situation include rehabilitation with an emphasis on dynamic stabilization by muscular strengthening if only mild instability is present.

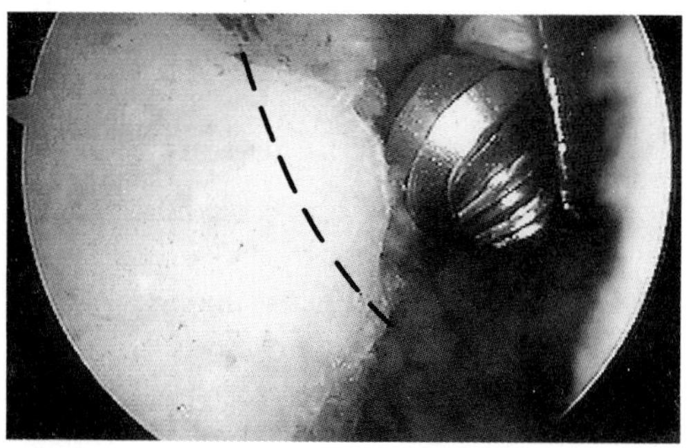

(a)

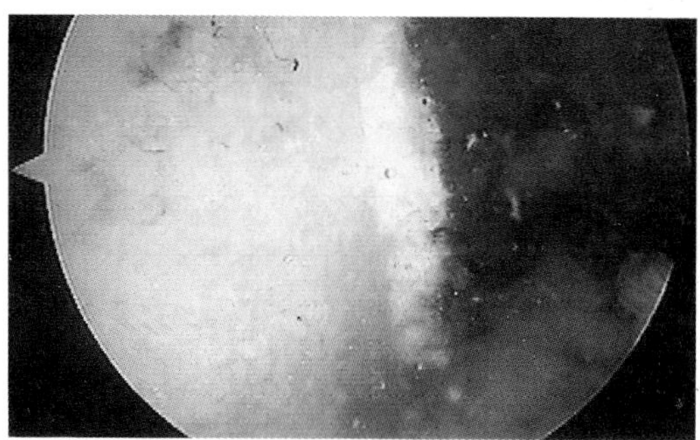

(b)

Fig. 28.4 Arthroscopic pictures of subacromial decompression. (a) Burr taking off bone; (b) the decompressed bony area.

If this fails, arthroscopic or open stabilization may be warranted.

Another cause of secondary impingement is primary rotator cuff failure from tensile overload. This failure occurs because of repetitive tensile overloading of the cuff as is seen in the deceleration phase of throwing. These forces encountered in athletic activity may ultimately exceed the ability of both the dynamic stabilizers to compensate, which may lead to secondary impingement phenomenon of the rotator cuff (Jobe & Glousman, 1991). Again, rehabilitation may be the first line of treatment; if this fails, arthroscopic debridement of the tensile tear is performed together with anterior stabilization and/or decompression of the coracoacromial arch as necessary.

Tensile lesions

The tensile lesions usually seen in the athlete's shoulder occur as undersurface rotator cuff tears and/or biceps–labral complex tears. The mechanism of injury in a primary tensile rotator cuff tear is deceleration of the rotator cuff as it resists horizontal adduction and internal rotation during the deceleration phase of throwing resulting in tensile and eccentric overload failure. Partial tears usually ensue secondary to repetitive microtrauma (Andrews & Angelo, 1991). These are found in the region of the undersurface of the supraspinatus tendon and may extend posterior to the area of the infraspinatus tendon. These tears may also be found isolated to the infraspinatus tendon and the posterior cuff and capsule.

The athlete may experience pain during the pitching motion. On physical examination, tenderness may be elicited over the supraspinatus and/or infraspinatus tendons; obvious weakness of the rotator cuff is not usually present. CT arthrogram or MRI may reveal a partial undersurface tear of the rotator cuff. Initially, the athlete is started on a rehabilitation programme with emphasis on strengthening the rotator cuff.

If there is no improvement over 2–3 months, arthroscopy may reveal a partial tear of the undersurface of the rotator cuff at its insertion into the humeral head. Arthroscopic debridement with a motorized shaver is performed to healthy bleeding tissue (Andrews *et al.*, 1985a; Andrews & Angelo, 1991). Inspection of the subacromial space is also performed. Frequently, there are no signs of impingement intraoperatively, but in chronic cases secondary impingement may be present with further tearing of the outer surface of the rotator cuff. In these cases, subacromial decompression with an acromioplasty should be performed.

Andrews *et al.* (1985a) reported on 34 athletes with partial tears who underwent arthroscopic debridement. 76% had an excellent result; 9% had a good result; and all were able to return to their previous athletic activities. 15% were rated as poor results and were not able to return to competitive throwing.

Debridement of partial rotator cuff tears appear to reduce the pain in the athlete's shoulder sufficiently to enable him or her to engage in a programme of progressive strengthening exercises (Andrews & Angelo, 1991).

Biceps–labral complex tears are thought to occur during the deceleration and follow-through phase of throwing. Large forces are placed on the proximal attachment of the biceps tendon as the humerus internally rotates at the same time as the biceps eccentrically contracts to decelerate elbow extension (Andrews *et al.*, 1985b, 1991). There may also be some type of concurrent entrapment of the biceps–labral complex associated with glenohumeral laxity.

Physical examination may reveal a popping or catching when the arm is in full abduction and external rotation brought out by circumducting the humeral head on the glenoid — the 'clunk test'. This test is performed with the patient in the supine position (Andrews *et al.*, 1991). The examiner's hand lies posterior to the humeral head applying an anteriorly directed force, while the opposite hand rests on the distal humerus, rotating the humerus. The patient's arm is brought into the full overhead position assessing for a clunk or grind in the shoulder suggesting a labral tear.

At arthroscopy, a tear of the labrum in the anterosuperior quadrant at the insertion of the long head of the biceps is evident. A partial tear of the biceps tendon near its origin may also be evident. Andrews *et al.* (1985b) suggest a mechanism for the anterosuperior glenoid labral tear. In 73 shoulder, arthroscopies performed in pitchers and throwing athletes with labral tears showed that 83% had glenoid labral tearing at the biceps–labral complex anterosuperiorly. Electrical stimulation of the biceps in five patients at arthroscopy produced tension in the biceps tendon and lifting up of the superior labrum off the glenoid. Andrews *et al.* hypothesized that this eccentric contraction may cause tearing of the anterosuperior labrum.

Treatment for this lesion usually entails conservative arthroscopic debridement of the labral tear, as well as the biceps tendon if it is partially torn (Andrews & Angelo, 1991). Infrequently, the tear may propagate into the superior attachment of the middle and inferior glenohumeral ligaments with subsequent instability present. If this is the case, the lesion should be repaired. Arthroscopic debridement is followed by rehabilitation.

Glenohumeral laxity

Most of the time, the diagnosis of shoulder laxity can be made on the basis of the history and physical findings. The athlete may have a history of a documented anterior dislocation with subsequent redislocations, or alternatively, the athlete may only present with the complaint of pain, clicking or the so-called 'dead arm' syndrome (Zarins & Rowe, 1984). In this syndrome, the athlete feels a sudden sharp or paralysing pain when the shoulder is forcibly, externally rotated in the abducted overhead position.

The most reliable finding on physical examination is the apprehension test, in which the abducted arm is rotated externally while forward pressure is exerted on the humeral head. This pushes the humeral head forward against the anterior capsule. If the patient experiences pain and apprehension, this suggests anterior instability.

Approximately one-half of the patients with shoulder subluxation are unaware of it (Zarins *et al.*, 1985). Therefore, physical examination, radiography and arthroscopy become important aids in the diagnosis (O'Brien *et al.*, 1983; Zarins *et al.*, 1985; Ellman, 1988; McGlynn & Caspari, 1991).

A decision must be made concerning the treatment plan. Athletes with mild instability may be tried with strengthening exercises first (O'Brien *et al.*, 1983) if this fails, then further intervention may be warranted. Those athletes with severe instability may certainly require an open stabilization procedure.

If there is an early true Bankart's lesion, arthroscopic repair may be performed as described by Caspari (1991), Johnson (1986) and Morgan and Bodenstab (1987) (Fig. 28.5). At the American Academy of Orthopaedic Surgeons Meeting in 1989, Caspari (1991) reported a 4% recurrence rate and a 4% one-time resubluxation rate for the arthroscopic Bankart's repair with 90% good or excellent results (Wallace, 1988). Regardless of this early enthusiasm for the arthroscopic repair of the unstable shoulder, most surgeons still do not recommend this procedure for those athletes going back to contact sports.

To date, limited experience exists regarding arthroscopic treatment of posterior instability. Treatment considerations are the same as for anterior instability (Schwartz *et al.*, 1987). Most athletes will respond to an aggressive exercise programme, especially those with generalized ligamentous laxity. Arthroscopy should be considered in those who fail an adequate trial of conservative therapy. Again, a thorough examination under general anaesthesia is mandatory. Arthroscopic debridement of labral lesions may decrease the athlete's pain sufficiently enough to allow him or her to return to competition. Reverse Bankart's lesion may be

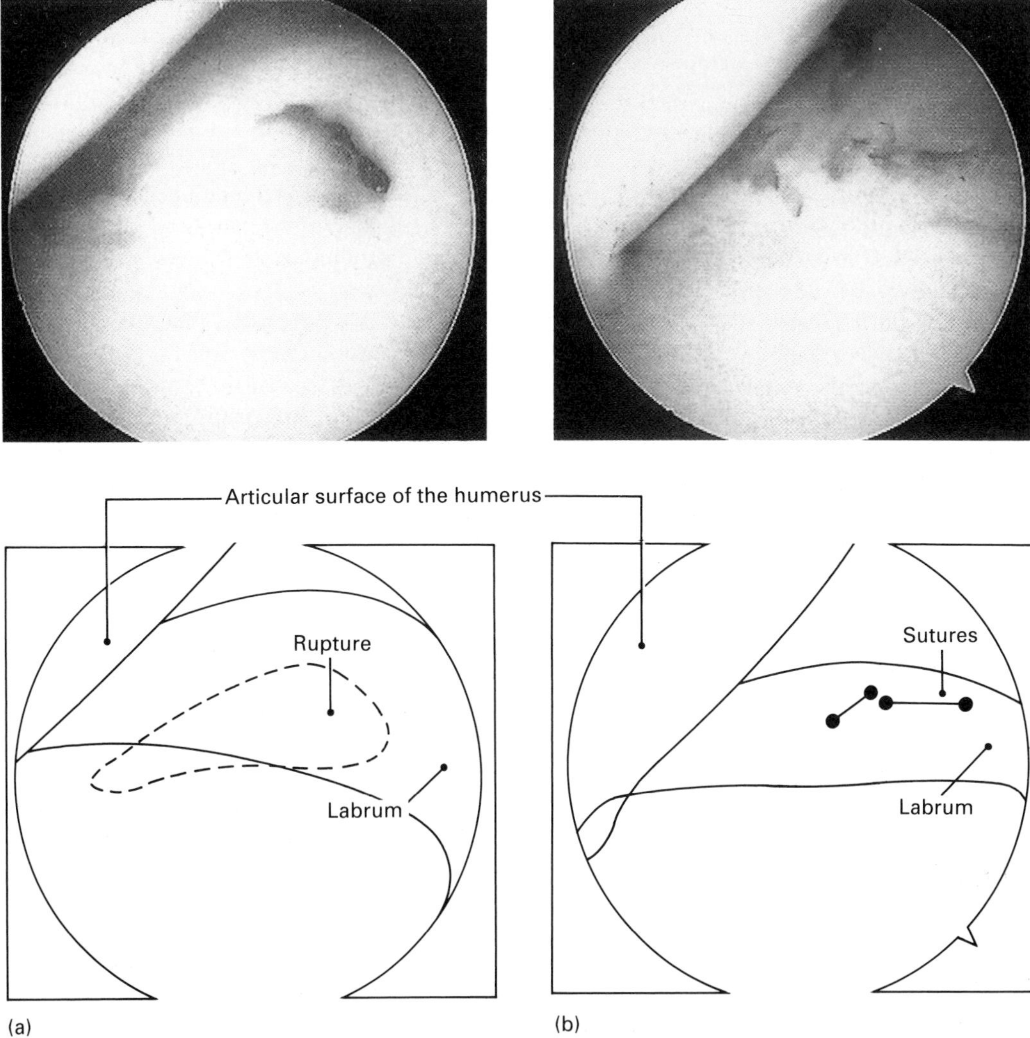

Fig. 28.5 Arthroscopic and line pictures of an anterior labral detachment (a) and repair (b).

repaired arthroscopically although most may require open stabilization procedures.

Glenoid labral tears

Not all labral tears are associated with instability (Ellman, 1988). A tear of the upper half of the labrum may occur with throwing and racquet sports or with some other type of deceleration injury. The mechanism of labral tearing can be due to repetitive overhead activity as in pitching, tennis, swimming, etc. (Andrews *et al.*, 1991). It may also be due to forceful entrapment of the labrum between the humeral head and the glenoid rim, such as a player diving to catch a baseball on the outstretched arm. A significant percentage of labral tears in the throwing athlete involve the anterosuperior portion near the insertion of the long head of the biceps tendon and are not associated with instability (Andrews & Gidumal, 1987). Pappas *et al.* (1983) noted a functional instability from the torn hypermobile labrum. There was no increase in glenohumeral translation, yet the patient felt insecure about their shoulder. They theorized that there was clicking, catching or locking in the joint secondary to the intermittent interposition of a partially attached fragment or bucket-handle tear between the glenoid and humeral head. One must be cautious that these functional tears may represent occult laxity and may lead to overt instability. Arthroscopy is indicated in the athlete with symptoms of catching, etc., who on physical examination may demonstrate a positive 'clunk test' (Andrews *et al.*, 1991). Labral pathology is debrided arthroscopically and the debridement should be carried out to a stable rim (Fig. 28.6).

Andrews *et al.* (1985b) reported on arthroscopy in 73 athletes with labral tears and found 83% with anterosuperior tears. After arthroscopic debridement, 88% had good to excellent results at 13.5 months follow-up.

Throwers' exostosis

The finding of a posterior glenoid exostosis in throwers with shoulder pain was first described in 1941 by Bennett, who studied a group of professional baseball players (in Andrews & Angelo, 1991). The exostosis is located at approximately the 8 o'clock position on the glenoid and is probably a secondary reaction associated with repeated microtrauma and tearing of the posterior and inferior capsule off its glenoid insertion (Andrews & Angelo, 1991). For many years it was thought that the exostosis was calcification in the long head of the triceps tendon insertion (Fig. 28.7). Personal open surgical inspection of this lesion by the senior author (J.R.A.) has proved that it is not in the triceps insertion in most cases.

The exostosis is visualized arthroscopically from the anterior portal using a 70° arthroscope. Resection is accomplished arthroscopically. Although there have been no published results of this procedure, arthroscopic resection had

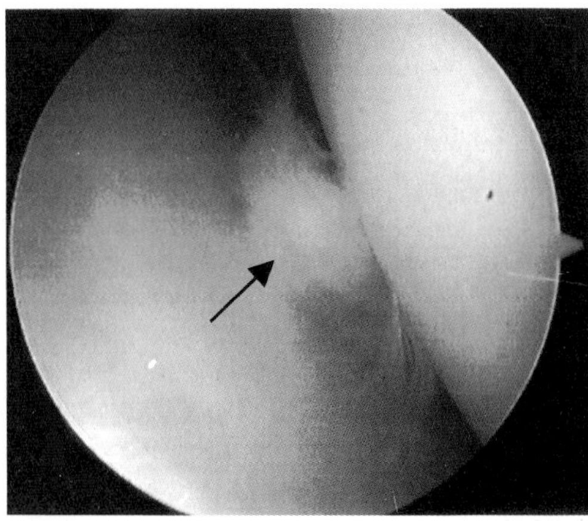

Fig. 28.6 Arthroscopic picture of a glenoid labral tear (arrow).

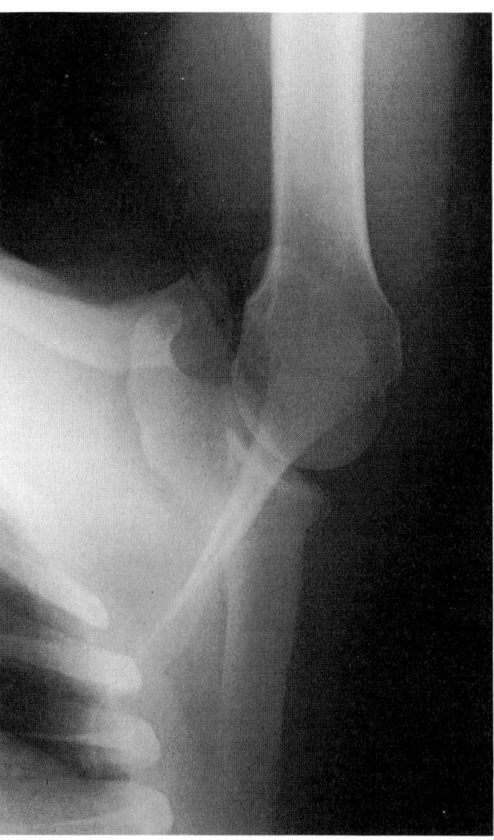

Fig. 28.7 Radiograph of a thrower's exostosis as seen in the Stryker view.

been performed on a number of pitchers with relief of their symptoms allowing them to return to competitive pitching.

Acromioclavicular joint injuries

Athletes who lift weights as part of their training programme and weightlifters are prone to acromioclavicular joint injuries. These include osteolysis of the distal clavicle secondary to longitudinal shear of compressive forces across the joint and partial or complete acromioclavicular joint separations secondary to post-traumatic injury to the joint. The athlete usually complains of a dull ache or pain over the acromioclavicular joint. Conservative treatment is tried first, consisting of non-steroidal anti-inflammatory medication, physical therapy, modification of physical and finally, steroid injection into the joint. If this fails, arthroscopic debridement of the acromioclavicular joint may be performed.

Valgus extension overload of the elbow

As a result of the extreme valgus forces transferred to the elbow from the trunk and shoulder during the pitching motion, a spectrum of injury across the medial aspect of the elbow occurs. Included are flexor/pronator mass tendinitis or medial epicondylitis, ulnar nerve neuritis, injury to the ulnar collateral ligament, and posteromedial olecranon osteophyte formation.

Evaluation of medial elbow pain in throwers requires a systematic and thorough elbow examination to elucidate the exact location of the injury. Initially, inspection of the elbow is important to compare the throwing elbow with the patient's non-throwing elbow. Frequently, hypertrophy of the musculature of the throwing elbow will be noted. The range of motion of the elbow is evaluated and may demonstrate a decrease in the extension of the affected elbow. Determining the specific location of tenderness is paramount in making the correct diagnosis as the structures on the medial aspect of the elbow lie in close proximity. Palpation of the medial epicondyle, the flexor muscle mass, the ulnar collateral ligament, the ulnar nerve and the posterior olecranon is necessary.

Valgus extension results from the centrifugal forces generated as the ball is accelerated causing extension and shear forces across the posteromedial aspect of the olecranon. The patient will complain of pain during the late cocking phase of throwing or during the deceleration phase of the pitching motion in advanced stages of the disease. On physical examination of the elbow, the location of the pain is on the posteromedial aspect of the olecranon. The ulnar collateral ligament is stable to stress testing unless injury has occurred to this ligament. The valgus extension overload test is positive and demonstrates pain on the posterior aspect of the olecranon with forceful extension of the elbow on valgus load applied by the examiner. Radiographs may demonstrate a posteromedial osteophyte on the olecranon in advanced stages of the process. Early radiographs may be normal. A CT arthrogram of the elbow will help demonstrate a posteromedial osteophyte or a loose body in the olecranon fossa which tend to occur frequently with valgus extension overload. The CT arthrogram will also help delineate the integrity of the ulnar collateral ligament.

Treatment consists of an initial trial of conservative therapy including physical therapy and anti-inflammatories. This period of active rest allows the patient to rehabilitate the arm and maintain conditioning but removes the repetitive trauma that the throwing motion causes in the elbow. If symptoms persist, or return when the patient returns to throwing, surgical treatment may be warranted. Arthroscopic evaluation of the elbow is performed with evaluation of the integrity of the ulnar collateral ligament by direct visual inspection and stress testing. Arthroscopic debridement of the posterior olecranon osteophyte and removal of loose bodies prevents impingement of the osteophyte on the olecranon fossa during elbow extension.

Ulnar collateral ligament instability

As the elbow is placed in the extreme valgus position during the throwing act, the resultant varus moment placed on the ulnar collateral ligament is approximately three times the force required to rupture the ulnar collateral ligament in the laboratory setting (W.P. Smutz *et al.*, unpublished data). This information indicates the dynamic stability imparted to the medial aspect of the elbow during throwing. With these large forces, the ulnar collateral ligament is exposed to repetitive microtrauma and prone to injury.

Using the motion–analysis technique with high-speed videography, the mean peak varus torque is calculated to 107 +/− 23 nM. Mean ultimate torque measured from cadaver tests was 32.9 +/− 5.4 nM. These results indicate that the ulnar collateral ligament is subjected to loads that exceed the maximum strength during each pitch. This supports the theory that injury or failure of the ulnar collateral ligament is a cumulative trauma injury and that some injury occurs to it during each pitch (Smutz *et al.*, personal communication).

The patient will notice pain during the late cocking and early acceleration phase of throwing. They may also describe a marked decrease in the velocity of their pitches and a loss of accuracy.

On physical examination, it is very important to locate specifically the tenderness on palpation. The course of the ulnar collateral ligaments runs from the medial epicondyle of the humerus to insert on the coronoid process of the ulna. Palpation of this area will reveal tenderness deep to the flexor/pronator muscle mass origin, which is also on the medial epicondyle of the humerus. Manual stress testing of this ligament is difficult to perform, and the subtle laxity difficult to detect clinically.

Following a 2–3 month period of active rest and rehabilitation of the elbow, if symptoms persist, further evaluation is necessary including a CT arthrogram of the elbow to determine if a complete tear of the ulnar collateral ligament exists. If the CT arthrogram is non-contributory regarding competency of the ulnar collateral ligament, diagnostic arthroscopy is indicated to evaluate and stress the ligament under direct arthroscopic visualization. If instability is demonstrated, an open reconstruction of the ulnar collateral ligament is indicated in patients who wish to continue on a competitive level. Conway *et al.* (1992) reported their 2-year results of reconstruction of the ulnar collateral ligament. Their follow-up showed 68% good to excellent results with this procedure, however the return of throwers to their previous level of competition was less successful.

Conclusion

Due to the many pathological conditions that often develop in the throwing athlete, it is obviously very important that concentrated attempts to prevent throwing injuries be made. Important in this effort include proper biomechanics, preseason and continuous maintenance conditioning programmes.

References

Anderson, T.E. & Ciocek, J. (1989) Specific rehabilitation programs for the throwing athlete. *American Academy of Orthopaedic Surgeons Institutional Course Lectures*, Vol. 38, pp. 487–91. CV Mosby, St Louis.

Andrews, J.R. & Angelo, R.L. (1991) Shoulder arthroscopy for the throwing athlete. In L.E. Paulos & J.E. Tibone (eds) *Operative Techniques in Shoulder Surgery*, pp. 79–84. Aspen Publishers, Maryland.

Andrews, J.R., Broussard, T.S. & Carson, W.G. (1985a) Arthroscopy of the shoulder in the management of partial tears of the rotator cuff: a preliminary report. *Arthroscopy* **1**, 117–22.

Andrews, J.R., Carson, W.G. & McLeod, W.D. (1985b) Glenoid labrum tears related to the long head of the biceps. *Am. J. Sports Med.* **13**, 337–41.

Andrews, J.R. & Gidumal, R.H. (1987) Shoulder arthroscopy in the throwing athlete: Perspectives and prognosis. *Clin. Sports Med.* **6**, 565–71.

Andrews, J.R., Kupferman, S.P. & Dillman, C.J. (1991) Labral tears in throwing and racquet sports. *Clin. Sports Med.* **10**, 901–11.

Åstrand, P.O. (1987) Exercise physiology and its role in disease prevention and in rehabilitation. *Arch. Phys. Med. Rehab.* **68**, 305–8.

Bigliani, L.U., Morrison, D.S. & April, E.W. (1986) The morphology of the acromion and its relationship to rotator cuff tears. *Orthop. Trans.* **10**, 216.

Bradley, J.P. & Tibone, J.E. (1991) An electromyographic analysis of the pitching motion. *Clin. Sports Med.* **10**, 789–805.

Caspari, R.B. (1991) Arthroscopic reconstruction for anterior shoulder instability. In L.E. Paulos & J.E. Tibone (eds) *Operative Techniques in Shoulder Surgery*, pp. 57–63. Aspen Publishers, Maryland.

Conway, J.E., Jobe, F.W., Glousman, R.E. & Pink, M. (1992) Medial instability of the elbow in throwing athletes. *J. Bone Joint Surg.* **74A**, 72–83.

Davies, G.J. (1984) *A Compendium of Isokinetics in Clinical Usage*. Simon & Schuster, Wisconsin.

Derscheid, H.L. (1988) Conditioning for the throwing student athlete. *Student Athlete* **1**, 6–8.

Ellenbecker, T.S., Davies, G.J. & Rowinski, M.J. (1988) Concentric versus eccentric isokinetic strengthening of the rotator cuff. *Am. J. Sports Med.* **16**, 64–9.

Ellman, H. (1988) Shoulder arthroscopy: current indications and techniques. *Orthopaedics* **11**, 45–51.

Feiring, D.C. & Derscheid, G.L. (1989) The role of preseason conditioning in preventing athletic injuries. *Clin. Sports Med.* **8**, 361–72.

Fleck, S.J. & Falkel, J.E. (1986) Value of resistance training for the reduction of sports injuries. *Sports Med.* **3**, 61–8.

Hawkins, R.J. & Kennedy, J.C. (1980) Impingement syndrome in athletes. *Am. J. Sports Med.* **8**, 151–7.

Jobe, F.W. & Glousman, R.E. (1991) Rotator cuff dysfunction and associated glenohumeral instability in the throwing athlete. In L.E. Paulos & J.E. Tibone (eds) *Operative Techniques in Shoulder Surgery*, pp. 85–91. Aspen Publishers, Maryland.

Johnson, L.L. (ed) (1986) *Arthroscopic Surgery, Principles and Practice*. Mosby, St Louis.

McGlynn, F.J. & Caspari, R.B. (1991) *Arthroscopic Findings in the Subluxation Shoulder*. Aspen Publishers, Maryland.

McKenzie, D.C., Taunton, J.E. & Clement, D.B. (1986) The prevention of running injuries. *Australian J. Sci. Med. Sport* **18**, 7–8.

Morgan, C.D. & Bodenstab, A.B. (1987) Arthroscopic Bankart suture repair: technique and early results. *Arthroscopy* **3**, 111.

O'Brien, S.J., Warren, R.F. & Schwartz, F. (1983) Anterior shoulder instability *Orthop. Clin. N. Am.* **18**, 395–408.

Pappas, A.M., Goss, T.P. & Kleinman, P.K. (1983) Symptomatic shoulder instability due to lesions of the glenoid labrum. *Am. J. Sports Med.* **11**, 279–88.

Schwartz, E., Warren, R.F., O'Brien, S.J. *et al.* (1987) Posterior shoulder instability. *Orthop. Clin. N. Am.* **18**, 409.

Silliman, J.F. & Hawkins, R.J. (1991) Current concepts and recent advances in the athlete's shoulder. *Clin. Sports Med.* **10**, 693–704.

Wallace, R.B. (1988) Application of epidemiological principles to sports injury research. *Am. J. Sports Med.* **16**(Suppl. 1), 22–3.

Zarins, B., Andrews, J.R. & Carson, W.G. (1985) *Injuries to the Throwing Arm.* WB Saunders, Philadelphia.

Zarins, B. & Rowe, C.R. (1984) Current concepts in the diagnosis and treatment of shoulder instability in athletes. *Med. Sci. Sports Exerc.* **16**, 444–8.

Further reading

Andrews, J.R. & Carson, W.G. (1984) The arthroscopic treatment of glenoid labrum tears in the throwing athlete. *Orthop. Trans.* **8**, 44.

Andrews, J.R., Carson, W.G. & Ortega K. (1984) Arthroscopy of the shoulder: technique and normal anatomy. *Am. J. Sports Med.* **12**, 1–7.

Åstrand, P.O. & Rodahl K. (1977) *Textbook of Work Physiology*, 2nd edn. McGraw-Hill, New York.

Fauls, D. (1985) General training techniques to warm up and cool down the throwing arm. In B. Zarins, J.R. Andrews & W.G. Carson (eds) *Injuries to the Throwing Arm*, pp. 266–76. WB Saunders, Philadelphia.

Fleisig, G.S., Dillman, C.J. & Andrews, J.R. (1989) Proper mechanics for baseball pitching. *Clin. Sports Med.* **1**, 151–70.

Glousman, R., Jobe, F.W., Tibone, J.E. *et al.* (1980) Dynamic electromyographic analysis of the throwing shoulder with glenohumeral instability. *J. Bone Joint Surg.* **70A**, 220–6.

Hurley, J.A. & Anderson, T.E. (1990) Shoulder arthroscopy: Its role in evaluating disorders in the athlete. *Am. J. Sports Med.* **18**, 480–3.

Yahiro, M.A. & Matthews, L.S. (1989) Arthroscopic stabilization procedures for recurrent anterior shoulder instability. *Orthop. Rev.* **18**, 1161.

Chapter 29

Injuries in Tennis

ROBERT P. NIRSCHL AND JANET SOBEL

All sport activities have positive and negative aspects. Tennis is no exception. The principles of treatment and prevention are often intertwined, especially those aspects of controlling overuse, and eliminating strength and flexibility deficits.

This chapter will review the issues specific to tennis. The wide variation in tennis activity invites an equally wide opportunity for a variety of injuries. As with other sport activities, if the individual's priority is to win, the injury potential is much higher. It is critical, therefore, to define and understand the goal of each individual participant.

Although the focus of this chapter is on the musculoskeletal system, it should be appreciated that a wide variety of problems do affect tennis players and play. These can include such wide-ranging possibilities as heat illness to drug use.

Goals of tennis

Tennis is a wonderful lifetime sport, and with appropriate supplemental exercises, can be an excellent tool for the achievement of consistent lifelong physical fitness. If the goal is, however, to win in a highly competitive atmosphere, the potential for fitness is often replaced by injury.

Other achievable goals of tennis include the development of highly sophisticated neuromuscular skill patterns and agility. The sport is also an excellent vehicle for social opportunity and teaches discipline, persistence and self-reliance. For the truly gifted, tennis offers the opportunity of financial rewards. Overall, tennis is a marvellous tool to achieve these goals in both youth and adulthood.

Demands of tennis

Tennis can be a stern taskmaster, and the imposed demands can challenge the individual both emotionally and physically. The coordination patterns of stroking one ball actually require the functions of running, catching, hitting and throwing. Learning these mechanical skill patterns can be frustrating, and the rigours of competition can challenge the strongest of egos.

Physical demands can result in a variety of deficiencies including acute injury, chronic overuse injury and musculotendinous imbalance predisposing to injury. The potential for injury is magnified by individual personal physical deficiencies brought to the sport by heredity, disease or prior injury. Common areas of tennis-imposed muscle–tendon imbalance include the elbow, shoulder, back and abdomen. Common acute injuries include ankle sprains, patellofemoral and meniscal knee problems, and muscle pulls of the back, abdomen and legs. Common overuse problems include tendinitis/tendinosis of the shoulder, elbow, patellar tendon, Achilles tendon and plantar fascia. In growing children, skeletal problems including apophysitis at the medial and posterior elbow, knee and os calcis are common. Osteochondritis of the elbow capitellum is not uncommon.

Prevention of injury

The overall concepts for the prevention and treatment of injury will be addressed in this chapter. The concepts of prevention take several forms. They are all designed to seek out and eliminate deficiencies or inadequacies in the player, equipment, technique, environment, or all of the above. All of these deficiencies can and do result in injury-produced overuse. The concepts of prevention include the following:

1 Fitness evaluation:
  (a) hereditary deficiency,
  (b) prior injury/disease,
  (c) performance capacity,
  (d) analysis of sports tendinitis/tendinosis-imposed body maladaptations, and
  (e) level of conditioning.

2 Training techniques.

3 Stroke mechanics.

4 Equipment:
  (a) shoes,
  (b) racquet,
  (c) grip size,
  (d) tennis balls,
  (e) playing surface, and
  (f) environment.

5 Counter force bracing.

6 Physiological considerations.

The following text will discuss these concepts in some detail. It should be noted that much biomechanical research needs to be done, as some of these conclusions are based on anecdotal evidence and intuitive reasoning. Nonetheless, the authors believe this discussion presents a solid base on which to expand our knowledge.

Fitness evaluation

As noted, tennis can impose substantial demands that either result in injury or the predisposition to injury through muscle–tendon imbalance. In addition, individual physical deficiency is often brought to the sport. Fitness evaluation is therefore a key ingredient in preventing injury and enhancing tennis performance.

In this regard, we have had an opportunity to play a role in the development of the United States Tennis Association (USTA) player development programme. It will be of interest to share some preliminary general fitness evaluation data on national level junior tennis players (16–18 years). The protocol includes testing for baseline conditioning, musculoskeletal durability and performance. This study focused on musculoskeletal durability with reference to individual physical hereditarial variations as well as tennis-imposed muscle–tendon imbalance and actual injury. Overall, of the first group of nationally ranked players who were tested, 70% were noted to have shoulder imbalances or injury. Elbow abnormalities, postural problems of the thoracolumbar area, abdominal problems, knee and ankle difficulties, and flexibility deficiencies were also quite common. The high incidence of shoulder problems in tennis is consistent with the reports of Kibler *et al.* (1988) and Priest (1988).

The message from this early preliminary data is quite clear. Even in élite, nationally ranked players, significant musculoskeletal deficiencies either resulting in, or predisposing to injury were present. It is likely therefore that in all tennis players, young and old, a significant percentage will have vulnerability problems that should be addressed before injury occurs. Resolution of these problems is undertaken by appropriate individual supplemental exercise programmes for strength, endurance, flexibility, aerobic and anaerobic capacity, agility and skill.

Training techniques

The majority of tennis players, whether adult or youth, do not participate in a meaningful, structured tennis training programme. The usual approach is merely to play. Adequate stroke mechanics may or may not be taught, and strategy for competitive play is sporadic. This typical approach often results in poor tennis mechanics, poor conditioning and muscle–tendon imbalance. All of these invite injury. If intense play, or a rapid escalation of frequency or duration of play, occurs (2–4 times·week^{-1}, 2–3 h sessions or greater), injury is common. Hard surfaces (cement or asphalt-based) are additionally punishing to the lower extremities. Use of a tennis backboard or a ball machine increases the number of ball impacts per unit of time, and also increases potential for overuse to the upper body.

Ideal training programmes include the following:

1 Obtain a quality fitness and performance examination such as the level III programme outlined in Table 29.1, adopted by our institution (Virginia Sports Medicine Institute) and the Lexington Clinic, as utilized in the USTA Touring Pro Program.

2 Obtain and perform supplemental exercises to eliminate deficiencies as identified in the fitness and performance examination (Nirschl & Sobel, 1988).

3 Implement equipment changes, counterforce bracing, or orthotics to supplement the deficiencies noted on the fitness and performance examination (Nirschl, 1973a; Sobel & Nirschl, 1981).

4 Start tennis training on a gradual basis (Dulany, 1986) for:

(a) stroke mechanics, and

(b) competitive strategy.

5 Although highly individualized, the following basic schedule for serious tennis play is suggested.

(a) Structured tennis programme 3 times·week^{-1} (2–3 h) with ample rest periods.

(b) Maintenance programme of supplemental exercises (1 h, 2 times·week^{-1}) after serious deficiencies have been eliminated by a quality medical rehabilitation programme (average achievement time 3 months) (Nirschl & Sobel, 1988).

(c) Random tennis play per skill level to a frequency and intensity that does not produce overuse injury.

(d) Fitness retesting is recommended every 6 months for competitive players to ensure that muscle–tendon imbalance is not recurring secondary to the imposed demands of the sport.

Table 29.1 Tennis fitness evaluation protocol.

History assessment
Musculoskeletal durability
varus valgus elbow angle
shoulder slope angle, scapular alignment and insufficiency
spinal postural alignment
Q angle (knees)
tibial os calcis alignment
foot posture
flexibility — shoulder, trunk, hip, knee and ankle
manual strength testing — shoulder, hip groups
grip strength (dynamometer)
grip (hand) size
Performance tests
upper body anaerobics (medicine-ball toss)
vertical jump
reaction time
hexagon test
fan ball drill
20-yard (18-m) dash
side-to-side shuffle
Baseline conditioning tests
submaximal aerobics
timed sit-ups
timed push-ups
sit–reach flexibility
lean body mass (calipers: three or six sites)
Isokinetic testing
Cybex 340 knee
Cybex 340 shoulder
Cybex 340 testing of clinically indicated areas

Stroke mechanics

As noted, a single tennis stroke encompasses all the attributes of a baseball game (e.g. running, catching, hitting and throwing). This is accomplished with the use of a 70 cm (28 in) lever (e.g. the racquet length). Frustration occurs often, as proper body position in relation to the ball requires speed and agility. In addition, the process of catching and hitting requires extreme focus on the ball–racquet interface, whereas the act of throwing requires some attention to the proposed target. Neuromuscular confusion is therefore commonplace, especially if attention to the target precedes the focus on the ball–racquet interface.

Tennis is further complicated by the variety of strokes involved. This variety includes ground strokes, volleying, half volleying, serves, overloads and lobs all with unlimited variation in spins, angles, velocities and grip positions.

INJURY-PRODUCING STROKE MECHANICS

In general, quality tennis players place high emphasis on the lower body (e.g. running and body balance). In contrast, inexperienced players place less or little emphasis on the lower body, and high emphasis on the upper body, thereby inviting arm overuse and injury (e.g. it is commonplace to run little and accept the ball in many arm overload positions). In addition to limited lower body speed and agility, inexperienced players lack the neuromuscular coordination for active use of the lower body and trunk so necessary for quality strokes. This coordination deficiency also invites arm overuse.

It should be noted that even with quality stroke mechanics (e.g. regional, national and élite tournament players) arm overuse does occur. In these instances of a large volume of play, a large repertoire of stroke variations including spins, and heavy punishing serves at high velocity are major contributors. It is also clear that today's high technology racquets allow players to 'cheat' on the time tested quality lower body stroke mechanics. This 'cheating of technique' by tournament (e.g. open body stances) as well as non-tournament players also invites arm overuse.

Equipment

SHOES

The tennis shoe is an extremely important part of tennis equipment. As noted, quality tennis play encompasses extremes of running with a high degree of agility in stop–start bursts. The shoe must accommodate to this activity while providing comfortable and adequate support. Tennis is also played on multiple surfaces (e.g. varieties of red and Har-Tru clay, rubber/asphalt, concrete, indoor carpet and grass). The outer sole must take into consideration these surface variations and indeed élite tournament players may have different shoes for these reasons.

A major problem is shoe fit. Indeed, the variation in individual foot size and anatomy seems infinite. Thus, a quality shoe in design terms may prove unsuccessful because of fit.

In general, the tennis shoe must be designed to accommodate side as well as forward and backward motion. The outer sole must adapt well to the playing surface and the midsole should absorb impact forces well. The insole should provide cushioned comfort and allow the opportunity to be replaced with a custom orthotic if need be.

In design, a firm heel counter, adequate toe box, multiple lacing system and a flexible forefoot are desirable.

RACQUETS

The selection of racquets incorporates the concepts of skill and tennis play as well as injury prevention. Powerful players with quality stroke mechanics often choose firm racquets with tight stringing to obtain additional ball control. Less powerful players often choose racquets and softer string tensions that deliver more ball velocity at the expense of control.

The needs of tennis play must be balanced against the needs of injury prevention. Although the data are clinical and anecdotal, it is our recommendation that the following racquet selection be utilized especially for symptomatic shoulder or tennis elbow injured arms.

1 Mid-sized racquet frame (580–710 cm^2 or 90–110 in^2 of hitting zone).

2 Graphite or graphite composite frame such as graphite plus fibreglass or kevlar); note that the majority of graphite composite racquets contain graphite as the major component.

3 Medium to moderate flexibility of the frame.

4 Medium to soft string tension.

5 Proper handle size.

The wide body technology of the 1990s has produced a new and exciting array of racquets which are lighter, stiffer and also impart greater energy into the ball. These racquets enhance the quality of play among all groups of players, novice to élite. This racquet technology appears, however, on the basis of anecdotal clinical observation, to have increased the incidence of arm injuries (e.g. tennis elbow and wrist).

The reasons for this apparent increased incidence of injury have not been investigated by scientific biomechanical analysis. It is our theory, however, that two explanations are likely. Firstly, as noted, these racquets allow a 'cheating of stroke mechanics' (e.g. high quality play is possible by use of arm strokes). Arm strokes invite injury. Secondly, the stiffness of wide body racquets likely imparts more energy to the arm (primarily torque rather than vibration). In view of the torque problem, we do not recommend a racquet hitting zone greater than 710 cm^2 (110 in^2).

The concept of vibration has been raised as a source of energy overload to the arm in association with ball impact. No scientific biomechanical data exists which has measured actual vibration energy in the arm. Theoretical considerations conclude that vibration is of much less importance than torque (twisting). There has, as well, been no medical clinical observations that suggest any aid in the prevention of treatment of elbow and wrist injuries by the use of antivibration devices. There is clinical observation, however, to support the concept of racquet change concerning wide body design, racquet stiffness, hitting zone size and string tension.

A final note in racquet selection concerns equipment size and weight. For best torsion control, a racquet handle size which fits the working size of the hand in our experience works best (see section on grip sizes). If error is to be made concerning grip size, it is best to err on the side of larger sizes (*re* torsion control). In growing children, suffice it to say, adult size equipment is inappropriate and potentially harmful.

PROPER GRIP SIZE

Regardless of which grip style is used (Eastern, continental or Western) problems stroking the ball properly will occur, unless the proper grip size is utilized. If the grip is too big, trouble occurs holding on to the racquet, especially on very hot days when hands sweat. Too small a grip, on the other hand, results in increased torque and can produce blisters.

For years, sporting goods store salesman and professional tennis shop assistants have fitted grips mainly on the basis of trial and error, asking how a particular grip 'feels'.

An accurate simple way to check grip size, is by the anthropometric palm crease factor. This method of grip size was developed by the senior author in 1973 (Nirschl, 1973b), and has stood the test of time. It is based upon anthropometric measurement of the working length of the hand. The length of the index and long finger divided by two equals the length of the ring finger. Measurement between the ring and long finger bisects the palm and the proximal palmar crease reflects to skin crease formed by the bend of the metacarpophalangeal (MP) joint. Using these parameters, measurement of the ring finger is ideal to determine proper grip size. The measurement (for example 10.8 cm (4.25 in) shown in Fig. 29.1) is the recommended grip size.

TENNIS BALLS

There are two basic types of tennis ball, vacuum hollow centre and hard core centre. Tennis balls may vary among manufacturers although there are official specifications from the tennis federations. The stiffness and elastic properties (coefficient of restitution of materials) and the outer 'fuzz' layer (regular and heavy duty) also

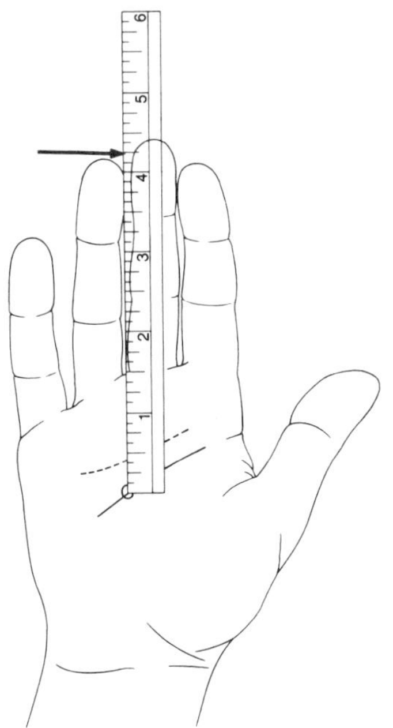

Fig. 29.1 Hand size measurement, Nirschl technique. Hand size measurement to determine proper grip handle size. Measure length of ring finger along the radial border from the proximal palmar crease to the ring finger tip. Measurement indicates working length of hand.

vary. In spite of slight variations, the usual fresh vacuum design balls are fairly consistent (56 g or 2 oz weight) and there is little to choose from in vacuum balls regarding prevention or treatment of injury.

Spent or 'dead' vacuum balls are another consideration. The impact forces are considerably greater and the opportunity for arm injury increases dramatically. This often occurs in practice sessions where a basket of 'dead balls' are hit in a short period of time.

Solid core balls, although long lasting, have also been noted to increase the incidence of arm symptoms.

It has also been observed that playing on wetter surfaces can increase the overuse phenomenon (e.g. moisture from watered clay surfaces is picked up by the ball increasing it's weight). In general, to prevent or treat overuse injuries of the arm, fresh vacuum balls are recommended.

PLAYING SURFACE

No discussion concerning the prevention of tennis injuries to the musculoskeletal system can be complete without court surface considerations. The size of a tennis court is universal, but the surfaces vary considerably, and surface variations affects not only the character of play, but the potential for injury. Injury prevention relative to the surfaces can be categorized as follows.

1 Consistent and unforgiving: (i) asphalt base; and (ii) concrete. These surfaces, also known as all-weather, have an essentially consistent surface dependent upon quality of construction and upkeep. The ball bounce is ordinarily not a problem, but speed of bounce and ball velocity often are. Late strokes are commonplace on these surfaces inviting arm overuse. Unforgiving surfaces are fatiguing and punishing to the legs and produce overuse problems to the legs (knees, shins, Achilles tendon and feet including stress fractures) are not uncommon. Adequate stroke mechanics to adjust to ball speed, and increased shoe padding plus adequate rest periods are recommended to prevent injury.

2 Inconsistent and unforgiving: indoor carpet. Indoor carpet is placed in this category as the usual situation, but depends upon the surface laid (e.g. concrete versus wood gymnasium floor), quality of taping job, and whether it is a travelling temporary or a permanent installation. All of the problems, as cited under category 1 may occur. In addition, bad bounces can increase the incidence of sudden arm overload and sticky surfaces can increase the potential of sudden unexpected stops (e.g. ligament sprains to knee and ankle).

3 Inconsistent and forgiving: (i) clay (red European type and Har-Tru). The velocity of the ball is less, therefore, stroke mechanics is less of a problem. Dependent upon upkeep, bad bounces are more prevalent. Hitting the tape with the ball or the foot can result in unexpected lurching and tripping of the body, and ball-producing injury. The forgiving surfaces are less likely to result in overuse injury to the legs. (ii) Grass. As with clay, the legs are better protected, but the ball velocity and bad ball bounces increase the incidence of arm problems.

Environment

Environmental factors are less of a direct threat to the musculoskeletal system. The major hazards in this category are heat and humidity with the resultant potential of heat exhaustion and ultimately heat stroke. At tournament level, there are times when the interest of the players come into conflict with the interests of the promoters.

At present, medical considerations have been subservient to the game in such areas as injury time out (e.g. play will be continuous), medical modification of the tennis match, and medical availability and consultation. For the good of the players and the game, the authors believe that amendments to the tennis rules of play need be implemented. Considerations in this regard include:

1 Cancellation of matches secondary to hot and humid weather.
2 Extension of the rest periods when environmental factors dictate.
3 Availability of sun-free enclosures during between-game change overs.
4 Specific accommodation for medical consultation and medical time outs during the course of play.

Counter force bracing

The term counter force bracing was introduced by the senior author (R.P.N.) in 1973 (Nirschl, 1973a,b). The concept of counter force bracing is to constrain the generation of internal muscle tension forces or prevent tendon migration. Applying a basically firm constraint in appropriate areas has been noted clinically to minimize the symptoms of medial and lateral tennis elbow. Analysis has also revealed biomechanical relevance including decreased angular acceleration and decreased muscle activity in the braced group (Groppel, 1986). The clinical success in pain relief has been reported by Froimson (1971) and the extensive use of the counter force concept attests to its wide acceptance. At present, counter force bracing is utilized at the elbow to prevent injury as well as being a treatment tool (Fig. 29.2). Overall, it has

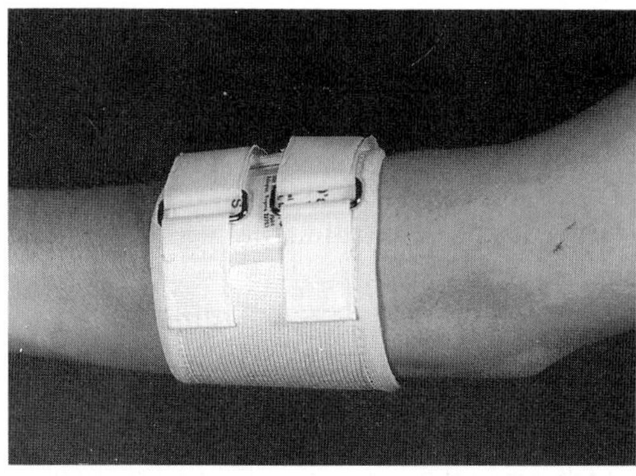

(a)

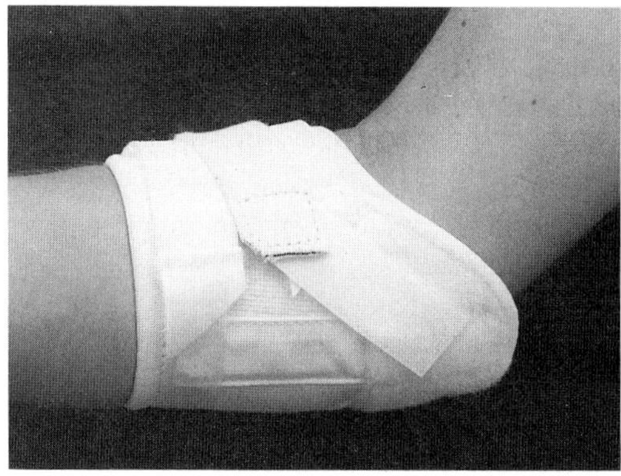

(b)

Fig. 29.2 Count R-Force elbow braces are used to decrease pain and control abusive force overloads. Adequate design includes multiple tension straps, wide dimensions, and curved contours to accurately fit conically shaped extremities. Local pressure points via solid materials or air cells are missed to avoid muscle imbalances. (a) Lateral elbow brace; (b) medial elbow brace. Courtesy of Medical Sports, Inc., Arlington, Virginia.

been clinically noted that a wide brace that controls all muscle groups in a comfortable balanced manner results in an effective control of pain in symptomatic elbow patients. This statement, although clinically evident needs clarification as the counter force principle has been altered by numerous manufacturers for reasons other than medical with resultant confusion and less than ideal success in many instances.

As noted in the sections on the demands of tennis and fitness evaluation, tennis imposes muscle imbalance maladaptations on the playing arm. These muscle imbalances and deficiencies have in the view of Kibler *et al.* (1988) and others, a direct relationship to fatigue, muscle–tendon overuse, and injury. The key concept in the counter force principle is to maintain effective (not excessive) constraint of internally generated tension on muscle–tendon units while maintaining essentially normal extremity function and muscle balance. To do otherwise, frustrates the rehabilitation process or invites injury. Braces which primarily constrain elbow, forearm or wrist motion or braces which actively seek muscle imbalance by concentrating pressure in one small area, either by pad or air cell do not adhere to the counter force principle.

Wrist abnormalities of the ulnocarpal and radiocarpal column are consistently controlled by wrist counter force braces that allow active finger and hand function.

In the lower extremity, shin splints, posterior tibial tendinitis, patellofemoral pain syndrome and plantar fasciitis are also aided by counter force bracing.

Metatarsalgia and symptomatic pronated feet are clinically aided by metatarsal pads and firm (not rigid) orthotics.

Common injuries

A wide variety of injuries occur secondary to tennis activities. As noted, however, many individual hereditarial and prior injury deficiencies are often brought to the sport. The most common musculoskeletal problems are as follows.

1 Tendon:
(a) tennis elbow tendinosis, lateral and medial,
(b) shoulder tendinitis/tendinosis (primarily the supraspinatus aspect of the rotator cuff),
(c) patellar tendinosis,
(d) Achilles tendinosis/peritendinitis,
(e) plantar fasciitis, and
(f) shin splint (posterior tibialis).

2 Ligament:
(a) wrist, triangular fibrocartilage and ulnar collateral ligament,
(b) ankle sprain (primarily lateral; anterior fibulotalar ligament),
(c) foot strain, fatigue, and
(d) knee instability (anterior cruciate ligament, collaterals).

3 Muscle:
(a) lumbar,
(b) calf (medial gastrocnemius),
(c) abdominal, and
(d) thigh (hamstring and adductors).

4 Joint:
(a) shoulder subluxation,
(b) wrist (distal radioulnar joint synovitis),
(c) knee (meniscal and patellofemoral),
(d) Wrist ganglion (radial carpal synovitis), and
(e) aggravation of pre-existent arthritis (neck, back, knee).

5 Apophysis:
(a) medial elbow (Little League elbow),
(b) knee, tibial tubercle (Osgood–Schlatter disease),
(c) os calcis (Siever's disease),
(d) vertebral (Scheuermann's disease), and
(e) posterior elbow (olecranon).

6 Skeletal elements:
(a) back, lumbar (spondylolysis),
(b) stress fracture of the tibia, and
(c) stress fracture of the metatarsals (foot).

7 Neural elements:
(a) ulnar nerve compression at elbow (neurapraxia),

(b) lumbar disc, and
(c) plantar neuroma (foot).

8 Skin:
(a) hand blisters, callouses,
(b) foot blisters,
(c) foot corns, callouses, and
(d) subungual haematoma (toe nail).

Overall, the injury experience at Virginia Sportsmedicine Institute has been equally divided between the upper and lower extremities. As noted, the lower extremity injuries are those typical of the running sports. The upper extremity problems are often more chronic, challenging and recalcitrant. The major recalcitrant problems in young players include (i) shoulder subluxation/tendinosis/tendinitis; and (ii) back and abdominal problems. Shoulder tendinitis is often associated with scapular weakness and subtle shoulder subluxation. Abdominal muscle pull and lumbar muscle–ligament strain often associated with thoracic kyphosis and lumbar lordosis are also quite common. Lumbar pars interarticularis stress fracture and lumbar disc disease must always be kept in mind, although statistically, these maladies are not common. As the individual matures to the later teenage years and adulthood, the problems clearly shift to the difficulties of tendon overload (e.g. tennis elbow and shoulder tendinosis). Meniscal and patellofemoral problems of the knee, and trunk problems (back and abdominal) are fairly common in the young adult to adult group as well.

Typical clinical presentations of common upper extremity tennis problems

The common chronic upper extremity problems most frustrating to both doctor and patient are the chronic overuse maladies of shoulder tendinosis/tendinitis, medial and lateral tennis elbow, and wrist problems of the radiocarpal and radioulnar columns. In the majority of instances, these problems are initiated by tennis play that is frequent, intense and of long duration (e.g. 2–4 times·week^{-1}, 2–3 h·session^{-1}) or with a sudden increase in activity after a lay-off of several months. The usual presentation of symptoms is gradual in onset after an intense session of practice (often in an attempt to change a stroke pattern). Poor stroke mechanics are often associated (e.g. inadequate elevation and poor lower body participation in the serve and overhead and late ground stroke patterns with excessive wrist snap) (Nirschl, 1973b, 1988; Kibler *et al.*, 1988). Young athletes often equate power with success and more likely than not, overhit most balls. Constant repetitive overload of this nature, not only incites symptoms of pain, but also induces muscle imbalances that further exaggerate pain symptoms and spread the area of injury vulnerability.

Shoulder tendinosis/tendinitis

The usual presenting symptom is pain with the activity of upward acceleration from the back scratch cocking position of the serve. The pain is characteristically located over the anterior rotator cuff and bicipital area with referred pain to the deltoid insertion on the proximal third of the humerus. Posterior pain over the infraspinatus insertion may be noted as well. Although rarely articulated by the patient, close questioning not uncommonly evokes the history of anterior subluxation of the glenohumeral joint. It is important, therefore, to perform subluxation tests designed to demonstrate anterior shoulder subluxation.

Clinical signs in the typical rotator cuff patient, reveal not only the classic areas of tenderness over the supraspinatus attachment point at the greater tuberosity, but stretched out and weak scapular muscles (positive rhomboid scapular winging) with tenderness over the levator scapulae attachment to the scapula and weak external rotator and abductor muscles (infraspinatus, supraspinatus, teres minor) (Kibler *et al.*, 1988).

Lateral tennis elbow tendinosis

The classical presenting symptom is pain just anterior and distal to the lateral epicondyle associated with wrist and finger extensor stress (e.g. drinking from a cup, shaking hands or hitting tennis backhands) (Nirschl, 1988). Wrist flexion or triceps–biceps activity causes no pain. Palpation over the extensor brevis origin causes exquisite pain, whereas palpation over the lateral epicondyle causes moderate or no pain. Resisted forearm pronation is usually painful, whereas supination is usually painless.

Medial tennis elbow tendinosis

The presenting symptom is pain at, and just distal to, the medial epicondyle associated with wrist flexion and forearm pronation stress (e.g. wrist flexor curls, shaving of the face, late tennis forehands or pronation and wrist snap with the serves). Palpation over the pronator teres and flexor carpi radialis at their attachment point to the medial epicondyle and just distal causes exquisite pain.

Associated findings may be a positive Tinel's sign at zone 3 of the medial epicondylar groove in the area of the ulnar nerve penetration through the flexor ulnaris arcade (e.g. neurapraxia of ulnar nerve) (Nirschl, 1988) (Fig. 29.3). In addition, close examination may reveal evidence of medial collateral ligament insufficiency as manifested by positive valgus instability testing or pain noted at the ligament attachment area on the medial epicondyle.

Medial epicondylar apophysitis (Little League elbow)

Medial apophysitis is the youth version of medial tennis elbow. Since the pathological changes occur at the medial epicondylar apophysis, however, the pain and palpable tenderness are located directly on the medial epicondyle. Pain is noted with valgus stress either by clinical examination or in the throwing/serve motion. Signs should also be sought on the lateral elbow, as osteochondritis of the capitellum can be a companion problem. X-rays may reveal fragmentation of the medial apophysis.

Wrist problems

Ulnar side wrist problems are quite common in tennis players. Indeed, since the introduction of wide body racquets, the incidence seems to have increased. In most instances, close

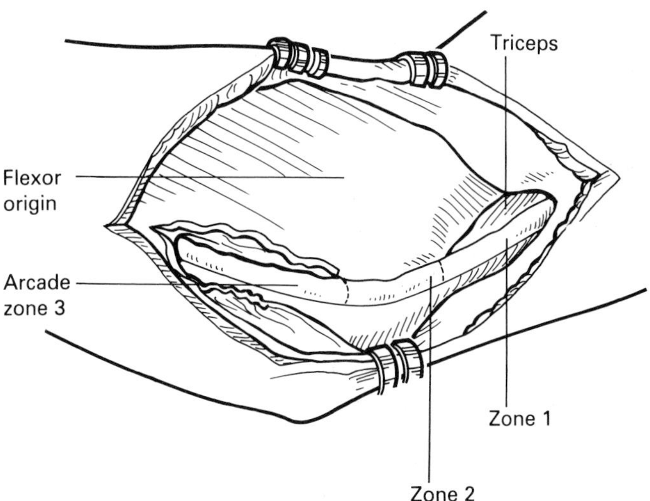

Fig. 29.3 Ulnar nerve zones at medial elbow medial epicondylar ulnar nerve zones. The most common ulnar nerve clinical problem is compression neurapraxia in zone 3. In this clinical circumstance surgical decompression is the treatment of choice. From Nirschl (1985).

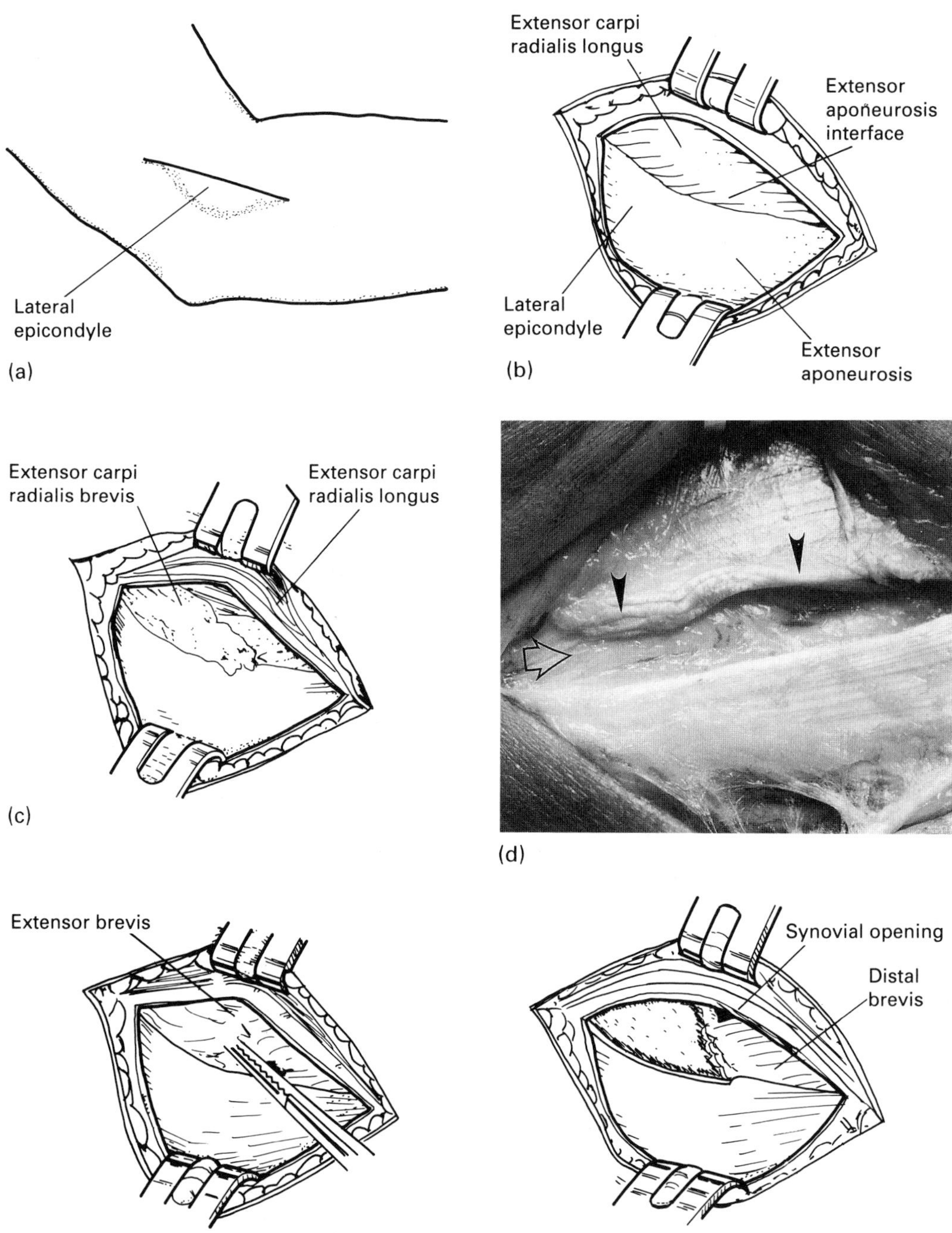
Lateral
epicondyle
(a)
Extensor carpi
radialis longus
Extensor
aponeurosis
interface
Lateral
epicondyle
Extensor
aponeurosis
(b)
Extensor carpi
radialis brevis
Extensor carpi
radialis longus
(c)
(d)
Extensor brevis
(e)
Synovial opening
Distal
brevis
(f)

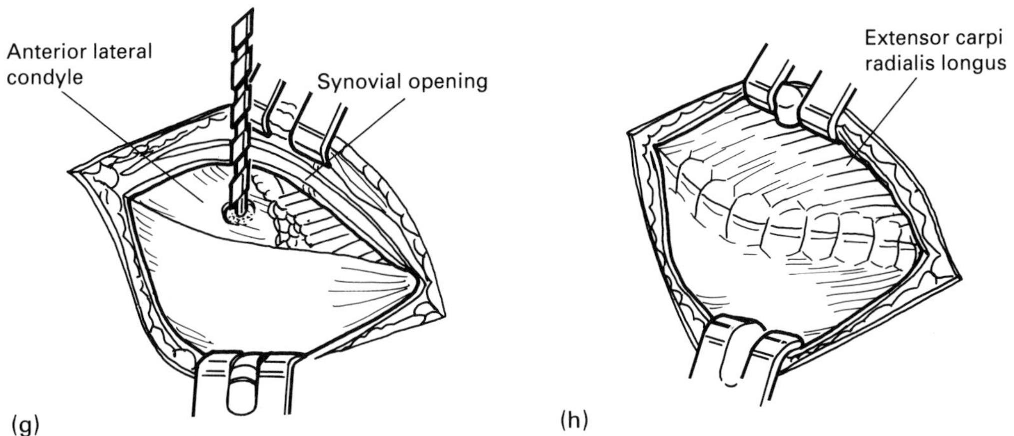

Fig. 29.4 (*Opposite*) Senior author's (R.P.N.) surgical technique for lateral tennis elbow tendinosis. (a) Incision is slightly anterior to lateral epicondyle and extends from the level of the radial head to 2.5 cm (1 in) proximal to the lateral epicondyle. (b) Interface between extensor carpi radialis longus and extensor aponeurosis is identified. (c) Incision in the extensor longus — aponeurosis interface is made. The extensor longus is 2–3 mm thick in this area. Do not make the incision too deep as origin of the extensor brevis will be distorted, thereby compromising the identification of the pathological areas. Extensor carpi radialis longus is retracted anteriorly and origin of extensor carpi radialis brevis comes into view. The normal brevis origin includes some attachment to the anterior edge of the extensor neurosis. The typical changes of greyish oedematous tendon alteration should also be visible without the use of optical assistance if the operative selection is correct. (d) Gross visual appearance of angiofibroblastic tendinosis. Open arrow identifies typical greyish homogeneous changes in extensor brevis characteristic of angiofibroblastic tendinosis. Black arrows identify edge of normal extensor longus. (e) Removal of angiofibroblastic degeneration of extensor brevis. In the typical case, the extensor aponeurosis and lateral epicondyle are not disturbed. (f) Final stage of angiofibroblastic resection. All pathological tissue is removed. A small opening in the synovium is made to inspect the lateral compartment but it is rare to identify any pathological changes. In approximately 35% of cases, some alteration is noted in the anterior edge of the extensor aponeurosis. This pathological change is removed if present. In 20% of cases, some lateral epicondylar exostosis is also noted. If exostosis is encountered a small section of the aponeurosis is peeled back and the exostosis removed. (*Above*) (g) Vascular enhancement. To enhance vascular supply, three holes are drilled through the cortical bone of the anterior lateral condyle to cancellous bone level. (h) Repair. The extensor longus is now firmly repaired to the anterior margin of the extensor aponeurosis. Because the extensor brevis is still attached to the underside of the extensor longus, it is unnecessary to suture the distal brevis. Note that a firm attachment of the extensor aponeurosis to the lateral epicondyle is maintained at all times. From Nirschl (1985).

questioning will reveal a wrist-orientated and rolling tennis stroke technique. Diagnostic considerations include a triangular fibrocartilage complex tear, synovitis of the distal radioulnar joint, tendinitis and/or subluxation of the extensor carpi ulnaris, and sprain to the ulnar collateral ligament.

Common problems on the radial side include ganglion or synovitis of the radial carpal joint, aggravation or pre-existent arthritis and less commonly a chronic scapholunate dissociation.

Exaggerated wrist positions, wrist roll with tennis spin shots, and a 'layed-back wrist' while executing forehand vollies are common aetiological factors in the incitement of ulnar column wrist abnormalities.

Basic treatment approaches

Although this chapter is dedicated to prevention, it seems appropriate to address the general aspects of treatment of the overuse problems so prevalent in tennis. The tennis elbow protocol utilized at Virginia Sportsmedicine Institute seems well suited for this purpose (Table 29.2) (Sobel & Nirschl, 1981).

Surgery

If a quality rehabilitative effort such as outlined in Table 29.2 fails, a surgical solution may be indicated (Nirschl, 1988). In general, the majority of tennis-related injuries are resolved by a quality rehabilitative programme. Those maladies most commonly presenting for surgery include:

1 Rotator cuff shoulder tendinitis/tendinosis.

2 Knee abnormalities (patellofemoral and meniscal).

3 Elbow (lateral and medial tennis elbow tendinosis) (Figs 29.4 & 29.5).

Overall, the variety of surgical problems can encompass all body areas from the fingers to the toes.

Postinjury prognosis for return to tennis

It is unusual not to be reasonably successful in returning an injured player back to tennis. Even in major ruptures of the shoulder rotator cuff, return is likely often within 6 months for recreational players if the acromion and deltoid do not undergo surgical disturbance. Major knee instabilities and recalcitrant lumbar disc syndrome would be more likely to preclude return. Even in these circumstances, surgery can often be restorative. The return to a highly competitive or world level is of course more difficult and more demanding than the regional tournament or recreational player. Even in the highly demanding group, however, success is not uncommon. Many of the principles for prevention are incorporated into the post-operative rehabilitation effort and are often a key to success. It is, of course, best to avoid injury by use of the preventive approaches addressed in this chapter.

Table 29.2 Tennis elbow rehabilitation protocol (Virginia Sportsmedicine Institute).

Rest phase — control pain (usually 1–2 weeks)
- avoid abusive activities in sports
- avoid abusive activities in daily living
- use counter force brace
- modalities of physical therapy (high-voltage electrical stimulation, ice and heat)

Anti-inflammatory medication
- aspirin or ibuprofen
- other non-steroidal anti-inflammatory agents (less commonly used)
- cortisone (oral or injection) if symptoms are of such severity to preclude compliance with the rehabilitative exercise programme

Start fitness programme at the time of rest phase onset

Start rehabilitative exercise when comfortable with required activities of daily living
- use counter force brace
- with elbow bent and arm supported start with 0.45 kg (1 lb) isotonic programme of wrist curls, supination and pronation, and ulnar and radial deviation daily
- at the same time, do tennis ball isometrics and finger extension against rubber band resistance
- progress to 1.35 kg (3 lb), then perform exercises with elbow straight and arm unsupported
- alternate isotonic weights with isoflex resistance system (tension cord) (Fig. 29.6)
- end-point of isotonic exercises is usually 2.3 kg (5 lb) 15 repetitions for women, and 3.6 kg (8 lb), 15 repetitions for men; painless anaerobic isoflex sprints, and dynamometer grip strength of dominant arm 10% greater than non-dominant
- *Note*: The arm and shoulder muscle groups are often weak in association with tennis elbow; check these muscle groups and if weakness is present, rehabilitation must also include, biceps, triceps, rotator cuff, and scapular muscle groups

Gradual return to tennis when rehabilitation end-points are reached. Continue maintenance supplemental exercises 2–3 times·week^{-1}
- use counter force brace for 3 months (minimum) or more
- check equipment and sports techniques and correct as indicated

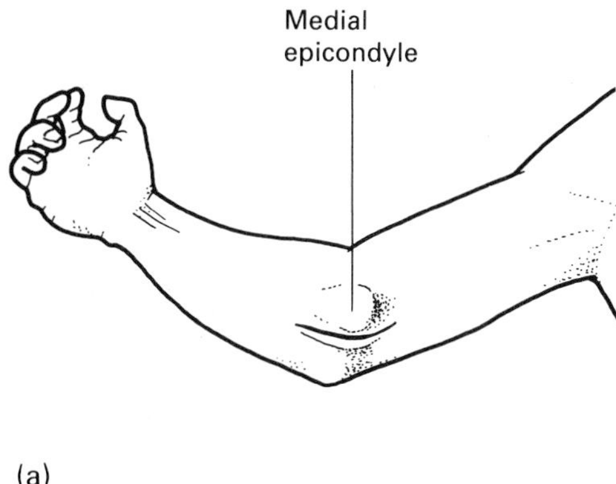

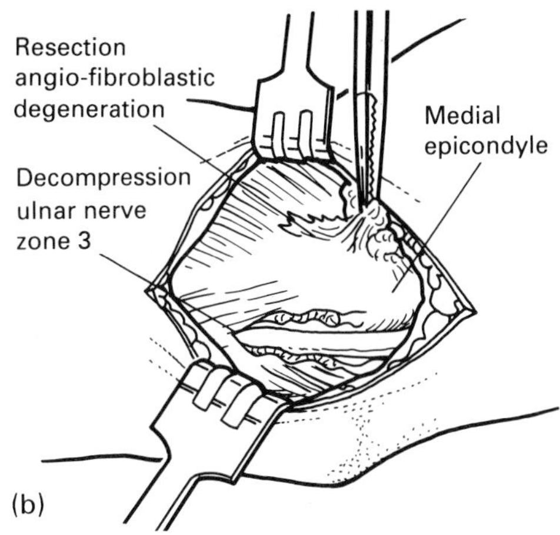

Fig. 29.5 Senior author's (R.P.N.) surgical technique for medial tennis elbow tendinosis and compression neurapraxia of ulnar nerve. (a) Incision is made as depicted. Care is taken to avoid harm to the sensory cutaneous nerve (medial antebrachial) just anterior to the medial epicondyle. (b) Resection of angiofibroblastic tendinosis. The angiofibroblastic changes are usually in the origin of the pronator teres and flexor carpi radialis. The pathological tissue is removed in longitudinal and elliptic fashion, leaving attachments of normal tissue intact. In 60% of cases, dysfunction of the ulnar nerve has been noted clinically; decompression of the ulnar nerve in zone 3 of the medial epicondylar groove is done. (c) Repair of medial tennis elbow. Repair of the common flexor origin is undertaken. Note that the medial epicondylar attachments of normal tissue are not disturbed. From Nirschl (1992).

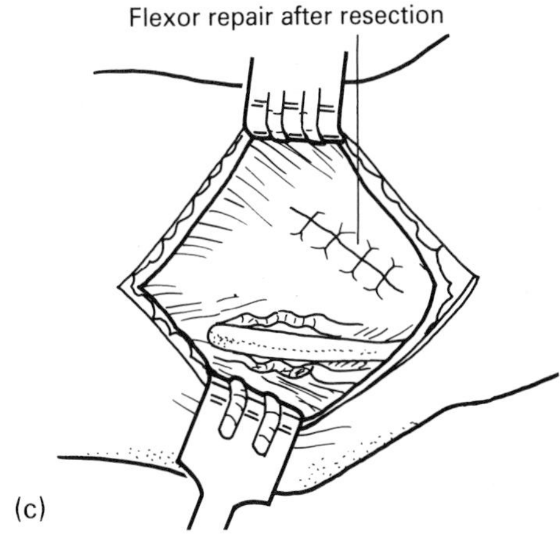

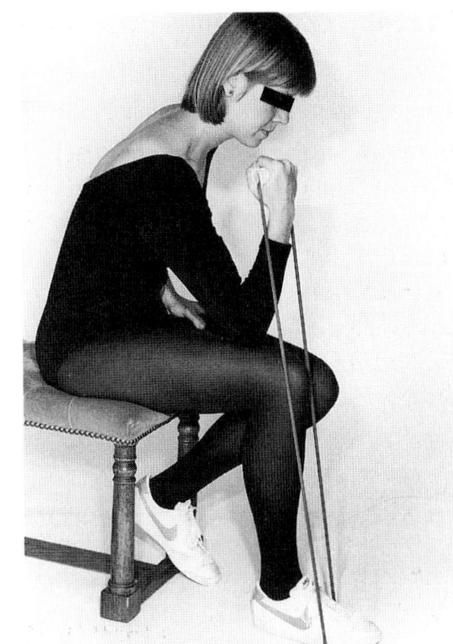

Fig. 29.6 Isoflex rehabilitative resistance exercises. Elastic tension cord resistance exercises in proper sequence with isometric, isotonic and isokinetic technique are important to the prevention, conservative treatment and postoperative rehabilitation of lateral, medial and posterior medial tennis elbow tendinosis. From Nirschl (1985).

References

Dulany, R. (1986) Tennis strokes. In F.A. Pettrone (ed) *American Academy of Orthopedic Surgeons Symposium on Upper Extremity Injuries in Athletes*, pp. 47–58. Mosby, St Louis.

Froimson, A. (1971) Treatment of tennis elbow with forearm support band. *J. Bone Joint Surg.* **43B**, 100.

Groppel, J. & Nirschl, R.P. (1986) A biomechanical and EMG analysis of the effects of counter force bracing on the tennis player. *Am. J. Sports Med.* **14**, 195–200.

Kibler, W.B., McQueen, C. & Uhl, T. (1988) Fitness evaluations and fitness findings in competitive junior tennis players. *Clin. Sports Med.* **7**(2), 403–16.

Nirschl, R.P. (1973a) Good tennis is good medicine. *Phys. Sports Med.* **1**(1), 26–37.

Nirschl, R.P. (1973b) Tennis elbow. *Orthop. Clin. N. Am.* **4**(3), 787–801.

Nirschl, R.P. (1985) Muscle and tendon trauma. In B.F. Morrey (ed) *The Elbow and its Disorders*, pp. 481–96. WB Saunders, Philadelphia.

Nirschl, R.P. (1988) Prevention and treatment of elbow and shoulder injuries in the tennis player. *Clin. Sports Med.* **7**(2), 289–308.

Nirschl, R.P. (1992) Elbow tendinosis/tennis elbow. *Clin. Sports Med.* **11**(4), 851–70.

Nirschl, R.P. & Sobel, J. (1988) *Supplemental Exercises for the Tennis Player. United States Professional Tennis Association Sport Science and Sports Medicine Guide*, Vol. 1, pp. 70–92. USPTA Publishers, Texas.

Priest, J.D. (1988) The shoulder of the tennis player. *Clin. Sports Med.* **7**(2), 387–402.

Sobel, J. & Nirschl, R.P. (1981) Conservative treatment of the tennis elbow. *Phys. Sports Med.* **9**, 42–54.

Chapter 30

Injuries in Badminton

UFFE JØRGENSEN AND PER HØLMICH

Badminton is primarily an indoor sport; however, as a recreational activity it is also played outdoors. Badminton is one of the most popular sports in the world, maybe because it is an enjoyable and social sport that can be played from childhood to old age, as well as a competitive sport played at different levels. In 1992 in Barcelona it was first played at the Olympic Games.

Badminton is played with a light-weight racket and a light-weight shuttlecock. It can be a game with quick movements and sudden changes of direction. At high levels it demands quick reactions, speed, coordination and a relatively good physical condition. The technique is easy to learn but a lot of skill and training is demanded to reach high levels.

The duration of a game is two or three sets, which takes from 15 min to 1 h. In tournaments there can be more than one game a day and often one player participates in single, double and mixed double games, which can result in many hours of badminton concentrated in only a few days. This organization of tournaments may explain many of the overuse injuries which are typical in badminton.

Badminton is looked upon by many as a low-risk sport, a statement previously based on experience and now confirmed by epidemiological investigations in different countries (Jørgensen & Winge, 1987; Backx *et al.*, 1989; van Galen, 1989). However, in contrast to other popular sports, only a few indepth studies have been done on injuries in badminton — on injury incidence and pattern, to identify possible risk factors and possibilities for injury prevention. No studies have been done on the effect of injury prevention in badminton.

Incidence of injuries

Overuse injuries are the most frequent type of injuries found in badminton. In Danish badminton 74% of the injuries were due to overuse, 12% were strain injuries, 11% sprains, 1.5% fractures and 1.5% contusions (Jørgensen & Winge, 1987).

The mean injury incidence in recreational and élite club badminton in Denmark was found to be 0.85 injuries·year^{-1} or 2.9 injuries·1000 h^{-1} of badminton (Jørgensen & Winge, 1987). In general, van Galen (1989) found a lower incidence in The Netherlands (1.6 injuries·1000 h^{-1}).

The incidence of injuries in badminton is low compared with other popular sports (Table 30.1). The injury incidences per year and per 1000 hours in Table 30.1 are from comparable studies made by the author and co-workers (Jørgensen, 1984; Jørgensen & Schmidt-Olsen, 1986; Schmidt-Olsen & Jørgensen, 1987; Winge & Jørgensen, 1989). The same registration method was used in all these studies (prospective self-registration of injuries — Jørgensen, 1984). Injuries were registered if they were as a result of badminton training or matches — if they handicapped play, required special treat-

Table 30.1 Sports injury incidence in comparable studies. From Jørgensen (1988) and E+1 98/96.

Sport	Injuries·year^{-1}	Incidence (injuries·1000 h^{-1})	Serious injuries·100 participants^{-1}
Badminton	0.85	2.9	0.4
Tennis	0.56	2.8	0.7
Soccer	1.36	4.1	3.9
Handball	1.11	8.3	2.9
Ice hockey	0.90	4.7	—
Volleyball	0.75	3.1	1.9

ment in order to play (i.e. special bandaging or medical attention), or if the injury made play impossible. Using a calculated index, the same ranking for risk of injury in different sports has been found amongst children by Backx *et al.* (1989).

Other studies confirm that badminton is a low-risk sport. In a report on sports injuries in The Netherlands (E+1 98/86), the average incidence of serious injuries necessitating hospital treatment per 100 participants was found to be 0.4 in badminton, compared to 0.7 in tennis and 3.9 in soccer (Table 30.1).

Gender

Men sustain more injuries than women in badminton (0.9 vs. 0.78 injuries·season^{-1}). The injury risk is higher for men particularly during matches (2.8 vs. 2.1 injuries·1000 match h^{-1}) (Jørgensen & Winge, 1987). A reason for this could be the greater intensity and faster speed found in men's badminton.

Playing level

Élite players sustain more injuries than other players from the same club who participate in club teams at recreational level (0.92 vs. 0.70 injuries·season^{-1}). However, when the time of exposure is taken into account the recreational players have a higher injury risk than élite players (3.1 vs. 2.8 injuries·1000 badminton h^{-1}) (Jørgensen & Winge, 1987). The higher number of injuries in élite badminton is explained by the greater exposure time, whereas the relatively higher injury risk of playing recreational badminton could be due to factors such training, fitness, technique, discipline connected with training and matches, and possibly equipment.

Training vs. matches

Contrary to most other sports (Ekstrand, 1982), élite badminton players have a greater injury risk during training than in matches (3.1 vs. 2.3 injuries·1000 h^{-1}). This may be due to players participating in other more dangerous sports during the training programme. Recreational players who had trained less had no difference in injury incidence (Jørgensen & Winge, 1987).

Both men and women, had a higher injury risk during training than in matches (men, 3.1 : 2.8 and women 3.1 : 2.1, respectively) (Jørgensen & Winge, 1987). Badminton players should probably just play badminton and not involve themselves in higher-risk sports, but this lack of alternative training could also influence the injury risk during matches.

Duration and costs of injuries

The mean injury time in badminton is relatively long (48 days), but the number of lost working days are low (2.4 days) (Jørgensen & Winge, 1987). This reflects the high level of overuse injuries in badminton. Although badminton injuries are seldom serious, the relatively high level of Achilles tendon ruptures means that they are comparatively expensive injuries (Lorentzon *et al.*, 1984).

Epidimology and type of injuries

Injuries to the lower extremities are most frequent. According to Jørgensen and Winge (1987), the lower extremities account for 58% of injuries, 31% are upper-extremity injuries and 11% are back injuries (Table 30.2). Foot and ankle injuries are the most frequent. Eye injuries seem rare in Denmark (Jørgensen & Winge, 1987), however, they are the third most common injuries in The Netherlands (E+1 31/86), and have previously been reported as a problem in badminton (Chandran, 1974).

Achillodynia seems to be the single most frequent injury, followed by tennis elbow, anterior knee pain (mainly patellofemoral pain syndrome and jumper's knee), plantar fasciitis and femoral muscle strains (Hensley & Paup, 1979; Jørgensen & Winge, 1987).

A well-known injury is rupture of the Achilles tendon sustained during badminton. However, this injury is rare in reported studies on organized club badminton. This can be explained by the fact that it is often older recreational players who rupture their Achilles tendon (Nistor, 1981). These players have stopped their competitive career and play badminton only as a recreational activity, 1–2 h·week^{-1}. The injury pattern in this group of players has not been investigated in an in-depth study.

Traumatic badminton injuries are, according to Lorentzon *et al.* (1984), most frequently caused by a sprain due to incorrect placement of the foot (40%) or by a strain due to excessive movement (38%) in the game. Less frequent injury mechanisms are stumbling due to imbalance or fast speed (14%) and contusion due to a strike (8%).

The overuse-injury mechanism in badminton is more speculative due to its multifactorial origin. In a study on élite badminton, Jørgensen and Winge (1989) put forward the following as central mechanisms of injury.

1 Achilles tendon injuries in badminton could

Table 30.2 The injury pattern in élite (n = 204) and recreational (n = 99) badminton.

	Élite players		Recreational players	
	Number of injuries	%	Number of injuries	%
Foot	26	13.8	3	4.4
Ankle	21	11.2	3	4.4
Achilles tendon	14	7.5	5	7.2
Crus	14	7.5	0	0.0
Knee	16	8.5	10	14.5
Femur	10	5.3	4	5.8
Groin	7	3.7	6	8.7
Lower extremity total	108	57.5	31	44.9
Back	23	12.2	7	10.1
Thorax	23	12.2		
Shoulder	15	8.0	7	10.1
Humerus	14	7.5	9	13.0
Tennis elbow	12	6.4	6	8.7
Lower arm	6	3.2	3	4.4
Hand	3	1.6	3	4.4
Upper extremity total	50	26.6	28	40.6
Eye	0	0	2	2.9
Others	7	3.7	1	1.5

be due to a combined effect of the special footwork demanded with fast, forward movements and stops with forceful heel strike and eccentric work by the triceps surae (TS), alternating with backwards toe running and concentric work of the TS, and backward or combined backward/sideward jumps with forceful eccentric work of the TS. Movements that produce alternating, fast-changing high tension in the Achilles tendon could produce microtrauma; if these are repeated frequently an injury could develop. Present badminton shoes do nothing to diminish this. They have a flat heel, low shock absorption and give no support to the foot.

2 The mechanism in patellofemoral pain syndrome could be similar to point 1, where the fast-changing eccentric/concentric work of the quadriceps in knee flexion and rotation can create high retropatellar stress.

3 Tennis elbow and other overuse problems in the arm and shoulder could be due to an incorrect emphasis in training. Functional studies of the strokes in badminton (Øsmosegård, 1983) have revealed that these are not primarily flexion/extension movements, but involve much more rotation than was previously believed, with the internal/external rotation of the shoulder as the greatest force-producing movement. Another possibility is that the greater degree of wrist motion in badminton compared to tennis could be of significance in the aetiology of tennis elbow in badminton players. Training has not previously taken this into consideration, so strengthening and stretching of these structures has been neglected.

General internal and external causes of overuse injuries have been described elsewhere (Lorentzon, 1988; Nigg, 1988), but specific causes in badminton could be:

1 Shoe–surface interaction (high friction, low shock absorption).

2 The badminton shoe (no heel support, low shock absorption, no heel elevation).

3 Inadequate flexibility and strength of the TS and the muscles involved in rotation during the badminton stroke.

However, the significance of these factors in badminton has not yet been studied.

Management of injuries

Achillodynia

Inflammation in the peritenon or bursae or tendinosus in the tendon are common reasons for pain in the Achilles region. The area may be warm, red and tender. The pain is often localized at the insertion of the tendon on the calcaneus or approximately 5 cm proximal to the insertion. When the retrocalcaneal bursa is inflammed, the symptoms are localized in the area just anterior to the distal part of the Achilles tendon (Kager's triangle, Fig. 30.1). Crepitus is sometimes felt, and in the more chronic stage a thickening of the tendon or the peritenon can be palpated. Functional pain is present on active plantar flexion against resistance and often also on forced passive dorsiflexion.

TREATMENT

It is always very important to analyse the injury mechanism, both the intrinsic and the extrinsic

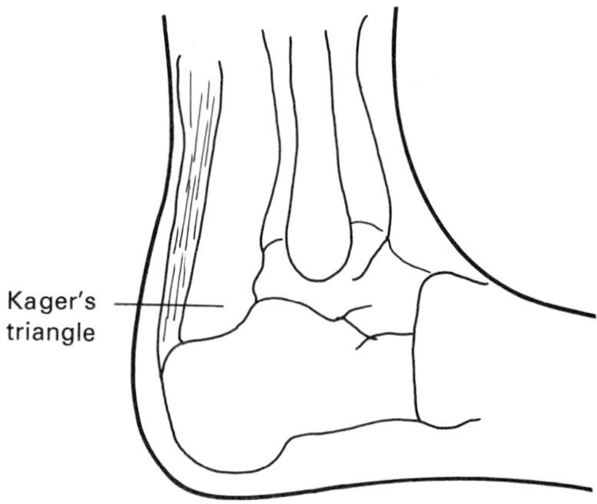

Fig. 30.1 In patients with pain at the distal insertion (the heel end) of the Achilles tendon, Kager's triangle is often too narrow. If it is, surgery with bone removel is often required.

factors, in order to choose the correct treatment. Whether a training error, tight muscles or insufficent footwear is involved, it is always mandatory that these problems are solved as part of the treatment. The symptomatic treatment is rest and limitation of activities, combined with ice, anti-inflammatory medication and stretching of the TS muscle and tendon. Sometimes different kinds of physiotherapy such as deep massage and ultrasound are useful.

If symptomatic treatment combined with correction of the factors that led to the injury is insufficient, it may be necessary to operate. Preoperative examination of the region with ultrasonography or magnetic resonance imaging (MRI) can be very helpful. At operation the paratenon is opened, any adhesions are divided, the bursae may be removed if they are the problem, and the upper posterior corner of the calcaneus can be removed. If areas of degeneration in the tendon are suspected, the tendon should be incised longitudinally and the degenerated tissue removed. Postoperative immobilization is rarely necessary, but care must be taken to ensure good healing of the skin before more extensive exercises are allowed.

REHABILITATION

After the initial improvement of symptoms, a gradual onset of rehabilitation can begin. This includes careful stretching of the TS, with both bent and straight knees, strengthening of the muscles in the whole lower leg with functional closed chain exercises, and exercises to stimulate proprioception, (e.g. one-leg balances with eyes closed or training on a wobble board).

Guided by the symptoms, jogging can usually begin after 3–4 weeks. If the tendon has been incised, jogging should begin very carefully after 6–8 weeks. Badminton is normally possible after 8–10 weeks.

PREVENTION

Strengthening of the muscles of the lower leg with functional closed chain exercises, and achieving a proper mobility of the ankle joint with stretching, are both very important factors in preventing achillodynia.

From working with élite badminton players, it is evident that even minor foot problems can cause disturbances in the movement of the Achilles tendon and thereby cause overuse problems. These problems grow with an increasing amount of training and matches. The shoes and insoles are very important and an early adjustment, either by getting a better shoe (stable with shock absorption) or by getting individually made soft insoles with shock-absorbing qualities, can prevent many overuse injuries.

Back pain

Badminton demands a very stable trunk as a basis for the movements of all four extremities. As the game consists of many torsions and rotations performed at a high speed, the muscles of the abdomen and back have to be well trained. It has been found that the quadratus lumborum muscle is often a site for pain as a consequence of overuse, and that the back extensors can also give rise to pain. The iliopsoas muscle is also a common cause of back problems in badminton; the psoas major originates from the lumbar vertebrae and inserts at the trochanter minor at the femur. If this muscle is tight it will indirectly cause an increased lumbar lordoses, thereby putting more load on the low back. The muscle can be tested with the Thomas test (Fig. 30.2) for tightness and pain, and the muscle can be palpated through the lower abdomen.

The treatment programme should include stretching exercises and multiple repetition exercises with low force (both concentric and eccentric) in the same directions.

PREVENTION

Possibilities for prevention include basic strength and stretching programmes for both the muscles of the back as well as the muscles of the abdomen (flexors, extensors and oblique muscles). These exercises are well-suited for

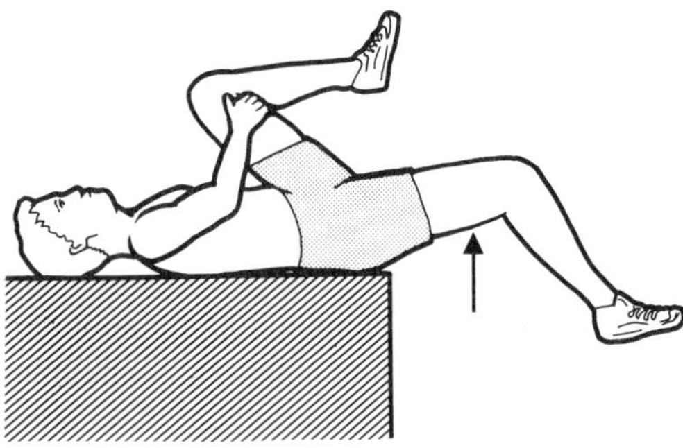

Fig. 30.2 Thomas's test shows a shortening of the iliopsoas muscle. It is positive if, at flexion in one hip, the leg of the other side moves upwards.

preseason training. Stretching of the iliopsoas muscles should be remembered at all times.

Overuse injuries to the foot

The high speed, frequent changes in direction and the multiple jumping characteristics of badminton demand a great deal from the feet. Badminton is played on a relatively hard surface and, as mentioned earlier, the footwear used is often insufficient in supporting and protecting the foot. In recent years some shoe manufacturers have started to use shock-absorbing materials, but the insoles, the construction of the heel support and the longitudinal stability still need further development. The main foot problems in badminton are plantar fasciitis, heel pain, sesamoid pain and callosities.

PLANTAR FASCIITIS

Pain in the plantar fascia is usually an overuse problem, but it can also be due to a sudden excessive loading of the foot. It occurs in both the high arched cavus foot and in the hyperpronation foot. The symptoms are pain at the tuber calcanei radiating forward in the plantar aspect of the foot (Fig. 30.3). There is pain when the fascia is stretched, both passively and during walking or running, especially when the big toe is dorsiflexed in the take-off. Tenderness of the fascia is present and sometimes crepitation or thickening at the insertion into the calcaneus can be palpated.

The treatment is ice, anti-inflammatory medication, relieving the tender area from pressure and correcting the factors that led to the injury. This means supporting the foot either by a shock-absorbing insole supporting the high arched foot or by correcting the excessively pronating foot with an insole and making sure that the shoe is stable and well-fitted. Stretching of the plantar fascia is important in both treat-

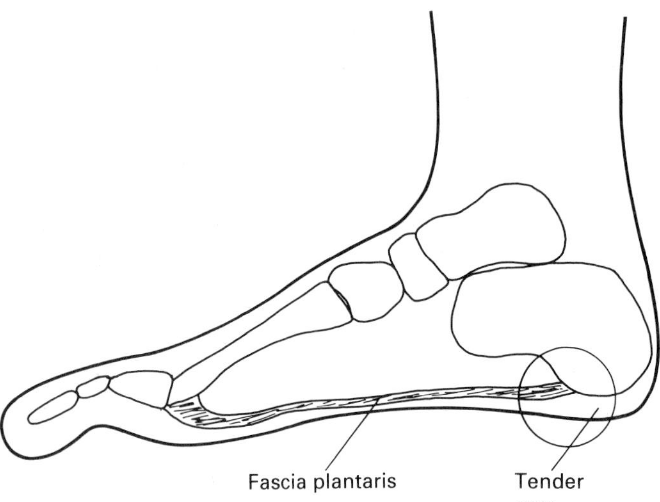

Fig. 30.3 In badminton players fasciitis plantaris is often localized at the insertion of the fascia on the calcaneous.

ment and prevention. In chronic cases, steroid injections around the fascia can be considered. Surgery is rarely necessary.

HEEL PAIN

Soft heel pads are a major problem in badminton accounting for a variety of overuse injuries. The shock-absorbing quality of the natural heel pad can be reduced significantly (Jørgensen, 1989) thereby leading to overuse problems in the other shock-absorbing systems of the body. In the heel itself, pain is a frequent problem.

A central factor in treatment is a shock-absorbing insole with a relatively rigid heel cup (Fig. 30.4) to support the heel pad and increase shock absorbency at heel strike. To prevent this problem, shoes should have an anatomically fitting heel counter and shock absorption. It is very important that this prevention is started in juvenile athletes.

SESAMOID PAIN AND CALLOSITIES

The sesamoids under the 1st metatarsophalangeal joint sometimes give rise to pain. It occurs most frequently in high arched feet. Sore callosities are most common under the metatarsophalangeal joints, especially under the 1st or 5th, and under the heel.

Both problems can be treated by correcting the function of the foot and distributing the weight evenly. This is done by using carefully made soft insoles and using well-fitting shoes. Even though it seems a minor problem, it is important that callosities are prevented and treated by regular foot care.

The sesamoids can develop both acute and stress fractures. These can be treated by either non-weight-bearing, an orthosis which decreases dorsiflexion in the first toe or by surgical removal of the fractured sesamoid.

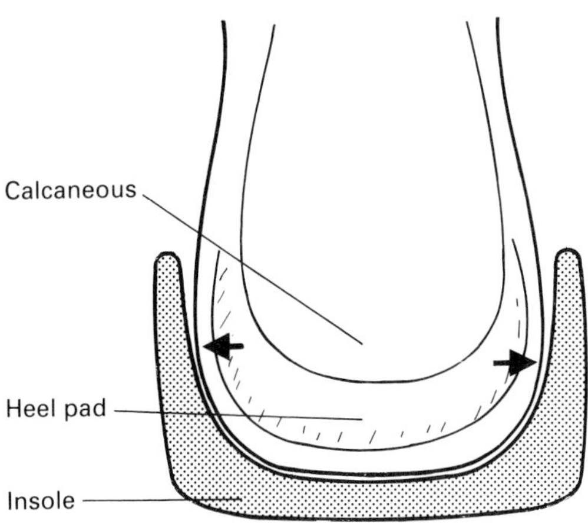

Fig. 30.4 External compression of the human heel pad by a well-fitted shoe or cup-formed insert increases the shock absorbency and protects the heel bone and the musculoskeletal system.

Jumper's knee

This term refers to a painful condition involving the proximal part of the patellar ligament and its insertion at the distal pole of the patella. Pain at the quadriceps tendon at the superior pole of the patella is also described as jumper's knee (Blazina *et al.*, 1973) (Fig. 30.5). Ferretti *et al.* (1983) also included the pathology of the bone–tendon junction of the patellar tendon on the tibial tuberosity.

Jumper's knee is believed to be a result of repetitive microruptures and sometimes macroruptures due to chronic overload of the ligament near or at the insertion. This has been confirmed histologically by several authors (Roels *et al.*, 1978; Basset *et al.*, 1980; Ferretti *et al.*, 1983; Kelly *et al.*, 1984).

Badminton is a sport with repetitive movements involving forceful concentric and eccentric quadriceps muscle action. This may be found in particular when the athlete moves towards the net to reach for the shuttlecock and then makes a very fast movement backwards to the backline of the field (Fig. 30.6). The change of direction consists of a decelerating eccentric contraction of the quadriceps which is changed to an explosive concentric quadriceps contraction to move backwards. The athlete suffering from jumper's knee describes a sudden pain at

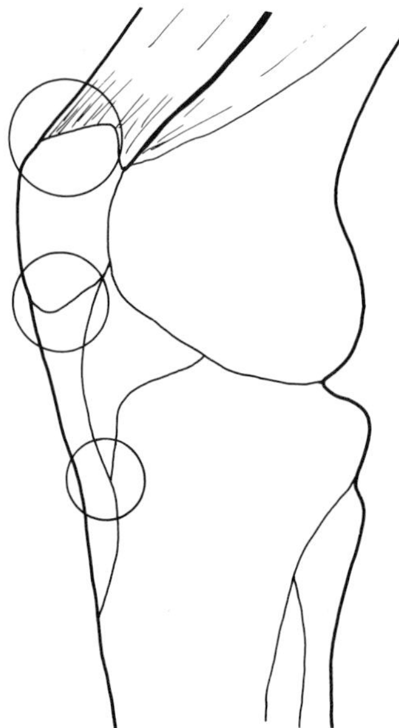

Fig. 30.5 Anterior knee pain in badminton players can either be at the three tendon insertions or of patellofemoral origin. The most typical tendon injury is jumper's knee which is caused by inflammation and probably partial rupture of the patella tendon insertion on the patella.

the moment of change in direction, often with a feeling of not being able to move backwards as forcefully as intended.

The element of jumping involved in a 'smash' or 'picking up' in the corners of the field can also cause pain.

At clinical examination, tenderness is found at the part of the extensor mechanism involved. Localization at the inferior pole of the patella is by far the most frequently found (Roels *et al.*, 1978; Jakob & Segesser, 1980; Karlsson *et al.*, 1991). Sometimes a minor swelling is found at the site of the pain and in chronic cases a firm nodule and sore swelling might be felt in the tendon. Generalized effusion of the knee joint is almost never seen.

TREATMENT

Due to lack of scientific evidence, the best course of treatment is debatable. The authors treat this injury by a modification or cessation of the activities which caused the pain. Ice and other symptomatic modalities can be used. An examination of a possible extensor mechanism malalignment should be done, and if present corrected with bandage and muscle training. The main element of the treatment is a programme of eccentric strength-rebuilding exercises as described by Stanish *et al.* (1985).

If this treatment fails after a training period of at least 6 months, surgery may be necessary. Ultrasonography, computed tomography or MRI are very helpful in confirming the operative indication and localizing the degenerated tissue in the tendon. At operation, the tendon is split longitudinally, the abnormal tissue is resected radically and the tendon is closed (Karlsson *et al.*, 1991). No immobilization is used postoperatively and a carefully planned and supervised training programme is undertaken. Running in water is possible after 3 weeks, jogging on a soft surface after 6–8 weeks and badminton after 8–12 weeks.

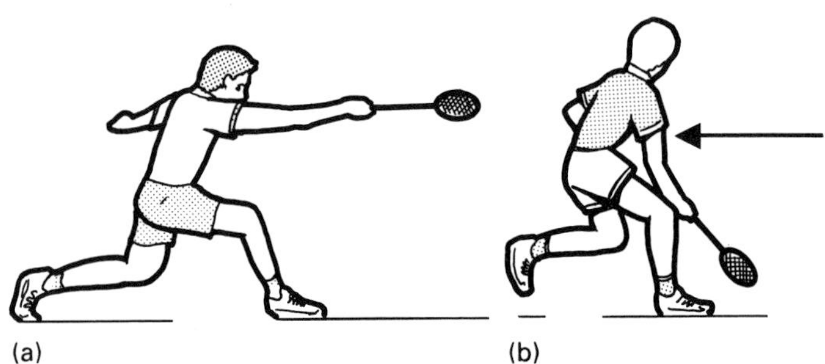

Fig. 30.6 Anterior knee pain can be provoked by multiple fast forward movements, sudden stops and backward movements, as a result of fast-changing concentric/excentric work of the extensor apparatus in particular.

PREVENTION

Coordination training of the lower extremities, where special attention should be given to the vastus medialis of the quadriceps muscle, can be used to help prevent jumper's knee and patellofemoral pain. Multiple closed-chain quadriceps exercises, with special emphasis on eccentric strength training and stretching the knee extensors should also be a part of the basic training programme.

Lateral epicondylitis

This is a painful condition at the origin of the extensor muscles of the forearm on the lateral humerus epicondyle. It is also known as tennis elbow. The condition is probably the result of longstanding overload with multiple microruptures in the musculotendinous junction of the wrist extensor muscles at the level of the lateral epicondyle (Nirschl & Pettrone, 1979).

The diagnosis is based on tenderness exactly at the attachment of the extensor aponeurosis to the lateral epicondyle (Fig. 30.7), pain on resisted active extension of the wrist with the elbow extended (Chard & Hazleman, 1989), and sometimes also pain on passive maximal flexion of the wrist on extended elbow. A decrease in flexion ability of the wrist on the affected side is often present. It is important to be very precise in the diagnosis since several other reasons for pain in the elbow region may exist (Table 30.3).

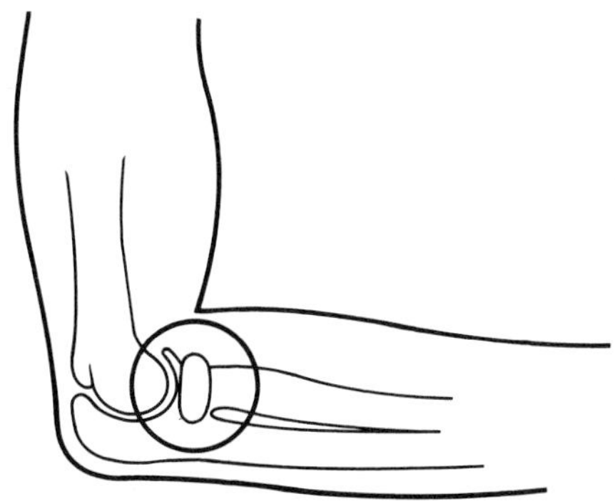

Fig. 30.7 Tennis elbow in badminton players can due to several mechanisms which result in pain at the lateral epicondyl. The aetiology of the pain should therefore be known before treatment is started.

TREATMENT

Treatment should start with a precise analysis of the injury mechanism to correct any technical errors or muscular weakness. Ice, rest, stretching exercises, deep massage and transcutaneous nerve stimulation (TNS) are useful. A gradual strength-training programme including both wrist extension, flexion and rotation can begin when the pain is controlled or as early as possible. An elbow band (4–6 cm wide) or a counterforce brace worn just below the elbow joint, where the circumference of the forearm is biggest, can often be helpful.

Cortisone injections can be used if exercises have limited effect after several months. Various operations can be performed in chronic cases when there is no response to a proper treatment regime.

The rotators of the forearm and the muscles of the shoulder and the upper arm are important in badminton so strength and flexibility exercises and a correct technique are important in preventing this injury.

Table 30.3 Differential diagnoses of lateral epicondylitis.

Cartilage lesion on the capitulum humeri or on the caput radii
Synovial plica
Degenerative changes in ligamentum annulare radii
Synovitis
Radial tunnel syndrome — entrapment
Chronic olecranon bursitis
Pain from trigger points in shoulder muscles such as m. supraspinatus
Cervical discus herniation
Degenerative changes in the cervical spine

Shoulder pain

The most important reason for shoulder pain in badminton players is secondary impingement due to glenohumeral instability (Jobe & Kvitne, 1979) or due to scapular instability (Kibler & Chandler, 1989). The main symptoms are complaints of pain on the anterior aspect of the shoulder. More specific pain in the affected weak and overworked muscles can be found. The impingement test with the arm abducted to 90° with flexed elbow and then brought passively into a maximal internal rotation is positive when it causes a subacromial pain (see Chapter 3, this volume). Sometimes a minor instability can be bound in the glenohumeral joint.

Treatment consists of specific strength and coordination exercises of the affected muscles. Both the muscles of the rotator cuff and the scapular stabilizers should be trained (Table 30.4).

An injection of cortisone in the subacromial bursa is sometimes useful, but must always be followed by a well-supervised training programme.

Specific attention to the muscles on the dorsal side of the shoulder girdle is important in a 'forward' motion sport like badminton in order to prevent overuse injuries to the shoulder. Ømosegård (1990) showed that in a group of Danish world-class players ($n = 21$) there was a major imbalance between the muscles on the anterior side of the shoulder girdle and those on the dorsal side, the anterior side being much stronger.

Table 30.4 Muscles of the rotator cuff and scapular stabilizers.

Glenohumeral muscles	Scapular stabilizers
M. supraspinatus	M. trapezius
M. infraspinatus	M. rhomboideus major
M. subscapularis	M. rhomboideus minor
M. teres minor	M. serratus anterior
M. biceps humeri	

Prevention of injuries

No studies have been published on the effect of injury prevention in badminton. Based on studies in soccer (Ekstrand, 1982), the known injury pattern in badminton and other possible injury mechanisms, the following measures could be taken.

1 Changes in the badminton shoe, with a higher heel (Lorentzon *et al.*, 1984), shock absorption and a stiffer, anatomically fitting heel counter (Jørgensen, 1989).

2 Adjustment of the friction between the shoe soles and playing surfaces (Mench & Jørgensen, 1983).

3 Specific badminton training including stretching and strengthening of the TS in particular and of the muscles involved in the internal and external rotation of the shoulder, elbow and wrist during badminton strokes.

Conclusion

Though badminton is one of the most frequently played sports in the world, there has been little sports-medicine research about it. Based on the few existing studies on injuries in badminton, it has been found that badminton, compared to other sports, is a low-risk sport dominated by overuse injuries. The injury duration is relatively long, although only a few working days are lost.

Anatomically, most injuries are localized to the foot and ankle; the single most frequent injuries are Achilles tendonitis and tennis elbow. Rupture of the Achilles tendon can occur, typically in older recreational players. When the time of exposure is taken into account, men are found to have a higher injury risk than women and recreational players a higher injury risk than élite players. Contrary to most other sports the relative injury risk is higher during training than in matches. Based on suggested causes of injury and injury mechanisms, together with the known injury pattern in badminton some preventive matters were suggested above.

References

Backx, F.J.G., Erich, W.B.M., Kemper, A.B.A. & Verbeek, A.L.M. (1989) Sports injuries in school-aged children, an epidemiologic study. *Am. J. Sports Med.* **17**, 234–40.

Basset, F., Soucacos, P. & Carr, W. (1980) Jumper's knee — patellar tendinitis and patellar tendon rupture. In *AAOS Symposium on the Athlete's Knee*. CV Mosby, St Louis.

Blazina, M.E., Kerlan, R.V., Jobe, F.W., Carter, V.S. & Carlsson, G.J. (1973) Jumper's knee. *Orthop. Clin. N. Am.* **4**, 665–78.

Chandran, S. (1974) Ocular hazards of playing badminton. *Br. J. Opthalmol.* **13**, 757–60.

Chard, M.D. & Hazleman, B.I. (1989) Tennis elbow — A reappraisal. *Br. J. Rheumatol.* **28**, 186–90.

E+1 98/86 (1986) *Sports Injuries in The Netherlands*. Report No. E+1 98/86. Ministry of Welfare, Health and Cultural Affairs, The Netherlands.

E+1 31/86. (1986) *Nature and Extent of Sports Injuries*. Report No. E+1 31/86. Ministry of Welfare, Health and Cultural Affairs, The Netherlands.

Ekstrand, J. (1982) *Prevention of soccer injuries*. Linkoping University Medical Dissertations No. 130, University of Linkoping, Sweden.

Ferretti, A., Ippolito, E., Mariani, P. & Puddu, G. (1983) Jumper's knee. *Am. J. Sports Med.* **11**, 58–62.

Galen, W. van (1989) Injuries in The Netherlands. In *Sports Injuries and their Prevention*. Proceedings of the third meeting, Papendal, The Netherlands, 1988.

Hensley, L.D. & Paup, D.C. (1979) A survey of badminton injuries. *Br. J. Sports Med.* **13**, 156–60.

Jakob, R.P. & Segesser, B. (1980) Extension training of the quadriceps — A new concept in the therapy of tendinosis of the knee extensor apparatus (jumper's knee) (in German). *Orthopäde* **9**, 201–6.

Jobe, F.W. & Kvitne, R.S. (1989) Shoulder pain in the overhand or throwing athlete: The relationship of anterior instability and rotator cuff impingement. *Orthop. Rev.* **18**, 963–71.

Jørgensen, U. (1984) The epidemiology of injuries in typical Scandinavian team sports. *Br. J. Sports Med.* **18**, 59–63.

Jørgensen, U. (1989) *Implications of heel strike: An anatomical, biomechanical, physiological and clinical study with focus on the heel pad*. Linkoping University Medical Dissertations No. 284, University of Linkoping, Sweden.

Jørgensen, U. & Schmidt-Olsen, S. (1986) The epidemiology of injuries in ice hockey. *Br. J. Sports Med.* **20**, 7–9.

Jørgensen, U. & Winge, S. (1987) Epidemiology of badminton injuries. *Int. J. Sports Med.* **8**, 379–82.

Karlsson, J., Lundin, O., Lossing, I.W. & Petterson, L. (1991) Partial rupture of the patellar ligament. *Am. J. Sports Med.* **19**, 403–8.

Kelly, D.W., Carter, U.S. & Jobe, F.E. (1984) Patellar and quadriceps tendon ruptures — Jumper's knee. *Am. J. Sports Med.* **12**, 375–80.

Kibler, W.B. & Chandler, T.J. (1989) Functional scapular instability in throwing athletes. In *American Orthopaedic Society for Sports Medicine 15th Annual Meeting*, Traverse City, Michigan, 19–22 June, 1989.

Mench, H. & Jørgensen, U. (1983) Frictional forces and ankle fractures in sports. *Br. J. Sports Med.* **17**, 135–6.

Nistor, L. (1981) Surgical and non-surgical treatment of Achilles tendon ruptures. *J. Bone Joint Surg.* **63A**, 394–9.

Lorentzon, R., Johansson, C. & Bjornstig, U. (1984) Fotbollen orsakar flest skador men badmintonskadan ar dyrast (Soccer causes most injuries, but badminton injuries are the most expensive). *Lakartidningen* **81**, 340–3.

Lorentzon, R. (1988) Causes of injuries: Intrinsic factors. In A. Dirix, H.G. Knuttgen & K. Tittel (eds) *The Olympic Book of Sports Medicine*, pp. 376–90. Blackwell Scientific Publications, Oxford.

Nigg, B.M. (1988) Causes of injuries: Extrinsic factors. In A. Dirix, H.G. Knuttgen & K. Tittel (eds) *The Olympic Book of Sports Medicine*, pp. 363–75. Blackwell Scientific Publications, Oxford.

Nirschl, R.P. & Pettrone, F.A. (1979) Tennis elbow: The surgical treatment of lateral epicondylitis. *J. Bone Joint Surg.* **61A**, 832–9.

Øsmosegård, B. (1983) *Kinetic Analysis of Badminton During Match or Match-like Situations* (in Danish). The Institute of Theoretical Physiology, University of Copenhagen, Denmark.

Øsmosegård, B. (1990) *Physical Training for Badminton Players* (in Danish). Tind Publishers, Denmark.

Roels, J., Martens, M., Mulier, J.C. & Burssens, A. (1978) Patellar tendinitis (jumper's knee). *Am. J. Sports Med.* **6**, 362–8.

Schmidt-Olsen, S. & Jørgensen, U. (1987) The epidemiology of injuries in volleyball. *Ugesk. Læger* **149**, 473–4.

Stanish, W.D., Curwin, S. & Rubinovich, R.M. (1985) Tendinitis: The analysis and treatment of running. *Clin. Sports Med.* **4**, 21–7.

Winge, S. & Jørgensen, U. (1989) Epidemiology of injuries in Danish championship tennis. *Int. J. Sports Med.* **10**, 368–71.

Chapter 31

Injuries in Squash

C. NIEK VAN DIJK

All common racquet sports are derived directly or indirectly from 'real tennis', their mother-sport and oldest of all racquet games. Squash owes its existence to racquets, and was probably born around 1865 at Harrow School in England where boys improvised in a small practice area with a soft 'squashy' ball while waiting to play tennis. Because of its historic association with aristocratic schools and the officer ranks of the British armed forces, squash used to be essentially an upper class sport. However, the last three decades has seen a spectacular increase in the popularity of the game. The limited amount of space and time required by the sport has been the fundamental factor in the development of squash into a highly popular recreational activity.

Countries like Australia, New Zealand, South Africa, Pakistan and more recently Japan count squash amongst their most practiced sports. Squash is played in practically all countries in Europe and in the UK alone more than 3 million people were registered squash players in 1985 (Halpin, 1985; Montpetit, 1990). Squash is often referred to as the fastest of all racquet sports. Contrary to many other racquet sports, the players share the same enclosed area (9.80 × 6.40 m) and are not separated by a net. The rubber squash ball (*c*. 41 mm diameter) is hit (directly or via other walls) towards the front wall at speeds of up to 230 km·h^{-1} (Chapman & Suderhoff, 1986).

Variants of the game include the American game of racquetball which is played with a larger, softer ball, and with shorter racquets.

Squash is a moderate to high intensity intermittent exercise that relies heavily on aerobic metabolism (Montpetit *et al.*, 1977; Montgomery *et al.*, 1981; Garden *et al.*, 1986; Merciez *et al.*, 1987). For professional and top amateur players, more than 50% of the rallies last longer than 10 s. The rest intervals fit a normal distribution with a mean duration of 8 s (Montpetit, 1990). The heart rate increases rapidly in the first minutes of play and remain stable at 150–170 beat·min^{-1} for the whole match for all levels of player (Montpetit *et al.*, 1977, 1987; Visser *et al.*, 1987). The thermal and metabolic response to squash is similar to that of moderate intensity running (Montpetit, 1990). Squash is a vigorous activity in which the two players, enclosed in the same area and hindered by a racquet in their hand, continuously have to adjust their rapidly changing movement patterns of repeated sprints and twisting movements.

The cause of injuries can be divided into three categories.

1 Impact from a racquet (either opponents or own).

2 Impact from the ball.

3 Other causes.

Numerous factors influence both the nature and the extent of injuries sustained. These can be broadly termed as host, exercise and environmental factors. Host factors include gender, age, experience, level of fitness and health status. Exercise factors include technique and duration and frequency of playing. Environmental factors include equipment, floor and wall surface, conditions and opponents behaviour, style and/or tactics.

At present there are no data in the literature that meet the strict criteria of epidemiological research. The problems in gathering information on injuries can be divided into three areas.

1 Definition of injury.
2 Description of population at risk.
3 Collecting of data in a systematic and organized manner (Maylack, 1988).

However, the studies that have been performed still give some useful indication of the incidence of injuries in squash.

Incidence of injuries

In 1978, Berson *et al.* reported on a retrospective survey of disabling injuries. A 'disabling' injury was arbitrarily defined as an injury incurred while playing squash, which then resulted in inability to compete for 14 days or more.

A questionnaire was circulated in a national magazine. There where 81 respondents reporting on a total of 131 injuries. Injuries to the lower extremities accounted for 54.2% of the total injuries. Of these injuries 38% were to ligaments, while 18% were ruptured Achilles tendons. Only one respondent reported a 'disabling' facial injury.

In 1981, Berson *et al.* reported on a random telephone survey of 200 squash players. The overall injury rate was reported at 45%. The injury incidence was calculated to be 8.8 (i.e. 8.8 injuries·100 players^{-1}·year^{-1}). In this survey, lower extremity injuries accounted for 45% of the total of reported injuries. Strains and sprains accounted for over one-third of all injuries. An exact percentage of facial injuries was not given, they were counted under 'other injuries' which comprised 18% of the total injuries.

Pforringer and Keyl (1978) reported on a survey in which questionnaires were sent to 30 squash centres, possessing a total of 8000 members. Information was provided on injuries sustained over a 12-month period. Minor or 'bagatelle' injuries were not reported. In all, 298 injuries were registered. This gave an injury incidence of 3.7 · 100 players^{-1}·year^{-1}. Lower extremity injuries accounted for 26.5% of the total, while strains and sprains made up 40% of this same total. Facial injuries comprised 50.7% of all injuries.

A further study by Keyl *et al.* (1980) reported on the results of a questionnaire sent to players who had sustained squash injuries. Again information related to a 12-month period. A total of 334 injuries were registered by 226 players. Lower extremity injuries accounted for 32.7% of the total and 67% of the injuries were strains and sprains. This time, 42.8% of the injuries were facial.

Van Dijk and Visser conducted a study in which questionnaires were distributed among 1000 players in 40 squash centres. There were 699 respondents (=70%). The injuries were distributed among all levels of experience of players with 56% admitted novices, 31% intermediate and advanced players and 13% top players. Slightly more than 50% of the injuries were direct contact injuries (ball or racquet). Novices and top players suffered these injuries four times more often than the intermediate and advanced players (van Dijk & Visser, 1985; van Mechelen & Hlobil, 1986). Of these injuries, 96% were bruises, contusions or small wounds. There were 20 eye injuries. Of the non-contact injuries, the most common injury was ankle distorsion (29%), followed by contusions (24%) and muscle injuries (23%).

Chard and Lachmann (1987) studied injuries treated in a sports clinic during an 8-year period. Squash provided 372 injuries, while 131 injuries relating to tennis and 128 injuries relating to badminton were treated during the same time frame. The fact that England and Wales have roughly similar numbers of tennis, badminton and squash players led the authors to the conclusion that individual squash players were approximately three times as likely to register with an injury in the sports clinic. However, the lack of data on the frequency of play prevents the calculation of an accurate comparative risk factor. In this study, 58% of the squash injuries involved the lower limbs. The majority of injuries affected the ankle (ankle distorsion), calf muscle, knee and lumbar region. Nearly one-third of all the patients studied in detail had taken up a racquet sport within the previous 3 months. Of the squash injuries, 25% occurred in players who played infrequently.

Nature and location of injuries

In the introduction it was stated that injuries can be sustained by contact with the racquet or ball, or through other causes.

Contact injuries

The players stand in close proximity and are not restricted to certain areas of the court and situations can arise where racquet swing, excessive, uncontrolled or otherwise, can make contact with themselves or their opponents. The racquet head speed may approach 161 $km \cdot h^{-1}$ (100 $mile \cdot h^{-1}$) (Maylack, 1988). Tables 31.1 and 31.2 show the nature and location of 1298 injuries caused by a racquet blow or a direct hit from a ball.

The most serious injury that can be caused by the impact of a squash ball is ocular damage. A squash ball will fit neatly into the confines of the orbital ring and can produce severe damage to the eyeball.

Easterbrook (1978) reported on 23 eye injuries

Table 31.1 Nature of 1298 injuries in 471 male and 228 female squash players caused by racquet blow or hit by a squash ball. From van Dijk & Visser (1985).

	Men			Women		
	Novice (n = 255)	Advanced (n = 160)	Top (n = 56)	Novice (n = 135)	Advanced (n = 55)	Top (n = 38)
Bruise	376	161	220	142	72	104
Contusion	29	23	1	3	1	2
Open wound	30	23	30	4	7	9
Fracture	3	3	1	0	0	0
Muscle injury	6	1	0	3	0	0
Concussion	1	0	0	1	0	0
Eye injury	9	3	2	3	2	1
Other	5	4	3	6	3	0
Total	459	218	257	162	85	117

Table 31.2 Location of 1277 injuries in 471 male and 228 female squash players caused by racquet blow or hit by a squash ball. The numbers are percentages. From van Dijk & Visser (1985).

	Men			Women		
	Novice (n = 255)	Advanced (n = 160)	Top (n = 56)	Novice (n = 255)	Advanced (n = 160)	Top (n = 56)
Head	19	21	27	17	18	19
Arms	27	19	35	33	16	15
Body	12	19	11	9	18	20
Legs	42	40	26	41	48	46

that he treated as an ophthalmologist in his practice over a 2.5-year period. Similar studies were performed by Littlewood (1982), MacEwen (1987) and Barrell *et al.* (1981). Injuries to patients wearing glasses tended to be more serious. Littlewood (1982) reported on 65 cases of traumatic hyphaemia treated in a university hospital and caused by sporting injuries. Of these, 29 (=45%) were caused by squash.

MacEwen (1987) examined the casualty records retrospectively over an 18-month period, thus discovering 246 cases of sport-related eye injuries. Squash was responsible for 19 (=7.7%) of these injuries, and most of the eye injuries were minor.

Barrell *et al.* (1981) identified the case notes of 118 sport-related eye injuries over a 2-year period. Of these, 58 occurred while playing squash. They estimated the rate of eye injury to be 5.2 eye injuries per 100 000 playing sessions. Further studies have been performed by a number of authors (Vinger & Tolpin, 1978; Clement & Fairhurst, 1980; Bankes, 1985). Bankes (1985) asked all ophthalmologists in England to report any ocular injuries sustained from squash during a 6-month survey period. A total of 339 players (278 men, 61 women) were reported. Injuries caused by balls outnumbered those caused by racquets by more than 2 : 1. In 40 cases, some degree of permanent visual impairment resulted (Bankes, 1985).

Vinger and Tolpin (1978) studied all ocular injuries caused by racquet sports treated in a surburban practise of five ophthalmologists during a 15-month period. They recorded 82 such injuries, broken down into 73 caused by tennis, six by squash, two by badminton and one by racquetball. One fact which emerged was that injuries seemed independent of the level of experience of the players. Clement and Fairhurst (1980) recorded all head injuries sustained during 10 658 competitive squash matches. The overall risk of injury per match was 0.6%. Racquet injuries accounted for 83% of the trauma. There were two eye injuries, giving a rate of 9.4 eye injuries per 100 000 competitive games.

Non-contact injuries

Of the acute non-contact injuries, ankle sprains are the most prevalent, followed by muscle injuries — mainly calf, hamstrings and back. Ruptured Achilles tendons provide a significant number (18%) according to Berson *et al.* (1978), who also concludes that older players run a greater risk of a serious injury than younger players. In particular, their survey showed a higher occurrence of orthopaedic injuries in the group of players over 40. In addition, the study by Pforringer and Keyl (1978) demonstrated a considerably increased rate of Achilles tendon injuries in players over 30.

Two special injuries are worthy of attention. Sherlock *et al.* (1987) reported on a patient with symptoms caused by a thrombosis of the carotid artery which he attributed to a game of squash. The likely mechanism appeared to be a stretching injury to the internal carotid artery as a result of extreme rotation and hyperextension of the neck.

Sheehan and Rainsbury (1987) reported a case of thrombosis of the inferior vena cava occurring in a previously healthy young man following a game of squash. They postulated that a tear in a small retroperitoneal vein was followed by a progressive ascending iliac vein thrombosis.

Of injuries caused by overuse, chronic back pain is the most prevalent followed by patellofemoral pain, chronic meniscal problems and chronic ankle pain. Chronic ankle pain usually results from ankle sprains. In a prospective study of 400 patients with ruptured lateral ankle ligaments (diagnosis confirmed with arthrography), the incidence of pain by palpation of the medial aspect of the ankle joint was 65% (van Dijk, 1990). At 6 months follow-up, 28% of patients still had complaints located on the medial aspect of the ankle. This was independent of the treatment (50% operative treatment, 50% conservative treatment with bandage). In an attempt to identify the cause of these medially located problems, a consecutive series of 30 patients was studied. These patients underwent operative repair of their acutely ruptured lateral ankle ligament complex. During this procedure an arthroscopy of the ankle joint was performed, whereby the medial aspect of the ankle joint was visualized. In 19 patients, a fresh injury of the cartilage was found. Most typically, the injury was located at the tip and/or anterior distal part of the medial malleolus, as well as on the opposed medial facet of the talus. In six cases, the cartilage destruction was such that a loose body had been formed. In most cases, the cartilage defect was associated with some synovitis or formation of fibrous tissue. The conclusion of the study was that in patients with rupture of one or more of the lateral ankle ligaments after an inversion trauma, an impingement occurs between the medial malleolus and medial aspect of the talus, which resulted in two-thirds of the patients in macroscopic damage to the cartilage. At 1 year follow-up nine patients complained of pain, swelling and/or stiffness located on the medial aspect of their ankle joint. Cartilage damage on the medial aspect of the ankle joint is the main cause of residual problems after lateral ankle ligament rupture.

In the upper body the main overuse injury involves the wrist. The pain is usually located over the dorsal wrist capsule and can be elicited by a forced dorsal flexion movement of the wrist. This is especially strong when this movement is performed while holding a relatively heavy racquet like a squash racquet, and hitting a relatively heavy ball like a squash ball. This repeated quick flick of the wrist exerts stress on the capsule and causes injury to the triangular shaped cartilage or chondromalacia. Therapy consists of some form of immobilization, non-steroidal anti-inflammatory drugs and, finally, change of stroke technique. The player should avoid making the stroke from the wrist. In particular and importantly, forced dorsiflexion movements must be abandoned. Helal (1979) reported on three squash players with chronic wrist injuries due to minor degrees of subluxation of the pisiform bone. Two of them also showed chondromalacia of the articular cartilage of the pisitriquetral joint. All three patients' conditions were relieved by excision of the pisiform bone (Helal, 1979).

Causes of injuries

The relatively high incidence of injuries in squash is the result of several factors. The first of these is the very nature of the game itself in which two players move around the same enclosed physical area, carrying a potentially dangerous racquet with them and continuously having to adjust themselves to rapidly changing strenuous movement patterns.

The rules of the game do provide for the player to stop the rally and ask for a 'let' (a replay of the point) if he or she feels playing on would endanger the opponent either with the racquet or ball.

Unfamiliarity with the rules (e.g. by beginners) increases the risk of such injuries considerably, especially when one considers that the speed of the game means that such a decision to stop must be more or less instinctive. Another aspect is the short time available for physical recovery in between two rallies. The time between games (1–1.5 min) is the only time for real recuperation. The combination of rapid bending and turning, overstretching and overstressing, multiple starts, sliding and loss of footing are the main causes of ankle, knee and back injuries. Injuries in beginners often arise from unfamiliarity with the game and its rules, faulty technique, inexperience and lack of physical condition. Injuries to top players are often caused by straining too hard, overtraining and an overexcessive desire to win.

Prevention of injuries

The measures mentioned in this article which can be taken to prevent squash injuries are based on facts which have been born from experience. There are but a few known studies (Bishop, 1981; Feigelman *et al.*, 1983) which actually try to evaluate the effect of preventive

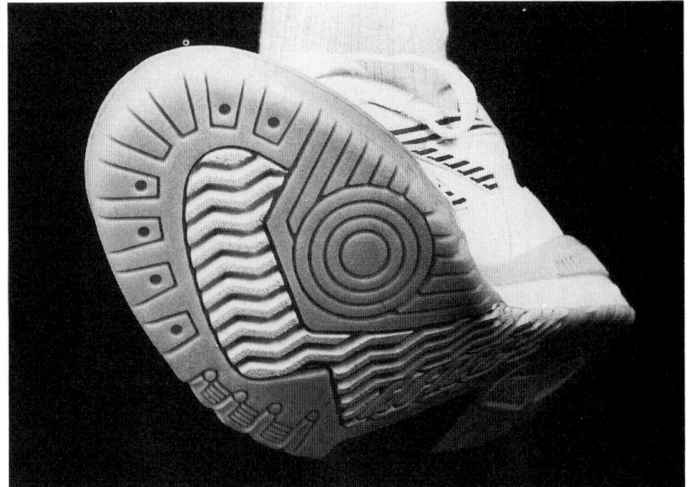

Fig. 31.1 Squash shoes must give sufficient support to the foot and the sole of the shoe should have shock-absorbing qualities. The underside of the sole should not have so coarse a profile that it unnecessarily hinders turning movements. It is for this reason that most squash shoes have a circular profile.

measures in squash. The main suggested preventive measures are:

1 Increased awareness, knowledge and application of the rules of the game.

2 Increased knowledge and skill in technique and tactics.

3 A good and balanced training schedule.

4 Wearing of correct and good quality footwear.

Squash shoes must give sufficient support to the foot and the sole of the shoe should have shock-absorbing qualities. The underside of the sole should not have so coarse a profile that it unnecessarily hinders turning movements. It is for this reason that most squash shoes have a circular profile (Fig. 31.1). The role of taping and bracing is still under dispute. In players with chronic instability there is definitely a role for these measurements (Fig. 31.2). A good warming up and limbering down and the taping of sensitive or vulnerable joints are also important.

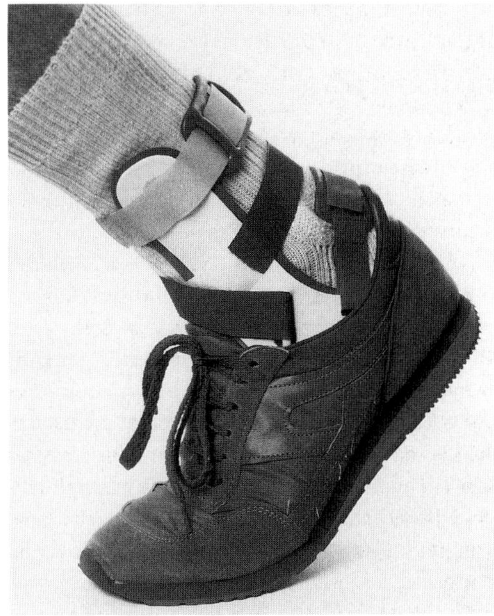

Fig. 31.2 The role of taping and bracing is still under dispute. In players with chronic instability there is definitely a role for these measurements in the prevention of recurrent sprains.

The prevention of eye injuries can be helped by the wearing of special eye protectors (Fig. 31.3). The unprotected eye is at great risk from injuries from both racquet and ball (Easterbrook, 1985). Standard spectacles or contact lenses offer no protection at all from injury: on the contrary they greatly increase the chance of a penetrating injury (Ingram & Lewkonia, 1973; Vinger & Tolpin, 1978; Gregory, 1986). Fiegelman *et al.* (1983) tested a variety of eye guards in the laboratory. All open (lenseless) guards failed

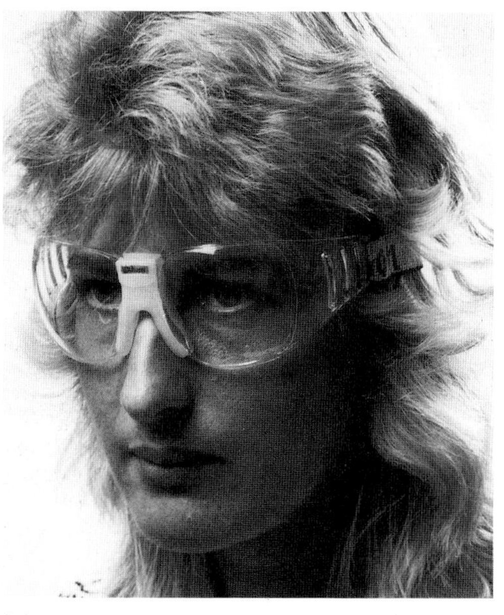

(a)

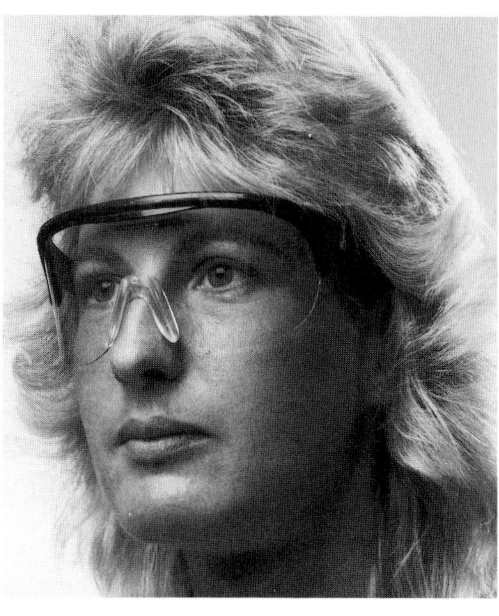

(b)

Fig. 31.3 The unprotected eye is at great risk from injuries from both racquet and ball. Standard spectacles or contact lenses offer no protection at all from injury; on the contrary they greatly increase the chance of a penetrating injury. Only polycarbonate plastic eye guards, as shown here, offer protection; the construction should be such that players performance is not hindered.

American and Canadian safety tests and the only lenses never to shatter were polycarbonate plastic ones. Despite some public awareness of the potential for eye injuries, nevertheless protective guards are rarely worn. The main reason appears to be that there is no form of protection which does not hinder player performance. Most players seem to judge that the small risk of a nonetheless devastating eye injury is outweighed by the advantages that would be conceded to their opponents (Verow, 1988). The final decision, therefore, must lie with governing bodies who must decide whether the frequency and severity of injuries necessitate legislation to enforce eye protection.

Conclusion

Squash is a moderate to high intensity intermittent exercise in which the injury incidence rate is above the injury incidence average taken over all sports. The average injury incidence rate seems to vary between 3.7 and 8.8 injuries$\cdot$100 squash players$^{-1}\cdot$year^{-1}. Just over 50% of the injuries are caused by racquet or ball contact. Most of these injuries are bruises, contusions or skin lacerations. The risk of eye injury would appear to be between 5.2 and 9.4 eye injuries per 100 000 competitive games. Just over 10% of these injuries result in some degree of permanent eye damage. Injuries in patients wearing glasses tend to be more serious. Polycarbonate plastic safety lenses are the only ones to offer sufficient protection to the eye. Of the non-contact injuries, over 70% involve the lower extremity. The most important prevalent injuries are ankle distorsion and muscle injuries to the calf, hamstrings and back. Injuries through overuse involve mainly the back, knee and ankle. In the upper body the most frequent injuries are to the wrist.

The main suggested preventive measures are:

1 Increased awareness, knowledge and application of the rules of the game.
2 Increased knowledge and skill in technique and tactics.
3 A good and balanced training schedule.
4 Wearing of correct and good quality footwear.
5 Prevention of eye injuries can be helped by the wearing of special eye protectors.

Concerning the eye protectors, the final decision must lie with governing bodies, who must decide whether or not the frequency and severity of injuries necessitate legislation to enforce eye protection.

References

Bankes, J.L.K. (1985) Squash rackets: a survey of eye injuries in England. *Br. Med. J.* **291**, 1539.

Barrell, G.V., Cooper, P.J., Elkington, A.R., Macfadyen, J.M., Powell, R.G. & Tormey, P. (1981) Squash ball to eye ball: the likelihood of squash players incurring an eye injury. *Br. Med. J.* **283**, 893–5.

Berson, B.L., Passof, T.L., Nagelberg, S. & Thornton, J. (1978) Injury pattern in squash players. *Am. J. Sports Med.* **6**, 323–5.

Berson, B.L., Roinick, A.M., Ramas, C.G. & Thornton, J. (1981) An epidemiologic study of squash injuries. *Am. J. Sports Med.* **9**, 103–17.

Bishop, P. (1981) Performance of eye protectors in squash and racket ball under impact. *Phys. Sports Med.* **6**, 434.

Chapman, A.E. & Suyderhoff, R.N. (1986) Squash ball mechanics and implications for play. *Can. J. Appl. Sport Sci.* **11**, 47–54.

Chard, M.D. & Lachmann, S.M. (1987) Raquet sports — patterns of injury presenting to a sports injury clinic. *Br. J. Sports Med.* **21**(4), 150–3.

Clement, R.S. & Fairhurst, S.M. (1980) Head injuries from squash: a prospective study. *N. Zeal. Med. J.* **92** (663), 1–3.

Dijk, C.N. van (1990) Arthroscopie van het bovenste spronggewricht (Ankle arthroscopy). In J.B. van Mourik (ed) *Letsels van de Enkle en Voet*, pp. 69–86. SCN Harem, The Netherlands.

Dijk, C.N. van & Visser, F.C. (1985) Hoe gevaarlijk is squash? (How dangerous is squash?) *Gen. Sport* **3**, 88–90.

Easterbrook, M. (1978) Eye injuries in squash: a preventable disease. *Canadian Med. Assoc. J.* **118**, 298–305.

Easterbrook, M. (1982) Eye injuries in squash and racketball: an update. *Phys. Sports Med.* **10**, 47–56.

Feigelman, M.J., Sugar, J., Jednock, N. *et al.* (1983) Assessment of ocular protection for racquetball. *JAMA* **250**, 3305.

Garden, G., Hale, P.J., Horrorks, P.M., Grase, J. & Hammond, V. (1986) Metabolic and hormonal responses during squash. *Eur. J. Appl. Physiol.* **55**, 445–49.

Gregory, P.T.S. (1986) Sussex eye hospital sports injuries. *Br. J. Ophthalmol.* **70**, 748–50.

Halpin, L. (1985) And still they come: the increase in squash players. In *Squash Rackets Association Annual*. Pelham Books, London.

Helal, B. (1979) Chronic overuse injuries of the pisotriquetral joint in racquet game players (Abstract) *Br. J. Sports Med.* **12**, 195–8.

Ingram, D.V. & Lewkonia, I. (1973) Ocular hazards of playing squash rackets. *Br. J. Ophthalmol.* **57**, 434–8.

Keyl, W., Pforringer, W. & Gast, W. (1980) Wie gefaerlich ist squash? (How dangerous is squash?) *Munch. Med. Wschr.* **122**, 1037–40.

Littlewood, K.R. (1982) Blunt ocular trauma and hyphaema. *Australian J. Ophthalmol.* **10**, 263–6.

MacEwen, C.J. (1987) Sport associated eye injury: a casualty department survey. *Br. J. Ophthalmol.* **71**, 701–5.

Maylack, F.H. (1988) Epidemiology of tennis, squash and racquetball injuries. *Clin. Sportsmed.* **7**(2), 233–43.

Mechelen, W. van & Hlobil, H. (1986) *Preventie van Sportletsels, deel 2, Sportspecifieke maatregelen* (Prevention of Injuries in Sport, Part 2, Sport-specific measurements). Werkgroep inspanningsfysiologie en gezondheidkunde Interfaculteit Lichamelijke Opvoeding, Vrije Universiteit, Amsterdam.

Merciez, M., Beillot, J., Gratas, A., Rochcongar, P. & Lessard, Y. (1987) Adaption to work load in squash players: laboratory tests and oncourt recordings. *J. Sport Med.* **27**, 98–104.

Montgomery, D.L., Malcolm, V. & McDonnell E. (1981) A comparison of the intensity of play in squash and running. *Phys. Sportsmed.* **9**, 116–19.

Montpetit, R.R. (1990) Applied physiology of squash. *Sports Med.* **10**(1), 31–41.

Montpetit, R.R., Beauchamp, L. & Leger, L. (1987) Energy requirements of squash and raquetball. *Phys. Sportsmed.* **15**, 106–12.

Montpetit, R.R., Leger, L. & Girardin, Y. (1977) Le racquetball, le squash et la condition physique (Raquetball, squash and physical condition). *Med. Quebec* **12**, 119–23.

Pforringer, W. & Keyl, W. (1978) Sportverletzungen bei squash (Injuries in squash). *Munch. Med. Wschr.* **120**, 1163–7.

Sheehan, N.J. & Rainsbury, R.M. (1987) Inferior vena cava thrombosis following a game of squash.

J. Roy. Soc. Med. **80**, 52.

Sherlock, D.J., Nightingale, S., Gardecki, T.I.M. & Hamer, J.D. (1987) Squash injury to the internal carotid artery. *Eur. J. Vasc. Surg.* **1**, 285–7.

Verow, P.G. (1988) Eye injuries in squash (Letter). *Br. J. Sports Med.* **22**, 81–2.

Vinger, P.F. & Tolpin, D.W. (1978) Racket sports: An ocular hazard. *JAMA* **239**, 2575–7.

Visser, F.C. & Mihciokur, M., Dijk, C.N. van, Engelsman, J. Den & Roos, J.P. (1987) Arythmias in athletes: comparison of stress test, 24 h Holter and Holter monitoring during the game in squash players. *Eur. Heart J.* **8**, 29–32.

Chapter 32

Injuries in Golf

WILLIAM J. MALLON AND RICHARD J. HAWKINS

Golf is a low-intensity sport which would not seem to be associated with a high risk, or a significant number, of injuries. In classifications of relative physical demands of various sports, it is usually near the bottom of any list (Michener, 1976).

However, golf is one of the most popular participant sports in the world. In the USA in 1989, 24.7 million people actively played golf (National Golf Foundation, 1989). In addition, golfers tend to be older than participants in most other sports which are usually played by teenagers or young adults. Among the 24.7 million participants, the National Golf Foundation determined that 6.6 million of the golfers were 50 years old or older (National Golf Foundation, 1989).

The mere quantity of participants, the fact that they tend to be older, and often not in good physical condition, suggests that the number of injuries relating to golf may still be high, despite the low demands placed on the body by the sport. Recent epidemiological work corroborates this hypothesis.

Epidemiology of injuries

It is well established that professional golfers play in spite of numerous ailments, some minor, some major. It has been estimated that over 50% of touring professionals have sustained some injury which required them to stop playing competitively, on the average, from 3–10 weeks (McCarroll & Gioe, 1982). In addition, amateur or recreational golfers also sustain a significant number of injuries. Over a 3-year period, McCarroll *et al.* (1990) and Mallon (1993) separately documented over 1200 injuries to this group.

A golf swing involves a significant rotatory torque of the trunk and requires both shoulders to be moved through a wide, rather unusual range of motion at very high speeds (Williams, 1967; Cochran & Stobbs 1968; Jorgensen, 1970; Milburn, 1982). Compared to professionals, weekend golfers do not place the same demands upon their bodies in terms of frequency of play and practice, yet their lesser demands are placed upon bodies not as well suited to the task as those of the professionals. In addition, it is well established that the techniques practised by recreational players are less refined and may place greater stress upon the musculoskeletal system during any individual swing (Abernethy *et al.*, 1990; Hosea *et al.*, 1990; Larkin *et al.*, 1990; Hosea, 1993).

Among professional golfers, McCarroll and Gioe (1982) found the low back to be the most commonly injured area in men, followed by the left wrist and shoulder (Table 32.1). Women professionals most commonly injured the left wrist, followed by the lower back (McCarroll & Gioe, 1982). Overall, the left wrist was the most common site of injury, followed by the lower back (they were virtually equal) and the left shoulder. Of approximately 300 professionals on the two tours, less than five play left-handed so it can be seen that the lead, or target-side,

Table 32.1 Injuries among professional golfers. From McCarroll & Gioe (1982).

	Men (n = 192)	(%)	Women (n = 201)	(%)	Totals (n = 393)	(%)
Left wrist	31	(16)	63	(31)	94	(24)
Lower back	48	(25)	45	(22)	93	(24)
Left hand	13	(7)	15	(8)	28	(7)
Left shoulder	21	(11)	6	(3)	27	(7)
Left knee	14	(7)	12	(6)	26	(7)
Left elbow	6	(3)	9	(5)	15	(4)
Left thumb	10	(5)	3	(2)	13	(3)
Feet	4	(2)	9	(5)	13	(3)
Cervical spine	9	(4)	3	(2)	12	(3)
Right wrist	3	(2)	9	(5)	12	(3)
Ribs	6	(3)	6	(3)	12	(3)
Right elbow	8	(4)	3	(2)	11	(3)
Right shoulder	1	(1)	9	(5)	10	(3)
Thoracic spine	8	(4)	0	(0)	8	(2)
Ankles	2	(1)	6	(3)	8	(2)
Groin	2	(1)	3	(2)	5	(1)
Left hip	4	(2)	0	(0)	4	(1)
Head	2	(1)	0	(0)	2	(1)

arm is most frequently injured. The incidence of injuries to the right arm in this study was quite low (McCarroll & Gioe, 1982).

McCarroll and Gioe (1990) performed a similar study of amateur golfers (Table 32.2). The low back and elbow were the most commonly injured areas; men sustaining injury to the back more commonly, while the primary site of injury among amateur women golfers was the elbow. In this study, the elbow involved is not mentioned. However, McCarroll and Gioe found that the lateral elbow was more frequently a source of injury than the medial elbow among amateur golfers.

Table 32.2 Injuries among amateur golfers. From McCarroll *et al.* (1990).

	Men (n = 584)	(%)	Women (n = 124)	(%)	Totals (n = 708)	(%)
Lower back	210	(36)	34	(27)	244	(35)
Elbow	190	(33)	44	(36)	234	(33)
lateral	160	(27)	34	(27)	194	(27)
medial	30	(5)	10	(8)	40	(6)
Hand and wrist	124	(21)	18	(15)	142	(20)
Shoulder	64	(11)	20	(16)	84	(12)
Knee	52	(9)	14	(11)	66	(9)
Neck	26	(5)	2	(2)	28	(4)
Hip	18	(3)	4	(3)	22	(3)
Ribs	16	(3)	6	(5)	22	(3)
Ankle	8	(1)	10	(8)	18	(3)
Foot	12	(2)	0	(0)	12	(2)
Head	12	(2)	0	(0)	12	(2)
Thigh	8	(1)	0	(0)	8	(1)
Face	6	(1)	0	(0)	6	(1)
Abdomen	4	(1)	0	(0)	4	(1)
Calf	4	(1)	0	(0)	4	(1)
Forearm	0	(0)	2	(2)	2	(0)

Jobe and Moynes (1982) and Jobe *et al.* (1986) reviewed his golf patient population. Of 412 injuries attributable to golf, Jobe found 85 of these to involve the shoulder, and felt that 79 of these 85 involved injuries to the rotator cuff. He did not discuss details of the remaining 327 patients. This is a higher proportion of shoulder injuries than found either by McCarroll and Gioe (1982), McCarroll *et al.* (1990) or Mallon (1993) but it should be remembered that Jobe has a specialized referral practice and is renowned as a shoulder surgeon.

Mallon (1993) reviewed golf injuries among recreational golfers and found that the majority of complaints involved the lower back (52%). Second in incidence were injuries to the elbow (24%). Shoulder (8%) and wrist (8%) problems followed in frequency of complaints (Table 32.3).

The term 'golfer's elbow' has been used to describe medial epicondylitis, apparently feeling that this is more common among golfers, while lateral epicondylitis, termed 'tennis elbow', is felt to be more common among tennis players. However, both McCarroll and Gioe (1982) and Mallon (1993) found that among professional and recreational golfers, lateral elbow pain was three times more common than medial elbow pain.

Stover *et al.* (1976) discussed stress syndromes from golf without performing a detailed epidemiological study. They felt that lateral epicondylitis occurred only in the right elbow from pronation while medial epicondylitis occurred primarily in the left elbow and attributed its origin to the supination required near and after impact.

The site of injury in golfers has been discussed in several articles, as referenced above. However, diagnoses of injuries at each site have not been specifically addressed. It is likely, however, that most golf injuries are joint sprains or musculotendinous strains, as is common in most repetitive sports (Garret, 1983).

Prevention of injuries

Warm-up and practice

Warming-up before playing a round of golf is advocated by most golf professionals (Palmer, 1963; Nicklaus, 1968; Player, 1974). All professionals warm-up by practising for at least 30 min before playing. Yet a large number of recreational golfers rarely practice any full shots prior to playing a round of golf. If they do warm-up at all, it often includes only striking a few putts on the putting green, which is the lowest intensity shot in golf, and hardly prepares the player for a high-intensity effort on his or her first full drive. In some cases, the

Table 32.3 Injuries among amateur golfers. From Mallon (1993).

	Men (n = 1160)	(%)	Women (n = 249)	(%)	Totals (n = 1409)	(%)
Lower back	617	(53)	111	(45)	728	(52)
Left elbow	273	(24)	68	(27)	341	(24)
lateral	131	(11)	49	(20)	180	(13)
medial	44	(4)	19	(8)	63	(4)
Left shoulder	101	(9)	10	(4)	111	(8)
Left wrist	71	(6)	35	(14)	106	(8)
Left ankle	34	(3)	7	(3)	41	(3)
Vision problems	28	(2)	6	(2)	34	(2)
Right hip	13	(1)	4	(2)	17	(1)
Left hip	10	(<1)	4	(2)	14	(1)
Right knee	7	(<1)	3	(1)	10	(<1)
Left knee	6	(<1)	1	(<1)	7	(<1)

golfer's failure to practice before playing is due to the lack of adequate practice facilities. However, in that case it is possible to warm-up with some stretching and swing exercises (Nicklaus, 1968).

Although the dogma of warming-up before playing is espoused by golf professionals, this has never been studied in golfers to determine if any physiological benefits actually occur which might decrease injury rates or improve performance. However, the physiological benefits of warm-up have been studied for other sports and other physical activities.

Among runners, Ingjer and Strømme (1979) compared an active warm-up to a passive warm-up of muscles (using hot showers) to no warm-up. They concluded that the active warm-up could substantially benefit athletic performance (Ingjer & Strømme, 1979). In a review article, Bennett (1984) concluded that high body temperatures permitted rapid rates of muscle contraction. However, this may also only affect performance and not injury development.

Safran *et al.* (1988) used a rabbit model to study the effects of isometric preconditioning on muscular injury. They concluded that physiological warming by isometric preconditioning was of benefit in preventing muscular injury by increasing the length to failure and the elasticity of the muscle tendon unit.

No studies have shown any detrimental effects from warming up before participating in sports, including golf. Thus, although specific studies have not been done, it appears likely that a short warm-up period before playing may benefit the performance of the golfer and possibly decrease their risk of injury.

Typical warm-up regimens begin with the player hitting golf balls on the driving range. A typical basket of practice balls contains approximately 50 balls and these can usually be hit in about 30 min. Most professionals recommend beginning with short pitch shots, which are played with a lofted club such as a wedge. These require only a short, low-intensity swing. After the player hits a few of these, they should then increase the length and intensity of the swing gradually. After the player has graduated to a full swing with a lofted club, he or she can then use the lower lofted clubs which hit the ball further, eventually building up to hitting the last few shots with a driver. As the clubs decrease in loft, the length of swing and the length of the shot both increase, and the intensity of effort increases concomitantly. Thus the longest shots should be hit only after fully warming-up with less lofted clubs.

Prior to beginning actual play, and after warming up by hitting full shots, most players will benefit from hitting some putts on the putting green and practising some short pitches around the putting green. Though it is unlikely that these shots will help avoid injuries, it is possible that they may improve the player's performance.

Madalozzo (1987) has stated that putting on the practice green or hitting a bucket of practice balls does not constitute a proper warm-up. He considers the definition of a warm-up to be a period of activity which gradually takes the body from a state of rest to an optimal working condition. He recommends beginning with activities which increase body temperature such as walking or a slow jog, followed by low-level calisthenics, stretching exercises and then specific golf-related activity such as hitting golf balls.

This approach is ideal. It cannot be faulted and Bennett's work on thermal dependence of muscle function supports it (Bennett, 1984). Similar methods are often used by many professionals, but the recreational player can rarely afford the time to perform such a lengthy warm-up. It is likely that beginning with short shots and increasing the length and intensity of the swing, as described above, will gradually raise the temperature of the golf-related muscles and constitute an adequate warm-up.

Technique training

One of the causes of injury in sports is usually considered to be poor techniques, although this has never been scientifically verified. In fact, it may be difficult to do so directly although indirect evidence of this can be deduced.

Jobe and Moynes (1986) compared biomechanical data of golf swings done by golf professionals and amateurs and found that the professionals used a much lower percentage of their maximal muscular output potential during their swing. This finding is supported by the work of Abernathy *et al.* (1990), Hosea (1993) and Hosea *et al.* (1990) who found that stress levels in the lumbar musculature were much higher among less skilled players. This is despite the fact, in both cases, that professionals tend to generate a higher velocity of the body segments and consequently more clubhead speed.

It is likely that this efficiency is due to the professional's use of a more refined technique. As they are using a lower percentage of their muscular potential, they will likely avoid the high stresses often associated with acute musculotendinous strains (Garrett, 1983). It does not, however, protect the professionals from chronic overuse injuries which may be the result of the high frequency with which they must practice and play to be successful.

In golf, development of proper technique can be done by several methods. There are multiple golf journals and magazines which discuss techniques. In addition, many golf professionals have written books on learning to play with proper swing mechanics.

The golf professional at most courses or clubs is usually available for golf lessons to instruct the less skilled player in the development of techniques which may make the player less susceptible to injury. In fact, if the player has a pre-existing injury or injury tendency, the professional may be able to help them design a swing which avoids stressing the affected body part. If a golfer truly wishes to spend time developing proper technique to improve his or her performance and decrease risk of injury, lessons from a golf professional are most likely the best method by which this can be achieved.

Flexibility conditioning

It has never been proved scientifically that one lessens the chance of injury or plays better golf by becoming more flexible. However, it seems that this would be the case because of the wide range of motion demanded of multiple joints during a golf swing.

During the backswing of a top calibre golfer, the trunk rotates 90° or more relative to the target line. This is usually termed the shoulder turn and is a combination of the hip turn, which occurs via pelvic rotation, and trunk rotation, which occurs primarily in the thoracic spine.

Also during the backswing, the shoulders must move through a wide range of motion (Jobe & Moynes, 1986). The left shoulder must flex from 50 to 80°, and then horizontally adduct almost 70°, to reach a position in which it crosses the chest. In addition, it also undergoes internal rotation. The right shoulder is abducted about 40°, and externally rotated about 90° (Jobe *et al.*, 1986).

Several of the above ranges of the trunk and the shoulders are close to the limits of the normal adult. The less flexible the golfer, the closer the above ranges will be to that golfer's maximum. Two alternatives then exist: (i) either the golfer will be forced to shorten his or her swing; or (ii) the golfer will still attempt a full-length swing, but with greatly increased muscle tension. While there is nothing inherently wrong with a short swing, if a golfer can increase flexibility, any lengthening of the swing will decrease muscle tension, as the range of joint motion achieved will be a smaller percentage of maximum. In general, most professionals feel that a lot of muscle tension is detrimental to the golf swing.

Nicklaus (1968) has described an excellent series of exercises to increase trunk flexibility, although he mentioned using them only as a warm-up series of stretching exercises (Jobe & Moynes, 1982). The exercises are as follows:

1 Trunk rotation with the club placed behind the lower back (Fig. 32.1).

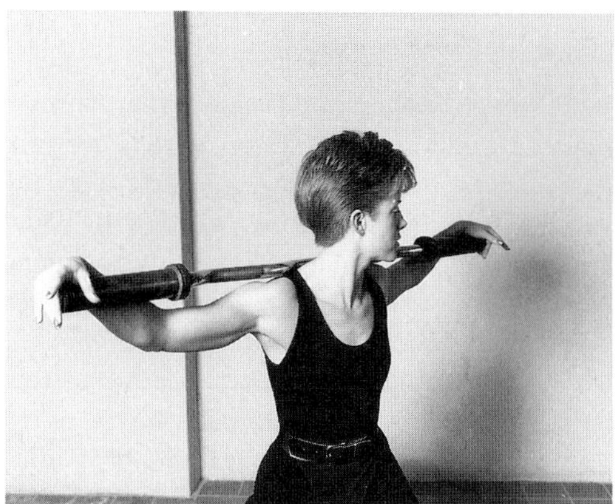

Fig. 32.1 Trunk rotation with a bar held over the shoulders. The trunk is rotated slowly in both directions. For increasing shoulder flexibility the exercise may also be performed with the club held behind the waist and the shoulders fully extended.

2 Trunk rotation with the club behind the back with the arms fully extended behind the back.
3 Trunk rotation with the club in front of the body with both arms elevated to shoulder height.

Trunk rotation is probably the key element to be developed in any flexibility programme for golf. Two excellent exercises for this are illustrated in Figs 32.1 and 32.2. Both involve placing a bar of some type over the shoulders. Both exercises are performed in the seated position. In Fig. 32.1, the trunk is slowly rotated side to side. In Fig. 32.2, the trunk is leaned towards the floor, and then, after returning to the upright, the body is leaned towards the opposite side. While the exercise can be performed with a broomstick or a golf club, a slightly weighted bar or stick, such as a barbell, will add a slight stretch at the end of the exercise as the weight will pull the body through the last few degrees of stretch. This should be performed very slowly to avoid injury.

Flexibility in the shoulders, which is also very important, can be developed in several ways. Jobe and Moynes (1986) have described a series of three exercises (Figs 32.3–32.5) which can be used to develop flexibility in the shoulders.

Perhaps the ultimate exercise for developing flexibility for golfers is to swing a weighted club. The player should attempt to maintain fairly good form, by not letting the left foot raise too high off the ground, nor rolling the weight to the outside of the right foot, and keeping the left arm fairly straight. If these parameters are maintained, the stretch will be placed entirely upon the trunk and shoulders, and flexibility will be developed in these areas.

Once again, it should be cautioned that

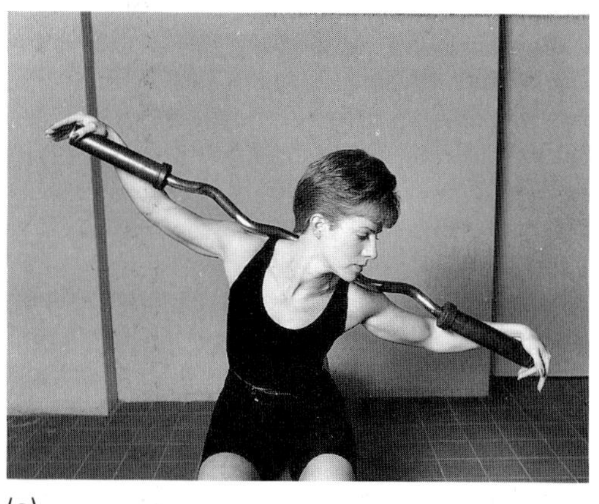

(a)

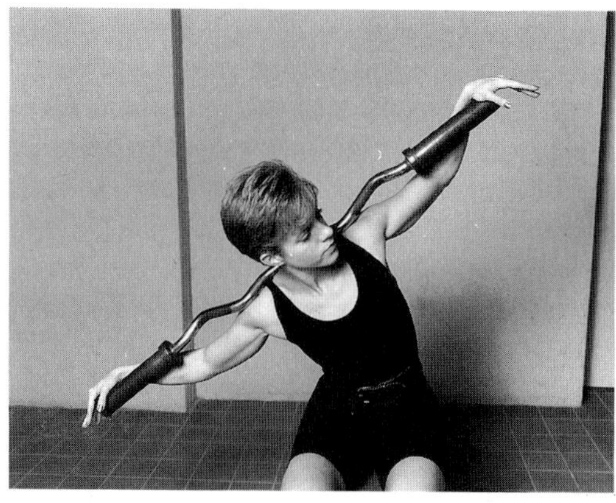

(b)

Fig. 32.2 Side bends. This exercise is performed to each side (a and b). The muscles exercised are the obliques and the erector spinae. These muscles will be alternately stretched and contracted.

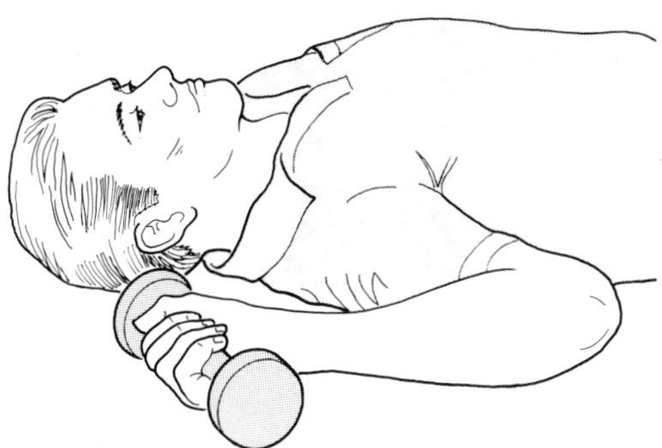

Fig. 32.3 Anterior rotator cuff stretching. While lying supine, a light weight (1–2 kg) is allowed to externally rotate the upper arm until a gentle stretch is felt in the anterior shoulder.

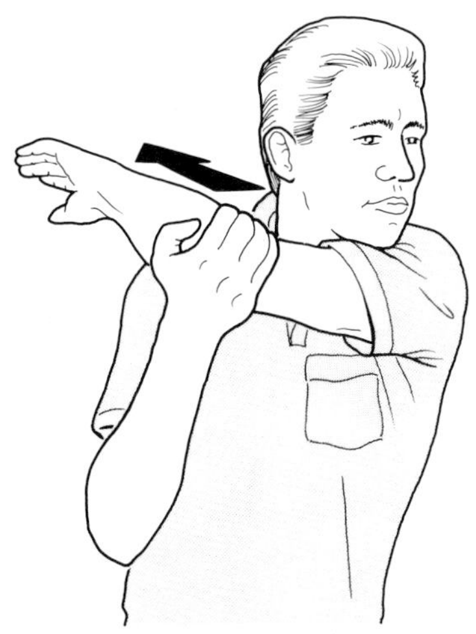

Fig. 32.4 Posterior rotator cuff stretching. The posterior cuff is stretched by gentle pressure from the opposite arm, as shown.

stretching exercises should be done slowly, so that the stretch at the end of the movement is a gentle one. Otherwise, injuries can result.

There are various stretching techniques which can be used, including statis stretches, ballistic stretches, and proprioceptive neuromuscular facilitation (PNF) (Sady *et al.*, 1982). PNF is a technique of therapeutic exercise which works muscles in diagonal patterns to take them from their fully lengthened state to

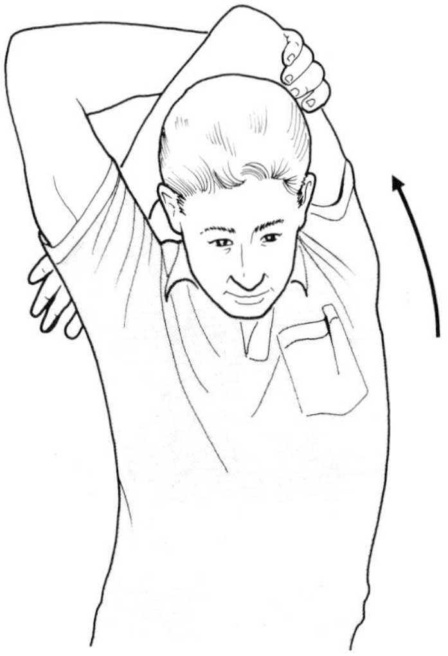

Fig. 32.5 Inferior rotator cuff stretching. The opposite arm applies gentle pressure to provide a stretch to the inferior cuff.

their most shortened state (Sobel, 1986). Sady *et al.* (1982) showed that PNF was the preferred method to increase flexibility. However, they also commented that there is conflicting evidence about this and that studies exist which show that any of the three is the superior method (Sady *et al.*, 1982).

Strength conditioning

As discussed earlier, the majority of injuries to golfers involve the back, elbow and wrist. Thus conditioning to strengthen the lower back and forearms should help decrease injury rates among golfers.

As with flexibility, it has never been proven that increased strength decreases an athlete's chances of becoming injured. However, this dogma has been repeated quite often and the hypothesis behind it is reasonable. In addition, it is unlikely that increasing the strength of muscle groups will increase the rate of injury from playing a sport, and the increased strength may be associated with improved performance.

The lower back can be exercised by the three stretching exercises mentioned above, but using a light barbell. These are variants of trunk rotations, one type of which is illustrated in Fig. 32.1. While the exercise causes a stretch on one side of the body (and eccentric strengthening on that side), the opposite side is contracting concentrically to work as a strengthening exercise.

To support the lower back, it is quite important to keep the abdominal muscles strong. The best exercise for this is termed a 'crunch' by body builders. It is actually an abdominal curl, in which, rather than doing a full sit-up, only the head and shoulders are curled up off the floor, while keeping the small of the back pressed firmly against the floor. This should be done with the feet elevated and not held down, the hip and knees flexed, and with the arms folded across the chest, rather than behind the neck. The beginning and ending movements are shown in Fig. 32.6. This exercise isolates the abdominal muscles while decreasing the use of the hip flexors, which can lead to further back problems by increasing lumbar lordosis.

The forearm muscles maintain the grip on the club and if not strong enough, they will be unable to maintain a firm grip as clubhead speed is increased. In addition, Jorgensen (1970) has shown that during the first part of the downswing the ability to maintain a torque on the grip by the wrists can increase clubhead speed. Increased forearm strength will also allow a firm grip to be maintained with a smaller percentage of grip strength. This will then increase flexibility in the wrists during the golf swing (Cochran & Stobbs, 1968). In addition, stronger forearm muscles may dissipate the shock of impact (from eccentric overload) which is likely responsible for many of the elbow injuries seen among golfers.

An excellent exercise to develop the forearms is simply to squeeze a rubber ball, performing many repetitions, up to 100·set^{-1}. Although in a different sport, this was the method used by Rod Laver to develop his left forearm perhaps enabling him to play tennis at championship levels.

Three weight exercises which can develop the forearm muscles are shown in Figs 32.7–32.9. These are the wrist curl, the reverse wrist curl and the wrist roller. In the first two (Figs 32.7 & 32.8) the barbell is lowered to the end of the fingertips and then the fingers curls the weight back into the palm, followed by the wrists curling up to lift the weight up another 3–5 cm. The wrist curl is performed with the forearms supinated while the reverse wrist curl

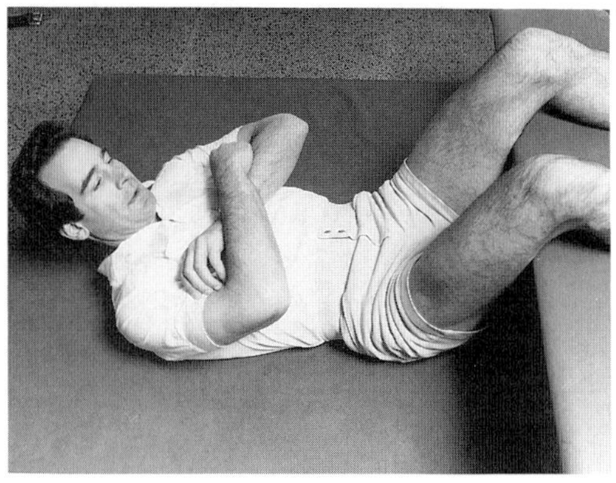
(a)

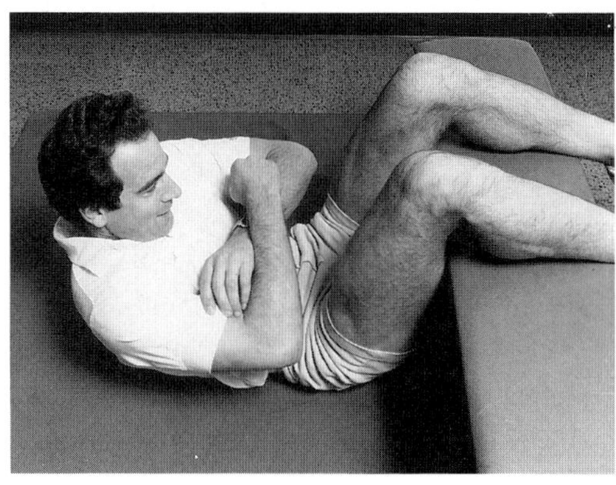
(b)

Fig. 32.6 Abdominal curl or 'crunch'. The upper body is slowly curled off the floor. The first movement is to curl the chin to the chest (a), then the shoulders slowly rise from the floor, and only at the end does the upper abdomen clear the floor slightly (b). This exercise should always be done slowly, with the knees flexed, and with the feet not held down.

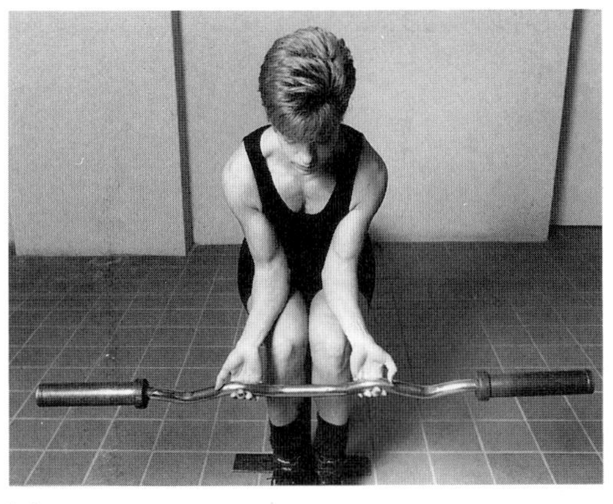
(a)

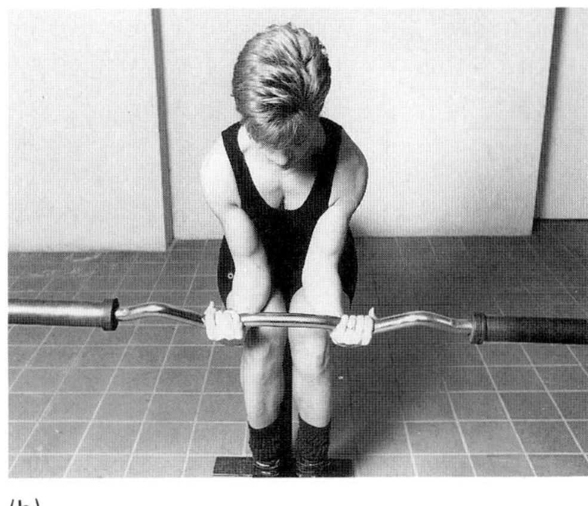
(b)

Fig. 32.7 Wrist curl. With the forearms supinated, a barbell (or dumb-bells) are curled up from the end of the fingers into the palm (a), and the wrist is then volar-flexed (b).

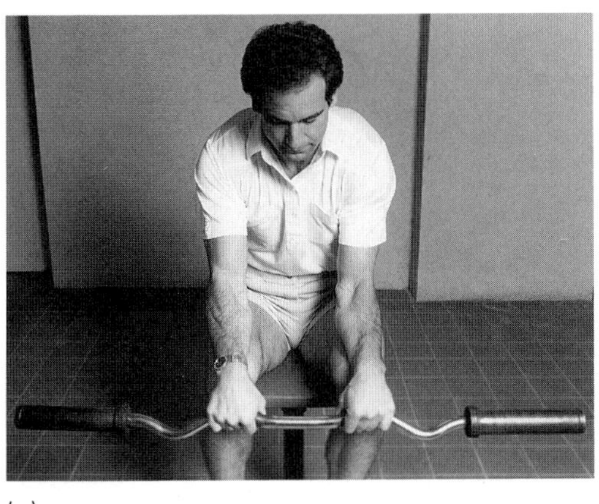
(a)

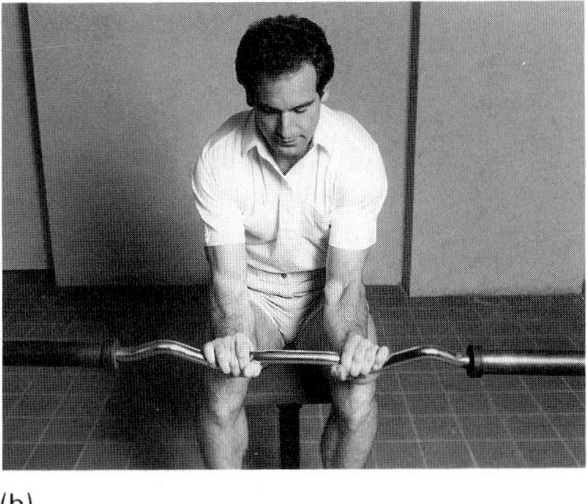
(b)

Fig. 32.8 Reverse wrist curl. With the forearms pronated (a), the wrist is then dorsiflexed (b).

is done with the forearms pronated. The wrist roller is performed by rolling the weight up all the way until the rope is fully wound around the bar (Fig. 32.9).

Treatment of golf-related injuries

The most common injuries among golfers occur in the back, elbow, wrist and shoulder, in that approximate order (McCarroll & Gioe, 1982; McCarrol *et al.*, 1990; Mallon, 1993). Treatment of those injuries begins with some form of resting for the injured part, at least initially.

As runners often cut down on their mileage when they are injured, so golfers must often be satisfied playing slightly less during their recuperation from an injury. One specific measure which often helps is to practise less than normal. Although practice is necessary for improvement, the continued stress of hitting balls repetitively places increased strain on the body and the duration of practice sessions may need to be decreased while injured.

Chronic injuries may necessitate some tech-

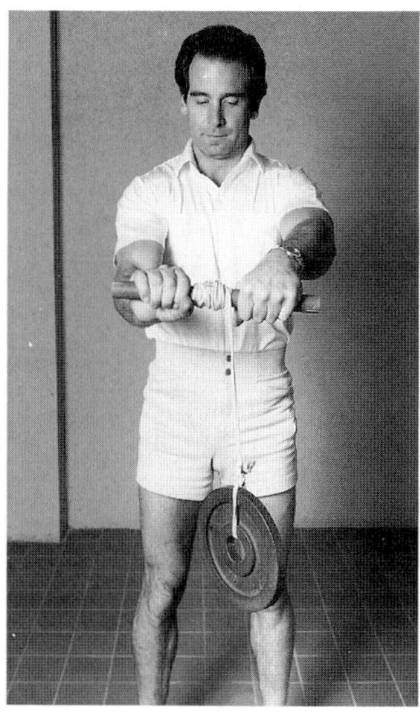
(a)

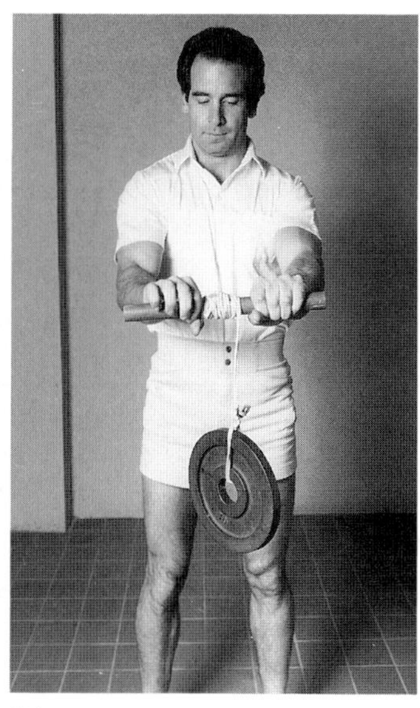
(b)

Fig. 32.9 Wrist roller. The weight held at the end of the rope is elevated by alternately volar flexing each wrist quickly. (a) Beginning, and (b) end of exercise.

nique changes and changes in equipment to allow the golfer to 'play around the injury'. Golfers with back pain will probably benefit from using one of the newer extra-long putters. These prevent the player from having to bend over from the waist, in a position which places extreme stress on the lumbosacral muscles and articulations.

There are three swing modifications which may help a player with back pain. One, the player may have to learn to swing with less torque in the back muscles. This is more of a 'classic' swing, as opposed to the modern swing, espoused by today's teaching professionals. The modern swing uses a large shoulder turn and minimal hip turn, usually with the left (or lead) foot kept relatively flat to the ground, creating excessive torque in the lower back muscles. The classic swing uses virtually equal amounts of hip and shoulder turn, with the player often rising up on the left toe. The second modification is a more upright stance, using more knee flex to reach the ball which golfer's with back pain will often benefit from. This takes stress off the lumbosacral area, but will necessitate a slightly flatter swing plane. Finally, players with back pain should learn to shorten their swings.

Players with elbow and wrist pain are difficult to treat. That is because impact, and the act of taking a divot, places a great deal of stress on the wrist and forearm musculature. If not playing competitively, a player may be able to play for awhile if he or she tees the ball up on all shots. While not legal for competition, this will avoid the jarring which occurs when a divot is taken. If the elbow or wrist pain is chronic, a player may need to change his or her swing to 'sweep' the ball off the turf, without taking a divot.

Shoulder pain in golfers usually results either from impingement or instability. Impingement usually occurs in the left shoulder in right-handed golfers. Golfer's with impingement syndrome will often benefit from shortening their swing and flattening their swing plane, to minimizing elevating their left arm. Golfer's with either impingement or instability symptoms while swinging will benefit from a shorter swing as this places less stress on the muscles about the shoulder.

In addition to swing and playing modifications, brief rest periods from the game, and decreasing the amount of playing and practice, treatment of golf-related injuries is similar to treatment of non-golf-related injuries. Nonsteroidal anti-inflammatory medication may decrease inflammation of soft tissues and promote more rapid healing. Cold therapy with ice packs will often serve the same purpose after playing and irritating the injured area. Back supports for players with chronic back pain may be necessary, although they will inhibit the swing to some degree. Golfers with wrist and elbow pain may benefit from using a wrist brace or forearm strap to take stress off the injured areas.

Conclusion

Though golf is a low-intensity sport, the number of players involved in the game, and the frequency with which they play, has led to a significant number of chronic injuries. The most frequently injured areas are the lower back, elbow and wrist.

Methods to decrease injury risk in golf include proper warming up before playing, and improving the technique of the golf swing to decrease stress on the musculoskeletal system. In addition, flexibility and strength conditioning should be performed as a training method for active golfers to also decrease the risk of injury.

References

Abernethy, B., Neal, R.J., Moran, M.J. & Parker, A.W. (1990) Expert–novice differences in muscle activity during the golf swing. In A.J. Cochran (ed) *Science and Golf*, pp. 54–60. E & FN Spon, London.

Bennett, A.F. (1984) Thermal dependence of muscle function. *Am. J. Physiol.* **247**, 217–29.

Cochran, A. & Stobbs, J. (1968) *The Search for the Perfect Swing*. Lippincott, Philadelphia.

Garrett, W.E. (1983) Strains and sprains in athletes. *Postgrad. Med.* **73**(3), 200–9.

Hosea, T.M. (1993) The golf swing: diagnosis, pathophysiology, and treatment of back problems. In W.J. Mallon, J.R. McCarroll & C.S. Stover (eds) *Medical Aspects of Golf*. FA Davis Co, Philadelphia (in press).

Hosea, T.M., Gatt, C.J., Galli, K.M., Langrana, N.A. & Zawadsky, J.P. (1990) Biomechanical analysis of the golfer's back. In A.J. Cochran (ed) *Science and Golf*, pp. 43–8. E & FN Spon, London.

Ingjer, F. & Strømme, S.B. (1979) Effects of active, passive, or no warm-up on the physiological response to heavy exercise. *Eur. J. Appl. Physiol.* **40**, 273–82.

Jobe, F.W. & Moynes, D.R. (1982) Delineation of diagnostic criteria and a rehabilitation program for rotator cuff injuries. *Am. J. Sports Med.* **10**(6), 336–9.

Jobe, F.W. & Moynes, D.R. (1986) *30 Exercises for Better Golf*. Champion Press, Inglewood, California.

Jobe, F.W., Moynes, D.R. & Antonelli, D.J. (1986) Rotator cuff function during a golf swing. *Am. J. Sports Med.* **14**(5), 388–92.

Jorgensen, T. (1970) On the dynamics of the swing of a golf club. *Am. J. Phys.* **38**(5), 644–51.

Larkin, A.F., Larkin II, W.F., Larkin, W.F. & Larkin, S.L. (1990) Annual torso specific conditioning program for golfers. In A.J. Cochran (ed) *Science and Golf*, pp. 61–3. E & FN Spon, London.

McCarroll, J.R. & Gioe, T.J. (1982) Professional golfers and the price they pay. *Phys. Sports Med.* **10**, 54–70.

McCarroll, J.R., Rettig, A.C. & Shelbourne, K.D. (1990) Injuries in the amateur golfer. *Phys. Sports Med.* **18**(3), 122–6.

Madalozzo, G.F.J. (1987) An anatomical and biomechanical analysis of the full golf swing. *Natl Strength Cond. Ass.* **9**(4), 6–8, 77–9.

Mallon, W.J. (1993) Epidemiology of golf injuries. In W.J. Mallon, J.R., McCarroll & C.S. Stover (eds) *Medical Aspects of Golf*. FA Davis Co, Philadelphia (in press).

Michener, J.A. (1976) *Sports in America*. Random House, New York.

Milburn, P.D. (1982) Summation of segmental velocities in the golf swing. *Med. Sci. Sports Exerc.* **14**(1), 60–4.

National Golf Foundation (1989) *Golf Participation in the United States*. National Golf Foundation, Florida.

Nicklaus, J.W. (1968) *My 55 Ways to Lower Your Golf Score*. Simon & Schuster, New York.

Palmer, A.D. (1963) *My Game and Yours*. Simon & Schuster, New York.

Player, G.J. (1974) *Gary Player: World Golfer*. Word, Waco, Texas.

Sady, S.P., Wortman, M. & Blanke, D. (1982) Flexibility training: Ballistic, static, or proprioceptive neuromuscular facilitation. *Arch. Phys. Med. Rehab.* **63**, 261–3.

Safran, M.R., Garrett, W.E., Seaber, A.V., Glisson,

R.R. & Ribbeck, B.M. (1988) The role of warmup in muscular injury prevention. *Am. J. Sports Med.* **16**(2), 123–9.

Sobel, J. (1986) Supplemental exercise program for throwing, swimming, and gymnastics. In F.A. Pettrone (ed) *Symposium on Upper Extremity Injuries in Athletes*, pp. 348–56. CV Mosby, St Louis.

Stover, C.N., Wiren, G. & Topaz, G.R. (1976) The modern golf swing and stress syndromes. *Phys. Sports Med.* **4**, 42–7.

Williams, D. (1967) The dynamics of the golf swing. *Q. J. Mech. Appl. Math.* **20**(2), 247–64.

Chapter 33

Injuries in Swimming

PETER J. FOWLER

Swimming at a competitive level places demands on the athlete which stress the muscles and tendon units of not only the shoulder but also of the knee, elbow, foot, ankle and back far beyond their natural limitations. Repetitive demands can predispose normal joints to injury. The enormous commitment made by top swimmers to their sport in terms of intensity and time spent in training is essential in order to achieve the desired level of success. Consequently, pain and injury are inevitable unless an equal commitment to prevention is made by the athlete, coach, trainer and sport physician.

Philosophies regarding training for the national calibre swimmer vary among coaches, but typically a swimmer in this group practises in the water a minimum of 5 days·week^{-1} often twice per day in sessions that are approximately 2 h in duration. A normal distance range is about 4000–8000 m·session^{-1}. The time spent in the water improves conditioning and technique while dry-land training increases strength and endurance.

Biomechanics

Familiarity with the biomechanics of the four strokes performed in competitive swimming is necessary so that those involved in the training and treatment of swimmers can contribute most effectively in both these areas. Keeping in mind that prevention of injury is as important as achieving speed and endurance, a good knowledge of the fundamental dynamics of each stroke is essential so that appropriate modifications and corrections can be recommended without compromising speed and efficiency.

Each of the four strokes, front crawl or freestyle, butterfly, backstroke and breaststroke, consists of four phases, (i) the reach or entry; (ii) the catch; (iii) the pull; and (iv) the recovery. The arms provide the majority (75%) of the propulsion in the front crawl, butterfly and backstroke whereas in the breaststroke arms and legs contribute equally. During the *reach* or entry phase, the arm reaches forward as it enters the water. In the *catch* phase which is similar in all competitive strokes, the swimmer begins to pull on the water. Here the elbow is flexed to approximately 100° and the shoulder begins to extend, horizontally abduct and slightly medially rotate. The *pull*, during which the swimmer sculls or pulls the water for the most efficient and forceful propulsion, varies slightly for each stroke. In this phase, except for the breaststroke, the arm starts at maximum elevation and ends in extension. The arm returns to start another pull in the *recovery* phase. Again with the exception of the breaststroke, the recovery is performed in the air.

Freestyle

Freestyle is the fastest stroke and the one most frequently used in practice. The hand enters the water with the palm facing downward, usually 30 cm in front of the shoulder, and reaches ahead until the arm is fully flexed.

A sculling motion initiates the pull phase and by rolling the torso about its longitudinal axis the arm is positioned deeper in the water where an S-shaped curving pull with the palm facing backward is produced under the torso. The recovery of one arm occurs simultaneously with the pull phase of the other arm and with a body roll which enables the arm to be released from the water and to sweep again into the entry position. Arm action is continuous with two to six vigorous flutter kicks per arm cycle.

Butterfly

In the butterfly stroke the arms and legs enter the water moving simultaneously during the pull and the recovery phases in a manner similar to freestyle. A dolphin motion with the whole body relieves stress on the shoulder. The legs also perform a dolphin kick, a flutter kick with the legs moving together.

Backstroke

In the backstroke, arm entry is performed with the shoulder in a fully elevated position. The arm enters the water straight and is enabled to produce an S-shaped pulling pattern to the side by the body roll. A flutter kick is used.

Breaststroke

In the breaststroke the arms, which are not allowed to pull below the waistline, move together during the pull and recovery phases. The whip kick which does not use natural musculoskeletal forces or motion at the knee joint, but is felt to be the superior kick in terms of speed and propulsion force, is performed. The legs are initially extended with the feet plantar flexed. The recovery begins with flexion of the hips and knees and ends with the feet dorsiflexed and external tibial rotation. The angle between the trunk and the thigh is 120°. As the knees extend, the feet are pushed outward and backward. The water is engaged with the soles of the dorsiflexed feet. Meanwhile the hip extensors drive the thighs toward the surface of the water and the legs are brought together with extension of the hips and knees. This action produces the maximal force of the kick. The feet are just a few inches apart while the knees are almost fully extended and the kick is completed with the feet in plantar flexion.

Shoulder injuries

Shoulder pain (swimmer's shoulder) is the most frequent complaint in the swimmer. Successful prevention requires the combined effort and cooperation of the athlete, coach and therapist. Rotator cuff pathology is the usual cause of the pain and is most often subacromial. This has been organized into three chronological stages by Neer and Walsh (1977).

Stage I, most often seen in athletes under 25, is oedema and haemorrhage.

Stage II: fibrosis and tendinitis develops in athletes over the age of 25.

Stage III is most often present in those over the age of 40 and involves the formation of bone spurs under the acromion and may be associated with complete tendon ruptures.

The aetiology of such cuff disorders in the swimmer is complex and may be a result of both anatomical features and biomechanical forces. Recent reports have quoted that 50% of swimmers have a history of shoulder pain (Richardson *et al.*, 1980) as compared to earlier surveys in the literature which reported this number to be 3% (Kennedy & Hawkins, 1974). This rise in incidence of swimmer's shoulder may be the result of an increase in training schedules. The best asset to both swimmers and coaches in reducing the incidence of swimmer's shoulder is an understanding of the factors involved.

The three main factors in rotator cuff tendinitis are (i) overwork, (ii) subacromial loading, and (iii) hypovascularity. The shoulder is the least stable joint and therefore the most vulnerable to injury with the strong, repeated overhead movements used. The muscles of the rotator cuff may work excessively hard merely to contain and stabilize the humeral head. This workload may fatigue these muscles and superior migration of the humeral head may result. This in turn increases subacromial loading which may then precipitate the onset of tendinitis.

The biceps and supraspinatus tendons insert on or across the humerus directly below the coracoacromial arch. When the arm is in abduction, forward flexion and internal rotation which is the position assumed in the catch phase of all competitive strokes, the head of the humerus moves under the arch and the tendons may be impinged here. This can result in a mechanical irritation and tendinitis which may further compromise the available space under the arch.

The functional relationship between arm position and blood supply to the supraspinatus and biceps tendons has been described by Rathbun and MacNab (1970). In adduction and neutral rotation, the tendons are stretched tightly over the head of the humerus and their blood supply is compromised. The vessels fill in abduction and circulation is restored. This 'wringing out' occurs in the area of the tendon most vulnerable to impingement and may contribute to early degenerative changes in the tendon as well as compounding the potential for damage by repetitive stress.

Again a knowledge of stroke mechanics as they relate to the factors contributing to tendinitis is important to the coach and trainer so that proper guidance can be available to the swimmer if modifications in technique are required to both treat and prevent injury. At entry and the first half of the pull phase the shoulder is in forward flexion, abduction and internal rotation. This forces the head of the humerus under the anterior acromion and coracoacromial ligament and may impinge the supraspinatus and the biceps tendon particularly in the fatigue situation.

Lateral impingement may be associated with the recovery phase of freestyle and butterfly strokes. The arm abducts in returning to the entry position and if there is associated internal rotation and/or horizontal abduction, the head of the humerus comes up against the lateral border of the acromion.

At the end of the pull phase, the shoulder is in adduction and internal rotation, a position which corresponds to the wringing out mechanism.

Biomechanical factors implicated in tendinitis seem to correlate with the freestyle arm position at the time swimmers experience pain. In a study by Webster *et al.* (1981), almost 50% of those with shoulder pain experienced it during the entry or the first half of the pull phase. 14% had pain during the second half of the pull phase, 23% reported pain during recovery and the remainder (17.8%) felt pain during the entire pull or recovery phase. Also some of these had pain throughout the entire stroke.

Clinically, tendinitis progresses insidiously with pain, which is often present at night or at rest becoming generalized about the shoulder. The athlete tends to avoid painful positions and develops subtle changes in stroke mechanics. All positions that aggravate symptoms will be modified despite the activities. The clinical classification of tendinitis is based on Blazina's categories for jumper's knee (Blazina, 1973) (Table 33.1).

Prevention of injuries

Table 33.2 summarizes a basic preventative programme (Fowler & Webster-Bogart, 1991). There are four principles basic to a preventive programme: (i) balanced muscle strengthening; (ii) flexibility; (iii) technique modification; and

Table 33.1 Clinical classification of tendinitis.

Grade I	Pain after the activity
Grade II	Pain during and after activity, not disabling
Grade III	Disabling pain during and after activity
Grade IV	Severe pain with daily activity

Table 33.2 Prevention of swimmer's shoulder.

Training regime	Gradually increase distance Gradually increase severity Place most vigorous sets at the beginning Proper warm-up and cool-down Warm-up after kicking sets
Strengthening	Include external rotators in dry-land sessions External rotator strengthening more than three times·week^{-1} Include exercises for the muscles surrounding the scapula No pain involved
Stretching	Under 15 years, single stretching Over 15 years pairs stretching Passive or PNF stretching only No ballistic stretching No pain involved
Stroke mechanics	Proper mechanics particularly during fatigue situations Proper body roll

PNF, proprioceptive neuromuscular facilitated.

(iv) avoidance of overwork. These can be readily incorporated into a training schedule as it begins. Any subsequent adjustments to the regimen should be made with these principles in mind.

Balanced muscle strengthening

In competitive swimming, both in pool and dry-land training, emphasis is naturally placed on strengthening the internal rotators and extensors important in propulsion (Fowler, 1988). An alteration in the balance of muscle strength between internal and external rotation, can result and contribute to tendinitis. A balanced exercise programme which includes strengthening of the external rotators as well as of the biceps and scapular muscles will help avert this imbalance. These exercises are simple to perform and require a minimum of readily available equipment such as surgical tubing, pullies, dental dam and free weights. The exercises are isotonic and eccentric to improve power and control in both prime mover and antagonist muscle functions. Also, they are performed in neutral, 90° of abduction and 90° of flexion to reproduce the arm position in the actual sport (Fig. 33.1). Biceps strengthening exercises should incorporate its functions as elbow flexor and forearm supinator and should be performed in several positions of shoulder range of motion as well. When doing weight-training, painful subacromial loading positions should be avoided. Paddles can produce increased leverage which may overload the rotator cuff muscles and should be used cautiously.

Flexibility

In 1985, Griep conducted a study which determined that regardless of gender or stroke most frequently used, those swimmers with restricted flexibility were more likely to develop tendinitis than those who enhanced their flexibility with a stretching programme.

Stretching should be included in the daily training warm-up routine. Pairs stretching is appropriate for those over 15 years of age as this group should be sufficiently mature to understand the dangers of these workouts (Fig. 33.2). If care is not taken to avoid overstretching of the soft tissues, irritation to the rotator cuff tendons can occur. Younger swimmers should stretch individually as illustrated (Fig. 33.3).

The stretching techniques employed by pairs are either passive or proprioceptive neuromuscular facilitated (PNF). In the former, the partner very slowly and gently stretches the swimmer to the pain-free limit and then holds this position. In the latter, the swimmer stretches to the pain-free limit. The partner maintains that position while the swimmer contracts against the resistance provided. These are repeated a variable number of times.

Modification of technique

Poor technique not only slows swimmers down

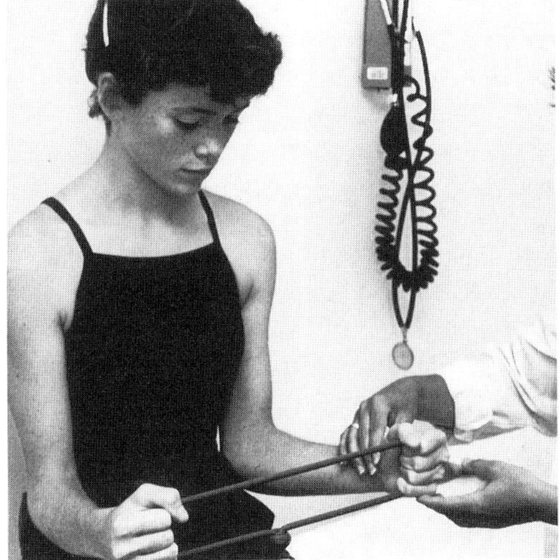

(a)

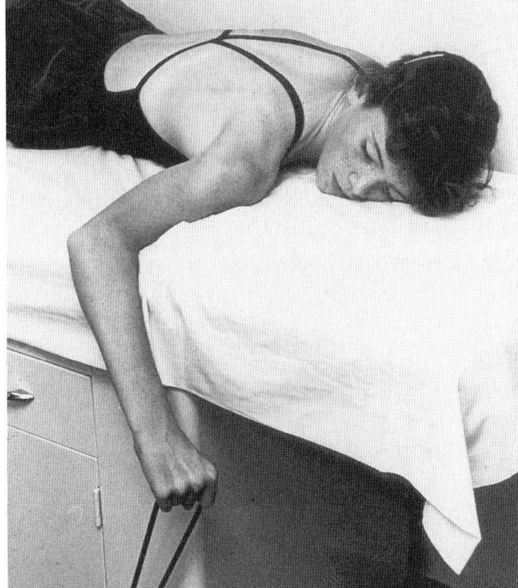

(b)

Fig. 33.1 External rotators are strengthened in neutral (a) and in 90° of abduction (b).

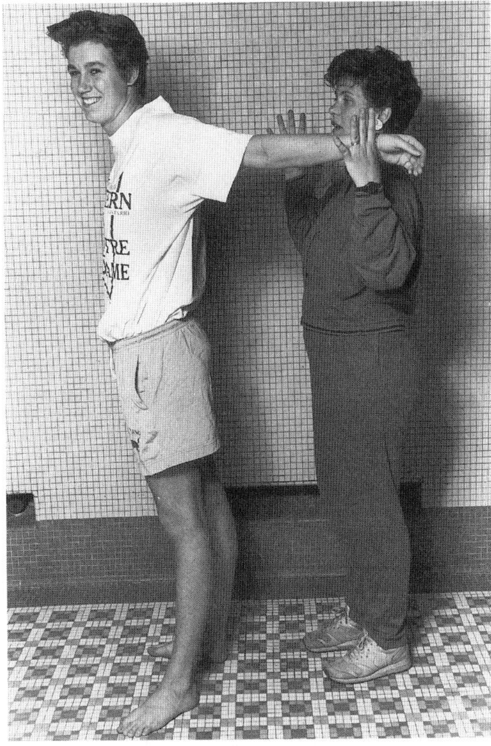

Fig. 33.2 A proper knowledge of technique is important in pairs stretching.

but can also be a cause of injury. Prevention of overwork and fatigue of the rotator cuff should be foremost in a coach's mind as training programmes are planned and the athlete's progress is monitored. Ongoing stroke analysis should be a routine process that can guide the swimmer away from errors that may contribute to tendinitis.

Of particular importance is the analysis of stroke mechanics during fatigue. Lateral shoulder impingement can be a result of insufficient body roll in freestyle or backstroke. A high elbow position during the recovery phase of the freestyle stroke must be achieved by body roll. Attempting to force the elbow into a higher position with muscle activity rather than sufficient body roll can induce subacromial impingement.

Overreach with excessive internal rotation

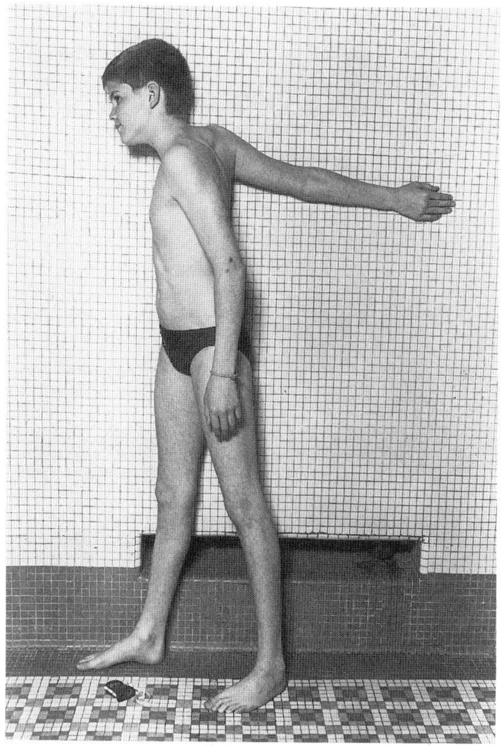

Fig. 33.3 Individual stretching is more appropriate for swimmers under the age of 15 years.

during the catch phase of all swimming strokes may cause undue subacromial loading and excessive activity for the cuff muscles to contain the humeral head.

The wringing out phenomenon is a result of the relationship between arm position and the blood supply to the supraspinatus and biceps tendon. In adduction and neutral rotation, the tendons are stretched tightly over the humeral head which compromises their blood supply. In abduction, the blood vessels fill and circulation is restored. This repeated hypovascularity which may contribute to early degenerative changes in the tendon can be intensified by excessive internal rotation. Changes to body roll, reach and the degree of shoulder rotation reduce the frequency and the length of time that the shoulder is in a precarious position.

Evidence as to the effect of breathing patterns on the incidence of tendinitis is contradictory. Breathing to alternate sides keeps the swimmer from leaning constantly on the same shoulder.

Avoidance of overwork

The demands on the swimmer should be increased gradually. Rigorous training sets before the athlete is ready or 'extra hard' practices at the beginning of training regimen can trigger the onset of tendinitis. Training sessions should be designed so that the difficult portion of the workout is completed early in the practice when the swimmer is rested. The workouts should be organized with a focus on providing the swimmer with relative rest to structures at risk. For example, after the difficult work has been completed, the practice can continue with emphasis on stroke drills, alternating stroke and leg work and start and turn techniques. Minimizing the potential for injury is dependent on proper instruction which will teach the swimmer to guard against fatigue and to be aware of the value of good stroke mechanics.

Knee injuries

Swimming injuries are not limited to the shoulder joint (Fowler & Regan, 1986). As mentioned earlier the whip kick subjects the knee to unnatural motion. The most common causes of knee pain in the swimmer are medial collateral stress syndrome, patellofemoral syndrome and medial synovitis. While Counsilman (1968) attributes to proper technique the fact that few of his swimmers developed painful knees, Kennedy and Hawkins (1974) believe that because of the severity and number of repetitions, the whip kick can subject all swimmers to knee pain in spite of good technique (Fowler, 1990). Suggestions by Kennedy and Hawkins include altering the training programme for breaststrokers so that the majority of it is devoted to other strokes and a period of at least 2 months·year^{-1} of total rest from swimming for élite competitive breaststrokers

(Fowler, 1990). An adequate warm-up period is advocated by Rovere and Nichols (1985) who recommend a minimum of 915–1370 m (1000–1500 yards) of warm-up before hard breaststroke training begins. As in all training, increase in distance must be gradual.

Important to note is the fact that anatomical problems such as ligamentous or significant patellofemoral instability may not be compatible with the performance of the whip kick at a competitive level. Recognition of these situations and communication among athlete, coach and physician are essential.

Elbow, foot, ankle and back injuries

In both the butterfly and the breaststroke, the arm pull is the main cause of elbow problems. Stroke modification is necessary if the swimmer is 'dropping' the elbow thereby pushing the water back less efficiently and requiring more force by the common extensor muscles. Applying eccentric loads will aid in both strengthening the muscles of the forearm and in increasing flexibility and endurance.

Foot and ankle pain in the swimmer is caused by tendinitis of the extensor tendons of the foot and ankle regardless of the stroke performed. Prevention involves routine stretching of the extensor tendons prior to practices.

A variety of lower back problems, including stress fractures of the pars interarticularis and frank spondylolisthesis may ensue from the lordotic attitude of the lower back further aggravated by the 'elbow up' position in the breaststroke. Similar back problems can be a result of inefficient and improper mechanics in the butterfly stroke. Again, conscientious and routine stretching prior to practice sessions as well as correcting amd modifying stroke techniques will contribute to the prevention of these conditions.

References

Blazina, M.E. (1973) Jumper's knee. *Orthop. Clin. N. Am.* **4**(3), 665–78.

Counsilman, J.E. (1968) *The Science of Swimming*. Prentice Hall, New Jersey.

Fowler, P.J. (1988) Shoulder injuries in the mature athlete. In W.A. Grana (ed) *Advanced Sports Medicine Fitness*, pp. 225–38. Year Book Medical Publishers, Chicago.

Fowler, P.J. (1990) Upper extremity swimming injuries. In J.A. Nicholas & E.B. Hershman (eds) *The Upper Extremity in Sports Medicine*, pp. 891–902. CV Mosby, St Louis.

Fowler, P.J. & Regan, W.D. (1986) Swimming injuries of the knee, foot and ankle, elbow and back. *Clin. Sports Med.* **5**(1), 139–48.

Fowler, P.J. & Webster-Bogart, M.S. (1991) Swimming. In B. Reider (ed) *Sports Medicine — The School-Age Athlete*, pp. 429–46. WB Saunders, Philadelphia.

Griep, J.F. (1985) Swimmer's shoulder: the influence of flexibility and weight training. *Phys. Sports Med.* **13**(2), 92–105.

Kennedy, J.C. & Hawkins, R.J. (1974) Swimmer's shoulder. *Phys. Sports Med.* **2**(4), 35–41.

Neer, C.S. & Welsh, R.P. (1977) The shoulder in sports. *Orthop. Clin. N. Am.* **8**(3), 483–591.

Rathbun, J.B. & MacNab, I. (1970) The microvascular pattern of the rotator cuff. *J. Bone Joint Surg.* **52B**(3), 540–53.

Richardson, A.B., Jobe, F.W. & Collins, H.R. (1980) The shoulder in competitive swimming. *Am. J. Sports Med.* **8**(3), 159–63.

Rovere, G. & Nichols, A.W. (1985) Frequency, associated factors and treatment of breaststroker's knee in competitive swimmers. *Am. J. Sports Med.* **13**(2), 99–104.

Webster, M.S., Bishop, P. & Fowler, P.J. (1981) *Swimmer's shoulder*. Undergraduate thesis, University of Waterloo, Ontario.

Chapter 34

Injuries in Cycling

CLAUDE E. NICHOLS

Cycling is a complex activity requiring the synchronous motion of multiple joints and the sequential firing of many muscle groups to propel the two-wheeled vehicle forward. The pedals spin around hundreds of thousands of times during a cycling season. This repetition, along with the complex muscle and joint interactions involved in every pedal stroke plus the subtleties of obtaining the proper fit and position on the bicycle, make the cyclist vulnerable to injury. These injuries are usually the result of training or equipment errors.

When examining an injured cyclist, both the cyclist and the bicycle must undergo a thorough evaluation. A quick review to note problems with the bicycle such as seat height, saddle position, stem length, handlebar padding, pedal type, shoe type and use of toe clips, should be performed. A riding history including the distance ridden per week, the type of riding, riding technique, cadence, climbing style and hand position is very important to establish the rider's habits. Often it is recommended that the cyclist visit a reputable bicycle shop for an expert evaluation of the fit of the rider to the bicycle because minor adjustments to the machine can often alleviate the complaints of the cyclist.

Bicycle fit

The proper fit of the bicycle to the rider is perhaps the most important aspect of injury prevention in the cyclist. To the uninitiated, the adjustments that cyclists make to assume their optimal riding position may appear trivial, but this attention to detail is imperative to injury-free cycling (Mayer, 1985).

Frame size

An issue that is frequently mentioned, but poorly addressed, is the frame size. The dimensions of the bicycle frame are dependent on the type of bicycle being ridden, the type of riding to be done and the rider's anatomy. The critical dimensions of the frame are the seat tube height (the actual frame size) and the top tube length. The height of the seat tube dictates the upper and lower limits of the saddle height which is an important factor in obtaining the correct fit. The top tube length indicates how far the rider will have to bend forward to grasp the handlebars in order to assume their riding position (Fig. 34.1).

There are several ways to determine the optimal frame size for a road bicycle. One rule of thumb is that the crotch should clear the top tube by 2.5–5 cm. For mountain bikes the difference is greater (7.5–15 cm) to allow for rapid mounting and dismounting (Fig. 34.2) (Mellion, 1991). Another method to determine the seat tube length of a road racing frame is to multiply the in-seam measurement (in cm) by 0.65 (Lemond & Gordis, 1988). These techniques, as well as more sophisticated devices, give the rider a general idea of the appropriate frame size for their anatomy and riding style.

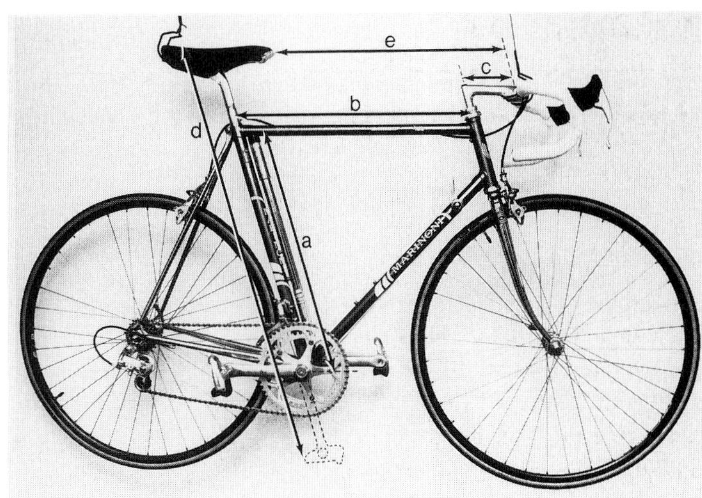

Fig. 34.1 Main dimensions of a bicycle: (a) seat tube length; (b) top tube length; (c) stem length; (d) seat height; (e) fore–aft position of saddle.

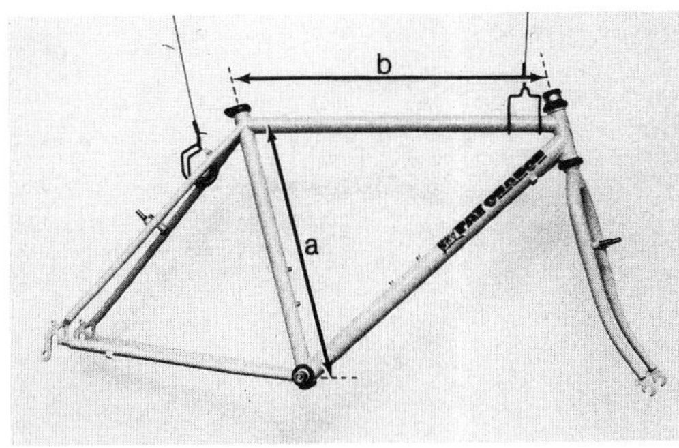

Fig. 34.2 Mountain bike frame: (a) seat tube length; (b) top tube length. Compare configuration with Fig. 34.1.

Seat height

The height of the seat is quite important because it dictates the range of motion of the hip, knee and ankle as well as affecting muscle activity during the pedalling stroke (Fig. 34.1).

Anecdotally, the appropriate saddle height is determined by sitting on the bicycle with the pedal at the bottom of the stroke, and the heel resting on the pedal with the leg straight. When the toes are on the pedal, the knee should be flexed approximately 15–20° (Dickson, 1985). There are formulae to determine the correct seat height such as the factor 0.833 × in-seam (Borysewicz, 1985) and values that are the result of scientific studies involving oxygen consumption (Nordeen-Snyder, 1977), electromyograph (EMG) activity (Gregor & Rugg, 1986), and pedal forces (Broker *et al.*, 1988). These formulae provide guidelines, but by no means determine the optimal seat height for everyone.

Saddle position

The fore–aft position of the saddle should permit the rider to position the *k*nee (tibial tuberosity) *o*ver the *p*edal *s*pindle (KOPS) with the crank in the horizontal position (Borysewicz, 1985). The KOPS rule has no biomechanical basis and may not be appropriate for all riders or riding positions, but it serves as a general guideline (Fig. 34.1).

Different frame geometries (road racing, touring, triathalon) have different seat tube angles which require fore and aft adjustments to achieve the proper alignment. Every saddle has rails which attach to the seat post, which also permit easy adjustment of the fore–aft position (Mellion, 1991). The saddle should be parallel with the ground.

Foot position

The ball of the foot should be positioned over or just anterior to the pedal spindle for optimal positioning and proper transmission (Lemond & Gordis, 1988).

Cleat position

For a fixed cleat–pedal interface, the clear position should be that which is most comfortable for the rider. This can be determined by riding with the cleat fastened securely, but not snuggly, and allowing it to seek the most comfortable position. Another technique for determining the appropriate position is the rotational alignment device (RAD) attachment that is part of the Fit-Kit protocol (Fig. 34.3).

Newer pedal design takes into consideration the foot's tendency to rotate on the pedal platform and have rotational capabilities built into the cleat–pedal interface. These pedals require proper placement of the cleat with respect to the ball of the foot and appropriate rotational alignment to prevent prerelease.

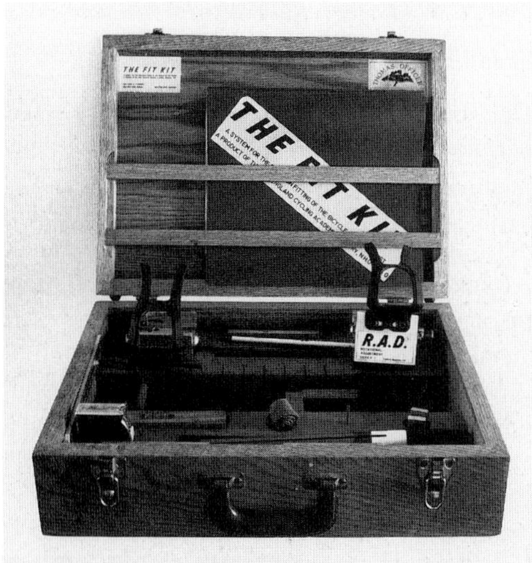

Fig. 34.3 Fit-Kit. A number of parameters are measured and appropriate sizing and position can be determined.

Stem length

Traditionally, stem length has been determined by that length which allows the handlebars to block the rider's view of the front hub (Borysewicz, 1985) or the distance from the rider's elbow to finger tips as measured from the nose of the saddle (Mellion, 1991). Recently, much attention has been given to upper body extension with some riders and authors advocating a more stretched out position to avoid lower back problems and promote a more aerodynamic position on the bicycle. This upper body extension is controlled by the fixed top tube length and the variable (up to 14 mm) stem length (see Fig. 34.1).

Stem height

For traditional drop handlebars the stem should be level or below (up to 5 cm) the saddle height. Recreational riders generally assume a more upright position requiring the higher stem height, while those riders who need to assume a more aerodynamic position need a lower (2–4 cm below saddle height) stem height (Borysewicz, 1985).

Gearing and cadence

The gear ratio dictates how far the bicycle will travel with one revolution of the pedals. Cyclists refer to gears as high or low, with high gears covering more distance with one revolution of the pedals and low gears propelling the bicyle smaller distances with one pedal revolution.

Generally, competitive cyclists attempt to maintain pedal revolutions of 80–100 r.p.m. on flat terrain (Hagsberg *et al.*, 1981; Faria *et al.*, 1982). This number of r.p.m. is termed the cadence. When climbing, the cadence drops to approximately 60–80 r.p.m. After trial and error, most cyclists assume that cadence which is physiologically most economical for them, which is usually approximately 70–90 r.p.m. (Coast *et al.*, 1986).

The importance of gearing and cadence is

noted when pedal forces are examined (Cavanaugh & Sanderson, 1986). A tendency to use higher gears implies higher forces must be applied to the pedals usually at a lower cadence. Implicit in this is that higher joint reaction forces are experienced by the hip and knee, along with a lower cadence. These higher forces have been implicated in overuse injuries in cyclists (Holmes *et al.*, 1990) and therefore should be avoided for prolonged periods of time. A lower gear ratio and a higher cadence are preferable as the forces across the joints are lower and therefore decreasing the likelihood of encountering injury (Davis & Hull, 1981; Ericson & Nisell, 1986).

Higher gearing is most suited to flat terrain and lower gearing being appropriate for climbing. Intermediate gears give the rider some leeway when riding on varying terrain.

Most modern bicycles are equipped with gearing that varies from 10 to 21 possibilities. Road racing bicycles are equipped with two chain rings on the crank set and a free-wheel or series of cogs on the rear hub that are from five to eight in number. Touring bicycles and mountain bikes have three chain rings. The different combinations of chain wheel–rear cog set-ups determine the gear ratios (Fig. 34.4). The size of the gear (measured in inches) can be calculated by dividing the number of teeth on the chain ring by the number of teeth on the rear cog and multiplying this by the diameter of the wheel. An easier method is to use a table.

Stretching

Flexibility of the cervical and lumbar spine, shoulders, hips and lower extremity musculature is essential to the cyclist (Anderson & Burke, 1990). Stretching prior to a ride prepares the muscle–tendon units for the repetitive work of the pedal stroke. Stretching after riding relieves tension in the fatigued muscles and promotes the quality of suppleness for which riders strive. Static stretches for the calves, hamstrings, quadriceps, shoulders and spine are a critical component in the prevention of injury to the cyclist.

Helmets

Head injuries present perhaps the most urgent risk to the cyclist regardless of age, skill or type of riding. The risk of dying from a cycling mishap is ultimately related to the severity of the head injury (Waters, 1986). It has been

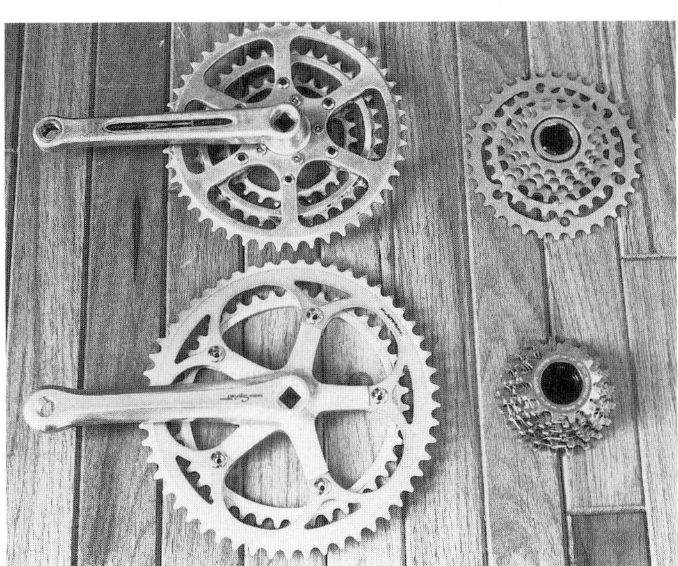

Fig. 34.4 Crank set and free-wheels. Top, triple chain wheel with wide ratio free-wheel. Bottom, double chain wheel with close ratio free-wheel.

speculated in one study that if the head injury could have been prevented, many of the fatalities could have been eliminated. Helmets have been shown to be effective in reducing the severity of head trauma in cycling mishaps, however, cyclists still balk at the idea of wearing them (Wasserman *et al.*, 1988). Common reasons for not wearing helmets include only going out for a short trip, the fact that helmets can be hot and uncomfortable and plain negligence.

Manufacturers have addressed some of these problems through cooperative efforts with cyclists. Material changes have made helmets lighter. Air flow through the helmet permits better cooling. In fact, helmet design has improved to the point where wearing one actually improves the cyclist's aerodynamics. Regrettably, they are still seen by some cyclists as unnecessary and cumbersome.

Presently the American National Standards Institute (ANSI) and Snell safety standards are used to judge whether a helmet meets the minimum standard of protection. Both hard shell helmets which are constructed of expanded polystyrene foam (EPS) with a hard plastic cover or soft shell helmets constructed of thick EPS, comply with these standards, and are available (Swart, 1990) (Fig. 34.5).

Helmet designs are constantly being reevaluated to optimize head protection. Whatever type of helmet is worn, it has been demonstrated that their use decreases the morbidity and mortality of head injuries sustained by bicyclists.

Specific injury sites

Neck injuries

Another problem that plagues the long-distance cyclist, especially the ultramarathoners, is neck pain. To assume an aerodynamic position on the bicycle, the cyclist strives to keep the back flat and parallel with the ground. This means that the head must be held up by the neck musculature to look down the road. 66% of cyclists reported neck and shoulder symptoms with 95% of these complaining of trapezius pain (Weiss, 1985).

Once again, bicycle fit can be a major cause of the problem (Burke, 1990f). An excessively long stem forces the rider to look up and extend the neck to visualize the road ahead. Even though this aerodynamic position is desirable, it can cause significant symptoms about the cervical spinal musculature. A shorter stem or upright handlebars achieve a more upright position thus relieving these symptoms. Changing position frequently, tilting and rotating the neck, wearing a lighter helmet, and

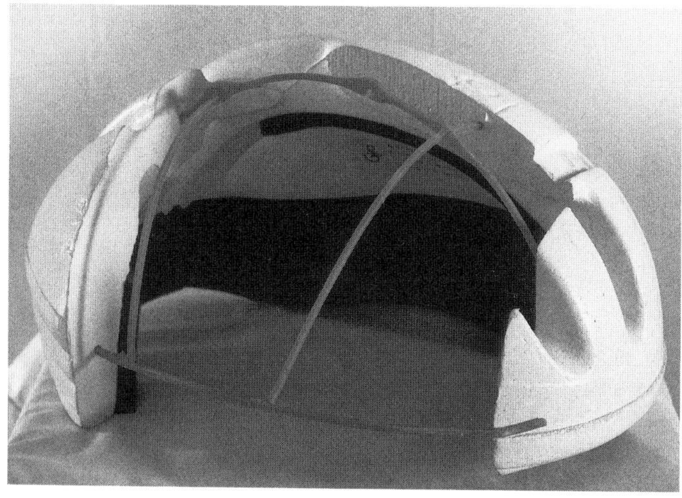

Fig. 34.5 Expanded polystyrene foam (EPS) helmet cross-section.

stretching and strengthening exercises are also helpful.

Low back injuries

One would hope that the mundane aches and pains of every-day living could be avoided when we engage in our recreational activities. This is not to be. Low back pain plagues the cyclist as it does individuals in all walks of life. The back muscles especially the latissimus dorsi, erector spinae and external oblique muscles as well as the trapezius are used for posture and stability during cycling (Burke, 1990a). Usually the dull ache riders experience in the lower back reflect overexertion or improper bicycle fit.

Stretching, abdominal muscle strengthening, as well as back muscle strengthening can help prevent back problems. Standing out of the saddle and stretching while riding can also help relieve minor aches during a ride.

Hand injuries

Another overuse injury frequently sustained by bicyclists is hand numbness. This is usually reported in long-distance cyclists as the insidious onset of numbness in the small and ring finger with progressive weakness in the intrinsic muscles demonstrated by grip weakness (Smail, 1975) and is due to ulnar nerve injury (Eckman *et al.*, 1975; Smail, 1975; Converse, 1979; Noth *et al.*, 1980; Frontera, 1983). The aetiology is thought to be compression of this nerve as it traverses Guyon's canal. The condition usually resolves spontaneously with rest, although it may take several months. The diagnosis can be confirmed with electrodiagnostic studies. Surgery is rarely necessary. Both sensory and motor branches of the ulnar nerve are usually affected in cyclists' palsy (Noth *et al.*, 1980).

Preventive measures include proper bicycle fit and riding position (Burke, 1990d). Leaning forward with too much weight on the hands can lead to compression of the soft tissues. Changing hand positions frequently on long rides, padded handlebar tape, padded cycling gloves and appropriately sized handlebars (width approximately shoulder width) and adjusting the stem height can also prevent the occurrence of this problem (Burke, 1981).

Buttock pain

The most common problem encountered by long-distance cyclists is buttock pain discomfort (Kuland & Brubaker, 1978; Weiss, 1985). The bicycle saddle inflicts repetitive trauma to the cyclists' hind parts causing a multitude of entities that have been described in the literature including peroneal nodules (Vuong *et al.*, 1988), ischaemic neuropathy of the sensory nerves to the penis (Bond, 1975; Powell, 1982; Desai & Gingell, 1989), pudendal neuritis (Goodson, 1981), urethritis (O'Brien, 1981; Herschfield, 1983), testicular torsion (Goodfellow, 1978), painless haematuria (LeRoy, 1972) and impotence (Solomon & Cappa, 1987). These conditions are usually the result of improper saddle selection, poor bicycle fit, incorrect saddle position or poor hygiene (Powell, 1982). 33% of cyclists in a survey of long-distance cyclists reported buttock pain (Weiss, 1985).

The appropriate saddle is one that is comfortable for the rider, yet is narrow enough to allow the thighs to glide over the surface as the legs move up and down. Modern saddle design includes gels and viscoelastic foams to allow better pressure distribution and optimize the rider's comfort. However, there is no one saddle that distributes pressure better or is more comfortable than others. It is a matter of personal taste (Fig. 34.6).

Saddle position has been implicated in the compression neuropathies about the groin. When the saddle is too far posterior, the nose of the saddle is tilted in either direction, or the seat height is excessive, the majority of the force is borne on the perineum by the narrow nose of the saddle compressing the dorsal arteries of the penis against the symphysis

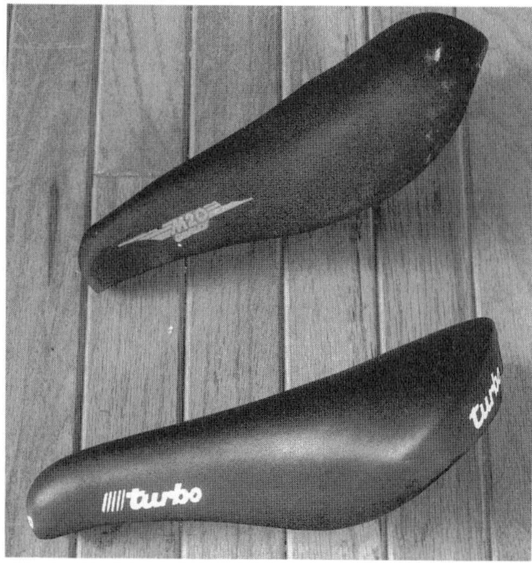

Fig. 34.6 Saddles. Top, 'anatomic' saddle with padding. Bottom, racing saddle.

pubis (Bond, 1975) leading to an ischaemic neuropathy and even vasogenic impotence. It is also believed that neural compression can occur leading to a similar presentation of penile anaesthesia. These complaints can be alleviated by adjusting the saddle position or by changing saddles or both.

Poor hygiene can result in rashes, boils and granuloma formation in the perineum. These problems can be avoided by wearing cycling shorts with chamois or synthetic liners which protect the groin region, and wick moisture, and by keeping the skin in this region meticulously dry and clean, and washing the shorts after every ride (Burke, 1990b). Drying cycling shorts in sunlight has been suggested to kill bacteria by utilizing the sun's natural ultraviolet radiation (Powell, 1986).

Peroneal nodules are felt to be endemic to professional and élite amateur cyclists. They are the result of repeated microtrauma and can be the source of significant disability sometimes requiring surgical excision (Vuong *et al.*, 1988).

Knee injuries

Weiss (1985) noted that knee problems occurred in 21% of the cyclists in his series of long-distance cyclists. This is understandable when the possible sources of knee pain are defined.

Firstly, the correct frame size and saddle height must be determined to allow the lower extremities to function optimally (Burke, 1990e). The fore and aft position of the saddle must allow the knee to assume the proper alignment with respect to the pedal.

Secondly, technique is quite important. The recommended cadence is between 80 and 100 r.p.m. When climbing, the pedal revolutions may drop to 60 r.p.m., but on flat terrain, a cadence less than 80 r.p.m. usually means that the cyclist is repetitively stressing the knee joint and is susceptible to overuse injuries.

Thirdly, equipment must be considered. The standard crank length is 170 mm with lengths up to 180 mm available. Longer cranks are thought to facilitate climbing and time trialling by increasing the length of the lever arm and allowing the cyclists to use larger gearing (Hull & Gonzalez, 1988). However, a longer crank arm also means a lower cadence and greater forces across the knee joint. In fact, longer cranks have been associated with knee problems in professional cyclists.

The shoe–pedal interface is another common problem encountered by the cyclist. The important aspect of this choice is to accommodate nature (Burke, 1990c). That is, the foot's natural tendency to out-toe or in-toe, should be reflected by the foot's position on the pedals. An 'unnatural' foot position can dramatically alter both knee and hip mechanics (Francis, 1986) and cause overuse injuries. Hence proper cleat alignment is mandatory in order to permit good form and avoid injurious stresses to the knee. Pedal systems with built in rotation have minimized the need for precise cleat alignment in the rotational axis and allow for the foot's natural tendency to rotate on the pedal (Fig. 34.7). Orthotics are occasionally useful to correct pronation of the foot on the pedal.

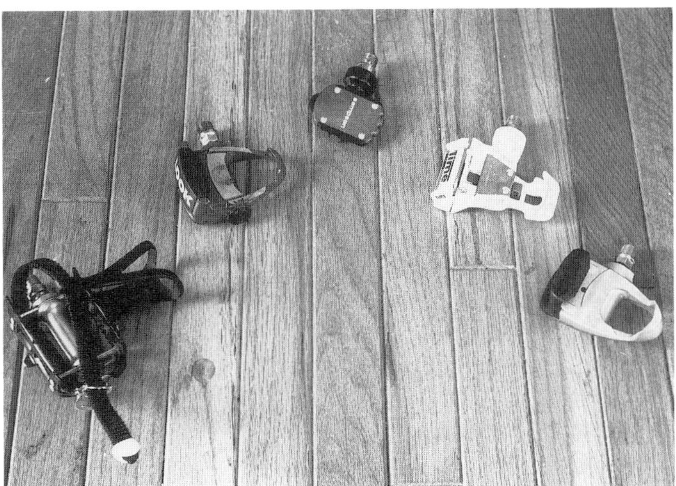

Fig. 34.7 Pedals, from left to right: one conventional pedal with toe clip; three styles of clipless pedals that allow rotation; and clipless pedal without rotation.

Holmes *et al.* (1990) classified knee pain in the cyclist according to the level of proficiency and the location of the pathology. Anterior and medial knee pain was related to the high repetitive stresses placed on the knee, whereas lateral pain appeared to be the result of alignment or technique errors. Entities commonly seen in cyclists with knee complaints, are patellofemoral pain syndrome, plica syndrome, hamstring tendinitis, patellar tendinitis and iliotibial band syndrome. These soft-tissue injuries reflect the fact that pedalling conditions such as load, seat height and shoe type, affect the level of muscle activity required to cycle. Meniscal and ligamentous injuries are uncommon (Fig. 34.8).

As in runners, overuse injuries about the knee in cyclists can usually be treated quite successfully in a conservative fashion after correcting the position of the rider. After an accurate diagnosis is made, these problems can be treated with non-steroidal anti-inflammatory medications, anti-inflammatory modalities such as heat and ice, and a rehabilitation programme based on the diagnosis.

Foot and ankle injuries

The gastrocnemius–soleus complex functions as both a knee flexor and ankle plantar flexor

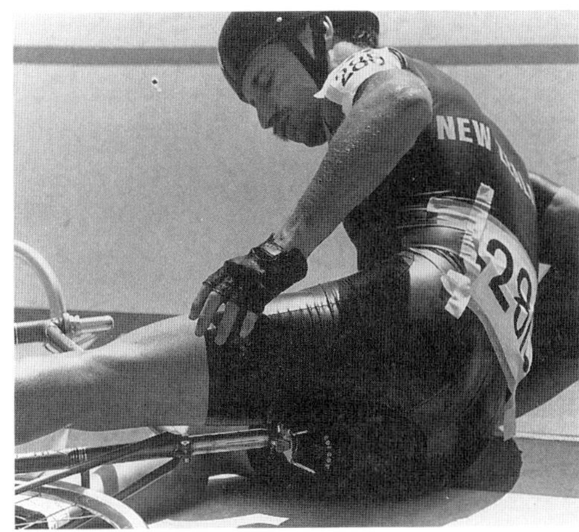

Fig. 34.8 Direct falls can cause more serious injuries. © IOPP/No 25789/Frame 11a.

during the cycling stroke. EMG analysis has shown that this muscle is active for approximately two-thirds of the pedal stroke (Jorge & Hull, 1986). This repetitive motion exposes this muscle–tendon unit to overuse that is usually manifested as Achilles tendinitis. This can be remedied by evaluating seat height and the foot position on the pedal as well as adjusting the cadence. Conservative measures such as non-steroidal anti-inflammatory medication, stretching and physical therapy modalities are effective. If symptoms persist, this might indicate microtears in the tendon's substance. Steroid injections are to be avoided.

Specialized footwear has been developed to improve the cyclist's power transfer to the pedals (Fig. 34.9). Stiff soled shoes provide a rigid platform for the foot to apply force to the pedals, thereby making the cyclist more efficient (Hull & Jorge, 1985). An intimate shoe–pedal interface also increases the efficiency of the cycling stroke by allowing the cyclist to apply useful force to the pedals during a greater duration of the pedalling cycle. The cycling shoe should have a stiff sole to protect the foot and improve efficiency, good ventilation to keep the foot cool, and a snug fit to avoid slippage. By using these parameters, the cyclist can avoid the common problems of soreness, overheating and blisters (Burke, 1990c). The numbness is usually the result of the injudicious tightening of the toe clip straps or ill-fitting shoes. This is remedied by loosening the straps slightly, using a clipless system, or by obtaining a better shoe fit.

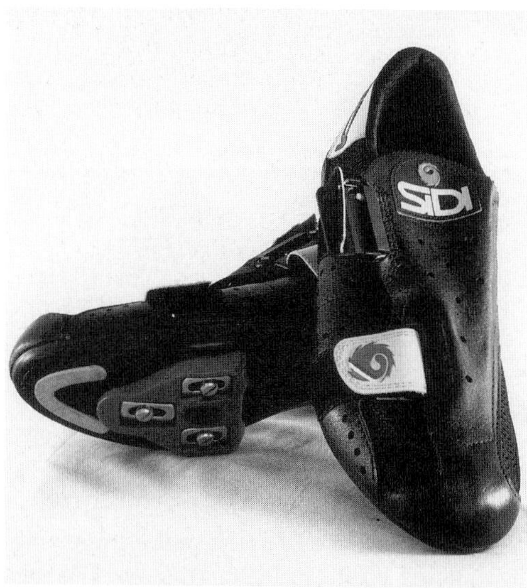

Fig. 34.9 Cycle shoes: these are notable for the light uppers and stiff soles.

Eye injuries

The cyclist's eye is quite vulnerable to injury. The range of difficulties range from drying out from wind exposure to foreign bodies. Sunglasses with shatter-proof lenses and plastic frames are available to offer protection not only from the drying effects of the air and particulate matter, but also from harmful ultraviolet radiation. Problems associated with excessive dryness or foreign bodies about the eye should be evaluated by an ophthalmologist (Schuller & Bruce, 1984; Powell, 1986).

Performance enhancers

Perhaps the most serious of the cycling-related injuries is death secondary to performance enhancers. Recombinant erythropoietin is a synthetic hormone developed to treat the anaemia of chronic renal failure (Scott, 1990). It acts by stimulating red blood cell production from bone marrow progenitors, thereby increasing the blood's ability to carry oxygen to tissues by increasing the haematocrit. Erythropoietin and blood doping (the transfusion of red blood cells) theoretically enhance performance in endurance athletes by improving oxygen transport (Cowart, 1989).

This technique of performance enhancing has been implicated in several cycling deaths over the past few years (Ramotar, 1990). Haematocrits greater than 55% are associated with risks including impairment of blood flow and rapid clotting which can lead to phlebothrombosis, myocardial infarction or stroke. The effect of the hormone is felt 5–10 days after the last dose. Endurance exercise causes dehydration which can result in haematocrits much greater than 55%, thereby exposing the cyclist to these potentially fatal risks.

Blood doping uses the athlete's own blood which is transfused 1–4 days before competition to enhance the oxygen supply to the exercising tissue. This technique is limited by the amount of blood that can be drawn off. Haematocrits over 60% would be difficult to achieve with blood doping alone, however with erythropoietin, levels up to 80% are theoretically possible. Neither of these techniques can be detected (Berglund *et al.*, 1989).

Another performance enhancer commonly involved in sports is the anabolic–androgenic steroid. There is no evidence that these anabolic steroids increase anaerobic power or capacity for muscular exercise (American College of Sports Medicine, 1987; Smith & Perry 1992). Endurance athletes are convinced however that anabolic–androgenic steroids allow them to train more intensely and more often than they would otherwise. The risks and side-effects of these medications is well-documented in the literature and methods of detection of anabolic steroid use are quite sophisticated.

Heat and hydration

The body, not being a particularly efficient machine, converts approximately 75% of all energy into heat. The primary mechanism to avoid overheating is through perspiring and the evaporation of sweat. To perspire, the cyclist must adjust fluid intake to match the fluid output, so that this heat removal can occur. Fluids should be consumed before the cyclist is thirsty and should be consumed liberally.

Early symptoms of hyperthermia problems include muscle cramps that occur immediately after exercise. Rest, massage and fluids are suggested.

Heat exhaustion is manifested as weakness, headache and central nervous system symptoms. Disregarding these warning signs can lead to the possible onset of the potentially fatal problem of heat stroke where the core temperature is elevated and disorientation or even coma can occur.

Heat exhaustion is treated by the careful administration of fluids and rest. Heat stroke is a medical emergency requiring cooling the victim to reduce their elevated core temperature, fluid resuscitation and often hospitalization (Sutton, 1984; Powell, 1986).

Conclusion

The repetitive motion of the pedal stroke, the subtle interplay of numerous variables related to the fit between rider and machine, the riding technique all expose the rider to various overuse injuries. Proper attention to equipment, fit, riding technique and flexibility can prevent most common complaints. The use of helmets, either hard or soft shell, is highly recommended to lessen the risk of catastrophic head injuries. Attention to detail can lead to many pleasurable miles of cycling.

References

American College of Sports Medicine (1987) Position stand on the use of anabolic–androgenic steroids in sports. *Med. Sci. Sports Exerc.* **19**(5), 534–9.

Anderson, B. & Burke, E.R. (1990) Loosen up! Simple stretches for stiff cyclists. *Bicycling* **31**, 130–3.

Berglund, B., Birgegard, G., Wilde, L. & Pihlstedt, P. (1989) Effects of blood transfusions on some hematological variables in endurance athletes. *Med. Sci. Sports Exerc.* **21**(6), 637–42.

Bond, R.E. (1975) Distance bicycling may cause ischemic neuropathy of the penis. *Phys. Sportsmed.* **3**, 354–6.

Borysewicz, E. (1985) *Bicycle Road Racing*. Vitesse Press, Vermont.

Broker, J.P., Browning, R.C. & Gregor, R.J. (1988) Effect of seat height on force effectiveness in cycling. *Med. Sci. Sport Exerc.* **20**(2) (Suppl.), 583.

Burke, E.R. (1981) Ulnar neuropathy in bicyclists. *Phys. Sportsmed.* **9**(4), 53–6.

Burke, E.R. (1990a) Back: The overlooked cycling muscles. *Bicycling* **31**(1), 84–5.

Burke, E.R. (1990b) Buttocks: Look back, something might be paining you. *Bicycling* **31**(5), 106–7.

Burke, E.R. (1990c) Feet: How to pacify a pair of barking dogs. *Bicycling* **31**(6), 84–6.

Burke, E.R. (1990d) Hands: Get a grip on several common problems. *Bicycling* **31**(4), 166–7.

Burke, E.R. (1990e) Knees: Your cycling future hinges on them. *Bicycling* **31**(8), 72–3.

Burke, E.R. (1990f) Neck: The pipeline to comfort and performance. *Bicycling* **31**(3), 106–7.

Cavanaugh, P.R. & Sanderson, D.J. (1986) The biomechanics of cycling: Studies of the pedalling mechanics of élite pursuit riders. In E.R. Burke (ed) *Science of Cycling*, pp. 91–122. Human Kinetics, Illinois.

Coast, J.R., Cox, R.H. & Welch, H.G. (1986) Optimal

pedalling rate in prolong bouts of cycle ergometry. *Med. Sci. Sports Exerc.* **18**(2), 225–30.

Converse, T.A. (1979) Cyclist's palsy. *N. Engl. J. Med.* **301**, 1397–8.

Cowart, V.S. (1989) Erythropoietin: A dangerous new form of blood doping? *Phys. Sportsmed.* **17**(8), 114–18.

Davis, R.R. & Hull, M.L. (1981) Measurement of pedal loading in bicycling: II. Analysis and results. *J. Biomech.* **14**(2), 857–72.

Desai, K.M. & Gingell, J.C. (1989) Hazards of long distance cycling. *Br. Med. J.* **298**, 1072–3.

Dickson Jr, T.B. (1985) Preventing overuse cycling injuries. *Phys. Sports Med.* **13**(10), 116–23.

Eckman, P.B., Perlstein, G. & Altrocchi, P.H. (1975) Ulnar neuropathy in bicycle riders. *Arch. Neurol.* **32**, 130–1.

Ericson, M.B. & Nisell, R. (1986) Tibiofemoral joint forces during ergometer cycling. *Am. J. Sports Med.* **14**, 285–90.

Faria, I., Sjajaard, G. & Bonde-Petersen, F. (1982) Oxygen cost during different pedalling speeds for constant power output. *J. Sports Med.* **22**, 295–9.

Francis, P.R. (1986) Injury prevention for cyclists: A biomechanical approach. In E.R. Burke (ed) *Science of Cycling*, pp. 145–84. Human Kinetics, Illinois.

Frontera, W.R. (1983) Case report. Cyclist's palsy: clinical and electrodiagnostic findings. *Br. J. Sports Med.* **17**(2), 91–4.

Goodfellow, R.D. (1978) Bicycle saddles and torsion of the testis. *Lancet* **i**, 1149.

Goodson, J.D. (1981) Pudendal neuritis from biking. *N. Engl. J. Med.* **304**, 365.

Gregor, R.J. & Rugg, S.G. (1986) Effects of saddle height and pedalling cadence on power output and efficiency. In E.R. Burke (ed) *Science of Cycling*, pp. 69–90. Human Kinetics, Illinois.

Hagsberg, J.M., Mullin, J.P., Giese, M.D. & Spitsnagel, E. (1981) Effect of pedaling rate on submaximal exercise responses of competitive cyclists. *J. Appl. Physiol. Resp. Environ. Exerc. Physiol.* **51**(2), 447–51.

Hershfield, N.B. (1983) Pedaller's penis. *Can. Med. Assoc. J.* **128**, 336–67.

Holmes, J.C., Pruit, A.L. & Whalen, N.J. (1990) Knee pain in cyclists. In *Abstracts of the American Orthopaedic Society for Sports Medicine*, pp. 12–13. Sun Valley, Idaho.

Hull, M.L. & Gonzalez, H. (1988) Bivariate optimization of pedalling rate and crank arm length in cycling. *J. Biomech.* **21**(10), 839–49.

Hull, M.L. & Jorge, M. (1985) A method for biomechanical analysis of bicycle pedalling. *J. Biomech.* **18**(9), 631–44.

Jorge, M. & Hull, M.L. (1986) Analysis of EMG measurements during bicycle pedalling. *J. Biomech.* **19**, 683–94.

Kuland, D.N. & Brubaker, C.E. (1978) Injuries in the bike centennial tour. *Phys. Sportsmed.* **6**, 674–8.

Lemond, G. & Gordis, K. (1988) *Greg LeMond's Complete Book of Bicycling*. Perigee Books, New York.

LeRoy, J.B. (1972) Banana-seat hematuria. *N. Engl. J. Med.* **287**(6), 311.

Mayer, P.H. (1985) Part 2: How to choose, adjust, and use a bicycle properly: Helping your patient's avoid bicycling injuries. *J. Musculoskeletal Med.* **2**(6), 31–8.

Mellion, M.B. (1991) Common cycling injuries: management and prevention. *Sports Med.* **11**(1), 52–70.

Nordeen-Snyder, K.S. (1977) The effect of bicycle seat height variation upon oxygen consumption and lower limb kinematics. *Med. Sci. Sports Exerc.* **9**(2), 113–17.

Noth, J., Dietz, V. & Mauritz, K.H. (1980) Cyclist's palsy: neurological and EMG study in four cases with distal ulnar lesions. *J. Neurol. Sci.* **47**, 111–16.

O'Brien, K.P. (1981) Sports urology: the vicious cycle. *N. Engl. J. Med.* **304**, 1367–8.

Powell, B. (1982) Correction and prevention of bicycle saddle problems. *Phys. Sportsmed.* **10**(10), 60–7.

Powell, B. (1986) Medical aspects of racing. In E.R. Burke (ed) *Science of Cycling*, pp. 185–202. Human Kinetics, Illinois.

Ramotar, J.E. (1990) Cyclists' deaths linked to erythropoietin? *Phys. Sportsmed.* **18**(8), 48–9.

Schuller, D.E. & Bruce, R.A. (1984) Ear, nose, throat and eye. In R. Strauss (ed) *Sports Medicine*, pp. 175–89. WB Saunders, Philadelphia.

Scott, W.C. (1990) The abuse of erythropoietin to enhance athletic performance. *JAMA* **264**, 160.

Smail, D.F. (1975) Handlebar palsy. *N. Engl. J. Med.* **292**, 322.

Smith, D.A. & Perry, P.J. (1992) The efficacy of erogenic agents in athletic competition. Part I: Androgenic anabolic steroids. *Ann. Pharmacotherapy* **26**, 520–8.

Solomon, S. & Cappa, K.G. (1987) Impotence and bicycling: a seldom reported connection. *Postgrad. Med.* **81**(1), 99–102.

Sutton, J.R. (1984) Heat illness. In R. Strauss (ed) *Sports Medicine*, pp. 307–22. WB Saunders, Philadelphia.

Swart, R. (1990) Soft shell versus hard shell helmets. *Cycling Sci.* **2**, 13–16.

Vuong, P.N., Camuzard, P. & Schoonaert, M.-F. (1988) Perineal nodular indurations ('accessory testicles') in cyclists: Fine needle aspiration cytologic and pathologic findings in two cases. *Acta Cytol.* **32**(1), 86–90.

Wasserman, R.C., Waller, J.A., Monty, M.J., Emery,

A.B. & Robinson, D.R. (1988) Bicyclists' helmets and head injuries: A rider-based study of helmet use and effectiveness. *Am. J. Publ. Health* **78**(9), 1220–1.

Waters, E.A. (1986) Should pedal cyclists wear helmets? A comparison of head injuries sustained by pedal cyclists and motorcyclists in road traffic accidents. *Injury* **17**, 372–5.

Weiss, B.D. (1985) Non-traumatic injuries in amateur long distance bicyclists. *Am. J. Sports Med.* **13**(3), 187–92.

Chapter 35

Injuries in Gymnastics

WILLIAM A. GRANA AND GARRON G. WEIKER

Just as figure skating is the premier sport in the Winter Olympics which combines athletic ability and aesthetics, gymnastics provides that particular combination of grace and skill in the Summer Olympics. Gymnastics is a prototype of the individual élite athlete's sport. Athletes begin at a very young age and continue into maturity, practising their sport for long hours at a very high level of activity. Wear and tear, as well as acute injury problems occur and are representative of the type of severe problems that all élite individual athletes face (Goldberg, 1989). The purpose of this chapter is to present a summary of our current understanding of these potentially serious problems in gymnastics competition and the preventative measures which are available.

Gymnastics began in Greece as a form of physical training for young men in preparation for combat. Eventually, gymnastics became a form of entertainment with travelling bands of acrobats entertaining local villagers. Tumbling was the mainstay of these activities. It was not until the time of Napoleon that the apparatus for gymnastics were developed. These devices were used to improve training methods and develop strength, power and riding ability. Ludwig Jahn in Germany and Pierre Ling in Sweden are credited with developing the pommel horse, the parallel bars and the rings. Modern gymnastics has evolved from this early form of military training to the highly stylized and rigorously controlled international, competitive sport it is today (Weiker, 1989).

Gymnastics in the USA is organized on several different levels. At the local level there are club and high-school teams which compete in local and interscholastic competitions and tournaments. At the college level, the National Collegiate Athletic Association (NCAA) sanctions gymnastics for men and women as an intercollegiate sport. Both individual and team trophies are awarded and this is a high level of gymnastics competition. However, the most highly organized programmes are those sanctioned by the US Gymnastics Federation. There are four classes of competition with the most advanced being class 1 with progressively decreasing levels of difficulty and complexity of routines down to class 4 which is the entry level stage of organized competition. In addition to the élite, club, high school and college programmes, there are a variety of programmes that are non-competitive with emphasis on the recreational and individual fitness aspects of participation (McAuley *et al.*, 1987; Weiker, 1989). The remainder of this chapter will focus on the risk factors, the specific injuries and the possible preventive measures that can be used to protect the competitive gymnast.

Epidemiology of injuries

Both acute and chronic or overuse problems are seen as a result of gymnastics participation. About two-thirds of the injuries are single episode, acute trauma while the remainder are chronic or overuse injuries (Snook, 1979;

McAuley *et al.*, 1987; Pettrone & Ricciardelli, 1987; Weiker, 1989). These latter injuries are frequently difficult to document because they may not keep an athlete out of training completely, but simply force them to avoid certain activities. The results of injury studies reported may, therefore, vary significantly with regard to overuse problems. On the other hand, these injuries, which are the result of repetitive microtrauma, may be more important because they predispose to recurrent or further injury and therefore should be documented. Gymnastics injuries are classified into the general categories of fracture, sprain, strain and contusion. Most studies have reported that sprains and strains are the most common injuries seen, although at least one study reported fractures of the wrist, fingers and toes as the most common (Snook, 1979; Garrick & Requa, 1980; Sands, 1981; McAuley *et al.*, 1987; Pettrone & Ricciardelli, 1987; Lindner & Caine, 1989; Weiker, 1989). About 25–30% of injuries occur in the upper extremity, about 15–20% to the trunk and spine and about 50–65% occur in the lower extremity (Snook, 1979; Sands, 1981; McAuley *et al.*, 1987; Weiker, 1989). Distribution of these injuries by type and anatomical area vary from one injury study to another and depend, to a great extent, on the level of competition, the degree of difficulty of the activities and the number of hours spent in training.

The most frequently injured anatomical areas are also reported variously in different studies. Lower extremity injuries are more common than upper extremity injuries (Fig. 35.1). The ankle is the most common site of injury, however this may simply reflect the ankle as a common site of injury in all sports. When age adjusted for controls, the incidence of ankle sprain in gymnastics is no different than in other populations of athletes. The knee is the most frequently seriously injured joint. In the upper extremity, shoulder, elbow and wrist injuries are common while in the axial skeleton, low back problems are common (Snook, 1979; Garrick & Requa, 1980; Sands, 1981; McAuley *et al.*, 1987; Pettrone & Ricciardelli, 1987 Lindner & Caine, 1989; Weiker, 1989).

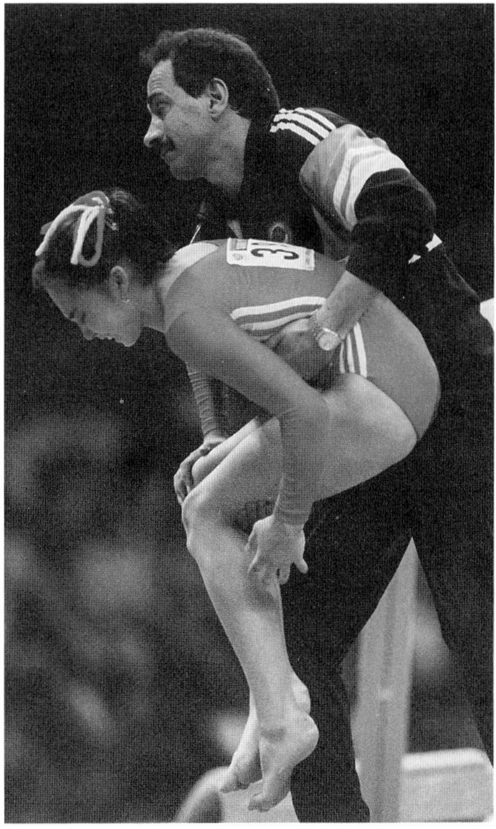

Fig. 35.1 Lower extremity injuries are frequent in gymnastics. © IOPP/S. Lyon.

Risk factors

The risk factors in gymnastics include the duration and frequency of practice which results in repetitive load application. Those events which involve repetitive impact loading result in more frequent acute or chronic injury. These events include the floor exercise as well as the dismount or landing portions of the beam, the bars, rings, horse and vault.

The duration and frequency of training seem to be related to the occurrence of injury, particularly the overuse type. In addition, the level of skill at which the gymnast competes is a factor. Both of these factors are documented in that the occurrence of injury increases as the degree of difficulty for the gymnastic event increases and as the gymnast ascends from the ranks of club gymnast to the élite level. As the gymnast becomes more skilled, there are more hours of practice, which means more exposure time, and a greater opportunity for injury. Practices may be 4–8 h a day, including related activities, such as warm-up and strength and conditioning routines. With this increase in practice time, there is an increased injury rate which is emphasized by Garrick and Requa's report that 95% of injuries occur during practice (1980). Insomuch as the coach determines the duration and intensity of the practice, as well as the spotting of athletes for jumping and vaulting activities, coaching philosophy becomes extremely important in the occurrence of injury. Misuse of equipment or inadequate spotting technique is also attributed as a source of risk.

The presence of safety equipment such as landing mats, foam pits and the repair of apparatus may contribute to injury as well. Thinner mats may result in more injuries than thicker mats.

In terms of the specific events, the floor exercise, which involves a great deal of tumbling, seems to be the most dangerous event. Twisting manoeuvres in the floor exercise are one of the most frequent causes of injury, particularly of the knee and the ankle. Another common mechanism of injury is during the dismount from the bars, the beam and the rings. Vaulting has consistently been reported as an event with few injuries, but that is probably because so little time is involved (Sands, 1981; McAuley *et al.*, 1987; Lindner & Caine, 1989). Until the trampoline was banned from competition, it was the event associated with the most frequent occurrence of serious injury (Hage, 1982; Torg & Das, 1985). In women's gymnastics the floor exercise, followed by the balance beam and uneven bars, in that order, are the most frequent sources of injury.

Another risk factor seems to be the anthropometric characteristics of the individual gymnast shown in a study of female gymnasts. Steele and White (1986) found that flexibility tests could be used to define those gymnasts who were at high risk for the occurrence of injury. On the other hand, another study by Lindner *et al.* (1991) indicated that withdrawal of a gymnast from activity cannot be predicted by physical make-up and performance capacities. Age alone, as well as the attendant psychosocial factors surrounding it, may be the most frequent cause of withdrawal from the sport (Steele & White, 1986; Lindner *et al.*, 1991).

Another risk factor is rapid periods of growth which may alter muscle function without adequate conditioning in the form of strength training to compensate for this. Gymnasts reach the élite level during their pubescence and especially female gymnasts, are affected by rapid periods of growth while they are trying to reach advanced levels of expertise in competition.

The level of difficulty of routines has increased in the last 25 years which results in greater risk and more frequent injury. Coaching techniques are also implicated in the occurrence of injury, particularly long practices with few rotations which leads to loss of concentration and inattentiveness (Pettrone & Ricciardelli, 1987; Caine *et al.*, 1989; Lindner & Caine, 1989).

Finally, because of the need for repetitive practices, it may be that lack of concentration also results in injury. Many injuries happen with moves that are basic or of moderate difficulty and have been a well established part of the athletes routine (Caine *et al.*, 1989). In addition, there is an increased risk when the gymnast is on the apparatus for an extended period of time. It appears that a loss of concentration is a major source of injury and therefore a key to injury prevention may be reorganization of the practice session (Lindner & Caine, 1989).

Another factor in the occurrence of injury is return to gymnastics before full rehabilitation has occurred. Reinjury rate is high, particularly for female gymnasts and coercion by coaches may be a cause of some of these problems. There is a high degree of pressure to return to practice because of the coaches insistence that required levels of expertise must be reached on a specific time schedule (Pettrone & Ricciardelli, 1987; Caine *et al.*, 1989).

Prevention of injuries

The prevention of injuries then would seem to focus on organization of practice schedules and provide for shorter practices and shorter workouts. There should be a shorter period of time on each apparatus with more frequent rotation in a practice environment in which the gymnast remains attentive. Emphasis for the younger athlete should be placed on strength training of those muscle groups that are most important in the activities of various events. Specifically, the quadriceps, hamstrings, calf muscles and the trunk muscles should be emphasized. A good deal of the responsibility then for the prevention of injuries must rest with the adults involved in the young gymnast's practice and competition. Coaches in particular must design their workouts to accommodate the above-noted risk factors. Coaches who allow athletes to continue to participate in an injured state should be condemned for this activity (Sands, 1981; Pettrone & Ricciardelli, 1987; Caine *et al.*, 1989; Lindner & Caine, 1989; Weiker, 1989).

Specific injury sites

Axial skeleton injuries

Most of the injuries in the axial skeleton are contusions or muscular strains which may be severe enough to limit participation but in general resolve quickly with little residual problem (Weiker, 1989). There are infrequent injuries to the skull as a result of 'missed moves' or falls from the bars or in the vault. However, these are unusual and have been minimized since the trampoline was banned from competition (Torg & Das, 1985). Head, neck and lower spine injuries have decreased dramatically by eliminating trampoline in competition particularly at the college level. Mechanism of injury was a fall in the centre of the trampoline on the top of the head resulting in forces which were dissipated through the cervical spine. This caused an unacceptable number of quadriplegia and quadriparesis injuries. Since the 1970s, trampolines are no longer used in the competitive arena and trampoline work for training is done with a safety harness and spotters (Hammer *et al.*, 1981; Hage, 1982; Torg & Das, 1985; Silver *et al.*, 1986b).

There are still isolated cases of cervical spine injury as a result of a missed move. The most common mechanism is a fall from the bars, when the gymnast misses a grasp and falls directly on the head. Injuries of the upper spine occurred primarily in the practice gymnasium as a result of failure of supervision. Of 31 spinal injuries, 28 were in the cervical region and three in the thoracolumbar region (Torg & Das, 1985; Silver *et al.*, 1986a; Goldstein *et al.*, 1991). The use of mini-trampoline and a somersault were also risk factors.

However, most cervical injuries are not fractures, but rather soft-tissue injuries which can be managed by support with a cervical collar, restriction of activity, local icing followed by heat and exercises to strengthen the paraspinous musculature. Fractures are managed in the appropriate manner for the level and type of fracture with fusion recommended for those injuries that fail conservative treatment with resultant instability and pain. Fusion is not a universal contraindication to return to competition but depends upon remaining mobility and residual deformity (Torg & Das, 1985; Weiker, 1989).

First rib fracture is uncommon but has been reported in gymnasts perhaps as a result of conditioning activities associated with gymnastics (Holden & Jackson, 1985; Proffer *et al.*, 1991). Fractures occur along the posterolateral aspect of the rib with the serratus anterior acting with the rhomboids and the trapezius to produce retraction and protraction as the major bending force (Proffer *et al.*, 1991). A bone scan is useful to document and localize these fractures. All of these athletes generally respond to conservative methods, although occasionally transaxillary resection of a portion of the rib may be necessary (Proffer *et al.*, 1991).

The thoracic spine has been implicated as a cause of back pain in both male and female gymnasts. Disc degeneration has been noted on magnetic resonance imaging (MRI) with 75% of those athletes evaluated showing change. Male élite gymnasts have a high risk of developing abnormalities of the thoracolumbar spine (Sward *et al.*, 1991).

The lumbar spine is the anatomical area of greatest interest (Micheli, 1985). Gymnasts get mechanical low back pain as do the general population. However, their abdominal strength and flexibility should protect them from such mechanical problems. More significantly, Jackson *et al.* (1976) noted that prevalence of spondylolisthesis in the female gymnast is four times that seen in the general population. They felt this high rate was due to the repeated impact forces and hyperextension of the lumbar spine experienced by female gymnasts (Jackson *et al.*, 1976, 1980; Ciullo & Jackson, 1985; Goldstein *et al.*, 1991). While abnormality of the spine seems to occur more frequently in the female gymnast than in other athletes, this seems to be related to the number of hours of training per week and the age of the athlete. Increasing age and level of expertise is associated with more frequent abnormality (Jackson *et al.*, 1976; 1980; Ciullo & Jackson, 1985; Micheli, 1985; Letts *et al.*, 1986; Goldstein *et al.*, 1991).

The occurrence of a pars defect is felt to indicate a stress reaction as a result of overuse (Jackson *et al.*, 1976; Ciullo & Jackson, 1985; Letts *et al.*, 1986). Back walkovers and lumbar hyperextension, done for many years, seem to lead to an increased risk in the development of the spondylolytic stress reaction (Hall, 1986). Moreover, these athletes are more likely to develop mechanical low back pain in their teenage years (Weiker, 1989).

MRI was found to be useful in the identification of these spinal problems, however a computed tomographic (CT) scan remains the procedure of choice for the detection of spondylolysis in the absence of spondylolisthesis. Radionucleotide bone scan is useful as a screening device for these spinal problems in the gymnast when plain radiographs are normal. A positive bone scan should lead to a CT (Ciullo & Jackson, 1985; Weiker, 1989; Goldstein *et al.*, 1991).

The detection of this problem depends on a high degree of suspicion, as well as the findings of pain on hyperextension, tight hamstrings and localized tenderness. Treatment is in a thoracolumbar orthosis with repeat scans at 3-month intervals. In addition, hamstring stretching, abdominal muscle strengthening and a graduated return to gymnastics with limited hyperextension is useful (Jackson *et al.*, 1976; Ciullo & Jackson, 1985; Micheli, 1985).

A second spinal abnormality is anterior wedging of a single vertebral body at the level of the thoracolumbar junction. The athlete has pain which is worse with flexion and occasionally on physical examination a bony gibbous will be detected. Treatment is an extension brace until the patient is pain free and there is no further progression of the deformity (Weiker, 1989).

Upper extremity injuries

Upper extremity problems are common in gymnastics because of the weight-bearing and impact-loading characteristics of the activity which places unine forces on the joints of the upper extremity. Flexibility is an important characteristic of a gymnast and all anatomical areas tend to be more flexible than in the non-gymnast. There is a strong tendency for the competitive gymnast to have hyperextension of the elbow, as well as generalized laxity of the shoulder. In addition, after an injury, it is extremely important that the greater than normal range of motion returns or the athlete will be unable to compete at the same level prior to the injury (Kirby *et al.*, 1981; Steele & White, 1986; McAuley *et al.*, 1987; Weiker, 1989).

Shoulder injuries: Acute and chronic instability of the shoulder is common in gymnasts because of the increased laxity noted above. Chronic recurrent subluxation of the shoulder is common and it appears to be related both to the sport and to the process of natural selection because of the premium placed on increased flexibility. Patients usually present with the sensation of the shoulder going out and with the more generic complaint of sudden pain, as well as weakness and heaviness of the involved extremity, the so-called dead arm syndrome. Patients respond well to conservative exercise and as in swimmers, surgery is a very last resort because of the propensity to interfere with regaining full range of motion. An exercise protocol for this problem encourages strength development in the shoulder girdle with special emphasis on internal and external rotation. Even though recurrent subluxation is common, recurrent dislocation is uncommon (Silvij & Nocini, 1982; McAuley *et al.*, 1987; Weiker, 1989).

Elbow injuries: Both acute and chronic elbow injuries have been reported as a result of gymnastics participation. The elbow is frequently subjected to axial loading as a result of weight-bearing activities in the vault and tumbling, as well as on the balance beam. A high percentage of these are fractures and dislocations. Emphasis in the management of these injuries is immediate anatomical reduction of the fracture or dislocation with early protective motion. If an athlete cannot regain a full range of motion as noted above, then it will be very difficult to return to the same level of competition. Passive motion should be avoided but active motion is essential to achieve full function (McAuley *et al.*, 1987; Lindner & Caine, 1989; Weiker, 1989).

Osteochondral injuries of the capitellum of the radial head are seen in skeletally immature patients. Aetiology is similar to that seen in the elbow and in Little League pitchers. There is an impact on the radial head of the capitellum with weight-bearing loads as a result of the vaulting activities of the athlete. Complaints are usually of pain with occasional mechanical locking. Physical examination is often unremarkable, although there may be a loss of full extension. Radiographs will often show the defect in the capitellum or radial head but if there is not an apparent abnormality then a bone scan followed by a CT scan may be useful to define the problem. Arthroscopy and debridement of the lesion is recommended, although careful follow-up of any recurrent symptoms is important because such a problem may result in a prognosis of continued degeneration of the lateral compartment of the elbow (Lindner & Caire, 1989; Weiker, 1989).

Wrist injuries: There have been a number of reports of fractures of the wrist or forearm which occur as the result of the use of the dowelled grip. Use of this device on the bars increases the grip strength and therefore allows more complex stunts to be performed. There is an increased velocity in giant swings and other manoeuvres, but also the inherent risk of locking on the bar. If the grip locks the hand to the bar, the body's momentum may continue and result in a fracture dislocation of the wrist or fracture of the forearm. These injuries are best prevented by careful maintenance of the equipment and the use of grips that are in good repair and properly fitted to the gymnast's hand. The grips used by men and women are different and fitted for the diameter of the bars that each uses. The smaller diameter bar that the men use is not suitable for the women's dowelled grip, and makes it more likely to lock on the men's bar (McAuley *et al.*, 1987; Lindner & Caine, 1989; Weiker, 1989).

A second set of problems seen in the wrist consists of a variety of overuse problems including stress reactions of the distal radius and the ulnar physis, impaction syndromes of the scaphoid and ulna, scaphoid stress fracture and avascular necrosis of the capitate, distal radial physeal arrest with secondary ulnar-positive variance, acquired Madelung's deformity and carpal chondromalacia. In addition, chronic soft-tissue inflammatory problems including ganglia impingement capsulitis, triangular fibrocartilage tears and chronic carpal instability may occur (Vender & Watson, 1988; Dobyns & Gabel, 1990).

Radial growth plate injury is very common in the skeletally immature female gymnast because of the activities of the floor exercise and the uneven bars. The appearance is of bilateral asymmetrical widening and irregularity of the distal radial growth plates with ill-defined cystic changes, sclerosis of the metaphyseal side of the physis and flaring of the metaphysis. These injuries have an appearance similar to that seen in rickets because of the shagginess and widening of the physeal line (Carter *et al.*, 1988; Vender & Watson, 1988; Dobyns & Gabel, 1990; Ruggles *et al.*, 1991).

In virtually all of these chronic problems, a cessation of the inciting activity is the key to the management of the problem. In addition to those injuries in which dorsiflexion reproduces the patient's symptoms, the dorsiflexion stop brace may help to limit the symptoms. By mechanical limitation of this motion, activity is allowed but extremes of motion do not occur and therefore the symptoms are less. Non-steroidal anti-inflammatory medication, local icing and strengthening of the forearm flexors is also useful (Carter *et al.*, 1988; Weiker, 1989; Dobyns & Gabel, 1990; Ruggles *et al.*, 1991).

Hand and finger injuries: Hand and finger fractures occur as a result of weight-bearing activity but none are unique, however there is a problem that is specific for the gymnast (Lindner & Caine, 1989). Chronic friction as a result of hours of practice on the various apparatus will result in thick palmar callouses which may tear as a result of their repetitive activity. Prevention is most important by keeping the hands clean and properly chalked or wearing grips that are properly fitted. Moisturizers and paring of thick callouses also helps to prevent cracking and decreases friction. With the acute episode, the gymnast should discontinue workout and ice the hand with careful hygiene of the wound. It usually takes several days for this to heal before beginning gradual resumption of activity (Weiker, 1989).

Lower extremity injuries

Knee injuries: Complaints of knee pain or injury vary from 14 to 24%. The knee is the most frequent site of major, disabling injury such as sprain, physeal fracture, patellar dislocation or subluxation, chondral fracture and acute and chronic tendonitis, and muscle–tendon unit strain (Garrick & Requa, 1980; Donati *et al.*, 1986; McAuley *et al.*, 1987).

Anterior cruciate ligament injury and more severe complex ligament instabilities occur as a result of dismount-type injury. Surgical reconstruction is a necessity if the gymnast intends to return to gymnastics. Bracing does not offer sufficient protection from the rotational forces generated in gymnastics and, therefore non-operative management is not an option. Early surgical reconstruction allows a successful return to competitive gymnastics in the majority of cases. The gymnast is a good candidate for progressive accelerated rehabilitation (Donati *et al.*, 1986; McAuley *et al.*, 1987; Weiker, 1989).

Patellar instability problems are also common as a result of the valgus and external rotation forces that occur in vaulting, floor exercise and dismounts. These problems are best treated by patellar buttress brace, as well as a patellofemoral exercise programme, anti-inflammatory medication and hamstring stretching. If recurrent instability occurs, appropriate realignment procedures may be necessary (McAuley *et al.*, 1987; Lindner & Caine, 1989; Weiker, 1989).

In the knee, a symptomatic medial shelf can

occur in gymnasts as a result of repetitive stress of landing on the knees and kneeling on the edges of the beam which cause a blunt trauma of the area of the medial shelf with subsequent oedematous, fibrosis and thickening. Arthroscopic management of this problem when it does not respond to non-steroidal anti-inflammatory medication and rest is the treatment of choice (Weiker, 1989).

Overuse problems, including quadriceps tendonitis, pesanserine bursitis, patellar tendonitis and iliotibial band tendonitis all may occur. In addition, strains of the hamstrings and quadriceps are also frequently seen. All of these overuse problems are related to the factors stated earlier, including lack of flexibility, repetitive stress and the intensity, frequency and duration of practice activities. Most of these problems can be treated with non-steroidal anti-inflammatory medication, local icing and other physical therapy modalities, as well as resistive exercise and the appropriate stretching (McAuley *et al.*, 1987; Lindner & Caine, 1989).

Lower leg injuries: A stress fracture can occur, particularly in the leg and the foot. These injuries are more common in female gymnasts and usually involve the distal fibula, middle third of the tibia and metatarsals of the foot. Diagnosis of these injuries may not be immediately apparent, particularly if plain radiographs are negative. A bone scan is useful in localizing and characterizing the problem as a stress reaction. Rest or alteration of practice routine is the best method of treatment and the athlete can frequently find that this may be a difficult problem. In the leg an ankle–foot orthosis for non-practice times with a bone stimulator incorporated may offer some benefit to the accelerated management of this problem (McAuley *et al.*, 1987; Lindner & Caine, 1989; Weiker, 1989).

Ankle injuries: Although ankle sprain may not be more common than it is in the general population, these injuries still occur and usually involve routine treatment (McAuley *et al.*, 1987; Lindner & Caine, 1989). Plain radiographs are taken to rule out a fracture and then a standard management consisting of rest, ice, compression and elevation is used to control the initial swelling and pain. An early return to motion, preferably in a supervised setting with a physical therapist or trainer is particularly beneficial. Taping and bracing are useful to improve support in proprioception while regaining a full range of motion, strength and balance. A functional protective brace on return to activity is an important art, as well as taping (Weiker, 1989).

Osteochondral fracture can occur after ankle sprain and must be considered in the differential diagnosis of chronic pain after ankle sprain. A bone scan and CT scan are useful in localizing this problem and ankle arthroscopy confirms the diagnosis and allows therapeutic measures to be instituted (Weiker, 1989; Grana, 1990).

A second complication is a recurrent subluxation of the peroneal tendons. This problem, when it occurs, usually does not resolve on its own and requires reconstruction of the peroneal retinaculum, as well as deepening of the peroneal groove behind the lateral malleolus. The most important factor in the diagnosis is to have a high index of suspicion because it is otherwise a relatively infrequent problem (Grana, 1990). In the gymnast, it occurs on landing with the medial forefoot on the edge of a mat and the heel in a crack or off balance. This results in inversion and dorsiflexion which places stress across the peroneal tendon retinaculum. In an acute dislocation, an initial treatment may consist of a period of casting and muscle strengthening exercises for the peroneal, as well as support of the ankle and pressure over the peroneal tendons with a felt pad. Further episodes of peroneal tendon dislocation should indicate the need for reconstruction of the retinaculum (Weiker, 1989; Grana, 1990).

Foot injuries: Foot injuries in the élite gymnast occur fairly frequently and include fractures, contusions of the heel pad and plantar fascial inflammation. Moreover, dermatological problems, such as blisters and callouses can also be a problem, just as they are in the hand. These injury problems must be recognized and treated early with healing and toughening of the skin (McAuley *et al.*, 1987; Lindner & Caine, 1989; Weiker, 1989).

Conclusion

A review of the gymnastics literature indicates that a variety of acute and overuse problems occur as a result of gymnastics competition. The problems seem to become more frequent as the level of expertise of the athlete increases, as well as the frequency, duration and intensity of workouts increase. Coaches and physicians must be aware of this in order to recognize problems early on. Certain problems, such as navicular stress fracture of the wrist, pars intra-articular stress fractures and other overuse problems, can be treated much better in the early phases and eliminate the potential for long periods of inactivity or disability if the coach recognizes the problem and takes the athlete in for treatment early. Allowing these problems to persist over a long period of time will result in long-term morbidity and sequelae which may result in an athlete being removed from the competitive arena.

References

Caine, D., Cochrane, B., Caine, C. & Zemper, E. (1989) An epidemiologic investigation of injuries affecting young competitive female gymnasts. *Am. J. Sports Med.* **17**(6), 811–20.

Carter, S.R., Aldridge, M.J., Fitzgerald, R. & Davies, A.M. (1988) Stress changes of the wrist in adolescent gymnasts. *Br. J. Radiol.* **61**, 109–12.

Ciullo, J.V. & Jackson, D.W. (1985) Pars interarticularis stress reaction, spondylolysis, and spondylolisthesis in gymnasts. *Clin. Sports Med.* **4**(1), 95–110.

Dobyns, J.H. & Gabel, G.T. (1990) Gymnast's wrist. *Hand Clin.* **6**(3), 493–505.

Donati, R.B., Cox, S., Echo, B.S. & Powell, C.E. (1986) Bilateral simultaneous patellar tendon rupture in a female collegiate gymnast. A case report. *Am. J. Sports Med.* **14**(3), 237–9.

Garrick, J.G. & Requa, R.K. (1980) Epidemiology of women's gymnastics injuries. *Am. J. Sports Med.* **8**, 261–4.

Goldberg, B. (1989) Injury patterns in youth sports. *Phys. Sportsmed.* **17**, 175–86.

Goldstein, J.D., Berger, P.E., Windler, G.E. & Jackson, D.W. (1991) Spine injuries in gymnasts and swimmers. *Am. J. Sports Med.* **19**(5), 463–8.

Grana, W.A. (1990) Chronic pain after ankle sprain. *J. Musculoskeletal Med.* **7**(6), 35–49.

Hage, P. (1982) Trampolines: an 'attractive nuisance'. *Phys. Sports Med.* **10**(12), 118–22.

Hall, S.J. (1986) Mechanical contribution to lumbar stress injuries in female gymnasts. *Med. Sci. Sports Exerc.* **18**, 599–602.

Hammer, A., Schwartzbach, A. & Paulev, P.E. (1981) Trampoline training injuries. One hundred and ninety-five cases. *Br. J. Sports Med.* **15**(3), 151–8.

Holden, D.L. & Jackson, D.W. (1985) Stress fracture of the ribs in female rowers. *Am. J. Sports Med.* **13**, 342–8.

Jackson, D.S., Furman, W.K. & Berson, B.L. (1980) Patterns of injuries in college athletes: a retrospective study of injuries sustained in intercollegiate athletics in two colleges over a two-year period. *Mount Sinai J. Med.* **47**, 423–6.

Jackson, D.W., Wiltse, L.L. & Cirincione, R.J. (1976) Spondylolysis in the female gymnast. *Clin. Orthop.* **117**, 68–73.

Kirby, R.L., Simms, F.C., Symington, V.J. *et al.* (1981) Flexibility and musculoskeletal symptomatology in female gymnasts and age-matched controls. *Am. J. Sports Med.* **9**, 160–4.

Letts, M., Smallman, T., Afansiev, R. & Gouw, G. (1986) Fracture of the pars interarticularis in adolescent athletes: A clinical–biomechanical analysis. *J. Pediatr. Orthop.* **6**, 40–6.

Lindner, K.J. & Caine, D.J. (1989) Injury patterns of female competitive club gymnasts. *Can. J. Sport Sci.* **15**(4), 254–61.

Lindner, K.J., Caine, D.J. & Johns, D.P. (1991) Withdrawal predictors among physical and performance characteristics of female competitive gymnasts. *J. Sports Sci.* **9**, 259–72.

McAuley, E., Hudash, G., Shields, K. *et al.* (1987) Injuries in women's gymnastics. *Am. J. Sports Med.* **15**(6), S124–31.

Micheli, L.J. (1985) Back injuries in gymnastics. *Clin. Sports Med.* **4**(1), 85–94.

Pettrone, F.A. & Ricciardelli, E. (1987) Gymnastic injuries: the Virginia experience 1982–1983. *Am. J. Sports Med.* **15**(1), 59–62.

Proffer, D.S., Patton, J.J. & Jackson, D.W. (1991) Nonunion of a first rib fracture in a gymnast. *Am. J. Sports Med.* **19**(2), 198–201.

Ruggles, D.L., Peterson, H.A. & Scott, S.G. (1991) Radial growth plate injury in a female gymnast. *Am. Coll. Sports Med.* **23**(4), 393–6.

Sands, W. (1981) Competition injury study: a preliminary report on female gymnasts. *US Gymnasts Fed. Technical J.* **7**, 114–18.

Silver, J.R., Silver, D.D. & Godfrey, J.J. (1986a) Injuries of the spine sustained during gymnastic activities. *Br. Med. J.* **293**, 861–3.

Silver, J.R., Silver, D.D. & Godfrey, J.J. (1986b) Trampolining injuries of the spine. *Injury Br. J. Accident Surg.* **7**(12), 117–24.

Silvij, S. & Nocini, S. (1982) Clinical and radiological aspects of gymnast's shoulder. *J. Sports Med. Phys. Fitness* **22**, 49–53.

Snook, G.A. (1979) Injuries in women's gymnastics: a 5-year study. *Am. J. Sports Med.* **7**, 242–4.

Steele, V.A. & White, J.A. (1986) Injury prediction in female gymnasts [Abstract]. *Br. J. Sports Med.* **20**, 31–3.

Sward, L., Hellstron, M., Jacobsson, B., Nyman, R. & Peterson, L. (1991) Disc degeneration and associated abnormalities of the spine in élite gymnasts. *Spine* **16**(4), 437–43.

Torg, J.S. & Das, M. (1985) Trampoline and mini-trampoline injuries to the cervical spine. *Clin. Sports Med.* **4**(1), 45–60.

Vender, M.I. & Watson, H.K. (1988) Acquired Madelung-like deformity in a gymnast. *J. Hand Surg.* **13A**(1), 19–21.

Weiker, G.G. (1989) Musculoskeletal problems and the gymnast. *Adv. Sports Med. Fitness* **2**, 177–200.

Chapter 36

Injuries in Weightlifting

MEINOLF GOERTZEN

Weightlifting has a long tradition. Already among the Greeks and in Egyptian mythology, stone-throwing and weightlifting were of high significance in the training of the body and of strength. And, although weightlifting was an Olympic discipline as early as the first modern Olympics in Athens in 1896, until today there remain many reservations against this sport, especially among Western nations.

Generally considered as a fringe sport practiced by unseemly 'colossi', Western sports physicians had very little appreciation of the movements, techniques and possible injuries relating to it. In contrast to this, it can no longer be dismissed in the 1990s as specific power training is part of almost every sport in modern sports theory and training doctrine. Other subdisciplines, e.g. body building and powerlifting, have also developed, not least within the framework of the fitness waves which have increasingly gained in significance over the last few years. These subdisciplines are certainly capable of being practised competitively.

Olympic weightlifting

There are 10 weight categories in Olympic weightlifting (52, 56, 60, 67.5, 75, 82.5, 90, 100, 110 kg and super heavy weight practised at over 110 kg body weight without limit). The competitions are held in the so-called Olympic duel and constitute 'snatching' and 'jerking'. Since the Olympic games in Munich in 1972, the weightlifting form 'pressing', which was practised until then, has been abolished due to medical intervention.

Snatching

In 'snatching', the weight is brought into an upward position without pause in a lifting movement with widespread arms (Fig. 36.1). A distinction is made here between the squatting technique and the jerking technique, the latter

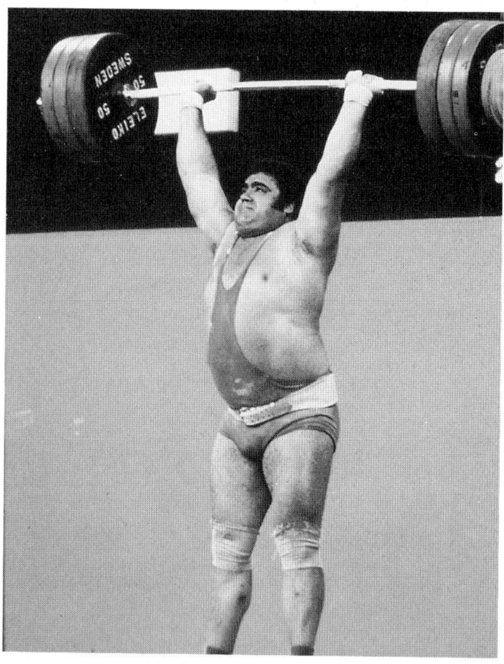

Fig. 36.1 The snatching technique.

being hardly practised any more today. In the squatting technique, the necessary holding of the weight with outstretched arms above the head is achieved by the athlete 'diving' into a squatting position at the moment when the weight reaches breast level during lifting (Fig. 36.2). During the straightening procedure, the lifter must bring the weight into an upward position keeping the arms outstretched. In the seldom practised jerking technique the lifter achieves a complete lifting of the weight by first introducing a jerk and then bringing the weight into an upward position (Fig. 36.3).

Jerking

In 'jerking', the weight is held at approximately shoulder width, brought up to the level of the breast in one movement and held in this position. This can be achieved with both the squatting and the jerking technique. In order to then bring the weight into an upward position a knee bend is introduced in order to achieve sufficient momentum for the last part of the lifting procedure.

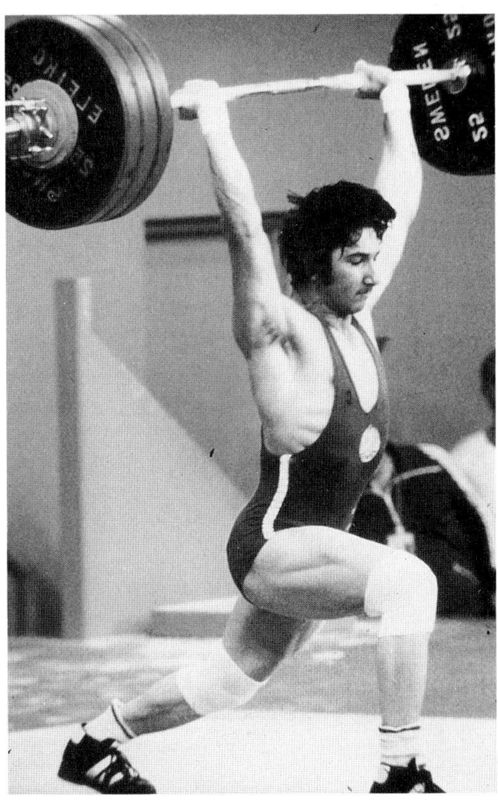

Fig. 36.3 The jerking technique.

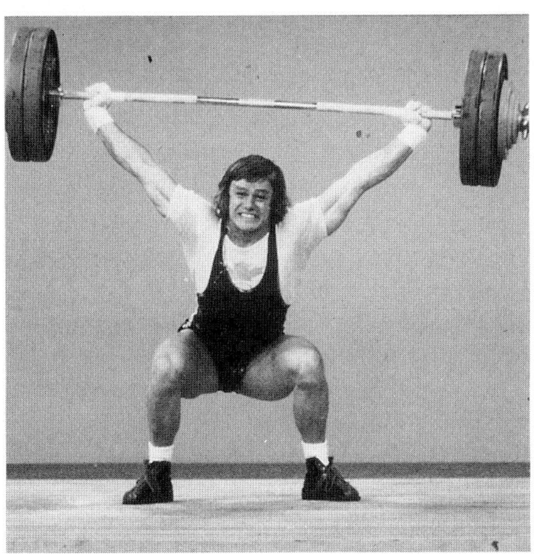

Fig. 36.2 The squatting technique.

Pressing

This technique was abandoned because degenerative spinal diseases were observed too often. The reason for these was seen in the jerky hyperlordosis movements of the lumbar spine mainly carried out during training; during these movements the weight, which was held at shoulder height, was brought into an upward position by the lifter whilst 'diving' during an extreme retroflexion of the spinal column (Fig. 36.4).

Sport equipment

The barbell is 2.2 m long and has a diameter within the holding area of 28 mm. It is equipped with rubber-covered metal weights on revolving sockets. These weights correspond

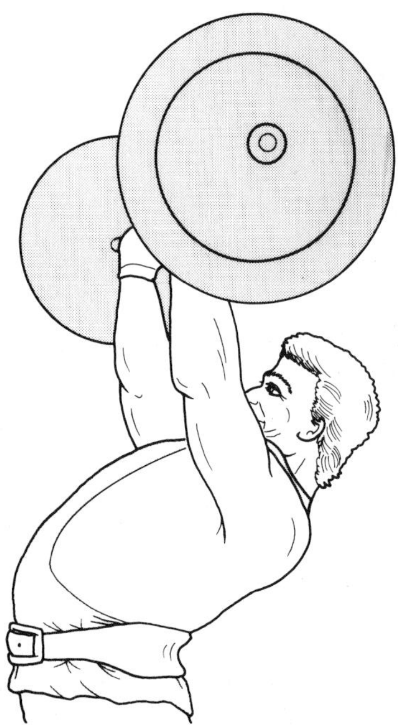

Fig. 36.4 During the pressing technique the spine can be brought in extreme retroflexion.

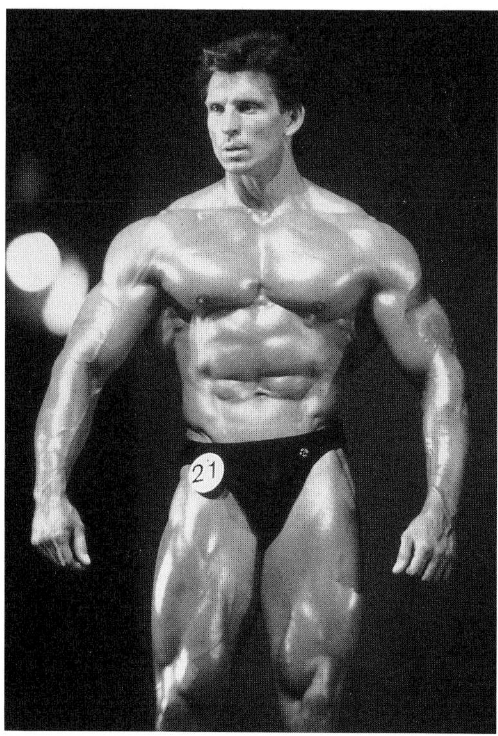

Fig. 36.5 A body builder's training is directed in exact correspondence to the proportion of the body.

to international norms and are available in weights of 1.25, 2.5, 5, 10, 15, 20, 25 and 50 kg. Many weightlifters wear leather belts around the waist. These have the function of providing a pneumohydrodynamic padding for extra stabilization of the lumbar spine.

In training and in competition, magnesia is rubbed into the inner surface of the hands in order to strengthen the grip. The wearing of wrist and knee joint bandages as well as thumb protective plasters is allowed. On the other hand, the wearing of bar belts for the protection of the inner surface of the hand is forbidden.

Body building

The aim of the body builder's training is directed solely towards the development of the muscles within an optimally balanced programme in exact correspondence to the proportion of the body (Fig. 36.5). For the most part, it is carried out in special studios with free-holding bars as well as with diverse power equipment.

Powerlifting

The aim of the powerlifter, on the other hand, is similar to that of the Olympic weightlifter and is directed towards lifting a maximum amount of weight. Powerlifting in its competitive form is constituted by three individual disciplines:

1 The squat-lift (Fig. 36.6).
2 The dead-lift (Fig. 36.7).
3 The bench-press (Fig. 36.8).

Methodologies of training

The specific training methodologies of these three power sports are quite different and their influence on the pattern of injuries is not

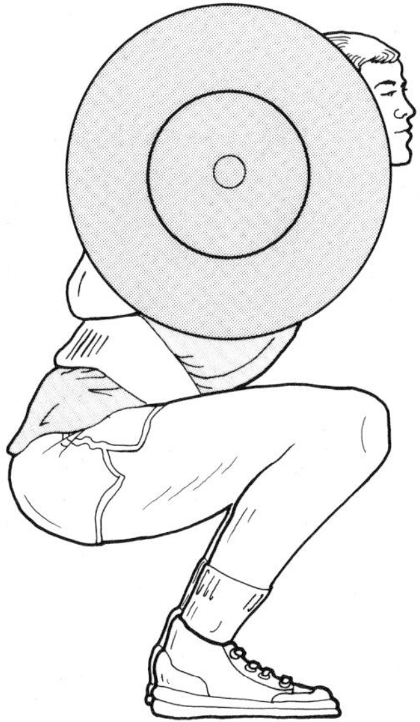

Fig. 36.6 The squat-lift.

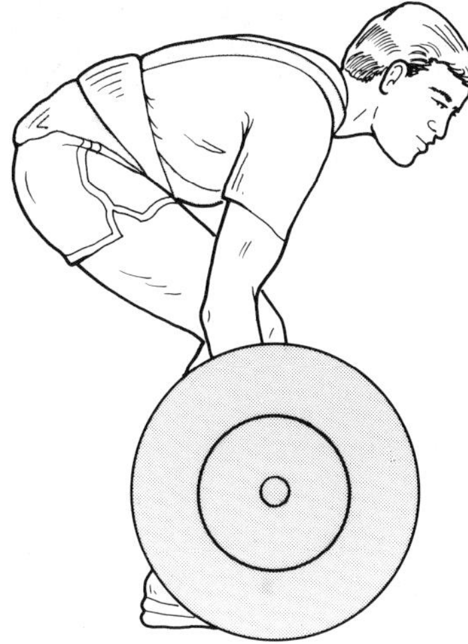

Fig. 36.7 The dead-lift.

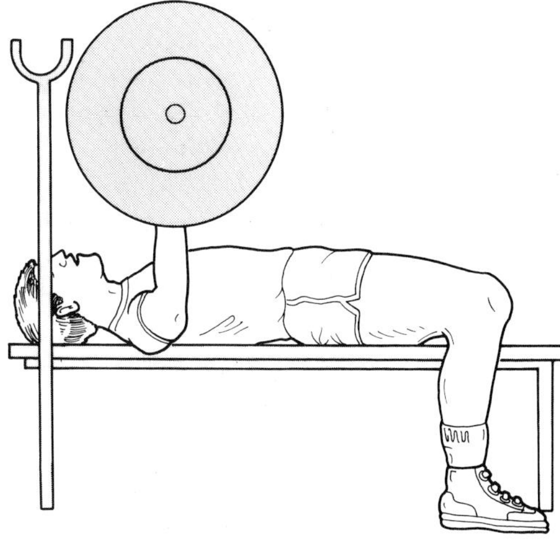

Fig. 36.8 The bench-press.

insignificant. Whilst the body builder and powerlifter prefer the methods of maximum expenditure of power with high intensity and few repetitions, most Olympic weightlifters give preference to weight strains which tend to be submaximum, as well as to many repetitions. Furthermore, body builders and powerlifters employ special strategies aimed towards total muscular exhaustion and thereby maximum muscle growth. To achieve this, they perform the following exercises, given in their order of significance:

1 *Forced repetitions*. After the end of a set, two or three repetitions follow with the help of a partner to the point where a movement can just be carried out.

2 *Burns*. Normally, six repetitions are carried out to the point where the muscles are fully exhausted. Typical burning muscle pains occur at this point. Subsequently, a further two to four repetitions are made, whereby execution of the movement is incomplete.

3 *Super-sets*. These are double-sets which are carried out one after the other without pause.

4 *Repetition after induced fatigue*. In this training procedure, especially circulating within body building, an antagonistic–agonistic muscle group is first exercised and then the main exercise for both muscle groups follows.

5 *Negative repetitions*. After the end of the set, a further two to three repetitions are made in order to bring the weight back to its starting position.

6 *Cheating repetitions*. Repetitions to the point of exhaustion and then aid from other muscle groups for completion of the movement. As a result of the proven unphysiological strains and the incorrect lifting techniques particularly employed during cheating repetitions, most injuries and overuse injuries are observed here. In the light of this knowledge, these repetitions now only play a very small role within the training of those practising power sports (Goertzen *et al.*, 1989).

Spectrum of injuries

Today, the health risks connected with Olympic weightlifting are relatively small when using corresponding systematic build-up training together with polished technical instruction, especially with regard to the occurrence of acute injuries of the postural and musculoskeletal systems. Observed injuries are mostly the later results of already existing overuse injuries. As a rule, acute injuries occurring in training or in competition afflict unpracticed athletes and can be traced to incorrect technical implementation, insufficient muscular preparation before training or insufficient warm-up.

Next to powerlifting, particularly more significant to injury is power training which is carried out in leisure time. The basic training of other sport disciplines which aim at an additional strengthening of the muscles also belongs in this category (Steinbrück, 1977). Systematic introduction to the associated bodily stresses and correct observation of training by specialized trainers are often lacking.

Happily, a change has occurred in the last few years and training now takes place less and less with free-holding bars and more with special power equipment. Power training equipment from diverse manufacturers allows for a measured strain within a guided movement. Furthermore, knowledge and experience within power training have increased among trainer and athletes alike, not least because of the information arising from various branches of the media.

Spinal column injuries

The spinal column and the knee joints belong to the regions of the body which are most injured by power athletes. In a study by Kotani *et al.* (1971), more than 95% of power athletes complained of pains in the lumbar region during their sport. Of these, 31% showed a spondylolysis/spondylolisthesis and 18% an axial deviation of the spinal column. Rossi (1978), Kulund (1978) and Goertzen *et al.* (1989) also found spondylolysis rates of over 30% in Olympic weightlifters and powerlifters, whereas Goertzen *et al.* (1989) could only prove spondylolysis/spondylolistheses in 4.6% of 358 body builders who had had an average of 4.5 training units·week^{-1} for over more than 3 years. The unanimous opinion is that cross-lifting or pressing, which are not practiced in body building and which have a great tangential stress on the pars interarticularis of the spinal column, are the main reasons for these changes to it.

Tusch and Ulrich (1974) showed the importance of correct lifting technique in their experimental investigations. During compression experiments on complete segments of the spinal column at an axial stress of maximum 1000 kg F (F, force), they were not able to induce any vertebral disc destruction. They estimated the strength of the vertebral tissue at approximately 1500 kg F. On the other hand, completely different biomechanical situations occur when the spinal column is in movement. By tilting the vertebral bodies against each other, tangential tensions arise on the convex side of the intervertebral disc which can exceed the level of axial stress by more than a factor of 8 (Nachemson, 1960, 1965). Granhed and Morelli (1988) calculated maximum stresses in the lower lumbar segment of up to 30 kN. Nevertheless, acute intervertebral disc prolapses remain an absolute rarity within the spectrum of injuries which befall power athletes.

Jaros and Cech (1965) have examined international class weightlifters involved in competitive sports for at least 8 years lifting a weekly quota of at least 10 000 kg *F*. Their radiological examinations did not show any increased rate of degenerative changes in the spinal column amongst weightlifters when compared to members of the normal population. On the other hand, in their examinations of previous weightlifters in age groups above 50, Granhed and Morelli (1988) determined a reduction of the intervertebral space in the lower lumbar segment in 62% of them.

Krahl (1975) could also confirm that degenerative disc lesions, spondylolyses and osteochondroses among top-class international weightlifters are comparatively seldom. In part, this result is most definitely due to the process of natural selection among top-class athletes. In particular phases of their training they must lift a daily quota of 70–90 t. Such enormous stresses however, can only be sustained without lasting damage when the correct lifting technique is employed.

The lifters always therefore attempt to distribute the weight evenly over the whole of the disc transverse section by stretching the spinal column. From the squatting position, the weight is lifted only by means of a slight forward bend. By holding the bars at the front, the power vector of the additional weight is much nearer to the pivot of the spinal column at L5–S1 during the entire exercise, whereby the resulting torque is considerably reduced in this segment than when holding the bars behind the head.

Lifting the bars in a forward position with the upper arm in as horizontal a position as possible also leads to a straightening of the thoracic vertebral column and an improvement of the intersegmental pressure transmission in this section. Furthermore, physiological adjustment of the lumbar spine is also triggered.

In comparison to athletes of other disciplines, in large numbers of weightlifters we find a restricted dorsal extension in the upper ankle joint. In these cases, the deep knee bend with a physiological position of the vertebral column is only possible when either the heels lift from the ground, which leads to unsteady footing, or with the feet fully placed on the ground, the trunk is more bent forward. This presupposes an increased bending of the hip and thereby leads to a delordosis of the lumbar spine. In any event, the torque in the lumbosacral transition increases significantly due to an extension of the lever arm. On the one hand, the delordosis has a pathogenic effect on the individual parts of the affected spinal segments due to high, punctuated stress peaks. On the other, an increased lordosis of the lumbar spine leads to an increased sliding together of the small articulations of the vertebral column and thus often to consecutive facet syndromes with pseudoradicular symptomatology of complaint.

A clean snatching through of the bar requires maximum technical skill, a skill which the athlete who only indulges in power training as a supplement to normal training cannot, as a rule, possess. The point of this training exercise is to accelerate as great a weight as possible above the head in as short a time as possible. For the non-specialist it therefore seems sufficient, at least with large weights, to carry out this exercise with the so-called snatching technique. The jerking of the displaced weight is only meaningful to the training method when special power in the shoulder girdle is required as an extra training objective (e.g. in throwing). Otherwise, the body extension achieved during displacement is sufficient, whereby a complete extension of the hips must be observed as well as that the athlete does not lift the heels from the ground until the end of the lifting phase.

In lifting the weight whilst standing, the original position of the body — with feet at approximately hip breadth with slight lateral rotation of the feet — need not be altered. In a technical displacement, this footing is altered at the end of the lifting phase, when the body 'dives' under the bar, for a rather broader one with more lateral rotation. With a good starting position, the feet are slightly more apart than hip breadth with slight lateral rotation, taking into account the anatomical torsion in the leg. Raising the heels is not useful because by doing so the stress to the ligamentum patellae is also increased (see patella tip syndrome). An athlete should not begin with snatching and displacing before mastering the knee bend technique and the stabilization of the spinal column in the individual, optimal position which is hereby necessary.

Knee injuries

PATELLA PAIN SYNDROME

In all power sports, the knee joint is the neuralgic point of the postural and musculoskeletal system with regard to overuse injuries. Complaints in the femoropatellar joint, specifically in the sense of a patellar chondromalacia, arise particularly frequently due to the enormous stresses caused by this type of sport and which are unavoidable in training and in competition. Causes for this are, in addition to congenital anomalies such as patella dysplasia and axial malposition, the frequent execution of deep knee bends with additional weight stress. Also to blame for this condition is the frequent catching of the bars whilst in the so-called 'half-stand'.

Frankel and Hang (1975) determined in their investigations concerning the pathogenesis of this typical power sport overuse injury, that with knee bends in excess of 40°, the forces effecting the femoral patellar gliding joint increase overproportionately. During a deep knee bend, peak stresses of up to 7.6 times that of the normal body weight can occur.

JUMPER'S KNEE

The formation of jumper's knee can also be seen as an expression of the discrepancy between the stress and the resilience of tissue. By this, we mean an insertion tendopathy of the knee extension musculature, which occurs often simultaneously in weightlifters and powerlifters at the upper or lower patellar role. The deep knee bend appears to be the main reason for triggering off these complaints. In contrast to this, training on the leg curler seems to cause less injury to the quadriceps muscle of the thigh whilst sitting, as well as to the ischiocrural muscles whilst reclining.

MENISCUS INJURIES

Meniscus injuries are occasionally observed, particularly among weightlifters as a result of a faulty technique. These occur mostly during diving into a squat during which a valgus stress with rotation of the knee joint ensues as a result of incorrect technical implementation.

Shoulder injuries

In contrast to Olympic weightlifters, the highest rate of injury for powerlifters and body builders is to be found in the upper extremities, particularly in the shoulder and elbow joints. Dominant are non-specific periarthritic shoulder complaints, impingement syndrome of the supraspinous tendon and insertion tendopathy of biceps and triceps brachial muscle of the arm as well as of the pectoralis major muscle. Powerlifters and body builders suffer from these complaints particularly frequently during back and neck pressing with excessive weights.

Overuse injuries observed among Olympic weightlifters in the form of an insertion tendopathy of the long biceps tendon and the supraspinous tendon are mostly caused by holding the horizontal bars too far behind the head, i.e. shifted behind the axis of the body. Inflammations of the bursa subacromialis are also observed. Should the bars fall behind the axis of the body, this can lead to traumatic anterior shoulder luxation. Arthrosis of the acromioclavicular joint or glenohumeral joint are not more often observed than in other sports.

Elbow injuries

Occurrence of ulnar epicondylitis of humerus can also normally be attributed to faulty barbell technique. This is very frequently observed in lifters after an unsuccessful attempt when the weight slips too far behind the axis of the body. Overuse reactions of the forearm extensors lead to complaints in the lateral epicondyle of humerus.

Hand injuries

Injuries and overuse reactions in the area of the hand are observed above all in training with free bars. Lesions of the articular disc occur during extreme overstretching with a simultaneous longitudinal force or hyperextension with additional pronation, e.g. when the horizontal bars slip (O'Donoghue, 1984). By means of a similar injury mechanism with dorsal flexion, pronation and additional radial abduction, luxations of the extensor carpi ulnaris tendon are observed.

A chronic hyperextension of the wrist and repeated severe muscle contractions, particularly whilst transposing the bars, lead to a tenosynovitis stenosans de Quervain. Other overuse reactions often observed in weightlifters are: tendinites of the flexor carpi ulnaris tendon and the finger flexor tendons caused by severe dorsal extension in the wrist and passage disabilities of the tendons in finger sections with tendon sheaths resulting in trigger finger due to an overtaxing of the tendons. Pain at the ulnar side of the wrist at the insertion to the collateral ligaments indicate a styloiditis ulnar.

Severe tensile effects of the flexor carpi ulnaris tendons caused by repeated, powerful bending movements in the wrist or by passive tension caused by extreme dorsal flexion of the hand increase the pressure in the pisotriquetral joint. This can lead to cartilage destruction and thereby to consecutive pisotriquetral arthroses with considerable pains in the hypothenar during powerful wrist bending. The resulting weakening of grip leads to considerable limitations in performance.

The most often occurring cause for carpal tunnel syndrome when observed in power athletes is a non-specific tenosynovitis resulting from extreme chronic strain on the flexor tendon and repetitive traumas of the tendon sheaths. The excessive stress at first induces an oedema of the paratenon. Through proliferation and scar formation, it can then lead to a permanent constriction of the median nerve in the carpal canal and its typical symptom form.

Dangles and Bilos (1980) also described appearances of compression of the nervus ulnaris with atrophy of the hypothenar as a result of a hypertrophy of the triceps muscle caused in training. Pressure and rubbing leads to blister and callous formation particularly on the palmar side of the metacarpophalangeal joint and in the region of the proximal phalanx as well as on the ulnar side of the thumb. Blister formation and deglovings which are often seen at these points are additionally favoured by increased sweating of the inner surface of the hand whilst practising the sport.

Muscle lesions

Favoured localizations for muscle injuries in power athletes are the musculature of the trunk and the long erector spinae muscles as well as the shoulder area (Klein *et al.*, 1979). The origin and insertion of the biceps brachii, serratus anterior and of the rhomboid muscles are also subject to a high susceptibility to injury. Stanish and Lamb (1978) report cases of paralyses of the serratus anterior muscle caused by traction injuries to the nervus thoracicus longus during transposition of the horizontal bar.

Muscle ruptures, particularly those in the region of the insertion to the triceps at the olecranon, are increasingly observed after an abrupt withdrawal of anabolics. Altogether, powerlifters show the highest rate of insertion tendopathy and muscle lesions of all power sports. Within the regions of the lower extremities the bandages used by powerlifters for stabilization lead, especially among women, to often observable ruptures of the smaller vessels caused by congestion and thereby to surface haematomas.

Signs of functional adaptation

After 3–5 years of systematic power training

by weightlifters, Koracenkov (quoted by Gekeler, 1975) could observe a clear enlargement of the diaphyseal diameters of the stressed tubular bones, the corticalis and the apophyses. In contrast to other sport disciplines, weightlifters showed the greatest bone density within the bounds of a functional adaptation of the tissue.

Nevertheless, individual stress fractures in the rib region and at the forearm are observed in cases of forced power training. Gumbs *et al.* (1982) attribute the continual switch between pressing and pulling stresses from the volar to the dorsal parts of the distal forearm bones as the causal mechanism in the emergence of distal forearm fractures. In particular, distal radial epiphysis fractures are seen among youths whose power training began too early and in incorrect doses (Ryan & Salciccioli, 1976).

Prevention of injuries

To the fore of prophylaxis for the described injuries and overuse injuries is the learning and practice of correct technique. Furthermore, injuries which are not fully healed as well as already existing infectious diseases present possibilities for the emergence of injuries and overuse injuries, and are therefore a contraindication to active weightlifting.

Degloving of the hand can be extensively avoided if the existing skin callouses on the metacarpophalangeal joint are regularly removed and smoothed out by the athletes. Insertion tendonopathies in the shoulder region and particularly in the epicondylitis humeri ulnaris can be extensively eliminated by observing the correct lifting technique. A dorsal transfer of weight behind the body axis must especially be avoided (Fig. 36.9).

Apart from the basic conditions necessary for the avoidance of overuse injuries to the spine, namely the exact observance of correct technique, correct development of the erector spinae muscles and the abdominal muscles is most important. As a preventive measure, the so-called pneumohydrodynamic padding should not only be provided for by a belt, but also by an adequate refinement of the abdominal muscles. As a preventive measure to overuse injuries of the knee joint, athletes having congenital anomalies and dysplasia in the femoral patellar joint should be informed before beginning achievement-orientated weightlifting that these changes predispose that athlete to damage and that he or she may therefore be well advised to reconsider. The same also applies for pronounced defective positions such as knock-knee and bow-leg.

In conclusion it must be said that muscle adaptation in cases of increased stress ensues much faster than adaptation of bradytrophic structures (cartilage, tendons, ligaments). A slow, gradually increasing rate of stress over a period of years also helps to minimize the emergence of acute injuries and overuse injuries. The above-mentioned points should communicate from an orthopaedic perspective how the stress to the musculoskeletal system can be held to a minimum, despite great amounts of additional external strain. Within the context of training, it is important to mention the principle of the variation of exercises as well as the equipment used and intensities within training respectively. In this way, the pathogenic summation of stress peaks typical to every form of power training exercise which is done monotonously, especially within powerlifting, can be reduced.

Reduction in flexibility, especially observed in power sports as a result of a one-sided muscle hypertrophy (especially restrictions in elbow flexion and extension, hip rotation and flexion as well as knee flexion), must be accompanied by consecutive stretch training and suitable, effective compensatory sports, especially those which serve to enhance the cardiocirculatory system.

As in contrast to weightlifters, an increasingly small number of body builders and powerlifters train under supervision, a further reduction in the rate of injury could certainly be achieved on a preventive basis by means of a substantial improvement of supervision

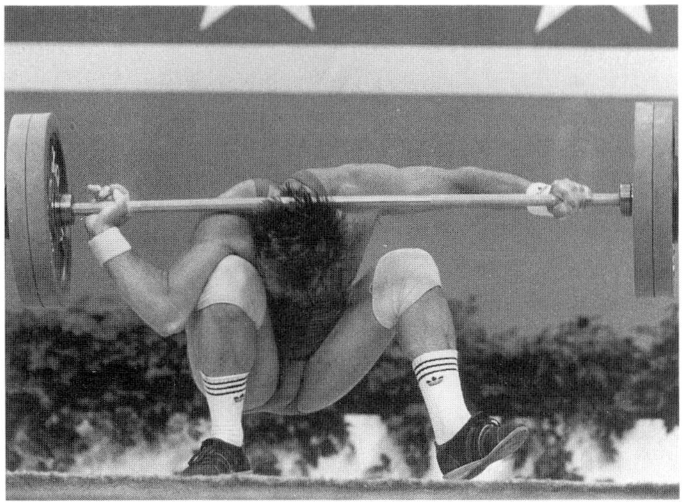

(a)

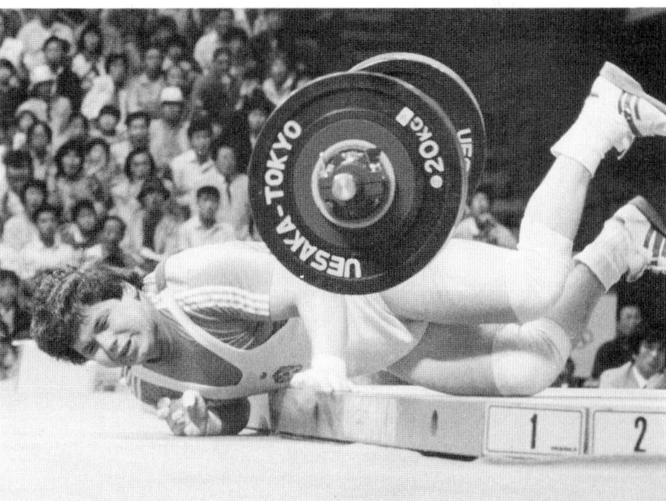

(b)

Fig. 36.9 The weights should be properly balanced to avoid injuries. © IOPP/T. Schmitt.

during training and an improved medical care tailored to the needs of the sport.

References

Dangles, C.J. & Bilos, Z.J. (1980) Ulnar nerve neuritis in a world champion weightlifter. *Am. J. Sports Med.* **8**, 443–4.

Frankel, V.H. & Hang, Y.S. (1975) Recent advances in biomechanics of sports injuries. *Acta Orthop. Scand.* **46**, 484–97.

Gekeler, J. (1975) Arthrose durch Hochleistungssport? (Arthritis in top-level sport?) *Therapiewoche* **29**, 4167–9.

Goertzen, M., Schöppe, K., Lange, G. & Schulitz, K.P. (1989) Verletzungen und Uberlastungsschäden bei Bodybuildern und Powerliftern (Overuse injuries in bodybuilders and powerlifters). *Sportverl. Sportschad.* **3**, 32–6.

Granhed, H. & Morelli, B. (1988) Low back pain among retired wrestlers and heavy weight lifters. *Am. J. Sports Med.* **16**, 530–3.

Gumbs, V.L., Segal, D., Halligan, J.B. & Lower, G.

(1982) Bilateral distal radius and ulnar fracture in adolescent weight lifters. *Am. J. Sports Med.* **10**, 375–9.

Jaros, A. & Cech, J. (1965) Die Wirbelsäule bei Gewichthebern (Spinal vertebrae in weightlifters). *Beitr. Orthop.* **12**, 653–60.

Klein, W., Schulitz, K.P. & Neumann, C. (1979) Orthopädische Probleme bei Bodybuildern (Orthopaedic problems in bodybuilders). *Sportmed.* **30**, 296–308.

Kotani, P.T. (1971) Studies of spondylolysis found among weight lifters. *Br. J. Sports Med.* **6**, 4–10.

Krahl, H. (1975) Aspekte der Tauglichkeitsbeurteilung im Leistungssport (Aspects of overloading in competitive sports). *Orthop. Praxis* **11**, 56–61.

Kulund, D.M. (1978) Olympic weight-lifting injuries. *Phys. Sports Med.* **6**, 111–18.

Nachemson, A. (1960) Lumbar intradiscal pressure. *Acta Orthop. Scand.* **43**, (Suppl.), 96–101.

Nachemson, A. (1965) The effect of forward leaning on lumbar intradiscal pressure. *Acta Orthop. Scand.* **35**, 314–19.

O'Donoghue, D.H. (1984) *Treatment of Injuries to Athletes*, 4th edn. WB Saunders, Philadelphia.

Rossi, F. (1978) Spondylolysis, spondylolisthesis and sports. *Ital. J. Sports Med. Phys. Fitness* **18**, 317–40.

Ryan, J.R. & Salciccioli, G.G. (1976) Fractures of the distal radial epiphysis in adolescent weight lifters. *Am. J. Sports Med.* **4**, 26–7.

Stanish, W.D. & Lamb, H. (1978) Isolated paralysis of serratus anterior muscle. A weight training injury. *Am. J. Sports Med.* **6**, 385–7.

Steinbrück, K. (1977) Sportmedizinische Probleme bei Gewichthebern (Sports medicine problems in weightlifters). *Sportarzt Sportmed.* **28**, 289–92.

Tüsch, C. & Ulrich, S.P. (1974) Wirbelsäule und Hochleistungssport (Spinal vertebrae and top-level sports). *Sportarzt Sportmed.* **9**, 206–8.

Chapter 37

Injuries in Wrestling

JACK HARVEY, RANDALL R. WROBLE AND SHAWN WOTOWEY

Wrestling is truly one of the oldest known sports and certainly one with the oldest record of injuries. In the 1990s, the sport still is one that presents the sports medicine team with frequent and varied challenges. In fact, at a large tournament it seems the sports medicine area turns into a war zone with a myriad of minor and serious injuries. The traumatologist of the team deals with acute injuries including fractures, sprains and dislocations. The team physician must be prepared to deal with infectious skin problems, head and spinal injuries and the usual systemic illnesses that affect all athletes undergoing a vigorous training or competition schedule. The athletic trainer must instil good nutritional habits, encourage good training techniques and rehabilitate injured athletes. Each team member is aware not only of treatment of injury but also has a desire to prevent as many injuries as possible.

Prevention of wrestling injuries will not just happen by itself. Injury rate reduction will require careful observation and analysis of the types and frequency of the injuries common in today's wrestlers. Consultation with exercise physiologists, nutritionists, biomechanists and other sports scientists will be necessary to develop and test new ideas. If these recommendations are sound, a reduction in one or more injury type will result.

Musculoskeletal problems

Epidemiology and risk factors

Not only is wrestling one of the most ancient sports, it also remains popular at the youth, high-school, college and senior level. Part of its popularity relates to the opportunity for participation by athletes of all sizes. In the USA alone, nearly 300 000 boys participate in high-school wrestling programmes. Thousands more from several hundred colleges participate at the university level. Despite this, in nearly all reports examining musculoskeletal problems in sports, injury rates in wrestling are significantly high and occasionally the highest among all sports. For example, in a 5-year study of 13 National Collegiate Athletic Association (NCAA) sports, wrestlers were injured at a rate of $10.03 \cdot 1000$ exposures^{-1}, the highest of all sports surveyed. Furthermore, wrestling showed the highest injury rate for both practices and competitions (Dick, 1988). In a high-school study, injury rates in wrestling over 2 years were second only to rates found in American football and were nearly double any other sport (Garrick & Requa, 1981). During the 1976 USA Olympic freestyle wrestling trials, 26.5% of wrestlers sustained an injury in just 2 days of competition (Estwanik *et al.*, 1978). In a 7-year review of college wrestling injuries, the most commonly injured anatomical regions were the knee, head, neck and face, shoulder, trunk and back, and ankle (Table 37.1) (Wroble & Albright,

Table 37.1 Percentage of injuries by anatomical region, University of Iowa, 1976–1977 to 1983–1984.

Site of injury	% of total
Head/neck/face	31.0
head	3.0
neck	12.0
ear	5.5
face	8.0
teeth	2.5
Upper extremity	22.0
shoulder	12.0
arm/elbow/forearm	5.0
wrist/hand	5.0
Trunk and lower back	10.0
Lower extremity	37.0
hip/thigh	4.0
knee	24.0
leg/ankle	8.0
foot	1.0

1986). The total injury rate was 176 · 100 wrestlers·year^{-1} or almost 2 injuries·wrestler·year^{-1}.

Why does wrestling have such a high injury rate? First, wrestling is a contact sport and unlike many other such sports, contact in wrestling occurs virtually 100% of the time. There is no question that this increases the at-risk period. Second, wrestling is also a collision sport. Collisions occur when a wrestler 'shoots' or attempts a take-down. Injuries occur during take-downs because of their explosive nature.

In an attempt to study the long-term consequences of wrestling injuries, Mysnyk and Albright (1989) conducted a study at the 1986 NCAA Wrestling Championships. Over 500 male volunteers were interviewed regarding their past and current musculoskeletal problems. In comparison to non-athletes, former wrestlers had three times as many neck problems and nearly four times as many knee problems (both statistically significant). Overall, 42% of former wrestlers had on-going musculoskeletal problems. The magnitude of both the acute and long-term problem mandates that research into injury prevention occur and that appropriate implementation of preventive programmes is initiated.

In two epidemiological studies, Wroble and Albright (1986) and Wroble *et al.* (1991) uncovered several factors which put wrestlers at high risk. For example, injury rates are much higher in matches (up to 40 times greater) (Wroble *et al.*, 1991) than practices, but nonetheless most wrestling injuries occur during practice reflecting the vast amount of time wrestlers spend in preparation for matches. Wrestlers are also at higher risk for injury early in the season, particularly in tournament competition. Tournaments may entail wrestling 3–6 times·day^{-1}, often with only an hour rest between matches. Because there are so many matches with resulting potential for aggravation, a minor injury can easily progress to a significant injury. It also seems that a wrestler with a previous injury is more susceptible to a reinjury. Indeed, we found a knee injury was twice as common in wrestlers who had previously hurt their knees (Wroble *et al.*, 1991). Whether the wrestler is attacking or defending can put that athlete at higher risk for certain types of injuries. While the attacking wrestler has a higher risk of neck injury, the defending wrestler has a higher rate of knee injury.

Once a wrestler has been injured and a plan for treatment is being developed, one must take into consideration an additional factor — non-compliance. An endemic problem among these athletes, we found non-compliant wrestlers had an injury recurrence rate over twice that of compliant wrestlers (Wroble *et al.*, 1991). Although virtually all wrestlers are highly motivated to return to action, this is a two-edged sword in that while they may perform beautifully in a rehabilitation programme, those who in their anxiety to return quickly to competition are non-compliant with medical advice are at tremendous risk of reinjury.

Prevention of injuries

Rules. The rules of wrestling serve to substantially reduce injuries by addressing several important areas. Conducting competition by weight class ensures that athletes are size-matched and injuries thus do not occur due to gross discrepancy in strength of competitors. The rules also require safety in positioning mats, scoreboards and tables during a competition as well as mandating medical staff be present at all events.

The most important wrestling rules, however, are those that prohibit dangerous and illegal techniques. A variety of holds are banned: (i) twisting of the fingers or toes; (ii) any hold with intent to injure or cause pain; (iii) holds that may cause dislocation; (iv) twisting of the neck or back; or (v) headlocks without an arm included (Fig. 37.1). Should these situations arise during a match, any advantage gained is nullified in the scoring and the referee takes one of the following actions. The referee may (i) break the dangerous hold without stopping the action; (ii) stop the action, break the hold, and award penalties: the opponent of the offending wrestler may be given one or two points and the offender is assigned a caution; (iii) if the wrestler is injured by the opponent's illegal action and is ruled medically unfit to continue, the wrestler at fault is disqualified; and (iv) a wrestler can be immediately disqualified for blatant unnecessary roughness. Referees are instructed in strict enforcement of these rules and penalties. Further education of referees into mechanisms of injury will enhance their ability to assess a potentially dangerous situation on the mat and to prevent injuries.

Equipment and the arena. Wrestler's equipment can serve a preventive function. Mouth guards have the potential to reduce dental injuries as well as lacerations to the mouth area. Head gear, used for ear protection, are recommended but not required at all levels of wrestling. They are not allowed in international competition. Use of properly fitting head gear diminishes the incidence of auricular haematoma and the ensuing cauliflower ear deformity. Medical personnel should press for requiring head gear use at all levels of amateur wrestling.

Although no epidemiological study has shown that knee pads prevent injuries, it has been our feeling that their use results in a lower incidence of prepatellar bursitis. Of course, knee pads and all other equipment must fit properly to function properly. Coaches and associated medical personnel can assist with this fitting. Team personnel should insist that no wrestling activity take place without proper protective equipment and further make sure that workout clothing is washed daily to minimize skin problems.

The wrestling facility and the wrestling mats

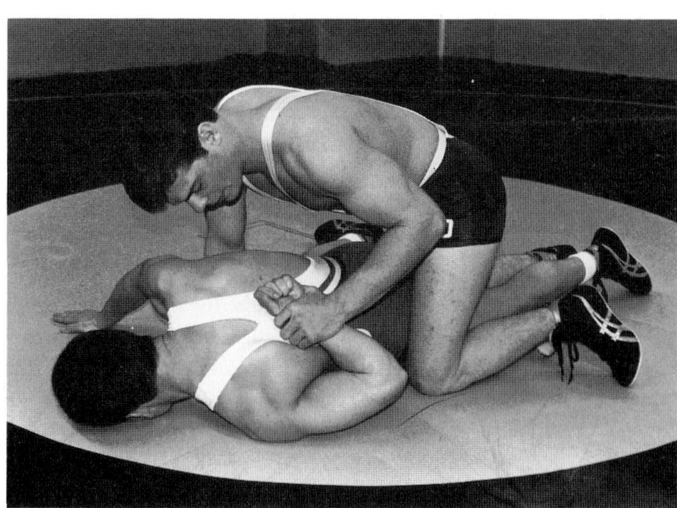

Fig. 37.1 The wrestler on top applies a hammerlock. With the elbow flexed more than 90°, injury potential is high and the technique is considered illegal. From Wroble *et al.* (1991).

can also be an area to approach prevention. The wrestling room itself should be designed so that participation occurs at an adequate distance from hazards such as walls or bleachers, or that padding is provided on all hazardous surfaces. During competition, wrestling mats must be bordered by a minimum protective area of 1.2 m. The same distance should be provided during practice. Furthermore, mats should be washed and disinfected daily and be in good condition with a smooth, non-abrasive surface.

Preseason examination. As with other sports, preseason examination and physical evaluation are key components of prevention. The preseason examination identifies conditions which preclude competition such as seizures, multiple concussions, unhealed fractures or sprains, or uncontrolled hypertension. This evaluation can also test for abnormalities which predispose to injuries such as inadequate muscle strength, lack of appropriate flexibility, or physiological hyperlaxity. We feel all wrestlers should receive a yearly preseason physical examination, and if possible body composition (percent body fat) evaluation, muscle function testing and measurement of aerobic and anaerobic fitness.

Since early season competition puts a wrestler at high risk for injury, we have recommended that scheduling of competitions, particularly tournaments, be postponed until optimum fitness levels have been reached and competitors can be assigned to appropriately matched skill levels (Wroble *et al.*, 1986). Because of the high injury rate during matches and tournaments, it is important to have a physician or trainer or both present at all competitions. In fact, in the ideal situation trained medical personnel would be present at all practices as well. Furthermore, protocols for emergency care of injured wrestlers need to be developed so that they can be implemented efficiently in any competitive environment.

Education. Coaches and wrestlers must be given education regarding the fundamentals of injuries and injury prevention. They must be made aware of high-risk factors and be versed in first aid. If they understand the importance of adequate treatment and rehabilitation in the avoidance of recurrent injuries, the medical staff's ability to prevent injuries is enhanced. Education promotes an alliance between the health-care provider and the athlete and results in a higher standard of care.

Training techniques. Factors in the training techniques of wrestlers (discussed below) impact on musculoskeletal injury prevention. Limited epidemiological evidence notwithstanding, conditioning is felt to be important in injury prevention. Improving cardiovascular endurance prevents fatigue of muscles which stabilize joints. Muscle strengthening also increases the size and strength of ligaments and tendons. Finally, flexibility increases muscle's ability to attenuate shock. Nutrition impacts on injury rates as a tired, malnourished wrestler cannot give peak performances and would appear susceptible to multiple problems. Coaching points such as teaching proper technique, using a good warm-up and stretch before practice, and off-season training which simulates the demands of wrestling, all increase wrestling safety. Finally, proper rehabilitation and reconditioning after an injury, supervised by the medical staff, can lessen the incidence of injury recurrence.

Specific injuries (Wroble *et al.*, 1991)

Head and neck. Although catastrophic or fatal head and neck injuries in amateur wrestling are rare (Rontoyannis *et al.*, 1988; Acikgoz *et al.*, 1990), only football had a higher rate of catastrophic injuries in the USA (Mueller & Cantu, 1990). Most of these serious injuries were caused by contact between head and mat. On the other hand, the much more common and much less severe head and neck injuries, including concussions and 'stingers', are more often caused by head/head, head/knee, or head/thigh contact during take-downs. Rules against slams tend to lessen the occurrence of high energy head/mat collisions, thus serving an important preventive function. Further research into the biomechanical properties of wrestling mats and the response of the mat to collision with a wrestler's head deserves attention to help in eliminating disastrous injuries.

Once the wrestler has sustained a significant head or neck injury, the highest priority lies in preventing an increase in severity. Measures required to accomplish this goal include automatic assumption of concomitant head and neck injury, meticulous examination and transport of the injured athlete, and prompt surgical evaluation in the more severely injured athlete. Proper management of acute neck injuries should be a thoroughly familiar procedure to all medical personnel involved in the care of wrestlers (including cardiopulmonary resuscitation training). Precise treatment protocols must be employed with strict return to action criteria. If the wrestler returns to action before pain, tenderness or range of motion have returned to normal, the likelihood of recurrence is high (Albright *et al.*, 1984, 1985). It is important to prevent recurrent neck injuries as repeated trauma appears to cause osteophyte formation, resultant foraminal narrowing and eventually permanent neurological loss (Fig. 37.2) (Reid & Reid, 1984; Wroble & Albright, 1986). Despite stopping the repetitive trauma of wrestling, 28% of ex-wrestlers with a history of neck injuries report continued symptoms (Mysnyk & Albright, 1989).

The auricular haematoma, an all too common wrestling injury, results from direct trauma to the ear, either on impact with another wrestler's head or knee causing the auricle to be compressed against the mastoid, or by abrasive, friction-causing forces as when wrestlers 'tie up' in the standing position. While most haematomas result when head gear are not worn, haematomas can and do happen while wearing head gear (Schuller *et al.*, 1988). We have found the most effective head gear is one that has four straps (chin, forehead, crown and occiput) and deep ear pieces (Fig. 37.3). We recommend that head gear be worn by all wrestlers at all practices and during competition if allowed. Treatment of the auricular haematoma is designed to decrease recurrence rates and prevent deformity. To be acceptable to wrestlers, treatment must allow immediate return to participation. We have found that this is best accomplished using the method described by Schuller *et al.* (1989). In this technique the haematoma is aspirated and cotton dental rolls are sutured to the lateral and medial aspects of the auricle. The wrestler is allowed to participate within 24 h. The authors of this study reported a recurrence rate of only 5%.

Facial injuries, most commonly lacerated eyebrows, corneal abrasions, nosebleeds and nasal fractures occur quite commonly in wrestling. In fact, in one study 18.4% of all wrestlers sustained injuries about the eye (Morton *et al.*, 1987). Face masks are available and are allowed in protecting a wrestler with such an injury at all levels up to international competition. While some authors advocate development of appropriate head gear to protect the face, athlete acceptance of such intervention would likely be low and if implemented would be found by some to be useful as a weapon.

Shoulder. Injuries to the shoulder come about by three principal mechanisms.

1 When being thrown to the mat from the standing position, wrestlers attempt to brace their fall by extending an arm, imparting force to the shoulder girdle severe enough to cause injury.

2 If the wrestler is unable to extend an arm, the fall may then be taken directly on the shoulder causing damage in this way.

3 Most importantly the wrestler, when attacking the opponent's legs, can become caught in a position with the body overextended. In this position, the head is down and the arm elevated above the head. The opponent's body is positioned upon the attacker's shoulder. As the opponent throws the hips back and increases the weight upon the shoulder, hyperflexion

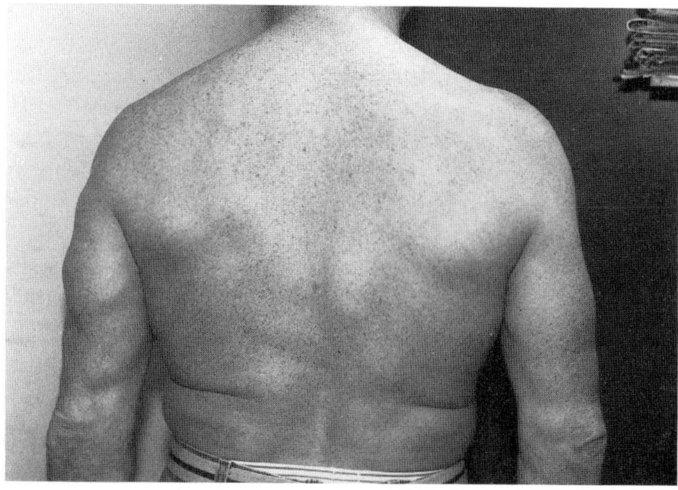

(a)

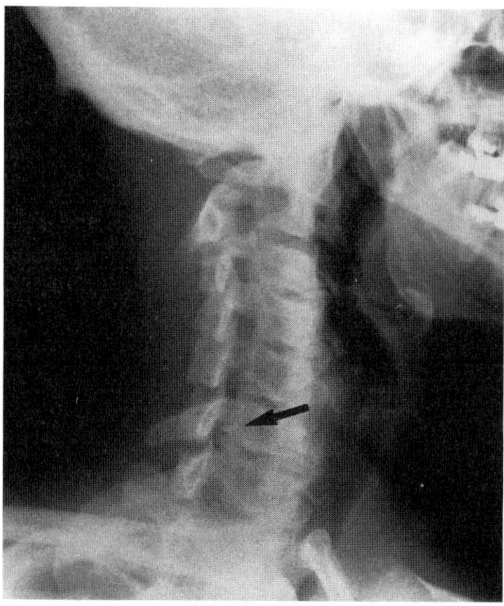

(b)

Fig. 37.2 A former college and international wrestler with permanent neurological loss after multiple neck injuries.
(a) Obvious triceps and supraspinatus wasting.
(b) Degenerative changes at multiple levels with large foraminal osteophytes seen on an oblique radiograph. From Wroble & Albright (1986).

ensues and anterior subluxation can occur (Fig. 37.4).

There are many wrestling holds which subject the shoulder to severe twisting and stretching. Fortunately, most are illegal and thus infrequently cause injury. Diminishing the incidence of shoulder injuries caused through direct mechanisms, however, may be accomplished by biomechanically more sophisticated mats designed to attenuate better the impact of a direct blow. Coaching helps in that observing proper take-down form will prevent the wrestler from getting in the shoulder flexed position (Horswill *et al.*, 1990) described above and lessen the chance for sustaining a shoulder subluxation. As with most injuries, proper rehabilitation and observance of return to action criteria can result in preventing recurrence of shoulder injuries.

Lower back. Lower back injuries are much less common and generally not as severe as those to the neck (Wroble & Albright, 1986). Problems such as pars interarticularis stress lesions, spondylolysis or serious injuries such as herniated discs or fracture have a very low incidence. Most low back injuries take place during take-downs. Wrestlers pull and push against one another with the lumbar spine in mild hyperextension. This extension, coupled with twisting, results in injury. Extension against resistance as in lifting an opponent off the mat is another common mechanism. Conditioning and stretching comprise the key elements in preventing back injuries. Patient education, discussing the nature of low back pain, its implications, and prognosis, allows wrestlers

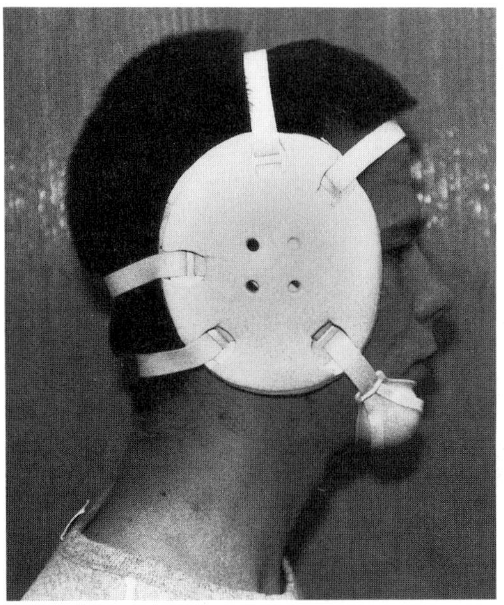

Fig. 37.3 The type of head gear that appears to be most effective in preventing auricular haematoma. Note the location and position of the four straps and the depth of the ear pieces. From Wroble *et al.* (1991).

to understand how to prevent activities predisposing to back injuries.

Knee. The knee is the most commonly injured anatomical region in wrestling and is involved in an even larger proportion of injuries causing more than 7 days time loss. Take-downs are involved in the majority of knee injuries, the defensive wrestler being more likely to sustain the injury. The most common injuries are prepatellar bursitis, medial and lateral collateral ligament sprains and meniscus tears (Wroble *et al.*, 1986). Lateral meniscal tears are proportionately more common in wrestling than in any other sport (Baker *et al.*, 1985).

Prepatellar bursitis can be caused by a single traumatic event or by chronic repetitive trauma. Conservative treatment is often effective but septic bursitis, which has a deceptively subtle presentation, must be ruled out in all cases with a substantial effusion (Mysnyk *et al.*, 1986). Repeated episodes may be diminished by requiring wrestlers to wear a knee pad with extra viscoelastic padding added anteriorly.

Meniscus injuries, the most common knee injury leading to surgery, occur most commonly via a twisting injury to a weight-bearing extremity. Collateral ligament sprains occur when a varus or valgus force is applied to the weight-bearing extremity of a defending wrestler. These mechanisms far more commonly cause injury than application of holds which intentionally apply twisting forces. The latter techniques are considered illegal and are penalized.

Careful initial evaluation of a knee injury

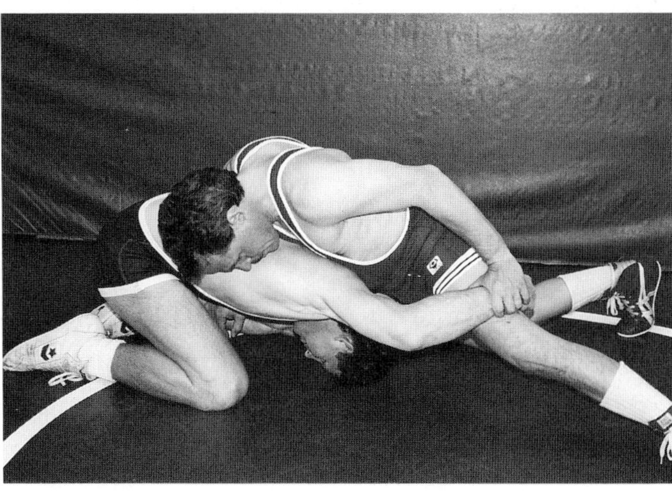

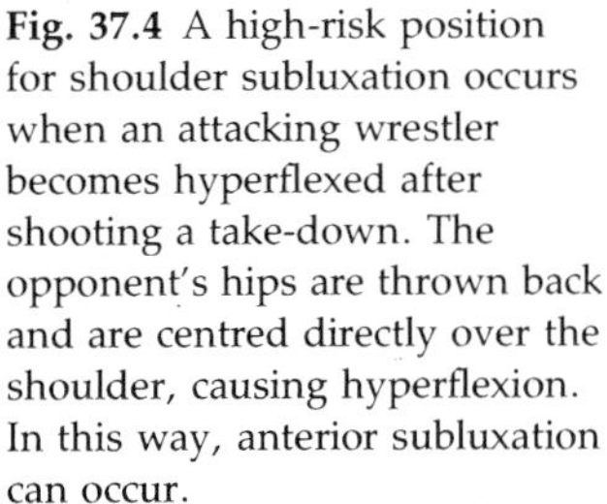

Fig. 37.4 A high-risk position for shoulder subluxation occurs when an attacking wrestler becomes hyperflexed after shooting a take-down. The opponent's hips are thrown back and are centred directly over the shoulder, causing hyperflexion. In this way, anterior subluxation can occur.

will allow exclusion of wrestlers from immediate return to participation when they are in danger of sustaining a more severe injury. Appropriate treatment and rehabilitation of knee injuries gradually phases in more and more strenuous wrestling activities — a functional progression. Return to the mat is always controlled and symptoms are monitored before introducing unlimited activities, reducing the incidence of reinjury.

Anterior cruciate ligament (ACL) injuries, while relatively uncommon, present another set of problems. Although some wrestlers may function reasonably well in the short term with ACL-deficient knees, many wrestlers will not have satisfactory function in their sport, and the majority will go on to have long-term problems. While we do recommend ACL reconstruction, functional bracing is an option for those who elect not to have surgery. Even though the objective value of functional braces has been difficult to demonstrate, most users at least seem to gain a sense of confidence. Any brace used must be protected so that it cannot cause injury to the opponent by sharp corners or exposed metal, etc. Knee braces are not allowed in international competition.

Ankle. Ankle injuries are moderately frequent, the most common being the anterior talofibular ligament sprain. Most occur during take-downs in one of two ways. First, when a wrestler attempts to throw the opponent, the attacking wrestler rises onto the toes and twists. A momentary loss of balance may then cause the attacking wrestler to 'roll over' the ankle into an inverted position. The second mechanism occurs to a defensive wrestler during a take-down. When the opponent has lifted one leg, all the support remains on a single foot. As the opponent attempts to bring the defensive wrestler to the mat by various combinations of changes in directions or trips, inversion stress can occur.

The design of the standard wrestling shoe affords little ankle protection. They have a rubber sole which has high friction with the mat, and the uppers consist of nylon, soft leather or suede, which offers little support (Fig. 37.5). In the future, wrestling shoes should be designed to provide more resistance to ankle eversion and inversion without compromising traction or diminishing plantar and dorsiflexion.

Medical problems

It is well known to team physicians caring for élite athletes that more medals are lost to illness than to injury. As athletes prepare for competition, travelling and training in foreign countries, they are exposed to new pathogens at a time when their bodies are stressed and ill equipped to deal with them. Upper respiratory

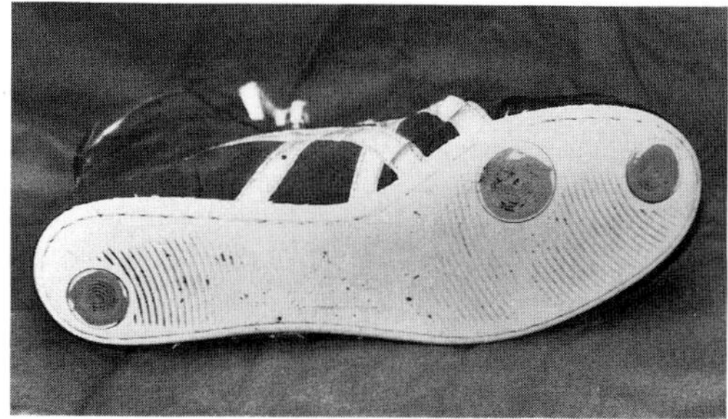

(a)

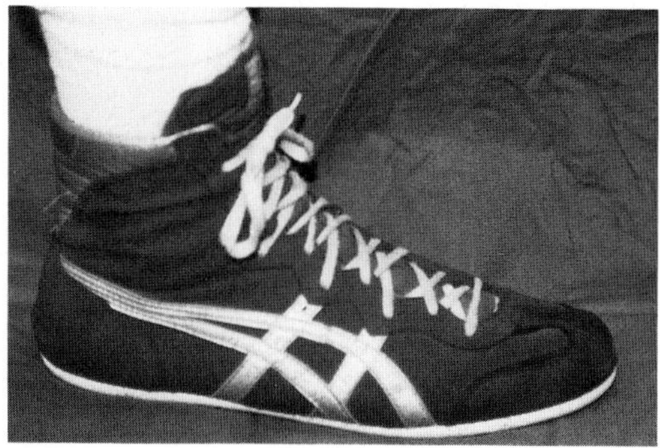

(b)

Fig. 37.5 A commonly used wrestling shoe. Note the high friction rubber sole (a) and the soft flexible nylon uppers (b). From Wroble *et al.* (1991).

illness saps strength, makes training difficult and is easily spread to other team members. Traveller's diarrhoea brings about rapid dehydration, loss of strength and endurance, and inability to train or compete. Travel to distant lands also creates a problem in adapting to time zones and the disorientation of circadian rhythm. Sleep deprivation makes for poor training.

In theory, prevention of these problems is not all that difficult. Team meetings emphasizing the importance of proper hygiene, adequate rest and preparation for changes in time zones, cultures and diet help prepare the team members for the stresses of the trip and competition. Athletes should begin adapting to different time zones days before departure. Meals, practice times and sleep should be adjusted to the new time zone so minimal adjustment is necessary upon arrival. The dehydration that occurs during air travel can be thwarted by consuming adequate fluids and, of course, avoiding alcoholic beverages. Keeping to the local customs and avoiding naps and meals at odd hours will allow the athlete to adapt quickly and efficiently to the new surroundings and be prepared for vigorous practice upon arrival.

Upper respiratory infections

These are usually viral and do not respond particularly well to any antibiotic regimen. Symptomatic therapy, good hydration, nutrition and adequate rest are the mainstays of treatment. Avoidance of the temptation to force training when the athlete is sick and not up to par is of utmost importance. In this scenario, hard training only brings about prolongation of the illness or onset of complications.

Preventing the spread of this type of illness among team members is also a necessary task. Good hygiene and some social isolation of the sick athlete are proper; however, the athlete's morale will suffer terribly if the coach and physician do not make several 'house calls' a day to look in on the sick athlete. Finally, it is the physician's duty to ensure that the athlete is not treated with any medications that will be positive on the antidoping test. Several prescription drugs and many over-the-counter medications used in upper respiratory tract infections are on the International Olympic Committee (IOC) list of banned medications.

Gastroenteritis

Gastroenteritis, or traveller's diarrhoea, is characterized by frequent loose, watery stools, abdominal pain, nausea and subsequent dehydration. Ingestion of contaminated food or water, such as eating or drinking from street vendors, is usually the culprit. A careful choice of sources is the best prevention. Avoid uncooked foods, salads or fruits and vegetables that cannot be peeled. Water should be obtained from a sterilized bottled source or rendered pure through boiling or iodine tablets. Avoidance of tap water for drinking, ice cubes or tooth brushing is encouraged unless the purity of local water is assured. The keystone of treatment is prevention of dehydration due to excessive fluid loss and inadequate replacement. Fluids should be copiously replaced with water or a sports drink containing electrolytes. Fruit juice, uncarbonated soda and clear soups are also good choices. Solid food should be withheld until bowel movements are reduced in frequency and volume. Medication such as PeptoBismol or bismuth subsalicylate, may be used prophylactically to prevent traveller's diarrhoea as can certain antibiotics such as doxycycline 100 mg b.i.d. and Norfloxacin 400 mg b.i.d.

Dermatology

Dermatological conditions may actually result in disqualification of the wrestler. Pre-event skin checks are required to identify staphylococcal, streptococcal and herpetic infections. These conditions are communicable through the direct skin-to-skin contact that occurs in wrestling. Prevention requires a high index of suspicion on the part of the wrestler, coach and team physician. Early identification of the problem and therapeutic intervention with appropriate medications are essential. Small lesions are usually amenable to covering with bandages and tape during the 2–5 days required for medication to be effective.

Furuncles and impetigo grow well on moist, sweaty, abraded skin. Good skin hygiene that includes daily or twice daily showers, frequent laundering of clothes and cleansing of workout mats is important in prevention. Pads, wraps or tape may provide good environments for these organisms to grow and furuncles need to be identified early. The sharing of sweaty nylon weight cutting suits and other workout gear is to be condemned. Areas of abraded skin need to be carefully monitored for the appearance of the typical honey-crusted impetigo lesions. Local care of furuncles should include sterile laceration and culture of the exudate, while impetiginous lesions need to be soaked and treated with antibiotic ointment. Both conditions require the administration of antibiotics (penicillin, resistant synthetic penicillin or a first generation cephalosporin) to be given orally for 7–10 days.

Herpes gladiatorum, a herpes simplex type I infection of the skin, is the most common and most contagious cutaneous infection seen in wrestlers. The highly contagious nature of this infection demands immediate cessation of practice and competition. Epidemics have been known to sweep through teams infecting up to half the team members before being brought under control. As with bacterial skin problems, early recognition is the key to prevention of such an epidemic. Wrestlers should be screened frequently by themselves, coaches and medical staff. Occasionally, a wrestler will report a burning or tingling sensation prior to the appearance of vesicles. The vesicles are small and fluid filled. Upon bursting they have a tendency to become secondarily infected. Sites of infection are usually the face, shoulders or arms and recurrences are not infrequent. Of special note is any infection involving the eye or tip of the nose which may progress to ophthalmic infection. This requires immediate ophthalmological consultation. Recurrence may be precipitated by sunlight, sickness or stress (i.e. competition).

Resolution of this viral infection is aided by the topical and oral application of acyclovir. Oral treatment with 200 mg given 5 times·day^{-1} for 14 days works well if initiated at the earliest symptoms. When lesions dry out and become crusty, the athlete is no longer contagious. Although no published studies are available, the prophylactic use of acyclovir in previously infected wrestlers under stress or to prevent the spread of a team-wide epidemic has some merit. During one team epidemic 28 wrestlers were treated prophylactically with 800 mg of acyclovir 2 times·day^{-1} with only one wrestler having a mild 2-day course of cutaneous herpes.

Human immunodeficiency virus (HIV) and hepatitis B virus

Finally, we must consider two life-threatening medical problems that loom in the future of wrestling. Both HIV and hepatitis B virus are well known to be transmitted in blood as well as in other body fluids. The combative nature of wrestling and the encouragement of intimate contact between contestants during a match allow adequate opportunity for cross-contamination of blood in bleeding athletes. HIV infection has been shown to be transmitted through blood to blood and blood to cornes contamination. Sweat has not been shown to be a route of transmission. These risks are not just theoretical, as a case of HIV transmission has been documented in the cross-contamination that occurred between two soccer players (Torre *et al.*, 1990). Observation of any wrestling tournament indicates a 30–40% rate of blood letting in some form. In practice, athletes always seem to have an abrasion, a small laceration or a bloody nose. The cavalier nature with which wrestlers are allowed to continue to compete or practice and the method of dealing with bleeding and blood products by mat officials, coaches and medical personnel invite disaster. The international wrestling community must take the immediate responsibility of dealing with this ever increasing problem now.

USA wrestling has become a vanguard in reacting to the problem of both HIV and hepatitis B cross-contamination in their athletes. A newly adopted programme involves education, body fluid precautions, rule changes and mandatory testing of national team members. Testing is also strongly encouraged in all international team members and associated health-care personnel. Education programmes will utilize brochures, articles in the national newsletter and videotapes for coaches' clinics. The former rule in international style wrestling that charged the injury time used to stop bleeding in lacerations and epistaxis against the total 2 min allowed each wrestler encouraged rapid and poorly executed first aid of bleeding injuries, and usually allowed no time for removal of blood from the wrestlers' bodies, uniforms and mats. The newly adopted rule does not charge either wrestler for injury time out when bleeding is involved. Careful first aid and decontamination are now required before the match can resume. All members of the USA national team will undergo yearly testing for both HIV and hepatitis B. Athletes found to be positive will be withheld from competition and training until their infectivity can be determined. Finally, precautions to protect wrestlers, officials and health-care attendants will be instituted and enforced at all USA wrestling sanctioned matches. The international governing body of wrestling, the Federation International Lutte Amateus (FILA), will be petitioned to also adopt such precautions.

RECOMMENDATIONS FOR HIV AND HEPATITIS B PRECAUTIONS IN WRESTLING

1 HIV and hepatitis B positive athletes and health-care attendants will be kept from competing and caring for injured athletes until their infectious status is determined.

2 At any time during a competition or training that an athlete bleeds, the action will be immediately stopped and adequate first aid and decontamination performed prior to allowing practice or competition to resume.

3 Decontamination must follow first aid of the bleeding athletes by careful removal of blood from the athlete's body, uniform and mats using a bleaching solution (one-quarter cup (60 ml) of household bleach in 4.5 l (1 gal) of water) and towels. Separate towels must be used for each athlete and upon completion all materials placed in special disposal sacks.

4 Officials, coaches and health-care attendants must wear disposable gloves during all first aid and decontamination procedures. Separate sets of gloves are to be used for each individual athlete. Gloves will also be disposed of in special sacks. If there is risk of blood spatter during the match or clean-up, goggles are strongly recommended for officials, coaches and health-care attendants.

5 All bloody dressings must only be handled with the gloved hand and properly disposed of after use.

6 In cases where possible cross-contamination has occurred, the HIV and hepatitis B status of both individuals must be determined immediately after the incident.

7 Teams should give careful consideration to competitions held where the viruses are found in epidemic proportions.

8 Testing of all competitors and mat-side attendants should receive strong consideration.

Athletic training

Training for wrestling is a never ending task. Rewards in terms of injury prevention and wrestling success can be obtained, however, by adherence to a good training programme. Deficits in flexibility, muscle strength and cardiovascular conditioning are major causes of poor wrestling performance and probably increase the risk of injury. A well-trained wrestler is more likely to be successful and less likely to be fatigued and suffer the setbacks of injury and illness.

Flexibility is paramount in that increased range of motion of a joint may decrease risk of sprains and strains. Development of flexibility is a slow process which requires daily maintenance. The recommended form of stretching is the sustained static stretch in which the athlete stretches a joint through its range of motion and holds the stretch for 10–20 s. This activity should be repeated several times. It is important that during the stretch the athlete does not push the joint to a range of motion that causes pain. Ballistic stretching should be avoided because of the definite risk of muscle injury. Every wrestler will benefit from a good overall flexibility programme but should pay particular attention to the shoulder girdle, groin, hamstrings and lower back.

The association between muscular strength and wrestling performance is obvious. All-round development can be accomplished through a general weight training programme, focusing both on concentric and eccentric exercises. Both free weights and machines can provide exercises important to the specifics of wrestling. The athlete's programme should focus on activities that require pulling and lifting similar to that required on the wrestling mat. Activities that will pay off on the mat include pull-ups, rowing, shoulder shrugs, back extension and leg press, leg adduction and bicep curls. The wrestler should be encouraged not only to have an off-season weight-training programme but to continue to work on strengthening throughout the season. The sport of wrestling alone is not enough to maintain strength without the addition of an in-season lifting programme.

The energy requirements for wrestling and training can be considerable. It is important that the wrestler be conscious of and in control of body weight. Maintaining a body fat percentage of 5–7% appears to provide optimal performance on the wrestling mat (American College of Sports Medicine, 1976). This requires careful attention to diet and exercise, the two variables which effect the wrestler's weight. A careful, well thought out plan will allow the wrestler to train effectively and require only small adjustments in weight prior to a competition. Attention to proper weight control will result in practices that are detrimental to the wrestler's performance and health (Morgan, 1970). Unfortunately, many wrestlers employ the 'yo-yo' method of dieting, relying on rapid weight loss in the last few days prior to competition. As competition nears, the wrestler who is several pounds over the required weight will, at that point, stop eating, start exercising more vigorously and, finally, use dehydration as a means of making weight. Dehydration can be brought about by exercise or the use of a thermal environment such as the sauna, or both. Other methods (not recommended) include the use of diuretics, laxatives and deprivation of fluid intake.

Several studies have shown that dehydration greater than 5% of the body weight results in decreases in muscular endurance and strength (Torranin *et al.*, 1979; Klinzing & Karpowicz, 1986; Horswill *et al.*, 1990; Webster *et al.*, 1990; Horswill, 1991). Although it would be ideal not to require any dehydration prior to a competition, wrestling tradition, the wrestler's poor planning or both, necessitate this at times. It is strongly recommended that no more than 2–3% of the body weight be reduced by dehydration. There are also individual differences in how dehydration affects various wrestlers. Some wrestlers seem to tolerate levels of dehydration better than others. However, no wrestler can participate effectively when more than 5–7% of the body weight is lost by rapid dehydration prior to the wrestling event.

Rehydration prior to competition can replenish the energy stores and improve performance if adequate time is available. Research studies show however, that at least 24–36 h may be necessary to restore strength and muscular endurance after a bout of acute dehydration (Allen *et al.*, 1977; Houston *et al.*, 1981; Horswill, 1991). Replenishment of muscle glycogen stores may require up to 48 h if the athlete has employed starvation techniques. The athlete therefore must realize that rehydration and refuelling immediately following weigh-in will help but will not totally correct the physiological disturbances that have resulted from fasting and rapid dehydration.

Proper recommendations on weight loss should be made to each athlete, attempting to minimize the health risks and to maximize wrestling performance. Minimal weight should be determined by body composition testing and the wrestler should be certified at a weight of no less than 5% body fat (American College of Sports Medicine, 1976). Weight loss should be accomplished at a rate of 1–1.4 kg·week^{-1} (2–3 lb·week^{-1}). We strongly recommend careful monitoring of the athlete's weight throughout the season to avoid the necessity of fasting and acute dehydration.

Conclusion

Few sports provide such a varied challenge to the sports medicine team as wrestling. Acute trauma, overuse injuries, medical illnesses and nutritional and training problems are all present in these athletes. The combative nature of the sport makes injury prevention a difficult problem. However, rule changes, monitoring of training and nutrition and management of medical problems are all areas that can result in lowering injury rates in wrestlers. The challenge for the wrestling team physician and trainer is to bring about these changes and so prevent many of their athletes' injuries.

References

Acikgoz, B., Ozgen, T., Erbeng, A., Peker, S., Bertan, V. & Saglem, S. (1990) Wrestling causing paraplegia. *Paraplegia* **28**(4), 265–8.

Albright, J.P., McAuley, E., Martin, R.K., Crowley, E.T. & Foster, D.T. (1985) Head and neck injuries in college football: an eight-year analysis. *Am. J. Sports Med.* **13**, 147–52.

Albright, J.P., VanGilder, J., El-Khoury, G.Y., Crowley, E. & Foster, D. (1984) Head and neck injuries in sports. In W.M. Scott, B. Nisonson & J.A. Nicholas (eds) *Principles of Sports Medicine*, pp. 40–86. Wilkins & Wilkins, Baltimore.

Allen, T.E., Smith, D.P. & Miller, D.K. (1977) Hemodynamic response to submaximal exercise after dehydration and rehydration in high school wrestlers. *Med. Sci. Sports* **9**, 159–63.

American College of Sports Medicine (1976) Position stand on weight loss in wrestlers. *Med. Sci. Sports* **8**, xi–xiii.

Baker, B.D., Peckham, A.C., Pupparo, F. & Sanborn, J.C. (1985) Review of meniscal injury and associated sports. *Am. J. Sports Med.* **13**, 1–4.

Dick, R. (1988) *National Collegiate Athletic Association Injury Surveillance System, 1982–1987*. NCCA, Kansas.

Estwanik, J.J., Bergfeld, J. & Canty, T. (1978) A report of injuries sustained during the United States Olympic wrestling trials. *Am. J. Sports Med.* **6**, 335–40.

Garrick, J.G. & Requa, R. (1981) Medical care and injuries surveillance in the high school setting. *Phys. Sportsmed.* **9**(2), 115–20.

Horswill, C.A. (1991) Does rapid weight loss by dehydration adversely affect high-power performance? *Sports Sci. Exchange* **3**, 30.

Horswill, C.A., Hickner, R.C., Scott, J.R., Costill, D.L. & Gould, D. (1990) Weight loss, dietary carbohydrate modifications, and high intensity physical performance. *Med. Sci. Sports Exerc.* **22**, 470–7.

Houston, M.E., Marrin, D.A., Green, H.J. & Thomson, J.A. (1981) The effect of rapid weight loss on physiological functions in wrestlers. *Phys. Sportsmed.* **9**, 73–8.

Klinzing, J.E. & Karpowicz, W. (1986) The effects of rapid weight loss and rehydration on a wrestling performance test. *J. Sports Med.* **26**, 149–56.

Morgan, W.P. (1970) Psychological effect of weight reduction in the college wrestler. *Med. Sci. Sports* **2**, 24–7.

Morton, K., Wilson, D. & McKeag, D. (1987) Ocular trauma in college varsity sports. *Med. Sci. Sports Exerc.* **19**(Suppl.), S53.

Mueller, F.O. & Cantu, R.C. (1990) Catastrophic injuries and fatalities in high school and college sports, fall 1982–spring 1988. *Med. Sci. Sports Exerc.* **22**, 737–41.

Mysnyk, M.C. & Albright, J.P. (1989) Relative risk and long term impact of injuries from amateur football and wrestling competition. Sports Medicine Symposium, Iowa City.

Mysnyk, M.C., Wroble, R.R., Foster, D.T. & Albright, J.P. (1986) Prepatellar bursitis in wrestlers. *Am. J. Sports Med.* **14**, 46–54.

Reid, S.E. & Reid, S.E. (1984) *Head and Neck Injuries in Sports*. Charles C. Thomas, Illinois.

Rontoyannis, G.P., Pahtas, G., Dinis, D. & Pournaras,

N. (1988) Sudden death of a young wrestler during competition. *Int. J. Sports Med.* **9**, 353–5.

Schuller, D.E., Dankle, S. & Strauss, R. (1989) A technique to treat wrestlers' auricular hematoma without interrupting training or competition. *Arch. Otolaryngol. Head Neck Surg.* **115**, 202–6.

Schuller, D.E., Strauss, R. & Dankle, S. (1988) Auricular injuries and the use of headgear in wrestlers. *Med. Sci. Sports Exerc.* **20**, S24.

Torranin, C., Smith, D.P. & Byrd, R.J. (1979) The effect of acute thermal dehydration and rapid rehydration on isometric and isotonic endurance. *J. Sports Med. Phys. Fitness* **19**, 1–9.

Torre, O., Sampietro, C., Ferraro, G., Zeroli, C. & Speranza, F. (1990) Transmission of HIV I infection via sports injuries. *Lancet* **335**, 1105.

Webster, S., Rutt, R. & Weltman, A. (1990) Physiological effects of weight loss regimen practices by college wrestlers. *Med. Sci. Sports Exerc.* **22**, 229–34.

Wroble, R.R. & Albright, J.P. (1986) Neck and low back injuries in wrestling. *Clin. Sports Med.* **5**, 295–25.

Wroble, R.R., Hoegh, J.T. & Albright, J.P. (1991) Wrestling. In B. Reider (ed) *Sports Medicine — The School Age Athlete*, pp. 520–58. WB Saunders, Philadelphia.

Wroble, R.R., Mysnyk, M.C., Foster, D.T. & Albright, J.P. (1986) Patterns of knee injuries in wrestling at the University of Iowa — a six year study. *Am. J. Sports Med.* **14**, 55–66.

Chapter 38

Injuries in Boxing

JEFFREY MINKOFF, BARRY G. SIMONSON AND GREGG CAVALIERE

Allegedly, boxing has a 9000-year-old history described by J.V. Frombach (Voy, 1990a). The word 'pugilism' derives from the Greek *pux* 'with clenched fist' (Elia, 1962). The Cretan and Aegean cultures were replete with boxing even prior to the Grecian era. Homer and Theocritus expounded upon the state of the art, describing opponents with leather wrist and hand strappings, who squared off for fights to the death. The ancient Romans, whose humour pitted heretics against lions were bemused by their droll innovations in pugilism; they added metal studs to the knuckle thongs and battled to the death in the arena. Forms of boxing were incorporated into the Olympics in the year 688 BC (Olympia 23) (Noble, 1987). Then, after centuries, the popularity of boxing waned during the rise of Christianity and the subsequent periods of chivalry. However, it flourished again during the seventeenth and eighteenth centuries as an art of self-defence, taught with other disciplines of that purpose, such as fencing (Voy, 1990a).

The origins of professional fighting are traceable to early eighteenth century London. Local brawlers would contend for a 'purse', the so-called 'prize fight' (Welles, 1969). Jack Broughton, a champion of the mid-eighteenth century, introduced the first official rules: the 30-s count, opponents returning to a neutral corner during the count, the use of a referee and a provision for the division of the purse (Voy, 1990a). Broughton also introduced the first padded glove (used only in sparring) (Voy, 1990a). This was the 'bare knuckle' era, which persisted for 150 years as an eyesore to upper class propriety. Still in the mid-eighteenth century, the Duke of Cumberland, disenchanted with boxing because he lost a large purse on a bet, appealed to Parliament for a ban. This was granted and not repealed until 1790 when King George III legalized boxing and made licensing mandatory (Voy, 1990a). In 1867, the old London rules were superseded by John Chambers' modifications: padded gloves, 3-min rounds, no wrestling and a 10-s count (Welles, 1969).

To attract the nobler classes, John Douglas, The Marquess of Queensberry, lent his title to Chambers' rules. Hence, modern boxing is predicated upon the Queensberry Rules. These rules, which encourage speed, agility and cleverness, as much as they do strength, led to the development of the so-called 'scientific fighter' (C. D'Amato, personal communication). Boxing in the USA has been a gateway from the ghetto. From its popularity in this country, beginning in the late nineteenth century, dominant talents have followed patterns of immigration, first the Irish, then the Jews and then the Italians. More recently, Blacks and Latins have pervaded the sport, leaving fans in constant pursuit of 'the Great White Hope'. The nominal purses of old London have grown to dollar amounts of more than seven figures, ample reason for frenetic concern when a planned fight is placed in jeopardy by an injury.

After a brief appearance in the Olympics of 1904, boxing was deleted from the games of

1912, and reinstated in the Olympics of 1920. Significant medical supervision for boxing was introduced in Berlin in 1936. At the 23rd Olympiad in Los Angeles (1984), 2672 years after the 23rd Grecian Olympics into which boxing was first introduced, 81 countries participated in the boxing competitions, featuring a staggering 357 boxers.

In the 1990s, the Amateur International Boxing Association (AIBA) is the embodiment of amateur boxing. Its philosophy is defence rather than offence, short bouts (only several rounds) and good sporting behaviour. The longer bouts (up to 12 rounds), 'win at all costs' attitude and large promotional influences of professional boxing result in totally different preparatory formats, styles and hype than those witnessed in the amateur ranks.

Fighter selection. Professional fighters are most often discovered through the Golden Gloves or the Olympics. Other sources of talent include spar-mates and the college ranks. It is interesting to note that professionals are not necessarily the 'best' fighters (Blonstein, 1969; C. D'Amato, personal communication). Remembering that to have commercial success a professional must have media appeal, it is not difficult to understand that a good fighter with a flair is a more likely professional prospect than a very good fighter with an insipid presentation.

What to look for in talent recognition. In asking managers and trainers what factors portray the greatest prospects, it became apparent that the most common responses related to observable but intangible characteristics. The foremost was dedication or a 'will to win'. The second was the ability to take a punch.

Equipment

Mouth guards

The combined responses regarding the use of mouth guards may be summarized as follows (Fig. 38.1):

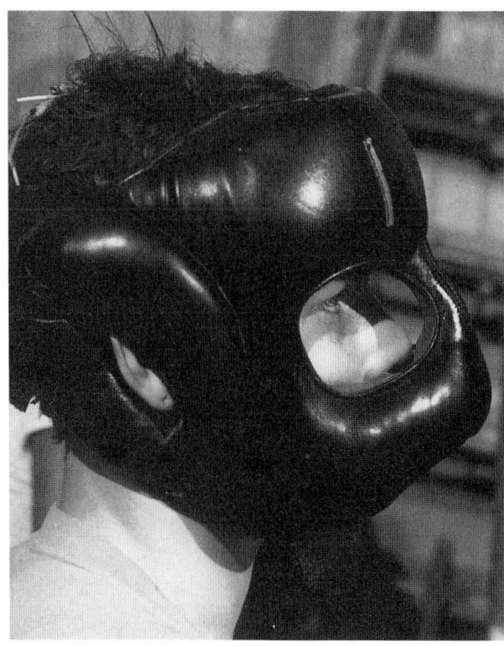

Fig. 38.1 A head guard offers protection to the nose, ears and mouth. However, it is not a supplement for mouth protection, even in sparring.

1 Custom mold varieties are best.
2 They do not compromise respiratory ability.
3 They help stabilize the jaw.
4 They prevent mouth cuts.
5 They prevent tooth breakage and loss.
6 They inhibit possible tracheal obstruction by broken teeth.

It would seem reasonable or even self-evident that mouth guards will help to protect the teeth from impact. In fact, mouth guards do much more than this. Hildebrandt (1982) indicates that not only will the occlusal surface (bite surface) of mouth protectors cushion the teeth from upward directed blows to the chin, but that the labial (lip) surface of protectors deflect forces aimed directly at the teeth and help prevent lacerations to the lips and cheeks. Forced occlusion upon unprotected teeth can result in their being fractured. Hildebrandt cites Osmanski (1976) and Sanders (1979) in support of the mechanism by which mouth guards also protect the head. The maintenance of disocclusion (an open bite) by the guards results in a decreased transmission of force from the mandible to the temporal bone. Hildebrandt cites Hickey *et al.* (1967) as having demonstrated, through *in vitro* studies, that mouth guards reduce recorded intracranial pressures when blows are delivered to the chin.

It follows that the effectiveness of mouth protectors, in serving the purposes indicated above, is a function of the fit and the material used. Furthermore, while serving their intended purposes, these protectors should not create any liabilities. With respect to these variables, it should be appreciated that there are three basic varieties of mouth guard (Hildebrandt, 1982). The stock form is the least effective because it does not conform to the player's bite and teeth, is cumbersome, and interferes with breathing and speech. Molded forms are the most commonly used. They are constructed of thermal or chemical setting materials (such as polyvinyl acetate–ethylene copolymer) which conform to the teeth. They are sometimes too bulky and do not conform properly to all dentitions, in which case custom mouth guards should be mandated. The latter are created by the dentist and almost never compromise breathing or speech (Hildebrandt, 1982).

Many have heard the expression 'glass jaw' referring to fighters who are easily subdued by punches to the jaw. Fractures of the mandible are not uncommon in boxing. Colpitts (1990) indicates that mandibular fractures are most frequent at the condylar process, then the angle and then the symphysis (Fig. 38.2). Ice packs and a Barton bandage are the immediate treatments. Surgery is often necessary to transfix the fracture.

Head gear and face protection

Contusion of the pinna are not infrequent occurrences in boxing. The formation of haematomas may herald serious injury. Blood or serum may collect between the perichondrium and the cartilage (Handler & Wetmore, 1982). When discovered acutely, seromas or haematomas should be aspirated promptly to avert permanent deformity or risk of infection. The application of a pressure dressing will inhibit a reaccumulation. The use of ear-guarded head gear helps prevent recurrent episodes which may lead to the so-called 'cauliflower' ear deformity with fibrosis and permanent thickening of the pinna (Handler & Wetmore, 1982) (Fig. 38.3).

Since modern head gear with ear flaps have eradicated the cauliflower ear, it would seem equally worthwhile protecting the boxer's eyes

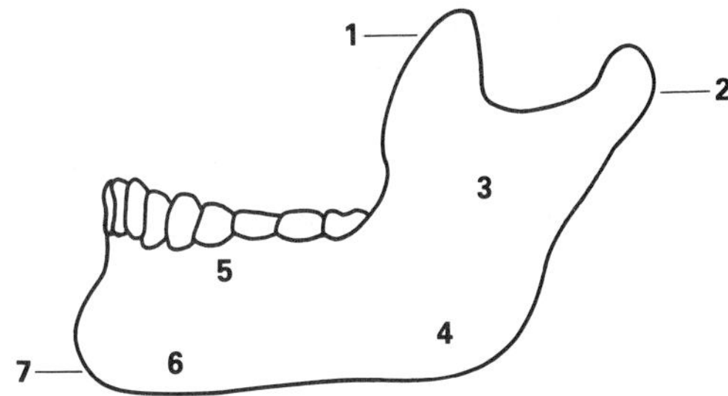

Fig. 38.2 Distribution and frequency of mandibular fractures in boxing. From Colpitts (1990). 1, coronoid process (2%); 2, condylar process (35%); 3, ramus (4%); 4, angle (20%); 5, alveolar process (4%); 6, body, (20%); 7, symphysis (14%).

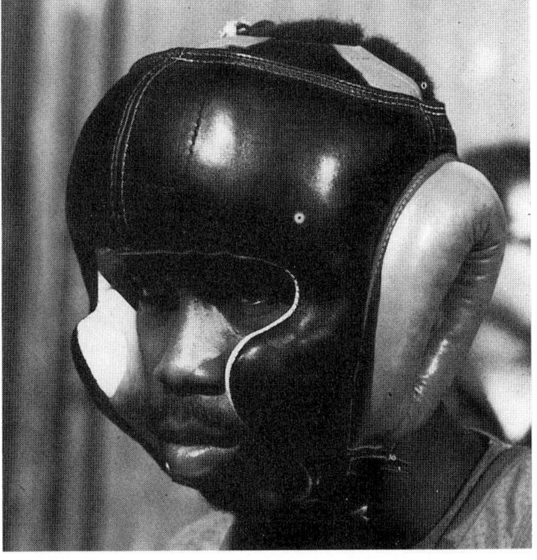

Fig. 38.3 Head protector with earflaps to prevent cauliflower ear. Compare with head protector with nose guard in Fig. 38.1.

and face. Though it would seem prudent to obviate fight delays due to facial cuts, a noteworthy objection to face masks by boxing experts (non-medical) was an anecdotal contention that glove to face contact promotes facial toughening and acclimatization to being punched.

Stimulated by this statement, a search was undertaken for pugilist volunteers for a skin biopsy. A single volunteer was found.

E.R. is a Black Latin professional in his early twenties. At the time of biopsy, he had fought in 20 professional bouts. He had never been cut, but had frequently had facial swelling about the cheeks and orbits. A several millimetre, full thickness skin biopsy was retrieved from the upper outer quadrant of the left eyebrow margin; this was considered to be a representative area in that it frequently receives jabs and is close to the area from which 'eye bleeding' is common (Fig. 38.4a,b).

The specimens were submitted to Dr Ackerman, Chief of Dermopathology at New York University Medical Center. Without having provided him with a history or designation of the purpose of the biopsy, the interpretation was as indicated in Fig. 38.4c (upper half).

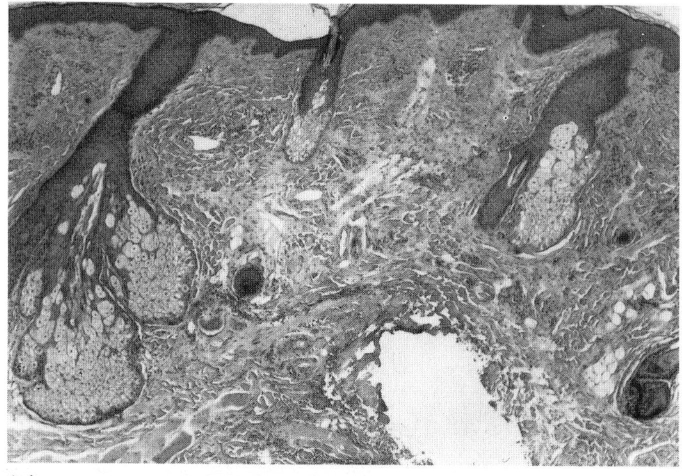

(a)

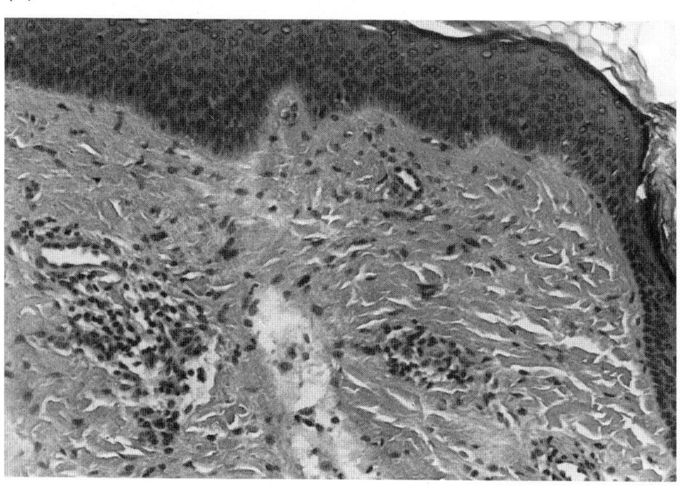

(b)

Fig. 38.4 (a & b) Low and medium power histophotomicrographs of the fighter's skin biopsy. There is *no* thickening of the epidermis. The dermis, on the other hand, is thickened with collagen and there are perivascular mononuclear cell infiltrates (H & E stain).

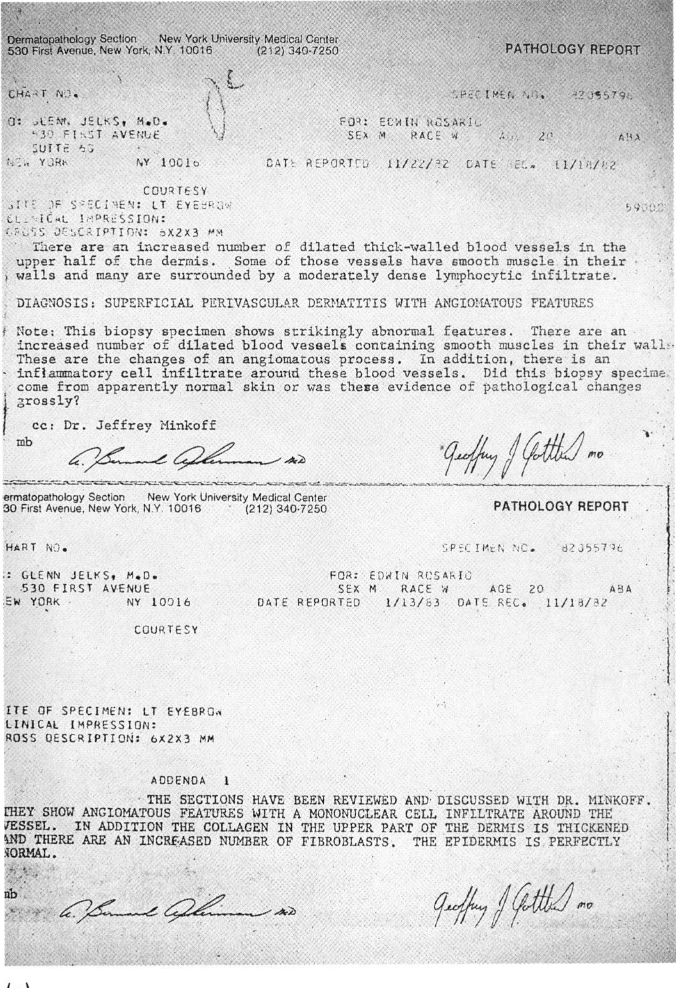

Dermatopathology Section New York University Medical Center
530 First Avenue, New York, N.Y. 10016 (212) 340-7250

PATHOLOGY REPORT

CHART NO. SPECIMEN NO. 82055796

O: GLENN JELKS, M.D.
530 FIRST AVENUE
SUITE 6G
NEW YORK NY 10016

FOR: EDWIN ROSARIO
SEX M RACE W AGE 20 ABA
DATE REPORTED 11/22/82 DATE REC. 11/18/82

COURTESY

SITE OF SPECIMEN: LT EYEBROW
CLINICAL IMPRESSION:
GROSS DESCRIPTION: 6X2X3 MM

There are an increased number of dilated thick-walled blood vessels in the upper half of the dermis. Some of those vessels have smooth muscle in their walls and many are surrounded by a moderately dense lymphocytic infiltrate.

DIAGNOSIS: SUPERFICIAL PERIVASCULAR DERMATITIS WITH ANGIOMATOUS FEATURES

Note: This biopsy specimen shows strikingly abnormal features. There are an increased number of dilated blood vessels containing smooth muscles in their walls. These are the changes of an angiomatous process. In addition, there is an inflammatory cell infiltrate around these blood vessels. Did this biopsy specimen come from apparently normal skin or was these evidence of pathological changes grossly?

cc: Dr. Jeffrey Minkoff

mb

---

ermatopathology Section New York University Medical Center
30 First Avenue, New York, N.Y. 10016 (212) 340-7250

PATHOLOGY REPORT

HART NO. SPECIMEN NO. 82055796

: GLENN JELKS, M.D.
530 FIRST AVENUE
EW YORK NY 10016

FOR: EDWIN ROSARIO
SEX M RACE W AGE 20 ABA
DATE REPORTED 1/13/83 DATE REC. 11/18/82

COURTESY

ITE OF SPECIMEN: LT EYEBROW
LINICAL IMPRESSION:
ROSS DESCRIPTION: 6X2X3 MM

ADDENDA 1

THE SECTIONS HAVE BEEN REVIEWED AND DISCUSSED WITH DR. MINKOFF. THEY SHOW ANGIOMATOUS FEATURES WITH A MONONUCLEAR CELL INFILTRATE AROUND THE VESSEL. IN ADDITION THE COLLAGEN IN THE UPPER PART OF THE DERMIS IS THICKENED AND THERE ARE AN INCREASED NUMBER OF FIBROBLASTS. THE EPIDERMIS IS PERFECTLY NORMAL.

mb

(c)

Fig. 38.4 (c) (*Top*) Initial pathology report, interpreted without a knowledge of the subject or the purpose of the biopsy. (*Bottom*) Final pathology report, interpreted with full knowledge of the intent and nature of the biopsy.

Dr Ackerman was then informed of the purpose of the biopsy and asked to address an interpretation to the issue of the effects of post-traumatic skin alterations. The second interpretation is indicated in Fig. 38.4c (lower half).

In a summary of head gear, Ryan (1987) indicated that such protection has the potential to half the estimated 453 kg (1000 lb) force deliverable by a strong punch. Nevertheless, the ability of head gear to inhibit serious brain injuries remains in doubt; this is because the most severe trauma is inflicted by rotational and angular accelerating blows which cannot be restrained by head gear (Jordan, 1987).

Fight shoe

The fight shoe has changed minimally in the twentieth century. The shoe is a soft leather high top with no heel and a leather or rubber sole (Fig. 38.5). Great uniformity exists amongst those questioned acclaiming the relative specificity of the shoe, which has the following features:

1 Its softness provides comfort.

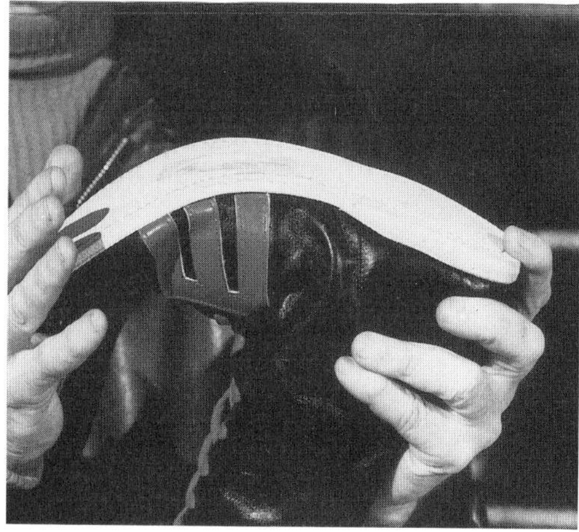

Fig. 38.5 Typical lightweight, high top, lacer fight shoe with soft sole and no heel.

2 Leather with no heel is lightweight.
3 The laces and high top character support the ankles.
4 The absence of a heel increases ballet-like balance.
5 The thin bottom permits a smooth shuffle on canvas.
6 The leather or rubberized sole on canvas provides the optimum degree of traction.

Points 5 and 6 would appear to be at cross purposes. The shoe compromises these features to some extent.

Gloves

In its formative years, boxing was performed with bare fists. The first transition came with the Queensbury Rules, which among other things, initiated the use of leather gloves (1894). What evolved was the bulky leather glove with one-piece stuffing that is used today. Different gloves are used for training as opposed to fighting (Fig. 38.6). Training gloves range from 340 to 510 g (12 to 18 oz). Fighting gloves range from 170 to 280 g (6 to 10 oz). The fighter therefore, will usually train with a glove heavier than that which is used in the fight. Heavyweights will train with 454 g (16 oz) gloves and lightweights with 340 g (12 oz) gloves. The majority of title fights uses 226 g (8 oz) gloves. Experiments (Unterhernscheidt, 1970) indicated that 170 g (6 oz) gloves could produce a peak force head acceleration 2.7 times greater than the more compressible 454 g (16 oz) gloves. It becomes obvious that old or poorly maintained gloves will influence the force of delivered blows.

The thumbless glove is an attempt to reduce eye injuries due to thumbing. Among the complaints registered about thumbless gloves have been:

1 More study is needed to determine efficacy.
2 There are too few eye injuries from the thumb

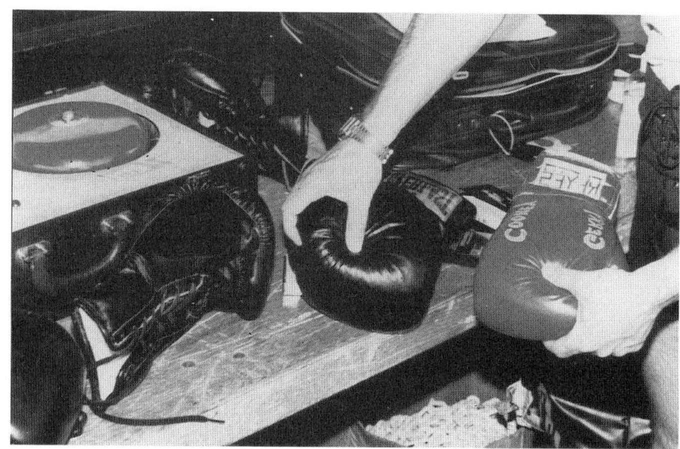

Fig. 38.6 Gloves. Fight gloves range from 170 to 280 g (6 to 10 oz). Training gloves range from 340 to 510 g (12 to 18 oz). Older gloves soften and may alter the force of the blow. (Note the difference in compressibility.)

to justify its existence (which is certainly far from the truth).

3 The New York State Commission's glove is a poorly structured version.

4 Many who have used it have complained of thumb cramping.

5 Reduces effective use of the hand in punching and parrying.

Training

A necessity for predicting when an injured fighter might be able to fight again after a lapse or injury is an understanding of both the injury recovery time and the usual preparation time for a bout. It should be recognized that preparation times are influenced by the condition of the fighter at the onset of training and the time elapsed since the previous fight.

When asked how many rounds were needed to prepare for the 'big fight' (professional), experts provided a range from 50 to 250 rounds with an average of 130 rounds. When asked the minimum time period needed for preparation, they indicated a range of from 4 to 8 weeks with an average of 5 weeks. The number of sparring rounds is usually escalated during training from two to three rounds on a given day early in camp to eight to 10 rounds as the fight approaches (for professional fighters). Sparring is not done every day. In all, sparring averages about four rounds·day^{-1} throughout the training camp.

There was virtually unanimous agreement that there exists a state termed 'overtraining'. Some described it as a weariness, others as a loss of drive, and most concurred that it represented a state of mind as opposed to an organic syndrome.

Those of us who have experienced lapses in otherwise routine physical endeavours have come to recognize that an edge has been lost upon return to activity. So too, is the case with the boxer. The experts suggested that from 2 months to a maximum of 5 months (average of 3 months) is the most time that may separate fights to prevent losing that needed sharpness.

Training equipment

There is relative uniformity of concurring opinion regarding the purpose of each of the training accoutrements.

1 The light or speed bag (Fig. 38.7a) serves to:
  (a) increase hand speed,
  (b) enhance coordination and reflexes, and
  (c) facilitate timing.

2 The heavy bag (Fig. 38.7b) serves to:
  (a) practice offence and defence,
  (b) increase punching power, and
  (c) increase stamina.

3 Rope jumping (Fig. 38.7c) serves to:
  (a) increase endurance,
  (b) increase leg speed, and
  (c) increase coordinated movements.

The most commonly employed cardioeffective methods were daily distance running (usually 8 km or 5 mile in professionals and much shorter distances in amateurs), wind sprints, cycling, rope jumping and sparring. It is traditional to do the running and calisthenics in the morning and the sparring in the afternoon.

Stretching is an important component in every programme designed by the respondents. It is interesting that the majority of the fight world denounces any but light weights and pullies for strengthening, and has an aversion to heavy weights and machine training.

Chasing chickens to gain quickness, as seen in the 'Rocky' movies, is not a typical training form, though it did have an ephemeral popularity in limited circles some decades ago. Push-ups for arm thrust and sit-ups to strengthen the abdominals are frequently practised.

There are several commonly accepted techniques for increasing hand/eye coordination (see section on vision training). As already indicated, the speed bag is one. The second is use of hand paddles (Fig. 38.7d). These are mitts of leather worn on the trainer's hands; the trainer then rapidly moves these 'paddles' high and low with the fighter attempting to hit them with gloved hands whenever they move. A third method is daily boxing with progres-

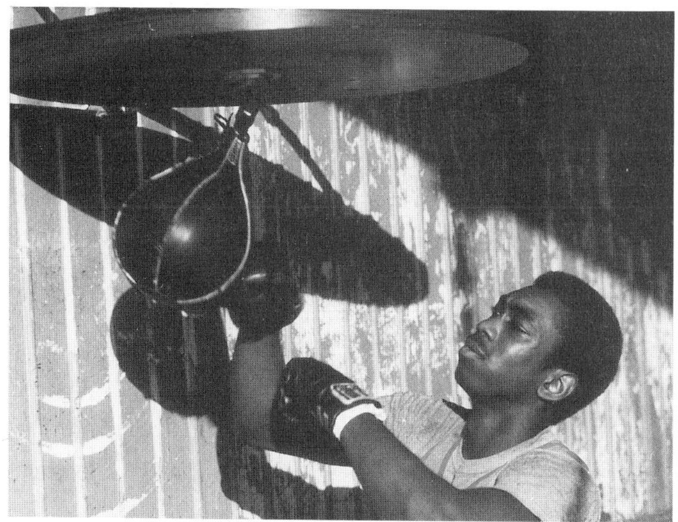

(a)

Fig. 38.7 (a) This light speed bag and the 'crazy speed' bag (not pictured here) are used to increase hand speed, coordination, reflexes and timing. (b) Heavy bag: this enhances offensive and defensive practice, punching power and stamina. (c) Rope jumping: this increases endurance, leg speed, and coordination.

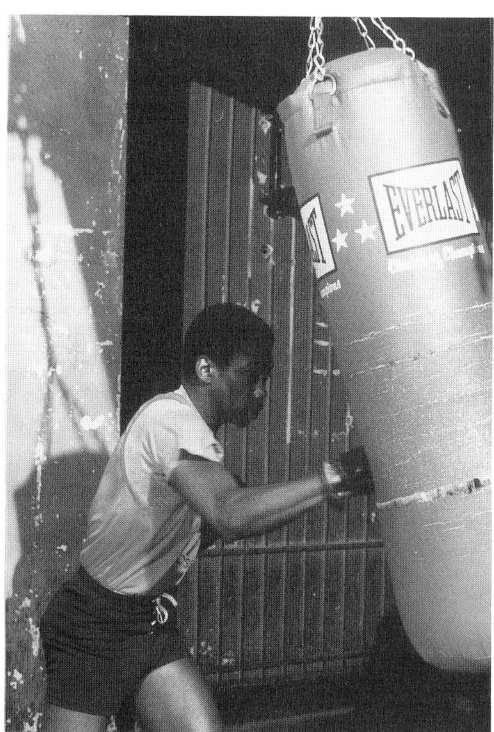

(b)

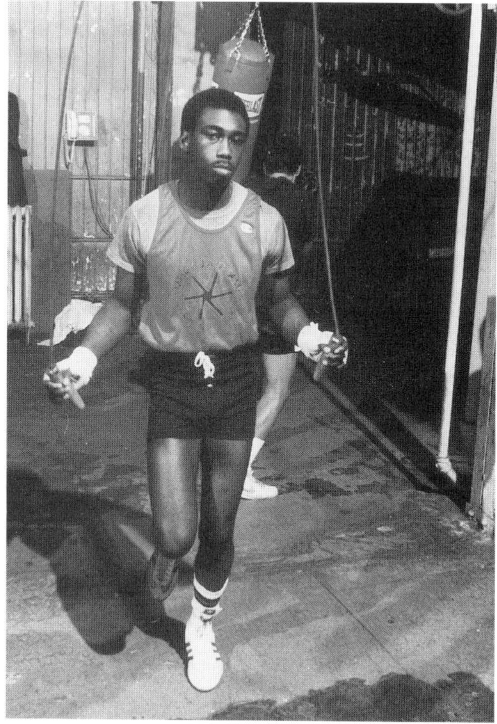

(c)

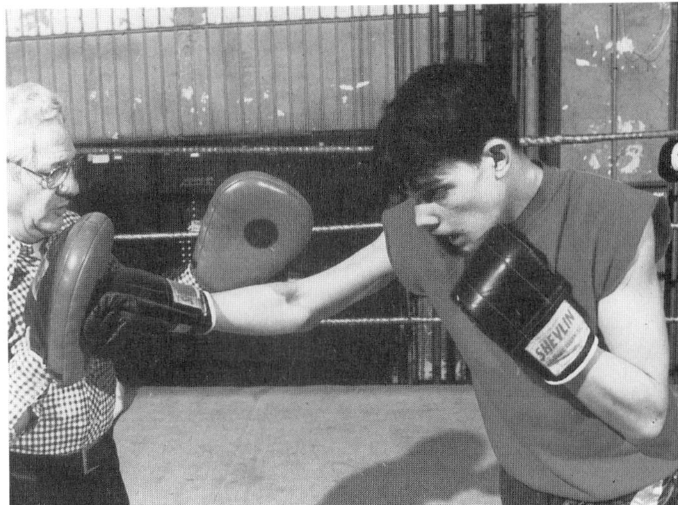

(d)

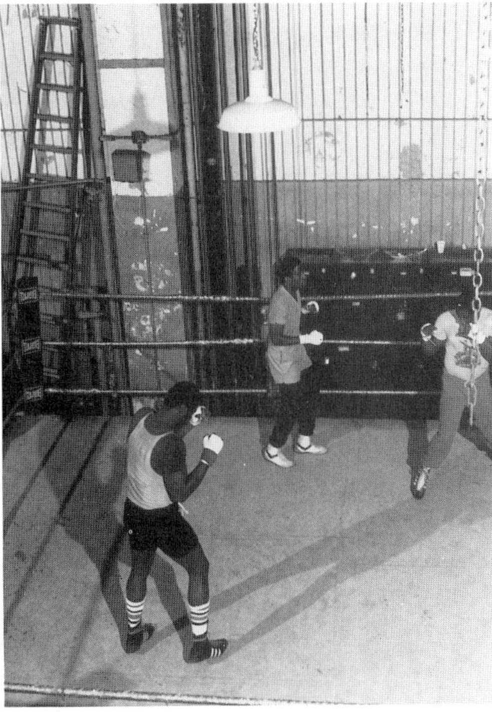

(e)

Fig. 38.7 (*Continued*) (d) Hand paddles are a means of increasing hand to eye coordination. The trainer rapidly moves the paddles to create split second targets for the fighter to punch or block. (e) 'Shadow boxing' is used by boxers to enhance ring movements and manoeuvres. Note that the traditional training gym is dark and has a well worn appearance.

sively faster sparring partners. Finding a proper array of partners makes the third method the most difficult to accomplish.

Arm weariness

Arm weariness is frequently found during boxing contests. Almost all boxers indicate having had an experience of arm heaviness or fatigue sometime in their career. Members of the boxing community consider the following measures as combatants to arm weariness:

1 Push-ups.

2 Sparring with heavy gloves.

3 Shadow boxing (Fig. 38.7e) with hands high.

4 The common visual cliché — running with hands in the air.

Nutrition

For major endurance events (such as marathoning), the final meal should be 2.5–3 h prior to competition with little fat and protein because they digest slowly (E. Colt, personal communication). The meal should contain light carbohydrate such as cereal. Carbohydrate administered too near the event may elevate blood glucose and insulin and lead to hypoglycaemic symptoms of subtle nature. It is popular to conduct boxing events in unusually hot atmospheres (such as Las Vegas, Nevada) where temperatures at fight time may approach 38°C (100°F). If the boxer becomes dehydrated, heat and exercise intolerance develop and the heart rate and body temperature rise. Adequate water and mineral replacement are essential to avert heat exhaustion, depletion of plasma volume, and stress to the cardiovascular system in addition to fatigue-induced defencelessness. Unfortunately, only small quantities of plain water are permitted during bouts.

The most dangerous of nutritional problems relate to fighter classes below heavyweights. In an effort to weigh in at an acceptable weight for their class, fighters often starve and dehydrate themselves in the few days prior to the weigh-in, thereby encouraging fatigue, danger and poor performance.

Efforts to lose or 'make' weight must be initiated weeks prior to a fight to avoid the problems associated with purposeful dehydration and starvation in the period just prior to the fight. The all too frequent use of saunas, rubber suits, saran wrap and diuretics are not only a danger, but they reduce work capacity; work capacity is reduced an estimated 40% with a 5% weight reduction by dehydration (Litel, 1990b). When starvation is added to dehydrating techniques, muscular work capacity decreases (quantity and duration), cardiac output diminishes, the extracellular fluid space contracts, there is an impairment of the thermoregulatory and glomerular filtration systems, and liver glycogen is depleted.

Ring design and ringside safety

Robert Voy, chairman of the USA Amateur Boxing Federation (ABF) Sports Medicine Committee (Voy, 1990b) states that amateur boxing is among the most medically supervised of sports by virtue of the threatened bans by medical associations. Knowing that the ring floor, posts and other accoutrements have been sources of injury, and that ring design has been a deterrant to expedient medical outrage, Voy (1990b) emphasizes the importance of the ring set up in preventing unwarranted disability. Figure 38.8 represents a prototypic ring design

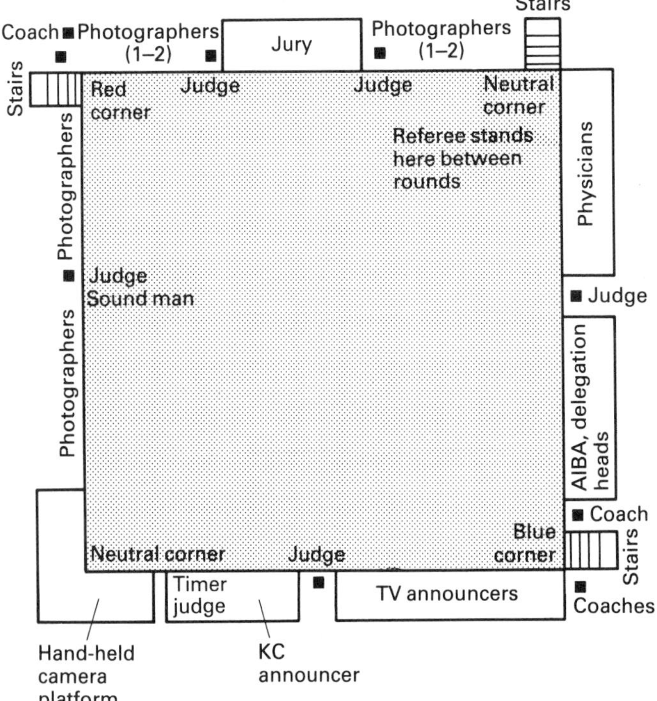

Fig. 38.8 Ring design as indicated in text. From Voy (1990b).

in amateur boxing. The area within the ropes is 148–186 dm^2 (16–20 ft^2) with a 0.6-m (2-ft) apron. It is well padded and contains no seams or defects in the ring-mat. The floor is a 2.5-cm (1-in) thick foam or ensolite pad overlayed upon a wooden base of at least 2.5 cm (1 in) in thickness. A thicker overlay might be too soft and cause injury to a knee or ankle. A tight canvas covers the mat. The ring-posts are padded with no exposed buckles and the four ropes are covered and made taut so the boxer cannot fall through them. A table large enough for a few physicians and their equipment is placed near a neutral corner which is accessed by stairs to allow a physician to quickly mount the apron.

Ringside management

Several entities are commonly handled at ringside by or under the scrutiny of the attending physician.

1 *Cuts*. The head guard has reduced the number of ring cuts. There are, nevertheless, certain common locations for cuts (Fig. 38.9) and some cuts mandate the termination of the bout. In general, cuts in or about the region labelled A in Fig. 38.9 are innocuous. However, cuts labelled B–E are 'fight-stoppers' and F is a potential fight-stopper for reasons indicated in Table 38.1.

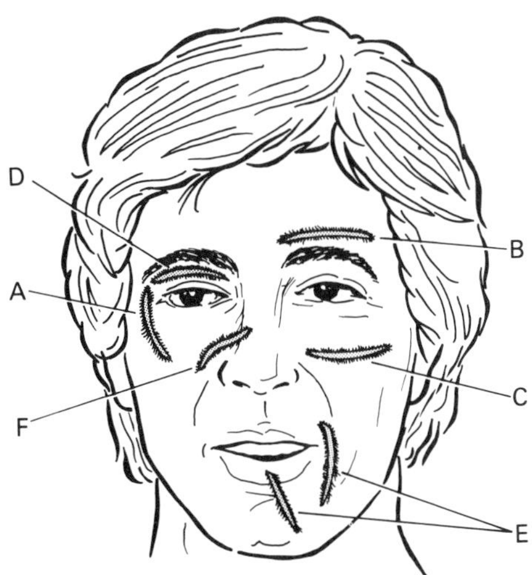

Fig. 38.9 Common locations for cuts from Voy (1990b). For an explanation of A–E, see text and Table 38.1.

2 *Nosebleeds*. In essence, uncontrolled epistaxis is reason to end a bout. If there are clots in the pharynx the fight must be stopped to avert aspiration (Voy, 1990b).

3 *Head injuries*. A boxer is considered 'stricken' (i.e. concussed) if disoriented, retrograde or antegrade amnesia is present, or has altered speech, or has impaired motor function, and/or has difficulty processing information. When such findings are present or if there are focal neurological abnormalities, the bout should be stopped and after evaluation, the boxer should be managed in accordance with Table 38.2.

If the boxer is unconscious, a more stringent vigil is applied as indicated in Table 38.3. The mouth piece should be removed to maintain the airway, taking care to keep the neck immobile in the event that a cervical fracture or sprain is present (Voy, 1990b).

Boxing injuries in general

It has been established that boxing has well entrenched traditions and patterns of training. The formats that have evolved are designed not

Table 38.1 Fight-stopping lacerations. Adapted from Voy (1990b).

Letter in Fig. 38.9	Reason to stop the bout
B	May jeopardize the supraorbital nerve
C	May extend to infraorbital nerve of nasolacrimal duct
D	May damage the tarsal plate
E	Vermillion border tears may extend and predispose to later tears with trauma
F	Stop if underlying nasal fracture

Table 38.2 Management guide for a stricken (unconscious) boxer. From Voy (1990b).

First step

1 Airway. Secure with airway if necessary. Check for cyanosis. Administer mask oxygen
2 Breathing. Check for abnormal pattern, regularity, etc.
3 Circulation. Check for pulse, rate, force

Have in mind a scale so that you can recall level of consciousness

1 Eyes opening: spontaneous (4), to voice (3), to pain (2), none (1)
2 Motor: obeys (6), local pain (5), withdrawal (4), flex with pain (3), extends with pain (2), none (1)
3 Verbal: oriented (5), confused (4), inappropriate words (3), odd sound (2), none (1)
4 A score of 15 is perfect, cautious care; if unconscious more than 2 min, remove to hospital

Assessment

1 Mild concussion. Stunned, dazed, 'out on feet', regains awareness and feels well after 1–2 min. Neurological examination is normal
2 Moderate concussion. Loss consciousness, mental confusion and retrograde amnesia, dizzy when erect, unsteady, ears ring. Ask the following 'cornering' questions for recall accuracy and memory lapse and time of unconsciousness
   (a) What is the last thing you remember before getting hit? Was it a right or a left? etc.
   (b) What is the first thing you remember after regaining consciousness?
3 Severe concussion. Remains unconscious, more than 2–5 min. The longer a boxer is unconscious, the greater the chance of subdural haemorrhage. When conscious, check for headaches, confusion, dizziness, retrograde and antegrade memory loss. If the boxer remains unconscious, place on stretcher or headboard with neck collar. Secure airway; helicopter or full siren ambulance to hospital immediately

Table 38.3 Protocol for head injury follow-up. From Voy (1990b).

Keep the athlete at rest for 24 h. No school, practice, competition or work

Clear liquids only for 8 h

You may allow the athlete to sleep, but check condition every hour while awake, and every 1–2 h while asleep. See that the athlete responds to a pinch or shake, and that colour, pulse and breathing are normal

You may give the athlete 1 Tylenol tablet, but not aspirin, every 4 h as needed for a headache; nothing stronger should be administered unless you are directed to do so by a physician.

Complications that should be brought to the immediate attention of a physician are:
1 Severe or prolonged headache that does not subside with a cool wet towel to the head or a Tylenol tablet
2 If the athlete vomits more than two or three times
3 If there is a convulsion (fit or seizure) or involuntary movements of the arms, face or legs
4 If the athlete complains of weakness or is unable to move one or both arms or legs
5 If there is difficulty with walking
6 If the athlete cannot be awakened easily or is lethargic
7 If there are peculiar eye movements, difficulty of focus, one pupil is much larger or different than the other or double vision
8 If the athlete displays any kind of repetitive behaviour, such as repeating the same word or phrase over and over again, or peculiar behaviour

only to garner victories but to protect the boxer. Boxers with inadequate preparation and conditioning are more likely to sustain injuries. While the most dreaded injuries are those of the brain; injuries to the eyes and viscera are of concern as well.

In a particular realm of amateur boxing (the Army), injury patterns may be representative of those with varied levels of training and conditioning. The USA Army has long been a proponent of amateur boxing. Enzenauer *et al.* (1989) and Enzenauer and Mauldin (1989) reported on hospital admissions for boxing injuries from the regular army and/or cadets of the Military Academy. The two studies assess more than 400 hospital admissions over a 6-year period. Head injuries represented almost 70% of admissions (and 80% of cadet admissions). The breakdown for other areas was as follows: upper extremity, 17%; torso, 7%; and lower extremities, 6%. These figures are almost identical to those of Oelman *et al.* (1983), who studied boxing in the British Army and found 35 hospitalizations·60 h^{-1} of participation· $boxer^{-1}$·$annum^{-1}$.

Oelman *et al.* (1983) evaluated all 'two or more' day admissions due to boxing of British Army personnel from 1969 to 1980 (as well as deaths and discharges between 1952 and 1980). Of 437 admissions, 67.7% were due to head injuries and 26% of these were coded as concussions. While there were no deaths in the 29-year period reviewed, discharges averaged $1 \cdot \text{year}^{-1}$; more than 50% were due to head injury (44% of which were haemorrhages).

Some of the above-indicated injuries may have been rendered as a result of illegal moves. Among the more common illegal moves with potential to produce injury are the following:

1 *Low blow*. Despite the use of a protective cup, a low blow can injure the testicles and momentarily disarm the recipient. A popular myth in the fight community it that low blows 'take something out of the boxer' (Fig. 38.10).

2 *Head butting*. In this manoeuvre, one boxer's head butts into the face of the opponent. This action often accounts for facial lacerations and nasal fractures.

3 *Rabbit punch* (Fig. 38.11). In this move, a punch is delivered to the back of the opponent's neck causing an acceleration of head and cervical contusion, either of which may daze the opponent.

4 *Kidney punch* (Fig. 38.12). Punches to the flank may damage the kidneys or other viscera, and again, may momentarily disable the recipient's defences.

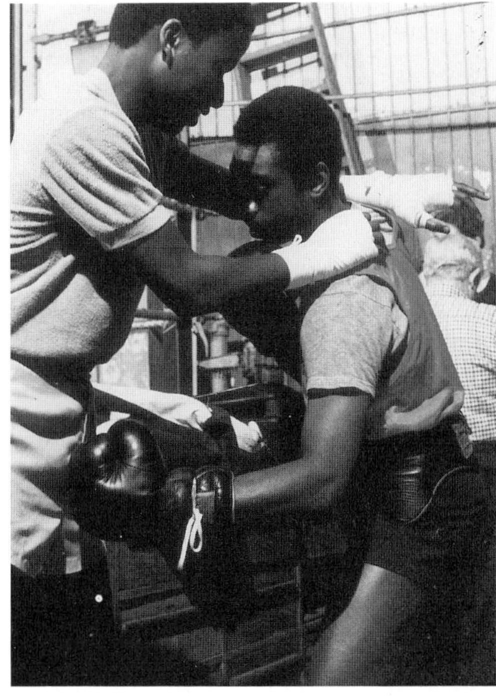

Fig. 38.10 The low blow.

5 *'Heeling'* (Fig. 38.13). In this manoeuvre, the

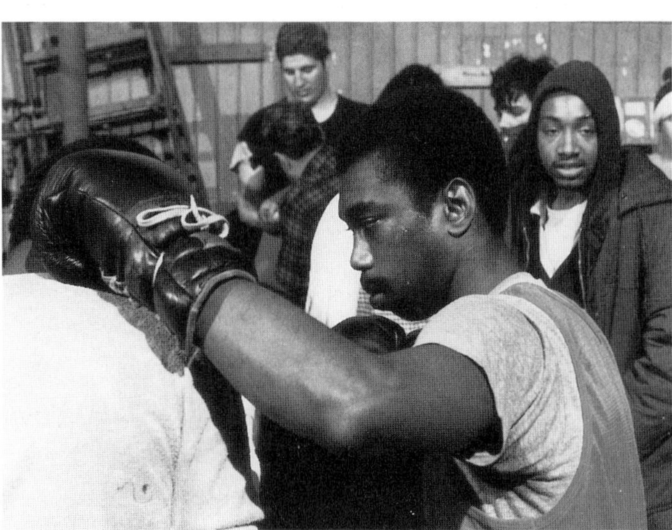

Fig. 38.11 Rabbit punch (hitting back of neck).

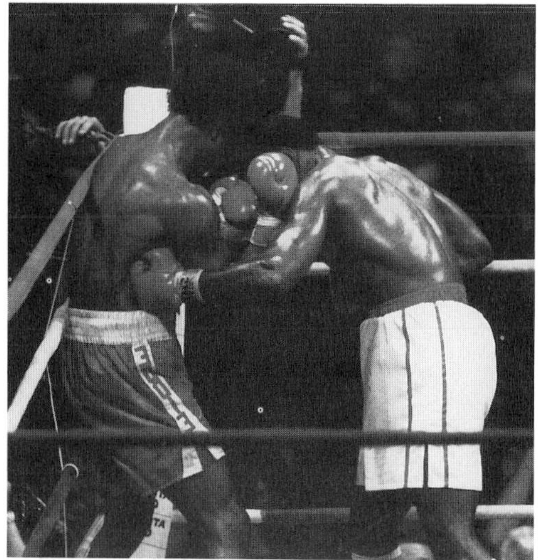

Fig. 38.12 Kidney punch (hitting flank area).

offender hits the opponent's face with an open glove, so that exposed laces can create facial cuts. Rules prohibit use of the open glove as well as exposure of laces.

6 *'Thumbing'* (Fig. 38.14). The thumb has been used to poke at the eye of the opponent to create laceration and/or penetrating injuries. This illegal action stimulated the movement for the development of the thumbless glove (see preceding section on gloves).

Ring-related deaths

In an assault upon boxing in 1983, George Lundberg, editor of the *Journal of the American Medical Association* (*JAMA*), indicated that '... boxing is an obscenity' and 'should not be sanctioned by any civilized society' (Lundberg, 1983). The statement was issued in the wake of a well-publicized ring death. Just two decades previously *JAMA* pointed out that boxing was only seventh on the list of hazardous sports and was below football and hockey (a statement made on boxing in *JAMA* on 21 July 1962). Reif (1981) created death risk charts which placed boxing below mountain climbing and scuba diving. In a defensive and paranoic act, the World Boxing Council (WBC) responded to the ring death of 1983 by reducing fights from 15 to 12 rounds. In the same year, Bert Sugar, publisher of *Ring Magazine* was quoted as having

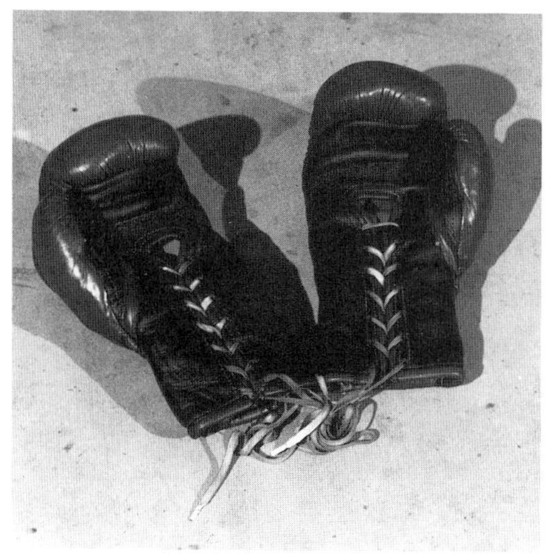

(a)

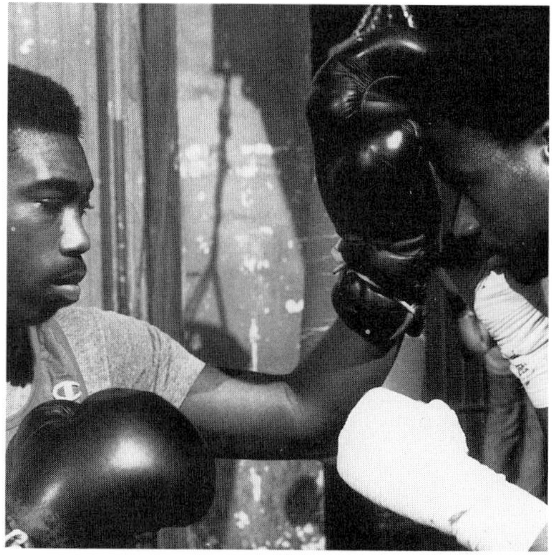

(b)

Fig. 38.13 (a) Laces on the palmar surface of the glove are capable of abrading an opponent's face. (b) Example of 'heeling' by which a boxer is coarsely running the laces of the glove across the face of the opponent.

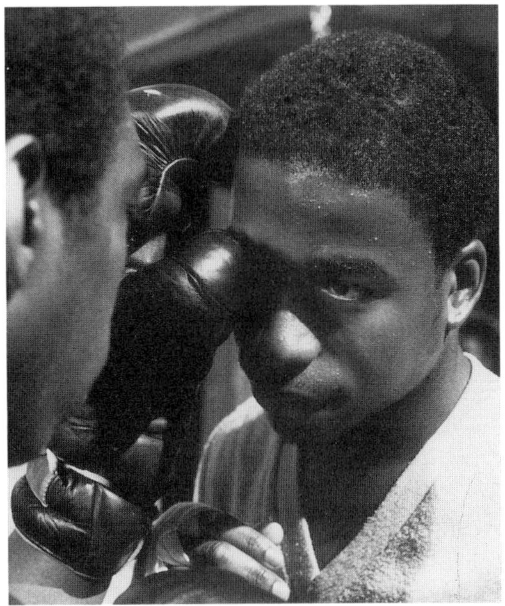

Fig. 38.14 'Thumbing' is an illegal action by which the fighter injures the eye of the opponent by poking the latter with the thumb of the glove.

said '... we have researched ring fatalities back to about 1918 and of the 439 ring deaths, only four came after the 12th round'. Nevertheless, in the mid-1980s, the World Boxing Association (WBA) also reduced their bouts from 15 to 12 rounds.

Ryan (1987) compiled reported mortality statistics on boxing from different sources covering different periods of the twentieth century. These are summarized in Table 38.4, and expanded adaptation of Ryan's.

The first observation to be made from Table 38.4 is that the annual fatality rate is not alarming by standards of some other sports. The second is that the rate has apparently progressively diminished despite improved reporting. If this trend is as it seems, it may be presumed that the reasons to be considered include:

1 Improved rules (more protective).

2 A trend toward reduction in the number of bouts fought or the frequency with which they occurred.

3 Better medical care (diagnostic and therapeutic).

The reality is that each of these have been realized progressively in the past few decades. Jordan (1987) suggests that recent data demonstrates a very low mortality rate when strict medical regulation is present. In New York State, for example, where medical regulation is particularly stringent 'only' one death was recorded for a 4-year period. Whether the single death should be considered a satisfactory rate is debatable, but in any case a well prepared medical system can only be a benefit (Jordan, 1987).

Neurological injuries

The review of neurological aspects of boxing by Guterman and Smith (1987) is among the finest and most comprehensive in the literature. It shall serve as a framework for this section on the mechanisms, sequelae, evaluation and testing of neurological disorders attributable to boxing.

Table 38.4 Ring fatalities, 1918–1985. Adapted from Ryan (1987).

Study period	No. of fatalities	No. of years elapsed (approx.)	Average no. of deaths$\cdot$annum^{-1} (approx.)
Jan. 1918–Jun. 1983	645	65	9.9
Jan. 1945–Jun. 1983	353	39	9.0
Jan. 1970–Dec. 1981	50	12	4.2
Jan. 1970–Dec. 1985	28	76	4.0

Mechanisms of injury

The mechanisms of acute brain damage are well depicted by Lampert and Hardman (1984) in the *JAMA* which crusaded the cause of boxing abolition throughout the 1980s.

Guterman and Smith (1987) make it clearly evident that brain lesions caused by acute and/or repetitious blows are localized within the depth of the brain as well as upon or within the cerebral cortices. Experiments using cats and rabbits (Unterhernscheidt, 1970) demonstrated that repeated subconcussive blows at intervals of 5–20 s produced severe vascular brain damage. The brain lesions were not observed in animals sacrificed immediately after the experiment but only in those sacrificed after several days or weeks. It was also interesting to note that five subconcussive blows were capable of producing foreleg paresis without loss of consciousness.

The kinematics of punching has been studied (Whiting *et al.*, 1988). Head acceleration tolerance has also been studied widely and has been graphed by two popular methods: the Wayne State curve and the Unterhernscheidt and Seller curve (Guardjian & Webster, 1958; Johnson *et al.*, 1975). Based on the former, the Gadd severity index was formulated to assign a numerical value to the severity of any head motion. From experiments of dummy and human boxing simulation, Johnson *et al.* (1975) determined by reference to the Gadd index that the unprotected boxer can exceed the limits of 'safety'. Johnson *et al.* pointed out the physics of head blow types. They indicate that for a solid sphere the local acceleration imparted by a blow to the head would be three or more times greater than that produced by a blow through its centre. For an ellipsoid, such as the human head, the factor is even greater. Johnson *et al.* performed studies on dummies, as well as upon volunteer human subjects, to determine that the unprotected head of a boxer will be subjected to blows which exceed the Gadd severity index (developed to determine safe limits for head concussion by the automobile industry) 'safety threshold' by as much as a factor of 4.

'The violence of a blow to the head is related to the velocity of the fist and the masses involved' (Unterhernscheidt, 1970). Clearly the factors concerned with the effects of the blow are numerous and include such variables as (i) the existing condition of the recipient mass (e.g. skull and brain), fighter weight, strength, hand size, and glove; and (ii) the size and compliance of the glove, speed of delivery, angle of blow, and number of repetitions are all factors to be pondered.

Well prior to the beautifully illustrated mechanisms of head trauma in boxers depicted by Lampert and Hardman (1984) (see below), a research physicist in the surgical physiology department at Oxford, mathematically deduced the mechanics of injury. Holbourn (1943) determined that shear strains were at the root of head injuries. His deductions were based upon five physical properties of the brain, not the least important of which were its incompressibility and its small modulus of rigidity (easy ability to change shape). Holbourn indicates that blows are analysable by their component forces, those which produce linear acceleration, and are not particularly injurious, and those which alter velocity about an axis: centrifugal, coriolis and rotational acceleration forces. The brain, argues Holbourn, does not rattle loosely in the skull to produce *coup/contrecoup* injuries. Since the brain is incompressible, no empty spaces ('rattling') can occur within the skull in response to a blow. While linear accelerating, centrifugal and coriolis forces are dismissed by Holbourn as relatively inconsequential, he asserts that rotational blows are particularly dangerous. The reason is that since no spaces can be formed, and therefore, since the brain cannot move away from the interior wall of the skull, the brain's only option in response to rotationally accelerating blows is to slide along the interior wall (Holbourn, 1943). Consequently, since the dura is firmly attached to the wall, the principal motion takes place between the dura and the arachnoid, stretching the cortical veins and, hence, producing subdural or subarachnoid haemorrhages. In support of his theory and as a counter to the *contrecoup* theory, Holbourn cited Denny-Brown and Russell (1941), who found that it was difficult to produce a concussion in cats when the head was fixed (i.e. when rotation was not possible). This information would lend support to the importance of strengthening the neck muscles. Holbourn's work was contemporary to that of Pudenz and Sheldon (1946), whose *in vivo* experiments dramatically complimented Holbourn's theory.

Unterhernscheidt (1970) indicates two kinds of impact to be considered, central and oblique. The impact of the former passes through the centre of gravity of the skull resulting in a simple translational acceleration. Oblique blows result in combined translational and rotational accelerations. Pure rotation may be induced by an upper-cut to the chin; while the skull rotates, the inertial brain does not, thereby tethering its suspensions and leading to the possible rupture of the bridging veins.

This is not to imply that the brain does not move within the skull to produce additional contusional damage (see Holbourn's theory above). In any case, it is an accepted tenet within the medical community of boxing that rotational acceleration of the brain produces its most serious injuries (Guterman & Smith, 1987). Guterman and Smith cite the report of Govons (1968), relating that rotation of the head is necessary to the production of loss of consciousness by a blow. Rotationally accelerating blows to the head can result in sudden death. Sudden death may also be caused by blows to the carotid sinus; and blows to the orbital region can lead to arrest by means of the Aschner–Dagnini reflex.

Pudenz and Shelden (1946) attempted to learn more about the response of brain movements to trauma by studying the macaque monkey whose calvaria had been replaced by lucite shells. A compressed air powered puncher was used to deliver physiological blows to the head and cinematography was used to record the results. Temporal and parietal blows rotated the brain through a combination of sagittal, horizontal and coronal planes creating a complicated brain excursion with striking sagittal and horizontal convolutional glide. Midline blows displaced the head through a sagittal arc with convolutional glide in the same arc. In each instance bleeding from the surface vessels could be observed through the transparent calvaria.

Clinical neurological syndromes of boxing

Guterman and Smith (1987) recognize the existence of numerous clinical syndromes brought to bear as a consequence of boxing. They include cerebrovascular syndromes, traumatic encephalopathies, amnestic states, midbrain syndromes, migraine headaches, cervical spine disorders and perhaps even tumours.

In the overview, brain injuries in boxing may be divided into acute and chronic varieties. Acute brain injury mechanisms are probably no better illustrated anywhere than in the article by Lampert and Hardman (1984) (Fig. 38.15). A flowsheet summarizing their concept of acute and chronic brain syndromes and the mechanisms by which they are produced is seen in Tables 38.5a & b.

ACUTE HEAD TRAUMA

The most definitive ending to a boxing match is a knock-out. Citing Estwanik *et al.* (1984), Jordan (1987) indicated that 8.7% of 547 bouts in the USA National Amateur Boxing Championships were stopped because of knock-outs or head blows.

The knock-out is essentially synonymous to a concussion and the latter is the most common acute neurological injury (Jordan, 1987). Concussion is not, however, synonymous to unconsciousness, but is, at the least, associated with no less than grogginess or dazing. Having examined injuries in 3000 amateur boxers, Blonstein and Clarke (1957) reported that about 1–2% had been severely concussed or knocked

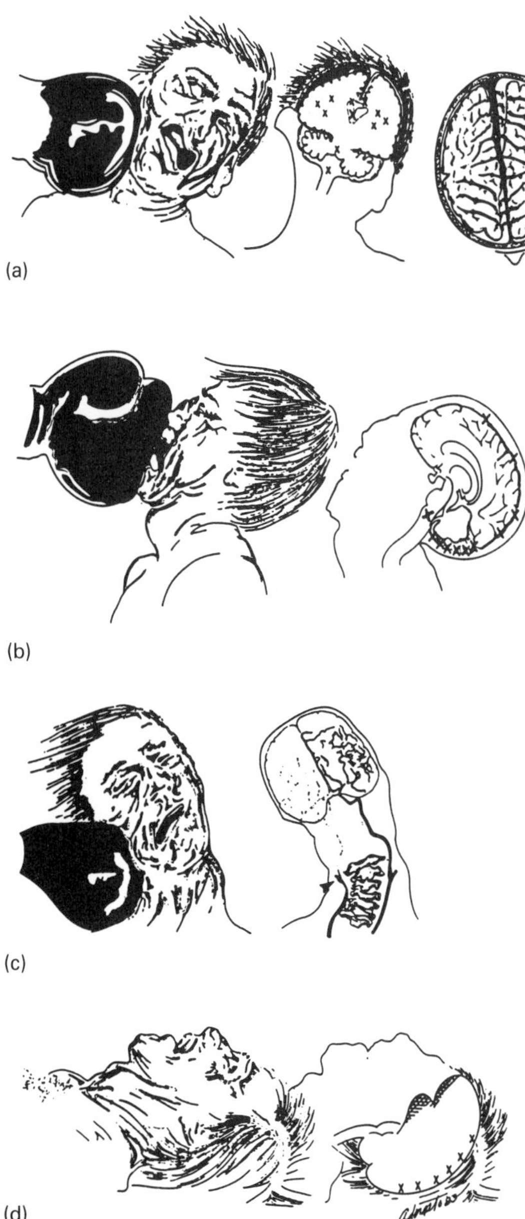

Fig. 38.15 Mechanisms of acute boxing head injuries. (a) Rotational (angular) acceleration causing rotational movement of brain resulting in subdural haematoma by tears of stretched veins and diffuse axonal injury by damage to long fibre tracts in white matter, corpus callosum and brain stem. (b) Linear acceleration of head causing gliding contusions in parasagittal regions of cerebral cortex, ischaemic lesions in cerebellum and axonal damage in brain stem. (c) Injury to carotid and compression of carotid sinus causes generalized ischaemia of brain. (d) Impact deceleration of head by falls against ropes or mat causes *contrecoup* lesions of orbital surface of frontal lobes and tips of temporal lobes as well as gliding contusions. From Lampert & Hardman (1984).

out more than once in a 7-month period, and that neurological and encephalographic testing was normal in all of them. Blonstein and Clarke (1957) recognized four categories of knock-out (concussion) severity:

1 No loss of consciousness:
(a) Type I — hypotomia and defencelessness; dazed.
(b) Type II — cannot recover before the end of the '10 count'

Table 38.5 (a) Acute brain syndromes in boxing as viewed by Lampert & Hardman (1984).

Cause	Entity	Components
Rotational (angular acceleration)	Subdural haematoma	Bridging cortical veins to superior sagittal space, most common cause of sudden death in ring
	Intracerebral haemorrhages	Vessels torn within the brain: parasagittal regions of cortex and subcortical white matter, deeper white matter, corpus callosum, and cerebellar peduncles
	DAI	Damage to white matter axons, easily missed on postmortem examination, can be caused by relatively mild trauma
Linear (translational acceleration)	Focal ischaemic lesions	Mostly in the cerebellum, manifest after several days, proportional to number of subconcussive blows
	Neck hyperextension	Medullopontine angle and retinacular substance, knock-out can result
	Ocular injuries	Most commonly retinal detachment
Carotid injury	Dissecting aneurysm Thrombosis Carotid sinus reflex	All may result in cerebrovascular accidents and/or loss of tone in neck musculature
Impact deceleration	'*Contrecoup*' contusions and haemorrhages	From hitting ropes or mat, orbital surface of frontal/tips of temporal lobes, subdural, subarachnoid haemorrhage possible
Cerebral oedema, ischaemia, herniation	Oedema	Can result from most of the above entities, can also result from secondary DAI or ischaemia
	Ischaemia	Vessels compressed by swelling
	Herniation	Brain herniates over tentorial edge and through foramen magnum, necrosis of inferior temporal lobes and cerebellar tonsils, death from midbrain and pontine ischaemia, surgical decompression life saving except when swelling due to cerebral oedema which has resulted from secondary DAI or ischaemia

DAI, diffuse axonal injury.

Table 38.5 (b) Chronic brain damage: dementia pugilistica in boxing as viewed by Lampert & Hardman (1984).

Cerebral atrophic changes	Ventricular enlargement, widened sulci, narrowed gyri	Consequent to axonal and neuronal degeneration
	Cavum septum pellucidum	Larger width and fenestrated
Cerebellar degeneration	Loss of Purkinje cells	Presumed due to tonsillar herniation with secondary ischaemia
Substantia nigra degeneration	Depigmentation of cells	Demonstrates predilection for brain stem injury; extrapyramidal, Parkinsonian findings; neurofibrillary tangles in degenerative cells
Cerebral 'tangles'	Cerebral neuronal degeneration	Especially in medial temporal cortex, a mygdaloid headeus and hippocampal gyrus

2 Loss of consciousness:

(a) Type I — briefly unconscious; quick recovery of faculties.

(b) Type II — prolonged unconsciousness.

Sercl and Jaros (1962) found that of 427 boxers with acute neurological symptoms, about 80% demonstrated resolution within minutes while about 20% had symptoms persistence for up to 24 h. The most common acute symptoms in descending order of frequency are: hypotomia, cerebellar and vestibular signs, and pyramidal signs (Jordan, 1987). Lampert and Hardman (1984) speculated that diffuse axonal injury (DAI) of the cerebral white matter, which results from acute head trauma, can accrue with repetition, ultimately to result in neurological deficits.

SUBDURAL AND EPIDURAL HAEMORRHAGES

Citing Guardjian and Webster (1958), Guterman and Smith (1987) indicate that subdural haemorrhages account for as much as 75% of acute brain injuries and the preponderance of boxing-related deaths. They result from disruption of the veins which bridge the subdural space. Epidural haemorrhages are much less frequently encountered as sequelae of boxing. Symptoms may become evident immediately or be delayed for days, weeks or months. Most fatalities occur within several days of the causative bout (Guterman & Smith, 1987).

CEREBROVASCULAR AND EMBOLIC SYNDROMES

Carotid artery thrombosis is also a syndrome known to be caused by boxing. Guterman and Smith (1987) cite multiple references, including Hughes and Brownell (1968), who determined that the syndrome derives from either direct blows to the neck or from stretching of the carotid on the side of the neck contralateral to the rotation of the head caused by an angular blow (e.g. glancing upper-cut). The syndrome characteristically presents with a progression of unilateral motor and sensory impairment or even acute hemiplegia.

According to Guterman and Smith (1987) cardiac arrhythmias leading to mural thrombi and embolic cerebrovascular accidents occur in boxing as a result of repeated blows to the chest.

BOXER'S ENCEPHALOPATHY

Pugilistic traumatic encephalopathy is a well-established entity, often satirically represented in cinema productions. Guterman and Smith (1987) contend that the encephalopathy is most common among second-rate fighters, and particularly those used extensively as sparring partners. Such individuals may enter amnestic states and/or be knocked out several times a day. Robert (1969), indicated that the severity of the condition correlates directly to the number of bouts, a fact later corroborated by Ross *et al*. (1983) and Casson *et al*. (1984). Critchley (1960) suggested that the incidence is greater among Caucasian than among Black fighters but offers no justifying explanation.

LaCava (1963) described a three-stage evolutionary process that typically follows the reversible prodrome of vertigo, ataxia, headache and amnesia, if the boxer continues boxing.

Stage 1 is variably reversible. It is hallmarked by euphoria and hypomania (a 'Mr Hyde' syndrome but without a loss of judgement). Gross motor functions remain intact but rope skipping, punch accuracy and intricate motor skills are impaired.

In stage 2, the hypomania is replaced by arrogance, irritability and a chauvinistic paranoia often related to impotence. A chronic amnestic state, resting tremor and shuffling gait, dysarthria and garbled speech are frequent findings.

Stage 3 typically appears a few years after the encephalopathic prodrome. Mentation slows, cognitive functions are impaired, hyperreflexia and mask-like facies herald the presence of both pyramidal and extrapyramidal disorders. A progression of psychiatric and neuromotor manifestations may be present at independent rates.

Ross *et al*. (1987) reassert that a wide spectrum of neurological dysfunction may be seen among boxers, and that the continuum extends from subtle, subclinical forms demonstrable only by neuropsychological testing, to flagrant 'punch-drunk' states with Parkinsonian and cerebellar manifestations. In today's boxing world, it is the earlier end of the spectrum which is most commonly encountered (presumably due to fewer bouts and more extensive evaluations). Whereas in the pre-World War II era a 200 match career was common, in the present era a total of 40–50 bouts would be on the excessive side.

Ross *et al*. (1987) essentially regard the neurological consequences of boxing to be a direct correlate of the number of bouts fought (particularly among professionals). Their general perceptions are summarized in Table 38.6.

Encephalopathic histology

It is within the realm of traumatic encephalopathy that the neuropathology of the boxer's brain is most appropriately discussed. Perhaps the most extensive neuropathological study was that of Corsellis *et al*. (1973). These authors reviewed the gross pathology and microhistology of 15 separate brains of ex-boxers.

While certain neurological sequelae attributable to boxing were defined in 1928 by Martland who coined the term 'punch drunk', it was probably not until Robert's report in 1969 that the danger of such damage was appreciated. Corsellis *et al*. (1973) chose to pursue studies of brain damage not hitherto based on more than

Table 38.6 Neurological sequelae in professional boxers. Adapted from Ross *et al*. (1987).

No. of bouts	Expectations
20–30	None or subclinical evidence of brain injury
25–50	No clinical dysfunction detectable *but* frequent CT and/or neuropsychological test abnormalities
>50	Many with clinical signs/ symptoms of brain injury and CT and/or neuropsychological test abnormalities

CT, computerized tomography.

a few necropsies. Despite the mean age of 69 and the frequency of alcoholism among the subjects, the findings to be described are to be considered the *sine qua non* for boxers' brains.

The more outstanding findings included the following. The septum pellucidum was often cavum and usually fenestrated (77% of the boxer versus 3% for the controls) (Fig. 38.16). The mean width of the septum was also greater in boxers (5.17 mm) compared to the controls (1.6 mm).

With respect to the pathology demonstrated, it was speculated by Ferguson and Mawdsley (1965) that destruction of the leaves of the septum pellucidum is a function of the recurrent elevations of intraventicular pressure (Guterman & Smith, 1987).

The finding of gliosis of the cerebellar and cerebral cortices is most evidenced in the lateral lobe and tonsillar region, a response to repeated concussions of these areas with bleeding (Fig. 38.17). There is a marked loss of Purkinje cells (often by more than 50%), the most sensitive cells to the effects of hypoexemia (Corsellis *et al.*, 1973; Guterman & Smith, 1987) (Fig. 38.18). The associated loss of cerebral tissue results in ventricular enlargement (hydrocephalus *ex vacuo*) and is due to boxing rather than aging (Corsellis *et al.*, 1973).

A facsimile of Parkinson's disease, boxer's

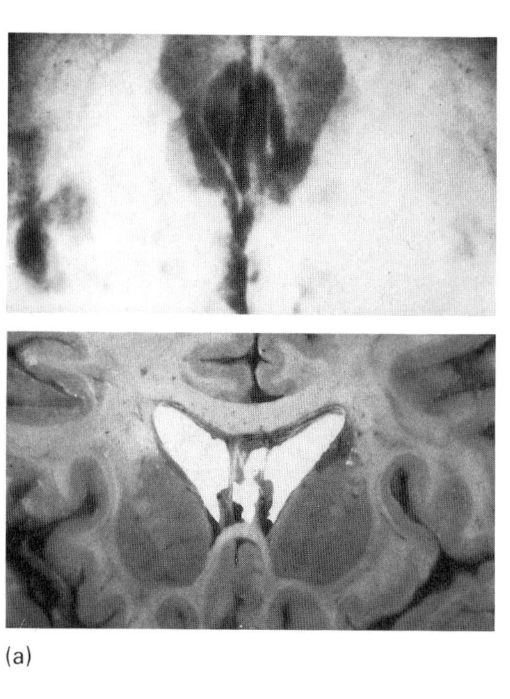

(a)

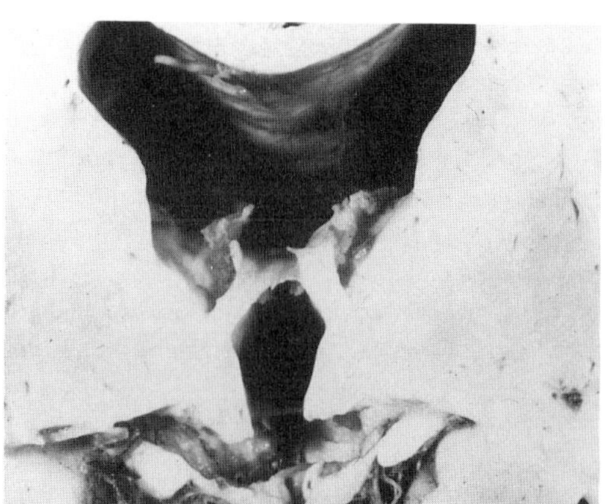

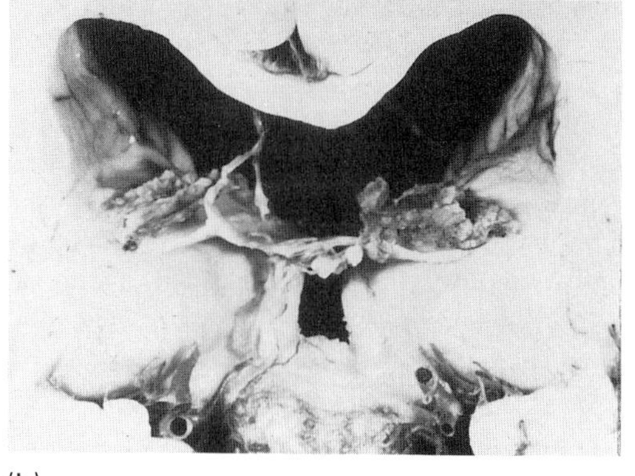

(b)

Fig. 38.16 (a) The pneumoencephalogram (*above*) demonstrates alteration of the septum pellucidum (broadened) and cavum in a former boxer. The hemispherical slice (*below*) shows the caval septum as well as fenestration of the right lamina. (b) The ventricles are just beneath the corpus callosum. The septum pellucidum is absent, destroyed beyond mere fenestration. Courtesy of J.N. Corsellis and associates.

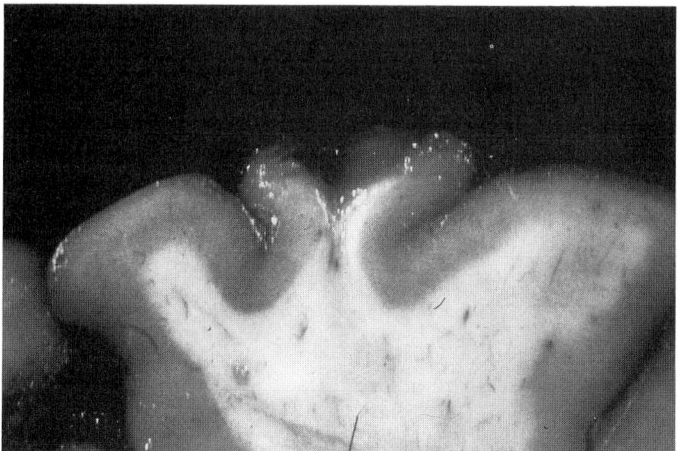

Fig. 38.17 Cerebral contusion: this gross section of cerebrum manifests evidence of contusion sustained any time from 6 weeks to years prior to death. Note the erythema at the superior margin of the specimen, and especially, the loss of grey matter on the crest of the gyrus. Courtesy of Dr M.P. Valsamis.

encephalopathy, is most characteristically represented by a loss and degeneration of pigmented neurones in the substantia nigra (Fig. 38.19), often associated with paired helical filaments within hydropic neurones, better known as neurofibrillary tangles (Corsellis *et al.*, 1973; Guterman & Smith, 1987) (Fig. 38.20). All of these findings correlate to the presence of extrapyramidal dysfunction. A similarity of these findings to those of an Alzheimer dementia, but possibly without the associated cholinergic dysfunction which exists in the former.

For nearly three decades, the neuropathological descriptions of Corsellis *et al.* (1973) remained largely unchallenged. However, the recent work of Roberts *et al.* (1990) refutes the basic distinction between boxer's encephalopathic dementia and Alzheimer's disease that had been alleged by their predecessors. Based on evaluations by Congo red and silver stains, Corsellis *et al.* reported that both dementias were characterized by neurofibrillary tangles but that dementia pugilistica failed to demonstrate the senile plaques characteristic of the other dementia. Roberts *et al.* re-examined the archival temporal lobe material from 14 of the cases studied by Corsellis *et al.* However, this time the material was studied by staining the β protein plaques with an antibody, after a pretreatment with formic acid. Diffuse plaques, similar to those of Alzheimer's disease, were thus disclosed. Both dementias are clearly related, each with temporal lobe concentrations of tangles, and each predilecting the pre α layer of Braak for destruction. In studies of brain-injured subjects unrelated to boxing, dementia is observed at a rate more than double that of the general population (Guterman & Smith, 1987).

Brain haemorrhages may emanate from trauma (as in a boxing injury) or from increased intracranial pressure (as in hyperextension or intracranial tumours), the latter type termed a Duret haemorrhage. Note in Fig. 38.21 the evidence for haemorrhage in the midbrain unaccompanied by increased cranial pressure, a consequence of a boxing injury. The aqueduct is uncompressed (M. Valsamis, personal communication).

Neurological findings

While neurological findings are a poor reflection of the degree of damage sustained, and more importantly, do not predict sudden death, there are rather characteristic signs attributed to dementia puglistica. Ross *et al.* (1983) have developed the following list:

1 Slow motor performance.

2 Clumsiness.

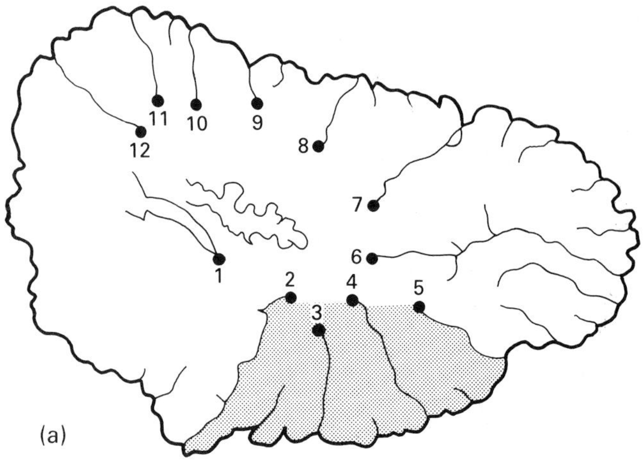

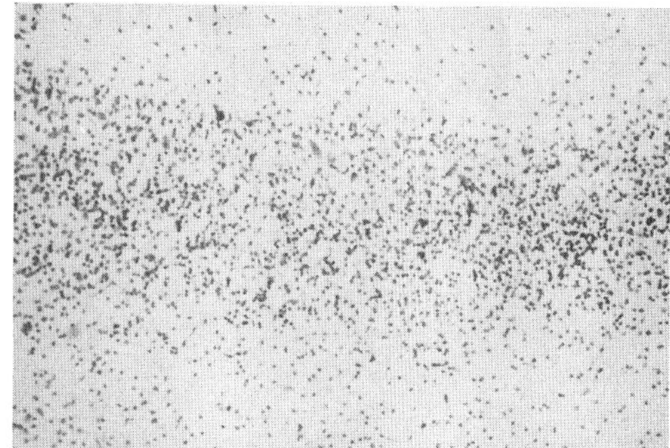

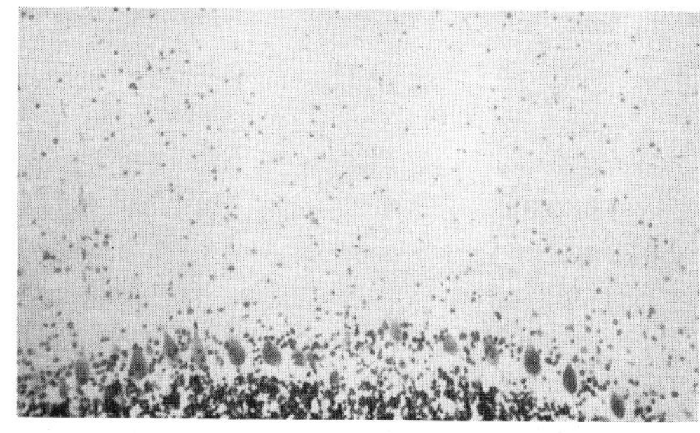

Fig. 38.18 (a) Cerebellum: this is a sagittal cerebellar map depicting the zones defined to acknowledge sites from which specimens were examined. (b) Cerebellum: the photomicrograph (*top*) demonstrated a paucity of pink Purkinje cells and reduction of the internal granular cell layer in the brain of a former boxer. (*Bottom*) The brain of a control subject with orderly alignment of Purkinje cells and a densely packed internal granular cell layer. Courtesy of J.N. Corsellis and associates.

3 Dysarthria.
4 Ataxia.
5 Tremors.
6 Rigidity.
7 Spasticity.
8 Memory loss.
9 Slow thinking.
10 Personality changes.

Ross *et al.* estimated that 17–55% of all professional boxers demonstrate one or more of these signs. While Robert (1969) found similar signs in 37 of 224 ex-professional boxers for about a 12% incidence.

Encephalopathic neuropsychological testing

Again, in conjunction with boxer's encephalopathy, it is appropriate to relate correlations of neuropsychiatric testing. Guterman and Smith (1987) review the results of several reported testings. Roberts (1969) reported that scores in the lower quarter for the Ravens non-verbal intelligence and the Mill Hill vocabulary tests correlated with a ring tenure in excess of 10 years.

Rimel *et al.* (1981) studied 538 non-boxers who had sustained head trauma causing unconsciousness for less than 20 min. When evaluated 3 months later, all had normal neurological examinations, but 79% complained of persistent headache, 59% of memory problems

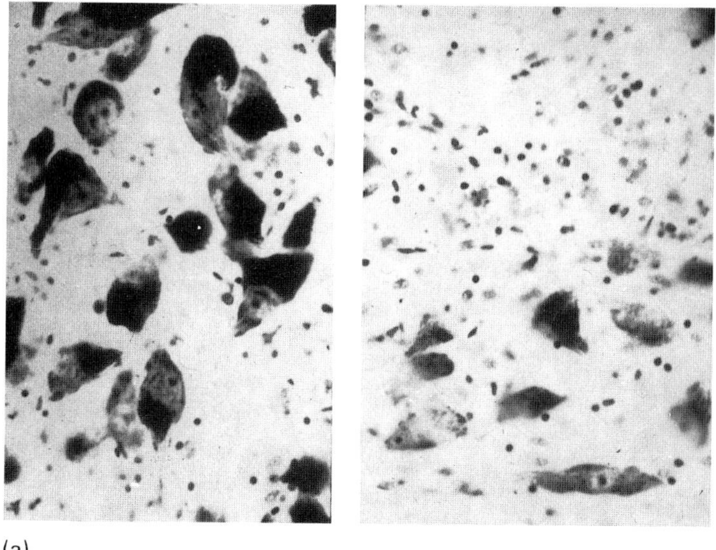

(a)

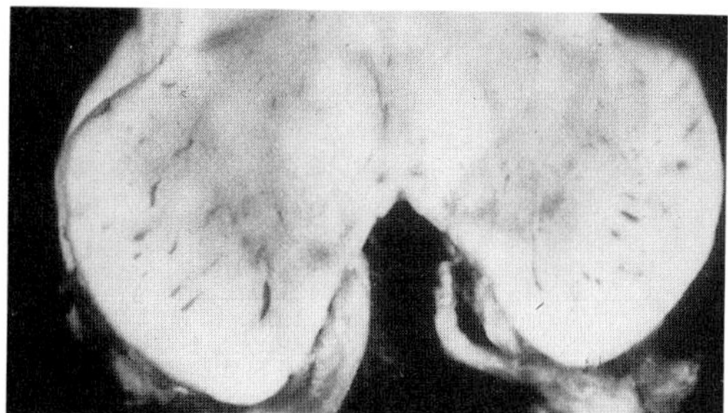

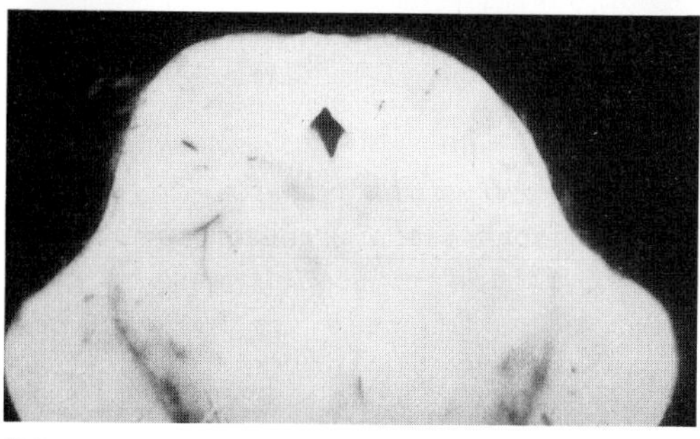

(b)

Fig. 38.19 (a) Substantia nigra photomicrographs: (*left*) a control subject demonstrating the neuronal cells capped with black neuromelanin pigment; (*right*) a boxer demonstrating neuronal pallor. (b) Midbrain slices: (*above*) a boxer demonstrating marked loss of nigral pigmentation; (*below*) a control subject demonstrating normal pigmentation of the substantia nigra. Courtesy of J.N. Corsellis and associates.

and nearly all demonstrated abnormalities on neuropsychological testing (Ryan, 1987).

Casson *et al.* (1984) reported the creation of an 'impairment index' which determined a percentage of abnormal tests among a neuropsychological battery and determined a correlation between the magnitude of abnormalities and the number of bouts. Correlations were more dramatic in the presence of computerized tomographic (CT) and electroencephalographic (EEG) abnormalities. Among the 38 boxers evaluated by Ross *et al.* (1983), every single one had more than one abnormal neuropsychological test score; more than 90% (15 boxers tested) scored abnormally on the 5-s recall Bender Gestalt test of visual memory and of 13 tested with the Wechsler memory test (verbal and visual), almost all scored abnormally on both components. Overall, 90% of those tested with memory tests scored abnormally. Of particular interest is that every boxer with either an abnormal CT scan or EEG had at least one abnormal memory test score. Conversely, all 12 boxers with impairment indices greater than 0.5 had an abnormal CT and/or EEG (as opposed to those with a lower index). Finally, impairment indices did not correlate positively with the number of bouts. Since no one neuro-

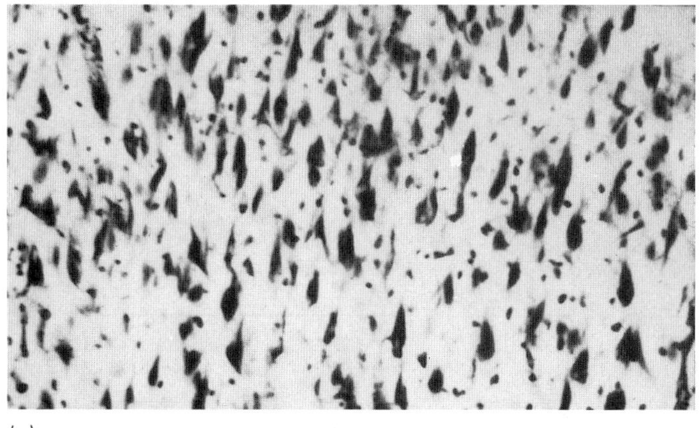

(a)

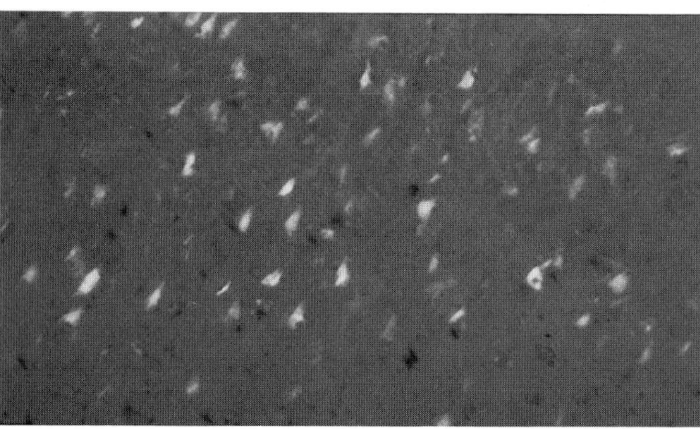

(b)

Fig. 38.20 Cerebral cortex: these photomicrographs demonstrate neurofibrillary tangles in the brain of a boxer. (a) The tangles are delineated in black by a bodian stain. (b) The presence of an amyloid material is evident as birefringent yellow dots (light areas) in a field stained with Congo red (dark background) and viewed under polarizing light. Courtesy of J.N. Corsellis and associates.

psychological test is a predictor of quantitative damage, it is recommended that multiple tests be administered.

The bottom line of neuropsychological testing, according to Guterman and Smith (1987) is that it has sensitivity but lacks specificity.

AMNESTIC SYNDROMES

Transient events, technically amnestic states, in which grogginess, confusion, and a slowing and impairment of motor function, have been noted among boxers (Critchley, 1960) and may represent the prodrome to a progressive encephalopathy (Gronwall & Wrightson, 1975). Guterman and Smith (1987) decry the all too frequent continuation of fights when one boxer has attained an amnestic state who becomes barely more than a 'reflex animal', with cervical hypotonia and incoordination adding physical defencelessness to that of mental ineptitude.

MIDBRAIN SYNDROMES

Midbrain syndromes characterized by ataxia, dysarthria, pyramidal tract signs and a loss of balance are known to occur, but are relatively rare consequences of boxing (Guterman & Smith, 1987).

HEADACHE SYNDROMES

Headaches, perhaps even true migraine types, have been known to occur in conjunction with

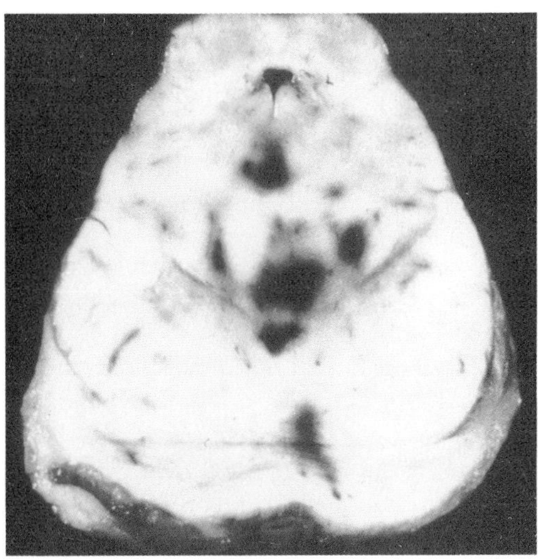

Fig. 38.21 Oblique section through brain; most superior are the inferior colliculi; most inferior are the pons and basilar artery. Note the dark blotches or haemorrhages in the midbrain just below the *uncompressed* aqueduct (see text). Courtesy of J.N. Corsellis and associates.

the afore-mentioned syndromes as well as independently of them. Elia (1962) reporting on an epidemiological survey, stated that 86% of boxers with a history of having been knocked out had suffered from persistent headaches. This is in comparison to a paltry 4% incidence among those who had never been knocked out. Obviously individuals with persistent headaches require an elaborate neurological and ophthalmological evaluation.

CERVICAL SYNDROMES

Knowing that punches can exceed the safety level of the Gadd severity index by large amounts offers an explanation of how upper cuts can cause hyperextension injuries of the cervical spine with dislocation. Bridging and other neck-strengthening methods are of little value in protection during amnestic periods when the cervical musculature is more flaccid.

A study of contact sport cervical injuries was undertaken at the Texas Institute for Rehabilitation and Research (Kewalramani *et al.*, 1981), classifying injuries by mechanism: ventroflexion, retroflexion and vertical loading. While ventroflexion injuries in collision sports are more frequently associated with severe neurological and osteoarticular deficits, such deficits might also derive from retroflexion injuries. Of 46 cervical cord injuries studied, one was sustained in boxing by the retroflexion mechanism.

Components of retroflexion injury to the cervical spine include the following.

1 Crowding of spinous processes/neural arches.
2 Intervertebral space (anterior) increased.
3 Retroluxation/dislocation.
4 Fracture of spinous process/neural arches.
5 Chip fracture anterior superior/inferior angle of vertebral body (teardrop injury).
6 Posterior atlanto-axial subluxation.
7 Possible absence of radiographical abnormality.

POST-TRAUMATIC TUMOURS

Head trauma was implicated in the development of the meningioma more than 50 years ago when Cushing and Eisenhardt (1938) reported the existence of an association, more than one-third of more than 300 cases of meningioma having had a history of head trauma; of these, 24 had swelling, a scar or a depressed fracture related to the tumour site (Walsh *et al.*, 1969). Preston-Martin *et al.* (1983) revealed that a history of boxing represented a significant risk factor for the development of a meningioma. Delays as long as 25 years are known to occur between a reported trauma and the detection of a meningioma (Walsh *et al.*, 1969).

Neurological testing (other than neuropsychological)

NEURORADIOLOGY: COMPUTERIZED TOMOGRAPHY AND PNEUMOENCEPHALOGRAPHY

Guterman and Smith (1987) indicate that there are three types of radiographical changes observe in boxers, (i) those indicating cerebral and/or cerebellar atrophy; (ii) those revealing a cavum septum pellucidum; and (iii) those demonstrating dilatation of the cistern of the lamina terminalis. Isherwood *et al.* (1966) and Guterman and Smith (1987) revealed a very high incidence of brain atrophy among boxers evaluated with pneumoencephalography (PEG) and CT respectively. The implications set fourth by Ross *et al.* (1983) and by Casson *et al.* (1984) were that boxers with abnormal CT scans were more likely to have neurological findings and that the abnormalities were more likely to be a function of recurrent knock-outs than of the number of career bouts.

Based upon the milestone article of Ross *et al.* (1983) in which CT abnormalities were graded (0–4) (and in which such abnormalities were found in 50% of boxers evaluated), Ross *et al.* (1987) have assembled tables correlating the number of bouts to CT findings, clinical symptoms, EEG, physical and neurological finds. A summary of these findings is found in Table 38.7 in which CT abnormalities are not distinguished by severity in the manner of Ross *et al.*

Not evident in Table 38.7 is that the CT abnormalities become more comprehensive as the number of bouts increases; neurological signs and symptoms did not correlate with CT evidence of cerebral atrophy, nor significantly, with the number of bouts.

The radiographical incidence of a cavum septum pellucidum has been variably reported. Of significance is that a cavum septum is more likely to be detected by PEG than by CT and that the incidence of this lesion is under 5% in the general population versus up to more than 50% in groups of boxers (Guterman & Smith, 1987).

MAGNETIC RESONANCE IMAGING

Magnetic resonance imaging (MRI) has enjoyed progressive popularity as a diagnostic modality for neurological disorders since the mid-1980s. A determination of its role in the evaluation of neurological disorders attributable to boxing has been tardy largely because the gathering of a large assemblage of boxers in a cost-effective manner in one centre with sophisticated MRI capability has been a logistical difficulty. Perhaps the most efficacious study to date has

Table 38.7 Correlations between number of bouts and CT, EEG, neurological signs and symptoms based on 38 boxers. Liberal adaptation from Ross *et al.* (1987).

		Abnormalities (%)			
Group	No. of bouts	CT	EEG	Symptoms	Neurological examination
1	0–49	33	18	29	27
2	50–99	60	17	40	17
3	<100	70	57	38	29

CT, computerized tomography; EEG, electroencephalography.

been that of Jordan and Zimmerman in New York City (1990), a neurologist and neuroradiologist respectively with a vast experience in the evaluation of boxers. Despite the affiliations with boxing, their study includes only 21 boxers, among which are both amateurs and professional (age range, 21–66 years), and some with and some without symptoms. The particular value of their study is that all 21 were subjected to both CT and MRI examinations, allowing a comparative evaluation of the two modalities. Jordan and Zimmerman ultimately concluded that with the possible exception of the acutely injured boxer, MRI was a more valuable test than CT. The reasons include (i) its multiplanar imaging ability; (ii) its ability to avoid false positive results due to artefacts from adjacent bone that were seen with CT; (iii) its ability to contrast brain and cerebrospinal fluid on T1-weighted images; (iv) its superior ability to image the brain surface; and (v) its ability to detect haemorrhages months after their occurrence. CT can detect them for only 1–2 weeks. A glaring deficiency of MRI at this time is its relative inability to detect haemorrhages within the first 48 h. Hence, for acute head trauma, CT is the initial procedure of choice, possibly to be followed up by MRI after 24–48 h. Jordan and Zimmerman caution that MRI is not a substitute for examination and EEG in terms of assessing brain function. Of the 21 boxers evaluated by CT and MRI, images of both tests were considered normal in 11 and abnormal in seven. MRI confirmed or enhanced findings present on CT when, detecting false positives due to artefact, and finding abnormalities missed by CT in several cases.

ELECTROENCEPHALOGRAPHY

Guterman and Smith (1987) point up the stark disparity in results of EEG correlations among investigators. For example, Beaussart and Beaussart-Boulenge (1970) found no abnormalities in immediate prefight and postfight tracings in more than 120 boxers. They provide one of the more interesting clinically based position statements attesting to the safety of boxing, especially considering the weight of evidence of its dangers at the time of publication. They evaluated 123 amateur boxers by physical examination and EEG immediately before and 10–15 min after the fights. They claimed to have found not one objective pathological change, even in cases where consciousness was lost. As strange and contradictory as these results might seem, they are not inconsistent with reports that EEG abnormalities may appear tardily (e.g. after hours or longer) (Larsson *et al.*, 1954). It is, however, more difficult to appreciate a consistent absence of clinical signs in those who lost consciousness. The authors conclude on the basis of their study that '... the ban on fighting for a certain period after ... knock-outs has no scientific justification'. Part of the basis of their conclusion was an observation of significant blood pressure variation in those who had lost consciousness. The authors presumed this to mean that reflex vascular phenomena rather than cerebral damage was responsible for the loss of consciousness, a throwback to the theories reviewed and largely dismissed nearly 20 years previously by Larsson *et al.* (1954). Prior to the study of Beaussart and Beaussart-Boulenge, Kaplan and Browder (1954) found no significant deviations in more than 1000 postfight tracings.

These results are in contradistinction to those of Busse and Silverman (1952) and of Larsson *et al.* (1954), each of these workers having found a high percentage of abnormalities in postfight tracings (Guterman & Smith, 1987). In the study by Busse and Silverman (1952), EEGs performed on knock-out victims revealed that 37% of those tested revealed abnormalities which could not be correlated to a severity of damage.

In a study conducted in the early 1950s, Larsson *et al.* (1954) conducted evaluations of two groups of amateur boxers, most with limited experience and all participating in bouts not exceeding three rounds. The boxers ($n = 75$) were examined in connection with 102 short matches. Of the 75 boxers evaluated, 44 underwent EEG examinations just prior to and within 30 min subsequent to the match. The remainder underwent EEG evaluation only after the bout. In the group which underwent prematch and postmatch EEG examinations, 30% of those knocked out or down, or who received hard blows, demonstrated pathological changes. 13% with seemingly less traumatic matches had such changes. In the group with only postmatch EEGs, the selection of which was based on having experienced an especially hard match, there was a 52% incidence of pathological findings. At the time of publication, Larsson *et al.* were in possession of Kaplan and Browder's contradictory manuscript (1954).

Trends from other studies suggested that the likelihood of an abnormal EEG increased with the number of bouts fought as well as their frequency (Guterman & Smith, 1987). Among the reasons offered for the less than dramatic correlation between the EEG and boxer's encephalopathy is that the former surveys the cortex while the pathology of the latter is often predominantly subcortical. A normal EEG may belie a significant pathology, but an abnormal EEG should preclude entry into the ring.

Specialized tests of a non-routine nature

SPECIAL ELECTROPHYSIOLOGICAL TESTING

The detection of traumatic encephalography by objective laboratory testing has been of limited success. Guterman and Smith (1987) suggest that topographical flash-evoked potential mapping and other electrophysiological measures more sensitive than EEG may be of value.

CEREBRAL BLOOD FLOW

Using a technique of Xenon-133 inhalation, Rodriguez *et al.* (1983) (Guterman & Smith, 1987) measured cerebral blood flow in a group of controls matched against amateur and professional fighters. While perfusion differences between controls and amateurs was nil, a reduction in flow (12%) was noted in professionals. In discussing this work, Guterman and Smith (1987) are at a loss to explain its significance or its particular involvement of the temporal and parietal lobes. The study does not correlate the findings with a quantitative analysis of cerebral atrophy. Neuropathologically, cortical atrophy is most marked in the lateral lobes (Corsellis *et al.*, 1973).

BIOCHEMICAL ASSAYS

A cytoplasmic enzyme of brain astrocytes and CK-BB (creatine kinase-brain band) has been demonstrated to be a sensitive indicator of cerebral injury (Phillips *et al.*, 1980). Brayne *et al.* (1982) found a significant correlation of the enzyme assay to the number of blows sustained by boxers.

Ophthalmological injuries

Courville (1942) presented the concept of *coup* and *contrecoup* injuries, concepts which pertain to the head and to eyes (Litel, 1990a). The volume of the eye cannot be changed, i.e. it is incompressible. Therefore it can sustain damage at the site of impact (*coup*) as well as at distant sites (*contrecoup*) from the shock wave transmission of the blow (Fig. 38.22) (Litel, 1990a).

The American National Society to Prevent Blindness secures eye injury data from the National Electronics Injury Surveillance System (NEISS). A 1981 NEISS survey reports that eye injuries contribute 2% of the total injuries reported in boxing.

Review of the files of the Eye Pathology Laboratory at the Massachusetts Eye and Ear Infirmary was undertaken to assess ocular sport injuries between 1960 and 1980 (Portis *et al.*, 1981). Only one of the 80 enucleations consequent to sports was due to boxing, while golf,

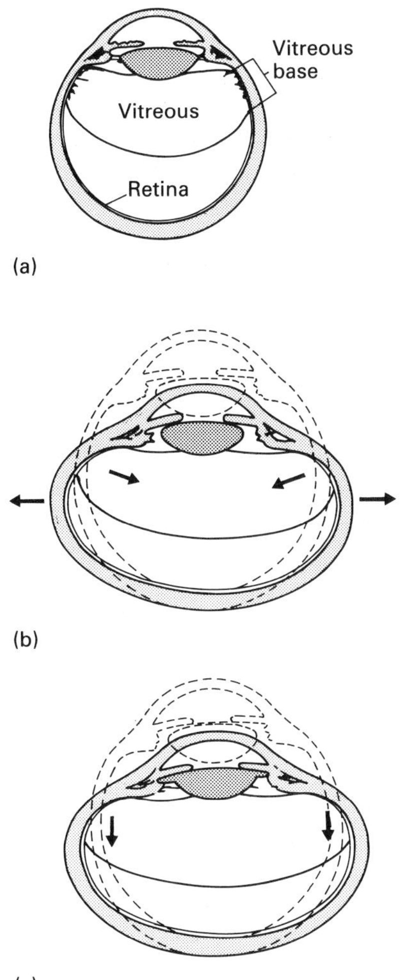

Fig. 38.22 Mechanisms of eye injury production. From Litel (1990a). (a) Unaltered eye; (b) *coup* injury mechanism; (c) *centrecoup* injury mechanism.

hockey and baseball accounted for 20 cases. Yet Vinger (1981a) vindicates boxing abolitionists, claiming boxing to be the only sport with an intent to cause injury. In an excellent book (1981b), he refers to the main eye afflictions of pugilism as angle contusion deformities and retinal tears, often asymptomatic until vision is lost from a later onset of glaucoma or long-standing retinal detachment.

It has been indicated that contusion angle deformities are typical ocular injuries among boxers. Tears of the ciliary body (an anterior chamber structure) result from a *coup* and result in recessed angles. About 10% of individuals with this problem will develop a post-traumatic glaucoma (Litel, 1990a). Most often, angle recessions occur in conjunction with hyphemas. Put another way, about 70–80% of eyes that have hyphema, have angle recession and 90% of hyphemas are caused by a tear of the ciliary body. Ophthalmoscopy is used to detect angle recessions (Litel, 1990a).

Retinal tears occur from globe distortion, traditionally a *contrecoup* mechanism whereby the abnormal stretch which results in tears or which detaches the retina from its contiguous tissues (most often the vitreous base). Vision loss may be temporary or permanent to varying degrees. Early surgery is the best treatment.

Other serious ocular injuries encountered with some frequency in boxing include subluxation of the lens which may result in late glaucoma or cataract formation, and blow-out fractures of the orbit (Litel, 1990a). The latter may be signalled by enophthalmos, diplopia (because of an entrapped orbital fracture), anaesthesia of the lower lid and cheek, and of course, X-ray evidence. The treatment is usually surgical (Litel, 1990a).

Among the more than 400 USA Army Hospital admissions studied by Enzenauer *et al.* (1989), 4% had an ocular injury as the primary cause of admission. The major diagnoses included open wounds of the adnexa, optic nerve injury, orbital floor fractures, eye avulsion and globe and retinal disorders. Hruby (1979) reported five cases of retinal detachment due to boxing, of which four went blind. During 40 years as a physician for the London Amateur Boxing Association, Blonstein alleged to have observed only four cases of detached retina (1969). Yet in a study of 55 former fighters with an average age of 59 years, angle deformities were observed by Palmer *et al.* (1976) in almost 10% and retinal detachments in 7%. A series of photographs depicting true and simulated pathology of boxers is demonstrated in Fig. 38.23.

Jones (1989) provides a perspective of the discrepancies which have existed with respect to frequency of ocular injuries in boxing. He cites Whiteson (1981) (Chief Medical Officer of the British Boxing Board of Control as well as of the WBC) as having suggested a meager incidence of retinal injuries occur in boxing and McCown (1959a,b) as having found less than 0.2% incidence of eye injuries in a large population of boxers. These are cited in comparison to the report of Giovinazzo *et al.* (1987) who found vision-threatening injuries in 58% of 74 professional boxers (see below). The discrepancy is largely explained on the basis of the more sophisticated ophthalmological examinations provided by Giovinazzo *et al.* In fact, Delrowe, a co-author of the work presented by Giovinazzo *et al.*, presented the alarming results of their study at a research meeting of the WBC (1987), where he discussed the implications with Whiteson. Most importantly, the implication to be appreciated from the disparate results of existing studies is the importance of creating a minimal standard of ophthalmological examination without which the prophylactic value of examinations is lost.

The ocular study reported by Giovinazzo *et al.* (1987) must now be considered the classical study by which others are to be measured. Giovinazzo *et al.* examined every seventh boxer seeking licensure in New York State. It is noteworthy that all examinees were allegedly asymptomatic and that no previous study undertook as extensive an eye examination. The examination included not only refraction, anterior segment slit-lamp study, applanation tonometry and gonioscopy, but also a dilated examination of the retina which included indirect ophthalmoscopy with scleral depression, and Goldmann three-mirror contact lens evaluation of the macula. Findings were matched against historical data for correlations. In all, 75 boxers were examined with an age range between 16 and 42 years. At least one pathological alteration was found in 66%. Vision-threatening injuries, i.e. those of the peripheral retina, macula, lens or angle, were present in 58%; and bilateral vision-threatening injuries were found in 28%. Of particular importance, according to the authors, was that many of the vision-threatening injuries were detected at a treatable stage.

With respect to specific lesions, it was noted that retinal damage increased significantly after six bouts or two losses (Fig. 38.24) and that peripheral retinal tears were present in almost a quarter of boxers examined. The contusion angle deformity, a characteristic lesion in boxers, was present in a little less than 20% or about at the same rate as in the study of Palmer *et al.* (16%) (1976).

Angle abnormalities, though alleged to result in glaucoma, had produced none in the study of Palmer *et al.* (1976). A 19% incidence of cataracts was observed by Giovinazzo *et al.* (1987), who did not ascribe any quantity to angle deformities but, who indicated that 13% were of a posterior subcapsular variety not previously reported.

Vision training

Excellence in sports is a multifactorial entity which includes talent, training, dedication and the avoidance of disability due to injury. Boxing is no different in these considerations, the latter of which being a major reason for having created the Spar Foundation.

Boxing, like virtually all sports, requires vision in order to perform. It is a given, therefore, that vision and participation in sports have a direct relationship. Yet vision, other than the ability to see, has been given little attention as a component among factors in sports excellence. Vision, however, is a component of talent and is to some degree trainable, as are the muscles of the body. Vision should not be construed to mean simple visual acuity (e.g. whether one has 20/20 eyesight). There are many subtleties of vision. In 1985, Blundell of Australia (1985) performed studies

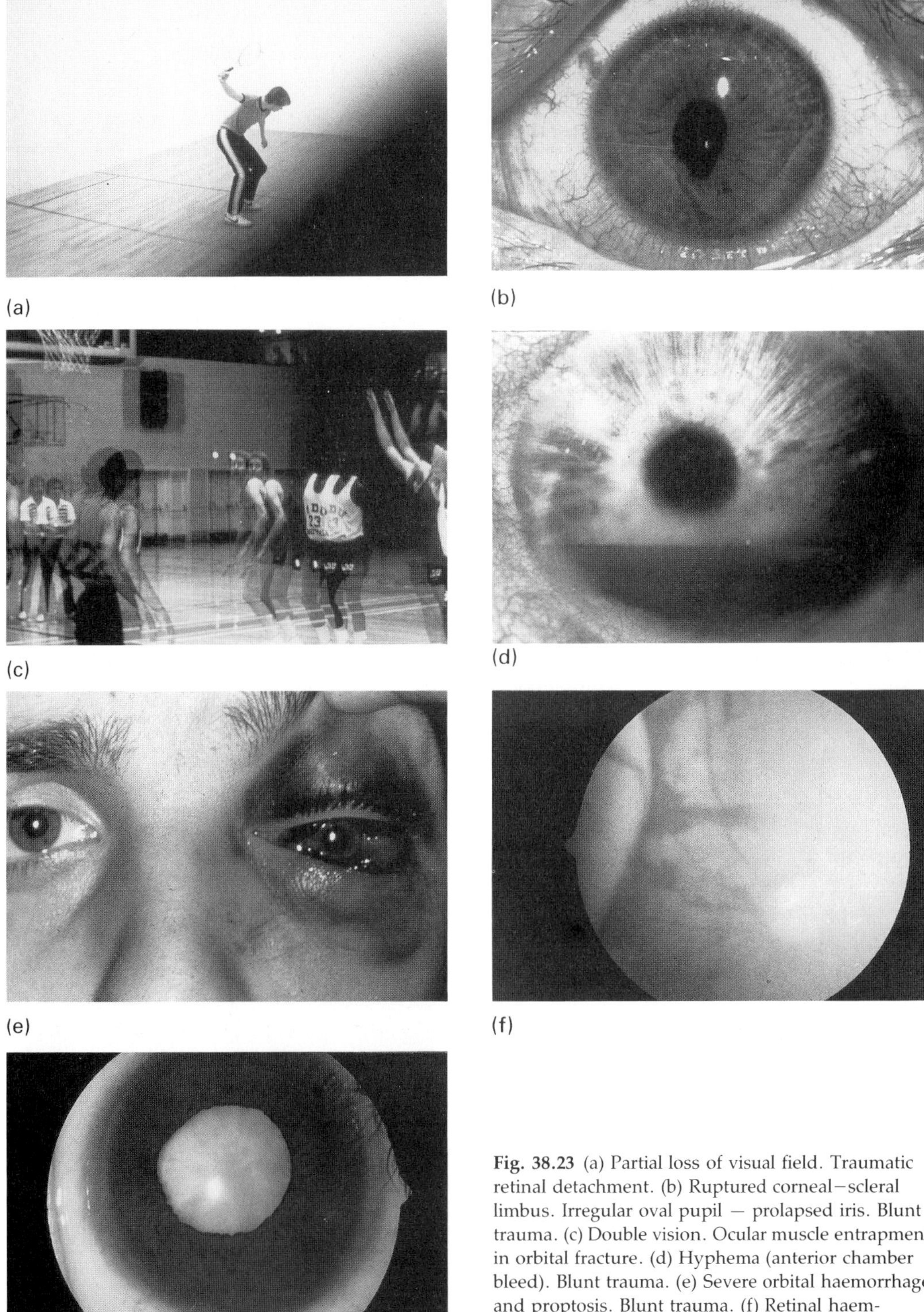

Fig. 38.23 (a) Partial loss of visual field. Traumatic retinal detachment. (b) Ruptured corneal–scleral limbus. Irregular oval pupil — prolapsed iris. Blunt trauma. (c) Double vision. Ocular muscle entrapment in orbital fracture. (d) Hyphema (anterior chamber bleed). Blunt trauma. (e) Severe orbital haemorrhage and proptosis. Blunt trauma. (f) Retinal haemorrhage/detachment. Blunt trauma. (g) Mature white cataract. Irregular pupil. Blunt trauma. Courtesy of the American Academy of Ophthalmology.

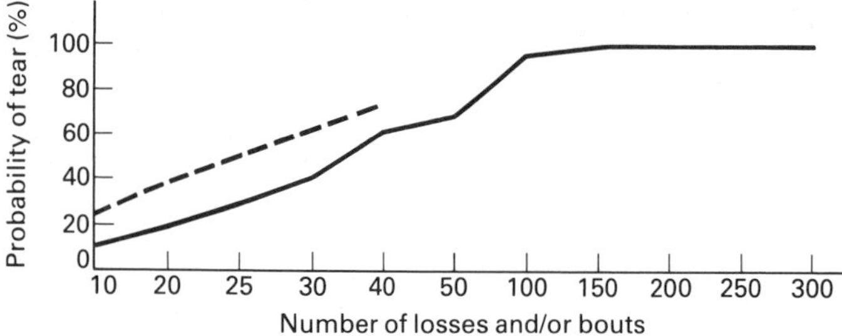

Fig. 38.24 Composite graphs adapted from the results of Giovinazzo *et al.* (1987), demonstrating the increasing probability of developing retinal tears as the number of bouts (———) and/or losses (– – – –) increases.

which proved that multiple visual parameters have an influence on athletic performance.

The role of vision in sports has been grossly understudied. Ophthalmologists have largely avoided sports vision research until recently, so that most of the studies to date have been undertaken by optometrists, or non-physician eye experts. In considering the visual aspects of sports, it became quickly evident that there are an almost overwhelming number of elements and variables.

First of all, it should be recognized that there are many types of vision. The simple eye chart (Snellen type) is too unsophisticated to help much with sports performance. Three-dimensional vision, visual speed, peripheral vision and contrast sensitivity, are among the specialized tests which may define sport-specific visual needs.

The type of sport being performed is very important with respect to which type of vision is being evaluated or trained. Running a sprint requires very little visual ability. Ice-hockey players need good peripheral vision, eye 'reading' speed and three-dimensional visual ability. In baseball, visual speed in a tunnelized form is needed to hit a ball pitched at high velocity, and better peripheral vision is needed on the side of the face turned toward the mound. A variable in this regard is the issue of training. For a given sport, we know that sport-specific training is helpful — but for some sports, visual training may be as, or more important than physical training.

Eye training for many sports, boxing included, may produce better performance results. While there is little, if any, objective evidence that visual training accomplishes this end, anecdotal evidence abounds. At the very least, such training seems to enhance the player's ability to concentrate. Examples of training techniques specific to a sport are provided in Figs 38.25 & 38.26. Spiral discs are used to train hockey goalkeepers (Fig. 38.25). Concentration upon the centre of the spiral allegedly leaves the goalkeeper with the illusion that the real puck is larger than it actually is. Figure 38.26 demonstrates a long tube along the length of which is a series of small light bulbs. A baseball batter, as an example, stands at one end, and a sequence of light is directed toward the player from the opposite end. One

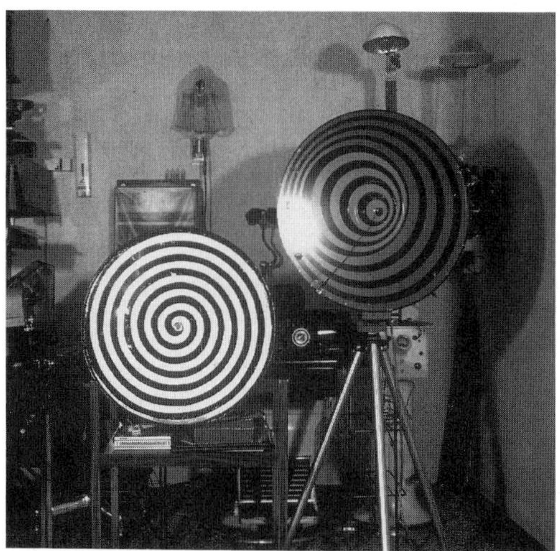

Fig. 38.25 Training spiral (see text).

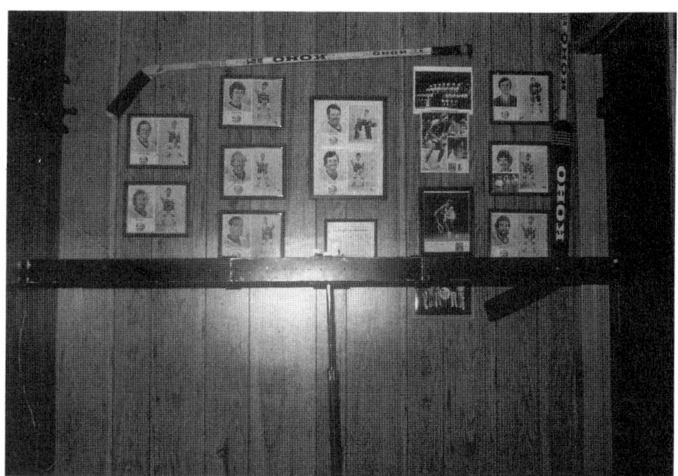

Fig. 38.26 Linear vision training device (see text).

light bulb after another is illuminated, so that the speed at which the sequence of lightings is propagated may exceed 160 $km \cdot h^{-1}$ (100 $mile \cdot h^{-1}$), likening it to a pitched fast ball. The player pushes a button when the impulse reaches his or her eye and the 'response time' is electronically recorded.

Whether such gimmicks help by increasing eye ability, by increasing concentration (as when learning how to speed read), or by increasing athlete confidence is not really known. In a way, boxing uses sparring and defence mitts to try to accomplish the same thing.

Thus far, an awareness has been developed of the complex role of vision in athletics, and of the possible need for 'eyerobics'. The relation of fitness to visual ability and boxer defence must still be considered, a subject which is quite controversial. In 1978, Bard and Fleury found that bicycle exhaustion had no effect upon three assigned mental tasks. In 1981, Fleury and Bard revealed vision was not affected by exhaustive activity in a very 'fit' population.

In 1986, Hancock and McNaughton revealed that fatigue impairs our ability to process visual information, and in 1987 Fleury and Bard did additional studies and restated that the physically fit can tolerate fatigue better than the unfit, having used vision as a test. The discrepancies amongst the studies cited are undoubtedly due to differences in the visual tests used, more sophisticated ones having evolved in the era of high-tech medicine. It should be understood that visual ability and athlete reaction are not totally integrated nor segregated entities. A recent study by Harbin *et al.* (1989) which set about evaluating oculomotor responses also reviews the subject of visual test components. First of all, they define response time as the speed with which an athlete can react to a stimulus (whether it is a punch or a pitched baseball). They define the oculomotor response time as a measure of the athlete's ability to repetitively analyse a complex stimulus and respond appropriately with a complex movement. In consists of a reaction time (the visual part) and a movement time (the muscle part). Reaction time is the time from a stimulus to the beginning of the muscle response. It has two components, a sensing time, which relates to visual ability, and a decision time which relates to the function of the brain. Visual reaction times are about 0.5 s. Movement time is the muscle part and extends from the end of the reaction time to the completion of the task (e.g. giving or ducking a punch).

Some years ago the senior author (J.M.) interviewed the great, now deceased, trainer, Cus D'Amato. In explaining why none of his many fighters were not knocked out during a more than 10-year period, D'Amato unwittingly revealed principles of reaction and response time improvement, i.e. visual training. He claimed that a gun fighter of the wild west would win a shoot-out if he learned to watch the shoulder of his opponents' gun-hand. Once the shoulder would move, the hand would follow next, and quickly. He repeatedly taught his fighters the same visual training tactic as a defensive protection, in a sense, increasing their visual concentration and response time.

To perform their study, Harbin *et al.* (1989) used a test board with coloured panels. The panels are linked to a colour television and a computer. When the television shows a colour (visual cue), the athlete steps on the panel of the same colour and the computer records the reaction time. Sequences of 30 colour flashes are made on the screen for each test. Football players, basketball players and others at the college and professional levels were tested before and after the season.

One result was that reaction times of college basketball players were improved after a season of playing. Élite athletes had superior oculomotor response patterns compared to less accomplished athletes (for sports studied). The implication of the result of preseason and postseason testing of the basketball players is that training can improve response. The issue is what training is best for any given sport.

Vision evaluation

The implications of a visual response enhancement programme, that might improve the defence of boxers, is self-evident. With evidence that even subconcussive blows can produce EEG abnormalities (LaCava, 1963) or accrued sequelae (Unterhernscheidt, 1970; Gronwall & Wrightson, 1975), the ability of the boxer to evade even one such blow every few sparring sessions or bouts, may well help to preserve the brain over the length of a career.

Thus far, the issue of fatigue as a deterrent to effective performance, and the supposition that visual training may improve performance (and defence, in the case of boxers) have been discussed. Visual testing may, in fact, have other roles with respect to boxing. It has been established in foregoing sections that no currently available diagnostic test is reliable in the early detection of brain damage (except in cases of acute severe head trauma and when an extensive battery of neuropsychological testing is performed). To a degree, the same may be said for the detection of ocular pathology when frequent and extensive testing (of a type discussed in the section on ocular pathology) is not performed.

With respect to other methods of screening that may provide an early (and perhaps ringside) suspicion of brain or eye pathology, special visual testing is, and has for several years, been a consideration by SPAR (Safety Performance Advancement through Research, a UCLA-based scientific foundation of the WBC). To this end, the foundation, in its efforts to underwrite research for the protection of boxers, provided a grant to determine the potential value of testing 'contrast sensitivity'.

Visual images can be broken down into basic sine wave components consisting of two elements: (i) spatial frequency, which corresponds to the size of an image; and (ii) amplitude, which corresponds to the contrast of an image.

The visual system uses different groups of nerve cells called channels, each sensitive to a narrow range of images, sizes and contrasts. An individual may be tested for ability in the various ranges by using a series of contrast images which the individual analyses by looking through a binocular system (Figs 38.27 & 38.28). Graphic displays of eye contrast performance are thus created (Fig. 38.29) to determine existing abnormalities for future comparisons. Contrast sensitivity provides a powerful measure of function because it tests all visual channels using different spatial frequencies of varying contrast in a manner similar to the way hearing is tested with different sound frequencies of varying volume.

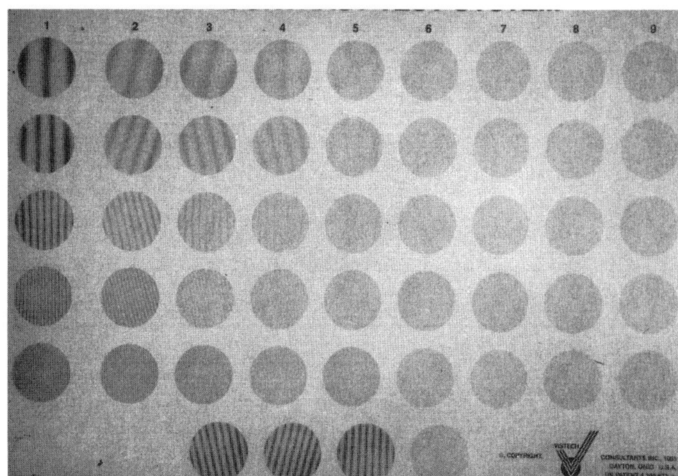

Fig. 38.27 Palette of contrast images used for testing contrast perceiving abilities of the subject.

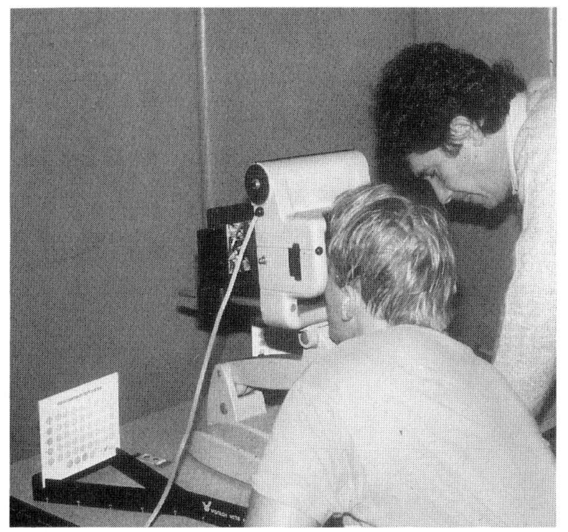

Fig. 38.28 Contrast image palettes are viewed by subjects through the pictured binocular viewer.

In professional basketball, there is one player known to the authors, whose shooting percentage drops dramatically each time he plays in a certain city where there is different illumination than in the rest of the league. This is probably due to the phenomenon of contrast sensitivity. An analogous circumstance in boxing may be in outdoor bouts at twilight, where the lighting is less uniform than it is with indoor fights. Preliminary testing revealed that a contrast test could be administered in a span as short as 20 s and might even be considered for use between rounds. Contrast sensitivity testing in boxing was considered worthwhile because contrast is critical to all visual function, is altered by brain and eye dysfunction, and because head stress may cause losses in the 6–12 cycles·degree^{-1} range. It was considered for use because contrast baselines may define normal, safe and abnormal levels of function; it may detect losses of protective visual reflexes, and might even reveal a return to normalcy in postknock-out states.

Studies were undertaken with the assistance of the USA Military Academy at West Point. The first phase dealt with determining the validity of visual screening for fatigue. The premise of the study was that fatigue can reduce a fighter's defences and the study used contrast sensitivity as a determinant. Subsequently, contrast ranges defining eye damage and brain damage will also be studied.

Thirty male cadets with no eye damage, a uniformly superior cardiovascular status, and perfect compliance were subjected to a modified Bruce protocol of graded treadmill exercise, used to bring the cadets to exhaustion. Each cadet was contrast tested before the treadmill and after exhaustion.

While there was a reduction in contrast ability after exhaustion, compared to the pre-

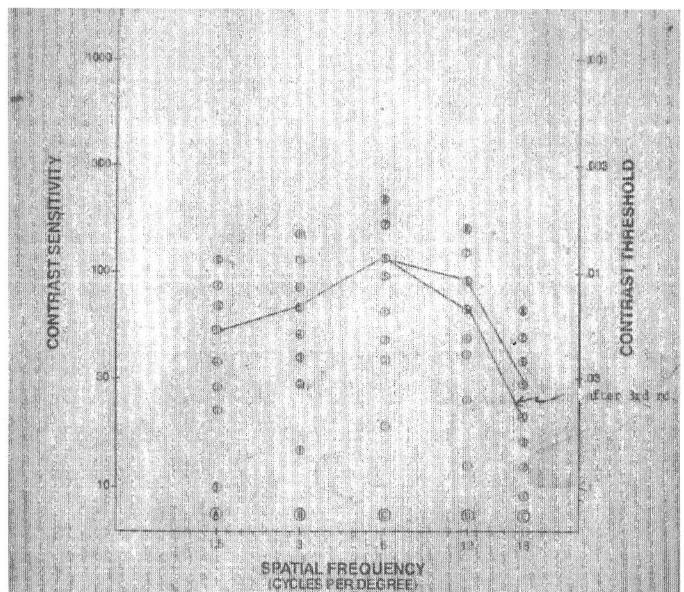

Fig. 38.29 Graphic results of contrast testing using the Vistech system.

treadmill tests, the differences were not statistically significant at a high enough level. Nevertheless, the implication of the trend, and its implication with respect to progressive fatigue and loss of defence during a bout was one of the inducements for the WBA to reduce championship fights from 15 to 12 rounds (based on a presentation of this data to the WBA in Costa Rica, October 1986). Permission has been pending to pursue visual testing in boxers before, during and after their bouts.

It seems clear that the role of 'special' vision as a diagnostic and therapeutic entity has not been worked out as yet. It also seems clear that it can and should play an important role in boxing, assuming its survival.

Orthopaedic injuries

McCown (1959a) reviewed the incidence of boxing injuries among professionals in New York State from 1952 through 1958 (Table 38.8). Apart from lacerations, contusions and concussions, it is apparent that musculoskeletal problems represent a small minority of the injuries. Many of the orthopaedic injuries in boxers are probably not reported. The present authors' experience with professional fighters over a few year span during which boxers were seen only occasionally, revealed a greater array of entities than those reported by McCown (1959a) over a 7-year period in an era when boxers fought more often and with less specialized medical screening.

Table 38.8 Incidence of boxing injuries in McCown's 1959 study of professional boxers in New York State, 1952–1958 (n = 11 173). From McCown (1959a).

Eye injuries	Cornea	13
	Retina	6
Orthopaedic injuries	Metacarpals	14
	Ankle	1
	Boxer's knuckle	18
	Shoulder dislocation	4

1 Injury to the pericostal muscles of the lower lateral rib area similar to that sustained by the American football quarterback who is hit when the arm is cocked, creating a sudden stretch of the ipsilateral torso.

2 Injury to the posterior rotator cuff muscles and rhomboids secondary to a forceful hook swing. While shoulder dislocations are reported occasionally, it must be presumed that there are many instances of shoulder instability with cuff or labral tears. This includes posterior instability fostered by missing the mark with a forceful punch, or punching an immovable object with recoil propagation of force to the posterior aspect of the shoulder.

3 Posterior impingement manifestations of the elbow related to sudden and exaggerated extension with jabbing.

4 Wrist pain with an ununited fracture of the carpal scaphoid.

5 A grade II rupture of the medial collateral ligament sustained by valgus leverage on the knee when being knocked over by an opponent's punch.

6 Transverse fracture of the distal phalanx of the thumb in a standard (not thumbless) glove.

7 A 'boxer's knuckle' unresolved with rest, splinting, and special padding. Successful surgery for this entity was described over 30 years ago by Gladden (1957). In this instance an instability of the third metacarpophalangeal joint was evident in addition to the typical thickening of the extensor hood tissues, retinacular rent, and varying degrees of articular surface dessication or fracture (see below).

8 Recently a WBA, WBC and USA Boxing Association title holder postponed a fight due to patellar tendinitis.

Hand injuries

When boxing was born during the first millennium BC the hands were wrapped with a 3-m long thong which extended up onto the forearm. This was later modified to a hard thong, thickened at the knuckle area. The Romans ultimately introduced the *'caestus'*, a sadistic modification of the antiquitous glove, which bore metal spikes about the knuckles. Boxing then largely disappeared from the annals of history until the nineteenth century when the 'bare-fisted era' became a vogue in England. Chambers not only offered 'his rules' but designed an animal hair-filled glove (1867). A foam rubber glove was introduced in this century and, in essence, has not been modified other than by its availability in different weights (Noble, 1987). Nowhere in this evolution of glove designs is there evidence of a scientific effort to preclude injury to the hand (nor reduction of impact to the opponent).

Noble (1987) concurs that boxing gloves have not evolved scientifically. In his study of 100 consecutive boxing hand injuries, he divided the hand and wrist into three zones each of which contributed an almost equal quantity of injuries (Fig. 38.30). Area A includes the 1st ray: thumb, metacarpal, greater multiangular and scaphoid. Injuries are sustained because the thumb is separate in most gloves and because the thumb cannot be locked in a fully fisted position. Abduction injuries are common. Area A accounted for 39% of all injuries. Area B includes the bases of metacarpals 2–5. This group accounted for 35% of the hand injuries in Noble's study, the majority of which were sprains of carpometacarpal junctions, often re-

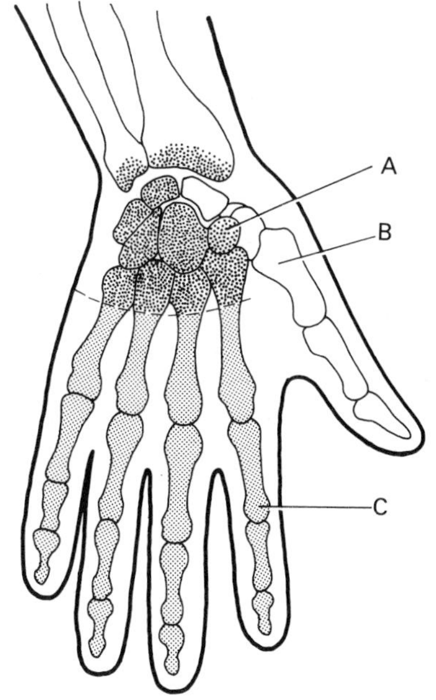

Fig. 38.30 Three areas of the hand involved in injuries recorded by Noble (1987). For an explanation of A–C, see text.

sulting in bossing. The mechanism again relates to the inability to make a firm fist (Fig. 38.31). Hook punches allow the hyperflexion flexes to act upon an inadequately supported wrist.

Area C, incorporating the distal portion of metacarpals 2–5 and the phalanges, accounted for 26% of injuries. Commonly seen in this group were metacarpal and phalangeal fractures and the ever common 'boxer's knuckles'. Fractures of the necks of metacarpals 4 and 5 are typical; (and are alluded to as 'boxer's fractures') as are boxer's knuckles involving metacarpals 2 and 3 (see below). Clearly, the present gloves allow stress concentrations in these areas. A summary of hand injuries observed by Noble is presented in Tables 38.9a–c (Noble, 1987).

The most serious hand injuries with respect to their potential to produce ultimate disability are the fractures and dislocations of the carpus. Ligamentous repairs and/or carpal fusions or fixations and grafting may be required, but can only be undertaken if the lesions are detected. Detection may require special radiography, i.e. cinetomoarthrography, stress views, bone scans, CT or MRI.

The 'boxer's knuckle', a seemingly innocuous entity at the outset, can progress toward becoming a disabling entity. Unfortunately, physicians often comply with the boxer's request to inject these knuckles with steroidal suspensions, allowing the boxer to continue participation, and at the same time, fostering a

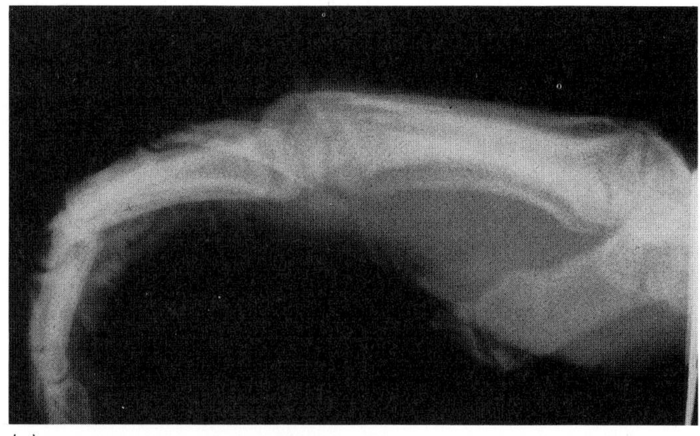

(a)

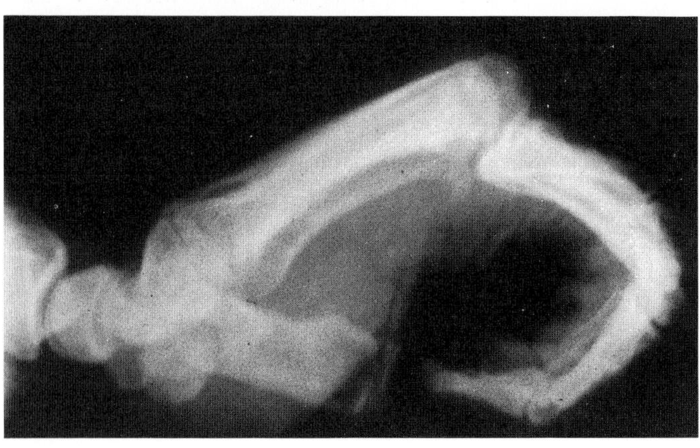

(b)

Fig. 38.31 Lateral X-rays of the hand wearing a standard boxing glove. (a) No problem is evident with hand in extension. However, with fist clenched (b), the 3rd metacarpal head stands proud and it is this joint which is most afflicted with 'boxer's knuckle'. Courtesy of Dr C. Melone.

Table 38.9 A Distribution of hand injuries by area (see Fig. 38.30). Adapted from Noble (1987).
(a) Injury distribution in area A.

Injury	No. and % (n = 100)
Tearing of ulnar collateral ligament of metacarpophalangeal joint of thumb	23
Injuries to carpometacarpal joint of thumb (traumatic synovitis, dislocation, Bennett's fracture)	10
Various fractures	4
base of metacarpal	2
base of proximal phalanx	1
shaft of metacarpal	1
Fractured scaphoid	2
Total	39

(b) Injury distribution in area B.

Injury	No. and % (n = 100)
Inflammation of carpometacarpal joint	12
Subluxation of one or more metacarpal bases	12
Dislocation of bases of metacarpals 2 and 3	1
Fracture/dislocation of bases of metacarpals 2, 3 and 4	1
Sprained wrists with diffuse swelling and tenderness (negative roentgenograms)	3
Fractures of base of metacarpal	6
Total	35

(c) Injury distribution in area C.

Injury	No. and % (n = 100)
Synovitis	12
Fractured neck of metacarpal	8
Fractured shaft of metacarpal	3
Fractured proximal phalanx	3
Total	26

progression of damage. The most comprehensive early description of the 'boxer's knuckle' was that of Gladden (1957) (Fig. 38.32).

Posner and Ambrose (1989) indicate that 'boxer's knuckle' is synonymous with rupture of the dorsal capsule of a metacarpophalangeal joint. They reported on six cases, five of which were sustained from punching with a clenched fist. In each instance there was an initial period of pain which resolved within days but with recurrence of pain and swelling after each sparring session. In each case, a palpable defect (in the dorsal capsule) was felt over the joint. After the failure of non-operative management, surgery confirmed the capsular rupture; and after surgery, boxing was forbidden for no less than 6 months.

In each case reported by Posner and Ambrose (1989), the location of the capsular tear was in the capsule of the metacarpophalangeal joint of either the index or middle finger. Evidently, this localization is due to the manner in which the punch is delivered to the impacting surface within the glove. Deficient padding may be a contributing factor. Professional fight hand wraps are flimsy, but not as limited as in the amateur ranks. In international amateur competition only a yard of muslim is permitted as a wrap.

Prevention of injuries

There is no stronger form of protective prevention than abstinence. The cry to abolish boxing has grown more vociferous in each of the past few decades. Recommendations to ban boxing are now voiced by the American Medical Association, the British Medical Association, the Canadian Medical Association, the Australian Medical Association and the World Medical Association (Enzenauer & Mauldin, 1989); but the century old tradition of modern boxing, thrill-seeking, a gladiator-fixated public, and the economic thrust of the sport have helped withstand the mounting attacks. For the time being, other protective measures must be sought.

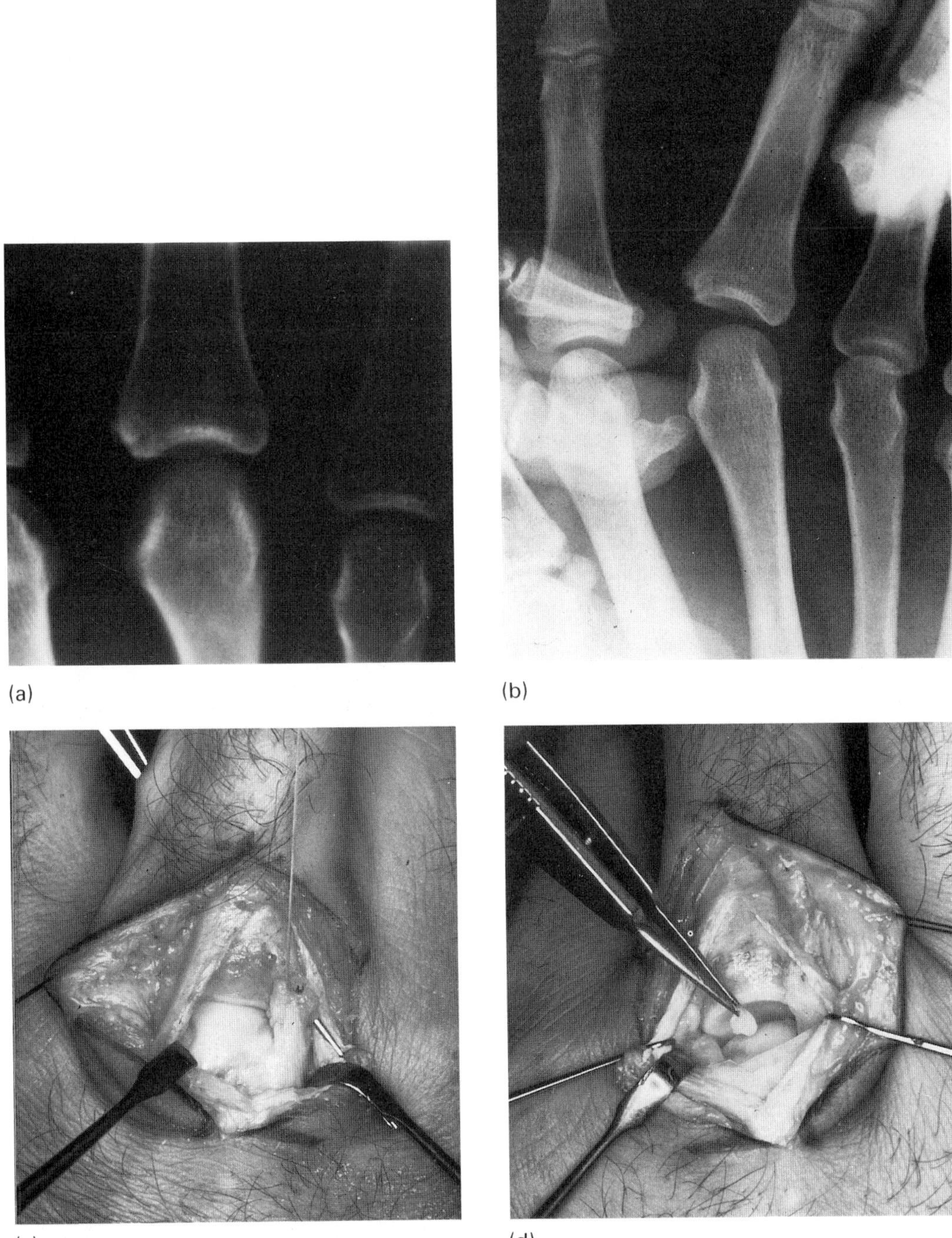

(a) (b) (c) (d)

Fig. 38.32 (a) Anterioposterior X-rays of a number 1 contender with 'boxer's knuckle'; close scrutiny and magnification demonstrates an irregularity of the radial side of the proximal phalanx near the 3rd metacarpophalangeal joint (left hand). (b) Stress views of the 3rd metacarpophalangeal joint reveals a severe sprain and laxity of the radial collateral ligament of the left hand. (c) Intraoperative photograph reveals reduction of avulsed fragment and reinsertion of radial collateral ligament with pin fixation. (d) A chondral body not infrequently found in the boxer's knuckle. Courtesy of Dr C. Melone.

Since the damage of greatest concern is concentrated on the brain and eyes, these structures should be the focus of prevention. To eliminate blows to the head would change the character of the sport, a prospect unlikely to find acceptability among its sponsors or spectators. The creation of protective equipment for these areas has long been considered. Head gear designed to reduce the force of blows to the head and ears has been used in sparring, the latter accounting for the majority of the pugilist's ring time. There is reasonable doubt as to the efficacy of such head gear. In fact, Guterman and Smith (1987) raise the prospect that such head gear is detrimental, providing unwarranted security and enlarging the target (head), to permit the reception of blows which might otherwise miss or harmlessly glance off the scalp.

It is abundantly clear that the eyes are at great risk in boxing, consequent to repeated blunt trauma; whether by a *coup*, *contrecoup* or equatorial expansion mechanism, the occurrence of retinal detachments and a gamut of adnexal pathology precludes fighting in most amateur and professional organizations. However, the pathology first must be detected, and by the appropriate examinations. Citing a survey by ophthalmologists, the British Medical Association reported that retinal detachments were the most frequently seen eye afflictions in boxing (46% among eye injuries reported) (Brayne *et al.*, 1982). Proper examinations can detect these commonly reported retinal detachments, and surgery can be performed to reattach them. Still, the reports of Maguire and Benson (1986) suggest that redetachments are realistic concerns. Risk to the eye is maximally reduced by not fighting again.

Moved by the alarming percentage of vision-threatening lesions detected in one or both eyes of boxers in a totally asymptomatic population, Giovinazzo *et al.* (1987) listed recommendations to promote ocular safety in boxing. These are adapted in Table 38.10.

The creation of eye protective equipment seems unacceptable. Its design would have to be such that transmission of force is not shuttled to the brain and skull. Only a full-scale helmet armed with a face shield or cage (as in ice hockey) would fit the 'protective bill', and obviously, this format is not practicable.

Table 38.10 Recommendations for ocular safety in boxing. Adapted from Giovinazzo *et al.* (1987).

There should be a registry for all amateur and professional boxers and sparring partners with a computerized data base to identify injury trends and their responses to rule changes and innovations

Ringside physicians should be meticulously educated with respect to boxing eye injuries and their detection and treatment

Define what injuries should stop a match

All organizations should use a thumbless glove. Ubiquitous rules should exist for ocular examination. Examination should include the same elements required by the Vision Safety and Performance Committee of the US Olympic Committee:
- (a) initial examination: visual acuity, visual fields, slit-lamp biomicroscopy, intraocular pressure measurement, gonioscopy, and a dilated vitreoretinal examination including ophthalmoscopy with scleral depression
- (b) repeat examinations: should be mandated whenever the following has transpired: (i) the passage of a year; (ii) six bouts; (iii) two losses; and (iv) the stoppage of a fight due to ocular injury
- (c) mandatory suspensions: 60 days for retinal tears that have been treated

An ophthalmologist should serve on every boxing advisory board

Taking into account the unlikely prospect that the basic format of the sport will change, modifications of equipment and/or rules are avenues to pursue. Equipment has changed little during the twentieth century. In the past decade, in particular, there has been a movement toward the thumbless glove, to avert both penetrating injuries to the eyes and abduction sprains and fractures of the thumb. Mandates for mouth protectors have reduced damage to the teeth and ostensibly to the brain. The creation of gloves of different weights may have been of benefit, but no study has proven it. Ear protectors for sparring (professionals) or for bouts (amateurs) have reduced the incidence of 'cauliflower ears'. The nature of the glove, inclusive of its construction materials, has been neither altered nor adequately studied to see if a glove can be created to minimize head impact while preserving the hand.

Rule modifications have been plentiful over the years. The limited allowable contact zone of the glove and the defensive emphasis of amateur boxing are positive examples. Rules imposed in the past few decades by professional organizations, such as the WBC, including a limit on fight frequency, no fights for specified periods after knock-outs, standardized medical evaluations for fighters, and others, have furthered the relative safety of the boxer. Certainly, if there are limits to the institution of true prevention, efforts should be directed toward the minimization of progression of pathology.

To inhibit a progression of pathology, the pathology must be detectable by available testing. Unfortunately, this is not always the case. Expertise of physicians, laboratories, neurological, neuro-ophthalmological and neuropsychiatric testing is not always available at the needed levels, especially in the Third World nations. Subtle pathology, furthermore, is not always detectable, even by the most sophisticated testing.

Guterman and Smith (1987) suggest that in addition to a thorough history taking and physical examination, necessary evaluations for boxers include an EEG with at least 16 channels recorded in both the waking and sleeping states, CT of the brain with and without contrast, and a formal battery of neuropsychological testing. They use the revised Wechsler adult intelligence scale, Boston naming test, controlled oral word association test, Benton visual retention test, Wechsler memory scale, Ravens coloured progressive matrices, trail-making and the Halsted–Raitan tests. In addition, Giovinazzo *et al.* (1987) indicate that the following ophthalmological tests be performed for thoroughness and is required by the Vision Safety and Performance Committee of the USA Olympic Committee:

1 Visual acuity.
2 Visual fields.
3 Slit-lamp biomicroscopy.
4 Intraocular pressure measurement.
5 Gonioscopy.
6 Dilated vitreoretinal examination with:
(a) indirect ophthalmoscopy, and
(b) scleral depression.

Guterman and Smith (1987) contend that such complete testing be performed at least yearly and that any evidence of irreversible neurological deficits ought to mandate the end of a fighter's career.

In view of the relationship between head trauma and the development of meningiomas, any boxer with focal neurological symptoms should be evaluated for brain tumour (Guterman & Smith, 1987).

Educational programmes for referees and ringside physicians are conducted within most fight organizations. Despite the education of these officials, fights are often allowed to progress even when a fighter has entered an amnestic state. The tools with which the boxer may protect against blows include a knowledge of defence and deflection, quickness of body and limb, and perhaps, strong neck musculature to damp the recoil of the head. However, when the fighter is fatigued or in an amnestic state, these protective tools are gone, even the energy-absorbing capacity of the cervical musculature.

Table 38.11 Medical organization and responsibilities to USA/ABF system. Adapted from Voy (1990b).

Ringside physician or osteopath
Ambulance available
Resuscitation equipment and stretcher
Crowd control: police or security
Medical treatment area
Referral hospital with CT scanner
Subspecialists on call, e.g. neurosurgeon
Physician evaluation of:
ring condition, paddings, etc.
boxer's head guards, gloves, genital cups
ringside table and chair with clear view

CT, computerized tomography.

Table 38.12 Examination of the head and face. Adapted from Colpitts (1990).

Airway injury may be heralded by stridor, subcutaneous emphysema in neck, or contusion over the larynx
Asymmetry of the face can be due to haematoma, facial fractures, ptosis and other neurological injuries
Fractures of the medial orbital wall will produce periorbital subcutaneous emphysema from ethmoid sinus air upon forced exhalation with the nostrils pinched
Malocclusion should raise suspicion of a fracture of the mandible or maxilla
The ears should be inspected for a fractured pinna or otorhoea
All facial fractures and all lacerations of the ear cartilage and the oral cavity require antibiotic treatment because they are either 'open' or 'dirty'

Clearly, the responsible intervention of fight officials can be improved upon. It would be of immense help, of course, if high-tech rapid methods of ringside testing could be performed which would reveal the presence of the amnestic state, grogginess or defencelessness and with which no official nor any contestant could argue.

The bottomline for boxers is that the more numerous the bouts and the more protracted the career, the greater is the likelihood of incurring irreversible neurological damage. Limiting the frequency of bouts (and sparring round) would constitute a great preventive measure. Discussions have ensued regarding the fixing of an age beyond which fighters must retire by mandate. This has held little appeal in the professional ranks.

Among the benefits of international amateur boxing is that compliance to one set of medical and protective rules is necessary for participation.

In testimony to the exceptional progress made by the amateur boxing organizations in preparing and training boxing physicians for their ringside duties are Tables 38.2, 38.3, 38.11–38.13, which have been extracted from the USA/ABF physician's certification manual (Voy, 1990b). These tables represent just a sample of the information contained within the manual.

Medical rules vary among professional organizations at state, provincial and international levels. The absence of a single unifying medical formula is a health detriment. In fact, the pro-

Table 38.13 Suggested list of items for physicians to carry when outside the USA on USA/ABF trips.

Diagnostic
- ophthalmoscope
- otoscope
- small flashlight or penlight
- stethoscope
- sphygmodynamometer
- thermometer
- nasal speculum

Instruments (a sterile suture kit is preferred. Disposable kits are available and acceptable)
- disposable suture kits
- forceps
- 'new skin' or collodion
- scissors
- steristrips
- sutures
- scalpels (disposable)
- sterile gloves
- non-sterile gloves

Orthopaedic
- finger splints
- adhesive tape
- ace bandage
- soft neck collar
- ankle splint (handy but not necessary)

Miscellaneous
- Betadine and/or alcohol sponges
- syringes
- needles
- anaesthetic (local), Xylocaine 1% or 2%
- airways, at least one large, one medium (adolescent size)
- oral screw
- tongue depressors
- plastic zip-loc bags (for ice bags)
- dressings
- eye patch
- sticking-plaster
- gauze sponge (4 × 4)
- roll-type gauze or Kling
- cotton-tip applicators, sterile and non-sterile
- razors (boxers must be clean shaven)

fessional organization with the most stringent and protective rules is at a potential disadvantage. A fighter of stature may be lost to that organization owing to its strict rules which prohibit fighting with a given disability that a competitive organization may deem an acceptable one.

What about mandatory counts? Is a 3-min round and 1-min hiatus the least dangerous format for boxers? Are the number of rounds a major, or even a minor, factor in the relative safety of the boxer? Such issues have never been truly explored by scientific or economic standards.

With respect to the hard-line abolitionists of boxing, the authors would concur that their arguments have cogency. The sport is unique in that its object is to inflict damage upon the foe. Brain and eye disease often result and may progress after the termination of a career. Most appalling of all is the spectre of sudden death.

On the other hand, it is a sport steeped in tradition with a major economic impact. Its contestants are not conscripted, but voluntarily participate for a variety of reasons which include escape from the ghetto, glory and financial reward. It is, indeed, a moving experience to hear the gratuitous speech of a boxer who has made it, claiming that even the risk of death was 'worth it' to side-step a community of drugs and to guarantee a life of security for parents, a wife, children and siblings. If there is a particular misgiving held by the authors in defence of this much maligned sport with a death-risk ratio less than mountaineering and hang-gliding (Reif, 1981), it is the lack of informed consent. To rectify this situation, the authors would suggest that each organization prepare a summary of published risks, liabilities and sequelae of boxing to be assimilated and signed by the prospective boxer (or guardians) prior to any formal participation. To more fairly segregate the differential bias which exists for amateur versus professional boxing, informed consent documents should be created based upon risk and morbidity statistics respective to each group. These documents should be re-evaluated for accuracy every few years.

References

Bard, C. & Fleury, M. (1978) Influence of imposed metabolic fatigue on visual capacity components. *Perceptual Motor Skills* **47**(3 Pt 2), 1283–7.

Beaussart, M. & Beaussart-Boulenge, L. (1970) 'Experimental' study of cerebral concussion in 123 amateur boxers, by clinical examination and EEG before and immediately after fights. *Electroenceph. Clin. Neurophysiol.* **29**, 529–30.

Blonstein, J.L. (1969) Boxing injuries. *J. Roy. Coll. Gen. Prac.* **18**, 100.

Blonstein, J.L. & Clarke, E. (1957) Further observations on the medical aspects of amateur boxing. *Br. Med. J.* **1**, 363–4.

Blundell, N.L. (1985) The contribution of vision to the learning and performance of sports skills: Part I: the role of selected visual parameters. *Australian J. Sci. Med. Sport* **17**(3), 3–11.

Brayne, C.E.G., Calloway, S.P., Dow, L. & Thompson, R.J. (1982) Blood creatine kinase isoenzyme BB in boxers. *Lancet* **ii**, 1308–9.

Busse, E.W. & Silverman, A.J. (1952) Electroencephalographic changes in professional boxers. *JAMA* **149**(17), 1522.

Casson, I.R., Sham, R., Campbell, E.A. *et al.* (1984) Brain damage in modern boxers. *JAMA* **251**, 2663–7.

Colpitts, R.W. (1990) Facial and oral injuries. In *USA/ABF Ringside Physician's Certificate Manual*, pp. 17–19. USA Amateur Boxing Federation, Colorado Springs.

Corsellis, J.A.N., Bruton, C.J. & Freeman-Browne, D. (1973) The aftermath of boxing. *Psychol. Med.* **3**, 270–303.

Courville, C.B. (1942) Coup–centrecoup mechanism of cranial cerebral injuries; some observations. *Arch. Surg.* **45**(1), 19–43.

Critchley, M. (1960) Medical aspects of boxing. *Trans. Med. Soc. Lond.* **76**, 12–26.

Cushing, H. & Eisenhardt, L. (1938) *Meningiomas: Their classification, Regional Behavior, Life History and Surgical End Results*. Charles C. Thomas, Springfield, Illinois.

Denny-Brown, D. & Russell, W.R. (1941) Experimental brain concussion. *Brain* **64**, 93–164.

Elia, J.C. (1962) Traumatic headache associated with the profession of boxing. *Headache* **2**, 138–46.

Enzenauer, R.W. & Mauldin, W.M. (1989) Boxing-related ocular injuries in the United States Army, 1980 to 1985, *South. Med. J.* **82**, 547–9.

Enzenauer, R.W., Montrey, J.S., Enzenauer, R.J. &

Mauldin, W.M. (1989) Boxing-related injuries in the US Army, 1980–1985. *JAMA* **261**(10), 463–6.

Estwanik, J.J., Boitano, M. & Ari, N. (1984) Amateur boxing injuries at the 1981 and 1982 USA/ABF national championships. *Phys. Sportsmed.* **12**, 123–8.

Ferguson, F.R. & Mawdsley, C. (1965) Chronic encephalopathy in boxers: Late sequelae of head injuries. In *Eighth International Congress of Neurology*, Vienna, pp. 81–4.

Fleury, M. & Bard, C. (1987) Effects of different types of physical acitivity on the performance of perceptual tasks in peripheral and central vision and coincident timing. *Ergonomics* **30**(6), 945–58.

Fleury, M., Bard, C., Jobin, J. & Carriere, L. (1981) Influence of different types of physical fatigue on a visual detection task. *Perceptual Motor Skills* **191**(3), 723–30.

Giovinazzo, V.J., Yannuzzi, L.A., Sorenson, J.A., Delrowe, D.J. & Cambell, E.A. (1987) The ocular complications of boxing. *Ophthalmology* **94**, 587–96.

Gladden, J.R. (1957) Boxer's knuckle. *Am. J. Surg.* **93**, 388.

Govens, S.R. (1968) Brain concussion and posture: The knockdown blow and the boxing ring. *Confinia Neurol.* **30**, 77–84.

Gronwall, D. & Wrightson, P. (1975) Cumulative effect of concussion. *Lancet* **ii**, 995–7.

Guardjian, E.S. & Webster, J.E. (1958) Head injuries in Sports. In *Head Injuries. Mechanisms, Diagnosis and Management*, pp. 348–56. Little, Brown & Co., Boston.

Guterman, A. & Smith, R.W. (1987) Neurological sequelae of boxing. *Sports Med.* **4**, 194–210.

Hancock, S. & McNaughton, L. (1986) Effects of fatigue on ability to process visual information by experienced orienteerers. *Perceptual Motor Skills* **62**, 491–8.

Handler, S.D. & Wetmore, R. (1982) Otolaryngologic injuries. *Clin. Sports Med.* **1**(3), 1431–47.

Harbin, G., Durst, L. & Harbin, D. (1989) Evaluation of oculomotor response in relationship to sports performance. *Med. Sci. Sports Exerc.* **21**(3), 258–62.

Hickey, J.C., Morris, A.L., Carlson, L.D. *et al.* (1967) The relation of mouth protectors to cranial pressure and deformation. *J. Am. Dent. Assoc.* **74**, 735.

Hildebrandt, J.R. (1982) Dental and maxillofacial injuries. *Clin. Sports Med.* **1**(3), 449–68.

Holbourn, A.H.S. (1943) Mechanics of head injuries. *Lancet* **ii**, 438–41.

Hruby, K. (1979) Netshautablosung Beim Boxsport (retinal detachment caused by boxing). *Klin. MBL. Augenheilk* **174**, 314.

Hughes, J.T. & Brownell, B. (1968) Traumatic thrombosis of the internal carotid artery in the neck. *J. Neurol. Neurosurg. Psych.* **31**, 307–14.

Isherwood, J., Mawdsley, C. & Ferguson, F.R. (1966) Pneumoencephalographic changes in boxers. *Acta Radiol.* **5**, 654–61.

Johnson, J., Skorecki, J. & Wells, R.P. (1975) Peak accelerations of the head experienced in boxing. *Med. Biol. Eng.* **13**(3), 396–404.

Jones, N.P. (1989) Eye injury in sport. *Sports Med.* **7**, 163–81.

Jordan, B.D. (1987) Neurological aspects of boxing. *Arch. Neurol.* **44**, 453–9.

Jordan, B.D. & Zimmerman, R.D. (1990) Computed tomography and magnetic resonance imaging comparisons in boxers. *JAMA* **263**(12), 1670–4.

Kaplan, H.A. & Browder, J. (1954) Observations on the clinical and brain wave patterns of professional boxers. *JAMA* **156**(12), 1138–44.

Kewalramani, L.S., Orth, M.S., Krauss, J.F. *et al.* (1981) Cervical spine injuries resulting from collision sports. *Paraplegia* **19**(Suppl.), 303.

LaCava, G. (1963) Boxer's encephalopathy. *J. Sports Med.* **3**, 87–92.

Lampert, P.W. & Hardman, J.M. (1984) Morphologic changes in brains of boxers. *JAMA* **251**, 2676–9.

Larsson, L.E., Melin, K.A., Nordstrom-Ohrberg, G., Silfverskiold, B.P. & Ohrgerg, K. (1954) Acute head injuries in boxer — clinical and electroencephalographic studies. *Acta Psych. Neurol. Scand.* **95** (Suppl.), 1–42.

Litel, G.R. (1990a) Eye injuries. In *USA/ABF Physicians Certificate Manual*, pp. 37–40. USA Amateur Boxing Federation, Colorado Springs.

Litel, G.R. (1990b) Fluid and electrolyte balance. In *USA/ABF Ringside Physician's Certificate Manual*, pp. 42–2. USA Amateur Boxing Federation, Colorado Springs.

Lundberg, G.D. (1983) The medical case for ending boxing. *JAMA* **249**, 2.

McCown, I.A. (1959a) Boxing injuries. *Am. J. Surg.* **98**, 509.

McCown, I.A. (1959b) Protecting the boxer. *JAMA* **169**(13), 1409–13.

Maguire, J.I. & Benson, W.E. (1986) Retinal injury and detachment in boxers. *JAMA* **255**, 2451–3.

Martland, H.S. (1928) Punch drunk. *JAMA* **91**, 1103.

Noble, C. (1987) Hand injuries in boxing. *Am. J. Sports Med.* **15**(4), 342–6.

Oelman, B.J., Rose, C.M.E. & Arlow, K.J. (1983) Boxing injuries in the army. *J. Roy. Army Med. Corps.* **129**, 32–7.

Osmanski, W.T. (1976) Teeth-fitted mouthguard can save a player's life. *Dent. Stud.* **54**, 35.

Palmer, E., Lieberman, T.W., Burns, S. *et al.* (1976) Contusion angle deformity in prize fighters. *Arch. Ophthalmol.* **94**, 225.

Phillips, J.P., Jones, H.M., Hitchcock, R., Adams, N.

& Thompson, R.J. (1980) Radioimmunoassay of serum creatine kinases BB as index of brain damage after head injury. *Br. Med. J.* **281**, 777–9.

Portis, J.M., Vasallo, S.A., Albert, D.M. *et al.* (1981) A review of cases on file in the Massachusetts Eye and Ear Infirmary pathology laboratory. *Intern. Ophthalmol. Clin.* **21**(4).

Posner, M.A. & Ambrose, L. (1989) Boxer's knuckle — Dorsal capsular rupture of the metacarpophalangeal joint of a finger. *J. Hand Surg.* **14A**, 229–36.

Preston-Martin, S.Y., Henderson, B.E. & Roberts, D. (1983) Risk factors for meningiomas in men in Los Angeles County. *J. Natl. Cancer Institute* **70**(5), 863–6.

Pudenz, R.H. & Shelden, C. (1946) Lucite calvarium. Trauma and brain movement. *J. Neurosurg.* **3**, 487.

Reif, A.F. (1981) Risks and gains (in sports). In P.F. Vinger & E.F. Hoerner (eds) *Sports Injuries, The Unthwarted Epidemic*, p. 88. PSG Publishing, Massachusetts.

Rimel, R.W., Giordani, B., Barth, J.T. *et al.* (1981) Disability caused by minor head injury. *Neurosurgery* **9**(3), 221–8.

Robert, A.H. (1969) *Brain Damage in Boxers*. Pitman, London.

Roberts, G.W., Allsop, D. & Bruton, C. (1990) The occult aftermath of boxing. *J. Neurol. Neurosurg. Psychiatr.* **53**, 373–8.

Rodriguez, G., Ferrillo, F. & Montano, V. (1983) Regional cerebral blood flow in boxers. *Lancet* **ii**, 858.

Ross, R.J., Casson, I.R., Siegel, O. & Cole, M. (1987) Boxing injuries: Neurologic, radiologic, and heuropsychologic evaluation. *Clin. Sports Med.* **6**(1), 41–51.

Ross, R.J., Cole, M., Thompson, J.S. & Kim, K.H. (1983) Boxers. Computed tomography, EEG and neurological evaluation. *JAMA* **249**(2), 211–13.

Ryan, A.J. (1987) Intracranial injuries resulting from boxing: A review (1918–1985). *Clin. Sports Med.* **6**(1), 31–40.

Sanders, B. (1979) *Pediatric Oral and Maxillofacial Surgery*. CV Mosby, St Louis.

Sercl, M. & Jaros, O. (1962) The mechanisms of cerebral concussion in boxing and their consequences. *World Neurol.* **3**, 351–7.

Unterhernscheidt, F.J. (1970) About boxing: Review of historical and medical aspects. *Texas Rep. Biol. Med.* **28**(4), 422.

Vinger, P.F. (1981a) Incidence of eye injuries. Ocular sports injuries. *Intern. Ophthalmol. Clin.* **21**(4), 30.

Vinger, P.F. (1981b) Treatment of eye injuries. In P.F. Vinger & E.F. Hoerner (eds) *Sports Injuries, the Unthwarted Epidemic*, p. 127. PSG Publishing, Massachusetts.

Voy, R.O. (1990a) A history of boxing. In *USA/ABF Ringside Physician's Certificate Manual*, pp. 107–9. USA Amateur Boxing Federation, Colorado Springs.

Voy, R.O. (1990b) Medical responsibilities of the ringside physician. In *USA/ABF Ringside Physician's Certificate Manual*, pp. 3–8. USA Amateur Boxing Federation, Colorado Springs.

Walsh, J., Gye, R. & Connelley, T.J. (1969) Meningioma: A late complication of head injury. *Med. J. Australia* **1**, 906–8.

Welles, M.M. (1969) Boxing. In *Encyclopedia Brittanica*, Vol. 4, pp. 39–43.

Whiteson, A. (1981) Injuries in professional boxing, their treatment and prevention. *Practitioner* **225**, 1053.

Whiting, W.C., Gregor, R.J. & Finerman, G.A. (1988) Kinematic analysis of human upper extremity movements in boxing. *Am. J. Sports Med.* **16**(2), 130–6.

Chapter 39

Injuries in the Martial Arts

GREG R. McLATCHIE, FRANCISQUE A. COMMANDRE, HERVÉ ZAKARIAN, PAUL VANUXEM, HENRI LAMENDIN, DENIS BARRAULT AND PHAN QUANG CHAU

The origins of the martial arts can be traced to China, Japan and other Asiatic countries. They have evolved to their present forms over several centuries. Although originally developed as self-defence or attack systems (*Mars*, the Roman god of war) they gradually evolved into sports, the characteristics of which include physical fitness *par excellence* and combinations of throwing techniques, locks against joints, strangle holds, punching and weaponry skills. They were introduced to the West at the beginning of the twentieth century and some are now admitted in the Olympic games, a recent example being Tae-Kwondo. Although judo was admitted to the Olympic games as far back as 1964 in Tokyo it is not by definition a martial art being invented in the 1860s by a Japanese college professor, Dr Jigaro Kano.

The very nature of these sports involves men, women or children attempting to overcome their opponent by the use of direct or indirect forces so that injury is an inherent problem with all martial arts. Injury situations should therefore be recognized so that the dangers can be reduced to an ideal minimum.

In all the martial arts there are three areas of participation where injury can occur.

1 Non-contact practice on one's own.

2 Striking objects.

3 Non-contact prearranged sparring, free sparring and competition.

Solitary practice

This can include the warm-up with flexibility exercises and Kata. Although these can be performed in groups, most problems are caused by injudicious or over enthusiastic warm-up and instructors should not push pupils past the limits of their flexibility by methods such as jumping on the knees during seated adductor muscle stretching or pushing on their back when stretching the hamstrings. Another frequent cause of adductor injury is doing forced splits, either fore and aft or sideways (Figs 39.1–39.4). The best method is to allow the pupil to set his or her own limits. If exercises are performed to the onset of discomfort and the position reached held for 10–15 s, progress towards flexibility will be quicker.

Injuries most prevalent in this group are strains and sprains yet few are reported (Birrer, 1982). Students continue to practise and in so doing may exacerbate a quite treatable acute injury which subsequently develops to a chronic problem.

Striking objects

This includes the use of punch bags, punch balls, Makiwara, sandbags and also Tameshiwara (breaking objects). Training is generally performed with the bare hands and feet. The commonest sites of injury are therefore to the hands and feet with nerve injury to the hand and fractures of bones in both hands

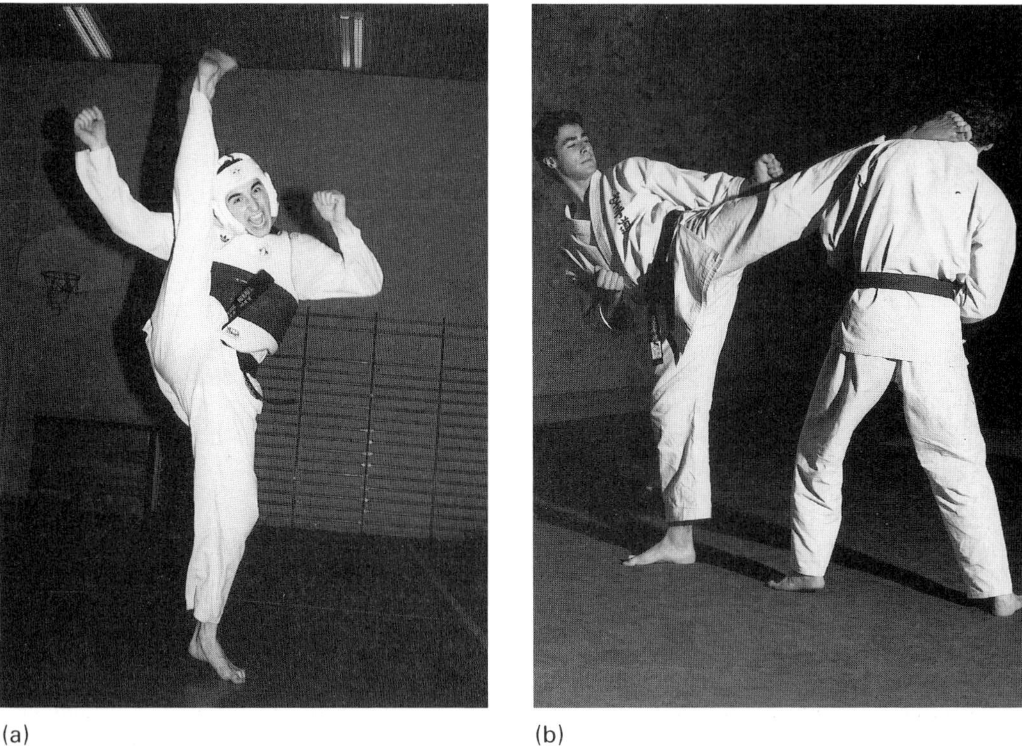

(a) (b)

Fig. 39.1 Splits can cause (a) adductor injuries; (b) groin injuries.

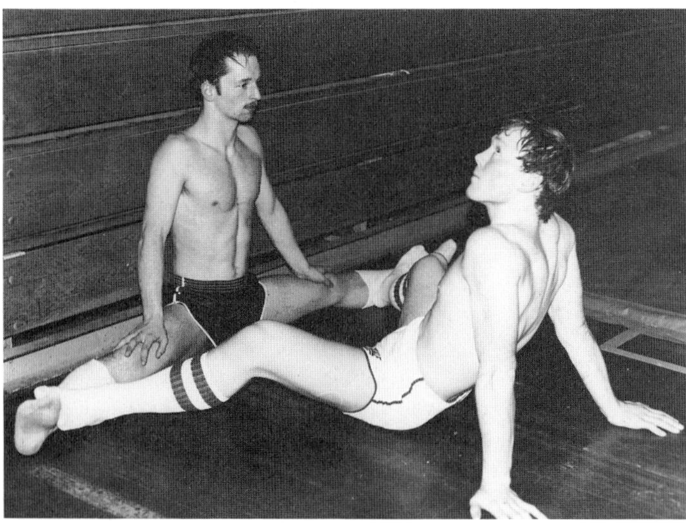

Fig. 39.2 Passive stretching can be carried out as shown — but it is very important to say when discomfort is reached and to train with a partner who is trusted.

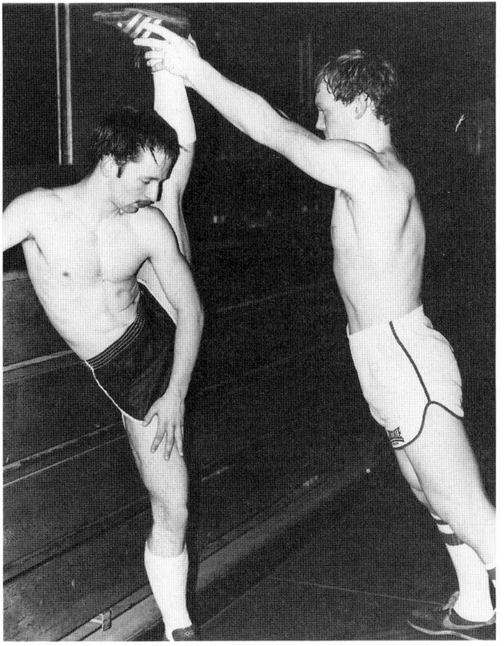

Fig. 39.3 Hypermobility can be achieved by careful, controlled and graded passive stretching.

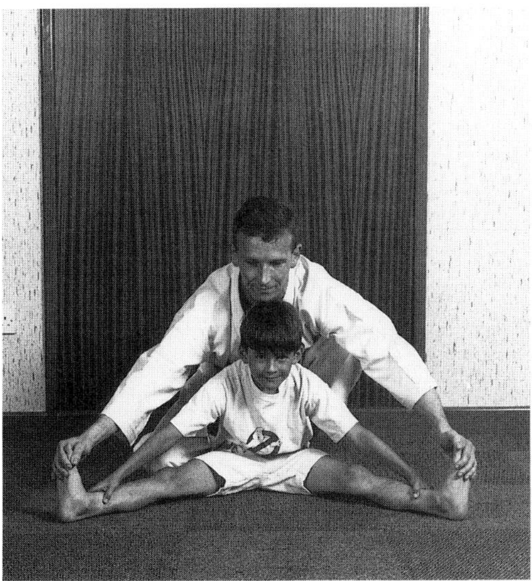

Fig. 39.4 Particular care is required when helping children to stretch.

and feet presenting a major risk (Nieman & Swan, 1971).

Protective changes are also known to develop, such as thickening of the skin over the little finger border of the hands and callouses on the knuckles. These can produce considerable discomfort and may even become infected (Sperryn, 1973).

Non-contact prearranged sparring, free sparring and competition

Similar injuries can result in these groups. It is only in prearranged matches that there is more control since each partner should know his or her role. In free sparring or competition, however, there are many variables which may predispose to injury (Kurland, 1980; Zemper & Pieter, 1989).

Tournament rules and officiating

The control exerted by the referee is immediate and important. The referee is in charge of the fight. The governing body exerts remote control in that it sets the rules and regulations with the referee interpreting and applying them. Experience is important for a referee because competitions can be very heated with considerable crowd participation. It is therefore vital that the referee sticks to the decisions made during competition and receives the support of the governing body so that the referee's decisions can be seen to be upheld.

Cheating

Any infringement of the rules is by definition cheating. Although violence in sport is generally regarded more as a problem in contact sports (like soccer or rugby football) it is also possible for violence to occur in combat sports and this should be regarded as cheating. For example, the use of any illegal technique infringes the rules. Furthermore because of the nature of the sport, serious injury can result.

Lack of protective clothing and equipment

The indoor training area should be well ventilated and illuminated and there should be adequate floor space to avoid collisions with other competitors. The use of sprung flooring in boxing rings has reduced the incidence of secondary head injuries in this sport when a boxer falls onto the ring after being struck and padded or matted flooring should be used for other combat sports (Fig. 39.5a)

There is also a considerable body of evidence that protective clothing reduces the number of injuries (McLatchie, 1977; Birrer, 1982; Barrault *et al.*, 1983; Lamendin, 1985; McLatchie *et al.*, 1987). This ranges from the use of mouth shields

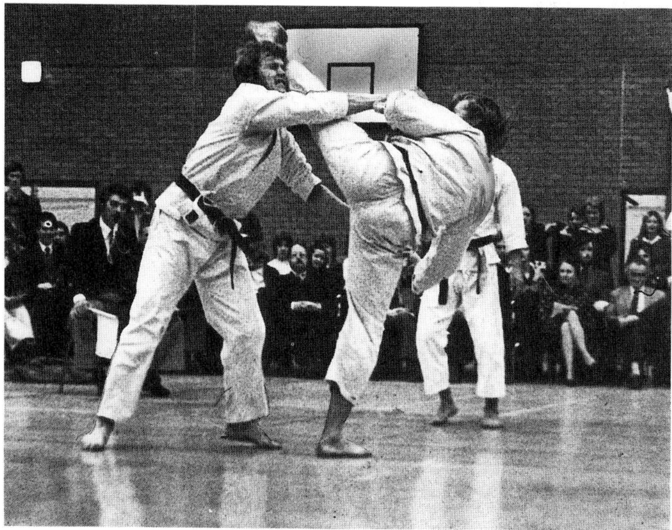

(a)

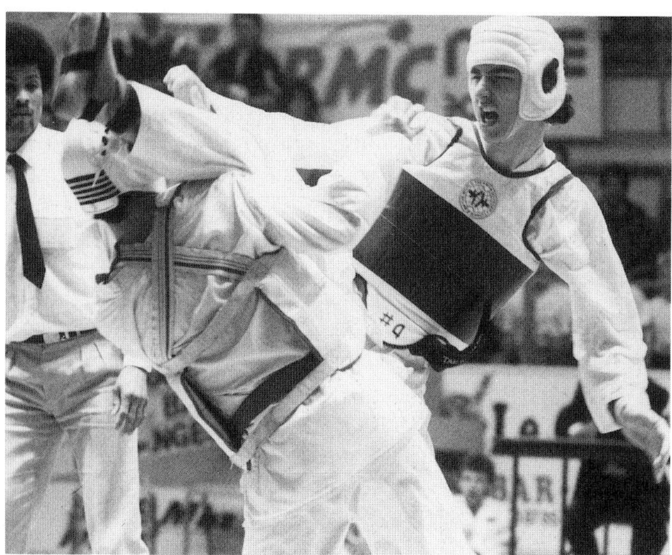

(b)

Fig. 39.5 (a) Lack of protective padding and the use of stone flooring were common causes of injury in the early 1980s in most countries. (b) Examples of protective equipment.

(Fig. 39.6) and protective padding (Fig. 39.5b) to wearing a head guard in sports like full-contact karate (an example learned from boxing). As a general rule, we would advise participants to wear such protection even in sparring.

Differences in body weight

Depending on the sport, the ideal should be that no competitor should outweigh the opponent by more than 3–6 kg (7–14 lb). Although this is not always possible in team martial arts competition referees should be aware of the dangers associated with weight disparity and their association with increased risk of injury.

Inexperience

Most injuries will occur in inexperienced fighters. However, when an injury does occur in an experienced fighter it is generally found to be more serious.

There are also situations where an experienced fighter will be sparring with a relative novice and the former must exercise great care for the novice may not anticipate the type of attack being launched and the novice's poorer reactions may lead to injury.

The sports

Most sports which derive from original combat are of three types.

1 Predominantly punching and kicking, like karate and Tae-Kwondo.

2 Predominantly grappling and throwing like aikido, jiu-jitsu and judo.

3 Weaponry, like kendo and the use of weapons in karate.

The reason for the division is that injury situations which arise are similar in each group. The types of injury also tend to conform although it must be emphasized that any injury can occur to any part of the body from any sport.

Punching and kicking arts

Karate

In modern Japanese, karate means empty hand. In its simplest sense this implies empty handed combat without the use of weapons. In a deeper sense there are strong religious convictions with implications of infinity of knowledge and self-discipline. The origins of the sport can be traced to China but modern karate is said to owe its development to the Ryukui islanders

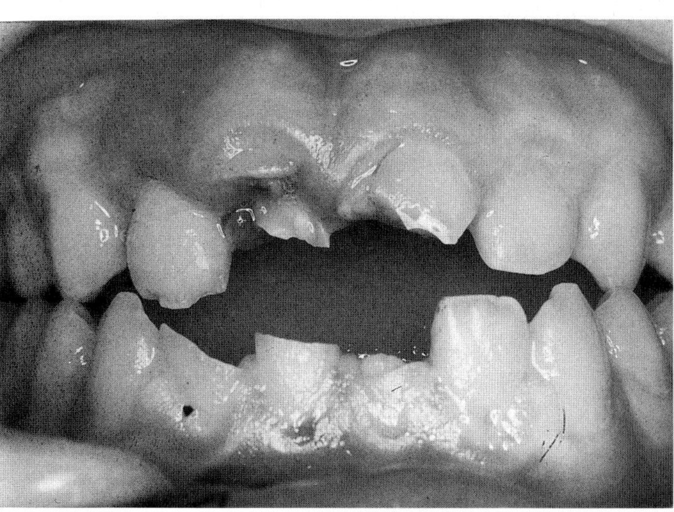

Fig. 39.6 Dental injury is a common result of trauma to the mouth and can be largely prevented by wearing gum shields.

who, when overrun by the Kyushu in 1609, cleverly circumvented the veto which banned weapons of any kind by devising an empty-handed form of combat so effective that a trained exponent could punch through the bamboo armour of his oppressors with his hardened fists, or dismount horsemen with high kicks. As practised today, it still has two distinct forms — the one a philosophical way of life linked strongly to the Zen religion; the other a practical martial art concerned with the acquisition of spectacular physical skills and historically linked to the ideal of bushido (the way of the warrior), the code of conduct of the samurai.

BUSHIDO

Bushido was a highly specialized code of honour and conduct which samurai warriors of feudal Japan were required and instructed to observe. Although it loosely related to chivalry, it dictated both how the fighting nobles should behave in battle and in their daily life. It was an unwritten code which had grown out of centuries of military life and for those who diligently adhered to its concepts it meant absolute loyalty to an immediate superior and therefore unquestioning obedience. The samurai had to be prepared to fight and die without the slightest hesitation. Obviously they were daunting adversaries.

The concept of bushido pervaded Japanese thinking and applied to many aspects of life especially during World War II. It also applied to the teaching and learning of martial arts. The acceptance of pain as being a necessary part of advancement in Japanese karate is one reason for the early experience in the West of a high injury rate in the sport. This principle has now gradually been eroded on common sense grounds. Injury causes valuable loss of time from work and sometimes more importantly from the sport itself.

FORCES IN KARATE

The peak velocity attained by a straight punch executed by a trained exponent is 56–64 $km \cdot h^{-1}$ with a force exerted of 3000 $N \cdot cm^{-3}$. These figures are proportionately higher for kicks. A velocity of 32 $km \cdot h^{-1}$ is sufficient to break a 5 cm block of wood and one of around 48 $km \cdot h^{-1}$ is sufficient to break concrete. The secret of the karate blow is the concentration of this energy in a small striking surface area, for example the first and second knuckles only (Fig. 39.7).

All karate exponents (karateka) are aware, however, that wood is easier to break than concrete. The reason for this is that only part of the energy is transferred to the target; the remainder is transferred to the striking fist where it is experienced as pain. Although wood will absorb most of the hand's kinetic energy, concrete obstinately refuses at least half of it. This may present a psychological problem to even the most hardened of karateka.

A further paradox is why the bones of the hand do not break when striking wood or concrete. This is because bone is much tougher than either, and provided the forces are directed along the lines of stress in the bone no damage will be sustained. Implicit in this is the posture of the striking hand or foot which must be correct if injury is to be prevented. This should

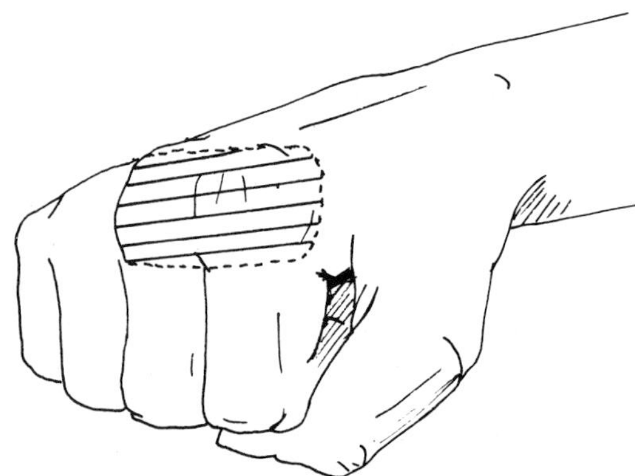

Fig. 39.7 The correct striking surface of the fist — the heads of the 2nd and 3rd metacarpals.

be remembered in all aspects of training and practice.

COMPETITION KARATE

This is a regular feature of modern karate which is increasing in popularity. Although once exclusive to men it now attracts women and children. Weight and grading categories have permitted a wide range of participation so that many exponents have opportunities to become winners. Most competitions are of three types.

1 Traditional.
2 Semicontact.
3 Full contact.

Traditional karate

This remains the most popular form. Contests last 2–3 min and blows are directed at specific targets on an opponent but are withdrawn just before or at contact. Points are scored on the basis of half points (waza-ari) or full points (ippon) depending on the style, quality and intensity of the technique. As body contact should be light or non-existent, difficulties occasionally arise in the scoring of competitions and referees should be aware of vulnerable areas of the human body so that fair scoring can be effected.

Semicontact competition

In some styles (e.g. kyokushinkai) the rules permit full contact to the body with punches and kicks. High kicks to the side of the head and sweeps or kicks to the legs are also allowed. A full point and subsequently a win is given for a good knock-down or a knock-out which is said to have occurred if the fighter is unable to stand up within 5 s of being knocked down. Half a point is given if the technique floors a fighter who is nevertheless able to get up again in 5 s. After each round, competitors are required to demonstrate their ability at wood breaking (tameshiwari) before progressing to the next. The weapons in order of use are the straight punch, the side of the hand, the elbow and each contest last 2–3 min. Most injuries in this type of competition occur to the limbs because of persistent low kicks (McLatchie, 1980; Amdriantsimahavandy, 1990).

Full-contact competition

This is a more recent development which bears many resemblances to Thai boxing. Blows of unrestrained velocity are directed with the hands or feet against the opponent. The contest is fought in rounds as in boxing and the winner is the fighter who accumulates most points or who succeeds in knocking out the opponent.

Tae-Kwondo

This is a Korean martial art similar in many ways to karate which was introduced as a demonstration sport in the 1988 Olympic Games in Seoul. Kicking techniques predominate in Tae-Kwondo and injury results when attacks are improperly blocked or inadequate protective equipment is used (Zemper & Pieter, 1989).

In both karate and Tae-Kwondo injuries occur to three main areas, namely the head (Figs 39.8–39.10) and neck, abdomen, trunk and limbs. Their prevention is discussed later in this chapter.

Reduction of injury (example of the Scottish karate injury register)

Over a 10-year period (1974–1983) split into three periods, all injuries sustained in traditional karate competitions were recorded (McLatchie, 1986). These are illustrated in Tables 39.1–39.4. After establishing the incidence of injury in the first year of the first 3-year period, preventive measures were introduced including the use of protective clothing in the form of gum shields, groin guards, knuckle pads, shin guards and foot pads as well as the introduction of padded flooring and the effects of these changes were audited during the period. In the second 3-year period, follow-

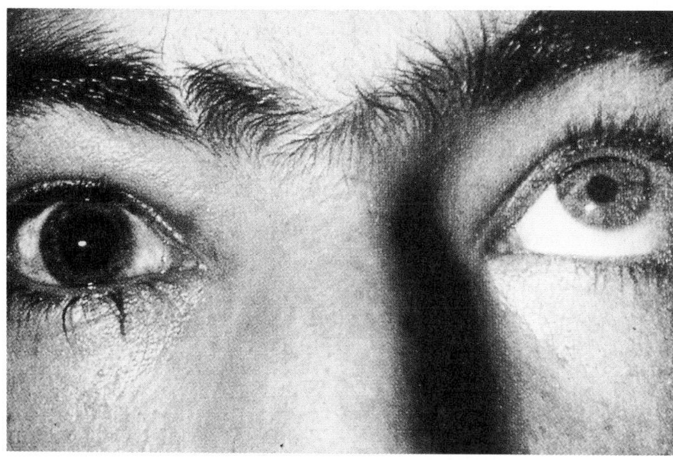

Fig. 39.8 Kicks or punches to the orbit have resulted in a blow-out fracture with paralysis of the upward gaze.

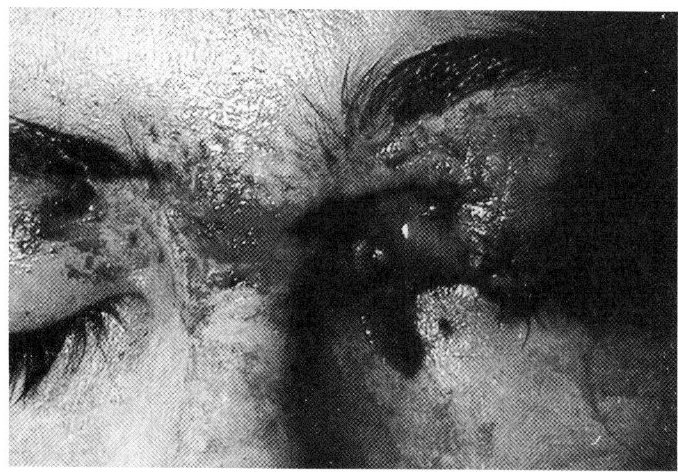

Fig. 39.9 Lacerations around the orbit are common sequelae to being struck with an ungloved fist.

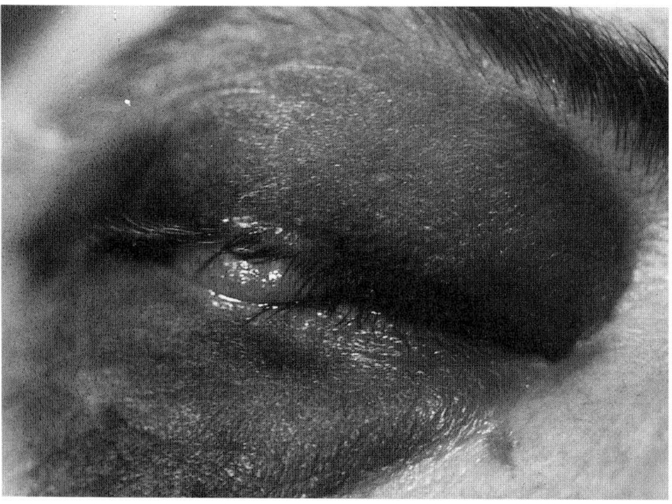

Fig. 39.10 A black eye with prolapse of the tear duct. This can be caused by punches or kicks.

Table 39.1 Injuries to the head and neck, 1974–1983, in the UK.

Injury	Number of cases		
	1974–1976	1977–1979	1980–1983
Epistaxis	91	17	20
Facial lacerations	110	33	15
Periorbital laceration (Fig. 39.9)	51	5	2
Head injury (PTA and other eye injuries, Figs 39.8 & 39.10)	170	83	45
Blows to the trachea	23	4	5
Cervical dislocation (C6–C7)	1	0	0
Maxillary sinus (rupture with pneumatocele)	2	1	0
Mandibular fracture	7	0	1
Malar fracture	8	2	1
Total	463	145	89

PTA, post-traumatic amnesia.

Table 39.2 Injuries to the trunk, 1974–1983, in the UK.

Injury	Number of cases		
	1974–1976	1977–1979	1980–1983
Rib fracture	35	22	16
Pneumothorax	15	3	2
Blows to solar plexus	185	115	70
Blows to testes	43	12	15
Splenic rupture	2	2	0
Acute traumatic pancreatitis	0	1	0
Total	280	155	103

Table 39.3 Injuries to the limbs, 1974–1983, in the UK.

Injury	Number of cases		
	1974–1976	1977–1979	1980–1983
Fractures	97	13	15
Karate thumb	27	5	4
Gamekeeper's thumb	15	5	3
Traumatic neurapraxia	27	5	7
Anterior tibial compartment syndrome	2	2	1
Retropatellar pain	35	21	18
Meniscus symptoms	80	52	32
Total	283	103	80

Table 39.4 Injuries in karate in the UK. Change in incidence over 10 years (13 566 contests).

	1974–1976	1977–1979	1980–1983
Total injuries	931	403	272
Number of contests	4003	3449	6114
Incidence	$1 \cdot 4\,\text{contests}^{-1}$	$1 \cdot 8.5\,\text{contests}^{-1}$	$1 \cdot 22\,\text{contests}^{-1}$

ing a reduction of injury, a national campaign in the UK was launched to educate referees and participants about the risk of injury, methods of prevention and immediate management. Equivalent weight classes were also introduced during this period (except in the team event) and the banning of dangerous techniques was introduced. The further recommendation, that there should be statutory medical control at all competitions where more than 20 participants took part, was supported by the Scottish Karate Board of Control.

The incidence of injury fell from one per four contests in the 1974–1976 period to one per eight contests in the 1977–1979 period. The effects of the changes introduced during these 6 years were further emphasized when during the period 1980–1983 injury rate fell to one per 22 contests.

From this study of over 13 500 karate contests, it is apparent that even in a combat sport (where injury may be intended and certainly accepted) the incidence can be considerably reduced by making the environment of participants safer, avoiding the use of dangerous techniques and providing adequate medical supervision and attention. There was no evidence from the study that the introduction of preventive measures in the form of protective clothing or coach and participant education adversely affected the fighters' performance. During the 10-year period of the study, Scotland won four European championships and the Great Britain team won the world championship on four occasions.

Introduction of safety measures

This has meant that karate fighters could train more regularly and have fewer absences from contests. This has allowed many to train towards their peak and compete more regularly in their chosen sport. The use of padded flooring has been extremely successful in reducing the number of head injuries which occur following sweeps, throws or even accidental contact.

If a fighter sustains a post-traumatic amnesia or a knock-out, the recommendation is that the athlete should not fight again for at least 3 or 4 weeks. The Karate Board of Control itself introduced a 3-month ban following a knock-out on the basis that some participants may feign unconsciousness to win a fight 'lying on his back'. In this way histrionics are avoided.

If a fighter has symptoms of a post-traumatic syndrome, the rule is that he or she does not return to the sport until the symptoms have resolved completely. If there has been a head injury severe enough to cause coma or lead to a neurosurgical procedure, such fighters should be advised to give up combat sport altogether. In all situations, those wishing to return to karate competition should be examined and certified fit by a neurologist when a serious head injury has been sustained.

Grappling and throwing arts

Judo

In the mid 1860s a Japanese college professor, Dr Jigaro Kano, began a detailed study of the fighting arts of the Orient and realizing that each school saw their concept as superior to the others synthesized what he had learned and called the art judo — the gentle way. He argued that the most efficient way of fighting was to use intellect, one's own personal ability and the opponent's mistakes to achieve superiority thus if an opponent threw a punch, that opponent could be thrown using his or her own momentum.

Judo is an extremely popular sport amongst adults and children and is a recognized Olympic sport. It involves rapidly changing one's centre of gravity to perform throws and also the use of ground work and locks to maintain an opponent in a helpless position. Locks against the joints and the application of strangles or chokes are characteristic of ground work and in experienced hands they can be applied as a throw is being completed so that the opponent is held firmly on the mat — a scoring position but also a potential injury situation (Barrault, 1986).

Aikido

This is a Japanese martial art which has been subsequently adapted and modified into various schools. It involves redirection of an attacker's energy with grappling and striking. It also involves some use of weapons. Again these areas are potential injury situations.

Jiu-jitsu

This Japanese martial art has uncertain origin and great antiquity. It involves throws, locks and holds with ancillary strikes to weaken or divert the attention of an opponent whilst a grappling technique is applied with the object of gaining a submission. Self-defence against weapon attacks are also taught. The art developed in several areas independently and there are therefore several different styles.

Particular injuries

Strangles and chokes can lead to unconsciousness through occlusion of the carotid arteries or trachea. Such episodes of unconsciousness after strangles should be treated subsequently in a similar manner to minor head injuries which can also result from poorly performed breakfalls or accidents with the various types of weaponry which may be used in demonstrations. The most commonly injured joints are the shoulders, elbows and fingers but mat burns, grazes and bruises are common. Fortunately, serious intra-abdominal injuries are rare.

Reduction of injury

Most injuries occur when:

1 A breakfall is poorly executed (Figs 39.11 & 39.12).

2 A limb lock over enthusiastically applied or not submitted to.

3 A choke or strangle is applied for too long.

The wrist, elbow and head are the areas most commonly injured after poor breakfalls and effective prevention lies in adequate warm-up and frequent falling practice. If an injury to a major joint (wrist, elbow, shoulder, hip or knee) does occur, the affected limb should be supported gently, either with broad bandages lightly applied or on pillows or sandbags until professional assistance is available. No attempts at heroic reductions of dislocated joints should be made unless specific expertise has been developed.

Weaponry arts

Kendo

Kendo is a traditional Japanese martial art now developed into a sport. The athlete always wears a protective suit and fights against an opponent using a bamboo sword (the shiai). The rules of kendo permit strikes to the head, the sides of the trunk, the back of the hand and the throat. The sport is characterized by explosive actions with rapid extension of the arms, legs and trunk. Most injuries are due to

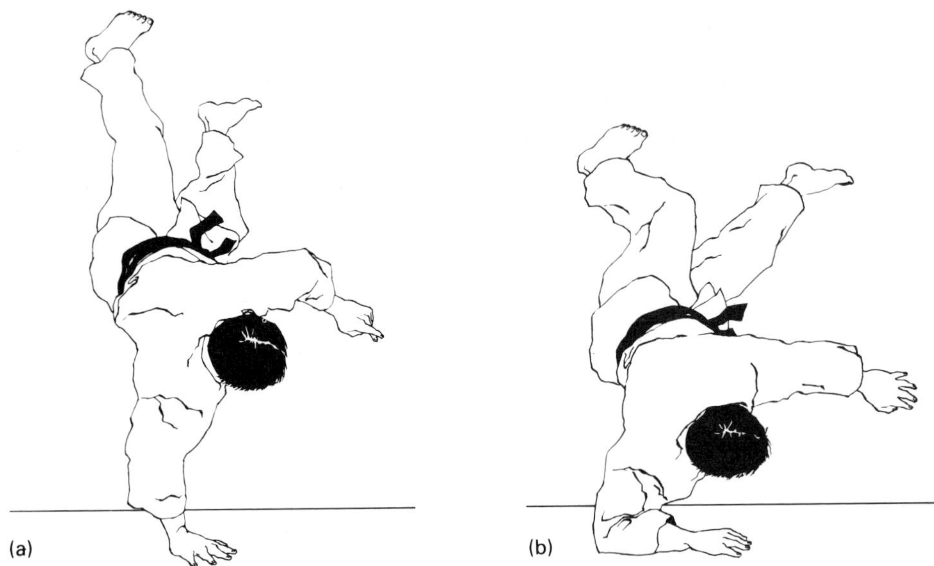

Fig. 39.11 A poorly executed breakfall: (a) a fall onto the outstretched hand can lead to a radial head fracture, and (b) forced flexion of the elbow can cause a fracture of the olecranon when it impacts on the floor.

strikes by the bamboo sword on the head, abdomen and arms (Ito, 1958). The commonest problems encountered are bruising, usually to the chest and upper arms and these are rarely troublesome in the long term.

In the last decade there have been two reports of death in kendo in Europe. Although these were described as accidents, the mechanism is worth noting for it emphasizes the importance of ensuring that protective equipment, if worn, is in good condition. It also emphasizes that frequent inspection and care of weapons is essential to prevent injury. In both cases, death was secondary to eye injuries when the shiai shattered and bamboo splinters penetrated the face guard and the orbit. One victim of such an accident died from a brain haemorrhage, the other from infection. In international fencing (where the foil may be regarded as being similar to a shattered shiai) the only two fatalities reported in the UK were both the result of penetrating injuries and major vessel haemorrhage. Such fatalities, although rare, emphasize the need for adequate protective clothing and an awareness amongst participants of the inherent dangers in the sport (Crawford, 1990).

Use of weapons in karate

One extension of karate is the use of Oriental farm implements as weapons, such as the rice flail. Extreme caution should be encouraged when the techniques of such implements are being taught. Strict control of the class and slow repetitive movements are recommended until mastery and coordination is achieved otherwise the inexperienced may find that their weapon is more injurious to themselves than to a possible opponent.

Prevention of injury

Prevention of injury depends on several factors.

Participant responsibility. People who present themselves to take part in martial arts should be in general good health. The responsibility is upon them to inform the coach or trainer of

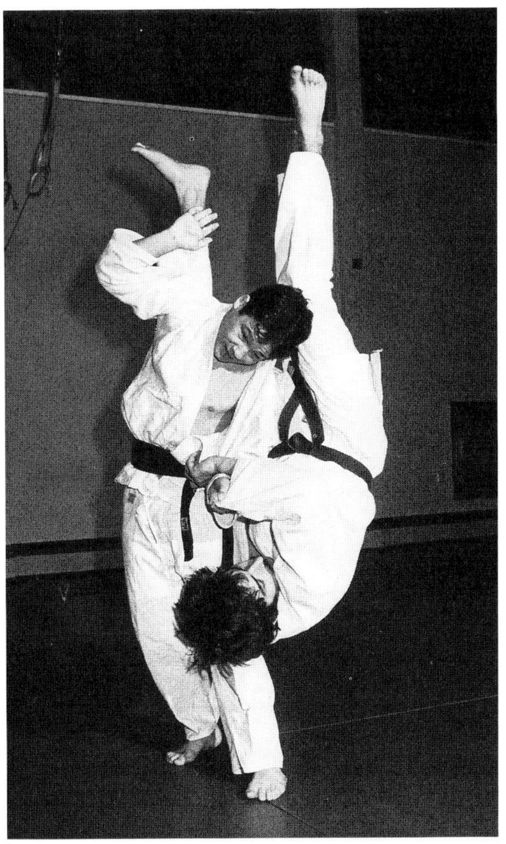

Fig. 39.12 Head or cervical injury can result from ineffective breakfalls.

any particular problems. Those who have pre-existing disease should have a medical examination carried out by a general practitioner to determine and evaluate their physical abilities to practise a martial art and also possibly to participate in competitions. At international level, medical examinations are mandatory in many of the martial arts.

Skill and injury prevention. In most studies done in groups of fighters, injuries are more common in unskilled people fighting or sparring. Although top-class athletes do become injured they are not so common although they are often severe. Skill, then, differentiates fighters from one another. Many talented athletes are naturally skillful but still develop superior skills by the repetition of preset movements. There is no doubt that injury could be prevented by increasing the skill level of most participants.

Flexibility. This aspect of training should not be neglected. Increased flexibility can be acquired with practice and increases the chances of developing good technique, improving the scoring repertoire in competition and possibly preventing injury. Flexibility exercises should be performed on a daily basis, morning and evening if possible, and certainly always before beginning a training session. Little energy is required for this and many of the movements performed stretch and prime the muscle groups ready for action. The exercises most commonly performed are of two types.

1 *Ballistic exercises.* These involve bobbing or bouncing up and down to stretch the required muscle group, sometimes with a partner. Although increased mobility is acquired, there is little control of the range over which the muscle has been stretched and injury is a possibility.

2 *Static exercises.* These are controlled stretching movements. The muscle group under attention is stretched until tightness is felt and the position held for several seconds. The muscles are then relaxed and the movements repeated. As the muscle warms up, the range of movement is gradually increased. There is less risk of injury in static stretching than in ballistic exercises but in practice combinations of both ballistic and static exercises are used. Both can be performed with a partner but he or she should always be someone who is trustworthy.

Strength. Whereas this may not be so important in punching sports there is little doubt that strength improves performance in the predominantly grappling sports such as judo, especially when coupled with skill and experience. The requirements for developing strength are high-resistance low repetition exercises. The training schedule should be at least 3 days$\cdot$week^{-1} — every day if the athlete has the time to recover and the commitment.

Endurance. The development of muscular endurance does much to prevent injury. If we examine injury statistics in combat sports, many occur when the athlete is tiring. This injury situation must be recognized by the referee for although a fight cannot be stopped just because one of the athletes is not as fit as the other, the referee can tighten his or her control of the competition to avoid injury if necessary. In martial arts, endurance is best built into muscles by circuit training exercises or road running. If weights are used in training the aim should be to use fairly light weights relative to ability to work fast with high repetitions. Short rests should only be taken between exercises and by doing this, recovery time will be eventually increased.

The warm-up. The warm-up period is important in the prevention of injury possibly for the following reasons.

1 Warm-up may increase the speed and force of muscle contraction.

2 Warm-up related to the particular activity seems to improve muscle memory and therefore coordination.

3 Warm-up may prevent injury to muscles, tendons and ligaments by prestretching these structures.

Guidelines for proper warm-up are as follows.

1 The warm-up should be strenuous enough to increase body temperature and cause light perspiration but should not lead to tiredness.

2 It should include strengthening and flexibility exercises.

3 It should include movements common to the sport to be undertaken.

4 It should begin 10–15 min before taking part in the exercise or competition proper.

5 The athlete should keep warm during the warm-up and especially afterwards by remaining active or wearing a light tracksuit.

6 At the end of the training session, light exercises should be carried out as part of the general cool-down before showering and changing.

Conclusion

Much has been done to make these potentially dangerous sports safer but there is still scope for improvement. With considerable potential for further prevention of injuries in combat sports. This would involve action for change in the philosophy of the referees to stop the competition at earlier stages to prevent a partially injured competitor becoming seriously injured. Action by the governing bodies of the sports is required to alter the rules to ensure that safer practices and equipment are adopted by players and officials, both in competition and in training. The accurate gathering of injury statistics and monitoring of potential injury situations is also an important new development which should receive further attention in order that the gains in safety already made can be consolidated.

Medical recommendations for reduction of injuries

1 A medical certificate of fitness to compete should be presented to the official before a contest as a prerequisite to entry.

2 Each fighter should carry a fight record in which previous performances and injuries are recorded.

3 A doctor should be present at all competitions.

4 Following an injury to the eye, ear or head, the competitor must be examined medically before fighting again. A minimum of 4 weeks should elapse before fighting after a head injury (knock-out, post-traumatic amnesia).

5 Equivalent weight classes should be encouraged. Ideally no fighter should outweight the opponent by more than 3 kg (7 lb).

6 Referees and instructors should be encouraged to learn first aid.

7 The governing body should issue a summary of the rules of the sport. They should be freely available to all members of the association.

8 Before competitions, a summary of the rules should be announced.

9 Suitable protective equipment must be worn as specifically recommended by the governing body in liaison with the medical officer to the sport.

References

Adriantsimahavandy, A. (1990) *La pathologie des extremites chez les karatekas* (Pathology of the extremities in karate athletes). Department Interuniversitaire Franco-Africain de Medecine du Sport, Marseille.

Barrault, D. (1986) Les luxations du coude au judo (Elbow dislocations in judo). *J. Traumatol. Sport* **3**, 130–5.

Barrault, D., Achon, B. & Solel, R. (1983) Accidents et incidents survenus au cours des competitions du judo (Accidents and injury during judo competition). *Symbioses* **15**, 144–52.

Birrer, R. (1982) Martial art injuries. *Phys. Sports Med.* **10**, 103–8.

Crawford, A.R. (1990). Medical hazards of fencing. In S.D.W. Payne (ed) *Medicine, Sport and the Law*, pp. 360–74. Blackwell Scientific Publications, Oxford.

Ito, K. (1958) Sports injuries in Kendo. *Saigai Igaku* **1**, 21.

Kurland, H.K. (1980) Injuries in karate. *Phys. Sports Med.* **8**, 80–5.

Lamendin, H. (1985) Prevention et protections buccodentaires des judoka (Prevention of injury to and protection of buccal dental area during judo). *Ceint. Noires France* **56**, 11–13.

McLatchie, G.R. (1977) Prevention of karate injuries — A progress report. *Br. J. Sports Med.* **11**, 78–82.

McLatchie, G.R. (1980) Injuries in karate — A case for medical control. *J. Trauma* **20**(11), 956–8.

McLatchie, G.R. (1986) *Prevention of injuries in combat sports. A ten year study of competition karate.* World Congress of Sports Medicine, Brisbane, Australia.

McLatchie, G.R., Brookes, N., Galbraith, S., Hutchison, J.S.F., Wilson, L., Melville, I. & Teasdale, E. (1987) Clinical neurological examination, neuropsychological testing, electroencephalography and computed tomographic head scanning in active amateur boxers. *J. Neurol. Neurosurg. Psychiatr.* **50**, 96–9.

Nieman, E.A. & Swan, P.G. (1971) Karate injuries. *Br. Med. J.* **1**, 233.

Sperryn, P.N. (1973) Traumatic bursitis in a boxer's hand. *Proceedings XVIII World Congress of Sports Medicine. Br. J. Sports Med.* **7**, 103.

Zemper, E.D. & Pieter, P.W. (1989) Injury rates during the 1988 US Olympic Team trials for taekwondo. *Br. J. Sports Med.* **23**, 161–4.

Chapter 40

Injuries in Rowing

ARTHUR L. BOLAND AND TIMOTHY M. HOSEA

While the origins of rowing are lost in time, since learning how to propel a boat through the water with an oar, rowers have concentrated on increasing speed and power. While many improvements have been technical leading to a more efficient transfer of effort to the oar, the rower has also developed training regimens designed to increase strength and endurance.

An élite rower develops absolute ventilation values comparable to élite endurance-type athletes, yet they must also have the motor coordination and strength to endure the gruelling 2000-m race (Hagerman, 1975). This strenuous activity demands intensive training and all too often leads to overuse injuries.

Learning to row

The mechanics of rowing differ slightly if an individual is using one oar (sweep) or two (sculling). However, the basic rowing stroke is divided into four phases: (i) the catch; (ii) the drive; (iii) the finish; and (iv) the recovery.

The catch occurs when the oar enters the water. At this point the ankles are dorsiflexed, the knees and back are flexed and the shoulders and elbows are extended. The oar is dropped into the water by lifting the hands while maintaining a flat line of pull from the wrists through the elbows to the shoulders (Fig. 40.1).

The drive is the power phase of the stroke. The back acts as a braced cantilever, transferring the power generated from the knees and hips extending through the upper extremity to the oar (Fig. 40.2). This power transfer requires fine coordination between the leg–back–arm linkage in order to maximize the effort and avoid injury. Late in the drive phase the elbow flexes bringing the oar handle into the body delivering the last bit of energy to the oar. At the completion of the drive phase the knees, hips and back are extended while the elbows and shoulders are flexed.

The finish occurs when the blade is removed from the water. At this event the hands are dropped and wrists dorsiflexed 'feathering' the oar, or flipping the blade from a vertical to horizontal position. This feathering enables the oar to move back to the position of the catch while minimizing the chances of striking the water with the blade and improving the aerodynamics by decreasing wind resistance (Fig. 40.3).

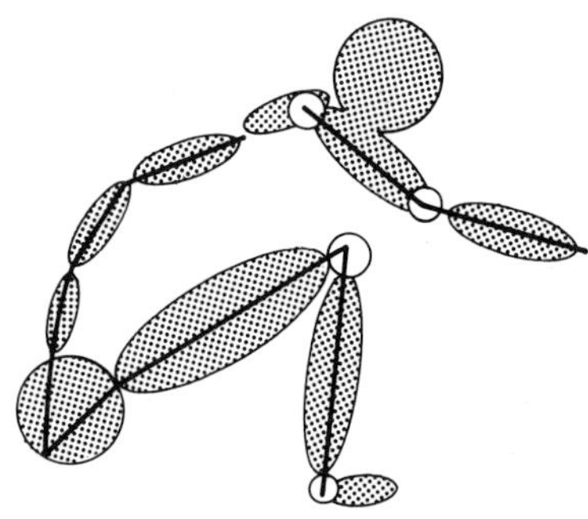

Fig. 40.1 The catch. The elbows and shoulders are extended with the knees and back flexed. The hands are raised and the oar placed into the water.

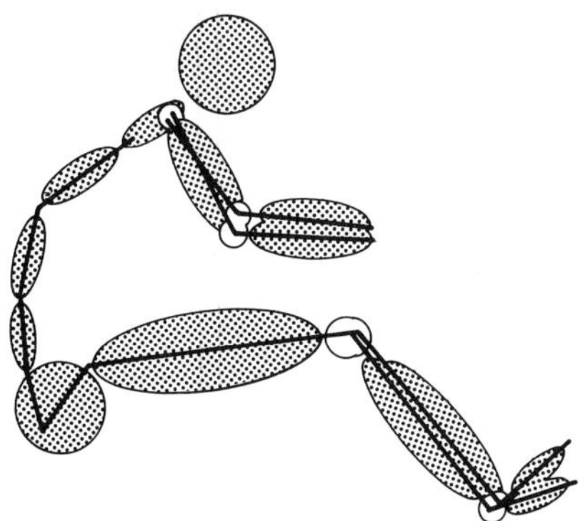

Fig. 40.2 The drive. The knees are forcibly extended with the back braced to transfer the force to the upper extremities and subsequently the oar.

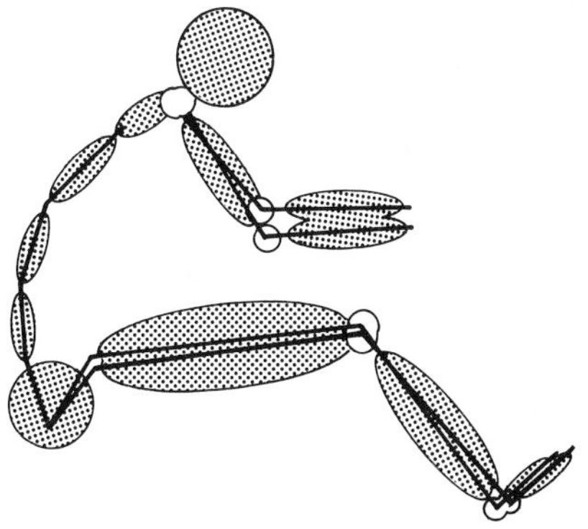

Fig. 40.4 The recovery. The knees and hip flex while the elbows and shoulders extend to return to the catch position and the next stroke.

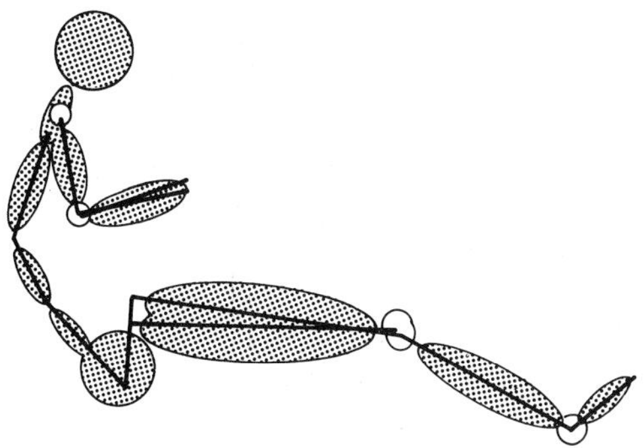

Fig. 40.3 The finish. The knees and back are extended, while the elbows flex to bring the oar into the body completing the drive phase by removing the oar from the water.

The recovery phase is initiated with the extension of the arms and shoulders and forward flexing the back. When the hands and the oar handle pass the knees, the hips and knees flex bringing the rower back into the position of the catch (Fig. 40.4).

Like a gait cycle, the rowing stroke is a continuous motion demanding precise interaction of the body segments. Failure to maintain proper technique may lead to an increased stress on the rower and a predisposition to injury. The novice should ensure proper technique and avoid common mistakes such as 'shooting the side', or failing to maintain the proper spinal angle and allowing it to increase during the drive thus increasing the lower back shear load (Fig. 40.5).

Another common error is 'falling into the catch', this occurs when the upper body hyperflexes and the head and hands drop, placing and trunk into a vulnerable position for injury and a mechanically poorer position from which to initiate the rowing stroke (Fig. 40.6).

This fine motor control is obtained by learning the proper stroke sequentially and progressing to a full stroke when each step is fully achieved. A beginner should first develop the necessary coordination between the back

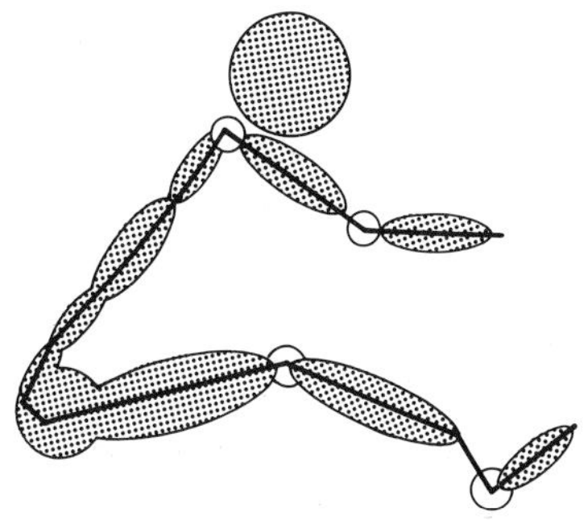

Fig. 40.5 Shooting the slide. The back fails to maintain the braced position, thus allowing the knees to extend with increased hip flexion and loss of force transfer to the oar.

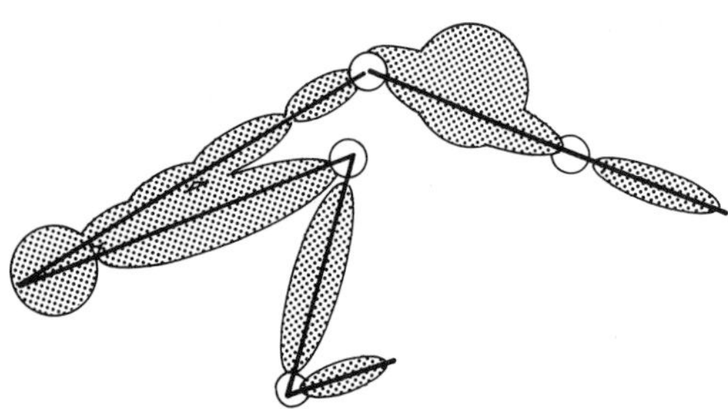

Fig. 40.6 Falling into the catch. The upper body and spine forward flexes causing the loss of mechanical advantage from which to begin a stroke.

and arms. This is accomplished initially by rowing with the legs extended and utilizing only the back and arms. Also during this time the oar should not be feathered in order to learn to keep the oar off the water. When this step is achieved, feathering the oar begins. The rower learns to incorporate the hands and wrists into the stroke, by feathering and squaring the oar at the finish and catch respectively. When this technique is fully controlled, the novice begins to use the legs, initially flexing the knees and hip one half of the total amount possible and progressing to full leg action as competence increases.

It is important during the novice training sessions to avoid fatigue which may lead to the development of poor mechanics. A typical early practice session would consist of four, 5-min segments for each of the above exercises culminating with 5 min of full leg action. This same format is utilized with a gradual increase in the length of time of full leg action as coordination and endurance improves.

Preparticipation screening

An injury survey of intercollegiate rowers from Harvard and Rutgers indicated a preponderance of back and knee injuries (Fig. 40.7) (Hosea *et al.*, 1989). As the rowing stroke and training regimen place a great deal of stress on the back and knees, the preparticipation screening should focus particularly on these areas.

A history of chronic lower back pain should elicit a thorough work-up in a potential rower. A significant spondylolisthesis of grade II or greater should be a relative contraindication to rowing, while those with a spondylolysis or grade I spondylolisthesis must be warned that rowing may aggravate this condition and cause pain. Individuals with active discogenic lower back pain should also not participate until the symptoms have abated and the abdomen and lower musculature have been reconditioned.

Many rowers have suffered a herniated disc during their careers and returned to active successful competition; however, a novice with a history of a herniated nucleus pulposus would be better served pursuing other aerobic activities which would not subject the lumbar motion segments to the extreme stress caused by rowing.

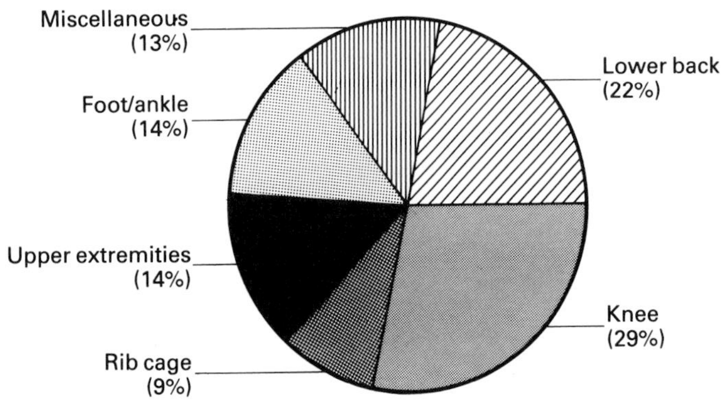

Fig. 40.7 Rowing injuries (Harvard and Rutgers Universities, 1983–1986). From Hosea *et al.* (1989).

Rowing entails the constant flexion and extension of the knee under load, causing significant loading of the patellofemoral joint. The training activities common in a rowing conditioning programme are designed to increase the strength of the quadriceps mechanism and include stair running, squat jumps and squat weight-lifting type activities. Thus individuals with chondromalacia and associated crepitus should avoid active participation in rowing. However, the rowing stroke, while requiring full flexion and extension does not require any twisting or lateral motion, enabling individuals with ligamentous instability of the knee to participate and succeed.

Common rowing injuries and their prevention

The rowing injuries of the men's and women's crew programmes of Harvard and Rutgers were compiled over a 3-year period. This survey revealed 180 injuries (47% male; 62% female). The vast majority of these injuries were overuse-related with the knee the most common site affected followed by the back (Table 40.1).

Table 40.1 Crew injury survey (n = 180). From Hosea *et al.* (1989).

Site of injury	Number
Knee (52)	
Chondromalacia	22
ITB syndrome	15
Patellar tendinitis	7
Meniscal tear	3
Pes bursitis	2
Hamstring tendinitis	2
MCL sprain	1
Back (39)	
Mechanical	29
HNP	5
Spondylolysis	5
Rib cage (16)	
Stress fracture	8
Costochondritis	4
Strain	3
Contusion	1
Upper extremity (25)	
Extensor tenosynovitis	8
Shoulder impingement	4
Flexor sheath tenosynovitis	4
Biceps tendinitis (elbow)	3
Thumb sprain	2
Carpal tunnel syndrome	1
AC separation	1
Anterior shoulder dislocation	1
Olecranon bursitis	1
Foot/ankle (25)	
Ankle sprains	12
Plantar fasciitis	3
Heel pain	3
Metatarsalgia	2
Peroneal tendinitis	2
Achilles tendinitis	1
Tarsal coalition	1
Club foot	1
Miscellaneous (21)	
Femur stress fracture	1
Greater trochanter bursitis	1
Shin splints	3
Hamstring strain	4
Stress fracture fibula	1
Plantaris rupture	1
Achilles tendinitis	1
Cervical strain	6
Quadriceps strain	3

AC, acromioclavicular; HNP, herniated nucleus pulposus; ITB, iliotibial band; MCL, medial collateral ligament.

Knee injuries

Reflecting the constant flexion and extension of the knee under load, the most common knee problems were chondromalacia and iliotibial (ITB) friction syndrome. The knee motion during a rowing stroke ranges from 110° of flexion at the catch to full extension at the finish. A rower with genu valgum or genu varum is predisposed to developing either chondromalacia or ITB friction syndrome respectively.

Chondromalacia commonly develops in individuals with increased femoral anteversion and/or patella malalignment. Individuals commonly present with anterior knee pain, which generally occurs with rowing, ascending or descending stairs or squatting activities. Occasionally, this anterior ache/throbbing pain is associated with an intra-articular effusion and intermittent episodes of knee buckling. Examination generally reveals patellar facet tenderness and on occasion crepitus with active knee extension. The rowing population will also generally present with a tight quadriceps mechanism and iliotibial band.

ITB friction syndrome occurs secondary to the pressure from the iliotibial band as it moves from a position anterior to the lateral femoral condyle in extension to one posterior in flexion (Fig. 40.8). The ITB is the tendinous extension of the fascia overlying the gluteus maximus and tensor fascia lata muscles and inserts into Gerdy's tubercle at the proximal lateral aspect of the lateral tibial metaphysis. While it sends fibres to the lateral intermuscular septum and lateral patella, the ITB glides freely anteriorly and posteriorly over the lateral femoral condyle. Repeated pressure from this gliding produces the painful syndrome (Boland, 1986). Ober's test for the ITB is usually positive. The pain is located over the lateral femoral condyle and may be associated with crepitus and/or localized swelling.

The treatment for both problems include rest, curtailing rowing, anti-inflammatory medication and a programme of specific stretching and strengthening exercises.

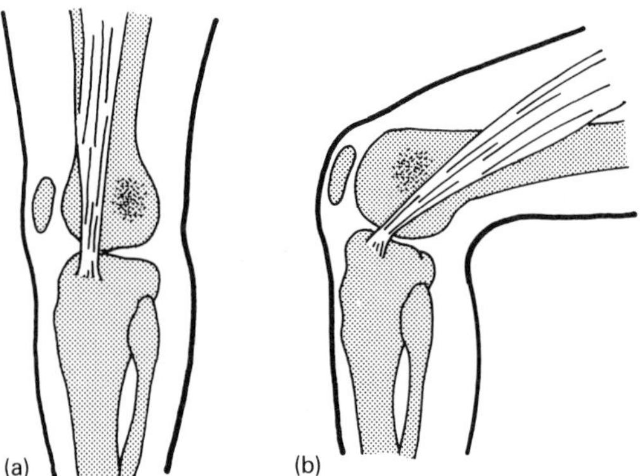

Fig. 40.8 Iliotibial band friction syndrome. With motion of the knee, the iliotibial band over the prominent lateral femoral condyle, which can produce pain, swelling and/or crepitus. With permission from Boland (1986). (a) Front view; (b) side view.

PREVENTION

Effective training for rowing entails a great deal of quadriceps strengthening activities, including squats, squat jumps, stair running as well as rowing. It is important that individuals with pre-existing severe patellofemoral crepitus and pain understand the risks associated with their participation.

To prevent the development of patellofemoral pain and ITB friction syndrome, we encourage a programme of vastus medialis obliquus strengthening exercises consisting of isometric as well as straight leg raising and short arc quads with progressive resistance at the ankle. In addition to vastus medialis obliquus strengthening a programme of quadriceps and ITB stretching is imperative. Quadriceps stretching may be accomplished either standing or lying prone, but must be performed with the hip extended. ITB stretch may also be performed either supine or sitting. It is important to stabilize the pelvis during this stretch and feel the stretch in the area of the greater trochanter. Finally, if the rower has femoral anteversion or external tibial torsion rotating the foot plate or shoe 'in the shell' to maintain neutral alignment of the patellofemoral joint would be helpful.

Low back pain

In our survey of rowing injuries, low back pain was a common complaint. Howell's study of élite oarswomen revealed an 82.2% incidence of low back pain compared to an age- and sex-matched incidence in the general population of 20–30% (1984). During the rowing stroke the lower back acts as a braced cantilever allowing transfer of the force from the leg drive to the oar. The trunk motion ranges from approximately 30° of flexion at the catch to 28° of extension at the finish (Hosea *et al.*, 1989). After the catch there is a rapid increase in the shear load affecting the lower back. This peak during the mid-drive is at 848 ± 133 N for males and 717 ± 69 N for females. During this time the compression load also increases to approximately seven times body weight for both men and women with an associated increase in the myoelectrical activity of the associated paraspinal musculature (Hosea *et al.*, 1987).

The loads placed on the lower back are similar to loads which produce pathological changes in cadaver studies (Adams & Hutton, 1988). These loads can produce not only a herniated nucleus pulposus but also defects in the pars interarticularis (spondylolysis and spondylolisthesis). Thus any rower who presents with low back pain must be carefully examined for signs of radiculitis and neurological deficits. If the pain is mechanical in origin, the neurological examination will be normal and the patient will generally improve with rest, heat, cessation of rowing, anti-inflammatory and antispasmodic medication. Return to rowing may occur when the pain and spasms have subsided and the patient has undergone a rehabilitation programme involving abdominal and paraspinal strengthening, as well as hamstring and lumbosacral stretching.

Patients with a neurological deficit should be followed very closely. Rowing must cease as well as other training activities while the standard initial treatment of rest, heat, analgesics and anti-inflammatories is started. We also routinely obtain complete lumbosacral radiographs. If after 2–3 weeks the symptoms and/or neurological deficits do not improve, further work-up is necessary with magnetic resonance imaging or computerized tomographic scan to further delineate the pathology. In the presence of a significant herniated nucleus pulposus return to élite levels of competition is difficult and often associated with recurrent painful episodes and may be best treated with laminotomy and discectomy.

Because spondylolysis and spondylolisthesis are also frequent problems in rowers, we routinely obtain oblique radiographs of the lumbar spine. A SPECT bone scan is also helpful in detecting a stress fracture of the pars interarticularis. Symptomatic individuals must stop rowing. Treatment is generally conservative although on occasion a lumbosacral antilordotic back brace may be helpful in controlling symptoms. Individuals with previously symptomatic spondylolysis or spondylolisthesis should be strongly discouraged from beginning a rowing programme.

PREVENTION

Prevention of low back pain in the rowing population depends on the development of proper technique, abdominal and lower paraspinal strengthening as well as lumbosacral and hamstring stretching. Technique development should be a progressive process beginning with use of the back and arm only with light pressure. The leg motion should gradually be incorporated into the stroke with a gradual increase in the rowing effort. The back must function as a braced cantilever and not be subjected to an increase in flexion during the drive phase, especially with exertion which would increase the anterior shear loading of the lumbar spine, thus placing it at risk.

In order to help support the lumbar motion segments the abdomen and lumbar paraspinals are strengthened with a programme of sit-up exercises and back extension exercises. Finally, the Williams flexion exercise programme which stretches the lower back with pelvic tilt, knee to chest and hamstring stretches is helpful to avoid injury.

Rib stress fractures

In 1985 Holden and Jackson reported a series of élite female rowers with stress fractures of the ribs. We have identified this problem in both sexes, confirmed by bone scan. They generally occur during the most strenuous rowing training period just before the competitive season. The pain is localized over the posterolateral area of a rib. On occasion there may be winging of the scapula. The pain is exacerbated during the drive phase of the rowing stroke. Pain can also be reproduced with deep inspiration and thoracic compression.

Biomechanical studies have predicted the highest bending stresses occur at the posterolateral segments of the ribs caused primarily by the serratus anterior as well as the rhomboids. Our analysis of the muscles found that they activate maximally at the catch and continue to the finish (Fig. 40.9) (Hosea *et al.*, 1989). This on and off muscle pattern leads to a fatigue mode of loading which may cause the stress fracture. Diagnosis is confirmed by a bone scan. Treatment consists of cessation of rowing and utilization of other forms of aerobic activity, such as a bicycle ergometer. Running tends to accentuate the discomfort. Symptomatic relief is provided with anti-inflammatory or analgesic medications. The rib stress fracture generally heals within 6 weeks when vigorous rowing can resume.

PREVENTION

No formal studies have addressed the question of preventing this stress fracture. However, we feel that a comprehensive programme of upper body and shoulder strengthening would be helpful. The programme should include progressive push-ups as well as pull-ups and bench pulls. The rower should start with 10 repetitions of very light weights and progress with resistance until it is difficult to complete three sets of 10 repetitions.

Wrist extensor tenosynovitis

This problem is associated with on-the-water rowing, generally in the cold weather of early spring, and is directly related to feathering the oar. At the finish of the stroke, the wrist is dropped, dorsiflexed and the oar is removed from the water and rotated parallel to the water during the recovery until the catch when the oar is rotated again to a perpendicular position and placed into the water. This action utilizes the abductor pollicis longus (APL), extensor pollicis brevis (EPB) and the extensor carpi radialis longus (ECRL) and brevis (ECRB). The ECRL and ECRB tendons pass beneath the APL and EPB and become compressed resulting in pain, swelling and frequently crepitus (Fig. 40.10) (Williams, 1977). Treatment consists of a cock up wrist splint, anti-inflammatory medication and physical therapy modalities.

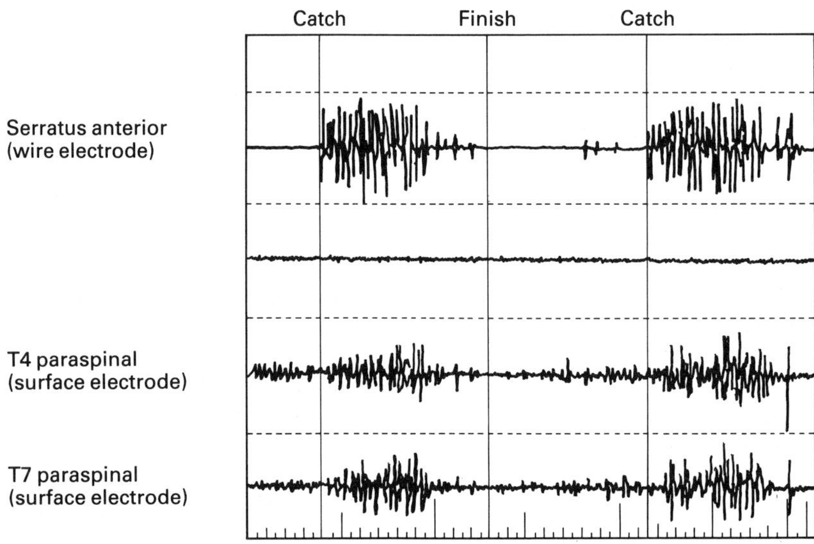

Fig. 40.9 Myoelectric activity of the serratus anterior and the thoracic paraspinal musculature during the rowing stroke. From Hosea *et al.* (1989).

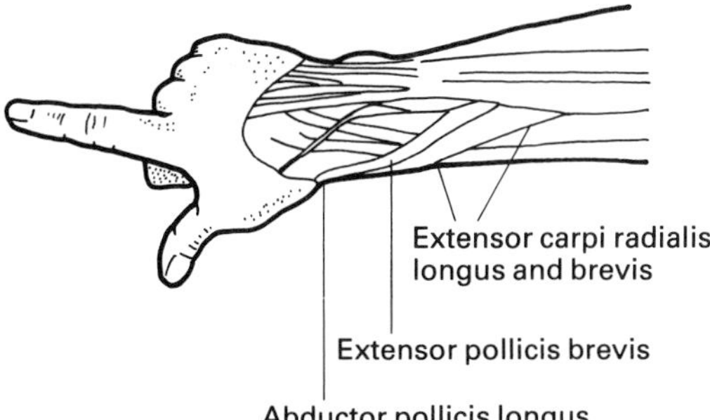

Fig. 40.10 Diagram of the distal forearm anatomy with abductor pollicis longus and extensor pollicis brevis overlying the extensor carpi radialis longus and brevis proximal to the extensor retinaculum. With permission from Williams (1977).

Generally, this problem will subside in 2–3 weeks with conservative measures. Steroid injection into the tendon sheath may be helpful in severe cases.

PREVENTION

This problem can be prevented by controlling and gripping the oar with the fingers, not the hand and relaxing the wrist as much as possible while feathering. In addition, it is important to keep the wrist and forearm dry and covered with layers when rowing in cold, wet conditions. Finally, wrist curls with a bar but no additional weight and sets of 20 or more repetitions are also helpful to improve wrist strength and prevent this problem.

Cross-training techniques

This sport is fortunate in that a rower is able to train utilizing essentially the same mechanics on the water as in a rowing ergometer. Lamb (1989) found that the back and leg forces were the same for both while there was some difference on the upper extremity activity as the ergometer has a fixed fulcrum during the stroke while the water creates an unsteady fulcrum.

Weight-training for rowing is designed to increase the strength of the major rowing muscles of the legs, back and arms. The leg exercises include the leg press, leg extension and squats with a bar. Back strengthening is performed with a back extension machine and cleans. Arm exercises include bench pulls, latissimus pull-overs and pull-ups. The strengthening programme begins with very light weights and sets of 10 repetitions. The resistance is slowly increased until it is difficult to complete three sets of 10 repetitions.

Cross-country skiing or a nordic track is an excellent cross-training device for a rower. It utilizes many of the same muscle groups in a rhythmic cyclic manner and improves the endurance and aerobic base of the rower without the same level of stress on the lower back and knee. While running is useful for aerobic conditioning it does not improve the muscular endurance of the rowing muscles. Hill or step running is an excellent exercise to develop strength and endurance in the hamstrings, quadriceps and gluteus maximus of the rower. However, this activity places a great deal of stress on the patellofemoral joint and should be avoided by those individuals with chondromalacia.

Conclusion

Rowing provides an excellent aerobic and anaerobic form of exercise. Competitive rowing demands a high level of conditioning and dedication. Injuries associated with this sport are generally overuse and stress-related. With proper technique, cross-training and a diligent stretching programme a large number of these injuries can be avoided. For those wishing to begin serious participation but with a pre-existing condition such as chondromalacia or spondylolysis, careful guidance is imperative, including discouraging participation altogether as appropriate.

Acknowledgments

The authors wish to acknowledge the assistance of Harry Parker, Harvard crew coach, in the preparation of this chapter.

References

Adams, M.A. & Hutton, W.C. (1988) Mechanics of the intervertebral disc. In Peter Ghosh, (ed) *The Biology of the Intervertebral Disc*, Vol. 2, pp. 39–73. CRC Press, Florida.

Boland, A.L. (1986) Soft tissue injuries of the knee. In J.A. Nicholas & E.D. Heishman (eds) *Spine and Lower Extremities in Sports Medicine*, p. 1003. CV Mosby, St Louis.

Hagerman, F.C. (1975) Teamwork in the hardest pull in sports. *Phys. Sports Med.* **3**(5), 39–44.

Holden, D.L. & Jackson, D.W. (1985) Stress fractures of the ribs in female rowers. *Am. J. Sports Med.* **13**(5), 342.

Hosea, T.M., Boland, A.L., McCarthy, K. & Kennedy, T. (1989) Rowing injuries. *Post Grad. Adv. Sports Med.* **3**(9), 1–16.

Hosea, T.M., Boland, A.L., Simon, S. *et al.* (1987) Myoelectric and kinematic analysis of the lumbar spine while rowing. *Am. J. Sports Med.* **15**(6), 625.

Howell, D.W. (1984) Musculoskeletal profile and incidence of musculoskeletal injuries in light weight common rowers. *Am. J. Sports Med.* **12**(4), 278.

Lamb, D.H. (1989) A kinematic comparison of ergometer and on water rowing. *Am. J. Sports Med* **17**(3), 367.

Williams, J.G.P. (1977) Surgical management of traumatic non-infective tenosynovitis of the wrist extensors. *J Bone Joint Surg.* **59B**(4), 408.

Chapter 41

Injuries in Canoeing and Kayaking

BO BERGLUND AND DON McKENZIE

Historically, both canoeing and kayaking originated in North America. The war and trading canoes of the Native Indians were adapted for use by the early settlers and the exploits of the 'Voyageurs' occupy a special place in Canadian history. The kayak has its origin in the Arctic and was developed by the Inuit people as a means to hunt fish and game, as well as to transport passengers and merchandise (Shephard, 1987). Canoeing and kayaking, both on flat and white water, became popular leisure sports in North America and Europe towards the end of the nineteenth century. In the beginning of this century, they developed into competitive sports in many countries and, as a consequence of the increased interest in canoe sport, the International Canoe Federation (ICF) was formed in 1924. The sport of canoeing, which includes both canoeing and kayaking, was admitted to Olympic competition in 1936 at the XIII Olympic Games in Berlin and, since then, flatwater racing has been a part of all summer Olympics. Whitewater racing, on the other hand, has been a part of the official Olympic programme only in 1972 and 1992, but will appear in the Olympic programme in Atlanta, 1996.

Canoeing is the national sport of several European countries and the recent growth of recreational and competitive canoeing and kayaking has not been matched by any other sport. It is attractive to all levels of participants as it represents a powerful blend of skill and aesthetics in a natural environment; for the competitive athlete there are severe physical demands that require optimal levels of strength, aerobic and anaerobic fitness and muscular endurance.

Although sprint racing and slalom competition have their place at the Olympic Games there are other popular forms of canoe sport. Marathon competitions occur at national and international regattas and involve distances from 10 km to several hundred-kilometre stage races (Paschke, 1987). Competitive events also occur in canoe sailing, canoe polo, outrigger canoe and the colourful dragonboat racing. Recreational canoeing and kayaking are becoming increasingly popular and can be enjoyed by enthusiasts of all ages. All canoe and kayak racing is sanctioned by the ICF which provides administrative and technical leadership for such activities throughout the world.

The Olympic events include canoe races for one (C1, Fig. 41.1) and two (C2) competitors over distances of 500 and 1000 m. Men's kayak is also raced at 500-m (K1 and K2) and 1000-m (K1, K2 and K4) distances. Women's events (K1, K2 and K4) all take place at the 500-m distance. This year (1994) will see the introduction of 200-m events at the World Championships and it is possible that this event will be introduced into Olympic competition, perhaps at the expense of the 500-m distance. All these races are flatwater events and, under ideal conditions, they are conducted without current or wind; the criteria for success is speed. In comparison, slalom events involve the descent

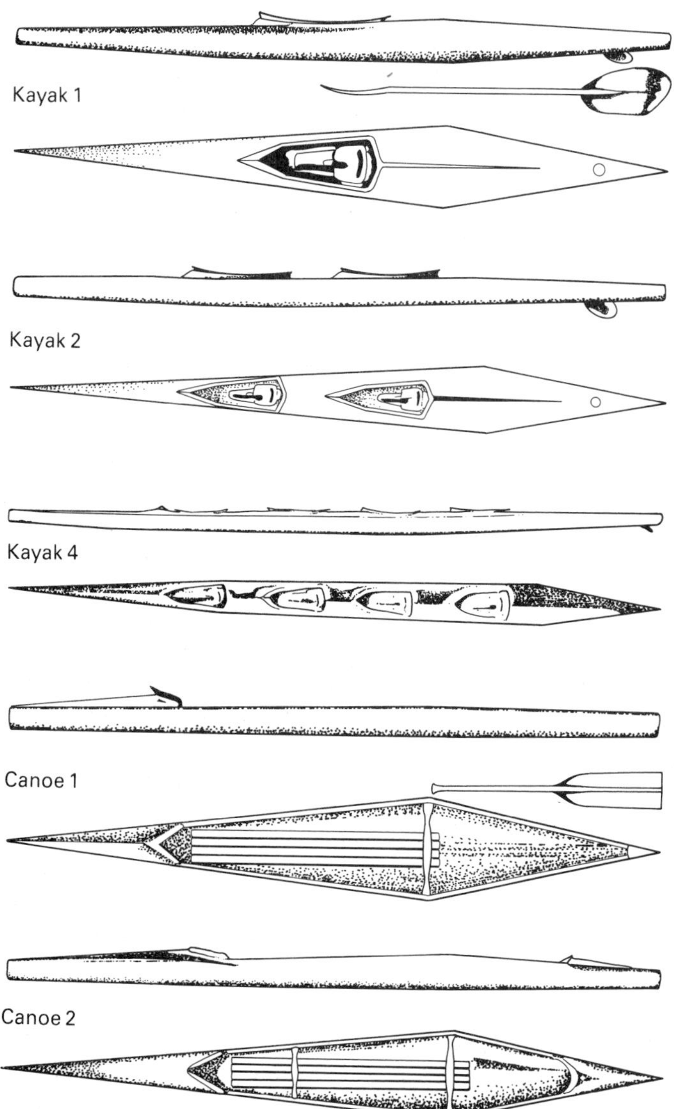

Fig. 41.1 Olympic racing canoes and kayaks. From Dal Monte *et al*. (1992).

of rivers, either natural or man-made, steep enough to produce strong currents and rapids and require the navigation of many gates in the fastest possible time. Although there are specific physiological requirements for white-water paddling, there is a much greater skill to conditioning ratio in this sport as compared to the flatwater competitions.

Common injuries

The physical demands of the sport necessitate formalized training programmes that are done on a year-round basis. This can result in injuries that occur both in the training facilities as well as on the water. The commonest musculoskeletal injuries are presented in Table 41.1.

Table 41.1 Common musculoskeletal injuries in canoeists.

Shoulder	Impingement syndrome, bicipital tendinitis, glenohumeral dislocations/subluxations
Forearm	Tenosynovitis of wrist extensor tendons, flexor tendinitis, carpal tunnel syndrome, forearm compartment syndrome
Back	Thoracic and lumbar muscle strain, lumbar disc herniation
Pelvic	Ischial bursitis, hamstring tendinitis, sciatic nerve compression
Miscellaneous	Peripatellar busitis, finger contusions, finger and heel calluses

Shoulder injuries

Impingement syndrome, both acute and chronic, is a constant source of lost training or missed competition. By the very nature of the canoe stroke the subacromial bursa and supraspinatus tendon are prone to impingement by the acromion process and coraco-acromial ligament. Figure 41.2 shows the proper technique of a flatwater canoe (C1) paddler. The top arm is placed in a position of forward flexion, abduction and internal rotation, and it is possible for these structures to be pinched on a repetitive basis. The kayak paddler also abducts and elevates the arm and can experience similar shoulder injuries. The mechanism responsible for this condition is overuse resulting in microtrauma causing local inflammation often associated with oedema. The muscular hypertrophy common in these athletes is a significant contributing factor in the development of this syndrome. Unfortunately this condition can become chronic as persistent inflammation can lead to fibrosis. Rotator cuff degeneration and tear, however, is very rare in this athletic population.

The most common presentation of acute impingement syndrome is early in the season when the on-the-water workouts begin. In the northern hemisphere, water training begins in the early spring and the environmental conditions can contribute to the development of this condition. Windy, cold weather does not allow for an adequate warm-up and balance can be compromised in these unstable boats leading to less than optimal technique. In the shoulder region, the bicipital tendon is also subjected to overuse and tendinitis of this structure is a common occurence.

Conservative treatment of impingement syndrome in competitive paddlers is usually all that is required; surgery for this condition in canoeists is rare. Common practice is to involve flexibility and strength training of all the rotator

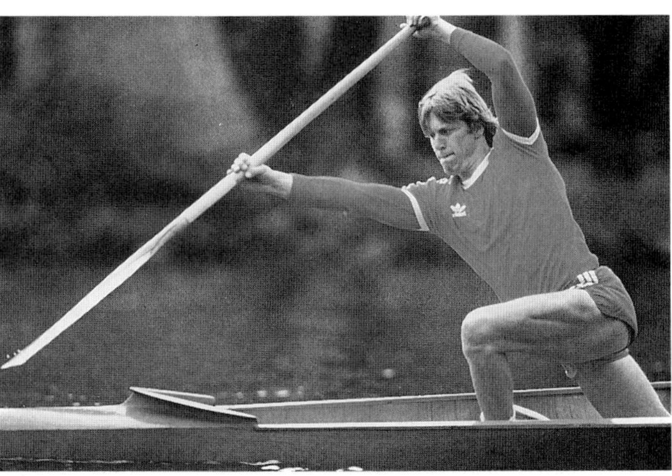

Fig. 41.2 Larry Cain, 1984 Olympic Gold and Silver Medalist (Canada), showing correct paddling technique for a flatwater canoeist.

cuff muscles as a preventive measure. Particular emphasis should be placed on the development of the strength of the external rotators. Testing with an isokinetic dynamometer has revealed that these athletes have exceptional strength in the movements of external and internal rotation of the shoulder. In order to prevent shoulder injuries one should strive for a ratio of external to internal strength of 0.7.

An analysis of the technical components of the stroke is warranted (Logan & Holt, 1985) and a reduction in the training volume and intensity may be necessary to allow the inflammatory reaction to subside. It is also necessary to consider the other accessory muscle involved in paddling as stroke mechanics are complicated and pathology in the shoulder may be a result of weakness and inflexibility of other muscles. Ice massage, non-steroidal anti-inflammatory medications (NSAIDs), physiotherapy, massage therapy and corticosteroid injections all have a role in the treatment of this disorder.

Whitewater paddlers are much more likely to experience shoulder dislocations and subluxations. Glenohumeral dislocation or subluxation occurs when a paddler is forced to brace strenuously downward to avoid capsizing. Frequently the shoulder is placed in a position of hyperabduction which levers the humeral head out of the glenoid fossa. The potential for this injury is greater in female paddlers who have less upper body muscle mass (Burrell & Burrell, 1982). Once again, shoulder-strengthening programmes form an integral portion of the training of these athletes.

Forearm injuries

Paddlers frequently suffer injuries to the forearm; the commonest injury being a tenosynovitis of the extensor tendons of the wrist. This is an overuse injury often seen with the initiation of on-the-water training. Traditionally, long distances are done early in the season and this excessive use can lead to an inflammatory condition. Windy conditions can also contribute to this injury as the athlete is forced to grip the paddle aggressively to control the boat and maintain proper technique. The control hand of the kayak paddler is most commonly affected as the wrist extensors of this hand are subjected to more use.

Several years ago there was a change in paddle shafts from wood to carbon fibre and the blade was altered to a 'wing' configuration. The harder shaft and altered stroke mechanics initiated by this new technology necessitated a period of adaptation. Many athletes fought the way the blade moved through the water and attempted to force the blade to follow their preconceived idea of where the blade was to travel. The result was a rash of forearm muscle strains and tendinitis.

Chronic tenosynovitis of the wrist extensor tendons with inflammation, crepitus, heat and swelling can be resistant to conservative management. Conservative treatment, including NSAIDs, subcutaneous heparin injections and physiotherapy, is useful but occasionally athletes must withdraw from the sport for extensive periods of time to allow this injury to heal. There have been cases where surgery is necessary so the athlete can return to competitive canoeing.

Aggressive gripping of the paddle is responsible for other forearm injuries. Flexor tendinitis is more common in the canoe paddler who must steer this rudderless boat with the bottom hand. Flexion of the wrist is necessary to perform the J stroke and, once again, the weather can play a role in the development of this injury. A cross-wind forces exaggerated wrist flexion and overuse initiates an inflammatory response. A tight grip of the paddle for a prolonged period of time can result in median nerve entrapment at the wrist. Tendon hypertrophy in these athletes may also play a role in the development of this exercise-related carpal tunnel syndrome. The classic signs and symptoms (pain, numbness and Tinel's sign) may be present in these athletes. Usually a looser grip and a paddle with a smaller diameter shaft will resolve this condition and further investigations and more aggressive therapy are seldom necessary.

Rarely, a tight grip, accompanied by intense activity, can result in a forearm compartment syndrome. Immediately post-exercise these athletes have very painful, tight, hard, flexor compartments with restricted wrist flexion and occasional numbness in the hand. Peripheral pulses are normal and the acute discomfort resolves within a few minutes. This condition can compromise training and treatment is directed at achieving a looser grip on the paddle and a change in the shaft dimensions. Massage therapy and a stretching programme for the forearms have both been useful adjuncts to the technical modifications.

Back injuries

The large muscles of the upper and lower back and shoulders provide the power in all canoe and kayak strokes and these muscles are subject to frequent strain (Walsh, 1985). Usually these injuries respond quickly to a period of modified activity, including specific flexibility exercises, and the athlete is able to return to training within a short period of time. The more serious injuries in this area occur in the weight room where maximal lifts generate tremendous forces in the thoracic and lumbar regions. The commonest injuries are to the rhomboid, trapezius, latissimus dorsi and serratus anterior muscle groups. Disc herniation and neurological involvement is rare in these athletes.

Pelvic injuries

Kayak paddlers spend a great deal of time sitting on a hard seat and with the rotation associated with each stroke considerable pressure is transmitted to the ischial tuberosities. The bursa that sits at the ischial tuberosity can become inflammed as can the origin of the hamstring muscles; pain in this area associated with longer periods in the kayak is a relatively common problem. Modifications of the seat with padding or even drilling holes in the seat to relieve pressure may help. Ice massage, hamstring stretching, physiotherapy and NSAIDs are useful therapeutic tools; corticosteroid injections into the bursa may be necessary to resolve this injury.

Sacral furunculosis can be a troublesome local lesion in kayak paddlers. These can be helped with meticulous attention to hygiene and washing and drying all paddling gear before it is used again. Topical and, occasionally, oral antibiotics are sometimes necessary in the treatment of these infections.

Compression of the sciatic nerve in the buttock with numbness to the foot is a chronic complaint which can be relieved by moving the position of the seat slightly, using appropriate padding, and maintaining the flexibility of the back, hamstring and gluteal muscles.

Miscellaneous conditions

The canoe paddler is subject to peripatellar pain in the 'down' knee and a chronic bursitis in this area has been reported. Modification of the block with special padding can resolve this injury.

Trauma with other boats, paddles, rocks, gates, etc. can result in lacerations, contusions and finger dislocations. Flatwater canoeing is a non-contact sport but there are occasions, particularly in distance races not conducted in lanes, where 'wash-riding' is employed; this can result in accidental contact and minor trauma. The slalom paddler is affected by a large number of variables and contact with rocks, gates or the side of the boat cannot always be avoided and a traumatic injury can occur.

All paddlers can form large calluses on the inside of the thumb where the paddle rubs; these can also form on the heel and dorsum of the foot from the foot strap. Careful maintenance of these calluses is necessary.

Medical problems

Canoeists face many of the usual problems

seen in sports medicine. They have a high energy demand and risk overtraining during periods of intense preparation for competition (Fry *et al.*, 1991).

Preparticipation screening

Training and competing at the élite level places a great deal of stress on the individual. Preparticipation screening of canoeists is therefore recommended and should consist of a medical history questionnaire plus a physical examination. A positive family history and/or cardiovascular symptoms such as chest pain, dyspnoea, dizziness and syncope should be followed by evaluation of physical status, an electrocardiogram (ECG) and echocardiography. Blood and urine tests, to determine haemoglobin and iron status or to detect unsuspected disease, are done routinely in several countries. Specific attention should be paid to the musculoskeletal system of these athletes. A detailed history and physical examination of the shoulder is necessary to assess range of motion, strength and muscle imbalance. If it is available, objective measurement of the strength of the internal and external rotators of the shoulder should also be done.

Environmental problems

The specific medical problems of canoeing are mainly related to environmental factors in connection with accidental turn-overs during training or competition. Many élite paddlers strive to train all year round on the water. During the winter the water is colder and there is an increased risk of hypothermia and drowning if the paddler should fall into the water. A sudden immersion can cause hyperventilation, bronchospasm and cardiac arrest due to the shock of cold water (Baker & Atha, 1981). Longer exposure results in loss of the capability to maintain thermoregulation and hypothermia can occur.

Therefore, when the water is cold, all paddlers are advised to wear adequate clothing (such as splash covers and wet-suits), floatation devices (such as a life-jacket) and to ensure that their boats have enough buoyant support. Although drowning is uncommon among élite paddlers (a major Swedish flatwater racing club has had two drownings in 30 years), it must be given serious consideration as a risk when training on cold water. A good method of prevention is to teach the paddlers that 'there are equal amounts of water close to the shore as in the middle of the lake'.

Heat produced during exercise in a hot, humid environment cannot be readily dissipated from the body. Therefore, during prolonged exercise in the heat there is a risk of developing fatigue secondary to hyperthermia. When accompanied by dehydration, heat exhaustion may lead to hypovolaemia, inability to provide both skeletal muscle and skin with oxygenated blood in required rates and heat stroke. This disorder is a potentially lethal condition characterized by disturbed consciousness and organ damage.

Another common environmental problem is solar radiation. During the summer months there is a considerable risk for sun-related medical problems due to increased exposure, diminished ozone levels and additional reflection from the water. Sunburn is a common problem and other solar-induced skin diseases, such as melanoma, are increasing in frequency, particularly in fair-skinned populations. Paddlers are prone to the development of pterygium, a growth of connective tissue that can extend over the conjunctiva. This ophthalmological condition is promoted by exposure to wind, water and the sun. Several cases of this condition have been reported in paddlers and excision of the lesion is necessary. Therefore, it is recommended that all paddlers wear sun protection (such as protective clothes, hats, sunscreens and sunglasses).

Common diseases responsible for turn-overs

Most turn-overs in élite paddlers are accidental but it is important to diagnose and treat diseases which can cause transient unconsciousness or an inability to maintain balance. It must be realized that these diseases are not dangerous *per se*, but may be hazardous due to the fact that they may lead to turn-overs. Most élite paddlers are young and healthy, but despite an excellent athletic profile they can have such underlying diseases. Many uncommon, mostly genetic, diseases may cause unconsciousness, but they will not be discussed here.

NEUROLOGICAL DISEASES

Exercise-induced syncope is a fairly common problem. It is the result of global cerebral ischaemia due to failure of cerebral perfusion. Perfusion failure during, or shortly after, a prolonged exertion, such as hard endurance training, may be related to cutaneous vasodilation while muscle blood vessels are still dilated, compromising cardiac output and resulting in syncope. Migrainous attacks (effort migraine) can occur after athletic effort of any kind. Many effort migraine attacks have only parts of the classic migraine. Severe headache, scotomas, occasional hyperventilation and nausea usually occur immediately after exertion. Focal neurological deficits are seldom seen. The symptoms may be precipitated by dehydration, excessive heat, hypoglycaemia and unaccustomed altitude. Effort migraine is more common in untrained athletes and tends to decrease provided physical fitness improves and other precipitating factors are avoided.

CARDIAC DISEASES

The Wolf–Parkinson–White (WPW) syndrome is an electrocardiographic syndrome due to the presence of a congenital anomalous atrioventricular conduction pathway. WPW syndrome is associated with attacks of tachycardia, sometimes very fast and of long duration. These attacks decrease cardiac output and symptoms such as dizziness and syncope may occur. At present, WPW syndrome can be treated successfully by pharmacological and surgical methods.

Paroxysmal atrial tachycardia (PAT) is a common type of cardiac arrhythmia seen in young adults. It is usually a benign re-entry arrhythmia with a duration from seconds to hours. During the attacks of tachycardia, cardiac output decreases and symptoms such as dizziness and syncope occur. PAT may be precipitated by dehydration, hypoglycaemia and drugs like β-stimulators and caffeine. This arrhythmia often diminishes with increasing age and absence of precipitating factors. PAT can be successfully treated with pharmacological agents, but several of these medications (especially β-blockers) decrease exercise capacity as well.

Hypertrophic cardiomyopathy (HCM) is the most common cause of sudden death in young athletes (Pelliccia *et al.*, 1991). It is a congenital disease with hypertrophy of the left ventricular wall, mostly the septum. The abnormal heart muscle can cause malignant ventricular arrhythmias and death. The symptoms are often few and may include accentuated dyspnoea, dizziness and syncope. However, sometimes sudden death is the first manifestation of the disease. About 30% of deaths in HCM occur during exercise, and the disease is therefore an absolute contraindication for exertional sports/training including canoeing and kayaking. HCM often causes ECG abnormalities and is diagnosed with echocardiography.

ENDOCRINE DISEASES

The type 1 diabetes mellitus is insulin-dependent and most often young individuals are affected. With proper insulin treatment many diabetic patients can participate on a high athletic level. The glycaemic control is, however, extremely important in paddlers since both hypoglycaemia and hyperglycaemia may lead to disturbed consciousness.

RESPIRATORY DISEASES

Exercise-induced asthma (EIA) is common in

the athletic population. Studies from many countries have demonstrated that approximately 10% of Olympic athletes have EIA. Usually paddlers do not have any specific problems controlling EIA. EIA which occurs on the water, however, may cause balance problems for the paddler especially if the EIA is severe and the paddler has problems finding the treatment (usually inhalers with β-stimulators/corticosteroids).

Specific problems for female paddlers

Female élite paddlers have the same medical problems as male paddlers. There are, however, two additional problems that must be stressed. As in other endurance sports, the hard training necessary for world-class canoeists may lead to disturbed menstruation and amenhorroea. Secondary to the low oestrogen levels there is a risk of development of osteopenia and stress fractures. Female athletes have a lower intake and larger losses of iron than do male athletes and therefore females run an increased risk of developing a hypochromic anaemia that decreases their performance. Iron-deficiency anaemia is most easily diagnosed by haemoglobin concentration and serum ferritin (an indicator of the iron stores). Regular check-ups are recommended. It must be emphasized that iron supplements will enhance performance in individuals who have iron-deficiency anaemia, but not in athletes with normal iron stores.

Doping

Canoe races in the Olympic Games have a duration from approximately 1.5 to 4 min. As described under physiological demands, élite canoeists need high aerobic, anaerobic and maximal power. Hence, there is a risk that doping agents or methods improving these capacities may also improve paddling performance. Regular doping controls, carried out by the ICF at World and Olympic Championships since the beginning of the eighties, have not yet resulted in a positive test. However, in the last few years testing has been carried out in connection with other international regattas and some cases of doping with anabolic steroids have been found. Recent documents also indicate that the use of doping substances in paddlers has been more comprehensive than expected in some countries (Berendonck, 1991). As a result of these findings the ICF has taken firm action against the use of forbidden substances and methods and has started up a comprehensive programme for out-of-competition testing of élite paddlers.

References

Baker, S. & Atha, J. (1981) Canoeists' disorientation following cold water immersion. *Br. J. Sports Med.* **5**, 111–15.

Berendonck, B. (1991) *Doping Dokumente. Von der Forschung zum Betrug*. Springer Verlag, Berlin.

Burrell, C.L. & Burrell, R. (1982) Injuries in whitewater paddling. *Phys. Sportsmed.* **10**, 119–24.

Dal Monte, A., Faccini, P. & Colli, R. (1992) Canoeing. In R.J. Shephard & P.-O. Åstrand (eds) *Endurance in Sport*, pp. 550–62. Blackwell Scientific Publications, Oxford.

Fry, R.W., Morton, A.R. & Keast, D. (1991) Overtraining in athletes. An update. *Sports Med.* **12**, 32–65.

Logan, S.M. & Holt, L.E. (1985) the flatwater kayak stroke. *Natl Strength Conditioning Assoc. J.* **7**(5), 4–11.

Paschke, W.S. (1987) *The World of Marathon Racing*. International Canoe Federation.

Pelliccia, A., Maron, B.J., Spataro, A., Proschan, M.A. & Spirito, P. (1991) The upper limit of physiological hypertrophy in highly trained élite athletes. *N. Engl. J. Med.* **324**, 295–301.

Shephard, R.J. (1987) Science and medicine of canoeing and kayaking. *Sports Med.* **4**, 19–33.

Walsh, M. (1985) Preventing injury in competitive canoeists. *Phys. Sportsmed.* **13**, 120–8.

Chapter 42

Injuries in Sailing

ROY J. SHEPHARD

Previous reports (Prevot & Auvinet, 1981; Plyley *et al.*, 1985; Shephard, 1990a,b) have reviewed the optimum characteristics of the successful competitive sailor. In contrast with many sports, the sailor is part of a complex human/machine system, and the primary energy source is found outside of the body (Gabillard, 1981). Apparently advantageous characteristics of the human operator (for instance, strong arms for manipulating controls such as rudders and sheets, and leverage for counterbalancing the boat) may be countered by adverse effects of these same characteristics upon other aspects of the system (for example, wind or water resistance). Moreover, the wind is a fickle source of energy. Strong gusts and squalls call for rapid decisions to avoid a danger such as capsizing, but under calm conditions the competitor must predict the course not only of her or his boat, but that of immediate rivals far into the future. Some events continue for many days, posing challenges of sustained vigilance (Levy, 1980; Gouard, 1981; Thomas, 1981) and circadian variations in both physical and mental performance (Shephard, 1984). Finally, the water is a hostile medium, presenting the discomfort of seasickness and the greater risks of hypothermia and drowning.

It is anticipated that the optimum body build and biomechanical and physiological characteristics would be rather specific, varying with wind conditions, type of craft, duration of event and crew position (Table 42.1). As the wind freshens, the primary demands shift from complex reasoning to the physical demands of handling ropes and counterbalancing the boat. A solo transatlantic crossing (Bennet, 1973; Urbanczyk, 1989) requires a very different type of sailor than the crew of a dinghy on a summer afternoon (MacBeth, 1983). To date, empirical observations have linked successful light wind performance only to an above-average resting blood sugar (Niinimaa *et al.*, 1977). Those with a high initial blood glucose may be more successful at sustaining cerebral function under conditions where glucose demand is increased (as in sustained anaerobic work). Under strong wind conditions, the skipper should be light (<60 kg), with quick reactions and an ability to communicate clear commands to crew members. Crew members should be heavy (>80 kg), but height does not give the expected advantage, perhaps because a tall person lacks the strength and tolerance of anaerobic metabolism to take full advantage of their greater leverage. One report has also linked aerobic power with the speed of a sailor's reactions to shifts of wind direction (Thomas, 1981).

The primary focus of this chapter is upon the prevention and treatment of medical problems associated with sailing and sailing events. Topics to be considered include recommendations for nutrition and training of the sailor, general health and safety precautions (including the maintenance of vigilance), potential musculoskeletal problems, exposure to sun, wind and water, seasickness, hypothermia and drowning.

Table 42.1 Optimum physical characteristics of international competitors, classified by type of vessel and crew position. From Shephard (1990b).

Category of craft	Canadian team				Participants in Montreal Olympics					
	Height (cm)		Body mass (kg)		Body fat (%)		Height (cm)		Body mass (kg)	
	Skipper	Crew	Skipper	Crew	Skipper	Crew	Skipper	Crew	Skipper	Crew
Board sailors (windsurfers)	—	172.3	—	65.7	—	14.3				
Finn	—	187.7	—	85.6	—	16.5	—	182.0	—	83.0
470	177.5	178.2	70.4	69.7	13.0	14.3	175.4	174.6	68.0	68.0
Flying Dutchman	181.6	183.7	74.8	85.4	14.3	20.0	177.8	183.2	73.8	83.2
Tornado	182.1	178.5	65.9	75.5	14.0	21.7	177.8	178.2	74.0	71.0
Star	183.1	179.9	91.1	86.5	16.5	16.0				
Soling	175.5	182.6	82.9	93.0	24.0	20.9	181.0	179.5	80.5	81.0

Nutrition and training

Nutrition

Participants in short- and medium-distance events must maintain sufficient plasma glutamine levels to sustain immune function, sufficient plasma glucose to maintain vigilance and cerebral function, and sufficient intramuscular glycogen to allow repeated anaerobic efforts by the skeletal muscles. To meet these objectives, the pre-race regimen should seek to overload muscle glycogen stores, using the techniques of the endurance competitor (Hultman & Greenstaff, 1992; Saltin & Hermansen, 1967), typically 3 days of a high-fat diet to deplete reserves, followed by a high carbohydrate intake (>600 g·day^{-1}) in the 3 days leading up to a key competition. Specific glutamine or carnitine supplements are sometimes suggested, but are probably not needed if the diet has an adequate content of high quality protein (>1.5 g·kg body mass^{-1}). Except in warm climates, fluid depletion is unlikely during competition. Carbohydrate can thus be administered as hypertonic solutions of glucose or glucose polymer, sweetened coffee or even as glucose-containing candy. A 500-ml dose of a polymer solution can be given 30 min before a race, and up to 150 ml in each succeeding 15-min interval, keeping watch for signs of gastric distention (and of bladder over-filling if the weather is cold).

Longer races can continue for as long as 50–60 days and body mass can decrease by as much as 10 kg (Lethuillier, 1983). If the route is through warm waters, the main cause is probably a cumulative mineral loss, with associated fluid depletion. Regular weighing of team members can detect and correct such problems at an early stage. Brisk breezes may mask a rapid rate of sweating in the tropics. In such a situation, sodium and potassium levels and the acid–base balance should be monitored, and the daily intake of salt should be increased. Leach (1978) has recommended regular administration of slow-release sodium tablets and the use of sea water for cooking.

Deep-water sailors face the occasional hazard of shipwreck, and life-rafts should carry at least a week's supply of emergency rations (60 MJ per crew member). If water is in short supply, urine production drops to the 'volume obligatoire' (850 ml·day^{-1} on a mixed diet, 550 ml·day^{-1} if starving and 150 ml·day^{-1} if energy needs can be met from carbohydrate). If no fresh water is available, body mass decreases by about 1 kg·day^{-1}. Water is drawn from the extracellular compartment and the kidneys attempt to normalize osmotic pressure by excreting minerals. However, osmotic pressure rises further, drawing fluid from within the cells. After 4 kg of fluid has been lost, both the kidneys and the circulation show signs of failure, but death is unlikely until 15 kg or more of water has been lost. Attempts to prolong survival by drinking sea water (Bombard cited by Mas, 1976) are generally unsuccessful. The salt content of the sea water shows some regional variation, but is usually about three times the plasma level. The ailing kidneys cannot excrete the excess of sodium ions, and the resulting rise in the osmotic pressure of the plasma and extracellular fluid merely draws additional fluid from the dehydrated cells (Mas, 1976; Shephard, 1982).

Training

Under light wind conditions, the prime basis of preparation of the sailor is practice in handling of the boat, and with the exception of tactics to augment blood glucose (discussed above), the sports physician can contribute little to the physiology of this process. Mental skills training, with a focus upon boosting feelings of readiness and confidence may help in meeting the psychological demands of high-level competition (Halliwell, 1989).

Under high and/or gusty wind conditions, possible tactics are to counterbalance the boat, or to reduce speed by spilling wind and reefing the sail. The counterbalancing force exerted by the sailor depends upon (i) body mass; (ii) the distribution of body mass (shoulders vs. legs); and (iii) the ability to sustain a 'hiking' position in the face of muscle fatigue and the accumulation of anaerobic metabolites. Overall body mass can be increased by soaking the clothing in water (increasing the risk of hypothermia), by over-eating (with an increase of body fat) or by progressive muscle-building exercises. Development of the shoulder muscles facilitates the handling of the sheet-ropes and maximizes leverage, but development of the thigh and abdominal muscles is also desirable to increase the tolerance of 'hiking'.

During the sailing season much of the necessary exercise can be obtained from sailing itself, but in countries such as Canada, the sailing season is short. International competitors must therefore adopt a land-based programme during the winter months in order to conserve (and if possible to develop) their physical condition (Clarke & Wright, 1973; Wright *et al.*, 1976). Normal circuit training (two 50-min sessions·week^{-1}) should be combined with two more specific weekly weight-training sessions (Table 42.2).

Wright *et al.* (1976) found that their regimen maintained aerobic power, decreased body fat and increased quadriceps girth, strength, muscular endurance and anaerobic capacity. Competitors were able to reach the same heart rate and oxygen consumption with a lesser production of lactate, thus conserving their muscle glycogen reserves. Tolerance of 'hiking' was also improved and there were substantial gains in competitive standings.

General health and safety precautions

Many of the precautions associated with organizing a major sailing event and optimizing the health of the competitors follow the principles associated with any type of athletic competition (Shephard, 1992), but additional

Table 42.2 Recommended programme of land-based training for sailors during the winter season. Based on recommendations of Wright *et al.* (1976).

Station	Activity	Repetitions
1	Sit-ups from a downward-sloping board with a 7-kg load behind the head	8 increasing to 15
2	Leg presses, lying on the back, elevating 100–150 kg by knee extension	15
3	Pulley work (both arms simultaneously): (i) raise arms above head, sagittal plane (ii) flex arms towards chest (iii) extend arms, frontal plane	50–100
4	Sit-ups from 'hiking' position with 7-kg load behind head	30 increasing to 50
5	Standard quadriceps exercises, unilateral loads of 35–50 kg	10, each leg in turn
6	Standard 'clean and press' manoeuvres at 45 kg progressing to 60 kg	10

Notes

1 Three circuits to be performed per day, with a 2-min interval between circuits

2 After 1 month, one of the 2-weekly strength sessions becomes a muscular endurance training session, with each item repeated three times before moving to the next station

3 After a further month, one of the two standard circuit training sessions is made into a muscular endurance session

4 Aerobic condition is improved by running 3–6 km at the best possible speed once or twice per week

challenges are imposed by the aquatic environment and the very limited space on most racing craft.

Event organization

Some yachting events attract large crowds, many in powerful boats. Regulation of traffic may thus be needed to avoid collisions and danger to competitors (Sleight, 1974). Alcohol consumption by spectators may be less easy to regulate than on land and any casualties are also less easy to evacuate (Galvin & Jelinek, 1989).

Sea rescue services should be well organized, and local hospitals and first-aid workers briefed on the appropriate treatment of hypothermia, drowning and other marine emergencies. In the Fastnet race of 1979, 15 people died and a further 179 had to be rescued, many by helicopter, because of inadequate information on weather conditions (O'Donnell, 1980).

Overall lifestyle

As in other sports where body mass confers a competitive advantage, there is a tendency for the sailor to accumulate body fat. The problem is exacerbated because the total energy demand under good weather conditions is quite light. One survey of national-level competitors (Plyley *et al.*, 1985) found an average aerobic power of only 45 $ml \cdot kg^{-1} \cdot min^{-1}$. Because the sport does not depend upon aerobic endurance, there is an increased risk that the competitor will be a smoker (Kavanagh *et al.*, 1993), and a high average age further augments the likelihood of significant coronary vascular disease (Mas, 1976).

Studies of mortality in athletes (Yamaji & Shephard, 1978; Polednak, 1979) have to date provided no specific information on prognosis in the sailor. The cardiovascular load involved in sail-trimming is not very high (Bernardi *et al.*, 1990), but the prolonged abdominal straining of 'hiking' seems likely to induce tachycardia and a rise of systemic blood pressure, augmenting the workload of the heart and predisposing to myocardial ischaemia. The preliminary medical examination should thus look carefully for cardiac risk factors, including early cardiac death in a near relative, cigarette smoking, obesity (determined from skinfold readings rather than body mass), hypertension, a low aerobic fitness level, and an abnormal resting or exercise electrocardiogram. Lipid screening is probably not warranted on all competitors, but is advisable if several other risk factors are present.

Counselling should be given to correct modifiable risk factors. Some sailors do now supplement on-water training with aerobic activity (Clarke & Wright, 1973; Dierck & Riechert, 1980; Wright *et al.*, 1976). Smoking cessation, a reduced intake of food and, where necessary, specific treatment of hypertension and hyperlipidaemia should also be arranged.

General health

The preliminary examination should ensure that the competitor is not only a competent swimmer and well-versed in lifesaving, but also has experience appropriate to the event in terms of navigational skills and communication techniques (Larson, 1974). A history of attacks of unconsciousness, whether from epilepsy or from cardiovascular problems, is a strong relative contraindication to involvement in sailing competitions (Dietz & Baker, 1974).

Balance and coordination should be good and reactions rapid. Good day and night vision are important in longer missions, as is the hearing needed to understand commands in a gale-force wind. Tolerance of solitude or the ability to work as a team also become vital on longer voyages (Leach, 1978; Levy, 1980). The ideal skipper is an introvert, with emotional stability, psychological endurance and dominance (Mas, 1976) plus a great tolerance of frustration (Thill, 1981, 1988). Particularly under foggy conditions, there must also be tolerance of sensory isolation and an ability to sustain vigilance in the virtual absence of external signals. Crew members, in contrast, can be extroverts, more spontaneous and impulsive, but willing to accept orders.

Prior to a major voyage, all the crew should receive a full schedule of vaccinations and innoculations (smallpox, yellow fever, cholera, typhoid, tetanus and poliomyelitis) in case injury or illness requires an unscheduled stop in a country where such infections are endemic (Leach, 1978). A thorough dental inspection is also a wise precaution. The vessel should carry a medical manual and a well-stocked medicine chest that includes at least two doses of papaveretum per crew member (Leach, 1978). An inflatable life-raft with appropriate survival kit (fishing equipment, knives, scissors, matches, cord, extra flares, a solar still, analgesics, antibiotics, lanoline, suture material, blankets and other necessities) should provide accommodation for the entire crew if the vessel founders (Leach, 1978).

As an event approaches, sailors face many of the health problems that are seen in other classes of competitor. A stress-related disturbance of immune function decreases resistance to respiratory viruses (Brenner *et al.*, 1993). The standard recommendation of avoiding others who are already infected (Shephard & Shek, 1993) may be difficult to implement in the confines of a small cabin. Potential preventive measures include a minimization of psychological stress (by such techniques as relaxation training and habituation to the competitive milieu), provision of a distraction-free environment that allows continued contact with home and family (Halliwell, 1989), maintenance of blood glucose and glutamine levels (important to lymphocyte proliferation) and possibly the administration of immunoglobulins to vulnerable individuals. If a long voyage is to be undertaken, it is particularly important to screen out as far as possible any individuals who are developing infections, as facilities for their treatment will be very limited while at sea.

Supplies of clean fresh water are very limited on a small boat, and there is a danger that inadequate washing of utensils and galley equipment may allow the transmission of gastrointestinal infections between crew members. There is increasing evidence of the bacterial contamination of estuaries and shallow sea water (Balarajan *et al.*, 1991). All water that is used in the galley should thus be boiled.

Disturbed sleep, shifts of circadian rhythm and the effects of either seasickness or the drugs used in its treatment can impair vigilance, increasing the risk of accidents and degrading competitive performance. If competition begins or is held in a foreign country, generous time should be allowed for the adaptation of the sailor's circadian rhythm to the new time zone (Shephard, 1984). Once adjustment to a given time zone has occurred, vigilance is at its poorest during the first watch. The skills of the calm-weather sailor are likely to reach their maximum in the late afternoon. Individuals vary in their hours of peak arousal, the 'larks' being at their best early in the morning and the 'owls' performing well in the late evening. Account should be taken of these interpersonal differences and an attempt made to adjust either watches or personal sleep schedules so that maximal wakefulness is achieved when sailing. In solitary, long-distance events, there is no such luxury. It has been argued that adverse placings result if a competitor takes more than 1 h of sleep at a time. Some contestants thus continue to control their vessels until they are totally exhausted. However, this is a dangerous practice and can lead to hallucinations, particularly in foggy weather. The optimum recommendation is probably to take at least three 2-h or two 3-h bouts of sleep in the course of a 24-h day (Lethuillier, 1983). Sleep should also be maximized prior to competition, and during an event it can be facilitated by an appropriate timing of anti-seasickness medicines.

Musculoskeletal and other injuries

The main muscular stress encountered by the sailor is the sustained isometric contraction of the quadriceps, the iliopsoas and (to a lesser extent) the abdominal muscles during 'hiking' manoeuvres (Rogge, 1973; Beillot *et al.*, 1979, 1981; Marchetti *et al.*, 1980). The whole weight of the body is in essence hanging upon the knees during this tactic (Newton, 1989). In Finn class vessels, the knees are commonly flexed to 90°, whereas Laser and Topper class vessels tend to be sailed with the knees almost fully extended (because of the short freeboard from the deck to the waterline). The body position also varies with the leg length of the sailor and the width of the deck. Effort is usually least at 60° of flexion (Rogge, 1973).

Laboratory simulation has shown peak heart rates averaging 137 beats·min^{-1}, and a peak blood pressure averaging 198/134 mmHg, corresponding to a sustained quadriceps contraction at 40% of maximal force (Niinimaa *et al.*, 1977). The manoeuvre induces a substantial short-term increase of blood glucose (to 6.5 mmol·l^{-1}) and a decrease of serum bicarbonate (to 21 mmol·l^{-1}) (Niinimaa *et al.*, 1977). During actual sailing, heart rates are quite variable, but again reach 140 beats·min^{-1} during 'hiking' (Bachemont *et al.*, 1981; Pudenz *et al.*, 1981).

One practical consequence of such heavy straining is anterior knee and/or low back pain. The former is often associated with the patellofemoral pain syndrome (Newton, 1989). Complaints are more frequent in Finn than in Laser sailors, but even in the latter type of craft as many as a third of competitors have pain at the beginning of the sailing season. Roughening of the articular surface of the patella can rarely be detected with radiography, but there is a typical history of pain when rising from a squatting position, when coming downstairs and when sitting for long periods (for instance, on an intercontinental airflight). There is often patellofemoral crepitus, pain when the patella is pressed upon the femoral condyles and during a lateral displacement of the patella. Genu recurvatum and a poor development of the quadriceps are predisposing factors. One immediate remedy may be to vary the pivoting point of the limbs during 'hiking'. This can be achieved by attaching foam-rubber planchettes to the rear of the thighs (Beillot *et al.*, 1981). In a longer term perspective, isotonic and/or isometric exercises should be introduced to develop the medial head of the quadriceps. The back pain also reflects muscle weakness, and prevention is mainly based upon a strengthening of the relevant muscles by squats and leg presses.

Accidents

In terms of other injuries, the most dangerous part of the voyage may be from the quay to the boat (O'Donnell, 1979). Over a 1-year period, water sports accounted for 43% of all recreational deaths in Scotland (Moncur, 1973). Boat propellers can cause fractures or amputations of the limbs which are rapidly fatal; it is vital that anyone operating power boats in the vicinity of competitions have adequate protection against dazzle from direct and reflected solar radiation (Sleight, 1974). A person who falls from a tender that is moving at high speed may force water into various body orifices, with attendant risks of sinusitis, otitis media, perforation of an ear drum, salpingitis and even rectal tears (Ramey, 1974). Spinal injuries and concussion are also possible if the falling body hits a rock (Paterson, 1971).

Other potential injuries (Winker, 1979) include cuts, grazes and burns from ropes or galley (Leach, 1978). When cooking at sea, it is a wise precaution to wear long oilskin trousers or a plastic apron. After cleaning with povidone-iodine, cuts can be closed using Steri-Strips; they should then be sprayed with Novecutane (a water-repellant acrylic resin/ethyl acetate preparation). Fractures from falls and concussion from a jibing boom are other hazards. Fractures require immobilization and adequate analgesics. If the leg is injured, evacuation will probably be required, and the same is a wise precaution if there has been more than a very transient loss of consciousness from concussion.

Exposure to sun, wind and water

Sunburn, herpetic blisters and a long-term risk of skin cancers (Gentile & Auerbach, 1987) are particular hazards of sailing. The light haze of many coastal areas masks the intensity of the ultraviolet irradiation, and burning is further concealed by the cooling effects of wind and water. An effective sunscreen must thus be applied liberally over all exposed areas of the skin surface (Leach, 1978).

Constant soaking of the hands with salt water leaches out the neutral oils. The skin becomes waterlogged and subsequently develops painful fissures. Frequent rubbing with lanoline helps to keep the skin soft and supple.

The air temperature at sea is usually lower than on land, and general body cooling is enhanced by a high wind velocity and by the relative motion of the boat. In winter weather, care must be taken to avoid frostbite of exposed skin (Reilly & Sanderson, 1981). Some sailors deliberately reduce the insulation of their clothing by soaking it to increase the effective body mass; spray often produces a similar effect. Chilling of the body is thus a frequent experience. It leads to a progressive deterioration of cognitive skills (DeFrancisco, 1993), strength, neuromuscular coordination and manual dexterity, with a decrease in the proprioception essential for accurate control of a vessel (Larin, 1990). Competitive performance thus decreases and accidents become more likely. As in other cold environments, the approximate impact can be estimated from the wind-chill index (Siple & Passel, 1945) and the duration of an event or a watch. Care must be taken to base estimates on marine, rather than on land, weather conditions. Protection against cold conditions rests on clothing that not only provides good insulation, but is adequately waterproofed and provides appropriate buoyancy if the vessel capsizes or sinks. Under very cold conditions, it is also advisable to shorten the length of watches (Leach, 1978).

Seasickness

Seasickness is that form of motion sickness associated with boats (Mas, 1976). It is thought to be caused primarily by a mismatching of neural input to the brain (Money, 1970; Shephard, 1974; Reason & Brand, 1975). If the sailor is resting in the cabin, the external horizon usually cannot be seen, and the mismatch is thus between the eyes and the vestibular system. When on deck, the mismatch is between the otoliths and the semicircular canals; a repetitive vertical motion causes the otoliths to detect an apparent cyclic change in the gravity vector, but the anticipated synchronized rotation does not occur (Reason & Brand, 1975; Reason, 1978; Pingree, 1989).

The main symptoms are nausea, malaise and epigastric discomfort or awareness. Of greater significance from the viewpoints of competition and safety in operation of a vessel, there may also be drowsiness, apathy, lassitude, a strong frontal headache, dizziness, spatial disorientation, anxiety and mental confusion (Money, 1970). Psychomotor manifestations include carelessness in the performance of routine duties, decreased muscular coordination and handgrip force, decreased performance on a pursuit meter, a decreased ability to estimate time and a decreased ability to carry out simple arithmetic (Money, 1970). Most people are aware of a decrement in their performance (Parrott, 1987). There is an associated oliguria (Taylor *et al.*, 1957), and an increased secretion of growth hormone, prolactin, antidiuretic hormone and cortisol (Eversmann *et al.*, 1978).

The incidence of seasickness varies from 15 to 66% of the population, being most frequently encountered by people in small vessels (Lawther & Griffin, 1986). It correlates closely with accelerations in the vertical axis (the heave of the boat), with only minor contributions from rotational motion (pitch and roll) (Lawther & Griffin, 1986). The critical frequency range is 0.05–0.5 Hz, with a peak susceptibility at 0.2 Hz. The probability of sickness also depends on the duration of exposure, the 'dose' being proportional to $t^{1/2}$ (Lawther & Griffin, 1986). Women are reportedly more susceptible than men (possibly because of hormonal differences), and the problem becomes less severe as a person becomes older; because they lack a functional vestibular apparatus, deaf mutes are immune to seasickness (Money, 1970). Susceptibility is greatly influenced by attitude and motivation (Reason & Brand, 1975), and symptoms are reputedly worsened by odours such as diesel fumes (Pingree, 1989). There may, finally, be circadian differences in susceptibility, corresponding to differences in sympathetic nervous system activation (McCauley *et al.*, 1979).

Given that the primary cause of seasickness is vertical motion, the most effective basis of prevention is to minimize such motion. Motion is likely to be least at the midpoint of the vessel, and susceptibility can be decreased fivefold by adoption of a prone position; intermittent recumbency can sometimes help a vulnerable individual (Money, 1970). Restriction of head movements only seems effective if dark goggles are used to limit vision. There have been claims that problems can be reduced by taking light carbohydrate meals with small amounts of liquid, but avoiding cerebral stimulants such as caffeine. Others maintain that the timing of the last meal has little impact on susceptibility. Likewise, although the seasick sailor may express a wish for fresh cool air, the ambient air temperature apparently has little influence on the course of the condition (Money, 1970). Adaptation occurs with repeated or prolonged exposure to the motion of the boat and is one of the most effective types of preventive therapy; however, a period of as long as 1 month may be required by very sensitive individuals (Pingree, 1989). Biofeedback training is also sometimes helpful, and uncontrolled studies have suggested benefit from acupuncture or localized applications of pressure (Weightman *et al.*, 1987; Pingree, 1989).

From a pharmacological point of view, seasickness is thought to develop when central cholinergic activity exceeds the counterbalancing influence of central adrenergic activity. The prime drugs used in treatment are thus anticholinergic agents such as hyoscine, antihistamine (H1 antagonists) such as cinnarizine (which probably also work via a cholinergic effect), and sympathomimetic drugs such as ephedrine (Pingree, 1989). Hyoscine is the most popular drug in both prevention and secondary treatment, although it is by no means 100% effective. It may be given orally (0.6 mg 6-hourly); an effect is then obtained within 1 h of ingestion (Pingree, 1989). If vomiting is severe, it may also be given intramuscularly (Graybiel & Lackner, 1987). Transdermal administration by adhesive patches (McCauley *et al.*, 1979; Homick *et al.*, 1983) is also gaining popularity. By this route, an effect is seen within 4 h, and it usually persists for 72 h. The transdermal route may be preferred if gastrointestinal symptoms have already developed. Patches are designed to deliver 0.5 mg, although absorption is subject to much inter- and intra-individual variation; key influences are environmental temperature, cutaneous bloodflow and the oiliness of the skin (Homick *et al.*, 1983).

Cinnarizine (Hargreaves, 1980) is typically administered as an initial oral dose of 30 mg, followed by 15 mg 8-hourly. It does not take effect for 2–5 h.

Both drugs cause a number of major side-effects, particularly at times of the day when sympathetic activity is reduced. Problems include sedation, a dry mouth, dilated pupils with blurring of vision, loss of memory and poor sustained attention. Occasionally, the patient develops visual hallucinations or a confusional state (McCauley *et al.*, 1979; Pingree, 1989). Given that many of these side-effects limit sailing ability, such drugs are unpopular in competitions and other situations where sustained vigilance is required. Since the drugs are sympathetic stimulants, care must also be taken that anti-doping rules are not violated.

Hypothermia and drowning

As noted above, the combination of a relatively

low metabolic heat production, a high speed of air movement over clothing, and a reduction of the anticipated insulation of the clothing by spray, fog, rain or deliberate wetting give some risk of impaired performance and hypothermia during normal sailing. However, this risk is greatly increased if the vessel is capsized (Keatinge, 1965, 1969). The thermal conductivity of water is some 25 times greater than that of air, so that even if the water temperature is as high as 20°C, a person who is immersed without special protection has a heat loss of 54 $kJ \cdot m^{-2} \cdot min^{-1}$. For much of the year, the water temperature in many parts of the world (0–10°C) is far removed from the thermally neutral zone (32–34°C), and both skin and core temperatures drop very quickly if the sailor is immersed.

The early reactions associated with sudden immersion pose significant threats to survival (Golden & Hervey, 1981; Tipton, 1989, 1993). An intense stimulation of cutaneous cold receptors causes a sensation of breathlessness, with reflex gasping and an inability to control breathing (Goode *et al.*, 1975; Cabanac, 1979). This makes swimming difficult and aspiration of water into the lungs becomes likely. It also becomes impossible to hold one's breath if attempting to escape from a submerged craft.

There may be an immediate bradycardia, but this is soon replaced by peripheral vasoconstriction, with an increase of both heart rate and systemic blood pressure. In individuals with some coronary atheroma, the combination of intense reflex stimulation with an increase of cardiac work can provoke premature ventricular contractions, myocardial infarction and (rarely) ventricular fibrillation or cardiac arrest ('hydrocution', Mas, 1976). An allergic type of reaction has also been described (LaHoute, 1979). This initial phase, which lasts at most 3 min, is probably the most hazardous component of immersion. The stimulus is a rapid decrease of skin temperature, rather than a decrease of core temperature, and the risk can be greatly diminished by a well-designed 'dry' suit that slows skin cooling.

Assuming the sailor survives the immediate cold shock, there is a progressive decrease of core temperature, with a slowing of muscle contractions, malfunction of the sensory receptors, uncontrollable shivering and a progressive clouding of consciousness. Early estimates of the rate of cooling and of survival times were based on the notorious Dachau 'experiments', where the majority of victims were pathologically thin. The survival of the well-nourished sailor is 2–3 times longer if exposed to the same water temperatures (Hayward, 1975). The rate of body cooling depends on many factors, including (i) water temperature; (ii) the insulation provided by any protective clothing; (iii) subcutaneous fat and unperfused muscle (Keatinge, 1969); (iv) posture (heat loss is minimized in the foetal position) (Hayward, 1975); (v) the extent of shivering (possibly depressed if intramuscular glycogen stores have already been depleted by 'hiking'); and (vi) currents and wave motion (which displace the film of warm water near the skin surface) (Steinman *et al.*, 1987).

There has been considerable discussion of swimming as a potential tactic for increasing body heat production; however, it is now agreed that the movement of the limbs increases heat loss, probably more from increased perfusion of the limb muscles and a resulting loss of insulation than from a stirring of the water in the immediate vicinity of the body (Hayward, 1975). Unless the shore is close at hand, the best plan seems to be to huddle in the foetal position and await rescue. Experiments in the USA navy (Molnar cited by Mas, 1976) suggest that the unprotected sailor can survive some 3 h in water at 10°C, and about 1.5 h at 5°C, although consciousness is usually lost more rapidly than this. Ventricular fibrillation becomes increasingly likely when the core temperature has dropped to 25–30°C.

A neoprene suit slows the rate of cooling by a factor of five at a water temperature of 5°C (Mas, 1976). Protection against hypothermia is sometimes better in a 'wet' than in a 'dry' suit (Goldman & Breckenridge, 1966; Allan *et al.*,

1986), but this advantage must be weighed against the potentially greater and more frequent dangers of an early cold shock response. The latter is best avoided by a dry suit with good wrist and neck seals (Tipton & Vincent, 1991). Uninsulated dry suits are the most comfortable form of cold protection to wear, and it has been argued that they provide adequate protection against hypothermia. Laboratory tests, however, have frequently lacked rigour, approval of a suit assembly being based upon the maintenance of core temperature without consideration of any increases in resting metabolism that may have been needed to assure this (Pasche, 1993). In the real world of the sailor, penetration of the clothing by cold water is greatly increased due to wind, waves, exercise, initial submersion and less than optimal sealing at the neck and wrists (Hall & Polte, 1956; Allan *et al.*, 1985, 1986). For example, Tipton (1991) found that a combination of a 15-s submersion, a light wind, small waves and periodic surface spraying decreased the effectiveness of a dry suit by 30% relative to specification.

Given that consciousness may be lost if rescue is delayed, it is important that the lifebelt is fully compatible with any immersion suit that is worn. The system should ensure self-righting, keeping the airways clear of the water and maintaining stability in a rough sea.

The colour of the clothing should be chosen with a view to facilitating rescue, whether the person is on the surface or submerged. Bioluminescent materials from marine animals have been suggested as a useful method of colouring garments (Dietz & Baker, 1974).

Conclusion

The physiological and psychological demands of sailing are highly specific to wind conditions, type of vessel, type of competition and crew position. Nevertheless, the sports physician can do much to maximize the physiological and psychological determinants of top performance. General health must be maximized, bearing in mind a number of aspects of sailing which threaten immune function and thus increase the risk of viral infections. Diet should seek to maximize intramuscular glycogen stores and to maintain blood glucose during competition. Training should extend over both summer and winter seasons, focusing on the development of the thigh and abdominal muscles, in order to minimize the risk of the lower back and patellofemoral pain that can result from prolonged 'hiking'. An aerobic training component should also be provided to minimize the risks of cardiovascular disease. Sailors must be protected against exposure to sunlight, cold winds and cold water. Vigilance must be sustained in the face of night watches and shifts of circadian rhythm. Advisors to the sailing team must, finally, have appropriate measures to counter seasickness in rough weather and to minimize the dangers of hypothermia and drowning if a vessel capsizes or is shipwrecked.

References

Allan, J.R., Higenbotham, C. & Redman, P.J. (1985) The effect of leakage on the insulation provided by immersion-protective clothing. *Aviat. Space Environ. Med.* **56**, 1107–9.

Allan, J.R., Elliott, D.H. & Hayes, P.A. (1986) The thermal performance of partial coverage wet suits. *Aviat. Space Environ. Med.* **57**, 1056–60.

Bachemont, F., Fouillot, J.P., Izou, M.A., Terkaia, M.A. & Drobowski, Th. (1981) Etude de la fréquence cardiaque en deriveur et planche à la voile par monitoring ambulatoire (Study of the heart rate in centre-board and sail-boarding by ambulatory monitoring). *Cinésiol.* **80**, 231–7.

Balarajan, R., Raleigh, V.S., Yuen, P., Wheeler, D., Machin, D. & Cartwright, R. (1991) Health risks associated with bathing in sea water. *Br. Med. J.* **303**, 1444–5.

Beillot, J., Rochcongar, P., Gouard, P., Simonet, J., Briend, G. & LeBars, R. (1979) Approache biomécanique de la position de rappel (Biomechanical approach to 'hiking'). *Lyon Mediterranée Méd.* **15**, 1279–83.

Beillot, J., Rochcongar, P., Gouard, P., Simonet, J., Briend, G. & LeBars, R. (1981) Le rappel sur Finn: approache biomécanique ('Hiking' on Finn craft: biomechanical approach). *Cinésiol.* **80**, 179–81.

Bennet, G. (1973) Medical and psychological problems in the 1972 single-handed trans-Atlantic yacht race. *Lancet* **ii**, 747–54.

Bernardi, M., Felici, F., Marchietti, M. & Marchettoni, P. (1990) Cardiovascular load in off-shore sailing competition. *J. Sports Med. Phys. Fitness* **30**, 127–31.

Brenner, I., Shek, P.N. & Shephard, R.J. (1993) Exercise and infection. *Sports Med.* (in press).

Cabanac, M. (1979) Temperature regulation. *Ann. Rev. Physiol.* **37**, 415–39.

Clarke, J. & Wright, G. (1973) Planned training programme for Sail Canada–Ontario Division. *Finnfare* **7** (Oct/Nov), 9–15.

DeFrancisco, P. (1993) Stress at work in cold climates – effects on performance. In *Proceedings, 9th International Congress on Circumpolar Health*, Reykjavik, June 1993, pp. S26–2. University of Reykjavik, Reykjavik.

Dierck, T.H. & Riechert, H. (1980) Belastung des Jugendlichen beim Optimistsegeln (Work rate of youngsters during 'optimist' sailing). *Dtsch. Z. Sportmed.* **31**(9), 262–7.

Dietz, P.E. & Baker, S.P. (1974) Drowning: Epidemiology and prevention. *Am. J. Publ. Health* **74**, 303–12.

Eversmann, T., Gottsmann, M., Uhlich, E., Ulbrecht, G., von Werder, K. & Scriba, P.C. (1978) Increased secretion of growth hormone, prolactin, antidiuretic hormone and cortisol induced by the stress of motion sickness. *Aviat. Space Environ. Med.* **49**, 53–7.

Gabillard, P. (1981) L'actualité en médecine appliquée à la voile (Current views on medicine applied to sailing). *Cinésiol.* **80**, 165–78.

Galvin, G.M. & Jelinek, G.A. (1989) The impact of the America's cup on Freemantle hospital. *Arch. Emerg. Med.* **6**, 262–5.

Gentile, D.A. & Auerbach, P.S. (1987) The sun and water sports. *Clin. Sports Med.* **6**, 669–84.

Golden, F.St-C. & Hervey, G.R. (1981) The 'afterdrop' and death after rescue from immersion in cold water. In J.A. Adam (ed) *Hypothermia Ashore and Afloat*. Aberdeen University Press, Aberdeen.

Goldman, R.F., Breckenridge, J.R., Reeves, J.E. *et al.* (1966) 'Wet' versus 'dry' suit approaches to water immersion protective clothing. *Aerospace Med.* **37**, 485–7.

Goode, R.C., Duffin, J., Miller, R., Romet, T., Chout, W. & Ackles, K. (1975) Sudden cold water immersion. *Resp. Physiol.* **23**, 301–10.

Gouard, Ph. (1981) La préparation scientifique de haut niveau en voile (Scientific preparation for high-level sailing contests). *Cinésiol.* **80**, 157–64.

Graybiel, A. & Lackner, J.R. (1987) Treatment of severe motion sickness with anti-motion sickness drug injections. *Aviat. Space Environ. Med.* **58**, 773–6.

Hall, J.F. & Polte, J.W. (1956) Effect of water content and compression on clothing insulation. *J. Appl. Physiol.* **8**, 539–45.

Halliwell, W. (1989) Delivering sport psychology services to the Canadian sailing team at the 1988 Olympic Games. *Sport Psychol.* **3**, 313–19.

Hargreaves, J. (1980) A double-blind placebo controlled study of cinnarizine in the prophylaxis of seasickness. *Practitioner* **224**, 547–50.

Hayward, J. (1975) Man in cold water, physiological basis for survival techniques. *Can. Physiol.* **6**, 89–90.

Homick, J.L., Kohl, R.L., Reschke, M.F., Degioanni, J. & Cintron-Trevino, N. (1983) Transdermal scopolamine in the prevention of motion sickness: Evaluation of the time course of efficacy. *Aviat. Space Environ. Med.* **54**, 994–1000.

Hultman, E. & Greenstaff, P.L. (1992) Food stores and energy reserves. In R.J. Shephard & P.O. Åstrand (eds) *Endurance in Sport*, pp. 127–35. Blackwell Scientific Publications, Oxford.

Kavanagh, T., Shephard, R.J., Mertens, D.J. & Thacker, L. (1993) *Masters competitions in preventive medicine*. Paper presented to the 3rd International Conference on Preventive Cardiology, Oslo, June 1993.

Keatinge, W.R. (1965) Death after shipwreck. *Br. Med. J.* **2**, 1537–41.

Keatinge, W.R. (1969) *Survival in Cold Water: The Physiology and Treatment of Immersion*. Blackwell Scientific Publications, Oxford.

LaHoute, L. (1979) *Differents aspects prophylactiques de la pathologie de windsurfing* (Different aspects of prophylaxis in the pathology of windsurfing). MD Thesis, La Riboisière, Paris.

Larin, Y. (1990) The sense of rudder and yacht's speed. *Finnfare* (Spring), 6–7.

Larson, L. (1974) *Encyclopedia of Sports Medicine*. Macmillan, New York.

Lawther, A. & Griffin, M.J. (1986) The motion of a ship at sea and the consequent motion sickness amongst passengers. *Ergonomics* **29**, 535–52.

Leach, R.D. (1978) The medicine of ocean yacht racing. *Br. Med. J.* **2**, 1771–3.

Lethuillier, D. (1983) *Pathologie médicale et traumatique des concurrents de 'la route de Rhum' 1982* (Medical pathology and traumatology of competitors in the 'Rum Route'). Memoire, Certificat d'étude specialisé de Biologie et Médecine du Sport, Hopital Pitié Salpetrière, Paris.

Levy, N.B. (1980) The psychology of sailing. *Psychiatr. Ann.* **10**, 51–3.

MacBeth, J. (1983) Studies of flow: Activity vs lifestyle in sailing. In M.L. Howell & J. McKay (eds) *Sociohistorical Perspectives*. University of Queensland, St. Lucia.

McCauley, M.E., Royal, J.W., Shaw, J.E. & Schmitt, L.G. (1979) Effect of transdermally administered scopolamine in preventing motion sickness. *Aviat. Space Environ. Med.* **50**, 1108–11.

Marchetti, M., Rigura, F. & Ricci, B. (1980) Biomechanics of two fundamental sailing postures. *J. Sports Med. Phys. Fitness* **20**, 325–32.

Mas, L. (1976) *Voile. Entrainement et Surveillance Médicale* (Sailing: Training and Medical Supervision). Editions Médicales et Universitaires, Paris.

Moncur, J. (1973) A study of fatalities during sport in Scotland (1969). *Br. J. Sports Med.* **7**, 162–3.

Money, K.E. (1970) Motion sickness. *Physiol. Rev.* **50**, 1–39.

Newton, F. (1989) Dinghy sailing. *Practitioner* **233**, 1032–5.

Niinimaa, V., Wright, G., Shephard, R.J. & Clarke, J. (1977) Characteristics of the successful dinghy sailor. *J. Sports Med. Phys. Fitness* **17**, 83–96.

O'Donnell, B. (1980) The Fastnet Race, 1979. *Br. Med. J.* **281**, 1665–7.

Parrott, A.C. (1987) Assessment of psychological performance in applied situations. In I. Hindmarch & P.D. Stonier (eds) *Human Psychopharmacology. Vol. 1. Measures and Methods*. John Wiley, Chichester.

Pasche, A. (1993) Use of human body temperatures for clothing evaluation. In *Proceedings of the 9th International Congress on Circumpolar Health*, Reykjavik, June 1993, pp. S26–4. University of Reykjavik, Reykjavik.

Paterson, D.P. (1971) Water skiing injuries. *Practitioner* **206**, 655–61.

Pingree, B.J.W. (1989) Motion commotion — A seasickness update. *J. Roy. Navy Med. Service* **75**, 75–84.

Plyley, M.J., Davis, G.M. & Shephard, R.J. (1985) Body profile of Olympic-class sailors. *Phys. Sportsmed.* **13**(6), 152–67.

Polednak, A.P. (1979) *The Longevity of Athletes*. CC Thomas, Springfield, Illinois.

Prevot, M. & Auvinet, B. (1981) L'actualité en médecine appliquée à la voile (Current views on medicine applied to sailing). *Cinésiol.* **80**, 153–260.

Pudenz, P., Dierck, T. & Rieckert, H. (1981) Die Herzfrequenz als Spiegelbild der Regattastrecke — eine experimentelle Studie ueber die Belastung beim Lasersegeln (Heart rate as the game plan of a regatta — an experimental study of work rate in laser sailing). *Dtsch. Z. Sportmed.* **32**(7), 192–5.

Ramey, J.R. (1974) Intrarectal tear with bleeding from water skiing accident. *J. Florida Med. Assoc.* **61**, 162.

Reason, J.T. (1978) Motion sickness: Some theoretical and practical considerations. *Appl. Ergonomics* **9**, 163–7.

Reason, J.T. & Brand, J.J. (1975) *Motion Sickness*. Academic Press, London.

Reilly, T. & Sanderson, F.H. (1981) Risks in selected outdoor water-based activities. In T. Reilly (ed) *Sports Fitness and Sports Injuries*, pp. 152–8. E & F Spon, London.

Rogge, J. (1973) Hiking in the laboratory. *Finnfare* **7** (Feb), 12–13.

Saltin, B. & Hermansen, L. (1967) Glycogen stores and prolonged exercise. In G. Blix (ed) *Nutrition and Physical Activity*, p. 32. Almqvist & Wiksell, Uppsala.

Shephard, R.J. (1974) *Men at Work. Applications of Ergonomics to Performance and Design*. CC Thomas, Springfield, Illinois.

Shephard, R.J. (1982) *Physiology and Biochemistry of Exercise*. Praeger, New York.

Shephard, R.J. (1984) Sleep, biorhythms and human performance. *Sports Med.* **1**, 11–37.

Shephard, R.J. (1990a) The biology and medicine of sailing. *Sports Med.* **9**, 86–99.

Shephard, R.J. (1990b) Sailing. In T. Reilly, N. Secher, P. Snell & C. Williams (eds) *Physiology of Sports*, pp. 287–310. E & F Spon, London.

Shephard, R.J. (1992) Medical surveillance of endurance sport. In R.J. Shephard & P.O. Åstrand (eds) *Endurance in Sport*, pp. 409–19. Blackwell Scientific Publications, Oxford.

Shephard, R.J. & Shek, P.N. (1993) Athletic competition and susceptibility to infection. *Clin. J. Sports Med.* **3**, 75–7.

Siple, P.A. & Passel, C.F. (1945) Measurement of dry atmospheric cooling in subfreezing temperatures. *Proc. Am. Physiol. Soc.* **89**, 177–99.

Sleight, M.W. (1974) Speedboat propeller injuries. *Br. Med. J.* **2**, 427–9.

Steinman, A.M., Hayward, J.S., Nemiroff, M.J. & Kubilis, P.S. (1987) Immersion hypothermia: Comparative protection of anti-exposure garments in calm vs rough seas. *Aviat. Space Environ. Med.* **58**, 550–8.

Taylor, N.B.G., Hunter, J. & Johnson, W.H. (1957) Antidiuresis as a measurement of laboratory-induced motion sickness. *Can. J. Biochem. Physiol.* **35**, 1017–27.

Thill, E. (1981) La constitution d'équipages en voile: Definition des profils psychologiques des barreurs et des équipiers (The constitution of sailing crews: definition of psychological profiles for helmspersons and crew members). *Cinésiol.* **80**, 193–200.

Thill, E. (1988) Evaluation longitudinale de traits de personalité de sportifs et de non-sportifs (Longitudinal evaluation of personality traits in athletes and non-atheletes). *Int. J. Sport Psychol.* **19**, 107–18.

Thomas, D. (1981) Effects of fatigue on vigilance in sailing. *Beam Reach* **11**, 12–13.

Tipton, M.J. (1989) The initial response to cold water immersion in man. *Clin. Sci.* **77**, 581–8.

Tipton, M.J. (1991) Laboratory based evaluation of the protection provided against cold water by two helicopter passenger suits. *J. Soc. Occup. Med.* **41**,

161–7.

Tipton, M.J. (1993) The concept of an integrated survival system for protection against the responses associated with immersion in cold water. *J. Roy. Navy Med. Service* **79**, 11–14.

Tipton, M.J. & Vincent, M.J. (1991) Protection provided against the initial responses to cold immersion by a partial coverage wet suit. *Aviat. Space Environ. Med.* **60**, 769–73.

Urbanczyk, A. (1989) Postawy, motywacje i oceny osobiste w samotnym zeglarstwie oceanicznym (Attitudes, motivations and personal opinions in ocean-going single-handed sailing). *Wychowanie fizyczne i sport (Warsaw)* **33**, 119–34.

Weightman, W.M., Zacharias, M. & Herbison, P. (1987) Traditional Chinese acupuncture: A potentially useful anti-emetic? *Br. Med. J.* **295**, 1379–80.

Winker, H. (1979) Traumatology in sailing and windsurfing. *Dtsch. Z. Sportmed.* **30**(6), 198–200.

Wright, G.R., Clarke, J., Niinimaa, V. & Shephard, R.J. (1976) Some reactions to a dry-land training programme for dinghy sailors. *Br. J. Sports Med.* **10**, 4–10.

Yamaji, K. & Shephard, R.J. (1978) Longevity and causes of death in athletes. *J. Hum. Ergol.* **6**, 15–27.

Chapter 43

Injuries in Equestrian Sports

JOHN LLOYD PARRY

Whilst dressage, show-jumping and 3-day eventing are the three competitive disciplines of the Olympic Games (Fig. 43.1), the diversity of horse-related sports is considerable. The number of participants, of all ages and experience, is also very large indeed.

The range extends from the thrill and speed of horse racing, through the nimbleness and skill of polo, to the fitness and endurance of long-distance rides. It is interesting to record that, in 1752, a wager struck in Ireland led to the first known jumping event for horses although, in Greece at the Olympic Games, horses had been ridden in a race in 648 BC (Holderness-Roddam, 1992). The present time has seen the development of vaulting (voltige) involving gymnastic feats on the horse, and pony clubs which develop the skills required for equestrian sports from an early age. Hunting has provided a suitable experience for horse and rider undertaking the high risks of cross-country riding in eventing (horse trials). The sport of carriage-driving is a logical development from the use of a horse as a means of transportation and for ceremonial duties.

The content and organization of many of these sports has evolved from the military background of certain equestrian disciplines. Whilst individual governing bodies provide their own regulations the overall control of the Olympic sports is the responsibility of the Fédération Equestre Internationale (FEI).

The risk of injury is naturally related to the type of sport, combined with the experience and skill of both horse and rider. However, it must not be overlooked that the behaviour of the horse can be unpredictable and this should be anticipated. Accidents to the young can be frequent and frightening and some horse-related injuries can be severe. Consequently, the suitability of the horse for its chosen task, the nature of the environment together with the teaching, supervision, fitness and diligence of the rider are of great importance in removing unnecessary risk factors. Of course, risk is inherent in most sports but it should be calculated as far as possible. In this context, the development of protective equipment is of great value, particularly in the prevention or amelioration of head injuries.

Aetiology and mechanism of injury

A fall from a horse is the most frequent cause of injury (Fig. 43.2) and sadly can prove fatal. A rider's head may be 3 m from the ground and the moving horse can attain a considerable speed which, for racing, has been estimated to be up to 60 km·h^{-1} (Miles, 1970). A rider will often be positioned with the head forward and Becker's principle states that the degree of this position is reflected in the number of head injuries sustained (Becker, 1959). During the fall, particularly with other horses in close proximity, there is the unpleasant hazard of a kick from a metal-shod hoof which can produce a force in excess of 10 kN (Firth, 1985). If the rider is not thrown clear, there is the danger of being

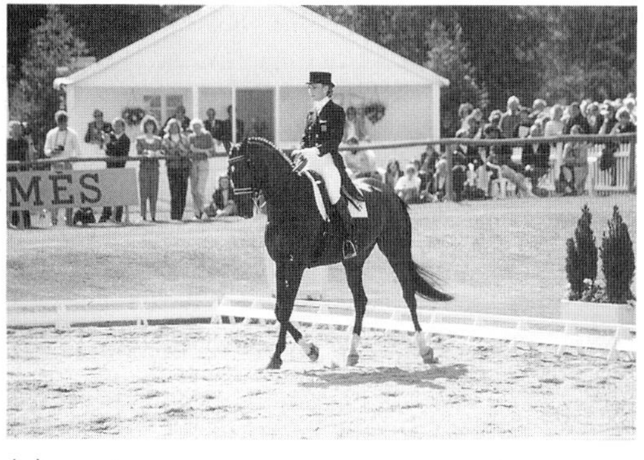

(a)

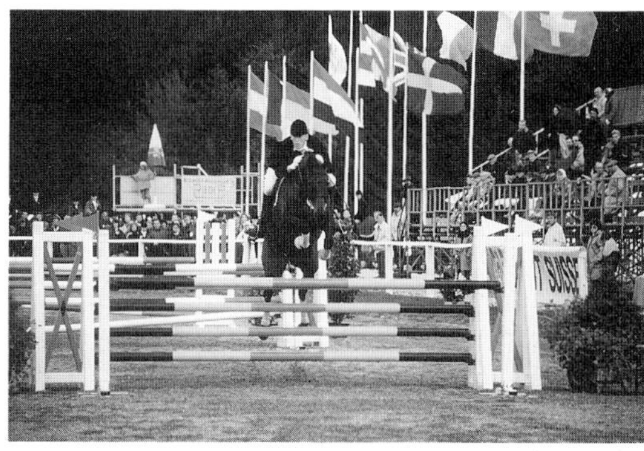

(b)

(c)

Fig. 43.1 Different types of equestrian sports: (a) dressage; (b) show-jumping; and (c) cross-country phase of a 3-day event at the Barcelona Olympic Games, 1992.

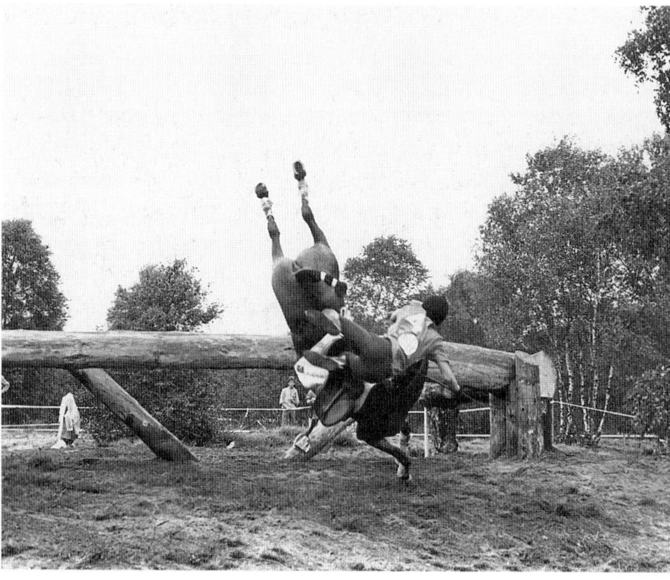

Fig. 43.2 The outcome of a fall may well be determined by whether the rider falls away from the horse.

trapped by the sheer weight of the horse, which may be up to 500 kg, and very severe or fatal injuries may be the consequence. Fortunately, this is uncommon and it is far more likely that the rider will be dislodged forwards over the horse's head and the arms used to break the impact of the fall. Soft-tissue injury or fracture of the upper limb may result but there is also a significant incidence of leg injury. Trampling may ensue whilst, in the stableyard, an unguarded moment may lead to an injured foot from stamping. The possibility of a bite may be instinctively recognized but the incorrect grip of reins or a leading rope is common and can lead to the loss of a finger or thumb (Regan *et al.*, 1991). Even when mounted, the nose and face can be in peril from an unexpected pitching forwards or the sudden elevation of the horse's head and neck. Further, if the rider is not using the correct stirrup and footwear then the foot may be trapped, and should the rider then fall dragging and serious injury can ensue (Gierup *et al.*, 1976).

Although a direct impact or blow is an obvious mechanism for injury, falls during cross-country riding can apply any vector to the

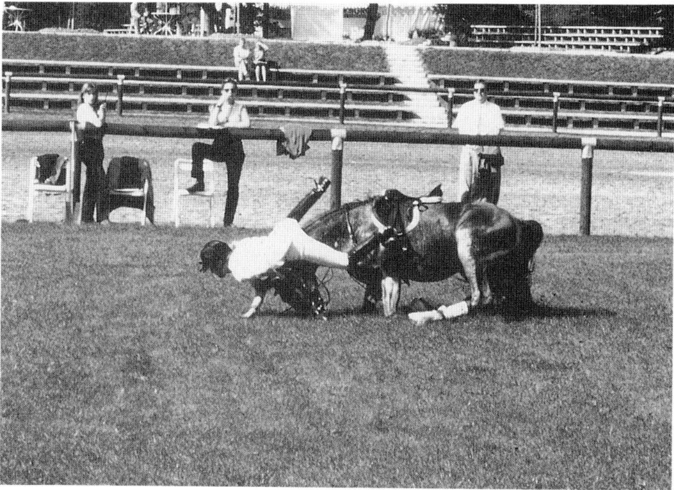

(a)

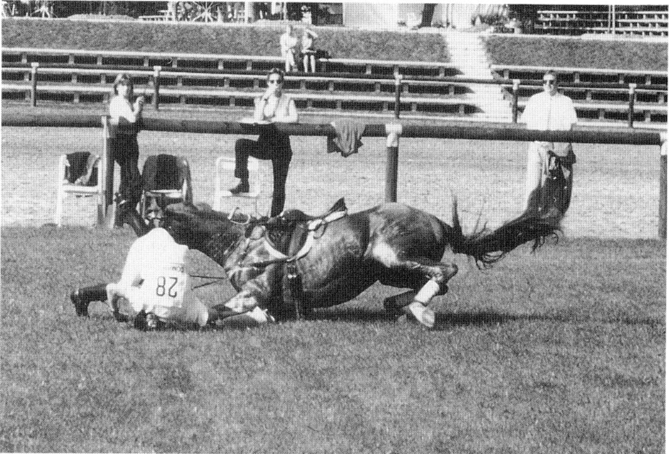

(b)

Fig. 43.3 Injuries to the head and neck are a great concern in horse-riding accidents.

spine with hyperflexion and extension, as well as lateral flexion and rotation (Firth, 1985). There must be a high index of suspicion for spinal injuries in such circumstances and those sustaining head injuries should be regarded as having an associated neck injury (Fig. 43.3).

An English study in 1991 analysed a small number of accidents and attempted to elucidate the cause (Silver & Lloyd Parry, 1991). It illustrated the case of a spinal injury to a 28-year-old woman who had hired a relatively unfamiliar 9-year-old mare of 14.2 hands and entered a sponsored ride for charity. In the previous week she had been unsaddled by the branch of a tree whilst on another horse. On this occasion, during a ride of several miles over obstacles, she was again dislodged as she pulled to one side of a fence, in order to avoid the rider ahead whilst bending low under a tree. She fell in a sitting position with her legs outstretched and immediately felt pins and needles and was aware of numbness from the waist downwards. She had experienced a similar fall previously and she had been kicked in the back 2 or 3 years before. A wedge fracture of L1 was later identified.

Incidence of injuries

During recent years increased attention has been focused on equestrian injuries, their incidence and early management. The frequency of head injury was emphasized by Barber (1973) at the Radcliffe Infirmary, Oxford; 67.2% of horseriders had such an injury. A survey analysing over 1000 riding accidents in 1987 by Whitlock (1988) in the West Midland region of England found that head (59 fractures) and face (99 fractures) injuries amounted to one third of the total. It is of concern that over 50% were aged 20 years or less in this survey, for Avery (1986), analysing children's accidents in south Warwickshire, England, had noted that 354 children attended hospital during 1980–1984 and 67 were admitted, of which 61.2% had head injuries. Bixby-Hammett, in summarizing studies of injuries and deaths associated with horseriding, estimated approximately 20% of the injuries occurred to the head and face (Bixby-Hammett & Brooks, 1990). Such figures indicate an area for concern, particularly given the emphasis from Nottingham (Muwanga & Dove, 1985), and earlier from Glasgow (Lindsay *et al.*, 1980) and Oxford (Ilgren *et al.*, 1984), of the serious nature of head injuries in horseriding and the need for adequate protection of this vulnerable area. Pounder (1984) noted that 14 out of 18 riding-related deaths in South Australia were the result of head injuries. The perusal of the medical examiner's records of 205 horse-related deaths in the USA showed that head injuries were the cause of over 60% of these deaths (Bixby-Hammett & Brooks, 1990).

Soft-tissue injuries are probably the commonest, although they are not usually specified, and had an incidence of 92% amongst professional rodeo riders (Griffin *et al.*, 1984). A survey in 1990 of 58 English riding accidents found 46% to have sustained tenderness and swelling, 19% tenderness and contusions, 12% cuts and lacerations with 3% having sprains and strains, and another 3% abrasions and grazes (A. Le Seuer, personal communication) (Table 43.1).

The upper limb is the most likely site of fracture. A large West Midlands survey (Whitlock, 1988) found 160 such fractures

Table 43.1 The types of injuries most frequently associated with riding accidents; percentages of all injuries found in a survey of 58 riding accidents, 1990 (A. Le Seuer, personal communication).

Injury	Percentage
Tenderness/swelling	46%
Bruises/contusions	19%
Fracture	12%
Cuts/lacerations	12%
Sprain/strain	3%
Internal head injury	3%
Abrasions/grazes	3%
Dislocation	3%
Other	1%

Table 43.2 Location of fractures found in a survey of horse-related accidents in the West Midlands, UK (n = 481) (Whitlock, 1988).

Location on body	Number
Head	59
Face	99
Clavicle	41
Upper limb	160
Spine	37
Pelvis	7
Lower limb	78

(24.32%) together with 41 fractured clavicles in the upper limb girdle. The lower limb fractures amounted to 78 (17.82%) with seven fractures of the pelvis (Table 43.2).

The severity of some horseriding injuries has already been noted and this survey identified 5.42% of the injuries were to the chest, including five pneumohaemothoraces, and 3.37% to the abdomen with 14 visceral ruptures. There was an incidence of 10.2% injuries (37 fractures) to the spine. It is important to note that if there is an injury to the spinal cord by a fracture-dislocation, it is most commonly to the lower cervical segments, particularly in flexion, or to the junction between the immobile dorsal spine and the relatively mobile lumbar spine. The elasticity of the spine in children may protect it from fracture but transient neurological symptoms may herald subsequent neurological signs and demands vigilance (Firth & Galloway, 1990).

In competition, an analysis of injuries sustained in eventing from accident report forms noted that concussion comprised 13.6% of the injuries, facial injuries 9.67%, with fractures and dislocations of the upper limbs 21.9%, injuries to the neck and back 19.6%, chest 7.5% and fractures and dislocations of the lower limb 3.5% (J. Lloyd Parry, unpublished data).

It is apparent that the problems encountered are principally those of trauma with the management of soft-tissue injuries being the most common. However, life-saving measures may have to be immediately instigated, particularly where there is high risk. The welfare of the horse is an essential part of advanced competition and attention is especially paid to the environmental conditions in these arduous disciplines.

At the present time drug abuse amongst riders has not been identified in international competition; the FEI is working in close collaboration with the International Olympic Committee in this respect.

Management and care of injuries

The care of the fallen rider requires training, planning and the highest standard of immediate communication. It involves teams ideally comprising doctors with trauma skills, paramedics, nurses and ambulance personnel. Adverse weather conditions may be encountered so that vehicles should have four-wheel drive capacity where difficult terrain is encountered (Fig. 43.4). The available equipment must include airway and ventilation items including endotracheal intubation and suction. Oxygen and nitrous oxide are likely to be standard items available on the ambulances. Fluids for infusion, together with giving sets, should include crystalloids and colloids in adequate quantities as internal or pelvic injuries may require considerable volumes. If a spectator collapses, there should be defibrillation facilities and a separate first aid base away from injured competitors.

The immobilization of fractures requires splints with traction available for certain lower limb injuries such as a fractured femur. Rigid cervical collars of various sizes are essential, although they must only be regarded as an adjunct to cervical immobilization and not as removing the need for manual immobilization (Fig. 43.5). Scoop stretchers or the Donway lifting frame are used in the UK for lifting into the ambulance or onto a vacuum mattress. The head and neck must be secured adequately prior to transportation and any pressure areas inspected and protected. At all times there

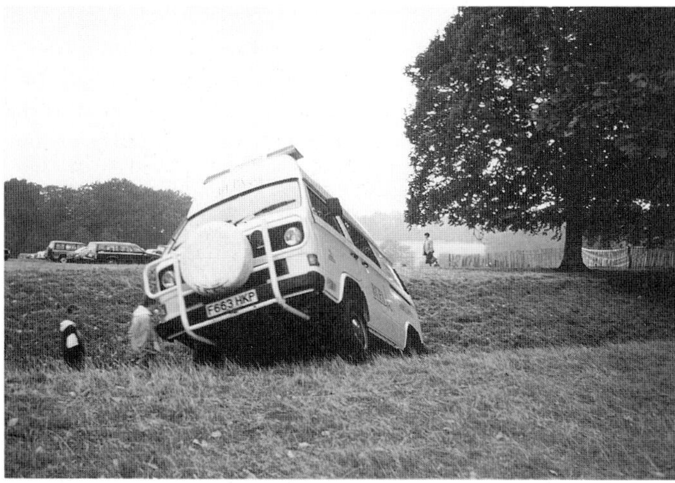

Fig. 43.4 Ambulances may have to tackle all types of terrain.

must be close observation and maintenance of the airway, for hypoxia is a deadly foe in the care of the severely injured.

The early diagnosis of concussion represents a formidable challenge and, if there is any doubt, the rider should not be allowed to continue in the competition. Any loss of consciousness or impairment of memory must be regarded as indicating an injury to the brain. The rider must be closely questioned and able to identify himself or herself, the horse, the locality and other details of the competition if mistakes are not to be made. It will also be necessary to re-evaluate the case at an agreed later time as other injuries may reveal themselves as normal composure returns. It is also wise to check tetanus immunization status in case of a significant but trivial wound.

Injuries require adequate recovery periods; that for head injuries being of prime importance. It is a matter for skilled judgement, but a minor injury certainly requires 1 day, although 1 week might prove to be of greater benefit. The danger of cumulative head injuries should

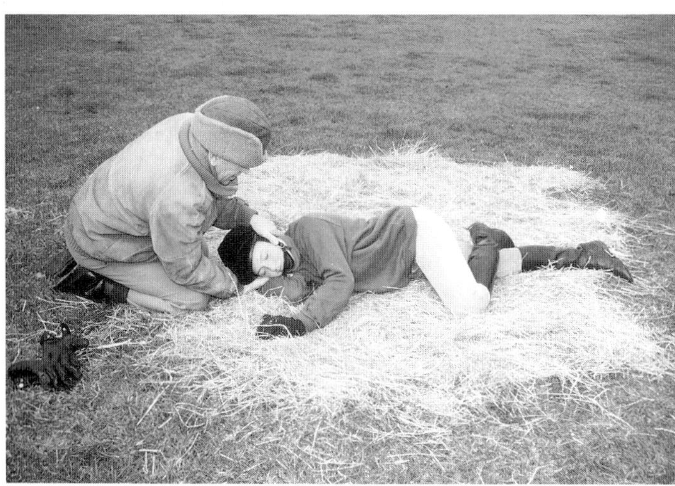

Fig. 43.5 If head and/or neck injuries are likely then manual immobilization must be instigated immediately.

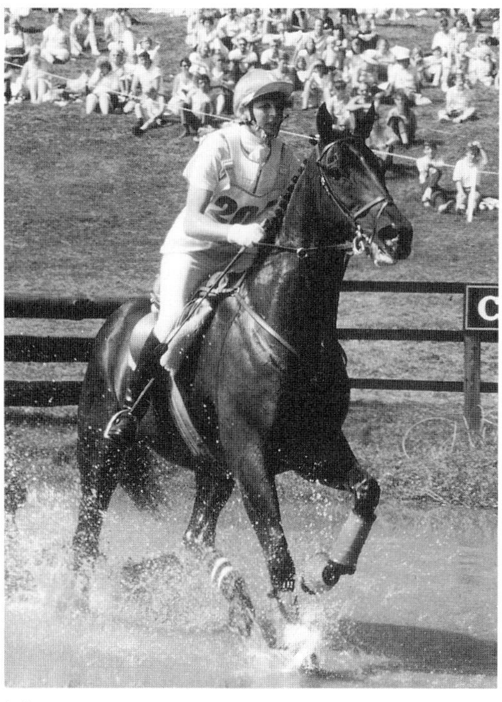

(a)

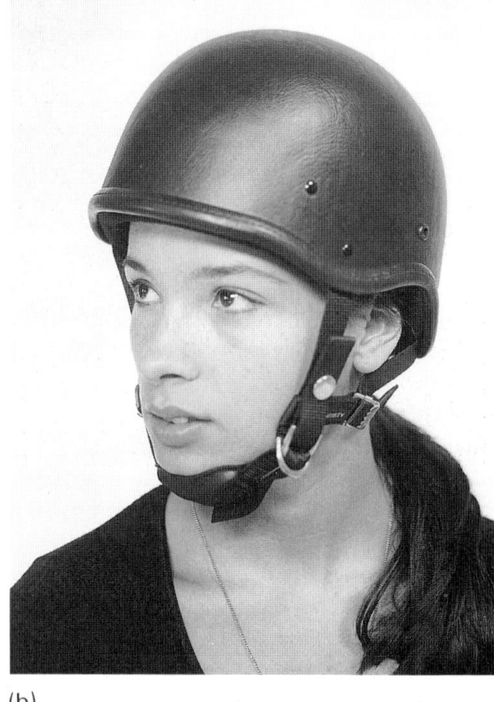

(b)

Fig. 43.6 Adequate head protection is vital; the rider in (a) is also wearing a body protector. (b) The present British Standard jockey skull cap (BS 4472). New specifications are imminent.

not be underestimated (Gronwall & Wrightson, 1975). Prolonged periods of unconsciousness should have neurological evaluation.

Although riders may not comply it is reasonable to suggest a fractured clavicle should be immobilized for 2 weeks and a similar period allowed for recovery. A comminuted fracture of the clavicle will require at least 6 weeks. The immobilization of dislocated shoulders varies between 1 and 6 weeks depending on different doctors and countries and whether it a first or recurrent dislocation.

Soft-tissue injuries may respond well to the conventional measures of rest, ice, compression and elevation. However, if drugs are to be used for pain relief then only those not prohibited for use in international competition should be chosen, with careful reference to the published lists, to allow further participation if possible. Physiotherapy has an important role in the early treatment and rehabilitation of injury and must be put in hand at the earliest opportunity. It is now customary to have physiotherapists available at the major 3-day events such as Badminton and Burghley in the UK.

Prevention of injuries

There can be no substitute for informed and adequate preparation of horse and rider if either recreation or competition is to be entered to its full extent and the risks successfully negotiated. Ideally, learning begins at an early age, informally growing up with horses and ponies and then undertaking formal instruction from qualified instructors in a safe environment. Unfortunately it is recognized that accidents can occur whilst under instruction so that the identification of competent instructors is essential and may well involve regulations. The British Horse

Society and the Pony Club are important institutions in the UK for the setting of standards and the monitoring of establishments and training. Similar organizations are found in many other countries. The Medical Equestrian Association (UK) now arranges training for doctors interested in providing medical cover at competitions as well as collating statistics on horse-related accidents and their prevention. The American Medical Equestrian Association collaborates with the pony clubs in the USA through their respective safety committees. It must also be recorded that both the Ireland and Northern Ireland Medical Equestrian Associations have close links with each other and the UK and a similar association has just been founded in Australia (HORSE) with possibly one to follow in New Zealand.

There is much to do and adequate head protection must be the immediate challenge (Fig. 43.6). There is no doubt that present head gear, properly secured, protects the head but there is concern that lateral and occipital protection should be improved. New materials may be the key to improving the absorption of energy and to exclude penetration whilst retaining a reasonable and wearable size, avoiding excessive weight and impaired ventilation.

Another field for development is the body protector (Fig. 43.6a). At present standards are in their infancy but UK manufacturers are now producing articles to the British Equestrian Trade Association (BETA) standards. It is essential that such garments should not be bulky as this would impede the flexibility of the rider, which would be a hazard in itself. It is thought that they have already proved their worth in preventing or reducing soft-tissue injury and possibly sparing ribs or vertebral processes from fracture. Certainly, it can make all the difference to the competitor required to ride again the same day or next — as in eventing, where dressage is the prelude to cross-country jumping which is followed by showjumping.

The use of mouth protectors is under consideration, given the high incidence of facial injuries, but face guards and knee pads are only considered to be for the protection of polo players at present.

The maintenance and proper condition and use of the reins (Fig. 43.7), saddle and other horse tack does not need any elaboration; nor should the use of suitable clothing particularly to protect the legs from being chafed. Proper footwear with a heel is mandatory if the foot is to be prevented from slipping through the stirrup iron (Fig. 43.8). Gloves, with a suitable

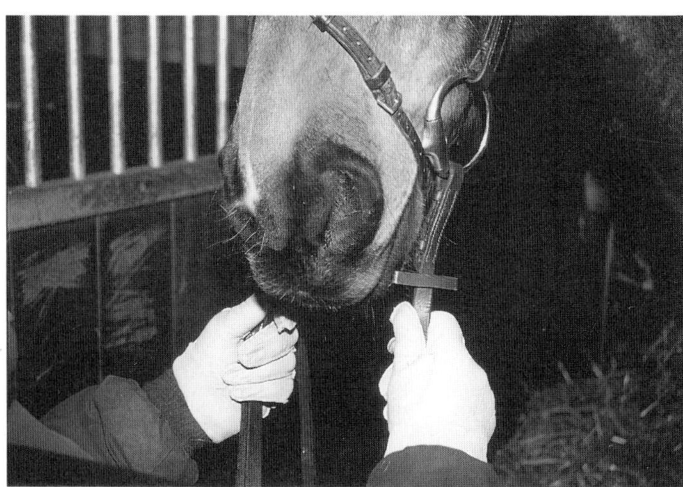

Fig. 43.7 Reins or ropes must not be wound around the fingers, but held in the palm of the hands.

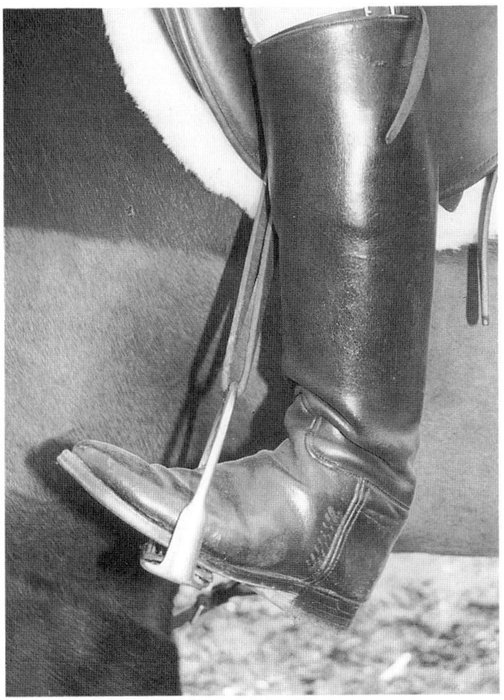

Fig. 43.8 The heel of the boot prevents the foot from sliding through the stirrup and becoming trapped.

gripping surface, can prove invaluable when leather reins become slippery.

It has been noted that riders who have had an accident may have sustained previous injuries. Consequently, it is of value to have a record of these injuries, particularly in the case of head injuries, readily available to the examining doctor. This measure has recently been introduced under the rules of the Governing Body of Horse Trials in the UK and competitors are required to carry a visible medical card, usually secured on the arm by a band, when jumping cross-country courses. The use of specified head protection and body protectors was already mandatory.

It may be that future attention can be paid to establishing exact and universal recovery periods for major injuries. Concussion currently has a rather arbitrary and possibly inadequate length of recovery time, and with the frequency and severe nature of such injuries, remains a cause for concern.

The prevention of horse-related injuries will owe much to the education of those who have the least knowledge and experience of horses. The example and conduct of the sporting fraternity cannot be underestimated, nor can the goodwill and dedication of the responsible equestrian and the motivated doctor. The best interests of the horse deserve no less for it has played a significant role in work, recreation and sport through the ages.

References

Avery, J.G. (1986) *Horse Riding Accidents*. Fact Sheets, Child Accident Prevention Trust, London.

Barber, H.M. (1973) Horseplay: Survey of accidents with horses. *Br. Med. J.* **3**, 532–4.

Becker, T. (1959) Das stumpfe schädel trauma als sportunfall (Skull trauma in sports injuries). *Unfallheidelkd.* **62**, 179.

Bixby-Hammett, D. & Brooks, W.H. (1990) Common injuries in horseback riding: A review. *Sports Med.* **9**(1), 36–47.

Firth, J.L. (1985) Equestrian injuries. In R.C. Schneider, J.C. Kennedy, M.L. Plant, P.J. Fowler, J.T. Hoff & L.S. Matthews (eds) *Sports Injuries: Mechanisms, Prevention and Treatment*, pp. 431–48. Williams & Wilkins, Baltimore.

Firth, J.L. & Galloway, N.R. (1990) Head injuries. In M.A. Hutson (ed) *Sports Injuries: Recognition and Management*, pp. 17–24. Oxford Medical Publications, Oxford.

Gierup, J., Larsson, M. & Lennquist, S. (1976) Incidence and nature of horse-riding injuries. *Acta Chirurg. Scand.* **142**, 57–61.

Griffin, R., Peterson, K.D. & Halseth, J.R. (1984) Injuries in professional rodeo. *Phys. Sportsmed.* **12**(10), 130–7.

Gronwall, D. & Wrightson, P. (1975) Cumulative effect of concussion. *Lancet* **ii**, 995–7.

Holderness-Roddam, J. (1992) *The New Complete Book of the Horse*. WH Smith, London.

Ilgren, E.B., Teddy, P.J., Vafadis, J., Briggs, M. & Gardiner, N.G. (1984) Clinical and pathological studies of brain injuries in horse-riding accidents: A description of cases and review with a warning to the unhelmeted. *Clin. Neuropathol.* **3**(6), 253–9.

Lindsay, K.W., McLatchie, G. & Jennett, B. (1980) Serious head injury in sport. *Br. Med. J.* **281**, 789–91.

Miles, J.R. (1970) The racecourse medical officer. *J. Roy. Coll. Gen. Pract.* **19**, 228.

Muwanga, L.C. & Dove, A.F. (1985) Head protection for riders: A cause for concern. *Arch. Emerg. Med.* **2**, 85–7.

Pounder, D. (1984) The grave yawns for the horseman. *Med. J. Australia* **141**, 632–5.

Regan, P.J., Roberts, J.O., Feldberg, L. & Roberts, A.H.N. (1991) Hand injuries from leading horses. *Injury* **22**, 124–6.

Silver, J.R. & Lloyd Parry, J.M. (1991) Hazards of horse-riding as a popular sport. *Br. J. Sportsmed.* **25**(2), 105–10.

Whitlock, M.R. (1988) Horse riding is dangerous for your health. In *Proceedings of the Second International Conference on Emergency Medicine, Brisbane*, p. 191. Australian College for Emergency Medicine.

Chapter 44

Injuries in Archery

DAVID L. MANN

Archery can be described as a static sport requiring strength and endurance of the upper body, in particular the shoulder girdle. Furthermore, it is characterized by the asymmetrical loads and forces placed on the body which contribute to the observed patterns of injury. During the course of an international event, a male archer will draw a 20–23 kg (45–50 lb) bow 75 times daily for 4 days. This is equivalent to 1545–1705 kg (3400–3750 lb) static force in a single day, which is a tremendous load to be placed on the bony, ligamentous and muscular structures involved. These figures have been somewhat diminished with the advent of the compound bow which is now recognized in international competition. The compound bow provides a mechanical advantage via a system of cables and off-set pulleys which allows the archer to achieve a greater peak drawing force (up to 27 kg (60 lb)) while only ·holding 60–75% of that peak force while aiming (Figs 44.1 & 44.2).

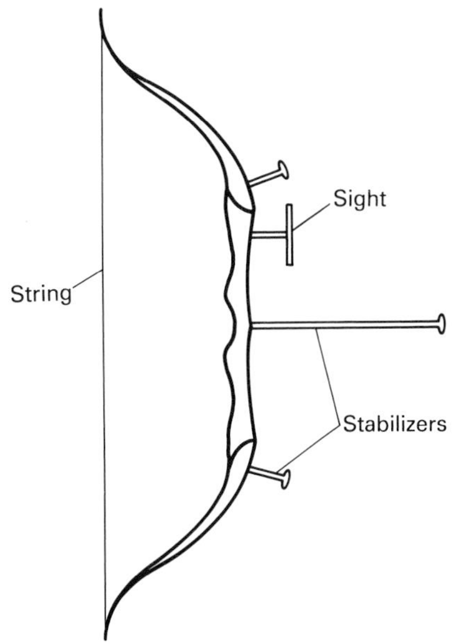

Fig. 44.1 Freestyle bow.

To understand the injury patterns in archery, it is necessary to review the normal shooting patterns that are involved. It is traditionally taught that the feet should straddle the shooting line at 90° to the target. However, many archers have adopted a more oblique stance, and this has implications regarding injuries (Fig. 44.3). Once the stance has been taken, the archer raises the arm in which the bow is held (bow arm) toward the target. The other arm holding the string (drawing arm) then draws the string back to the side of the face where it is said to be anchored in a position of full draw. Full draw is maintained for several seconds while the archer aims, followed by release of the arrow (Fig. 44.4).

As the archer is starting to draw the string back, the drawing arm is held at 90° or greater abduction and the shoulder is flexed across the body. During the drawing phase the arm maintains 90° or greater abduction as the arm unit extends across the body towards full draw. This action is referred to as horizontal extension

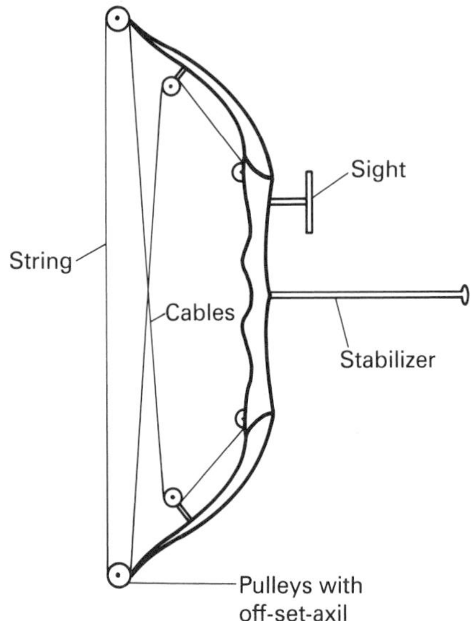

Fig. 44.2 Compound bow.

(Pappas *et al.*, 1985), and probably contributes to the shoulder injuries observed. Archers will often deviate from the stance and trunk position described above. In particular, the aforementioned oblique stance may be further augmented by the archer leaning back or away from the target.

There are further variations of this technique related to the equipment now used. The compound bow has greatly increased the archer's accuracy due to the greater force that can be applied to the arrow, resulting in the arrow travelling faster and therefore less affected by wind and other external factors. The basic technique of shooting a compound bow is similar to that of the traditional or freestyle method, except that the forces encountered during drawing and at full draw are quite different. The peak force during compound shooting occurs in the middle of the drawing phase, while it occurs at full draw in freestyle (Fig. 44.5). This may have implications in the injury patterns seen clinically. Another technical device utilized by compound shooters is the mechanical release (Fig. 44.6); this replaces using fingers to release the string. The release is held in the drawing-arm hand and is usually a rope and/or hook mechanism, although many designs are used. This device further increases accuracy and may decrease some of the finger problems seen.

Freestyle shooters commonly use a device called a clicker (Fig. 44.7). The clicker is a small strip of metal fixed to the bow under which the arrow is drawn. As the point of the arrow is drawn past the clicker, it snaps (or clicks) against the bow and the archer releases the arrow. The clicker ensures the arrow is drawn back exactly the same distance each time, as a small variation at the bow results in large variations at the target. The contrary effect of the clicker is that the archer must coordinate several factors for optimal accuracy. These include aiming, maintaining a rigid stance, holding a 20–23 kg draw weight bow at full draw, and gradually drawing the arrow past the clicker before releasing. This process typically takes 3–6 s per shot.

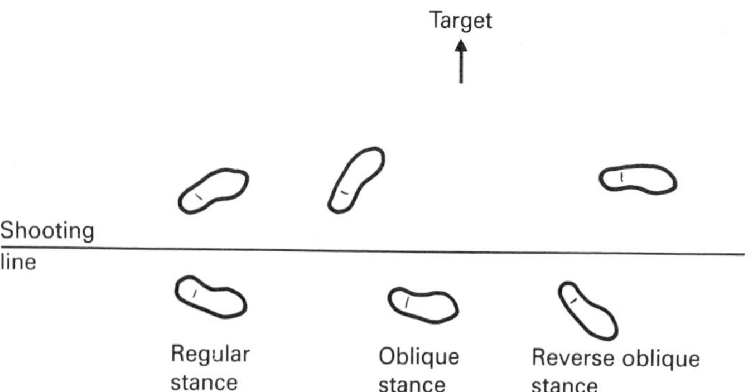

Fig. 44.3 Stance.

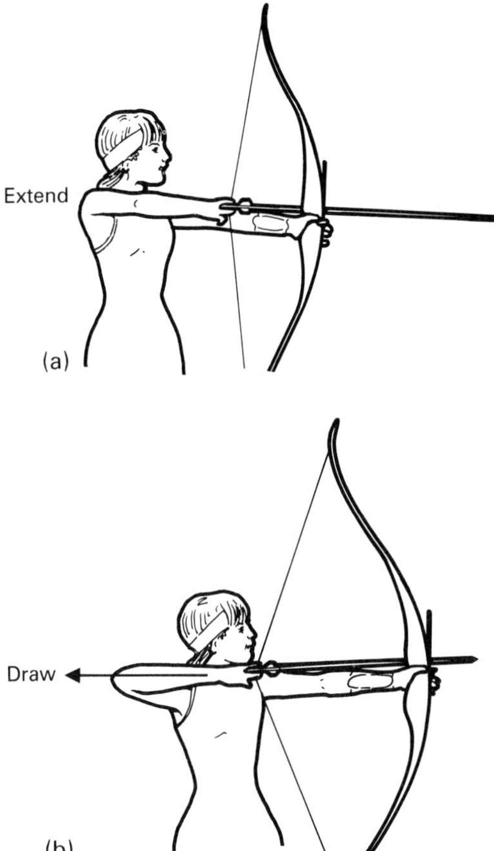

Fig. 44.4 (a) Archer about to draw back the string. The drawing arm is in a position of flexion/ abduction. (b) Archer at full draw. The drawing arm has completed the cross-extension motion.

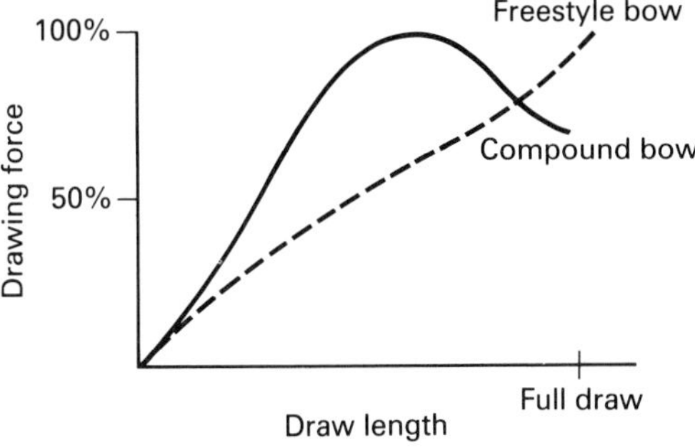

Fig. 44.5 The drawing forces of the freestyle and compound bows.

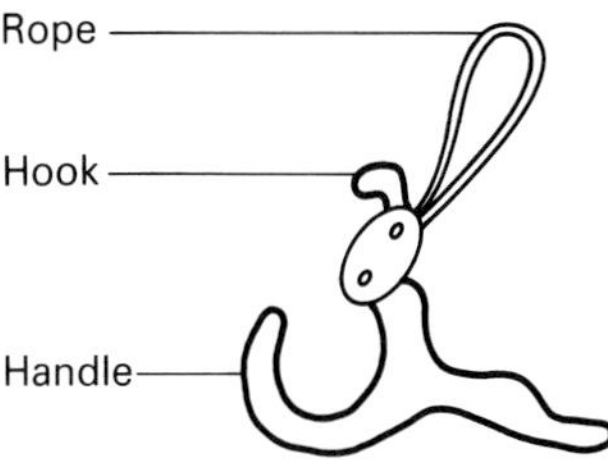

Fig. 44.6 The mechanical release. The release rope wraps around the bow string and is held by the hook. As the archer gradually pulls on the long end of the handle, the rope slips off the hook and the bow string is released.

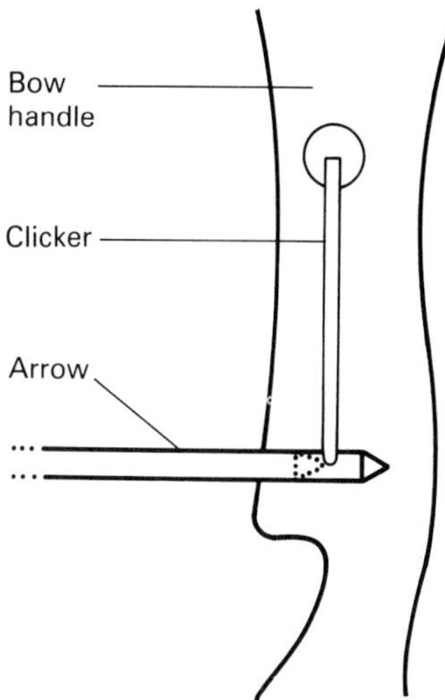

Fig. 44.7 The clicker. This is a flexible piece of metal, under which the arrow is pulled. As the arrow is pulled back past the point of the clicker, it 'clicks' onto the bow handle, indicating a consistent draw length has been achieved and the arrow is released.

Injury patterns

Very little has been published in the literature concerning the injury patterns in archery. In Mann and Littke's (1989) study 21 élite archers were studied and their shoulder injuries documented; the injuries were correlated to anatomical dissections. Injuries to the drawing-arm shoulder in female archers were found to be the most prevalent type of injury. It was suggested that the factors involved included lack of specific rotator cuff training, coupled with overtraining and inappropriate technique.

The remaining profile of archery injuries can only be based upon clinical experience. Shoulder injuries appear to predominate, followed by neck, back, hand and wrist injuries.

Mechanisms of injury

Shoulder injuries

The drawing-arm shoulder is the most likely area of the body to be injured in archery. Mann and Littke (1989) found that five out of nine élite female archers had significant shoulder pathology on examination. The mechanisms proposed are that during horizontal extension to full draw the coraco-acromial arch impinges upon the long head of the biceps (LHB) and supraspinatus tendons. This effect is accentuated as the drawing-arm elbow is elevated beyond 90° abduction (see Fig. 44.4), but cannot be eliminated with less abduction as determined by cadaveric examination (Mann & Littke, 1989). The repetitive motion of drawing the bow is obviously contributory. These mechanisms account for the anterior shoulder pain that is typical in drawing-arm injuries; the diagnosis being an impingement tendonitis of the LHB and/or supraspinatus.

A subgroup of drawing-arm injuries have been identified with posterior pain (Mann & Littke, 1989). This injury is not as disabling as its anterior counterpart, and probably relates to the relative weakness of the posterior external rotators of the rotator cuff group — infraspinatus and teres minor. In fact, muscle underdevelopment of this group was observed (Mann & Littke, 1989). This condition may also be attributed to posterior capsular inflammation or even osseous changes as suggested by Lombardo *et al.* (1977), but these are more typical in overhead baseball pitchers.

Neck and back injuries

The neck problems that archers complain about usually involve stiffness and soreness in the paracervical and upper shoulder muscle groups. The aetiology is probably due to asymmetrical positioning of the head and neck (see Fig. 44.4), coupled with muscle imbalance developed during drawing and maintaining full draw. This mechanism would be particularly troublesome to freestyle clicker shooters who must maintain a high degree of muscle tone in an abnormal position.

Back complaints typically involve the lumbosacral region, but can be located around the thoracolumber junction. It seems intuitively obvious that these problems will originate in the abnormal stance many archers assume (see Fig. 44.3). Symmetry of musculoskeletal function is a time-honoured principle, and is routinely violated in archery. It has been this author's experience that those archers with the most pronounced complaints also deviate the most from the usual stance. Stance positioning including rotation and/or leaning away from the target, or a combination of both, will probably be identified as significant causes of injury. The muscle imbalance and shortening that occurs after many years of archery, particularly if practised with poor positioning, can be considerable.

Hand and wrist injuries

Injuries to the hand and wrist are restricted to the drawing-arm release side. Blisters are encountered with excessive shooting and are managed in the usual way. Not infrequently a blister will appear during a competition, requiring it to be lanced, dressed appropriately and protected so that the archer can continue.

Freestyle shooters frequently develop finger hypertrophy, which is adaptive and usually asymptomatic. Occasionally the repetitive squeezing of the fingers together at full draw will result in digital nerve damage with decreased, or complete loss of, sensation distally. The solution is assuming proper hand position on the string, adding spacers between the fingers, using a longer bow and adding extra padding to the protective tab. The condition is usually reversible with these modifications, or cessation of shooting temporarily if necessary. The final problem seen is extensor digatorum tendonitis at the dorsum of the wrist. This injury is invariably seen in archers who maintain their release wrist in some degree of dorsiflexion, as a result of either inappropriate anchor position or not drawing the string back far enough. The key is prevention with proper full-draw positioning, as treatment of the acute injury is frustrating unless the archer will stop shooting for a period of time.

Management of injuries

The most common injury, and the most serious with respect to lost performance and potential for permanent damage, is drawing-arm anterior impingement with resultant tendonitis of the LHB and/or supraspinatus. This injury is recognized by the classic signs and symptoms of impingement syndrome (Jobe & Jobe, 1983; Neer, 1983). These include pain felt anteriorly with a dull, throbbing pain referred anteriolaterally, a painful arc sign, positive impingement sign (Hawkins & Kennedy, 1980) and pain with weakness to supraspinatus testing (Jobe & Moynes, 1982). Specific LHB tendonitis is detected by a similar pain pattern plus pain to direct palpation and discomfort to resisted supination or flexion with the elbow extended in the sagittal plane (Calliett, 1984). The mechanism of this injury has been described above, and several points of intervention can be planned.

The first point of intervention is an assessment of the archer's stance, and in particular whether he or she is leaning away from the target too much. By leaning back, the angle of the acromioclavicular ligament impinging on the LHB and supraspinatus tendons is increased. A similar result is obtained by raising the drawing-arm elbow (increasing abduction), and this position must also be reviewed. The final point to be considered is how much horizontal extension is achieved and whether it is sufficient to minimize the forces on the tendons to reduce injuries. Figure 44.8 demonstrates the differences between inadequate horizontal extension and more appropriate extension at full draw. This is particularly important for those with posterior drawing-arm shoulder pain, as full horizontal extension would minimize the tension on the infraspinatus and teres minor group. Those archers with dorsal wrist problems may also not be extended enough.

Muscle-strengthening programmes

If the stance and shoulder and elbow positions are acceptable, then the area of injury itself must be rehabilitated. Prior to any exercise programme, though, it is advisable to perform some stretching of the muscles in question. Stretching of the neck, shoulders and back is particularly important (Parker, 1988), and at least 10 min should be spent doing this prior to any exercises.

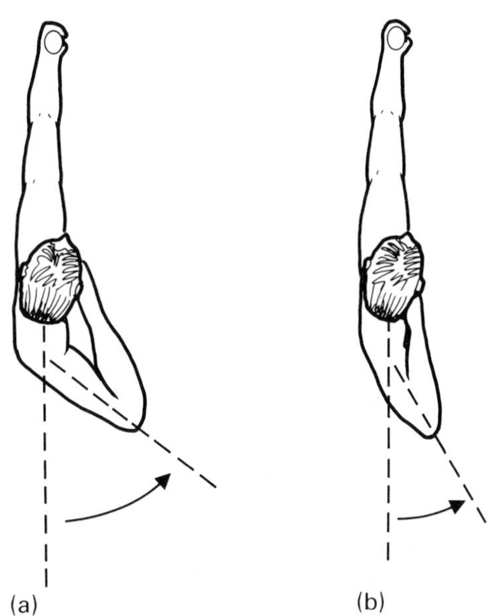

Fig. 44.8 Variations in horizontal extension. Looking from above, the angle between the line of pull and the drawing arm should be minimized. (a) Insufficient extension; (b) appropriate extension.

ROTATOR CUFF MUSCLES

It is recognized that the rotator cuff group functions synergistically to control the position of the humeral head in the glenoid fossa (Pappas *et al.*, 1985). By strengthening the cuff muscles, the humerus can be better depressed in the glenoid to minimize the trauma incurred by the tendons with repeated horizontal extension (drawing the bow). Once the injury is recognized, a rotator cuff-strengthening programme should be initiated.

The rotator cuff muscles can be relatively well isolated if particular attention is paid to body positioning, as determined by electromyographic (EMG) analysis (Townsend *et al.*, 1991). The exercises include scaption, external rotation, flexion, horizontal abduction in external rotation and press-ups (Figs 44.9–44.13). Either free weights or elastic tubing may be used as resistance; the latter having the advantages of being portable, adjustable and inexpensive. These exercises should be done daily with three sets of 15 repetitions each, with the resistance slowly increased as strength develops. However, emphasis should be placed on the endurance aspect of the rehabilitation, and additional repetitions and sets should be added before increasing the resistance to a significant degree.

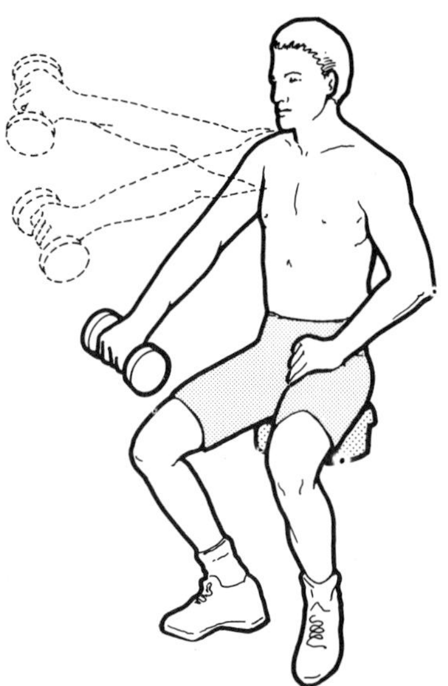

Fig. 44.9 Elevation of the arm in the scapula plane (scaption) with the arm internally rotated.

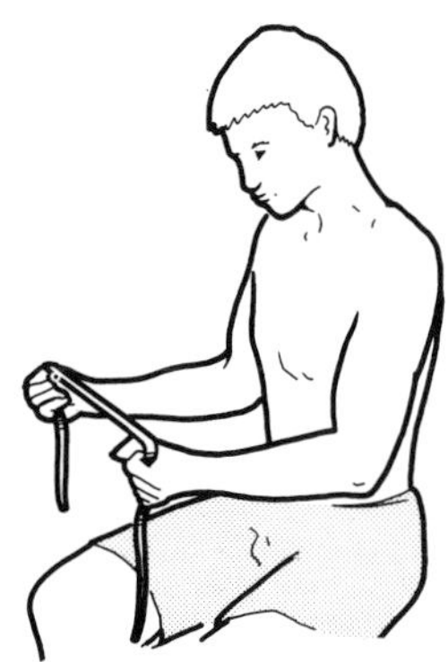

Fig. 44.10 External rotators.

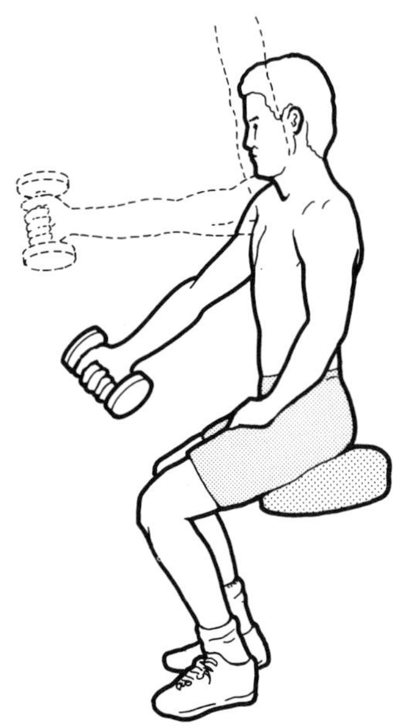

Fig. 44.11 Elevation of the arm in the sagittal plane (flexion).

PERISCAPULAR MUSCLES

Archery is unique in that the periscapular muscles are utilized to both maintain the full-

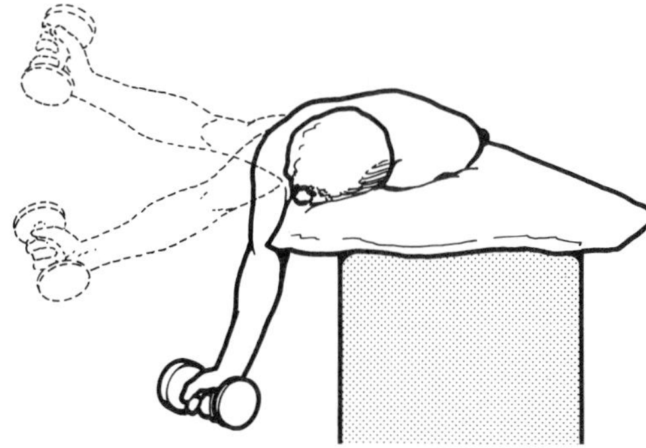

Fig. 44.12 Horizontal shoulder abduction with the arm externally rotated.

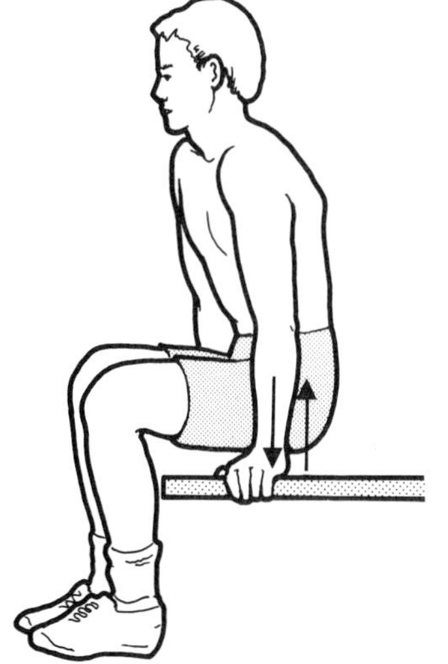

Fig. 44.13 Press-ups.

draw position and to gradually pull the arrow past the clicker in a slow, smooth and controlled fashion. The muscles in question include the serratus anterior, rhomboids, trapezius and latissimus dorsi. These muscles also need to be assessed and probably strengthened, with particular attention paid to the muscles that retract (pull towards the midline) the scapula — the rhomboids and trapezius. These muscle groups have also been isolated by EMG (Mosely *et al.*, 1992) and the specific exercises include scaption, press-ups, rowing and push-ups with a plus (Figs 44.9, 44.13–44.15). Supplementary exercises include military presses and pull-downs (Figs 44.16 & 44.17). The muscles are much larger and stronger than the rotator cuff group, and should be exercised by using greater resistance and fewer repetitions. A typical programme might be 8–10 repetitions with three sets done every second day. The resistance is gradually increased, keeping the repetition and sets constant. The resistance for press-ups and push-ups can be increased by wearing weight belts. The goal is to develop significant strength in these muscles, as opposed to the rotator cuff muscles which require both strength and endurance.

Female archers

Mann and Littke (1989) found that women have a much greater prevalence of drawing-arm shoulder problems. While this may simply be a sampling phenomenon, consideration should

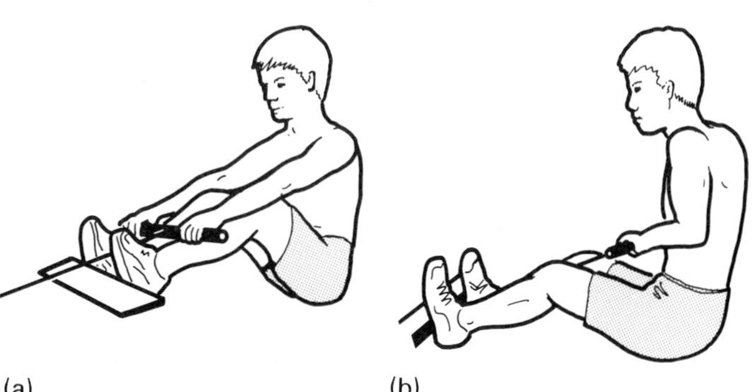

Fig. 44.14 Rowing exercise.

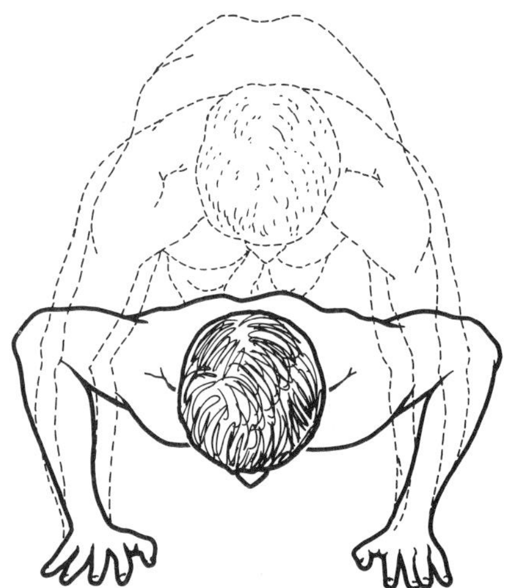

Fig. 44.15 Push-up with a plus: a normal push-up adding maximum shoulder and scapula protraction with elbows fully extended.

be given to its possible cause. The reason may be due to gender differences in strength; the weight of bows shot by women may simply be too heavy. However, in the study very few women actively followed a properly designed rehabilitative programme, so it would be wiser to initiate that first, although decreasing bow weight temporarily is a good option until strength can be regained.

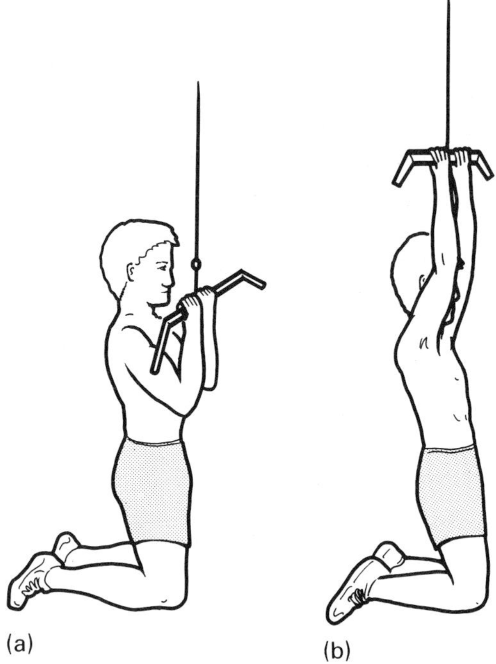

(a) (b)

Fig. 44.17 Pull-downs.

BACK MUSCLES

Another major area of injury requiring preventive and rehabilitative exercises is the back. Once again a significant proportion of these problems stem from poor stance which should

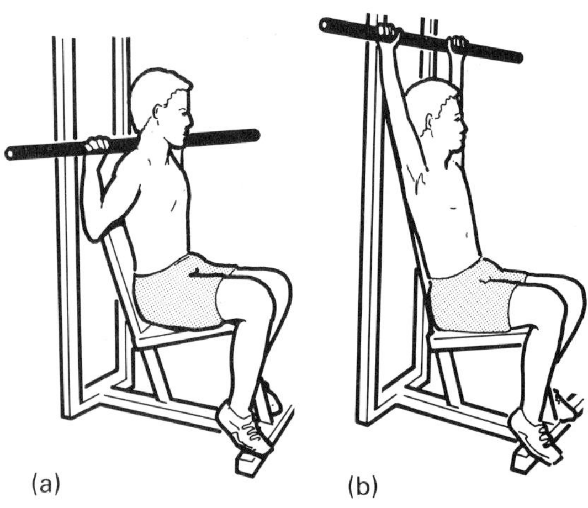

(a) (b)

Fig. 44.16 A military press.

be corrected. Excessive leaning away from the target and rotation is often observed. This leads to asymmetrical stresses being placed upon bony and ligamentous structures, as well as promoting muscle imbalance and soreness as the paraspinal muscles attempt to compensate for the primary asymmetry. Observing the archer with his or her back and shoulders exposed will demonstrate these features.

A stretching programme is of particular importance with these types of problems, as years of static asymmetric positioning results in a greatly restricted range of motion. Each archer will need to be assessed individually. However, there are several general stretches that can be advocated. The lumbar spine can be stretched specifically (Figs 44.18–44.20), with more emphasis placed upon stretching in flexion than in extension as excessive lordosis is more problematic in archery. The rotational manoeuvres should also be highlighted (Figs 44.21 & 44.22), particularly in those archers adopting an oblique stance. The hip flexor group should also be stretched, as tightness in these muscles accentuates lumbar lordosis (Figs 44.23 & 44.24).

After the problems of stance and flexibility have been addressed, the archer needs to strengthen the supporting musculature of the back. It has already been noted that the majority of injured archers suffer from excessive lordosis and/or rotation, so the abdominal muscles need to be emphasized. These muscles can be easily exercised by sit-ups (Fig. 44.25) and rotational variations of sit-ups (Figs 44.26 &

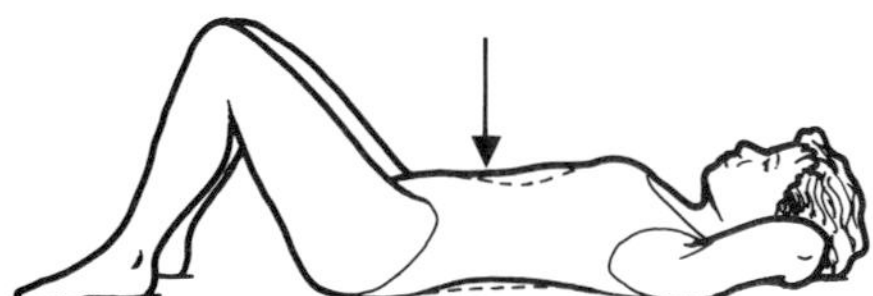

Fig. 44.18 Pelvic tilts.

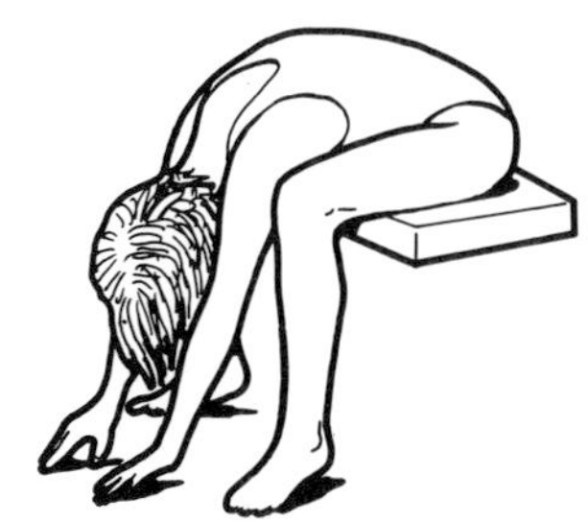

Fig. 44.19 A seated low back stretch.

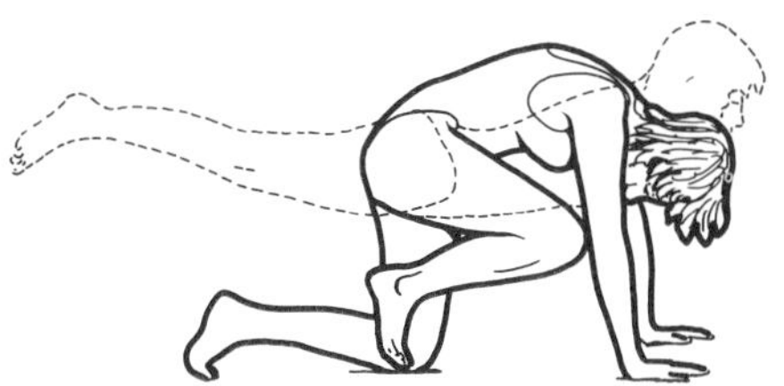

Fig. 44.20 A knee to chest stretch on all-fours.

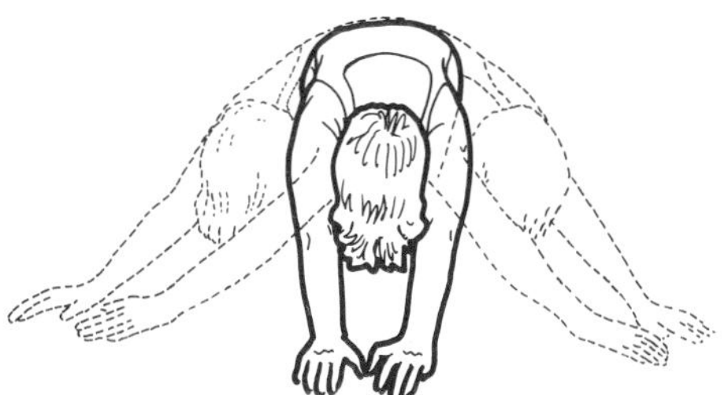

Fig. 44.21 A mid-back rotation stretch.

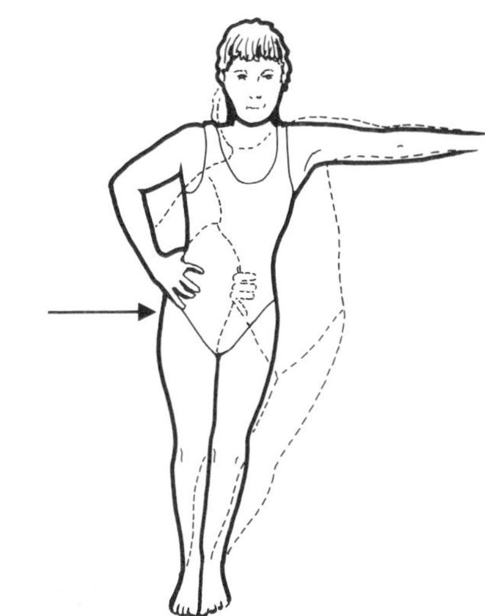

Fig. 44.22 A wall lean stretch.

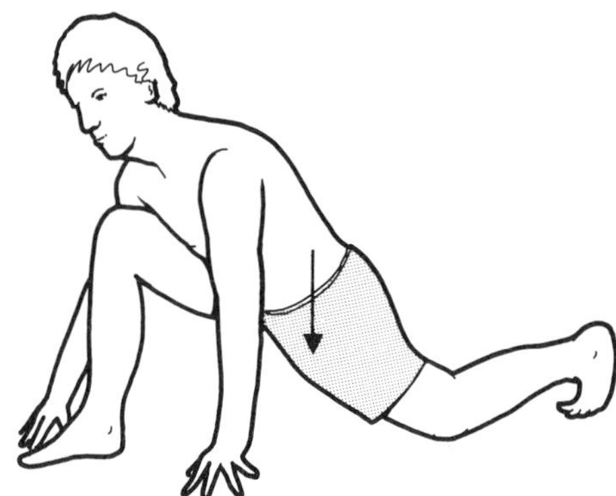

Fig. 44.23 A lower back stretch.

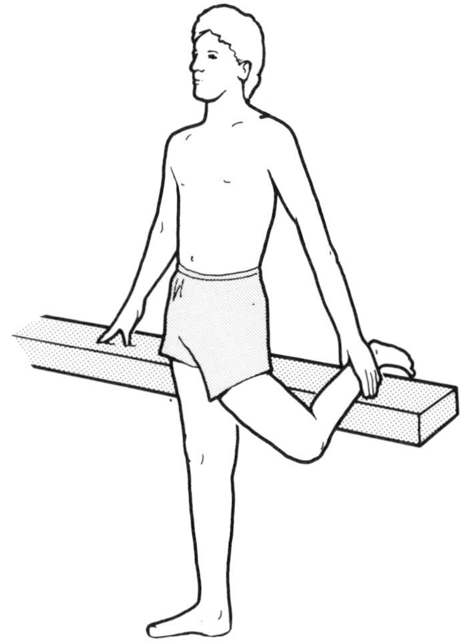

Fig. 44.24 A quadriceps stretch.

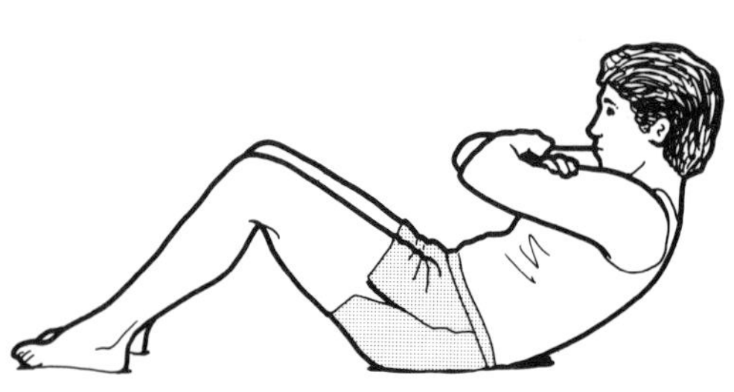

Fig. 44.25 Sit-ups.

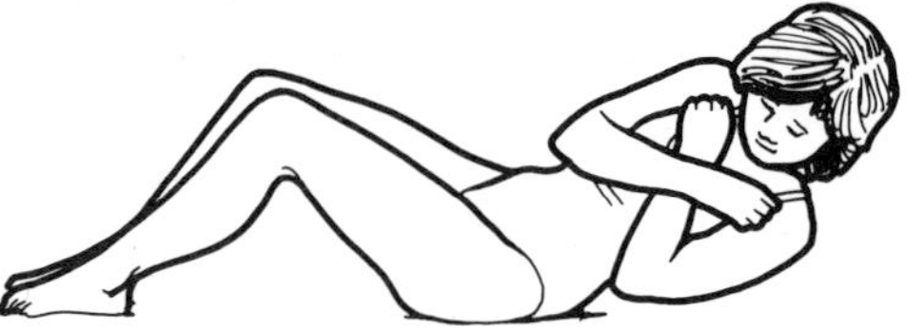

Fig. 44.26 Diagonal sit-ups.

44.27). The endurance training of these groups is important, so daily sessions with steadily increasing repetitions is the proper design. Start off with three sets of 20 repetitions each and increase by 5 repetitions every third session until 75 repetitions can be completed. Stretching the back in extension between sets will help to alleviate stiffness (see Fig. 44.20).

Back pain is a complex entity and its cause is often multifactorial. If symptoms are not resolving after 3 weeks of this exercise programme the archer should seek specialized help. This often means that the rehabilitation programme of stretching and strengthening needs to be reconsidered and individually designed to address the specific pattern of the injury that the archer is experiencing.

NECK MUSCLES

Archers also commonly complain of neck pain or stiffness. In searching for the causes in archers, once again attention must be paid to the way the head and neck are positioned,

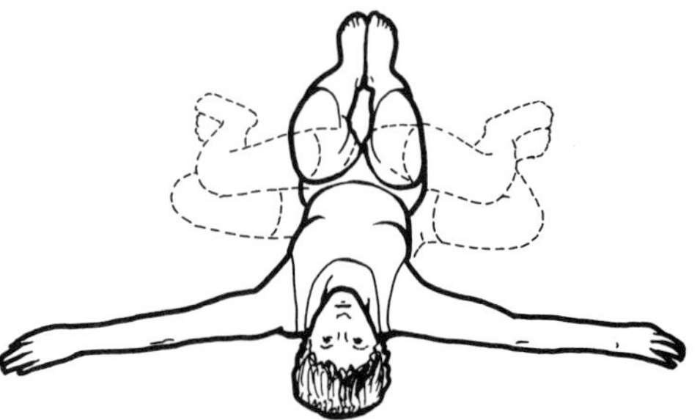

Fig. 44.27 Lower trunk rotation.

particularly at full draw. Several abnormal positions may be adopted, but the usual mistake is to try to bring the head to the string rather than the string to the head when anchoring at full draw. Freestyle archers will try and achieve a firm anchor point with their hand and string against their face. This position should be achieved with a minimum of head and neck movement, particularly if neck pain is becoming a problem.

The other major cause of neck pain is muscle imbalance and inflexibility due to asymmetrical positioning. Once again, passive and active range-of-motion exercises are the cornerstone for recovery, followed by appropriate muscle retraining. There may also be a role for manual therapy, modalities and medications if the symptoms are persistent or severe. Individual assessment is again indicated.

It should be emphasized that these strengthening rehabilitation programmes should be done bilaterally to achieve muscle balance and to counteract the asymmetrical nature of the sport.

Other treatment, including physiotherapy modalities (ice, ultrasound, etc.), anti-inflammatory medications, steroid injections and surgical options, are beyond the scope of this chapter. Every case must be reviewed individually, and these measures applied when clinically applicable.

Nevertheless, prevention is the key intervention in the management of most overuse injuries. By correcting stance errors, and strengthening the appropriate muscles at risk, injuries should be minimized.

Differential diagnoses must also be kept in mind. Many archers are in their thirties, or older, including at the élite international level, so degenerative changes should also be considered, such as rotator cuff tears and disc degeneration of the neck and back.

Conclusion

Archery is a unique sport that places asymmetric static loads on the shoulders, as well as the neck, back and drawing-arm hand and wrist. Particular attention should be paid to positioning and stance before initiating a preventive and rehabilitative programme. Prevention must address rotator cuff and periscapular strengthening and endurance around the drawing-arm shoulder, and flexibility and muscle imbalance around the neck and lower back.

References

Calliett, R. (1984) *Shoulder Pain*. FA Davis Co, Philadelphia.

Hawkins, R.J. & Kennedy, J.C. (1980) Impingement syndrome in athletics. *Am. J. Sports Med.* **8**(3), 151–8.

Jobe, F.W. & Jobe, C.M. (1983) Painful athletic injuries of the shoulder. *Clin. Orth. Rel. Res.* **173**, 117–24.

Jobe, F.W. & Moynes, D.R. (1982) Delineation of diagnostic criteria and a rehabilitative program for rotator cuff injuries. *Am. J. Sports Med.* **10**(6), 336–9.

Lombardo, S.J., Jobe, F.W., Kerlan, R.K., Carter, V.S. & Shields, C.L. (1977) Posterior shoulder lesions in throwing athletes. *Am. J. Sports Med.* **5**(3), 106–10.

Mann, D.L. & Littke, N. (1989) Shoulder injuries in archery. *Can. J. Sport Sci.* **14**(2), 85–92.

Moseley, J.B., Jobe, F.W., Pink, M., Perry, J. & Tibone, J. (1992) EMG analysis of the scapular muscles during a shoulder rehabilitative program. *Am. J. Sports Med.* **20**(2), 128–34.

Neer, C.S. (1983) Impingement lesions. *Clin. Orth. Rel. Res.* **173**, 70–7.

Pappas, A.M., Zawacki, R.M. & McCarthy, C.F. (1985) Rehabilitation of the pitching shoulder. *Am. J. Sports Med.* **13**(4), 223–35.

Parker, S. (1988) *Rotator Cuff Impingement Syndrome in Archery*. Federation of Canadian Archers, Ottawa, Ontario.

Townsend, H., Jobe, F.W., Pink, M. & Perry, J. (1991) Electromyographic analysis of the glenohumeral muscles during baseball rehabilitation program. *Am. J. Sports Med.* **19**(3), 264–72.

Chapter 45

Injuries in Alpine Skiing

ROBERT J. JOHNSON AND PER A.F.H. RENSTRÖM

The sport of Alpine skiing is actually only a very recent invention. Although cross-country skiing has existed for thousands of years in the Scandinavian countries, it is only during the past 50–60 years that Alpine skiing as we know it has developed. The firm attachment of the heel of the ski boot to the ski was the change which allowed this evolution. This seemingly minor alteration allowed the development of techniques which we now recognize as Alpine skiing. Previously, the front portion of the boot was the only attachment site. The provision of the rigid coupling between the ski boot and the ski has provided two major differences for participants. First, the firm attachment allowed much improved control of the ski by the skier (Fig. 45.1). This precipitated the development of skies with extremely hard, sharp edges. Second, it provided the potential for a marked increase in the production of lower extremity injuries by allowing the ski to act as a lever which bends or twists the leg which produces injury much more effectively than by the previous attachment methods. It is primarily because of this factor that cross-country skiing has had the reputation of being a relatively safe sport, while Alpine skiing has rightfully been considered a dangerous sport.

In Nordic countries, skiing of various forms has been an integral part of hunting, transportation, military activities, and perhaps even athletic contests for thousands of years. Undoubtedly injuries resulted, and quite probably initial studies concerning the mechanisms, treatment and prevention of these injuries began long before recorded history penetrated that part of the world. According to J. Waage (personal communication), it was not until 1894 that the Norwegian Trondheim Ski Club (founded in 1884) placed a rescue toboggan on its ski slopes to bring injured skiers down to the city.

The first medical publications about skiing injuries also came from Scandinavia in 1889. Between that year and 1901, Ekehorn described 11 femoral fractures from skiing falls (Ekehorn, 1901). Interestingly, he did not indicate what other fractures sustained in ski accidents were treated during that time at his hospital in Sundsvall, Sweden.

When vonSaar, in 1914, summarized information about skiing injuries, there were already about 40 published articles in Europe. When Petitpierre wrote his book on winter sports injuries in 1939, he referenced several hundred articles on skiing injuries.

In the USA, Ellison credited Brothers and Moritz with pioneering publications in the English language on the aetiology of ski injuries (Brothers, 1941; Moritz, 1943, 1959; Ellison, 1977). By repeatedly questioning patients concerning the direction in which their legs were twisted, both authors concluded that ankle fractures frequently resulted from external rotation. Each observer noted that an important factor involved in injury production was fixation of the ski to snow so that the continued motion of the falling skier imparted bending

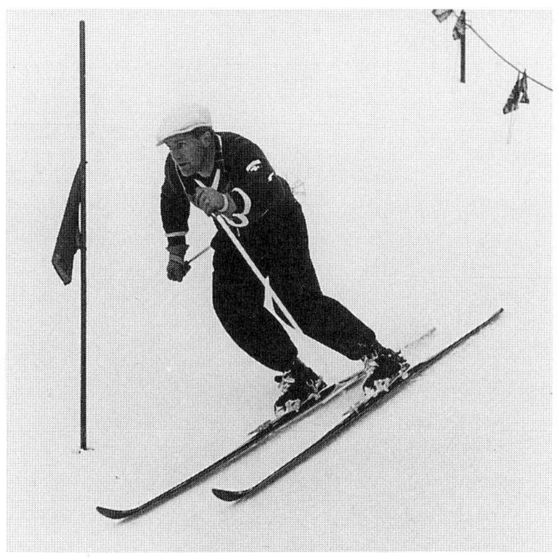
(a)

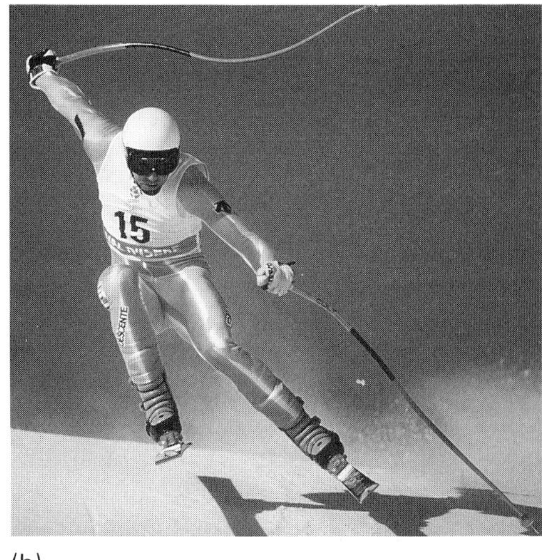

(b)

Fig. 45.1 The development and improvement of downhill skiing equipment has been dramatic from (a) the 1948 Olympic Games to (b) the modern Olympics. (a) © IOC, (b) © Allsport/C. Cole.

and twisting moments to the lower extremity. The 'elongation' of the foot by the ski magnified the loads transmitted to the leg.

Ellison (1977) observed that another factor besides fixation of the ski must be present to result in injury to the lower extremity, because many falls do not result in injury to the lower extremity, neither do they result in damage to the skier. He labelled the second factor 'enhancement', meaning that the pathological moments applied to the leg are increased by the continuing motion of the skier. If, for instance, a skier catches the inside edge of the right ski in a fall and the momentum causes the upper body to rotate to the left, enhancement will occur, and abduction and external rotation torques acting on the lower extremity will rapidly climb to intolerable levels. Injury will ensue unless the ski frees itself from the snow or the binding releases. If, however, the skier is able to rotate the trunk to the right during such a fall, enhancement will not occur and abnormally high loads will not be imparted to the bones and joints of the leg, thus avoiding injury.

In Ellison's study of 2140 ski falls recorded on slow motion movie film, 85% of all falls resulted in external rotation of the lower extremity (Ellison, 1973a). Less than 2% of the falls (four of the 2140) resulted in injury. In each of these instances, the excess moments occurred in external rotation. According to physicians experienced in ski injuries, excessive external rotation loading of the lower extremity is the most important factor in the production of ski injuries. However, other mechanisms do exist (including internal rotation of the tibia relative to the femur) which produce a significant number of injuries (Johnson *et al.*, 1974, 1979; Eriksson, 1976; Johnson & Pope, 1977; Marshall, 1977).

During the past 20–30 years, participation in downhill skiing has increased at least 40-fold in the USA, and recently has been estimated to be as high as 14 million skiers annually (Ellison, 1977; O'Malley, 1978). However, this figure, according to Cal Conniff of the National Ski Area Association (personal communication, 1983), is probably inflated, and the true number of skiers is closer to 8 or 9 million on an annual basis. It is estimated that the number of ski injuries in the USA has reached the staggering figure of 250 000–600 000·year^{-1} (Shealy *et al.*, 1973; Gutman *et al.*, 1974; Young *et al.*, 1976; Davis *et al.*, 1977; Ellison, 1977; O'Malley, 1978). Such injuries probably exceed 1 million per annum in the entire world.

Injury rates

The occurrence of Alpine skiing injuries is undoubtedly high compared to other recreational activities (Fig. 45.2). Most studies of injury rates are based on the number of injured skiers per 1000 skier days. Although this technique produces relatively inaccurate data concerning the number of injuries produced per time of exposure of a given population, it is the only commonly available method. The attempt made by investigators using this method is to establish, as accurately as possible, the number of skiers at risk each day. Often ticket sales are used to establish the population at risk, but this number can be misleading for the number of season pass holders and other skiers (ski instructors, patrol skiers and multi-day pass purchasers) who are not required to purchase a ticket each day, are not registered by this technique. Likewise, the purchase of a ticket does not imply equal exposure to risk by different skiers. Some individuals may ski continuously throughout the day, while others may only ski a few runs.

Another problem is that of the frequent failure of skiers to report even serious injuries to the ski patrol or to local medical facilities (Garrick & Kurland, 1971; Shealy *et al.*, 1973). In effect, any data reported by investigators of ski injury, is only the 'tip of the iceberg' because no studies have been devised that identify all of the injured skiers. It must be assumed that these unreported injuries could vary the studies presently available, but it is doubtful that they could make major changes in the primary conclusions of such investigations. Since there appears to be no practical way to identify and evaluate every injury, well-controlled and designed studies will have to continue in spite of this flaw.

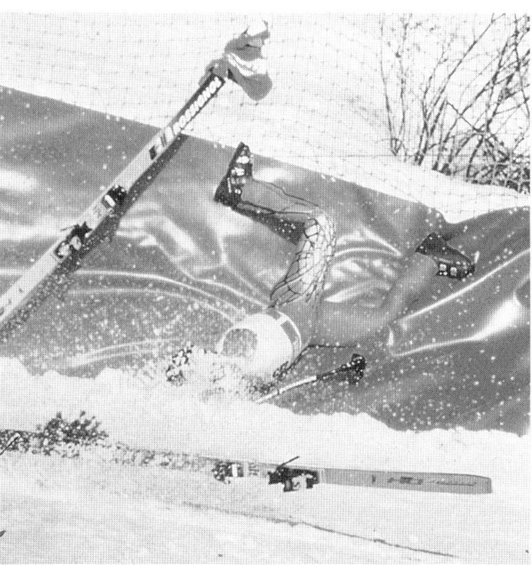

Fig. 45.2 The frequency of Alpine skiing injuries is high, and serious consideration should be given to prevention. © Vandystadt.

Table 45.1 reveals the reported injury rates (injuries·1000 skier days^{-1}) by several investigators over the years. Lamont showed a wide variation of injury rates in his review of the world literature (Lamont, 1991). Many of these papers do not have comparable results because of varying study design and a wide variation in the definition of any injury. Two recent prospective studies of a closed population used a very liberal definition of injury which revealed very high injury rates (Oliver & Allman, 1991: 24 injuries·1000 skier days^{-1}; Hauser, 1989: 17.3 injuries·1000 skier days^{-1}). In spite of these variations, a definite trend of improvement has been observed over the past 20 years. Our own data, and that of Young and Crane, have demonstrated that this trend has been slowing down during the last several ski seasons (Young & Crane, 1985). The reasons for the lack of improvement observed in recent years will be discussed at length in several sections of this chapter. Suffice it to state here that there is probably a rate of injury which will eventually be reached that cannot be improved. As long as

Table 45.1 Injury rates per thousand skier days.

Year	Author	Injury rate	Country
1959	Moritz	7.6	USA
1962	Haddon *et al.*	5.9	USA
1965	McAlister *et al.*	7.3	USA
1974	Johnson *et al.*	5.0	USA
1980	Johnson *et al.*	3.3	USA
1982	Crane *et al.*	3.5	USA
1982	Dubravcik *et al.*	2.7	Canada
1982	Korbel & Zelcer	1.4	Australia
1982	Ascherl *et al.*	2.2	West Germany
1982	Shealy	2.2	USA
1989	Johnson *et al.*	2.0	USA

Alpine skiing continues, there will undoubtedly be some injuries produced. The very nature of the sport which allows the individual to travel at relatively high speeds down slopes of varied degrees of difficulty and surface characteristics will continue to produce falls and collisions, a certain number of which will result in injury.

A mistake frequently made by investigators who treat ski injuries at a medical facility near a ski slope is that of apparent trends based on the incidence of injuries seen. Data generated from such studies may reveal a change in the number of certain injuries from year to year, but erroneous conclusions can result if the investigators use these data to project the population at risk. Only by accurately establishing the number of people skiing near the medical facility undertaking the investigation, can accurate estimates of the trends be established. For instance, an increase in the number of thumb injuries treated near a ski slope may rise rapidly during a certain period of time. This has too frequently resulted in the conclusion that such injuries are occurring more frequently to the population at risk, when in fact it really means that the population at risk has increased and the true rate of the injury has stayed the same, or even decreased somewhat.

Another confusing factor that has been discussed in the past has been the change in incidence of portions of the body injured overtime. Table 45.2 provides reported information concerning the relative percentage of lower extremity injuries compared to upper body (pelvis and above) during the years. Care

Table 45.2 Percentage of lower extremity injuries versus percentage of upper body injuries.

Year	Author	Lower extremity (%)	Upper body (%)
1955	Smith	80	20
1959	Erskine	79	21
1963	Kowalski	88	12
1972*		67	33
1978*		53	47
1981*		47	53
1985*		46	54
1990*		53	47

* From our own unpublished data.

should be taken by investigators from concluding that upper extremity injuries are thus increasing in incidence. These changes reflect the vast improvement in the ability of modern skiing equipment to protect the lower leg, and do not suggest that there has been an increase in the number of injuries to the upper body. Our own data have revealed that no significant increase in upper body injuries has occurred (Johnson *et al.*, 1989).

When closely evaluating the relative incidence of ski injuries from one year to the next, care must also be taken not to put too much emphasis on short-term trends. So many variables contribute to the generation of ski injuries that vast swings in certain injuries may occur from year to year, but when considered over a several-year period result in no significant changes. Likewise, our own study involving the evaluation of all injuries at a ski injury clinic at a Northern Vermont ski area has revealed a trend of decline, but only a few groups of injuries have actually been reduced at a statistically significant level (Johnson *et al.*, 1980, 1989). We observed that lower leg injuries have shown the greatest decline between 1973 and 1988 (Johnson & Ettlinger, 1982; Johnson *et al.*, 1980, 1989). Twist-related injuries have decreased markedly (i.e. spiral fractures of the tibia down 89%, and ankle sprains down 86%), while bending injuries have diminished at a slower rate (68%) (Johnson *et al.*, 1980, 1989). The true incidence of all upper body injuries did not change during the 15-year study period. Sprains of the ulnar collateral ligament of the metacarpal phalangeal joint of the thumb actually increased, but not at a statistically significant rate. Knee sprains, which have long been the most commonly reported injury to ski patrols and ski injury clinics near ski areas, declined somewhat, but unfortunately only minor (grades I and II) sprains to the medial collateral ligament decreased a significant amount (Johnson *et al.*, 1980, 1989).

Table 45.3 displays the changes observed in the incidence of injuries classically associated with skiing since the 1940s. Here again, the ability of modern ski boots and bindings to protect the ankle and tibia is indicated. However, the lack of improvement observed in the production of knee ligament sprains clearly reveals this to be the major problem still to be resolved in skiing safety.

Skier-related factors

Gender

In the past, several investigators established that females have a higher rate of injury than males (Smith, 1955; Rigos & Gross, 1957; Moritz, 1959; Haddon *et al.*, 1962; Howorth, 1965, 1980; Spademan, 1968; Arnold & Ackman, 1973; Ellison, 1973b; Garrick, 1973; Shealy *et al.*, 1973; Johnson *et al.*, 1974; Young *et al.*, 1976; Korbel & Zelcer, 1982). Other studies indicate

Table 45.3 Relative incidence of lower extremity injuries in skiing as a percentage of total injuries.

		Sprain		Fracture		
Year	Author	Foot and ankle	Knee	Foot and ankle	Tibial shaft	Total
1942	Moritz (1959)	35	19	11	3	68
1959	Moritz (1959)	30	23	11	3	67
1964	Harwood & Strange (1966)	18	22	8	16	64
1972	Eriksson & Johnson (1981)	12	20	7	11	50
1972*		6	21	1	6	34
1982*		4	28	3	3	37
1987	Johnson *et al.* (1989)	2	25	1	2	30

* From our own unpublished data.

that such differences do not appear to be significant when considering all injuries (Clayton, 1962; McAlister *et al.*, 1965; Marrocco & Warren, 1970; Young *et al.*, 1976; Criqui, 1977; Campbell *et al.*, 1982; Crane *et al.*, 1982). Selected injury types, however, occur more frequently to females than males (i.e. knee sprains and fractured ankles) (Campbell *et al.*, 1982; Johnson & Ettlinger, 1982; Young & Crane, 1985; Ellman *et al.*, 1989). Males more frequently sustain upper body injuries. Females do not sustain tibia fractures at higher rates than males (Johnson & Pope, 1977; Johnson & Ettlinger, 1982). The differences in incidence of injuries of various types between males and females are not clearly explainable. So many variables contribute to the generation of each injury that the variable of gender alone probably has little bearing on the production of a specific injury type. Besides the obvious difference in size and strength, factors such as aggressiveness and willingness to take risks may be partially responsible.

Skier ability

There is general agreement in the literature concerning the effect of skier ability on injury rates. It has been well established that far greater risk exists for the inexperienced skier. However, we have only recently observed the alarming fact that while less skilled skiers sustain relatively minor (grade I) sprains of the media collateral ligament of the knee at a higher rate than those with greater skill, they are no more frequently observed in the group of patients sustaining complete tears of the medial collateral and/or anterior cruciate ligaments than skilled skiers (Johnson *et al.*, 1980, 1989; Johnson & Ettlinger, 1982).

Skill acquisition

Numerous investigators have stated that all skiers should be encouraged to take lessons in order to minimize the risk of injury (Smith, 1955; Erskine, 1959; Earle, 1962; Haddon *et al.*, 1962; Kowalski, 1963; Howorth, 1965; McAlister *et al.*, 1965; Spademan, 1968; Arnold & Ackerman, 1973; Ellison, 1973b; O'Malley, 1978; Ekeland *et al.*, 1989, 1991). However, our own work (Johnson *et al.*, 1974) and that of Shealy *et al.* (1973) and Garrick and Requa (1977) suggested that ski lessons do not apparently have a positive effect on reducing the injury rate unless they are coupled with much skiing experience. We have postulated in the past that this possibly results from a rapid increase in the skiers' technical ability, thus allowing them to ski on terrain which is more difficult. Due to their lack of experience, they are unable to respond appropriately to the changes in terrain and snow conditions which in turn may lead to an accident. It appears that the variations in ski conditions can only be learned by repeated exposure. Thus, care should be taken by novice skiers, no matter how rapidly they develop specific skiing techniques, until they have skied for many days.

We found that the number of hours of ski instruction had no apparent benefit in a group of patients who had sustained lower extremity injuries, but we did observe that the total number of days skied was significantly less in that group of patients than our uninjured control population (Johnson *et al.*, 1974). It appears that changes in ski instruction, with more emphasis on proper equipment function and the proper means of falling and safety in general, may be necessary to improve the importance of ski lessons in assisting the beginner in avoiding injury. Eriksson (1976) reports that ski instructors in Sweden are urged to pay more attention to safety than those in the USA. For instance, skiers who present themselves to a ski class with bindings which appear to be unsafe to the instructor, are not allowed to take part in a lesson until they return with adequate equipment. He feels that the emphasis by instructors on such safety factors is one of several variables which contributed to a dramatic improvement in skiing safety observed in Sweden in the mid-1970s. More work is necessary in this area; certainly common sense would indicate that proper ski instruction should diminish the risk of injury.

Skier age

Numerous investigators have reported a strong correlation between youth and the risk of injury (Clayton, 1962; Earle *et al.*, 1962; Ellison *et al.*, 1962; Mclntyre, 1963; McAlister *et al.*, 1965; Harwood & Strange, 1966; Spademan, 1968; Arnold & Ackerman, 1973; Shealy *et al.*, 1973; Johnson *et al.*, 1974; Danielsson, 1976; Young, 1976; Johnson & Pope, 1977; Eriksson & Danielsson, 1978; Pechlaner & Philadelphy, 1978; Requa & Garrick, 1978; Garrick & Requa, 1979; Crane *et al.*, 1982; Moreland, 1982; Ungerholm *et al.*, 1983; Blitzer *et al.*, 1984; Ungerholm & Gustavsson, 1984). We observed, as Requa and Garrick had previously, that children under 10 years have the same risk of injury as adults (Garrick & Requa, 1979; Requa & Garrick, 1978; Blitzer *et al.*, 1984). The highest rate of injury in our study was to skiers aged 11–13 years, with children aged 14–16 in an intermediate category (Blitzer *et al.*, 1984). We concluded that several factors relate to the relatively high incidence of injury to children aged 11–16 years. These young skiers have sufficient skill to ski rapidly on relatively difficult terrain, but they frequently demonstrate poor judgement and recklessness. They have weaker bones than adults of similar size, and often ski on old, worn and obsolete bindings which function poorly, if at all in preventing lower extremity injuries (Johnson & Pope, 1977; Johnson *et al.*, 1974; Johnson & Ettlinger, 1982a; Lange & Asang, 1978; Blitzer *et al.*, 1984; Ungerholm & Gustavsson, 1984). Parents must realize that providing children with inexpensive, hand-me-down equipment is a practice contributing to injury risk. Children require the most modern, high-quality ski bindings available.

Skier size

The fact that the most common method of determining binding settings in the USA uses the skier's weight as the principal determinant means that skier size correlates to the ability of the tibia to resist fracture. The experience of many investigators shows a high correlation between small skier size and injury risk (Johnson *et al.*, 1974; Davis *et al.*, 1977; Campbell *et al.*, 1982; Crane *et al.*, 1982; Blitzer *et al.*, 1984).

Fatigue and conditioning

Fatigue is one of the most difficult variables affecting ski injury rates to evaluate. Several investigators were unable to prove conclusively that fatigue has an important role, noting that the majority of injuries occur in less than 3 h of skiing (Earle *et al.*, 1962; Haddon *et al.*, 1962; Spademan, 1968; Ellison, 1973b; Davis *et al.*, 1977; Ascheri *et al.*, 1982). In controlled studies (evaluation of population at risk as well as injured skiers), Young and Lee (1991), Young *et al.* (1976) and Criqui (1977) concluded that injury rates do increase late in the day, and thus fatigue is likely a factor (Crane *et al.*, 1982). Several other investigators stated that they believed fatigue was important, but presented no convincing data (Moritz, 1959; Marrocco, 1970; Westlin, 1976; Davis *et al.*, 1977; Reider & Marshall, 1977). Likewise, several authorities imply that preseason training may be effective in reducing injury occurrence in skiing (Kraus, 1961; Howorth, 1965, 1980; Johnson & Pope, 1977; Reider & Marshall, 1977; Jenkins *et al.*, 1985). Yet only Kraus (1961) made an attempt to present any data to confirm these observations. Unfortunately, he provided no information on the 'conditioning' programmes used, and no statistical information to prove his conclusion that proper conditioning is the single most important measure in preventing skiing injuries.

In spite of the confusion that results from a review of the literature on the subject of conditioning and fatigue, it seems only rational to conclude that these factors are important. Skiers often recall feelings of loss of control and discomfort while taking that 'one last run', it is therefore not difficult to construe that danger exists for the exhausted skier. Likewise, when skiers are well conditioned, they ski long and hard without fatigue.

Skiing requires sustained muscle contractions (skiing in a flexed hip and knee position), quick bursts of powerful but finely coordinated muscle contractions (reaction to sudden changes in snow conditions or terrain), and general flexibility and cardiopulmonary fitness. A myriad of exercise programmes with varying emphasis are presented annually in the popular skiing literature. We cannot recommend one programme that is particularly superior, but we believe that well-rounded training including endurance work (jogging, cycling, cross-country skiing, swimming) and isokinetic or isotonic thigh and hip muscular exercises, are a minimum. Stretching to increase the range of motion of the lower extremity joints which may tighten with the endurance work and weight-training together with agility drills may also be helpful.

Alcohol

Ascheri *et al.* (1982) report that it has been estimated that as high as 30% of injured skiers in Europe were impaired by alcohol at the time of their accident. However, in their own investigation only 9% of their injured skiers had consumed alcohol and most of that group was probably not legally intoxicated. It had been the authors' impression that very few skiing accidents are associated with alcoholic intoxication in spite of its availability at most ski areas. Throughout the years we had been aware of its presence associated with a few injuries, and thus elected to run a study concerning its presence in injured skiers. At our ski injury clinic we asked all injured skiers of legal age who presented themselves on the day of an injury to participate in a breathanalyser test. The majority consented to this procedure. After approximately 2 months of analysis, the study was discontinued because of the extremely low incidence of positive findings. No skiers were legally intoxicated, and very few had any measurable alcohol levels.

Skier attitudes

An intangible factor at work in the production of ski injuries is certainly the attitude of the skier. Injured skiers often express surprise that they have sustained an injury. Most would admit that skiing is potentially dangerous, yet they somehow believe that they are immune. Many skiers think that their bindings, which they understand were designed to prevent injury, will somehow magically function no matter how old, worn or mistreated they have been. These attitudes seem most common in the young aggressive skiers who, as has been stated earlier, have the highest injury rates.

It is perhaps the inherent danger in skiing which offers a challenge to individuals who are willing to take risks. These individuals often develop a high degree of skill, but also enjoy placing themselves in situations that constantly challenge their abilities. This in turn results in skiing at high rates of speed over challenging terrain. Although accidents may occur relatively rarely to such individuals, when they do happen they are often spectacular and all too frequently result in serious injury.

On the other hand, individuals intimidated by the challenges of skiing may also be at risk because of their fearfulness. The inability to 'relax' and enjoy skiing may result in a high number of slow speed falls due to the skier's fear. It is well recognized that falls of this type may result in loading configurations to which bindings are unable to respond.

One of the most important factors which may reduce the experienced skier's risk of injury may be common sense. The ability to judge those conditions which may be dangerous, and avoid them, is a major factor. This may best be expressed as being 'in control' at all times. Among factors involved in this concept are avoidance of trail and snow conditions above the skier's ability, resisting the temptation to join one's peers in reckless skiing activity, courteous consideration of other skiers, avoiding high speed in crowded areas, and constantly being alert for sudden unexpected behaviour on the part of others. These factors are very difficult to teach, but certainly are necessary if accidents and injuries are to be avoided. For example, present ski boots and skis have greatly improved the ability of even inexperienced skiers to rapidly attain the skills necessary to ski at high rates of speed. We have observed during the last few years an ominous tendency for a large segment of the skiing population to ski at speeds which are not only potentially dangerous to themselves but also to those around them. These individuals, often young, aggressive males, frequently exhibit poor judgement by skiing far too rapidly in crowded areas. The potential for collision with others or frightening slower beginners skiers has led to many accidents. Unfortunately, this type of discourteous and dangerous behaviour can only be controlled by literally placing 'traffic police' at strategic positions along crowded areas. Unfortunately, even such strict measures as removing the offending skier's lift passes has done little to eliminate this unnecessary hazard on the ski slopes.

Collisions

Injuries resulting from skiing accidents can be divided into two categories: (i) those resulting from falls on the snow surface; and (ii) those from impact with some object (i.e. trees, lift towers, other skiers, skis, slalom gates and others). It has been proposed that the more severe injuries result from collisions with such objects rather than falls on the snow (Johnson *et al.*, 1974; Shealy, 1982). In an investigation reporting on 3536 injuries at our ski injury clinic in northern Vermont, we evaluated many parameters of collision injuries (Jenkins *et al.* 1985).

We found as Lystad had that 18.5% of these injuries resulted from collisions with objects other than the skiing terrain (Lystad, 1989b). Collision injuries in general were less severe than non-collision injuries. However, collisions with trees produced a disproportionately high number of serious injuries. Contact with the skier's own ski during a fall resulted in 6.7% of all injuries, but these generally resulted in non-severe injuries, followed by collisions with other skiers (3.1%), lift towers, rocks, fences or poles (2.4%) and slalom gates (0.7%). Surprising among our findings was that the skill of most skiers injured in collisions was greater than that of the non-collision injury group and not different from a control population of uninjured skiers. Thus, the attainment of skill alone is not enough to ensure against such injuries. Relative to the population at risk, males tended to have a higher incidence of collision injuries than females with the exception of collisions with other skiers, where females predominated. Avoidance of reckless skiing habits, and using care when skiing near fixed objects are probably important factors in preventing these injuries.

Ski equipment

Bindings

From the standpoint of skiing safety, there can be no doubt that the binding is the most important factor. Our research has clearly shown that those injuries resulting from events where the ski was allowed to act as a lever to bend or twist the leg, have diminished very significantly during the last 15 years (Johnson *et al.*, 1980, 1989; Johnson & Ettlinger, 1982). At the same time, there has been little or no change in the rates of injuries sustained by parts of the body not potentially protected by properly functioning bindings. The improvements in binding-related injuries resulted primarily from modernization of binding design and function. We still recognize that the ultimate goal of the perfect ski binding has not been attained.

All bindings are designed primarily to secure rigidly the skier's foot to the ski during skiing manoeuvres. The modern ski boot and binding provide a comfortable means of allowing the skier to control precisely the edge of the ski. This requirement is called retention. Once it was recognized that rigid retention of the skier to the ski greatly increased the likelihood of injury to the lower extremity, efforts began to devise a system whereby the binding could release the skier's boot if it were subjected to loads which were high enough to pass the threshold of injury to the lower extremity. The secondary purpose of the binding consequently became safety.

It has been universally accepted by binding manufacturers that the breaking strength of the tibia is the design criteria used to produce release bindings. This undoubtedly developed because of the high incidence of fractures of this bone observed in the 1950s and 1960s. The spiral fracture of the tibia rapidly became known as the 'skier's fracture'. It is produced by rotation of the foot with respect to the tibia when the ski becomes incarcerated in the snow and acts as an extension of the skier's anatomy. It was only after the development of relatively high and rigid boots that the site of the fracture was raised from the ankle to the tibia. During the 1930s and 1940s, the classic skiing injury involved an external rotation fracture of the lateral malleolus (ankle fracture) due to the softer and lower boots used at that time. The binding device that engineers tried to develop would ideally provide a means of release that would respond to loads higher than the fracture threshold of the tibia in bending (transverse or oblique fractures at the boot top) and twist (spiral fractures along the shaft).

Conventionally, most binding manufacturers have elected to utilize bindings which release from side to side at the toe and upward at the heel. In forward lean, the boot pivots about a fulcrum located a short distance behind and under the boot toe, and during twist release the boot pivots about an axis located a short distance forward of the heel. Since the pivot point (axis of rotation) in twist is close to the axis of the tibia, the binding and the leg experience similar moments regardless of where the load is applied to the ski. However, the location of the fulcrum in forward lean (boot top) and the location of the forward lean release mechanism at the heel mean that tensile or compression loads on the leg will prevent the binding from sensing the true bending moment on the leg. The problem is made even more difficult by the load distribution on the leg which is not easily determined and not conventionally defined. These bindings that release in this fashion are termed 'two-mode release systems' (Fig. 45.3). These bindings account for the vast majority of those commonly in use in recent years. Manufacturers of these bindings make the assumption that skiers fall in such a manner as to require release in only the two directions allowed. Certainly most falls result in forward lean at the heel and/or a twist to one side or the other at the toe of the binding. However, bindings of this type are insensitive to other loading configurations which could result in injury. Several of our publications have expressed concern about this limitation of these binding designs, because certain injuries to the knee and tibia can occur due to loading of the leg by the ski in directions to which the binding is blind (Johnson *et al.*, 1979, 1980; Johnson & Pope, 1982; Eriksson & Johnson, 1981; Ettlinger & Johnson, 1982).

Another option available to binding manufacturers is to provide additional directions of release (backward lean at the toe, side-to-side at the heel, roll off the top of the ski, and shear from the top of the ski) to those existing in the common two-mode release systems. Any binding having one or more of these additional release directions is termed a 'multi-mode system'.

Many factors besides binding design play an important role in lower extremity injury in skiing. For instance, no binding can prevent an injury to the tibial shaft of a skier who strikes a leg against a tree. Likewise, the loads that cause injury may be passed directly from the boot to the leg, whether or not the ski is still attached to the boot. This appears to be especially true for the knee joint, where our statistics indicate

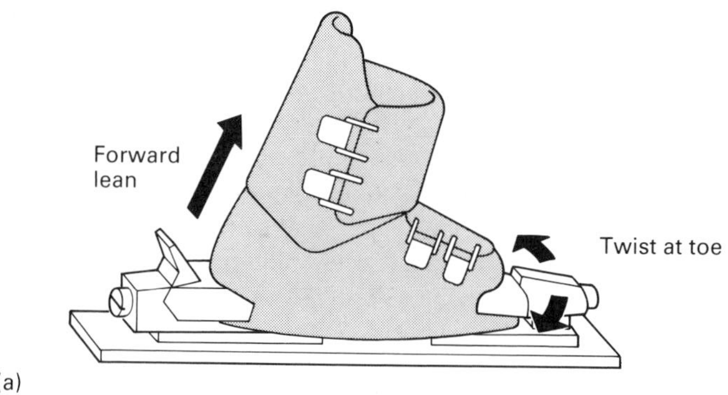

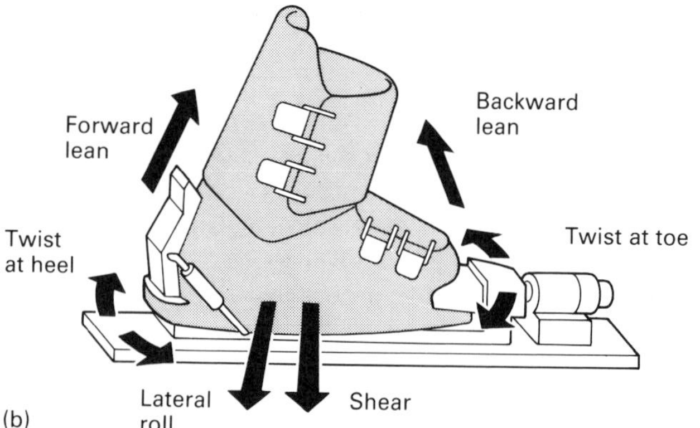

Fig. 45.3 Modern, well-adjusted and functioning ski bindings are essential. (a) Two-made release capability; (b) multimode release capability. From Peterson & Renström (1986).

that the injury rate has shown little improvement with the passage of time. Although the incidence of relatively minor knee sprains has decreased since 1980, we have observed a tragic increase in the incidence of severe knee sprains primarily to the anterior cruciate ligament (Johnson *et al.*, 1989).

At present the top models of all major binding manufacturers are excellent. We urge most skiers to seek bindings which allow an upward release at the toe, as well as the conventional side-to-side release at the toe. Modern boot-binding ski systems have proved to be effective in reducing the probability of ankle and leg injuries, if properly selected, installed, adjusted and maintained. Installation, adjustment and maintenance should be conducted by mechanics trained by the equipment manufacturers and using the proper tools, jigs, fixtures and testing equipment.

Recommendations

THE RELEASE SYSTEM

Daily inspection and routine maintenance are the responsibility of the skier. The following recommendations may, in our opinion, be of help in maximizing the reliability and useful life of the release system:

1 Read and save all manufacturers' literature.

2 Note the indicated release setting of each binding component. Check these values regularly.

3 Routinely lubricate all external surfaces of the binding with a thin film of silicone to prevent icing and corrosion, unless the manufacturer specifies otherwise.

4 Keep bindings covered when transporting them on a car top carrier to avoid exposure to corrosive salt or abrasive sand contamination.

5 Wash with water when contaminated.

6 Release all binding components in all directions of release each day before skiing.
7 Avoid walking in ski boots to reduce wear and contamination of critical surfaces that meet with the binding.
8 Clean the boot sole of ice, snow and contamination before entry into the binding.
9 Make sure the boot is properly buckled while skiing.
10 Check all equipment routinely for wear, damage, or missing parts.
11 Inspect the ski brake each day for proper function.
12 Return the equipment to a qualified mechanic prior to the beginning of each season for a complete inspection, including release tests with a mechanical testing device and maintenance to include lubrication if necessary.

Although lower leg injuries currently account for only 15% of all reported injuries, most of these injuries are serious, and have a significant medical and economic impact on the patient (Johnson *et al.*, 1989). Failure to follow these simple recommendations can, in our opinion, dramatically and unnecessarily increase the risk of injury.

SKI BOOTS

There can be no doubt that improvements in ski boot construction and design have contributed significantly to the protection of the foot, ankle and distal tibia. These changes have directly resulted in the reduction of injuries to these areas as presented in Table 45.3. Besides offering a protective shell for the foot and ankle region, the ski boot acts as an effective means of transferring those forces which the skier uses to control his or her progress down the slope from the upper body to the ski.

In most cases the boot is, in fact, an integral part of the system utilized to effect a release when, for instance during a fall, dangerous loads to the leg may result in injury. Thus, many of the characteristics of the boot including its stiffness, contour, length, height, coefficient of friction, wear and cleanliness, all affect the ability of a ski–boot–binding system to release properly during an accident.

Boot selection is equal in importance to binding selection. We believe that the major criteria in selecting a ski boot involves closely interrelated factors, including safety, performance and comfort. Because of the wide variation in the needs of various skiers, equipment manufacturers offer a wide variety of boots, none of which are the best for both performance and safety. The needs of a professional ski racer are quite different from those of a beginner. There is a wide variety of opinion as to what characteristics are most important from a performance standpoint. In general, racers prefer stiff boots, which for a beginner may be potentially more dangerous than a somewhat softer and more forgiving boot.

For all but the most skilled skiers, a mid-priced boot is probably all that is necessary since they are well padded and contoured, but tend to be less stiff than the most expensive models. Very inexpensive boots are to be avoided for they frequently fit poorly and tend to have little padding or contouring at the boot top. The boot must be comfortable and able to tolerate long periods of wear. We suggest keeping the boot tightly buckled while walking about and simulating skiing motion for as long as practical before deciding to buy. This allows the skier to discover pressure points which may not be apparent until the boot is worn for some time. Even so, it is not uncommon to discover a 'hot spot' the first time the skier wears the boot for most of a day. The response to such pressure points is often the loosening of the boot so that skiing can continue with less pain. This results in a dramatic reduction in ski control which in turn may lead to an accident. If pressure point pain is observed during use, most ski shops have the means of stretching the boot's shell or modifying and padding the boot's inner lining. Excellent advice on how to modify boots effectively can be found in popular skiing magazines. As the skiers' skills become more advanced, they may wish to move up to the more expensive, high-performance boots, but this should be done to improve skiing performance, and not just to emulate the world class skier seen in advertisements.

Two properties of the boot should be considered, the interface with the leg and the interface with the binding. Boots should be comfortable and fitted properly when purchased. Movement of the foot within the boot should be minimized by the use of modern fitting aids and proper size selection. The boot should distribute the load widely on the leg in both forward and backward lean. Pressure should not be concentrated, and the centre of pressure should not move down the leg during forward lean. Overall stiffness characteristics can be a matter of personal preference, but very soft boots may require lower release settings in forward lean than is the current practice. With respect to the binding interface, the boot should be hard, low in friction, and conform to the shape requirements of the binding manufacturer.

SKIS

The ski may produce injuries by acting as a lever to bend or twist the lower extremity in those instances when bindings do not release properly. Thus, its length may be a factor by increasing the potential lever arm. Young *et al.* (1976) noted no difference in the length of skis between a group of skiers who sustained lower extremity injuries and a group of uninjured skiers until they also considered the height and ability of the skiers. They then observed among injured expert skiers that longer skis were more prevalent. They made no comment concerning the effect of ski length on the production of leg injuries in less skilled skiers, but they did point out that this study was done in 1971 before short skis became popular. It is probably rare that the ski is incarcerated at the tip or the tail, thus allowing the full length of the ski from those points to the centre of rotation of the leg to act as a lever during an injury. However, inexperienced skiers may manoeuvre a short ski with less difficulty than a longer ski. Thus the use of graduated length of ski during instruction may result in fewer falls during the learning phases of skiing. This may consequently result in a reduced injury rate, but no statistical proof of this contention is known to the authors.

Before the last 10 ski seasons, runaway skis had been prevented by the use of a so-called safety strap. Thus, during a fall when the ski was released from the binding it remained attached to the skier via one of many flexible straps. In high speed tumbling falls, the safety strap thus kept the ski in close proximity to the falling skier. This could result in the ski striking the skier and producing lacerations, most frequently to the head and face. More recently, the need for safety straps has been eliminated by the use of retention devices known as ski brakes. These devices allow the fallen skier to separate from the released ski, but prevents the ski from travelling on down the slope. Shealy (1982) observed fewer face and head injuries and lacerations when the use of ski brakes became more prevalent and our own work has demonstrated a decrease in the incidence of lacerations from the ski edge (Johnson *et al.*, 1989).

SKI POLES

Many investigators have discussed the relationship of ski poles to the production of injuries (Ellison, 1977; Carr *et al.*, 1981; Ascherl *et al.*, 1982; Dubravcik *et al.*, 1982; Shealy, 1982; Young & Crane, 1985; Hauser, 1989). The majority of these injuries result in sprains of the ulnar collateral ligament (UCL) of the metacarpophalangeal (MCP) joint of the thumb when the skier's hand grasping the ski pole strikes the surface of the snow. Whether the pole abducts and extends the thumb directly, or simply aligns the thumb with the snow surface leading to extension and abduction after contact, is unknown. In either case, we advise the use of poles with a grip that allows the skier to easily discard the pole during a fall. Thus, the use of pole straps or moulded grips which retain the pole when the skier's hand is opened, should be avoided. Unlike Shealy (1982), we found no evidence that moulded grips were helpful in preventing thumb injuries (Carr *et al.*, 1981). Hauser (1989) has demonstrated that pole grips resembling a sabre hand guard may eliminate a large proportion of these common injuries.

To prevent the ski pole handle from penetrating an eye socket or causing blunt trauma to the chest or abdomen, the top of the grip should be larger than standard poles of the early 1980s. A broad smooth top to the grip, by distributing the load over a larger area, can reduce the risk of injury when the skier falls forward on a pole planted upright in the snow.

The business end of ski poles should not end in a pointed tip, but rather have cratered, serrated or multi-pointed tips. These allow good holding on ice and are safer by making puncture wounds less likely.

SKI CLOTHING

It has become obvious that a frequent contributor to the development of severe collision injuries following a high speed fall is the slipperiness of the skier's clothing. Tapper and Moritz (1974) revealed that between 1969 and 1972, 1.3% of the injuries reported at Sun Valley resulted when a simple fall resulted in a precipitous slide due to 'wet-look' clothing. At Sugarbush North, Vermont between 1972 and 1980, we observed that 12% of all injured skiers reported their injury occurred after sliding for some distance (Johnson & Ettlinger, 1982). We did not establish the coefficient of friction of the clothing worn. Vonallmen and Glenne (1978) reported that clothing with a coefficient of friction less than the tangent of the slope upon which a skier has fallen, will result in a terminal sliding velocity similar to that of an upright skier. Thus, they strongly urged skiers to avoid clothing with slippery surfaces.

Skiing injuries

Skiing injuries do not differ substantially from those produced in other athletic endeavours. However, the use of a ski which effectively lengthens the foot if the bindings fail to release and the speeds attained during skiing do result in somewhat different patterns of injuries. During an 18-year prospective study (1972/1973 to 1989/1990), we evaluated 6671 injuries at a clinic situated in the base lodge of a moderately sized northern Vermont ski area. Table 45.4 presents the incidence of each of the 20 most frequently observed injuries to the entire injury group. Table 45.5 provides a comparison of the relative ranking of the 10 most common injuries seen at our ski injury clinic in 1972/1973 versus 1989/1990. It must be understood that Tables 45.4 and 45.5 present the percentage of the total injuries observed and not the true injury rates based on the population at risk.

In the remaining section of this chapter we will present our observations concerning several of the more frequently observed injuries occurring in Alpine skiing. It is not our purpose

Table 45.4 Injuries treated at a moderately sized northern Vermont ski area from 1972 to 1990.

Injury	Total injuries (%)	No.
Knee sprains	22.8	1522
Thumb sprains	10.1	673
Lacerations	7.7	513
Shoulder contusions	4.9	327
Boot top contusions	4.2	278
Ankle sprains	4.0	265
Tibia fractures	3.4	230
Knee contusion	3.4	226
Leg contusion	3.1	208
Arm contusion	3.0	205
Shoulder dislocation	2.9	195
Trunk contusion	2.2	146
Concussion	2.1	143
Ankle fracture	1.6	110
Metacarpal fracture	1.6	109
Patellar injury	1.6	107
Back contusion	1.6	107
Clavicular fracture	1.5	97
Meniscal injury	1.4	96
Phalanx fracture	1.4	93
Total	84.5	5650

Table 45.5 Ten most frequent injuries observed at a moderately sized northern Vermont ski area.

Alpine injuries (n = 335) 1972/1973			Alpine injuries (n = 339) 1989/1990		
Injury	No.	% of all injuries	Injury	No.	% of all injuries
Knee sprain	67	20.0	Knee sprain	89	26.3
Leg contusion	35	10.5	Lacerations	27	8.0
Ankle sprain	32	9.6	Leg contusions	27	8.0
Laceration	26	7.8	Thumb sprain	23	6.8
Ankle sprain	23	6.9	Shoulder contusion	18	5.3
Thumb sprain	23	6.9	Shoulder dislocation	17	5.0
Tibia fracture	22	6.6	Knee contusion	13	3.8
Shoulder contusion	17	5.1	Arm contusion	11	3.2
Knee contusion	14	4.2	Back contusion	10	2.9
Ankle fracture	12	3.6	Metacarpal fracture	7	2.1

to provide details concerning the treatment of these conditions. Our main aim is to identify any observed peculiarities of injuries generated during Alpine skiing, and provide general information concerning the treatment and prevention of these injuries.

Knee injuries

There can be no doubt from a review of the literature and the material provided in this chapter that the single most important injury produced in skiing accidents is the knee sprain. Not only is this the most commonly reported injury, but it is also the most frequent one which results in prolonged disability for the skier. More surgery is required for the treatment of knee sprains than any other type of injury. Knee ligament sprains have accounted for 22.8% of all injuries seen at our ski injury clinic between 1972 and 1990 (Table 45.6). Of all injuries treated, 30% involved the knee. By far the most commonly injured ligament is the medial collateral (MCL), which was involved in just over 80% (1228) of our cases. Of these MCL sprains, 59.1% were grade I and 24.7% were grade II (American Medical Association, 1968). Complete tears of the MCL accounted for 16.2% of these injuries. Almost all of the grade III MCL sprains and a larger proportion of the grade II MCL sprains were associated with a complete tear of the anterior cruciate ligament (ACL) as well. 609 (38.9%) knees sustained a complete tear of the ACL with or without damage to other ligaments.

Table 45.6 Knee injuries (n = 6671) in a moderately sized northern Vermont ski area (1972/1973–1989/1990).

Knee injuries	No.	% of all injuries
Sprains	1522	22.8
Contusions	226	3.4
Patellar pain syndromes*	101	1.5
Possible meniscal tears	96	1.4
Lacerations sutured	35	0.5
Tibial plateau fracture	19	0.3
Patella fracture	6	0.1
Total	2005	30.0

* Chondromalacia, patellar subluxation and dislocation, other patella pain syndromes.

During the 1972/1973 season, the incidence of complete tears of one or more ligaments of the knee was 15% and during the 1989/1990 season it had risen to 65.6%. This ominous trend occurred in spite of the fact that the total percentage of knee sprains versus total injuries did not change significantly (Johnson *et al.*, 1989).

The distribution of injuries within the knee suggests a specific pattern of loading has occurred. For instance, valgus and external rotation have been shown to result in damage to the MCL, and if the distortion continues, eventually the ACL (Kennedy & Fowler, 1971). Hyperextension and internal rotation have been assumed to result in damage to the ACL, and appear to be capable of producing an 'isolated tear' of that structure (Marshall & Johnson, 1977). Much comment has been made about the impossibility of producing a truly isolated lesion of the ACL, and while this is technically probably true, we have observed a large number of instances where an ACL tear is not associated with any other significant damage to the knee.

After 1980 we observed a dramatic increase in the number of ACL injuries. In the early 1970s 'isolated' ACL sprains accounted for less than 1% of all skiing injuries. In recent years we have observed that approximately 15% of all ski injuries involve an ACL tear. In an investigation still underway, we observed some very significant differences between skiers with predominantly severe MCL injuries to those with isolated ACL injuries. A higher percentage of ACL injuries than MCL injuries resulted from backward falls. Individuals sustaining ACL injuries were more skilled and more often males than those sustaining MCL injuries. Those sustaining ACL tears wore higher and stiffer boots than those of the control population or those who sustained MCL injuries. From these factors and interviews with injured skiers, it became apparent that a previously unsuspected mechanism of injury was responsible for at least a portion of the 'isolated' ACL tears. In this configuration, the skier falls backwards while the upper shell of the boot in effect acts to produce an anterior drawer type of loading to the proximal tibia (Fig. 45.4). A second mechanism of injury of the ACL is shown in Fig. 45.5. If the skier is falling out of control, the only way the injury could be prevented would be for the toe of the boot to move upward from the ski or possibly by allowing the ankle to plantar flex. Unfortunately, the majority of bindings are incapable of releasing in this manner and modern ski boots have fixed dorsiflexion at the ankle (Johnson *et al.*, 1980). Thus, we believe that the combination of higher, stiffer boots and bindings incapable of releasing upward at the toes are at least in part responsible for the unfortunate increase in ACL sprains. It is now apparent that present skiing equipment is incapable of protecting the ACL and as far as the authors know, nothing is on the horizon which will allow for any improvement.

Aside from those few incidences where a true dislocation with vascular injury has occurred, most knee sprains can be treated as non-urgent. Much controversy exists concerning the ideal method of treating complete tears of major knee ligaments, especially the 'isolated' ACL sprains. It is not our purpose to discuss these complex opinions and options. However, the frequent occurrence of complete disruption of more than one major ligament in skiing accidents means that individuals often sustain injuries which will require surgery.

Physicians examining patients at or near a ski area face a unique situation in determining the correct method of initial treatment. The skiing population tends to be transient. Families or groups have usually travelled long distances for their ski vacations. It is the responsibility of the physician who initially evaluates the patient to make a definitive or at least a working diagnosis. If a major ligament disruption has been identified or strongly suspected, it is the physician's responsibility to initiate treatment that will avoid further damage to the joint and, in our opinion advise the patient to return to his or her home for consideration of the ultimate treatment within a practical length of time. Thus, splints, crutches and compression dressings are utilized. Convincing patients that they have sustained a significant injury is often difficult because they frequently observe that they were not moving very fast at the time of the accident, had pain only briefly, and noted very little disability immediately following their accident.

Very few knee sprains require urgent surgery. The old adage that knee ligaments can

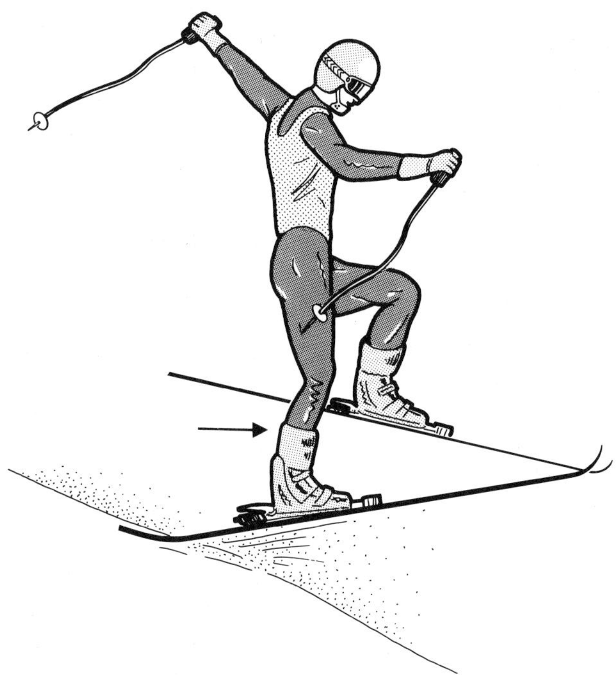

Fig. 45.4 The mechanism involved in the production of complete tears of the anterior cruciate ligament (ACL) which has been termed the boot-induced ACL injury mechanism. The skier comes down from a jump and lands on one ski when he or she are slightly off balance, with the upper body leaning backward. The tail of the ski hits the snow first, causing the ski to be driven into the snow quickly, allowing the boot top to drive the tibia shaft forward. At the moment of landing the skier's knee is in full extension and the opposite arm is thrown back in an attempt to regain balance. The actual injury to the ACL occurs at about the time the foot is driven flat on the snow (a few milliseconds after the situation that is depicted here). The fixed forward lean built into all modern ski boots is instrumental in the production of this type of injury mechanism. Redrawn from Feagin (1988).

best be repaired if operated immediately is a myth that we believe should no longer be believed. The majority of knee ligament surgery can be considered to be elective. This allows plenty of time for most patients to return to their homes where the inconveniences of surgery can be minimized. Thus, surgery, follow-up care and rehabilitation can then be accomplished by one physician, which we feel is an important advantage over emergency surgery far from home. Recent evidence strongly suggests that reconstruction of the ACL should be delayed for 2–3 weeks or at least until effusion and restricted range of rotation have been eliminated to reduce the risk of arthrofibrosis (Shelbourne *et al.*, 1991).

We believe that young, active patients who wish to continue high-risk sports which require contact, jumping, cutting and turning, are best served by reconstructions of complete tears of the ACL. The same is true when additional major structures such as collateral ligaments or menisci are also involved. We realize that this is a very controversial subject, and so the patient must be fully informed. Patients who are returning to their homes are urged to seek assistance from physicians they know and trust, and to follow the advice they receive from them.

Isolated tears of the menisci in the absence of significant ligamentous injuries are relatively rare in skiing, as can be seen in Table 45.4.

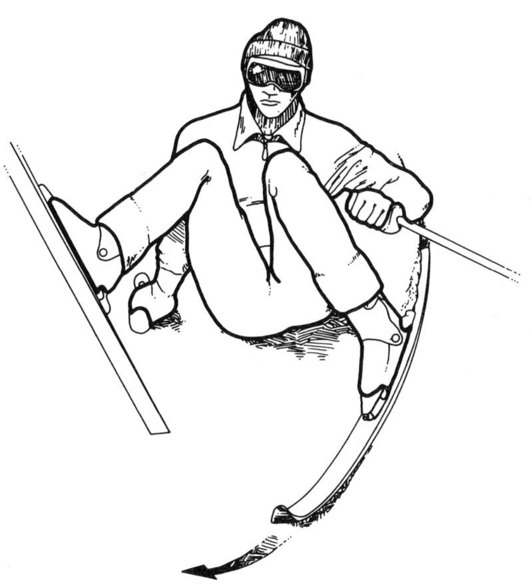

Fig. 45.5 An injury mechanism unique to skiing accidents: the 'phantom-foot' mechanism. As seen here, the skier has lost his balance and has fallen backwards. The right ski has left the surface of the snow, so only the inside edge of the portion of the ski behind the skier's left foot is in contact with the snow. As soon as this set of circumstances occurs, the ski carves a turn and produces an internal rotation of the tibia in relation to the femur. In all circumstances where we have evaluated films of this occurrence the knee is flexed to past 90°. This mechanism can produce isolated injuries to the anterior cruciate or injuries resulting in some damage to the lateral and posterior lateral aspects of the knee. This mechanism is probably more common than the boot-induced anterior drawer mechanism depicted in Fig. 45.4.

These injuries do occur and most often involve experienced skiers who are skiing hard in mogul fields. They result when the skier's leg is weighted in the compression phase of a rapid turn after coming down from a jump or over a mogul. It is not infrequent that such injuries occur even when the skier did not fall.

Unfortunately, there appears to be no major breakthrough in the methods available to diminish knee injuries in skiing (Ettlinger, 1989). It thus seems likely that the numbers and severity of knee injuries will not change in the foreseeable future. Hopefully, the work of individual researchers and organizations such as the American Society of Testing and Materials will continue to study the problem until factors capable of producing improvements are identified. In the meantime, the medical community will be required to deal with this epidemic situation.

Thumb injuries

Thumb injuries account for a significant proportion of all injuries reported in innumerable studies. Some authors have observed recent increases in the number of such injuries (Gutman & Weisbuch, 1974; Young & Crane, 1985), but our own observations, while noting some wide variations from year to year, have noted no significant trends (Johnson *et al.*, 1989). These injuries, which tend to be less devastating to the skier than major lower extremity injuries, are undoubtedly underreported to ski patrols and medical facilities evaluating ski injuries, and thus may well be the most common ski injury (Garrick & Kurland, 1971; Carr *et al.*, 1981). By far the most important injury in this group is sprain of the UCL of the thumb's MCP joint (Table 45.7). In our study this injury has accounted for 10.6% of all injuries between 1972 and 1982. During

Table 45.7 Thumb injuries (n = 500) at a northern Vermont, moderately sized ski area 1971/1972–1981/1982 (total injuries = 3690).*

	No.	% total injuries
MCP joint–UCL sprain, with or without fracture	391	10.6
Fracture phalanx	48	1.3
MCP joint sprain other than UCL	30	0.8
IP joint sprain	27	0.7
Dislocation carpometacarpal joint	4	0.1

* An additional 60 metacarpal fractures occurred, but the first metacarpal was not separated from the others in our data.
IP, interphalangeal; MCP, metacarpophalangeal; UCL, ulnar collateral ligament.

the 1979/1980 ski season, we observed that 34.8% of these injuries were grade I, 47% grade II and 18.2% grade III (Carr *et al.*, 1981). Of these sprains, 23.3% included an avulsion of a variable size flake of bone from the base of the first phalanx (Carr *et al.*, 1981). Such fractures were frequently present even in grade I sprains. Thus X-rays are advised even when the sprain appears to be minor. Mogan and Davis (1982) in a review of the literature, point out that the role of surgery in the treatment of complete lesions of the UCL of the MCP has become favoured. They suggest caution in vigorous examination of UCL sprains of the MCP for fear of converting a grade III injury from one which would have healed satisfactorily by conservative means to one which requires surgery. They point out that interposition of the adductor aponeurosis between the torn ligament ends may occur in some cases. They suggest a very gentle ulnar deviation of the joint to establish the presence or absence of even slight instability is all that should be done clinically. Attempts to deviate the thumb to the maximum amount allowed should be avoided. If even mild instability is present an arthrogram using 0.25 ml Renografin can establish whether or not the adductor aponeurosis is interposed. Surgery is suggested when this lesion is present, but protection of the joint with a cast is all that is required if the ligament ends are in contact (Mogan & Davis, 1982).

Finally, treatment of a sprain of the UCL of the MCP joint of the thumb need not cut short a ski vacation. A limited clinical evaluation including routine radiographs is all that is necessary by the primary-care physician. In most cases, a gauntlet cast molded to fit the patient's ski pole grip provides enough protection to allow the skier to ski safely even if a lesion which will eventually require surgery exists. Obviously, patients with marked swelling and pain should be splinted and advised to avoid further skiing. Definitive diagnosis and surgery can be provided by the patient's family surgeon upon returning home. Mogan and Davis (1982) feel that the interval between injury and surgery should be no more than 2–3 weeks, and sooner when possible.

Tibial fractures

Tibial shaft fractures came to be synonymous with the 'ski injury' in the 1960s. These injuries so impressed the skiing industry that the breaking strength of the tibia became the major criteria by which binding manufacturers design and adjust their devices. Thus it is not surprising that we observed an 88% decrease in the incidence of tibial shaft fractures between 1972/1973 and 1986/1987 (Johnson *et al.*, 1989).

Tibial fractures resulting from skiing accidents are in general the result of relatively low energy trauma. Thus comminution and open fractures are relatively infrequent. As we noted in 1977, most fractures of the tibia resulting from skiing injuries heal satisfactorily (Johnson & Pope, 1977). Internal fixation is rarely required in the treatment of these injuries. But short oblique fractures near the junction of the middle and distal thirds of the shaft and other unstable fractures do produce a challenge in maintaining length and alignment and avoiding delayed healing.

Lacerations

Although these annoying injuries are rarely serious, they frequently occur to the head and face and can be disfiguring. Almost invariably they result from a ski striking the skier after the bindings release in a fall. Since many of these lacerations occur during the tumbling stop of a high-speed accident, the ski patrol frequently describes these as 'egg-beater' injuries. The majority (85%) occur to the head and face area; most others involve the leg (Eriksson & Johnson, 1981). Most of these injuries are not serious and require simple suturing. The incidence of such lacerations has been reduced by the use of ski brakes (Johnson *et al.*, 1989).

Ankle fractures

Most ankle fractures result from external rotation of the ankle, produced by incarceration of an inside ski edge as the skier falls. The relative incidence of this injury has diminished in the past 15 years, but occasional severely comminuted ankle fractures are still observed. Fortunately, the majority of these injuries are minimally displaced oblique or spiral fractures of the fibular metaphysis beginning anterior to the ankle joint and extending posteriorly and upward. Interviews with skiers who sustained this injury frequently reveal that soft boots or deliberately loosened upper boot buckles to ease foot discomfort contributed to the injury. As in other equipment-related injuries, skiers who sustained these fractures frequently had their bindings set incorrectly or in poor functional condition (Johnson *et al.*, 1974). Prevention of this injury thus depends on proper boot fit, contour and padding, and proper binding function.

The majority of ankle fractures result in no significant displacement, and thus can be protected with plaster without reduction. Severe injuries with marked comminution and displacement, although rare, present a challenge to even the most skilled orthopaedic surgeon.

Shoulder injuries

Shoulder injuries include contusions, acromioclavicular separations, rotator cuff strains and glenohumeral dislocation (7.8% of all injuries at our ski injury clinic 1972/1973 to 1989/1990). The majority of these are relatively non-severe, but can be very painful. With the exception of shoulder dislocations, most result from direct trauma to the shoulder in forward falls. Rotator cuff injuries occur when the abducted glenohumeral joint is forced to the skier's side in spite of a strong contraction of the abductors, or by impingement of the cuff between the humeral head and the acromion, when forces are passed proximally along the shaft of the humerus during a fall on the elbow. In our experience almost all shoulder dislocations occur from falls which force the upper arm into abduction and external rotation rather than by catching the ski pole basket on vegetation as the skier is in motion.

Treatment of shoulder injuries initially requires support and rest with the exception of the glenohumeral dislocations. These latter injuries should be reduced as soon as the patient can be brought to the attention of a physician. If seen early, they can almost all be easily reduced by the common traction techniques.

Life-threatening injuries

Fortunately, life-threatening injuries are relatively rare. Head injuries, cervical fractures, cord injuries, haemopneumothorax and rupture of the viscera are all occasionally observed, and must be suspected. Most ski patrols are well trained and capable of handling all such emergencies. Primary-care physicians and facilities near ski areas should carefully rule out major injuries before discharging a patient, and be capable of rapid transport to a hospital when necessary.

Conclusion

In skiing, the high velocities to which the unprotected human body is exposed and the unnatural lengthening of the foot by the ski–binding–boot system generate large numbers of devastating injuries. As many as 30% of all ski injuries probably result from failure of the ski bindings to function properly. Thus, good binding design along with maintenance, mounting and settings must all be carefully considered and maintained at an optimal level if the risk of injury is to be reduced. Skiers who understand the risks involved in skiing and who consciously strive to minimize them by avoiding many of the common pitfalls discussed in this chapter can undoubtedly decrease the threat of injury to themselves. Although the treatment of skiing injuries requires no special knowledge from that required for the satisfactory management of other sports injuries, physicians who treat skiing injuries can better advise their patients on how to avoid further injuries by understanding all the relevant data. Not all risks can be removed from the sport of skiing, but a large proportion of the injuries which occur are simply unnecessary. Much is still to be learned before the breakthroughs necessary to prevent all or most knee ligament injuries are identified. This most challenging area of injury prevention will hopefully stimulate more research into possible improvements.

References

American Medical Association (1968) *Standard Nomenclature of Athletic Injuries*. Subcommittee on Classification of Sports Injuries, American Medical Association, Chicago.

Arnold, I.M.F. & Ackman, C.F.D. (1973) Skiing injuries in Canada: a coast-to-coast study. *J. Sports Med.* **1**, 31–3.

Ascherl, R., Schlemmer, H. & Lechner, F. *et al.* (1982) A ten year survey of skiing injuries. In W. Hauser, J. Karlsson & M. Magi (eds) *Ski Trauma and Skiing Safety*, Vol. IV, pp. 153–63. Technischer Uberwachungs, Verein Bayer, Munich.

Blitzer, C.M., Johnson, R.J., Ettlinger, C.F. *et al.* (1984) Downhill injuries in children. *Am. J. Sports Med.* **12**, 142–7.

Brothers, W.W. (1941) Ski injuries at Sun Valley. *Northwest Med.* **40**, 14–16.

Campbell, R.J., Ettlinger, C.H., Johnson, R.J. *et al.* (1982) High risk injury groups in downhill skiing. In R. Johnson, M. Lamont, W. Hauser & J. Karlsson (eds) *Ski Trauma and Skiing Safety*, Vol. III, pp. 126–34. Technischer Uberwachungs, Verein Bayern, Munich.

Carr, D., Johnson, R.J. & Pope, M.H. (1981) Upper extremity injuries in skiing. *Am. J. Sports Med.* **9**, 378–83.

Clayton, M.L. (1962) Ski injuries. *Clin. Orthop.* **23**, 52–66.

Crane, H.D., Young, L. & Cushing, W. (1982) The influence of equipment and ski factors on ski injuries with an update — 13 year study. In R. Johnson, M. Lamont, W. Hauser & J. Karlsson (eds) *Ski Trauma and Skiing Safety*, Vol. III, p. 134. Technischer Uberwachungs, Verein Bayern, Munich.

Criqui, M.H. (1977) The epidemiology of skiing injuries. *Minn. Med.* **60**, 877–88.

Danielsson, K. (1976) Swedish measures for reduction of skiing accidents with special reference to children. *Orthop. Clin. North Am.* **7**, 59–61.

Davis, M.W., Litman, T., Drill, F.E. & Mueller, J.K. (1977) Ski injuries. *J. Trauma* **17**, 802–8.

Dubravcik, P., Azpilberg, M. & Maistrelli, G. (1982) Pattern of skiing injuries at Mount Tremblant, a changing dimension. In W. Hauser, J. Karlsson & M. Magi (eds) *Ski Trauma and Skiing Safety*, Vol. IV, pp. 171–7. Technisher Uberwachungs, Verein Bayern, Munich.

Earle, A.S., Moritz, J.R. & Saviers, G.B. *et al.* (1962) Ski injuries. *J. Am. Med. Assoc.* **180**, 285–8.

Ekehorn, G. (1901) About ski fractures. *Nordiski Med. Arkiv* **34**, 1.

Ekeland, A., Holtmoen, A. & Lystad, H. (1991) Alpine skiing injuries in Scandinavian skiers. In C.D. Mote Jr & R.J. Johnson (eds) *Skiing Trauma and Safety: Eighth International Symposium, ASTM STP 1104*, pp. 144–51. American Society for Testing and Materials, Philadelphia.

Ekeland, A., Holtmoen, A. & Lystad, H. (1989) Skiing injuries in Alpine recreational skiers. In R.J. Johnson, C.D. Mote Jr & M.-H. Binet (eds) *Skiing Trauma and Safety: Seventh International Symposium, ASTM STP 1022*, pp. 41–50. American Society for Testing and Materials, Philadelphia.

Ellison, A.E. (1973a) *Ski Injuries* (film). Johnson & Johnson.

Ellison, A.E. (1973b) Skiing injuries (editorial). *J. Am. Med. Assoc.* **223**, 917.

Ellison, A.E. (1977) Skiing injuries. *Ciba Clin. Symp.* **29**, 2–40.

Ellison, A.E., Carroll, R.E., Haddon, W. & Wolf, M. (1962) Skiing injuries. Clinical study. *Public Health Reports* **77**, 985–91.

Ellman, B.R., Holmes, E.M. III, Jordan. J. & McCarty, P. (1989) Cruciate ligament injuries in female Alpine ski racers. In R.J. Johnson, C.D. Mote Jr & M.-H. Binet (eds) *Skiing Trauma and Safety, Seventh International Symposium, ASTM STP 1022*, pp. 105–11. American Society for Testing and Materials, Philadelphia.

Eriksson, E. (1976) Ski injuries in Sweden: a one-year survey. *Orthop. Clin. North Am.* **7**(1), 3–9.

Eriksson, E. & Danielsson, K. (1978) A national ski injury survey. In J.M. Figueras (ed) *International Series of Sports Science*, Vol. 5. *Skiing Safety*, Vol. III, pp. 47–55. University Park Press, Baltimore.

Eriksson, E. & Johnson, R.J. (1981) The etiology of downhill ski injuries. *Exerc. Sports Sci. Rev.* **8**, 1–17.

Erskine, L. (1959) The mechanisms involved in skiing injuries. *Am. J. Surg.* **97**, 667–71.

Ettlinger, C.F. (1989) What can be done about all the

knee injuries? *Skiing* **41**(7), 85–7.

Ettlinger, C.F. & Johnson, R.J. (1982) The state of the art in preventing equipment related Alpine ski injuries. *Clin. Sports Med.* **1**, 199–201.

Feagin, J.A. (ed) (1988) *The Crucial Ligaments*. Churchill Livingstone, New York.

Garrick, J.G. (1973) The mythology of ski injuries. *Phys. Sports Med.* **1**, 34–8.

Garrick, J.G. & Kurland, L.T. (1971) The epidemiologic significance of unreported ski injuries. *J. Safety Res.* **3**, 182–7.

Garrick, J.G. & Requa, R.K. (1977) The role of instruction in preventing ski injuries. *Phys. Sportsmed.* **5**, 57–9.

Garrick, J.G. & Requa, R.K. (1979) Injury patterns in children and adolescent skiers. *Am. J. Sports Med.* **7**, 245.

Gutman, J., Weisbuch, J. & Wolf, M. (1974) Ski injuries in 1972–1973. A repeat analysis of a major health problem. *J. Am. Med. Assoc.* **230**, 1423–5.

Haddon, W., Ellison, A.E. & Carroll, R.E. (1962) Skiing injuries. Epidemiologic study. *Public Health Reports* **77**, 975–85.

Harwood, M.R. & Strange, G.L. (1966) Orthopedic aspects and safety factors in snow skiing. *NY State J. Med.* **66**, 2899–907.

Hauser, W. (1989) Experimental prospective skiing injury study. In R.J. Johnson, C.D. Mote Jr & M.-H. Binet (eds) *Skiing Trauma and Safety: Seventh International Symposium, ASTM STP 1022*, pp. 18–24. American Society for Testing and Materials, Philadelphia.

Howorth, B. (1965) Skiing injuries. *Clin. Orthop.* **43**, 171–81.

Howorth, B. (1980) Conditioning for skiing (guest editorial). *Orthop. Rev.* **9**, 19–21.

Jenkins, R., Johnson, R.J. & Pope, M.H. (1985) Collision injuries in downhill skiing. In R.J. Johnson & C.D. Mote Jr (eds) *Skiing Trauma and Safety: Fifth International Symposium, ASTM STP 860*, pp. 358–66. American Society for Testing and Materials, Philadelphia.

Johnson, R.J. & Ettlinger, C.F. (1982) Alpine injuries. Changes through the years. *Clin. Sports Med.* **1**, 181–97.

Johnson, R.J., Ettlinger, C.F., Campbell, R.J. *et al.* (1980) Trends in skiing injuries. Analysis of a 6-year study (1972 to 1978). *Am. J. Sports Med.* **8**, 106–12.

Johnson, R.J., Ettlinger, C.F. & Shealy, J.E. (1989) Skier injury trends. In R.J. Johnson, C.D. Mote Jr & M.-H. Binet (eds) *Skiing Trauma and Safety: Seventh International Symposium, ASTM STP 1022*, pp. 25–31. American Society for Testing and Materials, Philadelphia.

Johnson, R.J. & Pope, M.H. (1977) Tibial shaft fractures in skiing. *Am. J. Sports Med.* **5**, 49–62.

Johnson, R.J. & Pope, M.H. (1982) Ski binding biomechanics. *Phys. Sportsmed.* **10**, 49–55.

Johnson, R.J., Pope, M.H. & Ettlinger, C. (1974) Ski injuries and equipment function. *J. Sports Med.* **2**, 299–307.

Johnson, R.J., Pope, M.H., Weisman, G., White, B.F. & Ettlinger, C. (1979) Knee injury in skiing. A multifaceted approach. *Am. J. Sports Med.* **7**, 321–7.

Kennedy, J.C. & Fowler, P.J. (1971) Medial and anterior instability of the knee: An anatomical and clinical study using stress machines. *J. Bone Joint Surg.* **53A**, 1257–70.

Korbel, P.J. & Zelcer, J. (1982) A controlled study of skiing injuries in Australia. In W. Hauser, J. Karlsson & M. Magi (eds) *Skiing Trauma and Skiing Safety*, Vol. IV, pp. 178–83. Technischer Uberwachungs, Verein Bayern, Munich.

Kowalski, R. (1963) Skiing accidents and their prevention. *Illinois Med. J.* **123**, 56–7.

Kraus, H. (1961) Prevention and treatment of skiing injuries. *JAMA* **169**, 1414–19.

Lamont, M.K. (1991) Ski injury statistics — what changes? In C.D. Mote Jr & R.J. Johnson (eds) *Skiing Trauma and Safety: Eighth International Symposium, ASTM STP 1104*, pp. 158–63. American Society for Testing and Materials, Philadelphia.

Lange, J. & Asang, E. (1978) Comparison of the shinbone loading capacities of children and adults. In J.M. Figueras (ed) *International Series of Sports Science*, Vol. 5. *Skiing Safety*, Vol. II, pp. 209–18. University Park Press, Baltimore.

Lystad, H. (1989a) A five-year survey of skiing injuries in Hemesdal, Norway. In R.J. Johnson, C.D. Mote Jr & M.-H. Binet (eds) *Skiing Trauma and Safety: Seventh International Symposium, ASTM STP 1022*, pp. 32–40. American Society for Testing and Materials, Philadelphia.

Lystad, H. (1989b) Collision injuries in Alpine skiing. In R.J. Johnson, C.D. Mote Jr & M.-H. Binet (eds) *Skiing Trauma and Safety: Seventh International Symposium, ASTM STP 1022*, pp. 69–74. American Society for Testing and Materials, Philadelphia.

McAlister, R., Brody, J.A., Hammes, L.M. *et al.* (1965) Epidemiology of ski injuries in the anchorage area. *Arch. Environ. Health* **10**, 910–14.

McIntyre, J.M. (1963) Skiing injuries. *Can. Med. Assoc. J.* **88**, 602–5.

Marrocco, G.R. & Warren, G.L. (1970) The causes of ski accidents. *Med. Bull. US Army* **27**, 10–15.

Marshall, J.L. & Johnson, R.J. (1977) Mechanisms of the most common ski injuries. *Phys. Sportsmed.* **5**, 49–54.

Mogan, J.V. & Davis, P.H. (1982) Upper extremity injuries in skiing. *Clin. Sports Med.* **1**(2), 295–308.

Moreland, M.S. (1982) Skiing injuries in children.

Clin. Sports Med. **1**, 241–51.

Moritz, J.R. (1943) Ski injuries: statistical and analytical study. *JAMA* **121**, 97–9.

Moritz, J.R. (1959) Ski injuries. *Am. J. Surg.* **98**, 493–516.

Oliver, B.C. & Allman, F.L. (1991) Alpine skiing injuries: an epidemiological study. In: C.D. Mote Jr & R.J. Johnson (eds) *Skiing Trauma and Safety: Eighth International Symposium, ASTM STP 1104*, pp. 164–9. American Society for Testing and Materials, Philadelphia.

O'Malley, R.D. (1978) Trends in skiing injuries: an 18-year analysis. *Phys. Sportsmed.* **6**, 68–76.

Pechlaner, S. & Philadelphy, G. (1978) Typical injuries caused by skiing equipment and methods to reduce them. In J.M. Figueras (ed) *International Series of Sports Science*, Vol. 5. *Skiing Safety*, Vol. II, pp. 131–8. University Park Press, Baltimore.

Peterson, L. & Renström, P. (1986) *Sports Injuries. Their Prevention and Treatment*. Martin Dunitz, London.

Petitpierre, M. (1939) *Winter Sports Injuries* (in German). Enke, Stuttgart.

Reider, B. & Marshall, J.L. (1977) Getting in shape to ski. *Phys. Sportsmed.* **5**, 40–5.

Requa, R.K. & Garrick, J.G. (1978) Skiing injuries in children and adolescents. In J.M. Figueras (ed) *International Series of Sports Science*, Vol. 5. *Skiing Safety*, Vol. II, pp. 5–10. University Park Press, Baltimore.

Rigos, F.J. & Gross, K.E. (1957) Ski injuries. *Northwest Med.* **56**, 1315–17.

Shealy, J.E. (1982) Two year statistical analysis of skiing injuries at 13 selected areas in the USA. In W. Hauser, J. Karlsson & M. Magi (eds) *Ski Trauma and Skiing Safety*, Vol. IV, pp. 207–16. Technischer Uberwachungs, Verein Bayer, Munich.

Shealy, J.E., Geyer, L.H. & Hayden, R. (1973) *Epidemiology of ski injuries: An investigation of the effect of method of skill acquisition and release binding used on accident rates*. Industrial Engineering Research Report.

Shelbourne, K.D., Wilckens, J.H., Mollabsky, A. & DeCarlo, M. (1991) Arthrofibrosis in acute anterior cruciate reconstruction. *Am. J. Sports Med.* **19**, 332–6.

Smith, V.D.E. (1955) Ski injuries — their prevention. *Bull. Am. Coll. Surg.* **40**, 289–90.

Spademan, R. (1968) Lower-extremity injuries as related to the use of ski safety bindings. *J. Am. Med. Assoc.* **203**, 103–8.

Tapper, E.M. & Moritz, J.R. (1974) Changing patterns in ski injuries. *Phys. Sportsmed.* **2**, 39–47.

Ungerholm, S., Engkvist, O., Gierup, J. *et al.* (1983) Skiing injuries in children and adults: a comparative study from an 8-year period. *Int. J. Sports Med.* **4**, 236.

Ungerholm, S. & Gustavsson, J. (1984) Skiing safety in children: a prospective study of downhill skiing injuries and their relation to the skier and his equipment. *Barnolycksfall vid Utforsakning Acta Universitatis Upsaliensis* **494**(IV), 1.

Vonallmen, B. & Glenne, B. (1978) Skiing accident dynamics. In J.M. Figueras (ed) *International Series of Sports Science*, Vol. 5. *Skiing Safety*, Vol. II, pp. 199–208. University Park Press, Baltimore.

vonSaar, G. (1914) *Sports Injuries* (in German). Enke, Stuttgart.

Westlin, N.E. (1976) Factors contributing to the production of skiing injuries. *Orthop. Clin. North Am.* **7**(1), 45–9.

Young, L.R. & Crane, H.D. (1985) Thumbs up: the changing pattern of ski injuries. In: R.J. Johnson & C.D. Mote Jr (eds) *Skiing Trauma and Safety: Fifth International Symposium, ASTM STP 860*, p. 382. American Society for Testing and Materials, Philadelphia.

Young, L.R. & Lee, S.M. (1991) Alpine injury pattern at Waterville Valley — 1989 update. In: C.D. Mote Jr & R.J. Johnson (eds) *Skiing Trauma and Safety: Eighth International Symposium, ASTM STP 1104*, pp. 125–32. American Society for Testing and Materials, Philadelphia.

Young, L.F., Oman, C.M., Crane, H. *et al.* (1976) The etiology of ski injury: an eight year study of the skier and his equipment. *Orthop. Clin. North Am.* **7**, 13–29.

Chapter 46

Injuries in Cross-Country Skiing

PEKKA KANNUS, PER A.F.H. RENSTRÖM AND MARKKU JÄRVINEN

Skis have been used for over 4500 years in Scandinavia, and until recently cross-country (Nordic) skiing was an important means of transportation during winter (Renström & Johnson, 1989). Until 1973, skis were made of wood and gliding capacity was limited. The development of skiing equipment has been rapid over the past 15 years with much more emphasis on arm strength and gliding than previously. In the 1990s, the racing skis are strong and ultra light (weight less than 500 g), made from fibreglass or graphite (Fig. 46.1). Also, ski poles, bindings and boots have changed to fulfil the demands of increasing speed on machine-made ski tracks (Fig. 46.2).

Cross-country skiing motion can be described in terms of a pulling and pushing phase, with forward extension and propulsion accomplished by the legs and arms (Renström & Johnson, 1989). The cross-country skiing stride consists of the overlapping kick, free glide, and poling phases. The traditional diagonal stride includes these three phases, as shown in Fig. 46.3a. In double poling, the skier uses the poles symmetrically to generate force for gliding (Fig. 46.3b).

During the 1984/1985 winter season, a revolutionizing change took place in competitive skiing as diagonal style was largely replaced by what is known as the skating technique (Kannus *et al.*, 1988) (Fig. 46.3c). This skiing style (known also as 'Siitonen step', Gertsch *et al.*, 1987) was first used with great success in long-distance ultramarathon competitions by a Finnish world cup winner Pauli Siitonen at the end of 1970s. The benefit was so drastic that only 5 years later, this skating technique had firmly rooted not only in competitive but also recreational cross-country skiing (Karvonen *et al.*, 1987).

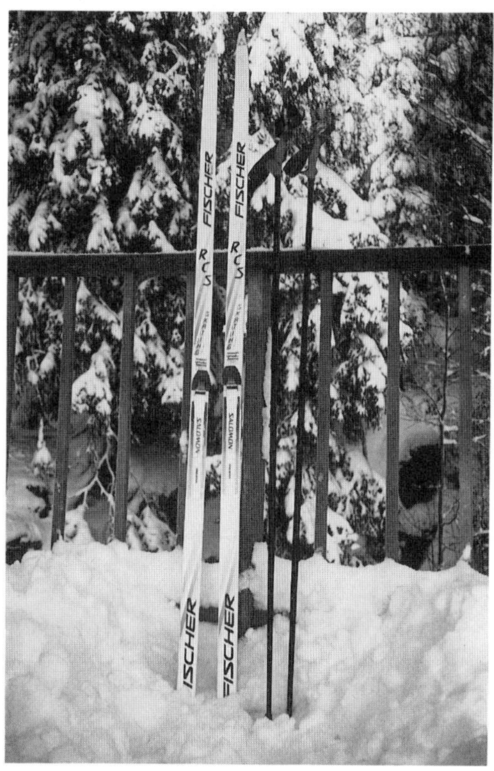

Fig. 46.1 Modern skating style cross-country skis with long poles. Courtesy of Dr P. Kannus.

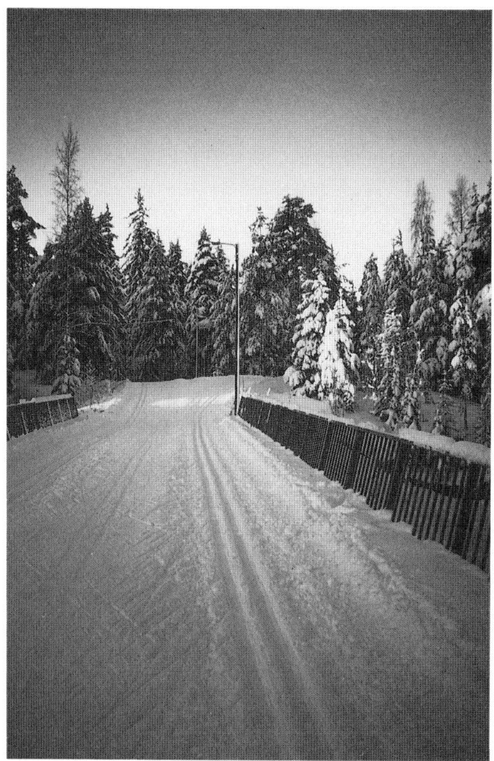

Fig. 46.2 A modern, machine-made ski trail with groomed tracks on each side and a well-packed area in the middle. Also lights are included making night skiing possible. Courtesy of Dr P. Kannus, Kauppi Cross-country Skiing Resort, Tampere, Finland.

Today, there are several variations to 'skate' with the skis. During 'marathon skating' one ski remains in the track as a gliding ski, and the other is edged at around 30° across the track to achieve a strong kick (Fig. 46.3c). At the same time as the skating ski is kicking the skier double poles forcefully. In 'V-skating', the legs alternate during the skating like a speed skater (Renström & Johnson, 1989). If there are no prepared tracks impressed on the snow but the snow is well packed, V-skating is the fastest way to move. In V-skating, there are different poling methods (double pole every other stride, double poling every kick, V-skate with diagonal alternative poling, and V-skate without poling) but no single method has been proven to be the most effective.

Cross-country skiing is one of the most popular competitive and recreational sports in Scandinavian countries (Eriksson, 1976; Orava *et al.*, 1985; Kannus *et al.*, 1988). The number of cross-country skiers in many other countries, such as the USA, Canada, Germany and Australia, has been reported to be growing steadily during recent years (Sherry & Asquith, 1987; Steinbruck, 1987; Hixson, 1989; Renström & Johnson, 1989). In the USA, for example, at the time of the 1932 Winter Olympics in Lake Placid, it was estimated that about 10 000 Americans were devotees of cross-country skiing; by the time the Winter Olympics returned to Lake Placid in 1980, the number had jumped to over 3 million; and in 1988, it was estimated that more than 7.2 million people were participating in this sports. Interestingly, today in the USA the popularity of cross-country skiing is growing at a faster rate than that of downhill skiing (Hixson, 1989).

In general, cross-country skiing is a safe sport, especially when compared with downhill skiing. The incidence of cross-country skiing injuries has been reported to be between 0.1 and $0.7 \cdot 1000$ skier days^{-1} (Eriksson, 1976; Westlin, 1976; Ellison, 1977; Lyons & Porter, 1978; Sandelin *et al.*, 1980; Boyle *et al.*, 1981; Clancy, 1982; Sherry & Asquith, 1987), while in downhill skiing it is $1-4 \cdot 1000$ skier days^{-1} (Westlin, 1976; Ellison, 1977; Sherry & Asquith, 1987; Johnson *et al.*, 1989). A comparative study of cross-country and downhill skiing injuries in one national park in Australia, revealed that the injury incidence was seven times lower ($0.49 \cdot 1000$ skier days^{-1}) in cross-country than in downhill ($3.54 \cdot 1000$ skier days^{-1}) skiing (Sherry & Asquith, 1987). In Finland, a similar comparative study revealed that the injury incidence was 13 times lower in cross-country skiing (Vuori *et al.*, 1988).

The injuries sustained in cross-country skiing can be defined as overuse or acute by nature. An overuse injury is usually considered to be a longstanding or recurring painful condition in the musculoskeletal system, which has started during training or performance due

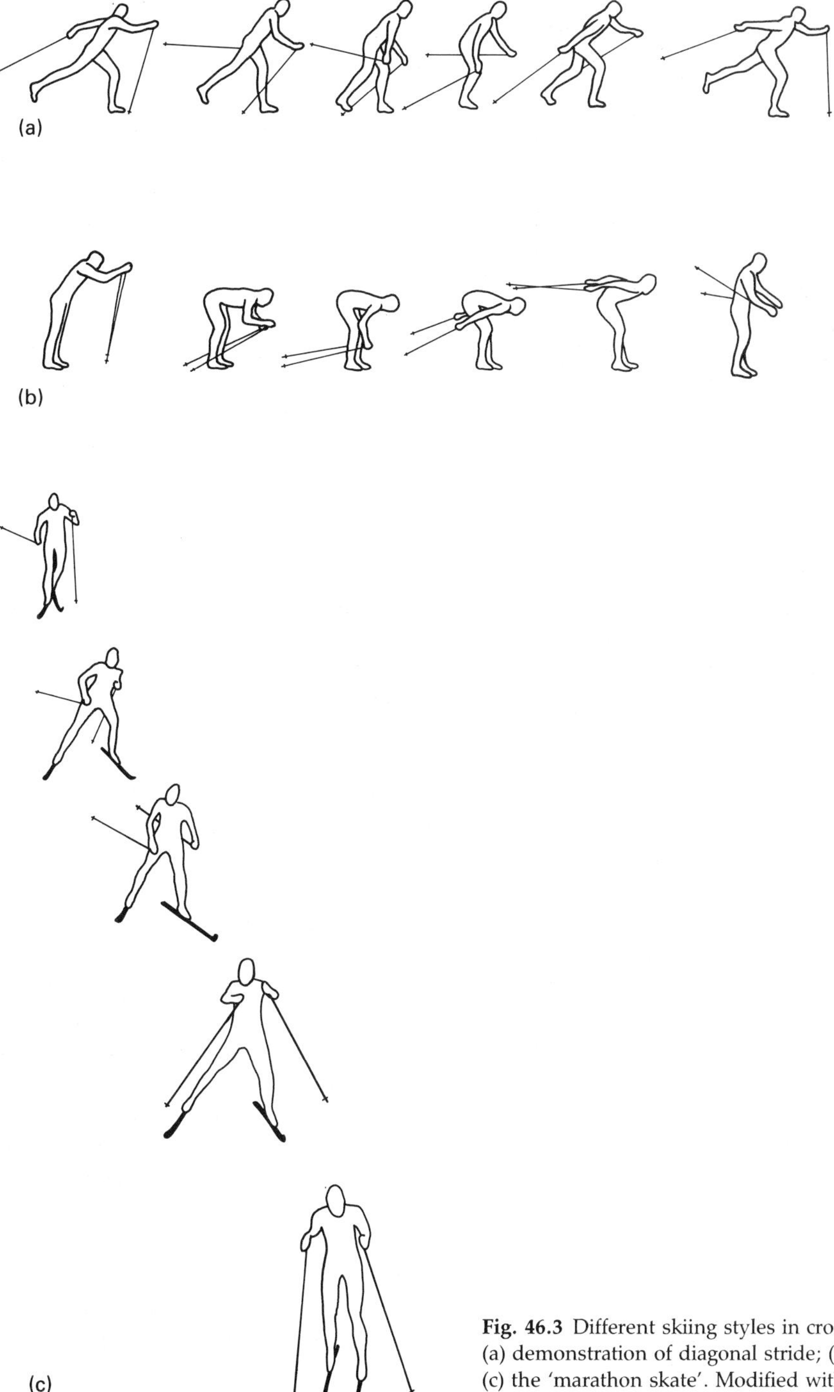

Fig. 46.3 Different skiing styles in cross-country skiing: (a) demonstration of diagonal stride; (b) double poling; (c) the 'marathon skate'. Modified with permission from Renström & Johnson (1989).

to repetitive tissue microtrauma (Orava, 1980). No single acute trauma is normally involved in the pathogenesis of an overuse injury. An acute injury is defined as a single impact macrotrauma, which, for example, can be a blow to the leg resulting in a fracture or a rotational injury of a joint resulting in a ligament sprain (Renström, 1988).

In cross-country skiing, approximately 40% of overuse injuries can be judged to be caused by the skiing itself, and about 60% are caused by forms of exercise and training other than skiing (mostly by jogging, running and jumping) (Orava *et al.*, 1985). Common predisposing factors are musculoskeletal malalignments, muscle weakness or imbalance, decreased flexibility, joint laxity, overweight, training errors (overload and too fast progression), faulty technique, and inadequate equipment.

Concerning acute injuries, the great majority of the accidents occur due to falls on downhill terrain, or on an icy or badly damaged lane of flat terrain (Boyle *et al.*, 1981, 1985; Steinbruck, 1987; Vuori *et al.*, 1988). Boyle *et al.* (1985) recorded in a prospective study the causes of accidents and injuries in cross-country skiing (Table 46.1). Injuries were often sustained by collision with some object other than the skiing surface. The most common mechanism for injury to the lower extremity was an external rotation–abduction moment applied by an entrapped ski to the leg. Also, forward falls were frequent. Other mechanisms are shown in Table 46.1. Vuori *et al.* (1988) observed that an actual collision with another skier is an uncommon cause of injury, but, as Renström and Johnson (1989) have pointed out, the fall of the skier may often occur when trying to avoid collision with another skier, especially on downhill terrain.

Table 46.1 Causes of accidents and injury in 43 cross-country skiers. From Boyle *et al.* (1985).

Cause of accident	Skiers	Cause of injury	Skiers
Loss of edge control	15	Impact with snow surface	21
Caught ski tip	10	Impact with object (tree, rock, pole, etc.)	10
Struck bare spot	3		
Deliberate fall	3		
Caught edge	3		
Slipped while standing	3	Twisted body part	3
Broke through crust	2	Impact with ski pole	1
Miscellaneous	4	Impact with another person	—
Total	43		43

Full understanding of reasons for injuries is fundamental when the preventive measures are planned.

Injuries in cross-country skiing

Overuse injuries

When the locations and types of overuse injuries are discussed, we must separate the problems occurring in diagonal and skating styles since their injury profiles may be different (Hixson, 1989).

During the seasons 1983 and 1984, when the diagonal style was still favoured, 75% of all injuries in the Swedish national cross-country team were overuse injuries and 25% traumatic injuries. The most common overuse injuries were medial tibial stress syndrome (shin splints), Achilles tendon problems and lower back pain. Other problems were knee pain (non-specific synovitis or extensor apparatus tendinitis), trochanter bursitis and iliotibial band friction syndrome (Renström & Johnson, 1989). Orava *et al.* (1985) analysed all the overuse injuries of Finnish competitive and recreational cross-country skiers (diagonal style) seen at two sports injury clinics between 1972 and 1983. Their findings are summarized in Table 46.2.

In addition to the above-mentioned findings, Renström and Johnson (1989), in good accordance with our own observations (Kannus *et al.*, 1988), have paid attention to several other overuse conditions seen in diagonal style cross-country skiing. They include triceps tendonitis;

Table 46.2 Typical overuse injuries associated with cross-country skiing. From Orava *et al.* (1985).

Cross-country skiing causes exertion injuries, which are most often located at:
- scapular and shoulder region
- lumbar spine
- ankle, foot and heel area

Most typical cross-country skiing injuries are:
- metatarsal pains
- retrocalcaneal bursitis
- tenosynovitis of big toe extensor
- entrapment of peroneal nerve (at the neck of the fibula)
- trochanteric bursitis
- pain of scapular muscles
- rotator cuff pain syndromes
- lumbar spine pains

Stress fractures caused by skiing are:
- metatarsal bone stress fractures
- sesamoid bone stress fractures (MTP 1st joint)

MTP, metatarsophalangeal.

lateral epicondylitis of the humerus; inflammation in the muscle insertions around the spinous processes in the lumbar and thoracic spine; instability at one or more spinal motion segments due to repetitive torsional load; patellofemoral pain syndromes; anterior compartment syndrome; tenosynovitis of the tibialis anterior and flexor hallucis longus tendons; tarsal tunnel syndrome; plantar fasciitis; nonspecific arthritis of the 1st metatarsophalangeal joint; and Morton's neuroma. We must remember, however, that it is difficult to differentiate which of these problems are due to skiing itself and which are mostly due to other training methods, such as running (Orava *et al.*, 1985).

Research results on the effect of skiing style on the number and types of overuse or acute injuries have been very scarce. At first the potential risks of the new skating style were much emphasized (Oja & Vuori, 1985; Dorsen, 1986), but with the growing use of the new technique many adopted a more positive attitude towards it. Regarding overuse symptoms, Mahlamäki *et al.* (1985) found in Kuopio, Finland that after the change-over to skating style, young competitive skiers suffered from fewer back and knee pains and from less muscle tension in the lower limbs, whereas complaints of the buttocks, hip, lower leg, arch of the foot and forefoot increased in number.

We performed a 2-year prospective follow-up (1985–1987) to find out if the change of skiing style affected the number and types of skiing injuries treated at our sports injury clinic (Kannus *et al.*, 1988). The results were quite dramatic. During the second skiing season (skating style) the number of overuse problems fell to half of that encountered in the first season (diagonal style). This was mainly due to the almost complete disappearance of overuse injuries of the lower and upper back, neck, shoulders and upper limbs. The number and types of overuse injuries affecting the lower extremities remained, however, essentially unchanged. We concluded that once the transition period of the change of skiing style had been overcome (new skis and boots, longer poles, etc.), the skating style in an athletic population seemed to be less stressful on the spinal segments and upper body than the conventional, diagonal style.

Acute injuries

To our best knowledge, our study has been the only one to evaluate the effect of the change in skiing style on frequency, types and sites of acute injuries (Kannus *et al.*, 1988). We found no changes. Half of the acute injuries involved the knee joint, and the most frequent single type of injury was a rupture of the knee ligaments. The high amount of acute knee sprains has been observed in many other studies, too (Westlin, 1976; Sandelin *et al.*, 1980; Boyle *et al.*, 1981; Clancy, 1982; Sherry & Asquith, 1987; Vuori *et al.*, 1988). The population at risk for an acute knee sprain has been observed to be the middle-aged female recreational skier (Fig. 46.4) (Eriksson, 1976; Eriksson & Danielsson, 1978; Kannus & Järvinen, 1986; Steinbruck, 1987; Vuori *et al.*, 1988). We assume that the modern skis made from fibreglass are often too slippery

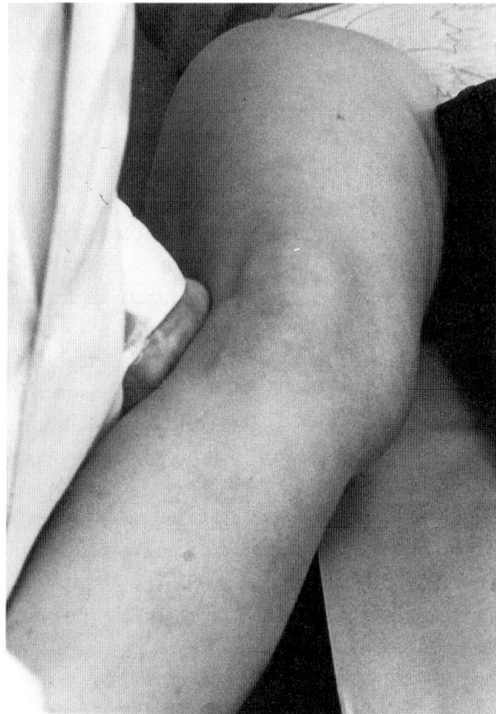

Fig. 46.4 41-year-old female recreational skier had a valgus distortion of the right knee while skiing on downhill terrain. The valgus stress test indicates a complete rupture of the medial collateral ligament.

Table 46.3 Acute cross-country skiing injuries during the 1979/1980 and 1980/1981 seasons in five ski touring areas in northern Vermont, USA (43 patients with 49 injuries) (Boyle *et al.*, 1985).

Upper extremity (41%)	
thumb sprains	6
shoulder dislocation	3
shoulder contusions	3
Colles' fractures	2
finger sprains (PIP joint)	2
elbow contusions	2
elbow fracture–dislocations	1
hand contusions	1
Total	20
Lower extremity (49%)	
knee contusions	4
ankle sprains	3
knee ligament total disruptions (MCL, ACL)*	2
knee ligament partial ruptures	2
hip contusions	2
leg contusions	2
hip, massive subcutaneous haematoma*	1
subtrochanteric femur fracture*	1
hamstring muscle strain	1
knee laceration	1
knee abrasion	1
patellar subluxation	1
patellar tendon open rupture*	1
tibia and fibula fracture	1
ankle fracture	1
Total	24
Head, face and trunk (10%)	
concussion	1
skull contusion	1
ear laceration	1
mandible fracture*	1
fracture of sacrum	1
Total	5

* Required surgery.
ACL, anterior cruciate ligament; MCL, medial collateral ligament; PIP, proximal interphalangeal joint.

when used on machine-made, often icy ski tracks. These conditions require better technique than the spare time female skiers usually have.

Other lower extremity traumas in cross-country skiing have been various as described in Table 46.3. In addition to knee injuries, Boyle *et al.* (1985) described ankle sprains, and hip and leg contusions occurring more than once in their series of 49 acute injuries. With the newest model of high skating style ski boots, the number of ankle sprains will decrease, but the number of knee injuries may increase, consequently. Renström and Johnson (1989) also pay attention to ankle and lower leg fractures, dislocation of the patella, hip fractures and hip and groin muscle–tendon strains, all of which may occasionally occur in cross-country skiing. Acute spinal traumas have been reported to be very rare in this sport (Frymoyer *et al.*, 1982).

Acute upper extremity injuries are quite common in cross-country skiing (Table 46.3) (Boyle *et al.*, 1981; Sherry & Asquith, 1987; Steinbruck, 1987; Hixson, 1989, Renström &

Johnson, 1989) representing approximately 30–40% of all acute traumas in this sport. Thumb and finger sprains (especially ruptures of the ulnar collateral ligament of the 1st metacarpophalangeal joint) (Fig. 46.5), distal radial fractures, shoulder dislocations and rotator cuff tears, acromioclavicular separations, and clavicular fractures are the most typical acute traumas in this part of the body.

Other types of acute injuries in cross-country skiing are rare. Such as neck sprains, head and face contusions, and ear or eye lacerations have been described. The most common cause of eye injuries is collision with frozen branches and twigs (Hixson, 1989).

Cold injuries

The potentially most serious injuries in cross-country skiing are due to cold and wind. Superficial frostnip is the phenomenon that turns a skier's nose, cheeks, ears, or tips of the fingers or toes white or blue–white. Once the skier goes indoors, where the usual interior temperatures prevail, the affected area thaws quickly, reddens and stings, but any blistering is minimal. Frostnip is also usual in female breasts and male genitalia in competitive skiers if tight racing suits are worn.

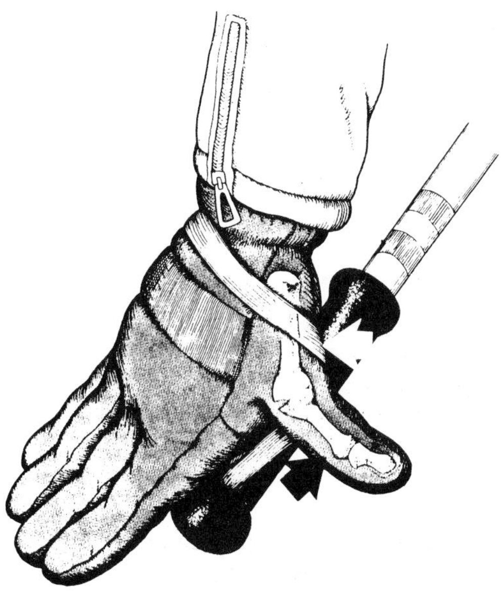

Fig. 46.5 Rupture of the ulnar collateral ligament of the 1st metacarpophalangeal joint is the most common acute upper extremity injury in cross-country skiing. If the rupture is complete, surgical treatment is required.

A more serious cold injury is frostbite. It affects the same area as frostnip, but involves deeper skin layers and is usually more painful. In a true frostbite, blistering occurs after the frostbitten skier returns to a warm environment. A frostbitten hand or leg can be warmed in the armpit or against the abdomen of the skier or another person. Rubbing of the damaged area is forbidden.

The most serious cold injury is hypothermia; that is, inability to maintain core temperature above 36.5°C. In hypothermia the core temperature is decreased usually due to a long exposure to cold, wet and/or wind. In cross-country skiing, this may be a problem in long ski marathons or ski tours, or in ski mountaineering. It is important to realize that freezing temperatures are not required for hypothermia to occur; prolonged exposure to cold, wet snow or even rain, can bring about the condition (Hixson, 1989).

Hypothermia always require immediate actions to return the core temperature to normal. Change of wet clothes, warm blankets, body contact and warm beverages should be done as for field emergencies. The patient should return to a warm environment immediately and hospitalized as soon as possible.

Prevention of injuries

The strategy in prevention of overuse, acute and cold injuries in cross-country skiing includes all efforts which can be made at individual, group and society level to minimize the number and seriousness of injuries. The connection of the preventive measures to skiing may be direct or indirect and the level of skiing may vary from mild recreational to strenuous professional.

Overuse injuries

At primary prevention of overuse injuries in cross-country skiing, individual efforts are of great importance. First of all, good basic physical fitness is a prerequisite for the musculoskeletal system to withstand increasing amounts of training and stress. This can be achieved only by regular exercise and general physical activity throughout the year. During the period of rehabilitation following illness or injury, or after a break in training, it is important that a reasonable level of basic physical fitness is reached before competition is resumed.

Warm-up exercises are designed to prepare the body for the ensuing sporting activity. Regarding injury prevention, the most common injuries to be prevented by proper warm-up are not only muscle strains but also tendon, ligament and other soft-tissue injuries and inflammations. After training or competition, cool-down exercises are desirable. Cool-down enhances the wash-out of the waste products of muscle metabolism (lactic acid, etc.) shortening the recovery time, respectively. It also offers a unique possibility to stretching exercises, since the muscle temperature is still high and stretching can be performed safely and easily.

Perhaps the most important preventive measure in overuse injuries is to progress slowly in training amount and intensity. The slow progression principle in injury prevention means that we allow the musculoskeletal system to adapt gradually to increasing or changing loads. This is especially true if the skiing style is changed from diagonal to skating, or vice versa. From this standpoint it is good that many, including top level, skiers use both techniques regularly. Musculoskeletal adaptation to stress is a slow but very potent process. Therefore, to avoid overuse symptoms, special attention is required from skiers and their coaches to understand the importance of slow progression. This concerns especially children and adolescents (Renström, 1988).

Preventive training of the musculoskeletal system is the key to both prevention of overuse injuries and to a successful recovery after an injury. Repeated, slowly progressive exercises will improve the mechanical and structural properties of the muscles, tendons, joints, ligaments and bones by increasing their mass and strength. Preventive training includes muscle training (strength, power and endurance), mobility and flexibility training, coordination and proprioceptive training, and sports-specific training (Peterson & Renström, 1986).

Preseason medical screening examination may be beneficial in prevention of overuse injuries in cross-country skiing. Such screenings should include a complete orthopaedic evaluation trying to discover possible risk factors, including overweight; previous musculoskeletal diseases like osteoarthritis, osteoporosis and chondromalacia; malalignments such as leg length discrepancy, scoliosis, joint hyperlaxity and foot hyperpronation; muscle weakness and imbalance; and decreased flexibility. Malalignment or leg length discrepancy corrections by individual shoe orthotics can be performed if necessary, not only to running shoes but also to skiing boots.

Technique and equipment. None of the previously mentioned measures can compensate the possible errors in skiing technique. If not properly loaded, the musculoskeletal system reacts by acute or subacute inflammation. If continued, the reaction changes from acute to chronic, which, in turn, is very resistant to any treatment effort. Proper skiing technique is best learnt in childhood. Adults are much more resistant to learning new tasks needing balance and coordination. It is of utmost importance to teach children all types of skiing so that they will learn to stress their body with various stimuli while skiing. Monotonous, asymmetrical and specialized training too early (one-sided skating style skiing only) is a great risk factor for overuse problems. By varying the exercise method, much larger amounts of total work can be carried out with less risk for injuries.

The errors in skiing technique may also occur because of poor and improper skiing equipment. Far too often the skis of a recreational skier are not properly waxed causing slipping in every kick. Very often the poles are too long causing overstrain to the upper extremities. Too long poles are an extremely common problem in competitive skating style skiers who have overestimated their racing performance.

In cross-country skiing, foot hygiene needs attention. In skiers, nail problems, as repeated small contusions of the toes against the inner side of the boot occur, are common. These can be prevented by toe boxes that are soft and spacious, as well as by proper nail hygiene (Renström & Johnson, 1989).

All of these previously mentioned individual preventive measures can be strengthened by secondary and tertiary efforts. This means continuous work in the field of rules, education, information and investments for safer skiing.

Acute injuries

In prevention of cross-country skiing injuries at individual level, it is important to stress the necessity of proper skiing equipment and technique. Slippery fibreglass skis with the wrong type of wax are often found behind a falling accident, especially in those older female spare time skiers. We assume that the non-releasable ski bindings of the cross-country skis are one of the major factors behind the great number of acute knee sprains in this sport and, therefore, we would like to see also releasable bindings in the future market. Several designs for releasable bindings are presently being developed, but at the present none of them are commercially available.

In order to prevent falls, recreational skiers should avoid the machine-made, fast ski trails, especially during icy conditions on downhill terrain. These places should be clearly marked on maps, trail guides and at the beginning of the dangerous part of the trail. Much can be done to improve the safety of the trails as well. Deep ruts and sharp turns should be omitted from the trail. The terrain adjacent to prepared tracks should be cleared of branches, brush, stones, rocks and low overhanging obstructions. The direction of skiing should be marked clearly by big signs at every entrance to avoid collisions with other skiers. Also, walking on the ski trail should, of course, be forbidden, and this should be clearly marked (Fig. 46.6).

In prevention of thumb sprains in inexperienced skiers, it is wise to avoid interlocking the pole strap into the hand in the standard fashion until the skiing skill develops enough to minimize the number of falls. This may also prevent a shoulder dislocation usually resulting from entrapment of the basket of the pole on a tree

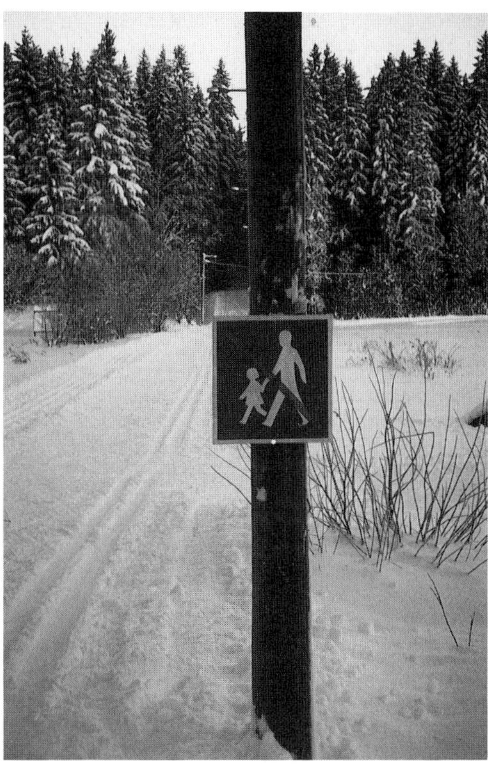

Fig. 46.6 A safe cross-country skiing trail is broad and well prepared with space enough for simultaneous diagonal and skating style skiing. Clear 'walking on the ski trail forbidden' signs should be located at every entrance of the trail. Courtesy of Dr P. Kannus, Kauppi Cross-country Skiing Resort, Tampere, Finland.

branch. To avoid eye injuries, the skiers can be advised to use goggles, even in the dark, and to be alert for small branches that might be difficult to see (Hixson, 1989).

At group and society level, skiing safety information and education in press, television and radio is of great importance. Preventive work performed in ski schools and clubs is, perhaps, even more important. Only through well-organized preventive work can encouraging results be expected.

Cold injuries

In prevention of cold injuries, common sense is by far the best weapon. Simply, skiers must avoid skiing in too cold, windy or wet conditions. This concerns especially long-distance ski tours.

Proper clothing can help a lot. Modern clothing is light and consists of several layers allowing the skier to add or subtract clothing as the temperature varies. The inner layer should transport perspiration away from the body, which can be accomplished with underwear made of polypropylene or other porous materials. A thin shirt should be worn outside the undergarment (Renström & Johnson, 1989). The outer layers should insulate but also allow moisture to escape. The clothes should be replaced when the skiing is stopped.

Racers often use one-piece suits made of thin, stretch materials which do not insulate well. Recreational skiers are encouraged to wear two-piece suits, which can be opened. The head and hands should be covered. People with easily frozen hands should use mittens rather than gloves. Overboots for cold weather and waterproof overboots for skiing in slush are very useful. In competitive skiers, protective bras for women and special polypropylene briefs with nylon wind shields for men are recommended. Woollen face masks leaving mouth and eyes open are commercially available. Protective glasses should be worn on sunny days when at high altitudes, and sometimes on very cold days as well (Fig. 46.7).

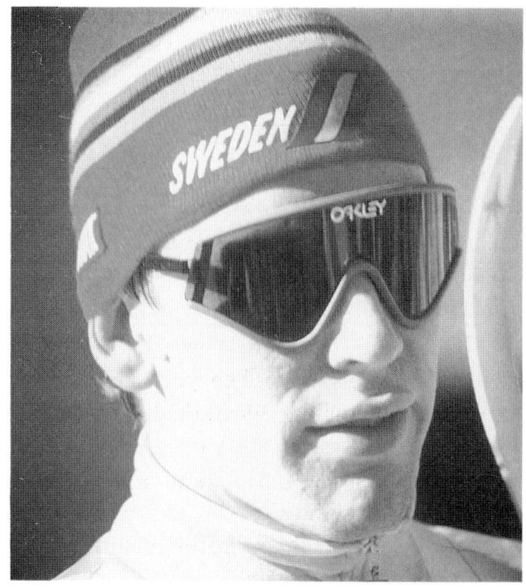

Fig. 46.7 Specially designed glasses protect the eyes from bright sunshine. Courtesy of Dr P.A.F.H. Renström.

Cold air may cause respiratory problems in cross-country skiing. Competitive skiers sometimes use a small heat exchanger which can be held in the mouth warming the air which is inhaled. They are effective even if unpleasant to wear.

At secondary and tertiary level of prevention of cold injuries, it is essential to have clear rules when training or competition has to be cancelled because of environmental malconditions. As mentioned, not only the temperature but also other weather factors should be taken into consideration. For example, the wind-chill factor is critical in cross-country skiing, since the wind has a marked effect on heat loss. If the thermometer reads $-7°C$ and the wind velocity is $32\ km \cdot h^{-1}$, the real exposure is comparable to $-23°C$ (Boswick *et al.*, 1983) (Table 46.4). This can be a real problem in long ski marathons, in which open fields or lakes may be crossed. In such conditions, an effective ski patrol system must be arranged to avoid major cold injuries (Sherry & Asquith, 1987).

Table 46.4 The temperature (°C) at different wind velocities ($m{\cdot}s^{-1}$).

No wind	5 $m{\cdot}s^{-1}$	10 $m{\cdot}s^{-1}$	15 $m{\cdot}s^{-1}$	20 $m{\cdot}s^{-1}$
0	−5	−15	−18	−20
−10	−21	−30	−32	−36
−20	−34	−44	−49	−52

Conclusion

Cross-country skiing, when performed at top level, is an extremely demanding sport on the cardiovascular system and on endurance of all large muscle groups in the human body. However, since the skiing speed can be adjusted within a very large scale according to individual performance capacity, this sport is also ideal for recreational athletes of all ages. In addition, cross-country skiing can play an important role in rehabilitation following many common medical problems and injuries. Because the movements are smooth, patients with musculoskeletal problems can often participate on flat surfaces.

The recent developments in skis, poles, boots, suits, ski tracks and skiing techniques have contributed to increased skiing velocities. This trend may be seen as an increased number of overuse injuries and acute injuries in this sport, even if in general cross-country skiing is a very safe sport if compared, for example, with downhill skiing (acute injuries) or running (overuse injuries).

Well-organized preventive work is needed to keep the injury incidences low so that the continually growing population of skiers can take all the benefits of this very enjoyable sport.

References

Boswick Jr, J.A., Danzl, D.F., Hamlet, M.P. & Schultz, A.L. (1983) Helping the frostbitten patient. *Patient Care* **17**, 90–115.

Boyle, J.J., Johnson, R.J. & Pope, M.H. (1981) Cross-country skiing injuries. A prospective study. *Iowa Orthop. J.* **1**, 41–8.

Boyle, J.J., Johnson, R.J. & Pope, M.H. (1985) Cross-country skiing injuries. In R.J. Johnson & C.D. Mote Jr (eds) *Skiing Trauma and Safety: Fifth International Symposium*, pp. 411–22. American Society for Testing and Materials, Philadelphia.

Clancy Jr, W.G. (1982) Cross-country skiing injuries. *Clin. Sports Med.* **1**, 333–8.

Dorsen, P.J. (1986) Overuse injuries from Nordic ski skating. *Phys. Sportsmed.* **14**, 34.

Ellison, A.E. (1977) Skiing injuries. *Clin. Symp.* **29**, 1–4.

Eriksson, E. (1976) Skiing injuries in Sweden: a one year survey. *Orthop. Clin. N. Am.* **7**, 3–9.

Eriksson, E. & Danielsson, K. (1978) A national ski injury survey. In R.J. Johnson & C.D. Mote Jr (eds) *Skiing Trauma and Safety: Second International Symposium*, pp. 25–31. Baltimore University Press, Baltimore.

Frymoyer, J.W., Pope, M.H. & Kristiansen, T. (1982) Skiing and spinal trauma. *Clin. Sports Med.* **1**, 309.

Gertsch, P., Borgeat, A. & Wälli, T. (1987) New cross-country skiing technique and compartment syndrome. *Am. J. Sports Med.* **15**, 612–13.

Hixson, E.G. (1989) Injuries to watch for this winter in cross-country skiing. *J. Musculoskeletal Med.* **6**, 56–66.

Johnson, R.J., Ettlinger, C.F. & Shealy, J.E. (1989) Skier injury trends. In R.J. Johnson, C.D. Mote Jr & M.-H. Binet (eds) *Skiing Trauma and Safety: Seventh International Symposium*, pp. 25–31. American Society for Testing and Materials, Philadelphia.

Kannus, P. & Järvinen, M. (1986) Role of sports in etiology and prognosis of surgically treated acute knee ligament injuries. *Int. J. Sports Med.* **7**, 39–43.

Kannus, P., Niittymäki, S. & Järvinen, M. (1988) Cross-country skiing injuries: Has the change of skiing style affected the frequency and types of skiing injuries treated at an outpatient sports clinic? *Scand. J. Sport Sci.* **10**, 17–21.

Karvonen, J., Kubica, R., Kalli, S., Wilk, B. & Krasicki, S. (1987) Effects of skating and diagonal techniques on skiing load and results in cross-country skiing. *J. Sports Med. Phys. Fitness* **27**, 473–7.

Lyons, J.W. & Porter, R.E. (1978) Cross-country skiing. A benign sport? *JAMA* **230**, 334–5.

Mahlamäki, S., Michelsson, J.-E. & Pekkarinen, H. (1985) Musculoskeletal symptoms caused by skating style skiing. *Finn. J. Sports Exerc. Med.* **4**, 110–13.

Oja, P. & Vuori, I. (1985) Skating style in cross-country skiing — skiers' experiences in winter 1985 (in Finnish). *Sport Sci. (Finland)* **5**, 226–31.

Orava, S. (1980) *Exertion injuries due to sports and physical exercise*. Academic Dissertation, Österbottningen Press, Kokkola, Finland.

Orava, S., Jaroma, H. & Hulkko, A. (1985) Overuse injuries in cross-country skiing. *Br. J. Sports Med.*

19, 158–60.

Peterson, L. & Renström, P. (1986) *Sports Injuries: Their Prevention and Treatment*, pp. 1–488. Martin Dunitz, London.

Renström, P. (1988) Diagnosis and management of overuse injuries. In A. Dirix, H.G Knuttgen & K. Tittel (eds) *The Olympic Book of Sports Medicine*, pp. 446–68. Blackwell Scientific Publications, Oxford.

Renström, P. & Johnson, R.J. (1989) Cross-country skiing injuries and biomechanics. *Sports Med.* **8**, 346–70.

Sandelin, J., Kiviluoto, I. & Santavirta, S. (1980) Injuries of competitive skiers in Finland: a three year survey. *Ann. Chirurg. Gynaecol.* **69**, 97–101.

Sherry, E. & Asquith, J. (1987) Nordic (cross-country) skiing injuries in Australia. *Med. J. Australia* **146**, 245–6.

Steinbruck, K. (1987) Frequency and aetiology of injury in cross-country skiing. *J. Sports Sci.* **5**, 187–96.

Vuori, I., Loponen, V., Rinne, M. & Oja, P. (1988) Cross-country and downhill skiing injuries in Finland in winter 1986 (in Finnish). *Finn. Med. J.* **43**, 1361–7.

Westlin, N.E. (1976) Injuries in long distance, cross-country and downhill skiing. *Orthop. Clin. N. Am.* **7**, 55–8.

Chapter 47

Injuries in Skating

DAVID L. MULLER, PER A.F.H. RENSTRÖM AND JOHN I.B. PYNE

Speed skating and figure skating have been part of the Winter Olympic Games since they began. These sports have been popular in countries with natural ice resources. In recent decades, they have also become popular in warmer countries that have built artificial ice tracks and skating rinks.

Speed skating is performed on 400-m long outdoor tracks with races varying from 500 to 10 000 m for men and 500 to 5000 m for women. Olympic or metric style races use time trials in which two skaters race at once against the clock. Recently, short-track skating has been introduced, with four to seven skaters per heat competing on an 111-m oval track.

Figure skating involves different events including singles, pairs skating and ice dancing. Each event emphasizes significant athletic skill, coordination and artistic presentation and are judged on technical merit and artistic impression. Acrobatic jumps and throws have been increasingly emphasized in singles and pairs and skating and are a major cause of injuries in competitive figure skaters.

Biomechanics and technique

Speed skating events involve a powerful start and then long skating strokes with constant repetition. Multiple factors are important for efficiency in speed skating. Factors such as air friction, ice friction, weather and air pressure will influence times and, thereby, drastically influence race outcomes (van Ingen Schenau *et al.*, 1989). Air pressure and therefore resistance, are reduced at high altitudes. The air pressure at the Medeorink in Alma Ata, former USSR at 1700 m is reduced by 20%. Maximum oxygen consumption has been shown not to be drastically altered at this altitude at the shortest distances (Malhotra & Gupta, 1976). These near optimal climate conditions coincide with the high number of world records set at the Alma Ata rink.

The goal of a speed skater at any level is to improve efficiency and speed by maintaining the trunk position as parallel to the ice as possible during a race (Fig. 47.1). This position places high strains upon the low back musculature. Variations in body positions and in anthropometric measurements have been shown to be different in élite versus less competitive skaters with the less competitive skater more upright (van Ingen Schenau & De Groot, 1983; De Boer *et al.*, 1986).

Techniques in speed skating are related to the event. With the Olympic or metric style, only two skaters are involved in each race and falls and collisions are less likely. Short-track skating on an 111-m oval is characterized by explosive pack starts and crowded tight turns with up to seven skaters per heat. There is a higher risk of falls, collisions and impact into the side walls.

The skating technique of figure skaters and speed skaters is remarkably different. Figure skaters perform forward and backward skating manoeuvres, jumps and spins. Pair skaters per-

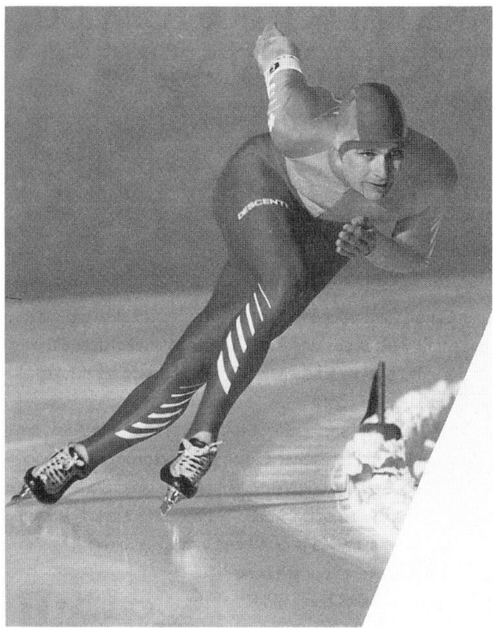

Fig. 47.1 Élite speed skaters maintain a parallel trunk position during the entire race.

form high-risk athletic manoeuvres involving lifts and throws. Ice dancers concentrate on speed, body angle and precise technique. Couples are judged on artistry, form, symmetry and musical interpretation.

Other types of skating which are not Olympic sports, include long-distance skating and in-line skating. Long-distance ice skating, on lakes and canals, is a recreational sport especially popular in Scandinavia and The Netherlands (Figs 47.2 & 47.3). The technique involves a more upright position using a stick or pole for balance, support and speed. In line skating was developed as an off-season training tool for ice hockey. In-line skating techniques can be modified to resemble various winter sports such as speed skating, figure skating, ice hockey, cross-country skiing and downhill skiing. This allows winter athletes to customize their off-season training to optimize benefits for their specific sport. In this fashion, in-line skating can be used to improve both technique and conditioning. Recreational in-line skating has undergone a popularity explosion in the USA and is now a common form of general fitness training.

During the off-season, skaters may train on roads, streets or bike paths using in-line skates. Most injuries are caused by an uneven skating surface. Stones, pot holes, sand and wet pavements cause many falls. Downhill terrain can be challenging, as high speeds can be obtained and braking is more difficult than with ice skates. The skaters stop by using friction bumpers on the back of the skate which are

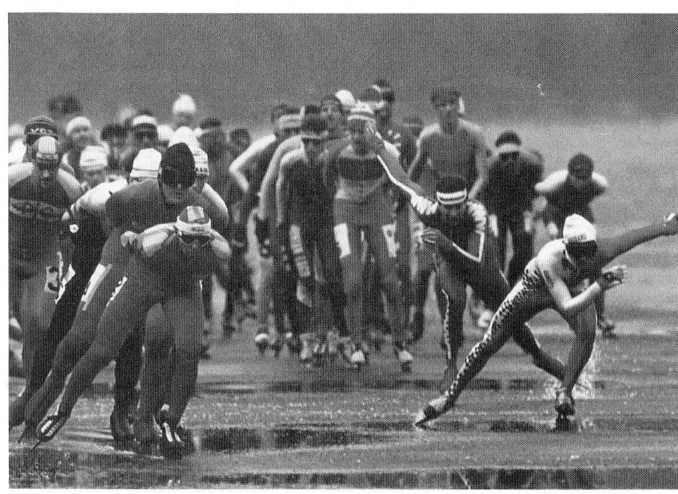

Fig. 47.2 Long-distance skating is both a recreational and competitive sport in Scandinavian countries and The Netherlands. Pack style races are common in this sport.

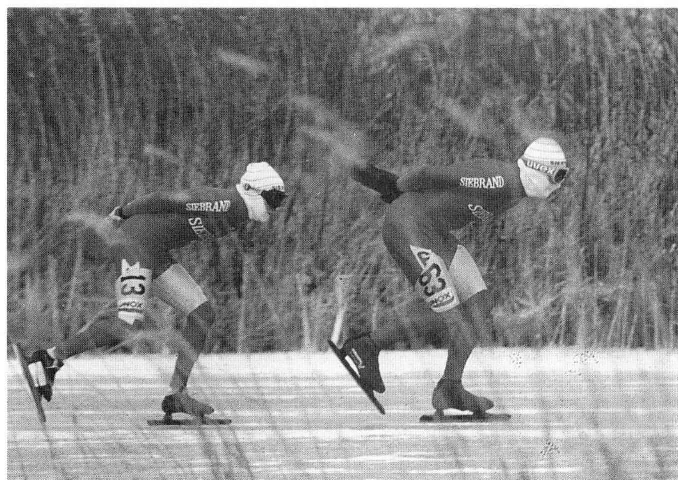

Fig. 47.3 The trunk position of these long-distance competitive skaters is more upright then that of an élite Olympic skater. Hats, gloves, masks and goggles are warn for protection from cold weather.

pushed against the pavement with the hip flexed and the leg extended in front of the skater (Fig. 47.4). Many skaters prefer to use a T-stop when travelling at faster speeds. To T-stop, the braking leg is dragged behind the skater with the skate perpendicular to the direction of travel. Serious falls can occur on hard pavements leading to fractures and contusions. These skaters, therefore, require more padding and prophylactic bracing than other types of skating.

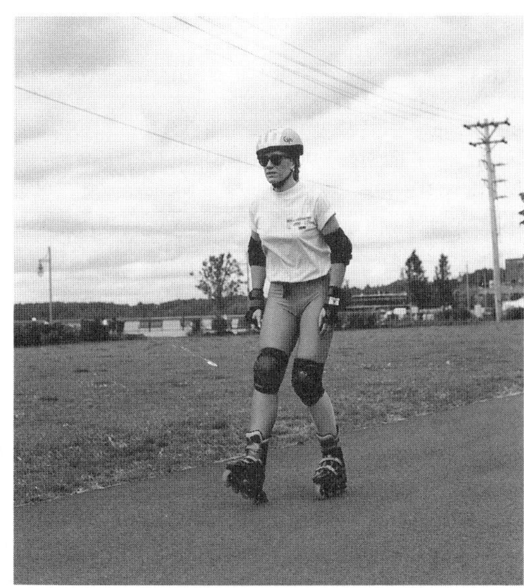

Fig. 47.4 Stopping with a friction bumper requires practice to help avoid high-speed falls and injury.

Equipment

The leather boots of speed skates are low cut and provide less ankle support than other skates. The speed skate blade is designed for maximal contact with the ice, being 37.5–40 cm (15–16 in) in length and flat along the length of the blade. The blade is 2–3 mm (1–1.25 in) wide and is sharpened without a hollow (Fig. 47.5).

The introduction of short-track skating has necessitated changes in the design of the speed skate. The short-track skate has a rock or crown along the length of the blade. The blade is not centred under the boot, but is positioned just to the left of centre in both the right and left foot. The heel post is higher, which allows a more acute skate to ice surface angle for tight turning. These two adaptations ensure that the boot does not make contact with the ice, result-

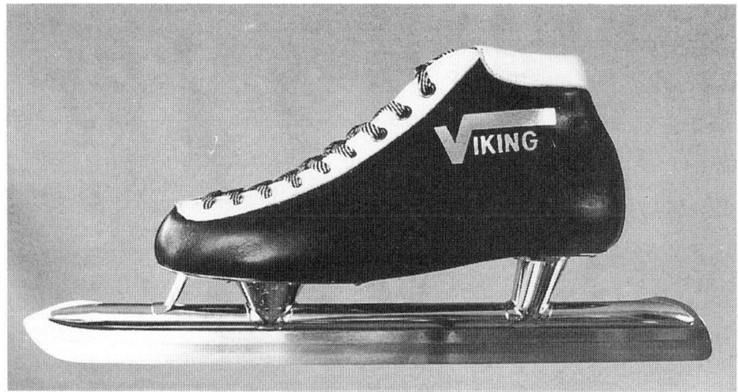

Fig. 47.5 The speed skate boot is low cut providing minimal ankle support. The long blade is designed for speed.

ing in a fall. Élite skaters will bend both blades to the left to allow tighter cornering.

Competitive speed skaters wear tight suits for minimum wind resistance during a race. These suits are thin and there is a risk of exposure to cold weather.

In short-track skating protective equipment is essential. A helmet is required as are leather gloves, knee pads and often shin pads. Recently, neck guards have been introduced to prevent lacerations. Short-track skating races are performed in indoor hockey rinks equipped with standard corner padding to cushion the falls of skaters.

Figure skating boots provide good support and a snug fit. The boot is in slight plantar flexion with a raised heel. The skate blade is approximately 4 mm (0.15 in) wide and has a slight crown or rock along its entire length. The front of the blade is moulded with a toe pick for starting and spins (Fig. 47.6).

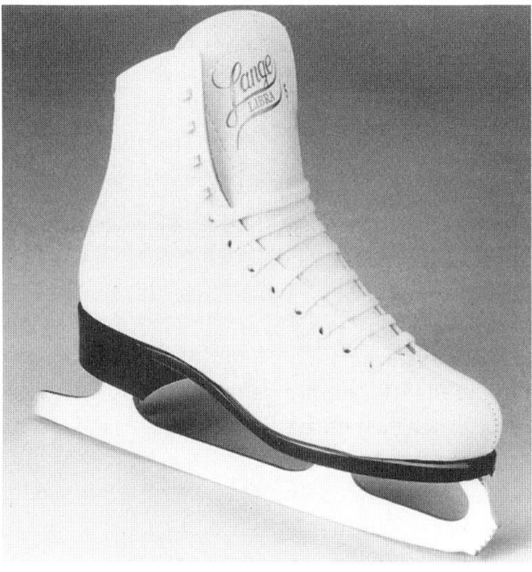

Fig. 47.6 A properly fitting figure skate can prevent many foot and ankle injuries to which figure skaters are susceptible.

The long-distance skater often wears a winter boot to which they strap the blades of a skate. Long-distance skaters carry ice spikes and a life line to be used in case of a fall through the ice. Long-distance skaters should wear helmets, elbow and knee pads for injury prevention.

The boots of in-line skates are either moulded plastic or leather and are very similar to hockey skate boots. Special racing skates are made which have a low cut boot and a longer blade similar to speed skates. The wheels are approximately 1 cm (0.4 in) in width and are arranged in a single line (Fig. 47.7). Recreational skates have three or four wheels and racing skates have five wheels. The quality of ball bearings and rolling resistance of the polyurethane determine the speed of an individual skate. Because of uneven wear, the wheels need to be rotated routinely. The hard plastic brake extends from the heel and needs to be replaced when worn down. Protective equipment designed for in-line skaters includes wrists guards, knee pads, elbow pads and helmets.

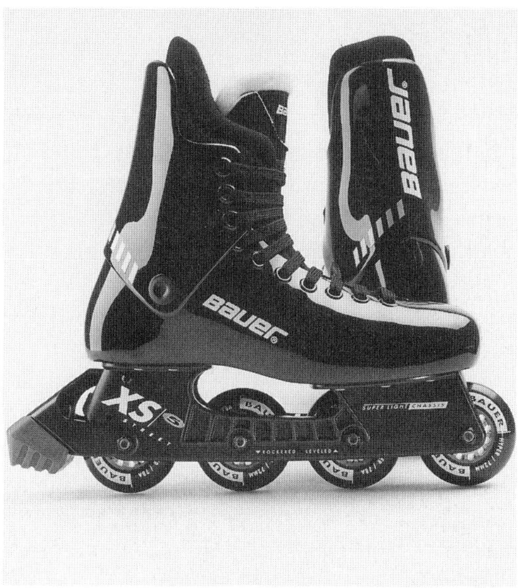

Fig. 47.7 In-line skates are usually made of moulded plastic and provide good ankle support. Racing skates are cut lower and have an additional wheel for speed.

Injuries in skating

Epidemiological studies on figure skaters indicate that competitive, recreational, and novice skaters are at risk for different types of injuries.

Figure skating injuries at public facilities have been shown by several authors to consist of fractures and lacerations due to falls. Williamson and Lowdon (1986) found an injury risk of one per thousand visits. Sixty percent of the injuries were fractures, of which 80% involved the upper extremity and 50% were distal radius fractures. The rest of the injuries were lacerations, two-thirds of which involved the hand. Seventy-five percent of the injured were novice skaters who had skated less than 10 times.

Garrick (1985) reported the injuries seen in a population of recreational figure skaters. Overuse injuries slightly outnumbered acute injuries and fractures represented only 8% of the injuries. The knee (30%), ankle (25%) and back (10%) were most commonly injured.

Several studies have looked specifically at competitive skaters (Smith & Micheli, 1982; Brock & Striowski, 1986; Smith & Ludington, 1989). An increasing incidence of injuries in these skaters has been observed which is believed to be related to the increased emphasis on difficult jumps. However, triple jumps are now also performed even at the novice level. Missed triple jump landings can cause tremendous rotational forces on the lower extremity. Repeated practising of the same manoeuvre leads to repetitive microtrauma and overuse injuries.

Brock and Striowski (1986) looked at injuries in nationally ranked Canadian figure skaters and found that 45% sustained a significant injury over a 1-year period. Overuse and acute injuries were equally seen. Sixty percent of acute injuries occurred during jumps. There were relatively few serious injuries, especially when compared to sports with similar training demands such as gymnastics. The study concluded that the overuse injuries were due to the minimal time spent stretching and could be prevented with better warm-up and flexibility exercises.

Ice dancers and pair skaters are at additional risk because of the potential for contact with their partners. Skate blade lacerations can occur during lifts and spins. Pair skaters perform numerous high-risk athletic moves involving lifts and throws. Smith and Luddington (1989) prospectively studied injuries in élite pair skaters and ice dancers. They found 33 significant injuries in 48 skaters over a 9-month period. The female pair skaters were at highest risk, with a rate of 1.9 significant injuries·skater^{-1}·year^{-1}.

There are no epidemiological studies on speed skating injuries and the sport is considered reasonably safe. Overuse injuries include groin strains and back pain related to the position of the skater with the back parallel to the ice. Collisions are rare in speed skating, but are much more common in short-track racing as is the potential for lacerations.

Injuries among long-distance skaters have been studied in Sweden with an injury incidence of 2.2 injuries·1000 skaters^{-1} (Eriksson *et al.*, 1977). The injuries were mostly in the arms and shoulders, with 50% being fractures. Eighteen percent were head injuries indicating that a helmet should be worn.

No epidemiological studies have been published on in-line skating injuries although clinical experience has shown us that distal radius fractures and contusions about the knee, hand and elbow are most common. Olecranon fractures are not uncommon. All could be prevented by wearing the recommended protective gear.

Prevention and care of injuries

Foot injuries

Skaters are frequently plagued by foot problems. Numbness and pain can simply be caused be wearing narrow boots, or boots too tightly laced. This pain usually disappears after the skates are taken off. Well-fitting skates and gradually increasing use of the skates can alleviate these problems.

Many problems are caused by poorly fitting skates. Hard corns, bursae and callosities are common. These soft-tissue problems are caused by irritation over bony prominences. These can usually be cured by appropriate padding to unload the irritated tissue. Occasionally, custom boots or supporting othotics are necessary.

Hammer toes are commonly seen in competitive skaters (Davis & Litman, 1979). These are usually caused by an incompetent transverse metatarsal arch. Callosities under the metatarsal heads, especially the second and third, are indicative of a transfer metatarsalgia and can lead to secondary hammer toes. Prevention is aimed at early use of a metatarsal bar when the callosities or hammer toes first appear.

Injuries to the foot also include stress fractures of the metatarsals. These should be treated with rest, and can usually be prevented by gradually increasing training duration and intensity. The amount of time spent practising jumping manoeuvres should progress slowly to prevent these types of fractures.

Ankle and Achilles tendon injuries

Anterior ankle pain can be caused by tibialis anterior or extensor hallucis longus tendinitis, or retinacular irritation. The most common cause is poorly fitting skates or skates too tightly laced. Compression of the tendon sheaths beneath the laces can lead to chronic irritation and inflammation. Well-fitting boots and appropriately padded boot tongues can prevent or treat this problem.

Achilles tendon injuries are common in skaters. Figure skaters are at high risk as tremendous forces are generated in the Achilles tendon as it works eccentrically in the landing of jumps. Older figure skaters are at increased risk for partial tears as the tendon degenerates and weakens with age. Adequate stretching and warm-up is helpful in preventing these injuries. A heel wedge can often be helpful.

Ankle sprains are not common, but do occur. The figure skater is at the highest risk, because of the torsional loads sustained while landing from jumps. However, the figure skater's boot usually provides adequate support to avoid these injuries. An ankle brace is sometimes needed to prevent recurrent sprains.

Lower leg injuries

Skaters are susceptible to lower leg overuse injuries. These include medial tibial stress syndrome (or shin splints), chronic anterior compartment syndrome and tibial stress fractures. These injuries are best prevented by preseason conditioning and gradual increases in training demands. Extensive off-season use of slide boards can cause compartment syndromes in speed skaters. Stretching and gradual increase in the use of these boards is important in prevention.

Knee injuries

Knee injuries are common in all kinds of skaters. Many are caused by falls onto the knee resulting in contusions, acute prepatellar bursitis, or less commonly, patella fractures. These can be prevented by the use of knee pads which are recommended for novice skaters, in-line skaters, short-track racers and figure skaters practising jumps. Twisting injuries are less common but can cause ligamentous or meniscal injuries. These are most often seen in figure skaters while landing from difficult jumps or throws. Short-track skaters are also at risk for these injuries usually caused by crashing into the boards or catching an edge. Cracks in the ice, not uncommon on natural ice, can cause serious knee injuries in long-distance skating. Good muscle strength and flexibility are helpful in the prevention of these injuries.

In competitive skaters, overuse injuries dominate over traumatic injuries. Patello-femoral pain syndrome and patellar tendinitis are the most common. These can be aggravated by the high knee flexion angle during skating, especially speed skating. Prevention and treatment are directed at quadriceps and hamstring strengthening and stretching.

Hip and groin pain

In speed skating, groin pain can be a problem, as the skaters rely on strong adductor groin muscles in the recovery from abduction and push-off. The most common problems are located in the adductor longus, but also rectus femoris and iliopsoas can be affected. Stretching of the groin muscles and tendons should be included in every warm-up for all types of skaters.

Long-distance skaters can sustain fractures of the femoral neck from a fall. This can be a very serious injury especially in young skaters, often resulting in avascular necrosis of the femoral head.

Back pain

The incidence of back pain is high in all kinds of skating. Speed skaters are especially at risk due to the need for the horizontal trunk position throughout a race. Low back pain can also occur in figure skating because of repeated jumping, twisting, hyperextension and lifting. Tight lumbodorsal fascia has been identified to be a cause of back pain in the younger skater (Smith & Micheli, 1982).

For prevention, a very careful stretching routine of the lumbar muscles should be included in all training programmes and in the warm-up before competitions for all skaters. Skaters need to emphasize training of these muscles to prevent injury. Speed skaters often use heat retainers, to keep the lumbar musculature warm during outdoor training and competition.

Upper extremity injuries

Wrist and lower arm fractures are by far the most common fractures seen in skaters because of falls onto outstretched arms. These are most commonly seen in inexperienced skaters and in-line skaters. Wrist guards are made for in-line skaters and should be worn at all times. Hand lacerations from skate blades are commonly seen in public skating rinks and gloves are recommended in crowded rinks. Gloves should be worn during in-line skating to protect against falls onto pavement or gravel.

Elbow injuries due to striking the olecranon during falls include acute olecranon bursitis and olecranon fractures. Elbow padding should be worn by all skaters at high risk for falls, especially beginners and in-line skaters. Shoulder injuries are not common but can result from a fall onto the shoulder. This can cause rotator cuff tears, acromioclavicular joint separations, clavicle fractures and shoulder dislocations. Prevention is aimed at avoiding falls.

Conclusion

Speed skaters, figure skaters, long-distance skaters and in-line skaters are at risk for numerous overuse and acute injuries. Most overuse injuries can be prevented by proper warm-up, stretching and conditioning. Skaters should gradually increase training duration and intensity. Properly fitting skates are crucial to avoid foot and ankle injuries. Many acute injuries can be prevented by wearing protective equipment in appropriate circumstances. Skating for a well-trained, well-equipped and experienced individual is a rewarding, enjoyable and relatively safe sport.

References

Brock, R.M. & Striowski, C.C. (1986) Injuries in the élite figure skaters. *Phys. Sportsmed.* **15**(1), 111.

Davis, M.W. & Litman, T. (1979) Figure skater's foot. *Minn. Med.* **62**, 647.

De Boer, R.W., Schermerhorn, P., Gademan, J., De Groot, G. & van Ingen Schenau, G.J. (1986) Characteristic stroke mechanics of élite and trained male speed skaters. *J. Sport Biomech.* **2**, 175–85.

Eriksson, E., Lofström, B., Räf, L. & Sartok, T. (1977) Injuries from long distance lake skating. *Nordisk Idrettsmedisinsk Kongress Beitostolen*, 27–30 March, pp. 142–9.

Garrick, J.G. (1985) Characterization of the patient population in a sports medicine facility. *Phys. Sportsmed.* **13**(10), 73.

Malhotra, M.S. & Gupta, J.S. (1976) Work capacity at altitude. In E. Jokl, R.L. Anad & M. Stoboy (eds) *Medicine Sport*, Vol. 9, p. 165. *Advances in Exercise Physiology*. Karger, Basel.

Smith, A.D. & Ludington, R. (1989) Injuries in élite pair skaters and ice dancers. *Am. J. Sports Med.* **17**(4), 482.

Smith, A.D. & Micheli, L.J. (1982) Injuries in competitive figure skating. *Phys. Sportsmed.* **10**(1), 36.

van Ingen Shenau, G.J. & De Groot, G. (1983) On the origin of differences in performance level between élite male and female speed skaters. *Hum. Movement Sci.* **2**, 151.

van Ingen Schenau, G.J., De Boer, R.W. & De Groot, G. (1989) Biomechanics of speed skating. In C. Vaughan (ed.) *Biomechanics of Sports*, p. 121. CRC Press, Florida.

Williamson, D.M. & Lowdon, I.M.R. (1986) Ice-skating injuries. *Injury* **17**, 205–7.

Index

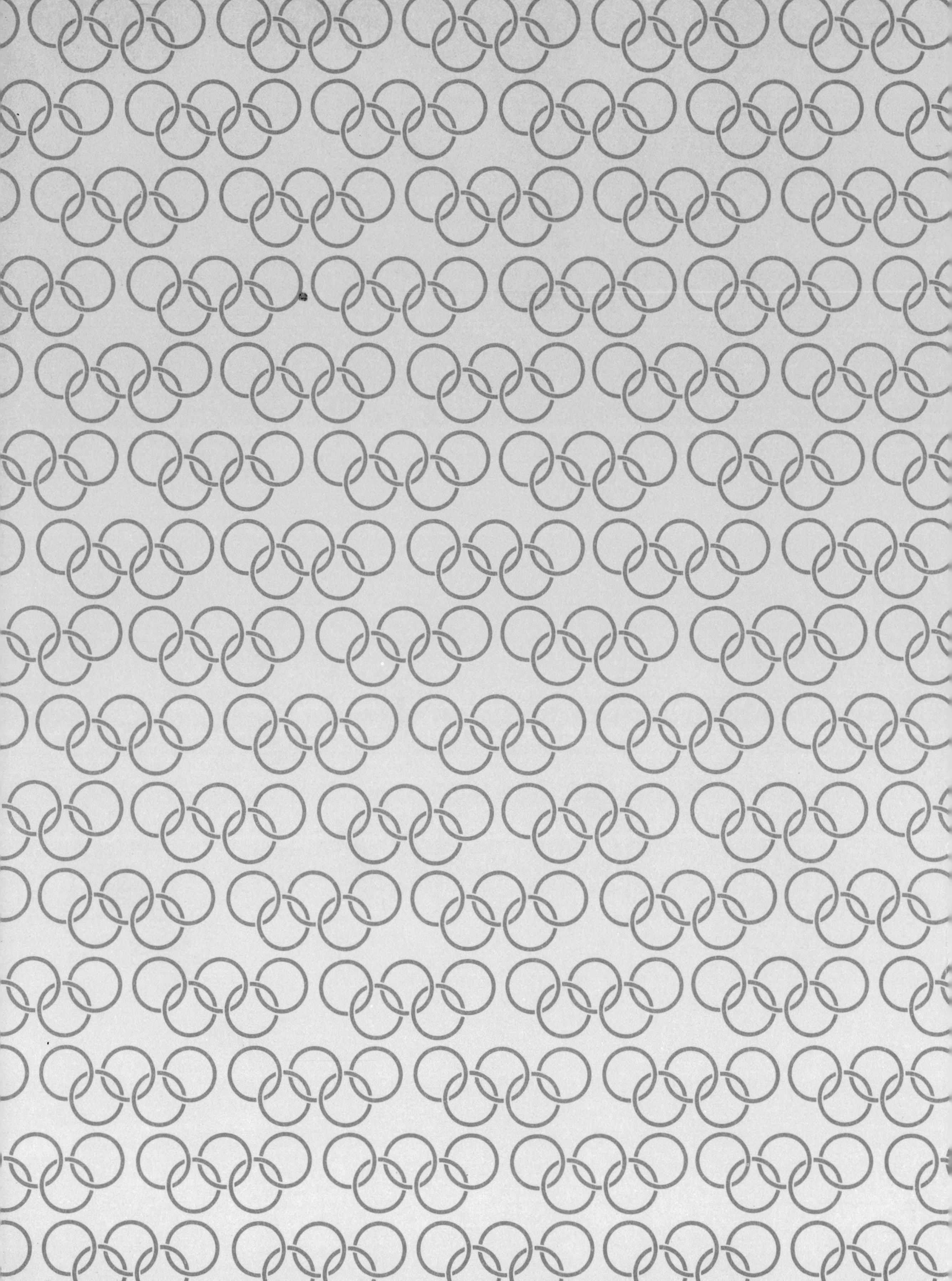